Essentials of
Physical Medicine
and
Rehabilitation

Essentials of Physical Medicine and Rehabilitation

Walter R. Frontera, MD, PhD

Earle P. and Ida S. Charlton Associate Professor and Chairman
Department of Physical Medicine and Rehabilitation
Harvard Medical School

Physiatrist-in-Chief
Department of Physical Medicine & Rehabilitation
Spaulding Rehabilitation Hospital

Physiatrist-in-Chief
Physical Medicine & Rehabilitation Service
Massachusetts General Hospital

Senior Physician and Chief
Division of Physical Medicine & Rehabilitation
Brigham & Women's Hospital
Boston, Massachusetts

Julie K. Silver, MD

Assistant Professor,
Department of Physical Medicine & Rehabilitation
Harvard Medical School

Medical Director, Spaulding/Framingham Outpatient Center
Framingham, Massachusetts

Associate in Physiatry
Physical Medicine & Rehabilitation Service
Massachusetts General Hospital

Associate in Physiatry
Division of Physical Medicine & Rehabilitation
Brigham & Women's Hospital
Boston, Massachusetts

Hanley & Belfus, Inc. / Philadelphia

Publisher: HANLEY & BELFUS, INC.
Medical Publishers
210 South 13th Street
Philadelphia, PA 19107
(215) 546-7293; 800-962-1892
FAX (215) 790-9330
Web site: http://www.hanleyandbelfus.com

Note to the reader: Although the information in this book has been carefully reviewed for correctness of dosage and indications, neither the authors nor the editor nor the publisher can accept any legal responsibility for any errors or omissions that may be made. Neither the publisher nor the editor makes any warranty, expressed or implied, with respect to the material contained herein. Before prescribing any drug, the reader must review the manufacturer's current product information (package inserts) for accepted indications, absolute dosage recommendations, and other information pertinent to the safe and effective use of the product described.

Library of Congress Cataloging-in-Publication Data

Essentials of physical medicine and rehabilitation / edited by Walter R. Frontera, Julie K. Silver.
    p. ; cm.
    Includes index.
    ISBN 1-56053-443-5 (alk. paper)
    1. Medicine, Physical. 2. Medical rehabilitation. I. Frontera, Walter R., 1955- II.
Silver, J. K. (Julie K.), 1965-
    [DNLM: 1. Musculoskeletal Diseases—rehabilitation. WE 140 E782 2002]
    RM700 .E84 2002
    617'.03—dc21

    2001051752

Printed in Canada

Essentials of Physical Medicine and Rehabilitation   ISBN 1-56053-443-5

Last digit is the print number: 9 8 7 6 5 4 3 2 1

Contents

Section 1   Musculoskeletal Disorders

Head and Neck

Shoulder

Section 2   Rehabilitation

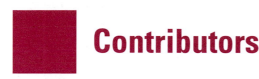

Contributors

Dorothy D. Aiello, PT
Senior Physical Therapist, Spaulding Rehabilitation Hospital, Framingham, Massachusetts; Laboratory Instructor, Northeastern University, Boston, Massachusetts

Venu Akuthota, MD
Assistant Professor, Physical Medicine and Rehabilitation, Northwestern University Medical School; Rehabilitation Institute of Chicago, Chicago, Illinois

Joseph T. Alleva, MD
Instructor, Physical Medicine and Rehabilitation, Northwestern University Medical School, Chicago, Illinois; Evanston Northwestern Healthcare, Evanston, Illinois

Michelle J. Alpert, MD
Instructor, Department of Physical Medicine and Rehabilitation, Harvard Medical School; Spaulding Rehabilitation Hospital and Massachusetts General Hospital, Boston, Massachusetts

Eduardo Amy, MD
Co-director, Sports Injuries Unit, Puerto Rico Olympic Training Center, Department of Physical Medicine, Rehabilitation and Sports Medicine, University of Puerto Rico, School of Medicine, San Juan, Puerto Rico

Karen Atkinson, MD, MPH
Department of Rheumatology, Massachusetts General Hospital, Boston, Massachusetts

Joseph F. Audette, MA, MD
Instructor, Department of Physical Medicine and Rehabilitation, Harvard Medical School; Spaulding Rehabilitation Hospital, Beth Israel Deaconess Hospital, Boston, Massachusetts

John Bach, MD
Professor of Physical Medicine and Rehabilitation, UMDNJ-New Jersey Medical School, Newark, New Jersey

Karen P. Barr, MD
Assistant Professor, Department of Physical Medicine and Rehabilitation, Eastern Virginia Medical School, Norfolk, Virginia

Peter K. Bienkowski, MD
Senior Medical Student, Dalhousie University Medical School, Halifax, Nova Scotia, Canada

Joseph Biundo, MD
Department of Physical Medicine and Rehabilitation, Louisiana State University Medical Center, New Orleans, Louisiana

Randie M. Black-Schaffer, MA, MD
Instructor, Department of Physical Medicine and Rehabilitation, Harvard Medical School; Clinical Associate Professor, Department of Rehabilitation Medicine, Tufts University School of Medicine; Spaulding Rehabilitation Hospital, Massachusetts General Hospital, Boston, Massachusetts

Philip John Blount, MD
Resident Physician, Physical Medicine and Rehabilitation, Charlotte Institute of Rehabilitation, Charlotte, North Carolina

William L. Bockenek, MD
Clinical Associate Professor, Physical Medicine and Rehabilitation, Charlotte Institute of Rehabiliation/Carolinas Medical Center, Charlotte, North Carolina

Joanne Borg-Stein, MD
Assistant Professor, Tufts University School of Medicine; Lecturer, Department of Physical Medicine and Rehabilitation, Harvard Medical School; Spaulding Rehabilitation Hospital, Boston, Massachusetts

Jay E. Bowen, DO
Clinical Chief of Sports Medicine, Kessler Institute for Rehabilitation, West Orange, New Jersey; Sports Medicine Fellowship Coordinator and Assistant Professor of Physical Medicine and Rehabilitation, UMDNJ-Newark Medical School, Newark, New Jersey

Jeffrey S. Brault, DO, PT
Instructor, Physical Medicine and Rehabilitation, Mayo School of Medicine, Rochester, Minnesota

Steven E. Braverman, MD, Lt. Colonel, US Army
Assistant Professor, Physical Medicine and Rehabilitation, Uniformed Services University of the Health Sciences, Bethesda, Maryland; Deputy Commander for Clinical Services, Moncrief Army Community Hospital, Ft. Jackson, South Carolina

Patrick Brennan, MD
Instructor, Department of Physical Medicine and Rehabilitation, Harvard Medical School; Spaulding Rehabilitation Hospital, Boston, Massachusetts

Jeffrey T. Brodie, MD
Attending Physician, Division of Orthopaedic Surgery, St. Joseph Medical Center, Baltimore, Maryland

Alexandra R. Bunyak, MD
Resident, Physical Medicine and Rehabilitation, Northwestern University Medical School; Rehabilitation Institute of Chicago, Chicago, Illinois

David T. Burke, MD, MA
Assistant Professor, Harvard Medical School; Director, Inpatient Traumatic Brain Injury Rehabilitation Program, Physical Medicine and Rehabilitation, Harvard Medical School; Director, Inpatient Traumatic Brain Injury Rehabilitation Program, Spaulding Rehabilitation Hospital, Boston, Massachusetts

Rene Cailliet, MD
Emeritus Professor, University of Southern California School of Medicine; Chairman (Retired), Department of Physical Medicine and Rehabilitation, USC School of Medicine; Currently Clinical Professor, UCLA School of Medicine, Los Angeles, California

Charles Cassidy, MD
Assistant Professor, Chief, Hand and Upper Extremity Surgery, Orthopaedic Surgery, Tufts University School of Medicine; New England Medical Center, Boston, Massachusetts

Heechin Chae, MD
Instructor, Department of Physical Medicine and Rehabilitation, Harvard Medical School; Spaulding Rehabilitation Hospital, Boston, Massachusetts

Jie Cheng, MD
Resident Physician, Spaulding Rehabilitation Hospital; Department of Physical Medicine and Rehabilitation, Harvard Medical School, Boston, Massachusetts

Andrea Cheville, MD
Department of Physical Medicine and Rehabilitation, University of Pennsylvania Health System, Philadelphia, Pennsylvania

Isaac Cohen, MD
Spine and Occupational Medicine Fellow (2000-2001), Spine Center; New England Baptist Bone and Joint Institute, Boston, Massachusetts

Earl J. Craig, MD
Clinical Assistant Professor, Department of Physical Medicine and Rehabilitation, Indiana University School of Medicine, Indianapolis, Indiana; Bloomington Hospital, Bloomington, Indiana

Alan M. Davis, MD, PhD
Assistant Professor, Division of Physical Medicine and Rehabilitation, University of Utah, School of Medicine; Active Staff, University Hospital and Salt Lake Regional Medical Center, Salt Lake City, Utah

David R. Del Toro, MD
Associate Professor, Physical Medicine and Rehabilitation, Medical College of Wisconsin; Froedtert Memorial Lutheran Hospital, Milwaukee, Wisconsin

Timothy R. Dillingham, MD
Associate Professor, Department of Physical Medicine and Rehabilitation, The Johns Hopkins University; The Johns Hopkins Hospital, Baltimore, Maryland

Alan F. Doyle, DO
Clinical Assistant Professor, Department of Neurology, University of Maryland School of Medicine; Baltimore Veterans Affairs Medical Center, Baltimore, Maryland

Sheila Dugan, MD
Physical Medicine and Rehabilitation, Rush Presbyterian Medical Center, Chicago, Illinois

Lester S. Duplechan, MD
Mayfield Clinic, Cincinnati, Ohio

Maury Ruben Ellenberg, MD, FACP
Associate Clinical Professor, Physical Medicine and Rehabilitation, Wayne State University, Detroit, Michigan

Erik R. Ensrud, MD
Neuromuscular Fellow, Department of Neurology, Harvard Medical School/Brigham and Women's Hospital, Boston, Massachusetts

Alice V. Fann, MD
Assistant Professor, Physical Medicine and Rehabilitation, University of Arkansas for Medical Sciences; Central Arkansas Veterans Healthcare System, Little Rock, Arkansas

Avital Fast, MD
Professor and Chairman, Physical Medicine and Rehabilitation, Albert Einstein College of Medicine/Montefiore Medical Center, Bronx, New York

Rosemarie Filart, MD
Assistant Professor of Physical Medicine and Rehabilitation, Johns Hopkins University Hospital, Baltimore, Maryland

Jason Tyler Franklin, DO
Instructor, Physical Medicine and Rehabilitation, Northwestern University; Northwestern University, McGaw Medical Center, Chicago, Illinois

Fae Helane Garden, MD
Associate Professor, Department of Physical Medicine and Rehabilitation, Baylor College of Medicine; Assistant Chief, Physical Medicine and Rehabilitation, St. Luke's Episcopal Hospital, Houston, Texas

Walter J. Gaudino, MD, MS
Assistant Professor, Physical Medicine and Rehabilitation, State University of New York, Stony Brook, New York

Michelle Gittler, MD
Associate Professor of Orthopedics, Department of Biological Sciences, Division of Surgery, University of Chicago; Schwab Rehabilitation Hospital, Chicago, Illinois

Mel B. Glenn, MD
Associate Professor, Department of Physical Medicine and Rehabilitation, Harvard Medical School; Spaulding Rehabilitation Hospital and Massachusetts General Hospital, Boston, Massachusetts

Paul R. Greenlaw, MD
Resident, Orthopedics, New England Medical Center, Boston, Massachusetts

Bertram Greenspun, DO
Clinical Associate Professor, Rehabilitation Medicine, Jefferson Medical College, Philadelphia, Pennsylvania

Navneet Gupta, MD
Resident Physician, Department of Physical Medicine and Rehabilitation, University of Arkansas for Medical Sciences, Little Rock, Arkansas

Farrukh Hamid, MD
Assistant Professor, Physical Medicine and Rehabilitation, University of Texas Southwestern Medical Center, Dallas, Texas

Todd E. Handel, MD
Director of Interventional Physiatry, Physical Medicine and Rehabilitation, Rehabilitation Hospital of Rhode Island, North Smithfield, Rhode Island

Toni J. Hanson, MD
Assistant Professor, Physical Medicine and Rehabilitation, Mayo Clinic, Rochester, Minnesota

Melvin L. Hecht, MD
Vice President, Medical Affairs, Youville Hospital and Rehabilitation Center; Harvard Medical School, Boston, Massachusetts

Howard J. Hoffberg, MD
Rosen-Hoffberg Rehabilitation and Pain Management Associates, Baltimore, Maryland

Joseph C. Honet, MD, MS, FACP
Professor FTA, Physical Medicine and Rehabilitation, Wayne State University School of Medicine; Chief, Physical Medicine and Rehabilitation, Sinai Grace Hospital of Detroit Medical Center, Detroit, Michigan

Thomas H. Hudgins, MD
Instructor, Physical Medicine and Rehabilitation, Northwestern University Medical School; Evanston Northwestern Health Care, Evanston, Illinois

Cristin Jouve, MD
Instructor, Physical Medicine and Rehabilitation, Harvard Medical School; The Spine Center, New England Baptist Hospital, Boston, Massachusetts

Darryl L. Kaelin, MD
Clinical Assistant Professor, Department of Physical Medicine and Rehabilitation, Indiana University Medical Center; Medical Director, Hook Rehabilitation Brain Injury Program, Center for Neurological Rehabilitation and Indiana Neurorestorative Center, Indianapolis, Indiana

Robert J. Kaplan, MD
Assistant Professor, Physical Medicine and Rehabilitation, Northwestern Medical Center; Rehabilitation Institute of Chicago, Chicago, Illinois

Ayal M. Kaynan, MD
Attending, Department of Surgery/Division of Urology, Morristown Memorial Hospital, Morristown, New Jersey

Florian S. Keplinger, MD
Assistant Professor, Department of Physical Medicine and Rehabilitation, University of Arkansas for Medical Sciences, Little Rock, Arkansas

Todd A. Kile, MD
Chair, Division of Foot and Ankle Surgery, Consultant, Department of Orthopaedic Surgery, Mayo Clinic Scottsdale–Mayo Clinic Hospital; Director, Foot and Ankle Fellowship, Mayo Clinic Scottsdale–Mayo Clinic Hospital; Associate Professor of Orthopaedic Surgery, Mayo Graduate School of Medicine, Scottsdale, Arizona

Ricardo Knight, MD
Instructor, Department of Physical Medicine and Rehabilitation, Harvard Medical School; Spaulding Rehabilitation Hospital and Massachusetts General Hospital, Boston, Massachusetts

Jason H. Kortte, MS, CCC-SLP
Speech-Language Pathologist, Good Samaritan Hospital, Baltimore, Maryland

Lisa S. Krivickas, MD
Assistant Professor, Department of Physical Medicine and Rehabilitation, Harvard Medical School; Director of Electromyography, Spaulding Rehabilitation Hospital, Boston, Massachusetts

Robert J. Krug, MD
Clinical Assistant Professor, Department of Medicine, University of Connecticut School of Medicine; Medical Director, The Rehabilitation Hospital of Connecticut; Chairman/Director, The Department of Rehabilitation Medicine, Saint Francis Hospital and Medical Center, Hartford, Connecticut

Tamara D. Lauder, MD
Assistant Professor, Departments of Physical Medicine and Rehabilitation and Neurology, Mayo Clinic-Mayo Medical School, Rochester, Minnesota

Elise H. Lee, MD
Physical Medicine and Rehabilitation, Harvard Medical School; Spaulding Rehabilitation Hospital, Boston, Massachusetts

Sammy M. Lee, DPM
Resident in Podiatry, Massachusetts General Hospital, Boston, Massachusetts

Ted A. Lennard, MD
Clinical Assistant Professor, Department of Physical Medicine and Rehabilitation, University of Arkansas for Medical Sciences, Little Rock, Arkansas; Private Practice, Springfield, Missouri

Paul Lento, MD
Assistant Professor, Physical Medicine and Rehabilitation, Loyola University Medical Center, Maywood, Illinois; Rehabilitation Institute of Chicago, Chicago, Illinois

Larry Z. Lockerman, DDS
Instructor of Clinical Surgery, Department of Surgery, University of Massachusetts Medical School; Medical Staff, Headache Disorder Chapter, University of Massachusetts Memorial Medical Center, Worcester, Massachusetts

Elizabeth Loder, MD, FACP
Instructor, Medicine, Harvard Medical School; Spaulding Rehabilitation Hospital, Boston, Massachusetts

Gerald A. Malanga, MD
Director of Spine Sport and Occupational Rehabilitation, Kessler Institute for Rehabilitation, West Orange, New Jersey; Associate Professor of Physical Medicine and Rehabilitation, UMDNJ-Newark Medical School, Newark, New Jersey

Katherine Mashey, MD
Assistant Director of the Podiatric Surgical Residency, Saint Francis Hospital and Medical Center, Hartford, Connecticut

Alec L. Meleger, MD
Clinical Instructor, Department of Physical Medicine and Rehabilitation, Harvard Medical School; Spaulding Rehabilitation Hospital, Boston, Massachusetts

Lyle J. Micheli, MD
Associate Clinical Professor of Orthopedics, Sports Medicine, Orthopedic Surgery, Harvard Medical School; Director of Sports Medicine, Boston Children's Hospital, Boston, Massachusetts

William Micheo, MD
Director and Associate Professor, Physical Medicine, Rehabilitation and Sports Medicine, University of Puerto Rico, Medical Science Campus; University Hospital, San Juan, Puerto Rico

Erasmus G. Morfe, DO
Resident Physician, Physical Medicine and Rehabilitation, Medical College of Wisconsin, Milwaukee, Wisconsin

Gregory J. Mulford, MD
Assistant Clinical Professor of Rehabilitation Medicine, Columbia University College of Physicians and Surgeons, New York, New York; Chairman, Rehabilitation Medicine, Morristown Memorial Hospital, Morristown, New Jersey

Scott F. Nadler, DO
Director of Sports Medicine, Associate Professor, Physical Medicine and Rehabilitation, UMDNJ-NJ Medical School; University Hospital, Newark, New Jersey

Shanker Nesathurai, MD, FRCP(C)
Chief, Rehabilitation Services, Department of Rehabilitation Medicine, Boston Medical Center; Associate Professor, Chairman ad interim, Physical Medicine and Rehabilitation, Boston University School of Medicine, Boston, Massachusetts

Ashok N. Nimgade, MD, MS, MPH
Research Fellow in Occupational Medicine, Harvard University, Boston, Massachusetts

Robert P. Nirschl, MD, MS
Associate Clinical Professor of Orthopedic Surgery, Georgetown University, Washington, DC; Director, Nirschl Orthopedic Sports Medicine Clinic/Virginia Hospital Center Arlington Sports Medicine Fellowship Program, Arlington, Virginia

Ryan C. O'Connor, DO
Assistant Professor of Physical Medicine and Rehabilitation and Team Physician, MSU Spartan Athletics, Michigan State University-COM; Ingham Regional Medical Center and Sparrow Hospital, East Lansing, Michigan

Michael D. Osborne, MD
Senior Associate Consultant, Department of Physical Medicine and Rehabilitation, Mayo Clinic, Jacksonville, Florida

Lora Beth Packel, MS, PT
Coordinator of Cancer Rehabilitation, University of Pennsylvania Health System, Philadelphia, Pennsylvania

Jeffrey B. Palmer, MD
Associate Professor, Physical Medicine and Rehabilitation, Johns Hopkins University; Good Samaritan Hospital, Baltimore, Maryland

Walter Panis, MD
Instructor, Department of Physical Medicine and Rehabilitation, Harvard Medical School; Spaulding Rehabilitation Hospital, Boston, Massachusetts

Paul F. Pasquina, MD
Director, Residency Training, Physical Medicine and Rehabilitation, Walter Reed Army Medical Center, Washington, DC; Assistant Professor of Neurology, Physical Medicine and Rehabilitation, Uniformed Services University of the Health Sciences, Bethesda, Maryland

Atul T. Patel, MD
Associate Professor, Rehabilitation, University of Kansas Medical Center, Kansas City, Kansas; Research Medical Center, Kansas City, Missouri

Inder Perkash, MD, FACS
Chief, Spinal Cord Injury Service, Veterans Affairs Palo Alto Health Care System; Professor of Urology, Physical Medicine and Rehabilitation, and Paralyzed Veterans of America Professor of Spinal Cord Injuries, Stanford University Medical School, Palo Alto, California

Edward M. Phillips, MD
Department of Physical Medicine and Rehabilitation, Harvard Medical School, Spaulding Rehabilitation Hospital, Boston, Massachusetts

Mahboob U. Rahman, MD, PhD
Instructor in Medicine, Rheumatology Unit, Department of Medicine, Harvard Medical School; Assistant in Medicine, Massachusetts General Hospital; Consultant Rheumatologist and Director of Rheumatology Training, Spaulding Rehabilitation Hospital, Boston, Massachusetts

James Rainville, MD
Assistant Clinical Professor, Department of Physical Medicine and Rehabilitation, Harvard Medical School; New England Baptist Hospital, Boston, Massachusetts

Edwardo Ramos, MD
Assistant Professor, Physical Medicine, Rehabilitation and Sports Medicine Department, University of Puerto Rico; University Pediatric Hospital, San Juan, Puerto Rico

Christopher R. Rehm, MD
Resident, Physical Medicine and Rehabilitation, Harvard Medical School, Boston, Massachusetts

Thomas D. Rizzo, Jr., MD
Assistant Professor, Department of Physical Medicine and Rehabilitation, Mayo Clinic, Jacksonville, Florida

Norman B. Rosen, MD
Rosen-Hoffberg Rehabilitation and Pain Management Associates, Baltimore, Maryland

Darren Craig Rosenberg, MD
Instructor, Physical Medicine and Rehabilitation, Harvard Medical School; Massachusetts General Hospital, Boston, Massachusetts; Spaulding/Framingham Outpatient Center, Framingham, Massachusetts

Leo M. Rozmaryn, MD
The Orthopaedic Center, PA, Rockville, Maryland

Seward B. Rutkove, MD
Assistant Professor of Neurology, Harvard Medical School; Beth Israel Deaconess Medical Center, Boston, Massachusetts

Francisco H. Santiago, MD
Attending, Physical Medicine and Rehabilitation, Bronx-Lebanon Hospital, Bronx, New York

Robert J. Scardina, DPM
Clinical Instructor, Orthopaedic Surgery, Harvard Medical School; Chief, Podiatric Division, Massachusetts General Hospital; Director, Podiatric Medical Education, Massachusetts General Hospital, Boston, Massachusetts

Walton O. Schalick, III, MD, PhD
Instructor, Division of Newborn Medicine, Department of Pediatrics; Assistant Professor, Department of History, Washington University; Attending Physician, Barnes-Jewish Hospital, St. Louis Children's Hospital, St. Louis, Missouri

Michael U. Schaufele, MD
Assistant Professor, Department of Orthopaedics and Department of Rehabilitation Medicine, Emory University; Emory University Hospital and Crawford Long Hospital, Atlanta, Georgia

Deborah Reiss Schneider, MD
Director, Physical Medicine and Rehabilitation Consult Service, Johns Hopkins Hospital; Instructor, Department of Physical Medicine and Rehabilitation, Johns Hopkins University; Staff Privileges at Johns Hopkins Hospital, Johns Hopkins Bayview Medical Center, and Good Samaritan Hospital, Baltimore, Maryland

Nutan Sharma, MD, PhD
Assistant in Neurology, Massachusetts General Hospital, Boston, Massachusetts

Andrew D. Shiller, MD
Medical Director, Outpatient Rehabilitation, Kent Hospital, Warwick, Rhode Island

Sarah Shubert, MD
Resident, Department of Orthopaedics, Tufts University; New England Medical Center, Boston, Massachusetts

Hilary Siebens, MD
Lecturer, Physical Medicine and Rehabilitation, Harvard Medical School; Massachusetts General Hospital and Spaulding Rehabilitation Hospital, Boston, Massachusetts

Julie K. Silver, MD
Medical Director, Spaulding/Framingham Outpatient Center, Framingham, Massachusetts; Assistant Professor, Department of Physical Medicine and Rehabilitation, Harvard Medical School; Associate in Physiatry, Physical Medicine and Rehabilitation Service, Massachusetts General Hospital; Associate in Physiatry, Division of Physical Medicine and Rehabilitation, Brigham and Women's Hospital, Boston, Massachusetts

Kenneth H. Silver, MD
Associate Professor, Chief, Division of Rehabilitation Medicine, Department of Neurology/Division of Rehabilitation Medicine, University of Maryland; Kernan Rehabilitation Hospital and Baltimore Veterans Affairs Medical Center, Baltimore, Maryland

Ajay Singh, MD
Clinical Director of Renal Division, Brigham and Women's Hospital, Boston, Massachusetts

Robert S. Skerker, MD
Attending, Department of Rehabilitation, Morristown Memorial Hospital, Morristown, New Jersey

David M. Slovik, MD
Associate Professor of Medicine, Harvard Medical School; Chief of Medicine, Spaulding Rehabilitation Hospital, Boston, Massachusetts

Rachael Smith, DO
Resident, Department of Physical Medicine and Rehabilitation, UMDNJ-NJ Medical School; University Hospital, Newark, New Jersey

M. Catherine Spires, MD
Clinical Assistant Professor, Associate Chair of Clinical Affairs, Physical Medicine and Rehabilitation, University of Michigan Health Care System, Ann Arbor, Michigan

Joel Stein, MD
Assistant Professor, Department of Physical Medicine and Rehabilitation, Harvard Medical School; Chief Medical Officer, Spaulding Rehabilitation Hospital, Boston, Massachusetts

Meryl Stein, MD
Resident, Department of Physical Medicine and Rehabilitation, Harvard Medical School; Spaulding Rehabilitation Hospital, Boston, Massachusetts

Sonja Stilp, MD
Resident, Orthopaedics and Rehabilitation, Loyola University Medical Center, Maywood, Illinois

Wayne Lawrence Stokes, MD
Assistant Professor, Orthopedics, Albert Einstein College of Medicine; Attending, Beth Israel Medical Center, New York, New York

Jeffrey A. Strakowski, MD
Clinical Assistant Professor, Department of Physical Medicine and Rehabilitation, The Ohio State University; Riverside Methodist Hospital, Columbus, Ohio

Cynthia C. Su, MD
Assistant Professor, Department of Physical Medicine and Rehabilitation, Eastern Virginia Medical School; Active Staff, Louise Obici Memorial Hospital, Norfolk General Hospital, Norfolk, Virginia

Mark A. Thomas, MD
Associate Professor of Rehabilitation Medicine, Albert Einstein College of Medicine/Montefiore Medical Center; Associate Chairman, Rehabilitation Medicine, Montefiore Medical Center, Bronx, New York

Ramon Vallarino Jr., MD
Assistant Clinical Professor, Physical Medicine and Rehabilitation, Albert Einstein College of Medicine, Bronx, New York

W. Alaric Vandam, MD
Moore Orthopaedic Clinic, Columbia, South Carolina

Yumei Wang, MD
Chief Resident, Department of Physical Medicine and Rehabilitation, Montefiore Medical Center, Albert Einstein College of Medicine, Bronx, New York

James E. Warmoth, MD
Professor, Past Chair, Physical Medicine and Rehabilitation, Medical University of South Carolina, Charleston, South Carolina

Jay M. Weiss, MD
Assistant Professor of Clinical Physical Medicine and
Rehabilitation, State University of New York at Stony
Brook; Medical Director, Long Island Physical Medicine
and Rehabilitation, Stony Brook, New York

Lyn D. Weiss, MD
Chairman, Director of Residency Training, Associate
Clinical Professor, Physical Medicine and Rehabilitation,
State University of New York at Stony Brook, Stony Brook,
New York; Chairman, Director of Residency Training,
Director of Electrodiagnostic Services, Nassau University
Medical Center, East Meadow, New York

David Wexler (Mr.), MD, FRCS (Tr & Orth) (Glasg)
Fellow in Foot and Ankle Surgery, Mayo Clinic, Scottsdale,
Arizona

Jane Wierbicky, RN, BSN
Registered Nurse, Department of Rehabilitation, Boston
Medical Center, Boston, Massachusetts

J. Michael Wieting, DO, MEd
Associate Professor, Director of Residency Training,
Consultant in Athletic Medicine, Department of Physical
Medicine and Rehabilitation, Michigan State University—
College of Osteopathic Medicine, East Lansing, Michigan

Sharon G. Willett, PTA, STS
Physical Therapy Associate Assistant, Virginia Sports
Medicine Rehabilitation Institue, Arlington,
Virginia

Faren H. Williams, MD, MS
Clinical Associate Professor, Department of Rehabilitation
Medicine, Jefferson Medical College; Albert Einstein
Medical Center and Moss Rehabilitation Hospital,
Philadelphia, Pennsylvania

Michael J. Woods, DO
Pioneer Spine and Sports Physicians, PC, West Springfield,
Massachusetts

Jeffrey L. Woodward, MD, MS
Private Practitioner, Springfield Physical Medicine and
Rehabilitation, PC; Staff, Cox Medical Center, Springfield,
Missouri

Anne Zeni, DO, PT
Assistant Professor, Sports Medicine Center, Departments
of Orthopaedic Surgery and Physical Medicine and
Rehabilitation, Medical College of Wisconsin, Milwaukee,
Wisconsin

Preface

From the beginning, it was our idea to create a book that covers a variety of medical conditions that the average internist/family practitioner, physiatrist, orthopedist, rheumatologist, and neurologist would encounter in his or her medical practice. We particularly wanted to emphasize the outpatient aspects of both musculoskeletal injuries and chronic medical conditions requiring rehabilitation from the perspective of a practitioner in an ambulatory setting.

Essentials of Physical Medicine and Rehabilitation covers many diagnoses in a deliberately succinct and specific format. This book is divided into two sections. The first section contains 91 chapters on specific musculoskeletal diagnoses. The second section consists of 54 chapters on common medical conditions that are typically chronic and benefit from rehabilitative as well as other interventions. Each chapter includes the same sections in the same order (Synonyms, ICD-9 Codes, Definition, Symptoms, Physical Examination, Functional Limitations, Diagnostic Studies, Differential Diagnosis, Treatment [Initial, Rehabilitation, Procedures, Surgery], Potential Disease Complications, Potential Treatment Complications, References). It is our hope that physicians in all specialties and allied healthcare providers will find that this book complements the excellent existing rehabilitation textbooks, and that it will be an efficient and useful tool in the office setting.

We are extremely grateful for the hard work of our colleagues who authored chapters and represent many different specialties and come from excellent institutions around the country. Their generous support of our work has made this book possible. We would like to specifically acknowledge the tremendous support of the faculty, residents, and staff in the Department of Physical Medicine and Rehabilitation at Harvard Medical School and Spaulding Rehabilitation Hospital. We would also like to thank the president of Spaulding Rehabilitation Hospital, John Cupples, and the Vice President for Non-acute Services of Partners Health Care, David Storto, who have unfailingly supported our academic endeavors.

Finally we would like to thank our talented illustrator, Suzanne Lennard, and the editors at Hanley & Belfus, Inc., Bill Lamsback and Tom Stringer, who were instrumental in bringing this book to publication.

Walter R. Frontera, MD, PhD
Julie K. Silver, MD

Dedication

To my mentors, teachers, colleagues, and students who have encouraged me to pursue an academic career with their enthusiasm for knowledge and learning.

Walter R. Frontera, MD, PhD

Throughout my life, I have been blessed with wonderful teachers who have devoted their lives to encouraging young people to pursue learning. I am particularly grateful to my greatest teacher, my father, who encouraged me to think critically and to pursue science and medicine. I am also eternally grateful to my mother and my husband for their unfailing support, a cherished gift.

Julie K. Silver, MD

SECTION 1

Musculoskeletal Disorders

1 Cervical Myelopathy

Avital Fast, MD
Mark A. Thomas, MD

Synonyms

Spondylosis

Neck arthritis

Osteoarthritis of the neck

ICD-9 Codes

721.0
Cervical spondylosis without myelopathy

721.1
Cervical spondylosis with myelopathy

723.0
Spinal stenosis in cervical region

723.1
Cervicalgia

723.4
Brachial neuritis or radiculitis nos; cervical radiculitis; radicular syndrome of upper limbs

781.2
Abnormality of gait

Definition

Cervical spondylotic myelopathy (CSM) is the most common spinal cord disease affecting middle-aged and elderly patients. The usual presentation is gradual paralysis over time. One or several spinal cord levels are compromised by degenerative changes in the spinal column. The condition tends to evolve gradually and is painless in many patients. CSM leads to gait dysfunction and functional decline in the upper extremities. The course of the disease is protracted and may result in significant disability.

The pathogenesis of CSM is complex and involves spinal cord compression and ischemia. Aging is accompanied by changes in the discs, ligaments, and bony structures of the spinal column. These changes can most severely affect one or multiple levels. Distortion of the spinal column may cause dynamic instability when the spine is flexed, extended, and rotated. This may lead to vascular insufficiency and ultimately ischemia.[1–4] The conservative management options are limited and do not affect the natural course of this condition. Surgical intervention, however, may arrest the condition and lead to gradual functional improvement.

Symptoms

CSM develops very gradually and subtly. The discrepancy between the patient's neurologic presentation and the paucity of pain may be quite striking. A minority of patients seeks help at an early stage due to radicular complaints. The patient may present initially with gait dysfunction, including complaints that the gait is not as smooth as it was, the base of support is wider, or that there are problems turning or changing directions. Later, the patient may start tripping or falling due to lower extremity weakness that may be combined with posterior column deficits. At times, vertigo or dizziness due to encroachment on the vertebral arteries further compromises the gait.

CSM may also present with slow and gradual development of weakness and clumsiness in the hands. Deficiencies in fine motor coordination may appear. Frequently these symptoms are accompanied by numbness in the hands although overt sensory deficits are not common.

Most patients do not present with a major complaint of neck pain, although when asked, many will recall past episodes of cervical pain.

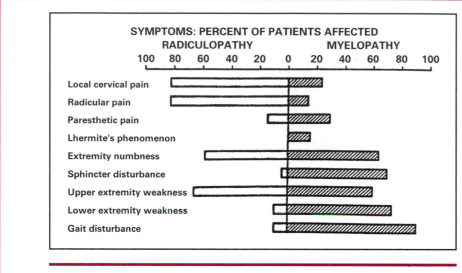

FIGURE 1. Symptoms at admission in radiculopathy and myelopathy groups. Included are all symptoms in all patients. Reproduced with permission; obtained from: Cervical spondylotic radiculopathy and myelopathy. Arch Neurol 1976;33: 618–625. Copyrighted (2000), American Medical Association.

Unlike cervical radiculopathy, CSM is relatively a painless condition in many patients (Fig. 1). Occasionally, patients may report feeling electrical sensations running down through the spine during neck flexion (Lhermitte's phenomenon).

Most patients maintain bowel and bladder function until late stages of the disease.

Rarely, the patient may spontaneously report the presence of fasciculations in affected muscles.[2,5–7]

Physical Examination

The essential elements in the physical examination are signs of lower motor neuron lesion in the upper extremities and signs of upper motor neuron lesion in the lower extremities. At times a mixture of upper and lower motor neuron signs may be elicited in the upper extremities. When CSM is accompanied by lumbar spinal stenosis, areflexia may be observed in the lower extremities.

Atrophy and weakness may be observed in the small muscles of the hands. Frequently the proximal muscles of the upper extremities are affected as well. Occasionally severe wasting akin to what is seen in severe peripheral neuropathy is apparent—amyotrophic hands. The clinical findings in the upper extremities may be symmetric or asymmetric, depending on the location and amount of nerve damage and atrophy. Long tract signs may be observed in the lower extremities: spasticity, hyper-reflexia and up-going toes. Decreased sensation to light touch, pain, and temperature may be observed (Fig. 2).

Most patients have a decreased cervical range of motion, especially in extension. In many patients the neck is permanently held in a flexed posture. As a result of this position the head does not reach the wall when the patient stands with the back to the wall. At times, this evolves into a fixed posture, and the patient cannot extend the head even to the neutral position.

Early on, while normal gait may be preserved, tandem gait becomes compromised or altogether impossible. As the disease progresses the gait becomes unsteady and the balance may be compromised. This leads to a wide-based jerky gait. Patients may have some difficulties in turning, and the turning is performed in a clumsy fashion.[3,8]

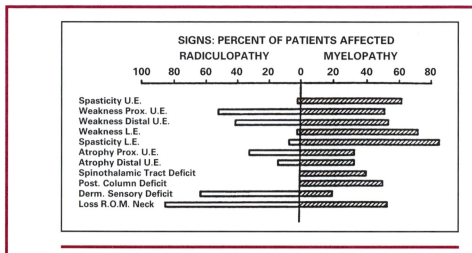

FIGURE 2. Physical findings at admission in radiculopathy and myelopathy groups. Included are all signs found in all patients. *UE* indicates upper extremity; *prox,* proximal part; *LE,* lower extremity; *derm,* dermatomal; *ROM,* range of motion. Reproduced with permission; obtained from: Cervical spondylotic radiculopathy and myelopathy. Arch Neurol 1976;33:618–625. Copyrighted (2000), American Medical Association.

Functional Limitations

Functional limitations depend on the degree of paralysis and associated symptoms, such as poor balance. Patients may resist going out because of the fear of falling. They may have difficulty going up and down stairs or even curbs. Lifting may become more difficult, and patients may be unable to unload groceries, lift small packages, etc. These limitations may affect home, as well as vocational, activities. Bowel and bladder dysfunction can be highly embarrassing and lead to social isolation.

Diagnostic Studies

Degenerative changes are commonly seen in the elderly (regardless of whether they are symptomatic), therefore, plain films are usually of limited value.

Dynamic studies (flexion and extension films) may reveal spinal segmental instability with excessive intervertebral movement (greater than 3 mm slip).[9] Quantitative methods are used to diagnose cervical spinal stenosis from plain films of the cervical spine. Using the lateral view, if the ratio between the sagittal diameter of the spinal canal (as determined from the posterior vertebral body cortex to the spino-laminar line) divided by the sagittal diameter of the vertebral body (at the same plane) is less than 0.82, then the patient has significant spinal stenosis.[10] This measurement technique, which eliminates magnification errors, is mostly helpful in identifying patients with developmental stenosis.

MRI may be the best diagnostic modality since it images the entire cervical spine. In patients with multilevel myelopathy, the cord appears in the sagittal views like a row of sausages, which can be easily identified. This shape is created due to cord impingement from the front by soft or hard discs and from the back by hypertrophied ligamenta flava. In the axial views the spinal canal diameter can be determined. A normal canal should have an anteroposterior diameter of at least 14 mm. The cord compression ratio (sagittal diameter divided by the transverse diameter × 100) and the cord sectional area may provide a good index of cord pathology. A cross-sectional area of less than 40 mm[2] is considered abnormal.[11,12]

The significance of an increased cord signal on MRI as a reliable prognostic indicator still remains controversial. Its presence, however, is indicative of cord atrophy, myelomalacia, edema, or gliosis. It is seen in T2-weighted images as hyperintensity within the cord parenchyma. The abnormal signal is usually found at the point of maximal compression or just below that area. Having a normal cord signal should not serve as a positive prognostic indicator and therefore should not rule out surgical intervention when indicated. On the other hand, increased cord signal does not necessarily predict poor outcome with conservative management.[12,13]

CT accompanied by myelography is generally only recommended in patients who are surgical candidates. Many surgeons feel comfortable enough to perform an operation in the absence of myelography and rely solely on MRI findings. On the other hand, some surgeons prefer to have this study done before operating since it provides superior bone details.

Electrodiagnostic studies such as somatosensory evoked potentials (SSEPs) and motor evoked potentials (MEPs) play a limited role from the diagnostic point of view. SSEPs may remain normal, even in individuals with symptomatic myelopathy. Serial evaluation of SSEPs and MEPs may have prognostic implications and may help in determining the management course. At times SSEPs may provide guidance to the surgeon and help exclude clinically silent cord compression from surgery.[14,15]

Differential Diagnosis

Amyotrophic lateral sclerosis	Inclusion body myositis[17]
Multiple sclerosis	Spinal radiculopathy
Syringomyelia	Polyneuropathy
Multifocal motor neuropathy[16]	Cervical spinal cord tumors

Treatment

Initial

CSM is a complex disorder with an unpredictable course. The natural history of CSM, though, is that it will worsen with time. Therefore, in medically stable patients, surgery is generally appropriate.

In elderly patients with significant co-morbidities, conservative treatment may be considered. The conservative approach should include patient education about the possible complications of cervical myelopathy. Additionally, lifestyle modifications should be addressed with particular attention given to avoiding activities in which prolonged cervical extension is required (e.g., painting a ceiling, placing items on high shelves).[18,19] The height of the computer should be adjusted, especially for patients with bifocal glasses. At the hair dresser the patient should face the sink and not get his or her hair washed with the neck hyperextended. When swimming, especially the breast stroke, a snorkel is highly recommended because it may help prevent repetitive hyperextension of the cervical spine. The headrest in the car should be adjusted so that it is in close proximity to the back of the head.

Cervical orthoses can be prescribed, especially in patients with severe narrowing of the spinal canal.

Analgesics, NSAIDs, and COX-2 inhibitors may be used to treat pain and inflammation. Local modalities such as heat and ice may also be used for pain.

Rehabilitation

Active cervical range-of-motion exercises should be discouraged. The normal aging process leads to restrictions in the cervical range, which may become beneficial, especially in patients with tight canal or narrowed intervertebral foraminae. Static neck exercises done in a neutral position may be safely recommended. These enable the patient to preserve his or her cervical muscle strength without jeopardizing the neural elements.

More aggressive strengthening exercises can be prescribed for the lower and upper extremity muscles. Physical therapy can focus on strengthening, and balance exercises may be done to help prevent falls.[2]

The physical therapist can also teach patients to use appropriate assistive devices (e.g., canes, walkers) to minimize the risk of falls.

Either a physical or occupational therapist may review the home environment for safety, and recommendations such as a raised toilet seat, grab bars in the bathroom, and a bath or shower seat can be helpful.

Procedures

The judicious use of epidural steroids may be advocated at times. This may bring temporary relief to some patients.

Surgery

Surgical intervention should be considered for patients with relentless progression manifested by functional deterioration. There does not seem to be a justification for prophylactic surgical intervention, even in patients with significant abnormalities in the neuroimaging studies.

Two basic surgical approaches exist: anterior and posterior. The surgical approach is influenced by the location of pathology, the number of levels involved, the presence or absence of cervical kyphosis, and the surgeon's comfort level with each approach. If the main pathology resides in the front (soft or hard disc) and when a significant amount of cervical kyphosis is present, the surgeon will likely choose the anterior approach. In patients with posterior pathology (hypertrophied ligamenta flava, thick laminae), the posterior approach is preferred. In patients with up to three level disease, the anterior as well as the posterior approach may be adopted. In patients with pathology in three or more levels, the posterior approach is preferable as the potential for significant complications and morbidity in this approach is lower.[2,20]

Patients who fail laminaplasty can undergo multiple laminectomies. Patients who successfully undergo surgery can expect stabilization of their neurologic condition and often can even improve their preoperative level of function.[2,20–22]

Potential Disease Complications

Paralysis is the primary disease complication. Additionally, bowel and bladder dysfunction may occur. In some instances, chronic intractable pain occurs, as well.

Potential Treatment Complications

Surgical complications are numerous and beyond the scope of this text. However, they should be discussed at length with the patient prior to operating. The risk for pseudoarthrosis rises when anterior cervical discectomy and fusion is attempted at three or more levels. In surgical fusions, many patients may develop clinically significant degenerative disc disease above or below the fusion.

Overly aggressive physical therapy may lead to clinical deterioration and paralysis.

Analgesics, NSAIDs, and COX-2 inhibitors have well-known side effects that most commonly affect the gastric, hepatic, and renal systems.

References

1. Hoff JT, Wilson CB: The pathophysiology of cervical spondylotic radiculopathy and myelopathy. Clin Neurosurg 1977;24:474–487.
2. Truumees E, Herkowitz HN: Cervical spondylotic myelopathy and radiculopathy. Instr Course Lect 2000;49:339–360.
3. Brain RW, Northfield D, Wilkinson M: The neurological manifestations of cervical spondylosis. Brain 1952;75:187–225.
4. Bohlman HH, Emery S: The pathophysiology of cervical spondylosis and myelopathy. Spine 1988;13:843–846.
5. McCormack BM, Weinstein PR: Cervical spondylosis. An update. West J Med 1996;165:43–51.
6. Long ML: Lumbar and cervical spondylosis and spondylotic myelopathy. Curr Opin Neurol Neurosurg 1993;6:576–580.
7. Macnab I: Cervical spondylosis. Clin Orthop 1975;109: 69–77.
8. Gregorius KF, Estrin T, Crandall PH: Cervical spondylotic radiculopathy and myelopathy. A long term follow-up study. Arch Neurol 1976;33:618–625.
9. Bernhardt M, Hynes RA, Blume HW, White AA: Current concepts review: Cervical spondylotic myelopathy. J Bone Joint Surg 1993;75-A:119–128.
10. Pavlov H, Torg JS, Robie B, Jahre C: Cervical spinal stenosis: Determination with vertebral body ratio method. Radiology 1987;164:771–775.
11. Mihara H, Ohnari K, Hachiya M, et al: Cervical myelopathy caused by C3-C4 spondylosis in elderly patients. Spine 2000;7:796–800.
12. Naderi S, Ozgen S, Pamir MN, et al: Cervical spondylotic myelopathy: Surgical results and factors affecting prognosis. Neurosurg 1998;43:43–49.
13. Matsumoto M, Toyama Y, Ishikawa M, et al: Increased signal intensity of the spinal cord on magnetic resonance images in cervical compressive myelopathy. Does it predict the outcome of conservative treatment? Spine 2000;25:677–682.
14. Tani T, Ishida K, Ushida T, Yamamoto H: Intraoperative electroneurography in the assessment of the level of operation for cervical spondylotic myelopathy in the elderly. J Bone Joint Surg 2000;82-B: 269–274.
15. Bednarik J, Kadanka Z, Vohanka S, et al: The value of somatosensory- and motor-evoked potentials in predicting and monitoring the effect of therapy in spondylotic cervical myelopathy. Spine 1999;24:1593–1598.
16. Taylor BV, Wright RA, Harper CM, Dyck PJ: Natural history of 46 patients with Multifocal motor neuropathy with conduction block. Muscle Nerve 2000;23:900–908.
17. Phillips BA, Zilko PJ, Mastaglia FL: Prevalence of sporadic inclusion body myositis in western Australia. Muscle Nerve 2000;23:970–972.
18. Samapth A, Bendebba M, Davis JD, Ducker TB: Outcome of patients treated for cervical myelopathy. A prospective, multicenter study with independent clinical review. Spine 2000;25:670–676.
19. Garvey TA, Eismont FJ: Diagnosis and treatment of cervical radiculopathy and myelopathy. Ortho Rev 199120:595–603.
20. Orr DR, Zdeblick TA: Cervical spondylotic myelopathy. Approaches to surgical treatment. Clin Orthop Rel Res 1999;359:58–66.
21. Tanaka J, Seki N, Tokimura F, Doi K, Inoue S: Operative results of canal-expansive laminoplasty for cervical spondylotic myelopathy in elderly patients. Spine 24: 2308-2312, 1999.
22. Hirabayashi K, Satomi K: Operative procedure and results of expansive open-door laminoplasty. Spine 1988;13: 870–876.

2 Cervical Facet Arthropathy

Ted A. Lennard, MD

Definition

Cervical facet arthropathy refers to any acquired, traumatic, or degenerative process that affects the normal function of the facet joints in the cervical region, often resulting in a source of neck pain and cervicogenic headaches. It may be a primary source of pain (e.g., whiplash) but often is secondary to a diseased or injured cervical disc.

Symptoms

Patients typically complain of generalized posterior neck and suboccipital pain but may present with localized tenderness over the posterolateral aspect of the neck. Pain provoked with cervical extension and axial rotation is common. These joints may refer pain anywhere from the midthoracic spine to the cranium, and often in the suboccipital region.[1–3]

Physical Examination

The essential element of the examination includes manual palpation of the spinal segments and elucidation of reproducible pain over the involved joints. Often the area of maximum tenderness is over the paraspinal muscles, which overlie the facet joints, and is precipitated by excessive cervical lordosis, causing abnormal joint forces. The fluidity of motion of the involved spinal area–cervical region may suggest extension pain with relief upon flexion.

Functional Limitations

When the cervical spine is involved, then cervical extension and rotation, overhead reaching, and overhead lifting may be difficult. This may interfere with activities such as driving, going to the theater, and brushing one's hair.

Diagnostic Studies

Fluoroscopic-guided intra-articular arthrographic-confirmed anesthetic injections are considered the "gold standard" for diagnosis.[4] Radiographic abnormalities on x-ray, CT, or MRI have not been shown to correlate with facet joint pain. A SPECT scan can be used in refractory cases of suspected

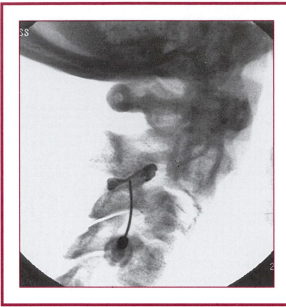

FIGURE 1. Lateral radiograph of a C2–C3 z-joint arthrogram using a lateral approach. (From Dreyfuss P, Kaplan M, Dreyer SJ: Zygapophyseal joint injection techniques in the spinal axis. In Lennard TA (ed): Pain Procedures in Clinical Practice, 2nd ed. Philadelphia, Hanley & Belfus, 2000, p 291.)

lumbar facet disorders to rule out underlying bony processes that may mimic facet pain (e.g., spondylolysis, infection, tumor). When positive, the scan may confirm the proposed diagnosis and determine which specific joint is affected.

Differential Diagnosis

Disc herniation

Internal disc disruption

Degenerative disc disease

Myofascial pain syndrome

Nerve root compression

Cervical stenosis

Spondylolysis/spondylolisthesis

Infection

Tumor

Treatment

Initial

Initial treatment emphasizes local pain control with ice, oral analgesics and NSAIDs, topical creams, local peri-articular corticosteroid injections, and avoidance of exacerbating activities.

Specialized pillows may be helpful, but rarely are cervical collars indicated.

Rehabilitation

Manual forms of therapy and low velocity manipulations (e.g., osteopathic manipulation) may be useful to patients with isolated facet disorders. In healthy patients with no associated spinal pathology (e.g., disc abnormalities, radiculopathy, stenosis, fracture), low velocity manipulations may be used on a limited basis in cases unresponsive to routine conservative care. Use in the cervical region should be approached with extreme caution and only performed by experienced practitioners.

Physical therapy may consist of passive modalities such as ultrasound; electrical stimulation, including TENS; traction; and diathermy to reduce local pain. However, these modalities have not been shown to change long-term outcomes. Regional manual therapy with facet gapping techniques can be helpful. Advancement into a flexion biased exercise program with regional stretching is the mainstay of rehabilitation. For recurrent episodes of pain, a change in daily/work activity, sporting technique, or other biomechanical adjustments may eliminate the underlying forces at the joint level.

Procedures

Intra-articular, fluoroscopic-guided, contrast-enhanced facet injections are considered critical for proper diagnosis and can be instrumental in the treatment of facet joint arthropathies. A patient can be examined both preinjection and postinjection to determine what portion of his or her pain can be attributed to the joints injected. Typically, small amounts of anesthetic and or corticosteroid are injected directly into the joint. Another step may be to perform medial branch blocks of the affected joints with small volumes (0.1–0.3 cc) of anesthetic. If the facet joint is found to be the putative source of pain, a denervation procedure using radiofrequency, cryotherapy, or chemicals (e.g., phenol) may be considered. Acupuncture may also be considered.

Surgery

Surgery is rarely necessary in isolated facet joint arthropathies. Surgical spinal fusion may be performed for discogenic pain, which may affect secondary cases of facet joint arthropathies.

Potential Disease Complications

Since facet joint arthropathy is usually degenerative in nature, this disorder is often progressive, resulting in chronic, intractable spinal pain. It usually co-exists with spinal disc abnormalities, further leading to chronic pain. This subsequently results in diminished spinal motion, weakness, and loss of flexibility.

Potential Treatment Complications

Treatment-related complications may be caused by medications: NSAIDs may cause GI and renal problems, and analgesics may result in liver dysfunction and constipation. Local peri-articular injections and acupuncture may cause local transient needle pain. Facet injections may cause transient local spinal pain, swelling, and possibly bruising. More serious injection complications may include infection, injury to a blood vessel or nerve, injury to the spinal cord, and an allergic reaction to the medications. Exacerbation of symptoms often transiently occurs postinjection. Cervical injections may also precipitate headaches.

References
1. Bogduk N, Marsland A: The cervical zygapophyseal joints as a source of neck pain. Spine 1988;13:610–617.
2. Dwyer A, Aprill C, Bogduk N: Cervical zygapophyseal joint pain patterns 1: A study in normal volunteers. Spine 1990;15:453–457.
3. Fukui S, Ohseto K, Shiotani M: Referred pain distribution of the cervical zygapophyseal joints and cervical dorsal rami. Pain 1996;68:79–83.
4. Bogduk N: International Spinal Injection Society Guidelines for the performance of spinal injection procedures. Part I. Zygapophysial joint blocks. Clin J Pain 1997;13:285–302.
5. Dreyer S, Dreyfuss P, Cole A: Posterior elements and low back pain. Phys Med Rehabil State Art Rev 1999;13:443–471.

3 Cervical Degenerative Disease

Avital Fast, MD
Mark A. Thomas, MD

Synonyms

Spondylosis

Arthritis

Osteoarthritis of the neck

ICD-9 Codes

721.0
Cervical spondylosis without myelopathy

721.1
Cervical spondylosis with myelopathy

722.4
Brachial neuritis or radiculitis; cervical radiculitis; radicular syndrome of upper limbs

723.0
Spinal stenosis in cervical region

723.1
Cervicalgia

723.4
Degeneration of cervical intervertebral disc

Definition

Cervical spondylosis encompasses the degenerative changes that occur in the spine (disc, vertebral body, and uncovertebral and facet joints). Cervical spondylosis may result in local pain, stiffness, and restricted cervical motion. In addition to degenerative changes related to age or trauma, genetics may play a role in the pathogenesis of cervical spondylosis, such as with chondrodysplasia or familial similarities in spinal shape and loading patterns.[1]

Cervical spondylotic radiculopathy is the clinical expression of nerve root compression or impingement due to hypertrophic degenerative changes of the cervical spine, including joints and ligaments, that follow disc dehydration and loss of disc space. This results in a narrowing of the neural foramen or lateral recess. Subsequent impingement of a cervical nerve root then results in pain, weakness, and sensory and reflex abnormalities in a specific distribution.

Degenerative spondylotic changes occur gradually and in a known sequence. Dehydration of the intervertebral disc results in loss of disc height. With this disc space narrowing, buckling of intralaminar ligaments takes place, and protrusion of the disc may occur. This change in the cervical spine configuration results in abnormal weight distribution and loading patterns with compensatory changes (e.g., sclerosis, osteophyte formation) in the vertebral body and facet and uncovertebral joints. Symptoms may relate directly to bony changes or abnormal load patterns and can also result from compromise of neural or vascular structures. Stenosis due to spondylosis may affect the spinal canal and provoke a myelopathy, or the neural foramen or lateral recess may be stenosed. When recess or foraminal stenosis occurs, the patient is at risk for radiculopathy (see Chapter 4). Uncovertebral osteophytes may compress nerve roots, particularly at the C4-6 levels due to root proximity to the spur at this level, the smaller AP diameter of the neural foramen, and the longer course of nerve roots relative to other cervical levels.[2] Asymptomatic spondylotic stenosis of the neural foramen places the patient at risk for radiculopathy due to compression when activities are performed that involve frequent lateral neck rotation or extension. Precipitating activities reported in the literature range from ballroom dancing to shampooing (salon sink radiculopathy).[3,4] Compromise of the anterior spinal artery or vertebral arteries may also produce an array of symptoms (see Potential Disease Complications later in the chapter).

Symptoms

Cervical spondylosis may cause neck pain, stiffness with loss of motion in one or more planes, and paraspinal muscle spasm. Nuchal or occipital headache may be present. Characteristic symptoms of cervical radiculopathy include arm pain, weakness, clumsiness, paresthesia, or hypesthesia occurring in a dermatomal distribution. Pain in the trapezius, paraspinal, and interscapular areas may also be noted. When symptoms persist, a chronic pain syndrome, including symptoms relating to lack of restorative sleep and depression, may develop. Much less common is pain in the chest (cervical angina), ear, or other craniofacial areas.[5]

Physical Examination

The diagnosis of cervical spondylosis can often be made on a clinical basis. Inspection of the spine may reveal an abnormal cervical posture. Straightening of the cervical lordosis may result from paraspinal muscle spasm, which may be noted on physical examination but is best seen from a lateral x-ray view (Fig. 1). Compensatory movement away from the site of nerve root impingement results in a postural asymmetry most readily seen from an anterior or posterior view. Palpation of the spinous processes, paraspinal muscles, and lateral neck muscles may disclose tenderness. Nuchal line or mastoid tenderness can be present when there is related muscle spasm. Muscles that are chronically in spasm may be tight and have a knotty or fibrous texture.

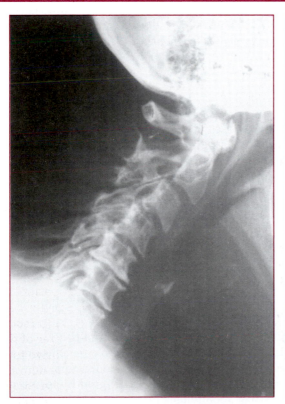
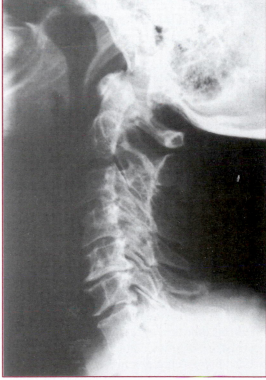

FIGURE 1. Cervical spondylosis. X-rays of the cervical spine, flexion and extension views. Note the loss of disc space, sclerosis, osteophyte formation, and changes in segmental alignment with motion.

Cervical active range of motion is generally reduced. It is important to note whether the loss of motion occurs in one or multiple planes. The speed and quality of cervical motion may also provide some insight into the severity of disease, and consequently the risk for disability. Patients will "splint" or restrict motion that provokes pain due to facet loading or nerve root impingement, thus restrictions in rotation, lateral flexion, and extension may indicate the site of pathology. Pain that is provoked by extension and axial rotation occurs when nerve root motion is restricted. This does not occur with a herniated cervical disc that does not impinge neural structures.[6]

The lower cervical segments, C5-7, usually demonstrate earlier and more severe degenerative changes than more proximal segments. Consequently physical examination for radicular findings most often demonstrates lower cervical root involvement. Related muscles can be weak, and occasionally fasciculations are present.

Provocatory positions or maneuvers, such as axial compression, may result in narrowing of the neural foramen and radicular symptoms. Positioning the neck in extension and rotation may have a similar effect. Pain with forward flexion may result from stretch of tight paraspinal/posterior muscles; however, when formication (a type of tingling paresthesia) is present (Lhermitte's sign), myelopathy is more likely. Radicular symptoms may ease when tension or compression of a restricted nerve root is decreased. For example, cervical flexion or flexion plus contralateral lateral flexion increases foraminal size, decreasing root compression; ipsilateral elbow flexion with shoulder abduction and flexion may reduce root tension (the abduction relief sign).[7]

Functional Limitations

Restricted cervical motion due to spondylosis can limit upward gaze and the ability to turn the head to look sideways or rearward. Driving, working overhead, swimming, and many other activities may be compromised for this reason. Motor and sensory changes may impair grip, handwriting, or other fine motor activities. Power grasp requires wrist extension and this, as well as any fine motor activity, often requires shoulder stabilization, which can also be affected when cervical roots are compromised.

Diagnostic Studies

The menu of diagnostic tests for cervical spondylosis includes plain radiographs, magnetic resonance imaging (MRI), computerized tomography (CT), Doppler ultrasound, and electrodiagnosis (electromyography and nerve conduction studies, somatosensory evoked potentials).

Plain films reveal spondylotic changes in many asymptomatic cervical spines. When a patient is symptomatic, however, AP and lateral views can provide insight into the severity of disc degeneration and vertebral hypertrophic changes. Oblique views allow visualization of the facets and neural foramina. Flexion-extension views are helpful when instability is suspected. It is possible to quantify foraminal stenosis by viewing plain radiographs. A 20% reduction of foraminal area occurs in conjunction with a 1 mm narrowing of the intervertebral disc space. When compared with normal segments, a 2 mm loss of disc height corresponds to a 30% to 40% foraminal stenosis and 3 mm of lost disc space corresponds to a loss of 35% to 45% of foraminal area.[8]

MRI studies of the cervical spine are good for delineation of soft tissues, including the intervertebral disc and spinal cord. They should be considered whenever neurologic changes are noted by history or physical examination. MRI can also provide insight into neurologic compromise before changes are clinically evident because the degree of cord signal hyperintensity on the T2 weighted images relates to both the severity of spondylosis and degree of ischemia caused by compression of the anterior spinal artery.[9]

MRI is usually the imaging study of choice; however, CT imaging is more appropriate when a fracture is suspected and plain films are inconclusive, or to determine the degree of osseous foraminal or lateral recess stenosis.[10] CT myelography may be considered when myelopathy is suspected (see Chapter 3).

Doppler ultrasound is a good method for examination of intertransverse flow of vertebral arteries.[11] It provides helpful information when there is symptomatic vertebrobasilar insufficiency and the level of spondylotic constriction is uncertain.

Electrodiagnostic studies are most useful for defining and locating a neurologic lesion. They supplement the clinical examination and imaging studies. They become particularly important in distinguishing peripheral nerve or brachial plexus lesions from radiculopathy when findings of weakness or sensory loss do not occur in a dermatomal distribution. In addition to providing useful information in the differential diagnosis, electromyography may help to determine the acuity, or chronicity, of the nerve lesion.[12]

Differential Diagnosis

Vertebral osteomyelitis

Epidural abscess

Tumor (particularly chordoma)

Radiculopathy due to other cause
   (for example, disc herniation)

Thoracic outlet syndrome

Peripheral nerve entrapment

Rheumatoid arthritis

Spondyloarthropathy

Cervical strain

Cervical sprain

Rotator cuff tear

Adhesive capsulitis

Glenohumeral ganglion cyst[13]

Treatment

Initial

With medical and rehabilitation management, most patients experience a good outcome as it relates to radiculopathy.[14] The prognosis for axial pain is not as favorable. When the patient is a candidate for cervical traction, the overall success rate is about 80%.[15] In general, two-thirds of patients with radiculopathy do well with conservative care, and one-third require surgical intervention.[14]

Pharmacologic management of cervical spondylosis and spondylotic radiculopathy should include nonsteroidal anti-inflammatory drugs (NSAIDs) including cyclooxygenase-2 (COX-2) inhibitors. Analgesics may be prescribed. Tricyclic antidepressants such as amitriptyline or, more commonly, nortriptyline (when the patient is elderly) may be used. There may be a role for brief, initial use of narcotic medication, but chronic use of narcotics should be discouraged. Muscle relaxants (e.g., eperisone,[16] diazepam, chlorazoxasone, or cyclobenzaprine) and adjunctive medication (e.g., acetaminophen or hydroxyzine) can be used to treat pain, stiffness, and restricted motion. Depending on the selection of medication(s), concomitant use of a stool softener, laxative, or antacid may be appropriate. Patients must be informed about medication-related sedation in order to avoid preventable injuries. The application of home modalities (e.g., heat, ice) and the use of counterirritants should be part of the initial patient education.

For some patients, particularly those with motion-related pain or significant muscle spasm, initial or intermittent use of a soft cervical collar or cervical pillow may be helpful. Long-term outcome studies comparing the use of a soft cervical collar to surgery and physical therapy show similar improvement in all groups after about 1 year.[17–19] There are no clear guidelines regarding the use of cervical collars or pillows. Anecdotal reports suggest that intermittent use may provide similar benefit to constant use and prevent the weakness, stiffness, and loss of motion that can occur following prolonged immobilization. A reasonable trial of soft cervical collar wear might be 3 hours of wear alternating with $\frac{1}{2}$ to 1 hour of free time with gentle active range of motion. The patient should be counseled regarding posture, movement, and activity as they relate to the pain—if it hurts, don't do it. Significant relief may be provided by shoulder abduction, particularly with lower cervical radiculopathy[20]; and this should be incorporated into the initial treatment when appropriate.

Epidural steroid injection can provide significant relief from radicular symptoms.[21] It is important to select patients carefully and to inject early in the course of the disease (prior to 4 to 6 months of disease duration).[22] See the Procedures section.

Rehabilitation

Patient education in the independent application of modalities and a home exercise program is the key element of patient management. Defects in posture or deficits in flexibility and strength of the cervical, scapular, and shoulder areas should be addressed. Education should also be provided about the natural course of the disease and the risk of serious injury with even minor neck trauma (e.g., incomplete cord syndromes).[23] The principles of motion economy (e.g., tool organization by frequency of use) and general safety (e.g., non-skid flooring and night lights) should be reviewed with the patient.

Manual or mechanical cervical traction may relieve radicular symptoms. It should be considered with the caveat that when there is chronic nerve root inflammation, resulting fibrosis can cause dural tethering and exacerbation of radiculopathy upon cervical distraction.[24] Gentle mobilization of the spondylotic cervical spine may provide symptomatic relief, but overt manipulation should be avoided due to the potential for serious vascular and neurologic complications.[20] Modalities (e.g., ice, electrotherapy, heat) can be useful to reduce or resolve muscle spasm, and transcutaneous electrical nerve stimulation (TENS) might provide relief from radiating or referred pain. Patients should be provided with adaptive equipment appropriate for their specific activities of daily living. For example, mirrors can supplement restricted cervical motion and the build-up of tool handles (e.g., utensils, pens) can compensate for loss of grip strength. If the patient uses a computer, the position of the monitor should encourage a neutral cervical posture. Appropriate ergonomic suggestions include the use of a slanted writing board, document holder, book stand, and telephone headset.

Procedures

Selective block of a nerve root, epidural steroid injection, facet block, or other injections is not commonly employed for spondylotic radiculopathy. Nonetheless, good pain relief has been reported—lasting up to 24 months for about 80% of patients treated by cervical epidural steroid.[25] If injection is considered, patients should be referred no later than 4 to 6 months after symptom onset[22] and specifically for the relief of radicular symptoms, rather than for axial pain.[26] For intractable head and neck or ear pain that relates to cervical spondylosis, facet block at the higher cervical levels may provide relief that has not been achieved through other conservative interventions.[5]

Surgery

While surgery is a common treatment modality when cervical spondylosis results in myelopathy, it is only considered for spondylosis alone or in combination with radiculopathy when the patient's symptoms cannot be managed conservatively. Stenosis of the lateral recess or neural foramen with intractable pain or progressive neurologic deficit, severe deformity, or instability may be indications for surgical intervention.[27] Success rates, as well as the definition of success, vary among authors, but the literature generally supports a surgical success rate of approximately 75% for long-term relief of symptoms.[28] A variety of surgical approaches and procedures are available, and controversy exists regarding which is optimal. All the diverse surgical procedures attempt to relieve compression or impingement of the spinal cord, nerve root(s), or spinal arteries (anterior spinal, vertebrobasilar) while providing a stable spine with as much residual motion as possible. Most techniques include anterior, posterior, or posterior plus anterior arthrodesis at one or more levels.[29,30] Generally central 1-2 level pathology is treated with anterior cervical discectomy and fusion. When three or more levels of contiguous pathology are identified, anterior cervical corpectomy or laminoplasty is common.[31] Posterior decompression with laminoplasty or anterior decompression procedures with corpectomy of the involved segment reportedly lead to similar results.[27] If degenerative changes are noted in the cervical segment adjacent to the symptomatic one, fusion should extend to that segment as well; otherwise, there is a significant risk for the rapid development of a new radiculopathy.[32]

Potential Disease Complications

The natural course of cervical spondylosis, with or without radiculopathy, is often one of slowly decreasing function.[28] Nonetheless, an acceptable quality of life can usually be maintained unless the patient suffers a significant complication of the disease or treatment.

The more common complications of cervical spondylosis are stenosis of the spinal canal, which can result in myelopathy, and lateral recess or neural foramen stenosis, which can result in radiculopathy. Uncinate osteophytes, or less commonly, facet osteophytes may cause compression of the anterior spinal artery and cord ischemia.[9] Spondylotic compression of the vertebral arteries may present with dizziness, impaired balance, and increased postural sway. It is not uncommon, and an estimated 17% of symptomatic vertebrobasilar insufficiency is due to cervical hypertrophic changes.[11] Minor injury of the spondylotic cervical spine may result in spinal cord compromise.[23] As with many conditions, complex regional pain syndrome type II (RSD) or chronic pain syndromes can be associated with cervical spondylosis or spondylotic radiculopathy.

Potential Treatment Complications

Analgesics, NSAIDs, and COX-2 inhibitors have well-known side effects that most commonly affect the gastric, hepatic, and renal systems. Treatment goals for cervical range of motion and posture should be realistic and recognize restrictions imposed by structural changes in the cervical spine. This patient population is often elderly with age-related changes in soft tissue as well as in the spine. Excessive exercise may lead to muscle strain and persistent pain. Potential complications resulting from the application of cervical traction include worsening of radiculopathy or provocation of a lumbar radiculopathy.[24] The equipment and application should minimize the risk of temporomandibular joint irritation. Prolonged or constant use of a cervical collar might result in muscle tightness and weakness. Misapplication of modalities may lead to complications such as a burn or lack of relief. Cervical manipulation can compromise vertebral or spinal artery flow, resulting in ischemia of the brainstem or spinal cord. Complications following cervical epidural steroid injection include arachnoiditis, infection, meningitis, and an acute block or compressive lesion of the spinal cord.[33] Direct cord damage has been reported following intrathecal perforation/cord penetration,[34] although this has only been reported to occur when patients are sedated and unable to report paresthesias or other neurologic changes during the procedure.

References

1. Yoo K, Origitano TC: Familial cervical spondylosis. Case report. J Neurosurg 1998;89(1):139–141.
2. Ebraheim NA, Lu J, Biyani A, et al: Anatomic considerations for uncovertebral involvement in cervical spondylosis. Clin Orthop 1997;(334):200–206.
3. Tsung PA, Mulford GJ: Ballroom dancing and cervical radiculopathy: A case report. Arch Phys Med Rehabil 1998;79(10):1306–1308.
4. Stitik TP, Nadler SF, Foye PM: Salon sink radiculopathy: A case series. Am J Phys Med Rehabil 1999;78(4):381–383.
5. Lamer TJ: Ear pain due to cervical spine arthritis: Treatment with cervical facet injection. Headache 1991;31(10):682–683.
6. Muhle C, Bischoff L, Weinert D, et al: Exacerbated pain in cervical radiculopathy at axial rotation, flexion, extension and coupled motions of the cervical spine: Evaluation by kinematic magnetic resonance imaging. Invest Radiol 1998;33(5):279–288.
7. Fast A, Parikh S, Marin EL: The shoulder abduction relief sign in cervical radiculopathy. Arch Phys Med Rehabil 1989;70(5):402–403.
8. Lu J, Ebraheim NA, Huntoon M, Haman SP: Cervical intervertebral disc space narrowing and size of intervertebral foramina. Clin Orthop 2000;(370): 259–264.

9. Misfud V, Pullicino P: Spinal cord MRI hyperintensities in cervical spondylosis: Aan ischemic pathogenesis?. J Neuroimaging 2000;10(2):96–100.
10. Kaiser JA, Holland BA: Imaging of the cervical spine. Spine 1998;23(24):2701–2712.
11. Jargiello T, Pietura R, Rakowski P, et al: Power Doppler imaging in the evaluation of extracranial vertebral artery compression in patients with vertebrobasilar insufficiency. Eur J Ultrasound 1998;8(3):149–156.
12. Ellenberg MR, Honet JC, Treanor WJ: Cervical radiculopathy. Arch Phys Med Rehabil 1994;75(3):342–352.
13. Uppal GS, Uppal JA, Dwyer AP: Glenoid cysts mimicking cervical radiculopathy. Spine 1995;20(20):2257–2260.
14. Sampath P, Bendebba M, Davis JD, Ducker T: Outcome in patients with cervical radiculopathy. Prospective, multicenter study with independent clinical review. Spine 1999;24(6):591–597.
15. Swezey RL, Swezey AM, Warner K: Efficacy of home cervical traction therapy. Am J Phys Med Rehabil 1999;78(1):30–32.
16. Bose K: The efficacy and safety of eperisone in patients with cervical spondylosis: results of a randomized, double-blind placebo-controlled trial. Methods Find Exp Clin Pharmacol 1999;21(3):209–213.
17. Persson LC, Moritz U, Brandt L, Carlsson CA: Cervical radiculopathy: pain, muscle weakness and sensory loss in patients with cervical radiculopathy treated with surgery, physiotherapy or cervical collar. A prospective, controlled study. Eur Spine J 1997;6(4):256–266.
18. Persson LC, Carlsson CA, Carlsson JY. Long-lasting cervical radicular pain managed with surgery, physiotherapy, or a cervical collar. A prospective, randomized study. Spine 1997;22(7):751–758.
19. Persson L, Moritz U. Neck support pillows: a comparative study. J Manipulative Physiol Ther 1998;21(4):237–240.
20. Fast A, Zinicola DF, Marin EL: Vertebral artery damage complicating cervical manipulation. Spine 1987;12(9):840–842.
21. Bush K, Hillier S: Outcome of cervical radiculopathy treated with periradicular/epidural corticosteroid injection: A prospective study with independent clinical review. Eur Spine J 1996;5(5):319–325.
22. Gnezdilov AV, Syrovegin AV, Ovechkin AM, Ivanov AM: The epidural administration of steroids and local anesthetics as the basis for the pathogenetic therapy of a radicular pain syndrome in the stages of its development. Anesteziol Reanimatol 1996;(3):28–32.
23. Chen TY, Dickman CA, Eleraky M, Sonntag VK: The role of decompression for acute incomplete cervical spinal cord injury in cervical spondylosis. Spine 1998;23(22):2398–2403.
24. LaBann MM, Macy JA, Meerschaert JR: Intermittent cervical traction: A progenitor of lumbar radicular pain. Arch Phys Med Rehabil 1992;73(3):295–296.
25. Grenier B, Castagnera L, Maurette P, et al: Chronic cervicobrachial neuralgia treated by cervical epidural injection of corticosteroids. Long-term results. Ann Fr Anesth Reanim 1995;14(6):484–488.
26. Ferrante FM, Wilson SP, Iacobo C, et al: Clinical classification as a predictor of therapeutic outcome after cervical epidural steroid injection. Spine 1993;18(6):730–736.
27. Grob D: Surgery in the degenerative spine. Spine 1998;23(24):2674–2683.
28. McCormack BM, Weinstein PR: Cervical spondylosis. An update. West J Med 1996;165(1-2):43–51.
29. Iwasaki M, Okada K, Tsumaki N, et al: Cervical spondylotic radiculopathy involving two adjacent nerve roots. Anterior decompression through a single intervertebral approach. Int Orthop 1996;20(3):137–141.
30. Ozer AF, Oktenoglu BT, Sarioglu AC: A new surgical technique: Open-window corpectomy in the treatment of ossification of the posterior longitudinal ligament and advanced cervical spondylosis: Technical note. Neurosurgery 1999;45(6):1481–1485.
31. Truumees E, Kerkowitz HN: Cervical spondylotic myelopathy and radiculopathy. Instr Course Lect 2000;49:339–360.
32. Hilibrand AS, Carlson GD, Palumbo MA, et al: Radiculopathy and myelopathy at segments adjacent to the site of a previous anterior cervical arthrodesis. J Bone Joint Surg Am 1999;81(4):519–528.
33. McLain RF, Fry M, Hecht ST: Transient paralysis associated with epidural steroid injection. J Spinal Disord 1997;10(5):441–444.
34. Hodges SD, Castleberg RL,, Miller T, et al: Cervical epidural steroid injection with intrinsic spinal cord damage. Two case reports. Spine 1998;23(19):2137–2142.

4 Cervical Radiculopathy

Isaac Cohen, MD
Cristin Jouve, MD

Synonyms

Cervical disc herniation

Radiculitis

Brachialgia

ICD-9 Codes

722.0
Displacement of cervical intervertebral disk without myelopathy

723.4
Brachial neuritis or radiculitis; cervical radiculitis; radicular syndrome of upper limbs

Definition

Cervical radiculopathy is characterized by signs and symptoms related to cervical nerve root dysfunction. The most common causes for cervical radiculopathy are nerve root compression from cervical disc herniation (most commonly posterolateral and rarely central) and cervical spondylosis (osteophytic spurs from the vertebral body, uncovertebral joint, facet joint, or a combination).[1,2] (See Figs. 1 and 2. See also Chapter 3.) Generally, there is no preceding trauma or inciting event. C7 is the most commonly affected nerve root, followed by C6, C8, and C5 in descending order of incidence.[2,3] Radiculopathies of the C2 to C4 nerve roots are felt to be uncommon and clinically difficult to distinguish from other sources of pain.

There are eight cervical nerve roots, and each cervical nerve root exits above the vertebra of the same numeric designation, except for C8, which exits above the T1 vertebra. The neuroforamina are bordered anteromedially by the uncovertebral joint, posterolaterally by the facet joint, and superiorly and inferiorly by the pedicles of the vertebral bodies above and below.

This chapter primarily focuses on cervical radiculopathy arising from extradural compressive pathology by disc material or osteophytes.

Symptoms

Patients usually present with neck and predominant sharp, radiating pain in the upper extremity—the specific distribution depending on the nerve root involved. Pain may refer into the shoulder; interscapular; suboccipital; and, rarely, chest wall regions. Interscapular aching is a common complaint at

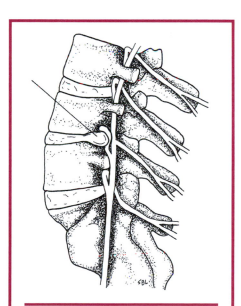

FIGURE 1. Typically, discs herniate posterolaterally and cause radicular symptoms when they compromise exiting nerve roots.

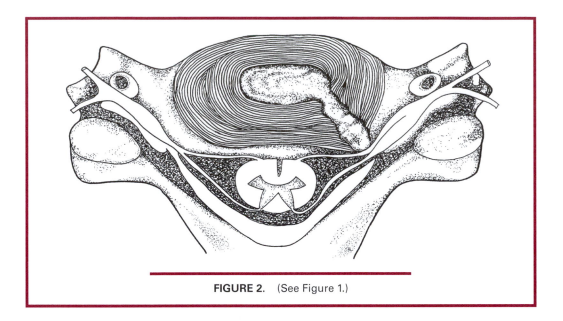

FIGURE 2. (See Figure 1.)

all cervical root levels and is of no localizing value.[4] Numbness and paresthesias are most commonly noted in the distal aspect of the dermatome involved. Neck movements and cough/Valsalva maneuvers commonly exacerbate pain. Patients may note weakness or inability to perform certain daily activities. A small percentage of patients will present only with weakness without significant pain or sensory complaints. Of the subjective complaints, the distribution of hand paresthesias appears to have the greatest localizing value.[4]

Bowel, bladder, and gait dysfunction are not features of a discrete radiculopathy, and the presence of these symptoms should alert the clinician to rule out spinal cord compression (i.e., cervical myelopathy).

Physical Examination

Although one should perform a thorough examination of the cervical spine, the main objective is to demonstrate specific nerve root level involvement. The clinician should observe the patient's gait, posture, and muscle bulk in the shoulder girdle and upper extremities. The bony and soft tissue structures of the cervical spine are palpated to assess for deformity and tenderness. Tenderness and muscle spasm are commonly present ipsilaterally. The cervical range of motion is assessed primarily to establish its relation to symptomatology, identify impairments, and establish a baseline for serial examinations. There is usually a reduction in cervical active range of motion, especially with extension, lateral bending, and rotation toward the symptomatic side, as these cause neuroforaminal narrowing and hence compression of the symptomatic nerve root.

TABLE 1

Root	Motor	Reflex	Sensory
C5	Deltoid, spinatii, biceps	Biceps	Lateral aspect of upper arm
C6	Biceps, brachioradialis, wrist extensors, pronator teres	Biceps, brachioradialis, pronator	Radial distal forearm and thumb, occasionally index finger
C7	Triceps, wrist extensors, pronator teres	Triceps, pronator	Posterior arm, dorsal forearm, middle and index fingers, occasionally index and ring fingers
C8	Intrinsic hand muscles	No reliable reflex is available	Medial forearm, fourth and fifth digits

The normal cervical range of motion is as follows:[5]

Flexion—45 degrees   Lateral bending—40 degrees

Extension—55 degrees   Rotation—70 degrees

A screening test of the shoulder involves asking patients to abduct their arms. If an abnormality is noted, then one should perform a more detailed assessment of the shoulder.

The neurologic examination should be directed toward looking for myotomal weakness, diminished/absent muscle stretch reflexes, and dermatomal hypesthesia of the involved root (Table 1). Comparison to the contralateral (uninvolved) side is helpful, and the distribution of motor weakness appears to be the most reliable physical examination sign for localizing the lesion to a single root level.[4] Myotomal weakness less than 3/5 is rare, given that all muscle groups in the upper extremity receive innervation from more than one root, with the possible exception of the rhomboids. Diminished muscle stretch reflexes can localize the level to one of two roots. The pronator reflex may be helpful to distinguish a C6 from a C7 root involvement when compared with the other reflexes.[6] Dermatomal examination of light touch and pinprick sensation should be performed at the distal aspect of the dermatome.

In addition to the gait examination, lower extremity muscle strength, deep tendon reflexes, plantar responses, and clonus should be tested to screen for myelopathy. There are several provocative/relief maneuvers[7-9] available to supplement the examination, and these appear to have a greater yield for the lower cervical nerve roots (i.e., C6 to C8). With Spurling's test (Fig. 3), the neck is laterally flexed and axially loaded. Reproduction of the patient's radicular symptoms is considered a positive sign. Having the patient elevate the hand above the head (shoulder abduction test) or providing gentle manual axial traction with the patient in a supine position (axial manual distraction test) are relief maneuvers that decrease nerve root tension and distract neuroforamina, respectively. These maneuvers do not localize the level of pathology, and their sensitivities are low (25% to 50%); thus they are less informative than nerve root tension signs with lumbar disc herniation.

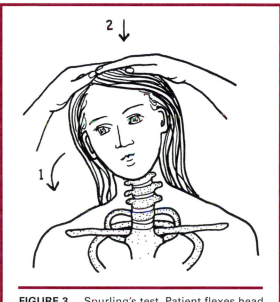

FIGURE 3. Spurling's test. Patient flexes head to one side (1), and examiner presses straight down on head (2).

Functional Limitations

Limitation of neck rotation secondary to pain may limit a patient's ability to drive and perform overhead activities. In addition, patients may experience weakness, clumsiness, and diminished grip strength. Triceps weakness may go unnoticed by a sedentary patient due to gravity assist in elbow extension. Pain commonly interferes with sleep, work, and social activities. Headaches may also be experienced, likely secondary to paraspinal muscle spasm and guarding.

Diagnostic Studies

Magnetic resonance imaging is the study of choice for evaluating cervical radiculopathy because it provides the best definition of the nerve root and herniation of the nucleus pulposus.[2,10] Plain radiographs should be performed in patients with a history or suspicion of trauma, infection, inflammatory diseases, or cancer. CT examination of the cervical spine is beneficial to rule out fractures and obtain further bony definition. All imaging studies require clinical correlation for meaningful interpretation, as radiologic abnormalities may be associated with minimal or no clinical pathology.

Electrodiagnostic testing (EMG and nerve conduction studies) is not necessary if the diagnosis of cervical radiculopathy is apparent by history, physical examination, and imaging studies. It may be useful to rule out neurologic conditions that mimic radiculopathy when clinical information is incomplete or discordant with the imaging studies.[11] The timing of EMG studies is important since evidence of denervation in peripheral muscles may not appear until 3 to 4 weeks after the onset of symptoms.

Differential Diagnosis

Neurologic

- Syringomyelia
- Intramedullary tumor
- Cervical myelopathy
- Motor neuron disease
- Plexopathy
- Thoracic outlet syndrome
- Peripheral nerve entrapment (median, ulnar, radial)

Musculoskeletal

- Cervical spondylosis
- Inflammatory spine disease
- Infection
- Tumor (extradural, Pancoast)
- Primary shoulder disease
- Myofascial pain syndrome
- Tendinitis (epicondylitis, De Quervain's tenosynovitis)

Other

- Angina pectoris/myocardial infarction

Treatment

Initial

The initial treatment focuses on patient education and control of pain and inflammation. The patient should be informed that most patients (70% to 80%) have good to excellent outcomes with conservative management[3,12–17] and that most of the pain subsides within several weeks. Nonsteroidal anti-inflammatory drugs (NSAIDs), including cyclooxygenase-2 (COX-2) inhibitors, may be used to decrease pain and inflammation, and, if necessary, a short course of tapering corticosteroids may be prescribed. Non-narcotic analgesics may be used for pain. Narcotic analgesics are infrequently needed and are usually prescribed for a few days to 1 to 2 weeks.

Patients should be encouraged to maintain their normal activities of daily living and may perform light stretches and apply ice to their necks. Although soft cervical collars are frequently prescribed for short courses, there is a risk of cervical soft tissue contracture and disuse weakness.

Rehabilitation

A multitude of treatments have been empirically prescribed for cervical disc herniation, including heat, cold, massage, mobilization, immobilization, traction, manipulation, trigger point therapy, acupuncture, and transcutaneous electrical nerve stimulation (TENS). However, the paucity of well designed (randomized, controlled, prospective) studies in the literature makes it difficult to assess their efficacy and whether they affect the long-term outcome.[12–17]

Supervised physical therapy is generally not necessary in treating cervical radiculopathy if the patient's pain resolves and the patient makes a functional recovery. However, patients who have persistent impairments or disability (e.g., difficulty with cervical range of motion or arm weakness) may benefit from a course of physical therapy involving progressive stretching and strengthening exercises of their cervical paraspinal, shoulder girdle, and low back muscles.[18,19]

A workstation evaluation may be beneficial in order to facilitate recovery and/or the return to work. The focus should be on improving posture and keeping the head and neck in a neutral position. Ergonomic equipment may include a telephone headset, slanted writing board, document holder, and book stand.

Procedures

If the aforementioned treatments do not alleviate the patient's pain, the clinician may consider referral for a cervical epidural steroid injection. A clinician who is experienced in this procedure should perform this injection; either a translaminar or selective nerve root block technique may be used. The efficacy of cervical epidurals is not known because prospective, randomized, controlled trials are lacking. Uncontrolled studies in the literature have reported good to excellent results in 41% to 75% of patients.[20–23]

It is unclear how many injections a patient may receive and how often they may be performed. Clinicians usually perform up to three injections in a 6- to 12-month period that are at least 5 to 7 days apart in order to assess the efficacy of the previous injection. It is prudent to weigh the risks and benefits in each patient when considering repeat injections, taking into account medical risk factors such as diabetes, hypertension, and congestive heart failure.

Surgery

Indications for surgery are threefold: (1) progressive weakness, (2) myelopathy, or (3) intractable pain despite aggressive conservative management.

Both anterior (anterior discectomy with or without fusion) and posterior (foraminotomy) approaches have been documented in the surgical literature to have good outcomes.[1,24] The approach in a given patient depends on the nature of the anatomic lesion and the preference of the surgeon.

Potential Disease Complications

Possible complications of cervical radiculopathy are persistent or progressive neurologic weakness, residual neck pain, chronic pain syndrome, myelopathy (rare, usually associated with spondylosis or large central disc herniation).

Potential Treatment Complications

NSAIDs may produce gastropathy, hyperkalemia, renal toxicity, hepatic toxicity, exacerbation of asthma, drug–drug interaction, bleeding, and CNS effects. The use of steroids (short course) may result in mood changes, fluid retention, hypertension, hyperglycemia, gastropathy, and suppression of hypothalamic–pituitary–adrenal axis. Cervical collars may cause disuse weakness of the cervical muscles, decreased range of motion, and reinforcement of the sick role. Traction and exercise can exacerbate symptoms. Manipulation also may exacerbate symptoms and may result in recurrent disc herniation, worsening weakness, carotid dissection, stroke, and quadriplegia. Epidural injection may produce vasovagal reactions, temporary exacerbation of symptoms, spinal headache, epidural hematoma, infection, allergic reaction, neural damage, and cardiopulmonary arrest. The side effects of narcotics are constipation, nausea, vomiting, sedation, impaired mentation/motivation, suppression of endogenous opioid production, tolerance, addiction, biliary spasm, and respiratory depression. Surgery carries the risks of infection; neurologic damage to the spinal cord, nerve roots, or peripheral nerves; nonunion of fusion; hardware loosening, migration, or failure; persistent neck and arm pain; and accelerated degeneration of level adjacent to fusion.

References

1. Ahlgren BD, Garfin SR: Cervical radiculopathy. Orthop Clin North Am 1996;27(2):253–263.
2. Malanga GA: The diagnosis and treatment of cervical radiculopathy. Med Sci Sports Exerc 1997;29(7)Suppl:S236–S245.
3. Caplan LR, et al: Management of cervical radiculopathy. Eur Neurol 1995;35:39–320.
4. Yoss RE, et al: Significance of symptoms and signs in localization of involved root in cervical disc protrusion. Neurology 1957;7:673–683.
5. Bates B: A Guide to Physical Examination and History Taking, 5th ed. Philadelphia, JB Lippincott, 1991, p 472.
6. Malanga GA, Campagnolo DI: Clarification of the Pronator reflex. J Phys Med Rehabil 1994;73:338–340.
7. Fast A: The shoulder abduction relief sign in cervical radiculopathy. Arch Phys Med Rehabil 1989;70:402–403.
8. Davidson RI, et al: The shoulder abduction test in the diagnosis of radicular pain in cervical extradural compressive monoradiculopathies. Spine 1981;6(5):441–445.
9. Viikari-Jutura E, et al: Validity of clinical tests in diagnosis of root compression in cervical disease. Spine 1989;14(3): 253–257.
10. Ellenberg MR, et al: Cervical radiculopathy. Arch Phys Med Rehabil 1994;75:342–352.
11. Wilbourn AJ, Aminoff MJ: AAEM Minimonograph #32: The electrodiagnostic examination in patients with radiculopathies. Muscle Nerve 1998;21:1612–1631.
12. Goldie I, Landquist A: Evaluation of the effects of different forms of physiotherapy in cervical pain. Scand J Rehabil Med 1970;2-3:117–121.
13. Heckman JG, et al: Herniated cervical intervertebral discs with radiculopathy: An outcome study of conservatively or surgically treated patients. J Spinal Dis 1999;12(5):396–401.
14. Honet JC, Puri K: Cervical radiculitis: Treatment and results in 82 patients. Arch Phys Med Rehabil 1976;57:12–16.
15. Martin GM, Corbin KB: An evaluation of conservative treatment for patients with cervical disc syndrome. Arch Phys Med Rehabil 1954;35:87–92.
16. Saal JS, et al: Nonoperative management of herniated cervical intervertebral disc with radiculopathy. Spine 1996; 21(16):1877–1883.
17. Sampath P, et al: Outcome in patients with cervical radiculopathy: Prospective, multicenter study with independent clinical review. Spine 1999;24(6):591–597.
18. Rainville J, et al: Low back and cervical spine disorders. Orthop Clin North Am 1996;27(4):729–746.
19. Tan JC, Nordin MD: Role of physical therapy in the treatment of cervical radiculopathy. Orthop Clin North Am 1992; 23(3):435–449.
20. Slipman CW, et al: Therapeutic selective nerve root block in the nonsurgical treatment of atraumatic cervical spondylotic radicular pain: A retrospective analysis with independent clinical review. Arch Phys Med Rehabil 2000;81:741–746.
21. Shulman M: Treatment of neck pain with cervical epidural steroid injection. Regional Anesth 1986;11:92–94.
22. Rowlingson JC, Kirshblum LP: Epidural analgesic techniques in the management of cervical pain. Anesth Analg 1986;65:938–942.
23. Warfield CA, et al: Epidural steroid injection as a treatment for cervical radiculitis. Clin J Pain 1988;4(4):201–204.
24. Dillin W, et al: Cervical radiculopathy—A review. Spine 1986;11(10):988–990.

5 | Cervical Sprain/Strain

Joseph T. Alleva, MD
Jason Franklin, DO
Thomas H. Hudgins, MD

Synonyms

Acceleration/deceleration injury

Whiplash syndrome

Whiplash associated disorder

Flexion/extension injury

Cervical soft tissue injury

Myofascial neck pain

Cervical myofascial pain syndrome

ICD-9 Codes

847.0
Sprains, and strains of other and unspecified parts of back

Neck; anterior longitudinal (ligament), cervical; atlantoaxial (joints); atlanto-occipital (joints); whiplash injury

Definition

Cervical sprain/strain typically refers to acute pain arising from injured soft tissues of the neck. This includes muscles, tendons, and/or ligaments. Although often associated with discogenic, neurologic, and facet symptoms, the name per se excludes these entities. The most common event leading to such injuries are motor vehicle collisions. The mechanism of injury is complex. Basically, the head and neck acceleration lag behind vehicular acceleration when struck. Eventually head and neck acceleration is two to two and a half times greater than the maximum car acceleration. This subsequently results in dramatic deceleration.[1,2]

Many factors have been associated with worse outcome in acceleration/deceleration injuries involving motor vehicles. Rate of recovery seems to be related to sociodemographic variables. Older women tend to have a worse prognosis than younger women and men in general. Crash-related factors associated with a worse outcome include occupancy in a truck, being a passenger, colliding with a moving object, and getting hit head-on or perpendicular.[3] A high intensity of neck pain, a decreased onset of latency of the initial pain, and radicular symptoms are also prognostic with worse outcomes.[4] Since many of these injuries result in patients initiating litigation, this too is a poor prognostic indicator.

Signs and Symptoms

The most common presentation of patients with cervical sprain/strain is non-radiating neck pain (Fig. 1). Patients will also complain of neck stiffness, fatigue, and worsening symptoms with cervical range of motions. It often extends into the trapezius regions and/or interscapular region. Headache is probably the most common associated symptom, originating in the occiput region and radiating frontally. Increased irritability and sleep disturbances are common. Paresthesias, radiating arm pain, dysphagia, visual symptoms, auditory symptoms, and dizziness may be reported.[4,5] In an isolated cervical sprain/strain injury, these symptoms are generally absent; however, if present, alternative diagnoses should be suspected. Myelopathic symptoms such as bowel and bladder dysfunction and weakness must be investigated.

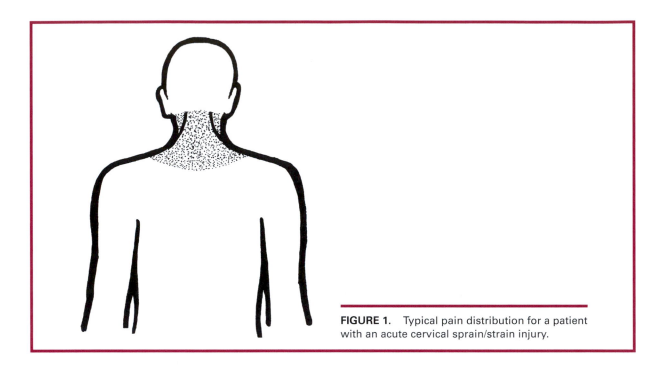

FIGURE 1. Typical pain distribution for a patient with an acute cervical sprain/strain injury.

Physical Examination

The primary finding in a cervical sprain/strain injury is a decrease and/or painful cervical range of motion. This may be accompanied by tenderness of the cervical paraspinals, trapezius, occiput, and/or anterior cervical musculature (i.e., sternocleidomastoid) (Fig. 2).

A thorough neurologic examination should be performed to rule out myelopathic and/or radicular processes. In an isolated cervical sprain injury, the neurologic examination should be normal.

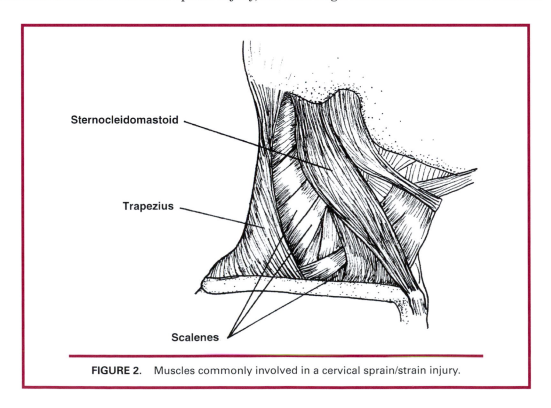

FIGURE 2. Muscles commonly involved in a cervical sprain/strain injury.

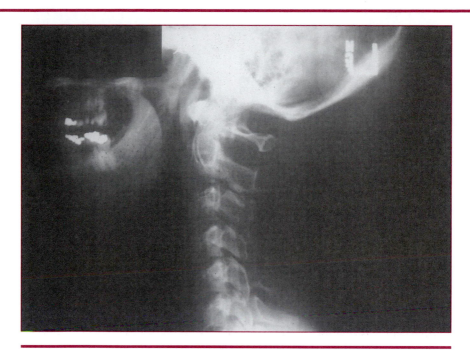

FIGURE 3. Cervical spine x-ray showing straightening of the spine and loss of the normal cervical lordosis.

Functional Limitations

Restricted range of motion of the cervical spine may contribute to difficulty with daily activities such as driving. Patients often complain of neck fatigue, heaviness, and pain with static cervical positions such as reading or working at the computer. Sleep may be affected as well.

Diagnostic Studies

It is generally accepted that x-rays should be obtained in patients involved in a traumatic event who have altered consciousness; are intoxicated; or who exhibit the following on physical examination: cervical tenderness, focal neurologic signs, and decreased cervical range of motion.[6] Although the clinician may commonly see straightening of the cervical lordosis on lateral cervical x-ray, it is not a diagnostic finding (Fig. 3). This is instead thought to be related to spasms of the paracervical musculature.

Studies such as MRI scans, CT scans, and electrodiagnostics are typically utilized to rule out alternative or co-existing entities.

Differential Diagnosis

Occult cervical fracture or dislocation
Cervical discogenic pain
Cervical herniated disc/radiculopathy
Cervical facet syndrome
Cervical spine tumor
Cervical spine infection

Treatment

Initial

Initial interventions utilized in patients with cervical sprain/strain have not been rigorously tested. Patient education is critical for a realistic expectation of resolution of symptoms. In most cases, symptoms will resolve within 4 to 6 weeks. In some cases, however, healing may be delayed up to 6 to 12 months.

It is reasonable to recommend rest within the first 24 to 72 hours of injury. The detriments of prolonged bed rest and/or the use of cervical collars have been clearly described and, in fact, may promote disability.[7] The use of NSAIDs/COX-2 inhibitors, muscle relaxants, and analgesic medications on a judicious basis is accepted to promote early return to activity.[8] Muscle relaxants and/or low-dose tricyclic anti-depressants (e.g., nortriptyline or amitriptyline 10 to 50 mg hs) are also used to help restore sleep if this is an issue. High doses of methylprednisolone have been used but are not currently considered the standard of care in cervical sprain/strain injuries.[9]

Rehabilitation

Although no one mode of rehabilitation has been proven effective, early mobilization/return to function is the key. Cervical manipulation, massage, and mobilization on a limited basis are geared toward correcting segmental restrictions and restoring normal range of motion. Such approaches have been shown to be more effective than passive modalities with regard to range of motion and reduction of pain.[10]

Modalities such as ultrasound and electrical stimulation can be tried for pain control.

Cervical traction done either manually (by a physical therapist) or with a mechanical unit (often done with an over-the-door unit at home) may be tried if there are no contraindications (e.g., fracture).

Strengthening and stretching exercises for muscles with a tendency for tightness and inhibition, respectively, should be utilized in conjunction with the aforementioned techniques. Muscle imbalances must be addressed, and weak muscle groups such as the scapular stabilizers (middle lower trapezius, lower trapezius, rhomboids, serratus anterior, and levator scapulae) should be strengthened. This is typically done after muscles with a tendency for tightness (upper trapezius, sternocleidomastoids, scalenes, latissimus dorsi, and pectoralis major and minor) are stretched.[11] Cumulative data suggests that utilizing such an approach for cervical sprain injuries produces long- and short-term benefits.[6] The overall treatment goal is to achieve an independent, customized home exercise program so that the patient can become active in his or her own treatment.

Ergonomic alterations, such as the use of a telephone headset and document holders, may also aid in recovery.

Procedures

Trigger point injections are a reasonable adjunct to decrease pain so that patients may participate in physical therapy. The upper trapezius, scalenes, and semispinalis capitus are the most common muscles to have trigger points after acceleration/deceleration injuries. Other cervical muscles that tend to develop trigger points after such injuries are the splenius capitus, longus capitus, and longus colli.[12] Botulinum toxin injections may be useful as well.[13] Facet injections, epidural injections, and cervical traction may be instituted for conditions that are often associated with cervical sprains/strains, such as cervical radiculopathy and facet syndrome.

Surgery

Surgery is not indicated.

Potential Disease Complications

The main complication from the injury itself is chronic intractable pain, leading to permanent loss of cervical range of motion and functional disability.

Potential Treatment Complications

Analgesics, NSAIDs, and COX-2 inhibitors have well-known side effects that most commonly affect the gastric, hepatic, and renal systems. Muscle relaxants and low-dose tricyclic anti-depressants can cause sedation. Overly aggressive manipulation or manipulation done when there is a concomitant unidentified injury (e.g., fracture) may result in serious injury. Injections are rarely associated with infection and allergic reactions to the medications used.

References

1. Bogduk N: The anatomy and pathophysiology of whiplash. Clin Biomechanics 1986;1:92–100.
2. Stovner, L: The nosologic status of the whiplash syndrome: A critical review based on methodological approach. Spine 1996;21:2735–2746.
3. Harder S: The effect of sociodemographic and crash related factors on the prognosis of whiplash. J Clin Epidemiol 1998;51:377–384.
4. Radanov, B, Sturzenegger M: Long term outcome after whiplash injury: A 2 year follow-up considering reatures of injury mechanism and somatic, radiologic and psychosocial findings. Medicine 1995; 1974;281–297.
5. Norris S: The prognosis of neck injuries resulting from rear-end vehicle collisions. J Bone Joint Surg (BR) 1983;65:608–611.
6. Spitzer W, Skovron M: Scientific monograph of the Core Back Task Force on Whiplash Associated Disorder: Redefining whiplash and its management. Spine 1995; 20(Suppl):S1–S5.
7. Mealy K, Brennan H: Early mobilization of acute whiplash injury. Br Med J 1986;292.1656–1657.
8. McKinney L: Early mobilization of acute sprain of the neck. Br Med J 1989;299:1006–1008.
9. Pettersson K, Toolanen G: High dose methylprednisolone prevents extensive sick leave after whiplash injury. A prospective, randomized, double blind study. Spine 1998;23:9844–9989.
10. Rosenfeld M: Early intervention in whiplash associated disorder. Spine 2000;25:1782–1787.
11. Janda V: Muscles and cervicogenic pain syndromes. In Grant R (ed): Physical Therapy of the Cervical and Thoracic Spine. New York, Churchill Livingstone, 1988, pp 153–166.
12. Simons D: Travell & Simon's Myofascial Pain and Dysfunction: The Trigger Point Manual, vol I. Upper Half of the Body, 2nd ed. Baltimore, Williams & Wilkins, 1999, pp 278–307, 432–444, 445–471, 504–537.
13. Freund JB, et al: Treatment of chronic cervical-associated headache with botulinum toxin A: A pilot study. Headache 2000;40:231–236.

6 Cervical Stenosis

Alec L. Meleger, MD

Synonyms

Cervical spondylosis

Cervical degenerative disease

Cervical radiculopathy

Cervical myelopathy

Cervical osteoarthritis

ICD-9 Code

723.0
Spinal stenosis in cervical region

Definition

Cervical stenosis is a disorder of the spine that can be congenital or acquired (Fig. 1). The congenital type is commonly due to the short pedicles rendering the spinal canal to be smaller than normal.[1] The small spinal canal of the acquired type can be due to the bulging or protruding degenerating intervertebral discs, hypertrophic arthritic zygapophyseal (facet) joints, and/or hypertrophic ligamentum flavum. On radiographic imaging, these degenerative changes are present in 25% to 50% of the population by the age of 50 and increase to 75% to 85% by 65 years.[2-4] Cervical stenosis affects individuals of different ethnic and racial backgrounds. Ossification of the posterior longitudinal ligament is a well-known cause of cervical stenosis in individuals of Japanese descent.[5] Diminution in the size of the neural foramina commonly occurs in the cervical stenosis.

Symptoms

Symptomatic presentation of cervical spinal stenosis can differ from patient to patient depending on the pathology and the anatomic structures involved. Intervertebral disc degeneration and zygapophyseal joint arthritis commonly present with axial neck pain. Patients with cervical foraminal stenosis may complain of radicular arm pain as well as of paresthesias, dysasthesias, numbness, and/or weakness of the arm(s). On the other hand, patients with cervical central canal stenosis can present with myelopathic symptoms of upper and lower extremity spasms; bladder and bowel dysfunction; unsteady gait; and weakness, paresthesias, and/or numbness of the lower extremities. Men may complain of erectile dysfunction.

Physical Examination

The physical exam of a patient with the cervical stenosis associated with myelopathy should be consistent with upper and/or lower motor neuron findings. Lower motor neuron findings are more commonly seen in the upper extremities, and consist of muscular atrophy, decreased reflexes, diminished muscle tone, and weakness. Decreased sensation to light touch and pinprick and a positive Spurling's sign (radicular pain on axial loading of an extended head rotated toward the involved extremity) can also be detected. Lower extremity exam is more consistent with upper motor

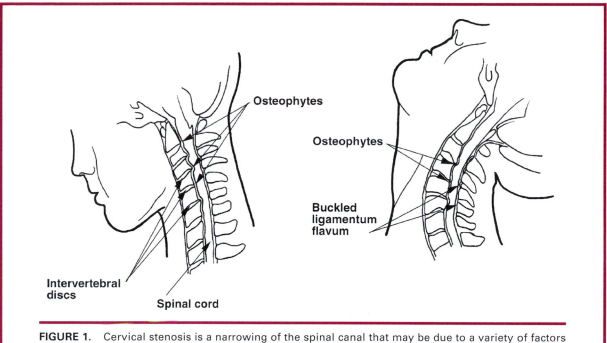

FIGURE 1. Cervical stenosis is a narrowing of the spinal canal that may be due to a variety of factors (e.g., congenital narrowing, osteophyte formation, hypertrophy of the ligamentum flavum).

neuron findings in the presence of cervical stenosis with myelopathy. Increased reflexes, sustained or unsustained clonus, spasticity, weakness, decreased sensation, and neurogenic bowel and bladder can be seen. Lhermitte's sign (a shock-like sensation that the patient reports going down the back when the neck is flexed) (Fig. 2) can sometimes be elicited.[6] Please refer to Chapter 1 on myelopathy for more detail.

Functional Limitations

The functional limitations are dependent on the extent of neurologic involvement. Pain may limit dressing, bathing, and work-related and recreational activities. Weakness may cause someone to have difficulty with walking, lifting and carrying. Balance may be impaired due to both weakness and sensory deficits, putting the patient at risk for falls. The fear of falling alone may cause someone to limit his or her activities and become more socially isolated. Bowel and bladder incontinence further adds to a patient's anxiety about going out in public. Sexual performance may be affected in both sexes due to pain and in men who have erectile

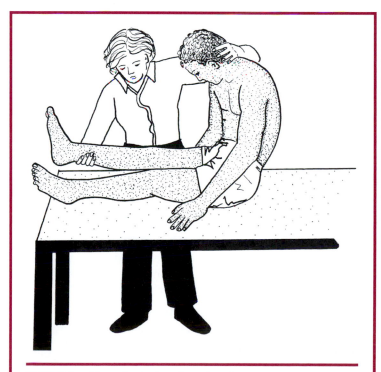

FIGURE 2. Lhermitte's sign. Examiner flexes patient's head and hip simultaneously.

dysfunction. Depression may ensue when pain becomes chronic or there is significant loss of sleep or ability to function. In extreme cases, paraplegia or quadriplegia may limit nearly all activities.

Diagnostic Studies

Facet and uncovertebral joint arthropathy, intervertebral disc space, and neuroforaminal size can be evaluated with cervical spine x-rays. Nerve root impingement, intervertebral discs, thecal sac, spinal cord, and ligamentum flavum are evaluated by MRI or CT. Myelography can further be used to assess spinal and foraminal stenosis in functional positions (i.e., upright, flexion, and extension). Somatosensory evoked potentials (SSEPs) can often confirm the presence of myelopathy, and electromyography any peripheral nerve root involvement.[7]

Central spinal canal stenosis is diagnosed by measuring the cervical sagittal diameter. The latter is defined as the anteroposterior diameter measured from the posterior aspect of the vertebral body to the most anterior point on the spinolaminar line. Stenotic central canals are less than or equal to 13 mm in anteroposterior diameter.[8]

Differential Diagnosis

Cervical intraspinal neoplasm	Spinal cord injury
Cervical intraspinal abscess	Arteriovenous malformation
Multiple sclerosis (spinal)	Thoracic outlet syndrome
Cerebrovascular accident	Idiopathic brachial neuritis
Syringomyelia	Brachial plexopathy

Treatment

Initial

Conservative treatment is generally undertaken in the absence of clinical evidence of cervical myelopathy (patients with suspected cervical myelopathy should be referred immediately to a surgeon). Relative rest of no longer than 2 to 3 days' is initially recommended. For severe cervical and/or radicular pain, a soft neck collar can be prescribed for a few days with subsequent self-weaning by alternating periods of collar removal.[9]

Initial analgesics of choice are nonsteroidal anti-inflammatory drugs (NSAIDs), including cyclooxygenase-2 (COX-2) inhibitors, which when taken at regular intervals may show some effect in cervical as well as in radicular pain. More than one family of nonsteroidals should be tried before deeming them ineffective. COX-2 inhibitors are recommended for the elderly and patients with history of peptic ulcer disease or renal insufficiency. A short course, 2 weeks, of mild opioids and muscle relaxants may benefit some patients. For radicular symptoms of moderate severity, a 1-week course of oral steroids is recommended. Oral prednisone can be prescribed on a tapering schedule starting with 60 mg and followed by 10 to 20 mg decrements every 1–2 days. Persistent radicular pain can be treated with neuropathic pain medications such as gabapentin, clonazepam, tricyclic antidepressants, and others.

Self-application of ice or heat for cervical pain and trancutaneous electrical nerve stimulation (TENS) for radicular symptoms can be of benefit to some patients.

Depression and loss of sleep should be addressed and treated appropriately in conjunction with pain management.

Patient education about the nature of cervical stenosis, its worrisome signs and symptoms, and the importance of staying active is of paramount importance. While advising patients to remain active, care should be taken with activities that may put them at risk (e.g., activities that may result in a fall with a subsequent further compromise of the spinal canal such as horseback riding, climbing ladders, etc.) Patients should also be advised to avoid the extremes of cervical flexion and extension (e.g., as occurs when painting a ceiling or swimming the butterfly stroke).

Rehabilitation

Physical and occupational therapy should focus on keeping patients as active as possible while educating them about activities that might place them at risk for further injury. All clinicians should avoid manipulation of the cervical spine. Cervical traction may also be tried in the absence of myelopathy or ongoing numbness and/or weakness of the upper extremities. With passing of the acute phase, a program consisting of stretching and static neck exercises should be undertaken. Once the pain free range of motion is achieved, dynamic neck strengthening is initiated.[10] Upper body conditioning may also be beneficial. Eventually, patients should be graduated to a home exercise program.

Depression and anxiety can lead to symptom magnification and should be addressed by a behavioral specialist. Cognitive therapy, biofeedback, self-hypnosis, and relaxation techniques must always be considered as part of the pain management armamentarium.

Procedures

A trial of epidural steroid injections is advocated for acute or subacute radicular symptoms of severe intensity unresponsive to more conservative measures. Patients without central spinal canal compromise and chronic severe radicular symptoms may be candidates for a spinal cord stimulator trial. Arthritic cervical facet joints, which are innervated by medial branch nerves, can be another source of pain. Diagnostic medial branch nerve blocks can be performed, and if found positive, are then followed by radiofrequency nerve lesioning.

Surgery

Immediate surgical intervention should be sought if the patient has symptoms of progressive weakness, bladder and/or bowel incontinence, unsteady gait, and/or upper motor neuron findings. A surgical specialist should also assess intractable pain of 3 months duration that is unresponsive to conservative treatment. Decompressive single or multi-level laminectomy, discectomy, foraminotomy, and/or cervical fusion using bone graft or instrumentation are the common surgical procedures. Referral to a surgical specialist should be considered for intractable radicular symptoms.[11,12]

Potential Disease Complications

If left untreated, continued pressure on the exiting cervical nerve root(s) and the cervical segment of the spinal cord may lead to progressive weakness, loss of sensation, dysfunction of the bladder and bowel, quadriplegia, or paraplegia.

Potential Treatment Complications

Aggressive/improper physical or occupational therapy can cause injury to the cervical spine and the surrounding structures. Cervical traction may promote signs of radiculopathy or myelopathy. Chronic use of a cervical collar will cause the neck muscles to weaken.

Analgesics, NSAIDs, and COX-2 inhibitors have well-known side effects that most commonly affect the gastric, hepatic, and renal systems. These medications are to be used cautiously or avoided in patients with a past history of peptic ulcer disease or with decreased renal function. COX-2 inhibitors may cause fewer of the undesired effects. All of the neuropathic pain medications have a significant side effect profile; gabapentin tends to show better tolerance. The most common side effects are sedation, dizziness, and gait imbalance. Continued use of opioids can lead to physiologic dependence, tolerance, dose escalation, sedation, constipation, etc. Objective evidence of improved function is required for their continued prescription. The most serious complication generally associated with oral steroids is avascular necrosis. However, this is a rare complication, particularly in the absence of long-term use.

Epidural steroid injections carry a small risk of a postdural puncture headache. In the majority of patients, these headaches are self-limiting and respond well to bed rest, hydration, and caffeine. Epidural blood patch is performed in cases when these are severe or longer lasting. Both epidural injections and surgical intervention carry a rare risk of intraspinal infection, intraspinal hematoma, and nerve and spinal cord damage.

References

1. Epstein JA, Carras R, Hyman RA, Costa S: Cervical myelopathy caused by developmental stenosis of the spinal canal. J Neurosurg 1979;51:362–367.
2. Bohlman HH, Emery SE: The pathophysiology of cervical spondylosis and myelopathy. Spine 1988;13:843–846.
3. Adams CBT, Logue V: Studies in cervical spondylitic myelopathy: I–III. Brain 1971;94:557–594
4. Connell MD, Wiesel SW. Natural history and pathogenesis of cervical disc disease. Orthop Clin North Am 1992; 23:369–380.
5. Ono K, Yonenobu K, Miyamoto S, Okada K: Pathology of ossification of the posterior longitudinal ligament and ligamentum flavum. Clin Orthop Rel Res 1999;359:18–26.
6. Clark CR: Cervical spondylotic myelopathy: history and physical findings. Spine 1988;13:847–849.
7. Yiannikas C, Shahani, BT, Young RR: Short-latency somatosensory-evoked potentials from radial, median, ulnar, and peroneal nerve stimulation in the assessment of cervical spondylosis. Comparison with conventional electromyography. Arch Neurol 1986;43:1264–1271.
8. Matsuura P, Waters RL, Adkins RH, et al: Comparison of computerized tomography parameters of the cervical spine in normal control subjects and spinal cord-injured patients. J Bone Joint Surg 1989;71:183–188.
9. Persson L, Carlsson C-A, Carlsson JY: Long lasting cervical radicular pain managed with surgery, physiotherapy, or a cervical collar: a prospective, randomized study. Spine 1997;22:751–758.
10. Levoska S, Keinanen-Kiukaanniemi S: Active or passive physiotherapy for occupational cervicobrachial disorders? A comparison of two treatment methods with a 1-year follow up. Arch Phys Med Rehabil 1993;74:425–430.
11. Orr RD, Zdeblick TA: Cervical spondylotic myelopathy: Approaches to surgical treatment. Clin Orthop Rel Res 1999;359:58–66.
12. Edwards RJ, Cudlip SA, Moore AJ: Surgical treatment of cervical spondylotic myelopathy in extreme old age. Neurosurgery. 1999;45(3):696.

7 Cervicogenic Vertigo

Joanne Borg-Stein, MD

Synonyms

Cervicogenic dizziness

Neck pain associated
with dizziness

ICD-9 Codes

386.10
Peripheral vertigo,
unspecified

386.11
Benign paroxysmal
positional vertigo

723.1
Cervicalgia

780.4
Dizziness and giddiness;
lightheadedness; vertigo

Definition

Cervicogenic vertigo is the false sense of motion due to cervical musculoskeletal dysfunction. The symptoms may present secondary to post-traumatic events, with resultant whiplash or postconcussive syndrome. Alternatively, cervicogenic vertigo may be part of a more generalized disorder, such as fibromyalgia or underlying osteoarthritis. Cervicogenic vertigo is believed to result from convergence of the cervical nerve inputs as well as the cranial nerve input and their close approximation in the upper cervical spinal segments of the spinal cord.[1,2]

Symptoms

Patients with cervicogenic vertigo experience a false sense of motion, often a whirling or spinning sensation. Some patients experience sensations of floating, bobbing, tilting, or drifting. Others experience nausea, visual motor sensitivity and ear fullness.[3] The symptoms are often provoked or triggered by neck movement and/or sustained awkward head positioning.[4–6] Cervical pain or headache may interfere with sleep and functional activities.

Physical Examination

The essential elements of the examination include a neurologic examination and an ear and eye examination for nystagmus. The results of these examinations are typically normal. Abnormalities in any of these aspects of the examinations indicate a need to exclude other otologic or neurologic conditions, such as Meniere's disease, benign paroxysmal positional vertigo, or stroke.[7] Musculoskeletal functioning is typically abnormal, generally with restrictions of cervical range of motion and palpable trigger points. At the end ranges of cervical motion, symptoms of vertigo may be elicited. A careful cervical examination should be performed, including range-of-motion testing and palpation of the facet joints, to assess for mechanical dysfunction. Myofascial trigger points should be sought in the sternocleidomastoid, cervical paraspinal, levator scapula, upper trapezius, and suboccipital musculature. Palpation in these areas can often reproduce the symptoms experienced as cervicogenic vertigo.[8]

Functional Limitations

Functional limitations may include difficulty with walking, balance, or equilibrium.

Diagnostic Studies

Cervicogenic dizziness is a clinical diagnosis. Testing may include cervical x-rays to rule out cervical osteoarthritis or instability. Cervical magnetic resonance imaging (MRI) is indicated if cervical spondylosis is suspected or to rule out a cervical radiculopathy or other pathology. Brain MRI/MRA (magnetic resonance angiography) may be ordered to exclude vascular lesions or tumor (e.g., acoustic neuroma).

Differential Diagnosis

Meniere's disease

Benign paroxysmal positional vertigo

Labyrinthitis

Vestibular neuronitis

Cardiovascular causes: arrhythmia, carotid stenosis, or postural hypotension

Migraine-associated dizziness

Progressive dysequilibrium of aging

Treatment

Initial

Initial treatment involves patient reassurance and education. Nonsteroidal anti-inflammatory drugs (NSAIDs, including COX-2 inhibitors) are useful for pain control for those who have underlying cervical osteoarthritis. Muscle relaxants, such as cyclobenzaprine, carisoprodol, or low-dose tricyclic antidepressants, may be used at bedtime to facilitate sleep and muscle relaxation for myofascial pain.

Rehabilitation

Rehabilitation is aimed at reducing muscle spasm, increasing cervical range of motion, improving posture, and restoring function. Modalities (e.g., ultrasound, electrical stimulation) may be useful to reduce pain. A physical therapist with experience and training in manual medicine, myofascial and trigger point treatment, and therapeutic exercise should evaluate and treat the patient to restore normal cervical function. Occupational therapy can improve posture, ergonomics, and functional daily activities.[9] Anyone suffering from cervicogenic vertigo should have a workstation evaluation if possible. A physical or occupational therapist can do this by using photographs of the patient at work. Recommendations to improve head and neck posture for office workers include using a telephone headset, slanted writing board, book stand, and document stand.

Procedures

Trigger point injections (TPIs) with local anesthetic are often helpful to decrease cervical muscle pain (Fig. 1). The clinician should locate those trigger point areas that reproduce the patient's symptoms. Acupuncture with an emphasis on local treatment of muscle spasm may be an alternative to TPI.[10,11]

Surgery

No surgery is indicated for treatment of this disorder, unless there is co-existent neurologically significant cervical stenosis or disc herniation.

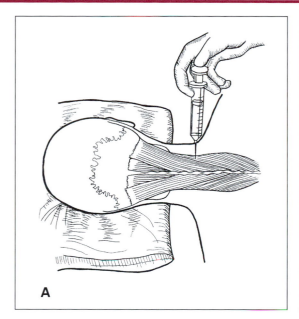
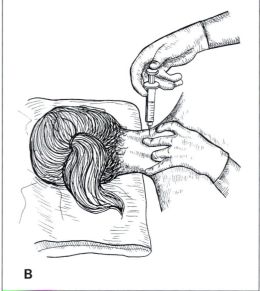

FIGURE 1. Injection of the lower trigger point area in the splenius cervicis muscle. *A*, Location where the needle penetrates the muscle. *B*, Injection of the trigger point as diagrammed in *A*.

Potential Disease Complications

The major complications are inactivity, deconditioning, falls, fear of going outside the home, anxiety, and depression. Chronic intractable neck pain and persistent dizziness may persist despite treatment.

Potential Treatment Complications

Side effects from NSAIDs may include gastric, renal, hepatic, and hematologic complications. Muscle relaxants and tricyclics may induce fatigue, somnolence, constipation, urinary retention, and other anticholinergic side effects. Local injections, if improperly executed, may result in intravascular injection, or pneumothorax. Transient localized post-injection pain and/or ecchymosis may occur.

References
1. Norre M: Cervical vertigo. Acta Oto-Rhino-Laryngologic Belgium 1987;25:495–499.
2. Revel M, Andre-Deshays C, Mingeut M: Cervicocephalic kinesthetic sensibility in patients with cervical pain. Arch Phys Med Rehabil 1991;72:288–291.
3. Karlberg M, Magnusson M, et al: Postural and symptomatic improvement after physiotherapy in patients with dizziness of suspected cervical origin. Arch Phys Med Rehabil 1996;77:874–882.
4. Jongkees L: Cervical vertigo. Laryngoscope 1969;79:1473–1484.
5. Praffenrath V, Danekar R, Pollmann W: Cervicogenic headache—the clinical picture, radiological findings, and hypotheses on its pathophysiology. Headache 1987;25:495–499.
6. Sjaastad O, Frediksen T, Praffenrath V: Cervicogenic headache: diagnostic criteria. Headache 1990;30:725–726.
7. Froehling DA, Silverstein MD, et al: Does this dizzy patient have a serious form of vertigo? JAMA 1994;271:385–388.
8. Travell J, Simons D: Myofascial Pain and Dysfunction, vol. I, 1999.
9. Karlberg M, Persson L, Magnusson M: Impaired postural control in patients with cervico-brachial pain. Acta Otolaryngol 1995;520(Suppl):440–442.
10. deJong P, de Jong M, et al: Ataxia and nystagmus induced by injection of local anesthetics in the neck. Ann Neurol 1977;1:240–246.
11. Carlson J, Fahlerantz A, Augustinsson L: Muscle tenderness in tension headaches treated with acupuncture and physiotherapy. Cephalalgia 1990;10:131–141.

8 Occipital Neuralgia

Todd E. Handel, MD
Robert J. Kaplan, MD

Synonyms

Cervicogenic headache

Occipital myalgia-neuralgia syndrome

Occipital headache

Occipital neuropathy

Arnold's neuralgia

Third occipital headache

Cervical migraine.

ICD-9 Code

723.8
Other syndromes affecting cervical region; occipital neuralgia

Definition

Occipital neuralgia occurs when there is pressure on the greater and/or lesser occipital nerve(s), resulting in posterior occipital headaches. A variety of disorders can generate pain in the upper cervical spine, craniocervical junction, and occipital region. Although references to occipital neuralgia have been documented in the clinical literature for more than 175 years, information regarding its etiology, epidemiology, natural course, and prognosis is limited. It does appear, however, that injuries, such as whiplash sustained in a motor vehicle accident, may predispose to occipital region pain syndromes.[1]

This chapter delineates occipital neuralgia from cervicogenic headache and defines it as pain in the distribution of the greater and lesser occipital nerves.

The *greater occipital nerve* is the largest purely afferent nerve in the body, innervating the posterior skull from the suboccipital area to the vertex. It is formed from the posterior division of the second cervical nerve. Within the substantia gelatinosa of the spinal cord, the afferent fibers from this nerve lie in close approximation to the nucleus and spinal tract of the trigeminal nerve. Rather than exiting through a discrete spinal foramen, the nerve leaves the bony spinal column between the arch of the atlas and axis. It travels inferolaterally toward the area of the C2–C3 zygapophyseal (facet) joint and then curves around the inferior oblique capitis muscle to ascend toward the occiput deep to the semispinalis capitis muscle. It pierces either through the tendinous insertion of the trapezius muscle[2] or between the trapezius and semispinalis muscles to reach the subcutaneous tissue of the occipital area. The site of perforation through these muscles is located just medial to the occipital artery.

The *lesser occipital nerve* forms from the anterior divisions of the second and third cervical nerves. It ascends along the posterior margin of the sternocleidomastoid muscle, where it provides sensory fibers to the area of the scalp lateral to the greater occipital nerve.

Symptoms

Occipital neuralgia may occur as an intermittent (paroxysmal) or a continuous headache. In continuous occipital neuralgia, the headaches may be further classified as acute or chronic.

Paroxysmal occipital neuralgia describes pain occurring only in the distribution of the greater occipital nerve. The attacks are unilateral, and the pain is sudden and severe. The patient may describe the pain as sharp, twisting, a dagger thrust, or an electric shock. The pain rarely demonstrates a burning characteristic. Although single flashes of pain may occur, a volley of attacks presents more frequently. The attacks may occur spontaneously; however, specific maneuvers applied to the back of the scalp or neck regions, such as brushing the hair or moving the neck, may provoke attacks.

> **BOX 1.** Sites of Compression of the Greater Occipital Nerve/Dorsal Ramus of C2
>
> The lateral articular masses of C1/C2
>
> The atlantooccipital membrane
>
> Tendinous origin of the trapezius muscle at the suboccipital base
>
> Inferior oblique capitis muscle
>
> The C2–C3 facet Intermediate or deep suboccipital muscle layer

Acute continuous occipital neuralgia often has an underlying etiology. The attacks last for many hours and are typically devoid of radiating symptoms (e.g., trigger zones to the face). The entire bout of neuralgia will continue up to 2 weeks before remission. Exposure to cold is a common trigger.

In *chronic continuous occipital neuralgia*, the patient may experience painful attacks that last for days to weeks. These attacks are generally accompanied by localized muscle spasm. The reported pain is usually a steady, sharp aching pain or pressure originating in the suboccipital region and spreading forward to the temples and vertex and auricular or orbital region. Pain due to irritation of the occipital nerves is not, however, confined to the posterior part of the skull. Referral of the pain into facial areas (trigger zones), particularly above and behind the orbit, is a common feature and occasionally the principal complaint. Associated complaints of scalp tenderness in this same area, most noticeable when the patient brushes the hair or wears hair rollers, are also common. Similarly, pain may increase with pressure of the head on a pillow. Prolonged abnormal fixed postures that occur in reading or sleeping positions and hyperextension or rotation of the head to the involved side may provoke the pain. The pain may be bilateral, though the unilateral pattern is more common. Often, a previous history of cervical or occipital trauma or of arthritic disease of the cervical spine is obtained. Occasionally, patients may report other autonomic symptoms concurrently such as nausea, vomiting, photophobia, diplopia, ocular and nasal congestion, tinnitus, and vertigo.

Physical Examination

The primary finding in occipital neuralgia is pain with palpation of the occipital nerves. Occasionally, there is hypesthesia or allodynia in the distribution of the occipital nerve. Local muscle spasm, frequently with palpable trigger points and taut bands, is often present.[3] Cervical range of motion may be restricted. Neurologic exam, including strength, sensation, deep tendon reflexes, and cerebellar function, is typically normal. An abnormal neurologic exam should alert the clinician that an alternative or underlying associated disorder might be present.

Entrapment of the nerve near the cervical spine should result in increased symptoms during extension or rotation of the head and neck. Compression of the skull on the neck (Spurling's maneuver), especially with extension and rotation of the neck to the affected side, may reproduce or increase the patient's pain if cervical degenerative disease is the cause of the neuralgia. Pressure over both the occipital nerve at the superior nuchal line and near the C2–C3 facet joints should cause an exacerbation of pain in such patients, at least when the headache is present. Entrapment of the nerve as it passes through the tendinous insertion of the trapezius muscle on the skull is less likely to exacerbate symptoms during extension or compression of the head on the neck. Symptomatology is more likely to occur during flexion of the neck and on palpation of the nerve at the superior nuchal line. Even if the actual pathology is in the cervical spine, tenderness over the occipital nerve at the superior nuchal line is usually present. This finding is of prognostic importance when attempting to determine where a nerve block should be performed.

Functional Limitations

Depending on the etiology of the occipital headache, patients may encounter significant problems with sleeping, reading, working at a computer terminal, or performing activities requiring prolonged or repeated cervical spine extension and loading.

Diagnostic Studies

The diagnosis of occipital neuralgia is generally made clinically; however, diagnostic nerve blocks with local anesthetic may be required to obtain a definitive diagnosis. The relief of pain after a diagnostic anesthetic block at the site of maximal tenderness or at the site of the occipital groove is generally confirmatory of the diagnosis of occipital neuralgia.[4]

X-rays are done to exclude other diagnoses or to provide rationale for underlying associated conditions (e.g., arthritis). If plain films are ordered, they should include an open-mouth view to evaluate the C2 facet joints and flexion views to determine whether hypermobility of C1–C2 is present. This may help determine the cause of the nerve entrapment. It is important to note that radiologic degenerative changes of the cervical spine do not necessarily correlate with the patient's symptoms and exam findings.

Cervical MRI can markedly enhance visualization of the paravertebral and occipital soft tissue structures to rule out other causes of cervical pain and headaches.[3]

Differential Diagnosis

C2–C3 subluxation/arthropathy

C2–C3 radiculopathy

Migraine headache

Cluster headache

Tension-type headache

Tumor (e.g., posterior fossa)

Congenital or acquired abnormalities at the craniocervical junction (e.g., Arnold-Chiari malformation or basilar invagination)

Rheumatoid arthritis

Atlantoaxial subluxation

Cervical myelopathy

Pott's disease/osteomyelitis

Paget's disease

Treatment

Initial

Initial treatment focuses on decreasing stress and muscle tension and improving posture. Moist heat may be used to decrease muscle spasm and relieve pain. Others may benefit from ice to the occipital region (20 minutes, 1 to 3 times daily).

TABLE 1. Pharmacologic Treatment of Occipital Neuralgia

Medication	Dosage	Common Side Effects
NSAIDs	Variable	GI bleed, dyspepsia, nausea, headache, dizziness, rash, fluid retention, urticaria, hepatotoxicity, and acute renal failure.
COX-2 inhibitor Refecoxin (Vioxx) Celecocib (Celebrex)	Celebrex—100 mg BID or 200 mg PO QD Vioxx—12.5 mg to 25 mg QD	Dyspepsia, nausea, abdominal pain, constipation, anorexia, elevated liver enzymes, acute renal failure, anaphylaxis, and agranulocytosis.
Tricyclic antidepressants Amitriptyline Nortriptyline Imipramine	Start at 10 mg QHS and titrate to 75 mg QHS or until clinical response	Dry mouth, constipation, urinary obstruction, sedation, postural hypertension, decreased seizure threshold.
Carbamazepine (Tegretol)	Start at 100 mg BID; titrate to 400 mg BID	Sedation, unsteadiness, nausea, blurred vision, seizures, hepatitis, aplastic anemia
Gabapentin (Neurontin)	Start at 300 mg QD; titrate to 1200 mg TID	Somnolence, dizziness, ataxia, fatigue, nystagmus, tremor, blurred vision, myalgia, weight gain, nausea, amnesia, leukopenia.
Mexiletine	Start 150 mg QD × 3 d, then 300 mg QD × 3 d, then 10 mg/kg QD	Dyspepsia, dizziness, tremor, coordination problems, insomnia, diarrhea, palpitations, nervousness, headache, tinnitus, depression, rash, dyspepsia, dry mouth, anorexia, fatigue, arrhythmia.

Pharmacologic treatment with NSAIDs/COX-2 inhibitors can be used to decrease pain and inflammation (Table 1). Analgesics may also be used for pain. Tricyclic antidepressants have been tried with some benefits as well.[5] Although not well reported, muscle relaxants may prove useful. Anticonvulsants such as carbamazepine and gabapentin have been used for many types of neuropathic pain with good results. Mexiletine may be advocated in refractory cases of occipital neuralgia. For acute occipital neuralgia associated with cervical strain/sprain injury (see Chapter 5), the patient may wear a soft cervical collar during the acute phase only to reduce exacerbations of painful paroxysms. Electrical stimulation (TENS) may prove beneficial in subacute or chronic cases. Proficient clinicians may utilize acupuncture and massage. Patients who present with concurrent depression or anxiety should be treated with appropriate medications and/or psychotherapy. Similarly, treating sleep irregularities is important.

Rehabilitation

The incorporation of stretching and strengthening exercises for the paracervical and periscapular muscles may be appropriate for the patient with subacute or chronic occipital neuralgia, particularly if the condition is provoked by cervical spine or trunk movement. Postural training and relaxation exercises should be incorporated into the exercise regimen. Principles of ergonomics should be addressed if worksite activity is limited by pain exacerbations (e.g., utilizing a telephone headset, document holder).

Manual therapy, including spinal manipulation and spinal mobilization, has been used to treat patients with cervicogenic headaches. Some studies have shown a transient improvement in pain and an increase in function, but these have not been proven in well-designed randomized controlled trials. Any spinal manipulation should be done with caution because there are serious risks if done improperly or if an underlying injury is ignored (e.g., cervical fracture).[3] Anecdotal reports support a trial of cervical traction in some cases.

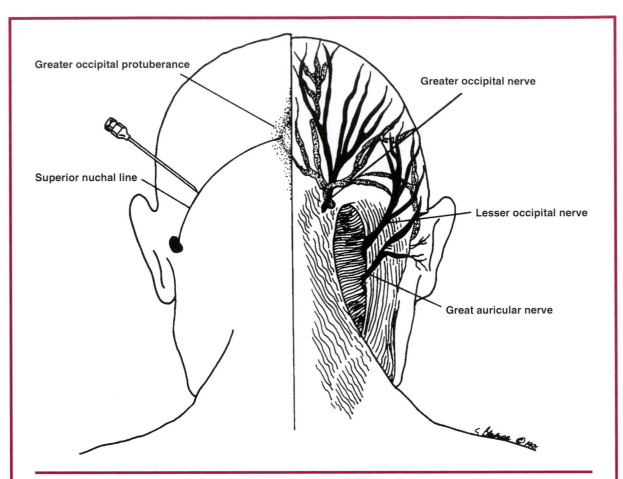

FIGURE 1. To perform the greater occipital nerve block, the occipital protuberance and mastoid process are identified by palpation on the involved side of the skull. Using an imaginary line between these two points, the greater occipital nerve lies on the medial one third of this line. The posterior occipital artery can be palpated as it transverses the superior nuchal line. Then under sterile conditions, using a 1- to 1½-inch needle and a local anesthetic solution (e.g., 1% lidocaine), advance the needle down to the occipital bone and the groove, and then slightly withdraw. Inject in a fanlike manner both medially and laterally approximately 1 to 2 cc. The local anesthetic may be combined with a corticosteroid. Immediate anesthesia and pain relief should occur.[5] The lessor occipital nerve can be anesthetized using almost the same technique. Using the same imaginary line between the mastoid process and the occipital protuberance, locate the junction of the middle and outer third of the line directly over the superior nuchal line, and inject the lessor occipital nerve, using the same injection technique.[5] Postinjection care can include local heat or ice and analgesics if there is excessive soreness.

Procedures

Blockade of the greater or lesser occipital nerve with a local anesthetic is diagnostic and therapeutic (Fig. 1). Pain relief can vary from hours to months. In general, at least 50% of patients will experience more than 1 week of relief after one injection. Case reports of isolated pain relief for greater than 17 months have been achieved after a series of five blocks.[3] The addition of a cortisone preparation is controversial, but it may provide additional benefit.[10]

Surgery

Patients with occipital neuralgia rarely require surgery, and the results are quite variable.[6,7]

Potential Disease Complications

Occipital neuralgia is generally a self-limiting diagnosis, but in some cases it may progress to a chronic intractable pain syndrome. In refractory cases, it is critical to rule out more ominous conditions. Patients involved in litigation or who have psychosocial stresses or vocational disputes may have a poorer outcome.

Potential Treatment Complications

The use of NSAIDs/COX-2 inhibitors has a number of well-established side effects, as do tricyclic antidepressants (see Table 1). The anesthetic block of the greater or lesser occipital nerve is considered relatively safe. Potential complications include bleeding, infection, paresthesias and nerve injury, and headache exacerbation. Care must be given not to puncture the posterior occipital artery. If the artery is punctured, then pressure should be applied vigorously.

References
1. Loeser J: Cranial neuralgias. In Bonica's Management of Pain, 3rd ed. 2000, pp 855–866.
1. Hammond SR, Danta G. Occipital neuralgia. Clin Exper Neurol 1978;15:258–270.
2. Sjaastad O, Saunte C, Hovdal H, et al: "Cervicogenic" headache: A hypothesis. Cephalalgia 1983;3:249–245.
3. Pollmann W, Keidel W, Pfaffenrath G: Headache and the cervical spine: A critical review. Cephalalgia 1997;17:801–816.
4. Anthony M: Headache and the greater occipital nerve. Clin Neurol Neurosurg 1992;94:297–301.
4a. Sjaastad O, Fredriksen TA, Pfaffenrath V: Cervicogenic headache: Diagnostic criteria. Headache 1990;30;725–726.
5. Lennard TA, Shin DY: Shoulder and chest wall blocks. Pain Procedures in Clinical Practice, 2nd ed. Philadelphia, Hanley & Belfus, 2000, pp 87–95.
6. Magnusson T, Ragnarsson T, Bjornsson A: Occipital nerve release in patients with whiplash trauma and occipital neuralgia. Headache 1996;36:32–33.
7. Rizzo MDT (ed): Head Injury and Post Concussive Syndrome. New York, Churchill-Livingstone, 1996, pp 168–171.
10. Antony M: Cervicogenic headache: Prevalance and response to local steroid therapy. Clin. & Exper. Rheum. 2000;18(2 Suppl 19):S59–S64.
13. Dugan MC, Locke S, Gallagher JR. Occipital neuralgia in adolescents and young adults. N Engl J Med 1962;267:1166–1172.
14. Schultz DR. Occipital neuralgia. J Am Osteopath Assoc 1977;76:335–343.
15. Bogduk N: The anatomy of occipital neuralgia. Clin Exper Neurol 1981;17:167–184.
16. Diamond S, Freitag FG: Headache following cervical trauma. In Tollison CL, Satterthwaite JR (eds): Painful Cervical Trauma. Philadelphia, William & Wilkins, 1992, pp 381–394.
17. Cicala RS, Jernigan JR: Nerve blocks and invasive therapy. In Tollison CD, Kunkel RS (eds): Headache: Diagnosis & Management. Philadelphia, William & Wilkins, 1993, pp 357–368.

9 Temporomandibular Joint Disorders

Larry Z. Lockerman, DDS

Synonyms

TMJ

Temporomandibular Joint

TMD

Temporomandibular Disorders

ICD-9 Codes

524.60
Temporomandibular joint disorders, unspecified

848.1
Jaw (sprain/strain); temporomandibular (joint) (ligament)

Definition

The abbreviation TMJ is commonly used to describe a diagnosis affecting the temporomandibular joint. However, TMJ really refers to the joint itself, and temporomandibular joint dysfunction (TMD) includes a collection of symptoms that refer to intrinsic and extrinsic temporomandibular joint conditions. The term is often used in a generic manner for facial pain that is not directly caused by pathology of the teeth and gums. A variety of pain disorders can refer pain to the temporomandibular joint region, and a thorough history of the pain and an examination are critical.[1,2]

Studies report that approximately 28% of the population exhibit signs of TMD that consists of TMJ and muscle of mastication tenderness. Of these, 14% had a restricted range of motion of the mandible, and only 1% had severe symptoms. Symptoms predominate in women (5:1) between the ages of 15 to 45 years.[3] Trauma is perhaps the most common cause of TMD (Figs. 1 and 2).

Within the TMJ there is a biconcave cartilage disc that normally moves with the mandibular condyle in the fossa. The TMJ has two types of movements. The first one third of opening is rotational and the last two thirds of opening includes rotation and translation. The innervation of the TMJs and supporting structures is primarily from the trigeminal and facial nerves.

Symptoms

Symptoms of TMD are varied and may at first seem unrelated. A common complaint is TMJ noise, such as popping, clicking, grinding, and crepitation. Pain in and around the TMJ is also common. Headaches may vary in location and are generally worse with chewing. Neckaches may also be present. Facial pain, earaches (including tinnitus), dysphagia, and photosensitivity have all been reported as well. Full excursion of the TMJ may not be possible, and in severe cases, patients complain that their jaw is "locked." TMD may be associated with sleep disturbance due to chronic pain.

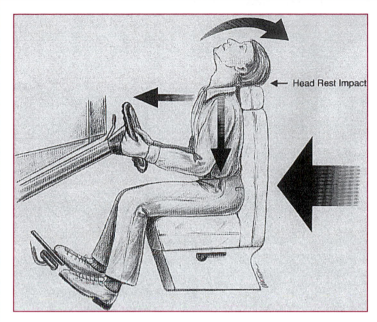

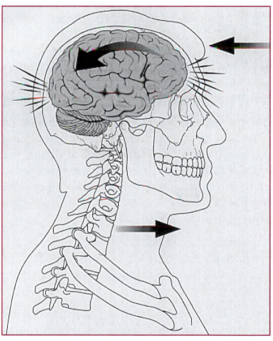

FIGURE 1 *(Left)*. The total duration of impact in rear-end motor vehicle accidents is 0.1–0.2 seconds. (From Windsor RE, Lox DM: Soft Tissue Injuries. Philadelphia, Hanley & Belfus, 1998, with permission.)

FIGURE 2 *(Right)*. Acceleration of various body parts can occur with no direct head trauma causing headache, face pain, and TMJ symptoms like tenderness and joint clicking. (From Windsor RE, Lox DM: Soft Tissue Injuries. Philadelphia, Hanley & Belfus, 1998, with permission.)

Physical Examination

The diagnosis is made by observing the range of motion of the mandible and with palpation of the musculoskeletal structures of the face and head. It is essential to determine whether the patient has an intrinsic TMJ problem. Both a TMJ exam and muscle exam are necessary (Table 1).

The translation can be felt by placing a finger over the TMJ (slightly anterior to the tragus of the ear) and asking the patient to open wide.

The clinician places a finger over the TMJ (slightly anterior to the left and right tragus) and asks the patient to open and close, feeling for crepitus, clicking, and full excursion.

TABLE 1. The Two-Minute TMJ Examination

Screening for TMD does not have to be a long, drawn-out affair. The following simple procedures will help to indicate whether there is a need for a dental consultation to rule out TMD as a contributing factor to the patient's pain complaints:

1. Maximal mouth opening
   a. Normal opening is approximately the width of three fingers without pain.
   b. Mandibular opening should be relatively straight without deviation.
2. Joint noise
   a. Popping, clicking, or grinding in one or both of the TMJs in the presence of facial pain, headaches, or neckaches is significant.
   b. Joint noise can be confirmed by patient report, manual palpation of the TMJs, or use of a stethoscope.
3. Pain on palpation of the masseter, temporalis, or intraoral muscles.
4. Otologic examination
   a. Excessive ear wax bilaterally or unilaterally in the absence of obvious pathology.
   b. Pain in the external auditory canals distal to the TMJs on insertion of the otoscope in the absence of obvious pathology.

From Windsor RE, Lox DM: Soft Tissue Injuries. Philadelphia, Hanley & Belfus, 1998, with permission.

Have the patient clench into his or her natural bite position, and note whether it causes pain. Measure the millimeter opening between the upper and lower incisal edges of the incisor teeth while the patient is opening as much as possible. Normal opening is approximately 38 to 45 mm, or the space three or more of the patient's fingers between the incisor teeth. Note whether the patient states that the mandibular opening feels restricted, and observe if the mandibular opening deviates to one side. With the patient's teeth slightly apart, ask the patient to move in left and right lateral directions, and record if the movements are the same. If there is limited opening, a deviation to one side, and limited lateral movement in the contralateral direction, there may be a disc displacement with no reduction in one joint.

If the disc in the TMJ is partially displaced (anterior disc displacement with reduction) or if there are arthritic changes, clicking and crepitus sounds can be heard or palpated as the disc clicks into its normal position with jaw opening. There will also be a click as the disc slips out of its normal position on closing. If the disc is fully displaced (anterior disc displacement with no reduction), there is no clicking and there is limited opening with an opening shift toward the locked side and no lateral movement to the contralateral side. Full lateral and protrusive movements with limited opening might be due to muscle spasm.[3]

The clinician should gently press his or her fingers on both masseters (slightly below the cheek), temporalis muscle (temple region), insertion of the sternocleidomastoid (slightly below the mastoid), and the suboccipital area (slightly below the bony ridge). Any sensitivity with palpation should be noted.

The neurologic exam including deep tendon reflexes, sensation, and strength in the upper extremities is typically normal. Cervical range of motion may be limited, particularly in post-traumatic injuries with a concomitant whiplash injury.

Functional Limitations

Functional limitations include pain that may limit talking and eating. In patients with chronic pain, sleep may be affected. Depression may also contribute to dysfunction in patients with chronic pain.

Diagnostic Studies

A plain x-ray can screen for major arthritic changes. Oral surgeons, many dentists, and some hospitals have a panoramic x-ray machine that can visualize the TMJ. Only MRI imaging can visualize the disc and provide a definitive diagnosis of the disc position. MRI imaging is generally not required for non-locking joints that click.

Differential Diagnosis

Trauma to the face causing muscle injury

Fractures

Tumors

Infected teeth and gums

Acute trismus or muscle spasm (not intra-articular joint pathology)

Facial nerve injuries

Cervical whiplash

Headaches (e.g., migraines)

Treatment

Initial

There are different philosophical approaches among clinicians in managing TMD. Some dentists try to calm symptoms with oral appliances and have the patient wean off of daytime use of the appliance within a few months. Others believe that permanent bite changes are necessary for long-term relief and will grind the bite surfaces of the teeth to "balance the bite." This approach is very controversial since it may not resolve the symptoms.

Acute pain with full lateral mandibular excursive and protrusive movement is treated as an acute muscle spasm. Recommend eating soft food with small bites. Moist heat and ice massage may help reduce pain. NSAIDs/COX-2 inhibitors may reduce pain and inflammation. Muscle relaxants may decrease spasm.[4] Low-dose tricyclic anti-depressant medication has been found to be useful in chronic pain. Massage and static exercise (place hand under chin and open downward with pressure against the hand for a few seconds at a time for six times, six times a day [called 6 × 6 exercise]).[5] If pain does not resolve quickly and/or the patient complains of continued "locking," an intraoral orthotic designed to relax the muscles and decrease inflammation can be prescribed.

Chronic pain (more than 3 months) management with abortive medications (such as NSAIDs, benzodiazepine, and narcotics) has risks of rebound headache. Sleep patterns must be reviewed, and a pain diary is helpful. If the generator of the pain cannot be determined, then prophylactic medications should be used (such as tricyclic anti-depressants, selective serotonin reuptake inhibitors, and gabapentin).[6]

If the problem persists for several weeks with no reduction in symptoms a referral to a clinician with expertise in managing TMD is necessary.

In some instances, altering a patient's bite may be necessary. This may include orthodontic work with appliances and braces or restorative dental work such as crowns.

Unilateral restricted translation of TMJ and limited opening with a deviation or acute inability to close (mouth open wide), called an open lock or subluxation, must be examined by a practitioner with expertise in managing TMJ disorders to "unlock" the joint.[7]

Painless joint noise with a normal range of motion in an adult is usually not treated. Growing children with joint noise should consult an orthodontist to determine whether there is a relationship between the joint noise and a possible malocclusion.

Rehabilitation

Physical or occupational therapy can be ordered to improve posture, reduce muscle spasm, and educate the patient on appropriate exercises. Modalities to reduce edema, muscle spasm, and increase circulation are also beneficial. Commonly prescribed modalities include ultrasound and electrical stimulation.

Application of cold on muscles with spasm followed by gentle stretching and massage can reduce pain. If there is intrinsic TMJ pathology, opening the mouth to stretch facial muscle is contraindicated.[4]

Rehabilitation may also include referral to a speech and language pathologist, dietitian, or massage therapist. Biofeedback may also be helpful.

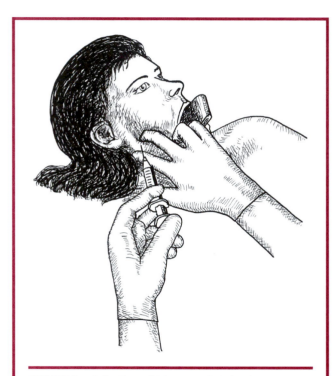

FIGURE 3. Injection of trigger points in the masseter muscle. The muscle is stretched by a prop between the upper and lower teeth. Ask the patient to point with one finger to the area of most intense pain. Then palpate for a taut band. Once localized, under sterile conditions, using a 30-gauge, 1-inch needle, inject approximately 0.1–0.3 cc of a local anesthetic (e.g., 1% lidocaine) into the muscle in several areas of this same site (puncture the skin only once). This should be accompanied by needling of the entire taut band to mechanically break up the abnormal and sensitized tender tissue. It is generally not advisable to inject local steroids into the muscle. This may be repeated in several areas during a single procedure visit. Additionally, this procedure may need to be repeated on several occasions depending on the patient's symptoms and reported relief from the treatment.

Procedures

An injection into the TMJ to unlock the disc may be necessary along with manual unlocking of the joint by a qualified clinician.

Muscle trigger point injections with lidocaine into the masseters, temporalis, sternocleidomastoid, and trapezius muscles can help ease localized and referred pain (Fig. 3).[7]

Diagnostic and therapeutic injection of the greater occipital nerve (suboccipital area) can also be helpful in some cases (see page 42).

Surgery

Surgery should only be considered as a final resort after x-ray and MRI imaging documents a diagnosis of intra-articular joint disease and all other treatment options have failed to give significant relief.

Potential Disease Complications

When an acute locked TMJ becomes chronic, it may become permanent. In some patients, the pain level is tolerable. Arthritic changes can exacerbate symptoms, causing secondary headache, facial pain, earaches, and neckaches. Chronic facial pain can interfere with normal sleep and cause symptoms of depression.

Potential Treatment Complications

Oral appliances used 24 hours a day for many months might create a permanent bite change. When this occurs, the patient cannot bring his or her teeth fully together when clenching. If not properly managed, this may increase symptoms. Athletic mouth guards bought in stores (also called boil and bite appliances) may aggravate TMD.

Analgesics, NSAIDs, and COX-2 inhibitors have well-known side effects that most commonly affect the gastric, hepatic, and renal systems. Surgery has well-known side effects of infection, injury to a blood vessel, or nerve.

References
1. Okeson J: Bell's Orofacial Pain. Chicago, Quintessence Publishing, 1995.
2. Okeson J (ed): Orofacial Pain: Guidelines for Assessment, Classification, and Management/the American Academy of Orofacial Pain. Carol Stream, IL, Quintessence Publishing, 1996.
3. Kaplan A, Assael L (eds): Temporomandibular Disorders: Diagnosis and Treatment. Philadelphia, W.B. Saunders, 1991.
4. Travel J, Simons D: Myofascial Pain and Dysfunction: The Trigger Point Manuel. Baltimore, Williams & Wilkins, 1983.
5. Wright EF, Schiffman EL: Treatment alternatives for patients with masticatory myofascial pain. JADA 1994;126(7):1030–1039.
6. Robbins L: Management of Headache and Headache Medication. New York, Springer-Verlag, 1993.
7. Friedman M, Weisberg J: Temporomandibular Joint Disorders. Chicago, Quintessence Publishing, 1985.
8. Assael L: Atlas of the Maxillofacial Surgery Clinics. Philadelphia, W.B. Saunders, 1996.

10 Trapezius Sprain/Strain

James E. Warmoth, MD
Meryl Stein, MD

Synonyms

Nonarticular rheumatism

Trapezius myositis

Myofasciitis

Fibrositis

Fibromyalgia

Tension neckache

Trapezium sprain/strain

Myofascial shoulder pain

ICD-9 Codes

847.0
Neck (sprain/strain); whiplash injury

847.1
Thoracic (sprain/strain)

847.9
Unspecified site of the back (sprain/strain)

Definition

Trapezius sprain/strain describes a condition whereby the trapezius muscle or one of its parts is injured. This is also commonly referred to as trapezius myofascial pain and dysfunction. Interestingly, myofascial pain in general most commonly involves the trapezius muscle—any one of its three parts.[1]

The term "trapezius myositis" is used to describe muscular hyperirritability when histologic evidence of inflammatory change is present.[2] In the past, when this term was more commonly used, it defined myalgias of nonarticular rheumatic origin.[3]

There are numerous causes of trapezius sprain/strain, including trauma (e.g., injuries from falls or car accidents, such as whiplash), chronic injury due to overload (e.g., injury in workers who repetitively lift heavy loads), ergonomically improper positioning (e.g., office workers who tilt their head to the side when using the phone), and skeletal variations (e.g., leg-length discrepancy or short arms).

In general, repetitive tasks involving the upper extremity produce pain, especially when the tasks require the arm to be abducted and in forward flexion.

Symptoms

The upper, middle, and lower trapezius fibers can function independently in various actions that contribute to neck, scapula, and arm movements. Patients report an annoying deep ache and focal tenderness in the portion of the muscle involved. If one of several trigger points is involved, this ache is often associated with referred pain in a characteristic pattern. The intensity of the pain varies depending on mechanical stressors, impaired sleep and fatigue, metabolic and nutritional inadequacies, and psychologic factors. Although weakness or limited range of motion does not characterize trapezius sprain/strain, testing may be hindered by the patient's protective splinting due to pain or fear of pain.

Physical Examination

The bilateral trapezii form a large diamond shape, with the origin of the muscle, being the base of the skull, ligament, of the neck, and spinous processes of C1 to T12 (Fig. 1). The upper fibers insert on the outer third of the clavicle. The medial fibers, which go from C6 to T3 spinous processes to the acromion and the superior lip of the spine of the scapula, are followed by the lower fibers that insert at the medial end of the spine of the scapula.[4]

With such a wide origin, the trapezius helps with several movements. In general, the trapezius muscles support the shoulders by holding the scapulae posteriorly; consequently, weak trapezii result in drooping shoulders.[5] The upper fibers flex the neck toward the ipsilateral side, raise the point of the shoulder, and rotate the scapula upward by turning the glenoid cavity upward. The middle fibers retract and adduct the scapulae as well as assist in the flexion and abduction of the shoulder. The lower portion of the muscle depresses the scapula and helps it rotate upward.[6]

On examination, contralateral head and neck rotation produces pain at near full range, and head to shoulder movement is moderately impaired.[7] Palpation and inspection of the neck and upper back and observation of the patient's posture, body symmetry, and movements are the essential elements of the exam. Strength, range of motion, sensation, and deep tendon reflexes should all be normal. Finally, the evaluation of possible trigger points with notable spot tenderness, taut bands, and characteristic referred pain patterns are important to identify because when present they are a factor in determining treatment.

The more serious diagnoses (e.g., referred visceral pain) can generally be readily excluded because they do not affect neck or shoulder range of motion or produce local tenderness.[8]

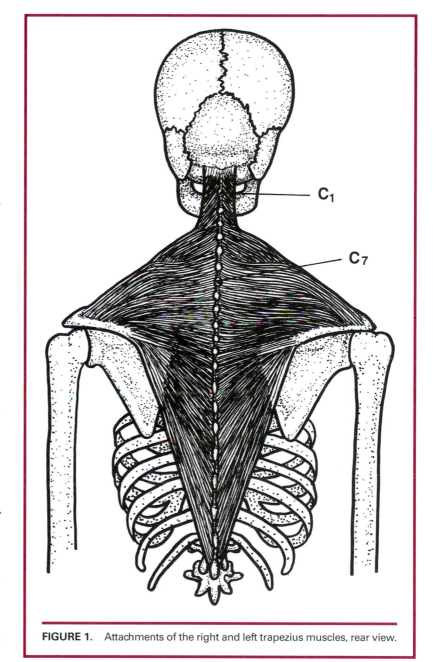

FIGURE 1. Attachments of the right and left trapezius muscles, rear view.

Functional Limitations

Pain and tenderness of the trapezius may interfere with a number of activities of daily living as well as avocational and vocational activities. Typing and use of the computer; driving; and activities requiring sustained shoulder elevation, such as telephone use, may be hindered. Likewise, participation in many sports, such as basketball, tennis, and golf, may be compromised.[9]

Diagnostic Studies

Trapezius sprain/strain is a clinical diagnosis based on physical exam and history. Radiographs and diagnostic tests are not performed, except to rule out other conditions.

Differential Diagnosis

Cervical radiculopathy

Supraspinatous, infraspinatous, rhomboid, levator scapulae sprain/strain (muscles that overlap the trapezius muscle may be the site of involvement)

Intramuscular abscess or tumor

Acute neck stiffness (e.g., torticollis involving the splenius cervicis or levator scapulae muscles)

Spinal accessory nerve entrapment

Cervical facet syndrome

Cervical arthritis

Treatment

Initial

It is important to begin with patient education regarding proper posture and positioning both at home and work. Encourage the patient to identify and correct likely sources of injury in his/her routine and environment. Tight bra straps, backpacks, and heavy coats and other clothing or accessories result in continuous microtrauma that can damage the muscle and associated soft tissues. Postural abnormalities must also be corrected (e.g., comfortable adjustable chair for work, telephone headset).

It may be worthwhile to provide lifts for leg-length discrepancies; ensure that existing canes are proper lengths; advise proper sleeping positions and pillow heights; and determine appropriate seating height and armrest height for various activities such as typing, driving, or using the telephone. These modifications can frequently be done on the initial office visit.

Medications such as NSAIDs/COX-2 inhibitors may be used for their analgesic and anti-inflammatory benefits. Muscle relaxants, used sparingly and primarily in evening doses, can also be helpful. Low-dose tricyclic antidepressants taken in the evening may also be used to help with sleep and pain. Cervical collars are generally not indicated since they promote muscular weakness. Moist heat, such as a hot shower, can help to reduce muscle spasm and pain.

Rehabilitation

The goal of physical or occupational therapy is to provide a supervised environment to work on posture, range of motion, and strength. The therapist can also be helpful in making job-related recommendations. A visit by the therapist to the worksite can be useful to identify the modifications necessary to ensure that the injury is not perpetuated and does not recur. Alternately, the patient may bring in photos of the worksite.

Modalities that may be useful include moist heat with a hydrocollator pack, ultrasound, and electrical stimulation. Deep tissue massage and spray and stretch techniques with a vapocoolant are also helpful. Instruction in body mechanics and postural alignment are staples of therapy. An appropriate home exercise program of stretching as well as general conditioning is also helpful in achieving symptomatic relief. Jogging, for example, can aggravate trapezius trigger points.[10]

Procedures

Trigger point injections can be very helpful in this condition (Fig. 2). Acupuncture may also provide substantial relief. More recently, botulinum toxin has been injected into the trapezius muscles to treat symptoms associated with whiplash injury.[11]

Postinjection care may include spray and stretch with a vapocoolant by the clinician and avoidance of aggressive use of the injected muscles by the patient. Heat or ice may be used depending on the patient's preference.

Surgery

Surgery is not an indicated treatment for trapezius sprain/strain.

Potential Disease Complications

Persistent shoulder pain can significantly compromise a person's functional status because he or she will avoid any task reproducing the discomfort. This could lead to significant personal and occupational disability. Ultimately, this forced isolation can produce depression or chronic pain behaviors, which are further disabling. Early intervention and therapy can help to avoid this.

Potential Treatment Complications

Because treatments for trapezius sprain/strain are relatively benign, complications are few. The most serious complication is a pneumothorax that could

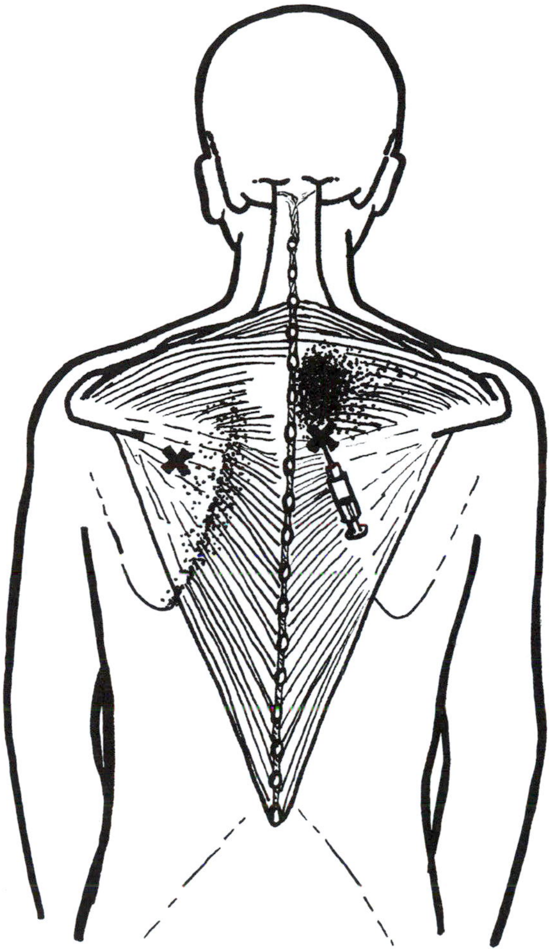

FIGURE 2. Ask the patient to point with one finger to the area of most intense pain. Then palpate for a taut band. Once localized, under sterile conditions, using a 27-gauge, 1½-inch needle, inject approximately 0.1–0.3 cc of a local anesthetic (e.g., 1% lidocaine) into the trapezius muscle in several areas of this same site (only puncture the skin once). This should be accompanied by needling of the entire taut band to mechanically break up the abnormal and sensitized tender tissue. It is generally not advisable to inject local steroids into the muscle. This may be repeated in several areas during a single procedure visit. Additionally, this procedure may need to be repeated on several occasions depending on the patient's symptoms and reported relief from the treatment.

result from a trigger point injection because the trapezius lies almost directly over the lung. Therefore, efforts should be made to insert the needle superficially. More commonly, patients complain of postinjection tenderness over the site—discomfort that generally resolves in a day or so. Additionally, infection and bleeding are remote complications of trigger point injections. Acupuncture has no significant side effects when sterile needles are used. Botulinum toxin is generally very safe to use in the trapezius muscles but may become less effective with repeated injections due to antibodies that develop. More commonly, adverse drug reactions limit the complete treatment. NSAIDs can cause gastrointestinal distress or, rarely, hemorrhage, and renal insufficiency. COX-2 inhibitors may cause fewer gastric side effects. Muscle relaxants and tricyclic antidepressants can cause somnolence and therefore should primarily be prescribed for evening use.

References

1. Sola AE, Rodenberger ML, Gettys BB: Incidence of hypersensitive areas in posterior shoulder muscles. Am J Phys Med 1955;34:585–590.
2. Travell JG, Simons DG: Myofascial Pain and Dysfunction. Baltimore, Williams & Wilkins, 1983, p 180.
3. Licht S: Therapeutic Heat. New Haven, CT, Elizabeth Licht, Publisher, 1958, p 2150.
8. Hadler NM: Medical Management of the Regional Musculoskeletal Diseases: Backache, Neck Pain, Disorders of the Upper and Lower Extremities. Orlando, FL, Harcourt Brace Jovanovich, 1984, p 118.
4. Basmajian JF: Muscles Alive, 4th ed. Philadelphia, W.B. Saunders, 1976, p 189.
5. Moore KL: Clinically Oriented Anatomy, 3rd ed. Baltimore, Williams & Wilkins, 1992, p 530.
6. Hollinshead WH: Functional Anatomy of the Limbs and Back, 4th ed. Philadelphia, W.B. Saunders, 1976, p 102.
9. Broer MR, Houtz SJ: Patterns of Muscular Activity in Selected Sport Skills, An Electromyographic Study. Springfield, IL, Charles C. Thomas, 1967.
10. Travell JG, Simons DG: Myofascial Pain and Dysfunction, The Trigger Point Manual. Baltimore, Williams & Wilkins, Baltimore, 1983, p 198.
11. Freund BJ, et al: Treatment of chronic cervical-associated headache with botulinum toxin A: A pilot study. Headache 2000;40:231–236.

11   Acromioclavicular Injuries

Thomas D. Rizzo, Jr., MD

Synonyms

Acromioclavicular joint injuries

Acromioclavicular pain

Acromioclavicular separation

Separated shoulder

Acromioclavicular osteoarthritis

Atraumatic osteolysis of the distal clavicle

ICD-9 Code

831.04
Closed dislocation acromioclavicular joint

840.0
Acromioclavicular (joint) (ligament) sprain

Definition

The acromioclavicular (AC) joint is a diarthrodial joint found between the lateral end of the clavicle and the medial side of the acromion.[1] The joint is surrounded by a fibrous capsule and stabilized by ligaments. The acromioclavicular ligaments cross the joint. Three ligaments begin at the coracoid process on the scapula and attach to the clavicle (trapezoid and conoid ligaments) or the acromion (coracoacromial ligament). This complex provides passive support and suspension of the scapula from the clavicle while allowing rotation of the clavicle to be transmitted to the scapula.[1,2]

Injuries to the AC complex are graded I through VI (Table 1).

At no time is the coracoacromial (lateral) ligament disrupted; therefore, the fibrous connection between anterior and posterior emanating structures of the scapula persists.[3] In rare instances there is an intra-articular fracture of the distal clavicle in addition to the ligamentous injuries.[4]

Symptoms

Patients will often provide a history of trauma to the shoulder or to the vicinity of the AC joint. Participants in contact or collision sports (e.g., football, downhill skiing) are particularly susceptible. Patients seek care because of pain in the anterior or superior aspect of the shoulder.[2] The pain may radiate into the base of the neck, the trapezius or deltoid muscles, or down the arm in a radicular pattern.[2,3]

Patients may describe pain brought on by activities of daily living that bring the arm across the chest (e.g., reaching into a jacket pocket) or behind their back (e.g., tucking in a shirt). Pain can also occur with shoulder flexion (reaching overhead) or with adducting the arm across the chest.

Physical Examination

Appropriate examination for suspected acromioclavicular injuries includes an examination of the neck and the shoulder joint and girdle to eliminate the possibility of a radiculopathy or of referred pain. Patients will have normal neck and neurologic exams. The presence of neurologic or vascular injury suggests that a greater degree of trauma has been sustained.[3]

TABLE 1. Grades of Acromioclavicular Joint Injuries and Treatments

Grade of Injury	AC Ligament	CC Ligament	Clavicle Displacement	Treatment
I	Sprain	Intact	Mild superior displacement	Conservative
II	Torn	Sprain	Definite superior displacement	Conservative
III	Torn	Torn	25%–100% increase in CC space	Controversial
IV	Torn	Torn	Posterior displacement	Surgical
V	Torn	Torn	100%–300% increase in CC space	Surgical
VI	Torn	Torn	Subacromial or subcoracoid location	Surgical

AC =Acromioclavicular; *CC* = Coracoclavicular

On inspection, there may be a raised area at the AC joint. This is caused by depression of the scapula relative to the clavicle or swelling of the joint itself. This area is commonly tender to touch. On active range of motion the patient may complain of pain or wince near the extreme of shoulder flexion.

Joint range of motion is typically within normal limits. Supporting the arm at the elbow and gently directing the arm superiorly may decrease the pain and allow for more complete assessment of the patient's shoulder range of motion. The pain may get worse as the shoulder is further flexed, whether it is done actively or passively. This is in distinction to impingement syndromes, which often hurt at a point in the arc of motion but are painless as the patient proceeds. Pain is typically absent with isometric manual muscle testing of the rotator cuff. Rotator cuff injuries will be painful with activation of the muscles of the rotator cuff. These problems are best identified with the shoulder in a neutral position since the muscles are in a lengthened position and are easily made symptomatic.

Special tests to identify AC joint pathology all attempt to compress the joint. The most common test is cross-body adduction test (Fig. 1). The shoulder is abducted to 90 degrees and the elbow is flexed to the same degree. The clinician then brings the arm across the patient's body until the elbow approaches the midline (or the patient reports pain).[2]

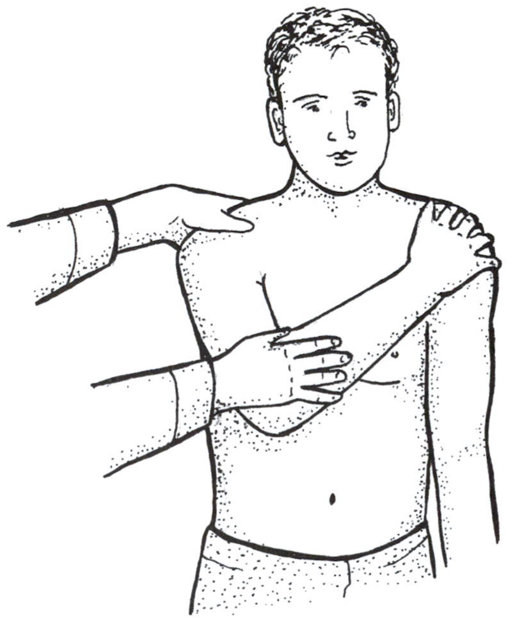

Other tests help to differentiate between impingement syndrome and AC joint pain. If the shoulder is passively flexed while internally rotated, the greater tuberosity can pinch (impinge) the suprasinatus tendon and subacromial bursa. The same test done with the shoulder externally rotated will compress the AC joint without impinging the subacromial space.[6] In the active compression test the shoulder is flexed to 90 degrees and then adducted to 10 degrees. The patient first maximally internally rotates the arm and then tries to flex the shoulder against the clinician's resistance. This puts pressure on the AC joint and may reproduce pain if pathology is present. The test is repeated with the shoulder in full external rotation. This will put stress on the biceps tendon and its labral attachment while excluding the AC joint.[7]

FIGURE 1. Cross-body adduction test. Testing for a sprain of the acromioclavicular joint.

Functional Limitations

Reaching up, reaching across the body, and carrying heavy weights are limited because of pain. Patients may have no pain at rest and little to no pain with many activities. Patients may complain of difficulty with putting on a shirt, combing their hair, and carrying a briefcase or grocery bag. Most recreational activities will be limited as well. Sleep may be affected due to pain.

Diagnostic Studies

Radiographs are important in most cases and should be done to rule out fracture as well as to assess the severity of the injury (Fig. 2). Views should include AP, lateral Y view, and an axillary view. It is important

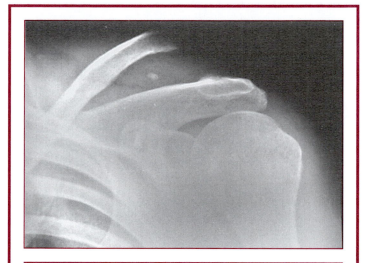

FIGURE 2. Grade III acromioclavicular joint dislocation. There is marked superior displacement of the distal clavicle relative to the acromion and coracoid processes. (From Katz DS, et al: Radiology Secrets. Philadelphia, Hanley & Belfus, 1998, p 445.)

to let the radiologist know that injury to the AC joint, not just the shoulder, is in question. Stress or weighted views are usually not helpful and cause undue pain without improving the diagnostic yield.[2,8] Overpenetration of films may make their interpretation difficult.[3]

A 15-degree cephalad AP view helps to diagnose sprains, whereas the 40-degree cephalic tilt AP should be used for suspected fractures of the clavicle. If the fracture is medial to the coracoclavicular ligaments, both an anterior and a posterior 45-degree view should be obtained.[3] Typically, the decision to obtain these views will be made by the radiologist.

Certainly, if there are concerns about a fracture or arthrosis and the x-ray images do not provide confirmation, further imaging with a bone scan[2,3] or MRI may be indicated.[9]

Differential Diagnosis

Fractures of the acromion or distal clavicle

Rotator cuff tears[2,4,10]

Tendinitis of the long head of the biceps[2]

Calcific tendinitis

Adhesive capsulitis

Glenohumeral arthritis

Shoulder impingement syndrome

Tears of the glenohumeral labrum[7]

Ganglia and cysts in the AC joint[2]

Arthritis (e.g., rheumatoid, crystal induced and septic)

Distal osteolysis of the clavicle[2]

Tumors[2]

Cervical radiculopathy

Referred pain may come from cardiac, pulmonary and gastrointestinal disease[2]

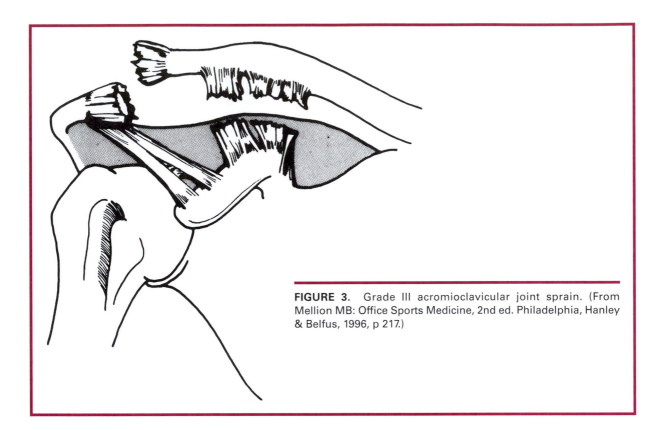

FIGURE 3. Grade III acromioclavicular joint sprain. (From Mellion MB: Office Sports Medicine, 2nd ed. Philadelphia, Hanley & Belfus, 1996, p 217.)

Treatment

Initial

Initial treatment will depend on the degree of injury and the patient's activity and goals.

Type I and II injuries are exclusively treated non-operatively, whereas types IV, V, and VI require surgery. Treatment of type III injuries is controversial (see Table 1).

The initial phase of treatment includes rest, ice, and possibly a sling or brace for 1 to 6 weeks, (2 to 3 weeks average). Over-the-counter or prescription non-narcotic analgesics are usually sufficient. NSAIDs/COX-2 inhibitors can be used for pain and inflammation. Injections into the joint can also be done in the initial phase of treatment for immediate pain control and diagnosis.

Rest should be relative—that is, the patient should avoid aggravating activities and should not be immobilized if at all possible.

Ice massage can be done over the painful area for 5 to 10 minutes every 2 hours, as needed. An ice pack can be used for 20 minutes at a time and also can be repeated every 2 hours. The usual precautions regarding the use of ice should be followed.

Type I and II sprains can be treated with a sling to help support the arm and shoulder. This should be used symptomatically and discontinued for painless activities and when the patient's pain is under control.

Type III injuries have been treated operatively and non-operatively (Fig. 3). The majority of orthopedists favor non-operative treatment as a rule, even in throwing athletes.[3,8,11,12] One study suggested greater long-term satisfaction in patients who had surgery but showed no difference in range of motion or strength.[13] The majority of patients have no long-term difficulty with non-operative management. There are also reports of high complication rates with surgery.[3] Surgery may be considered in symptomatic individuals with type III injuries and those who do not respond to conservative measures.

One approach is to treat conservatively with relative rest, support, modalities, medications for symptoms, and a gradual return to activity over 6 to 12 weeks. If there is a significant limitation in function, including avocational or sport activities, or if the patient is not progressing as expected, further evaluation is warranted.[3] Unlike musculotendinous injuries, delayed surgery does not lead to poorer outcomes.

Rehabilitation

Physical or occupational therapy can be ordered to assist with patient education; pain control; and in later stages, gradual range of motion and strengthening exercises. Modalities to control pain can include, in addition to ice, ultrasound or phonophoresis with 10% lidocaine. Alternatively, interferential current (IFC) can be used. As pain is controlled, motion can be obtained in a pain-free range. Codman's and pendulum exercises can progress to active or active-assisted range of motion to restore shoulder flexion and abduction, both individually and in combination. In the initial phase of a rehabilitation program, it is reasonable to avoid painful positions or movements. These typically include extremes of flexion—even when done passively—and adduction across the chest. When the shoulder is pain free and has full range of motion, rehabilitation can progress to gradual strengthening and return to activity. A typical shoulder rehabilitation program can be used.

Procedures

Patients with AC joint pain due to type I or mild type II injuries can receive injections and return to play or work immediately with little risk of injury as long as they have full functional range of motion and symmetric[2] strength. For diagnostic purposes, a local anesthetic injection may confirm the diagnosis of a type 1 sprain[2] if the patient has complete pain relief immediately following the

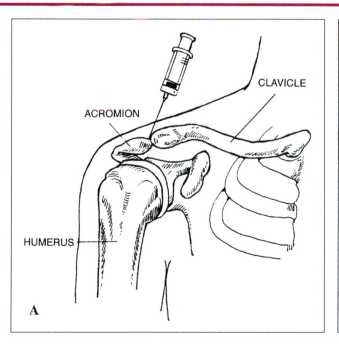
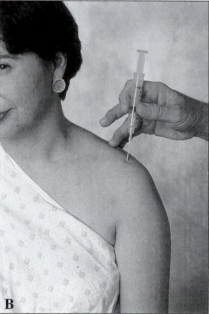

CLAVICLE

ACROMION

HUMERUS

A

B

FIGURE 4. Internal anatomic (*A*) and approximate surface anatomic (*B*) sites for injection of the acromioclavicular joint. (From Lennard TA (ed): Pain Procedures in Clinical Practice, 2nd ed. Philadelphia, Hanley & Belfus, 2000, p 129.)

injection. Intraarticular injection of a combination of a local anesthetic and a corticosteroid may give immediate and longer-acting relief. Injections into the joint can be done for higher-grade injuries as well to give quick symptomatic relief. However, this is not a substitute for relative rest in more seriously injured joints (type II and higher), and 1 week of avoiding provocative maneuvers is advised.[2]

With the patient sitting or supine and the shoulder propped under a pillow, under sterile conditions, using a 25-gauge, 1½-inch disposable needle and a local anesthetic or anesthetic/corticosteroid combination, the AC joint is injected (Fig. 4). Typically a 1 to 3 cc aliquot of solution is injected (e.g., 1 cc of 1% lidocaine mixed with 1 cc of betamethasone). Keep in mind that the AC joint is small and superficial.

Post-injection care should include local icing for 10 to 15 minutes and patient instruction to avoid aggravating activities for at least 1 week.

Surgery

Type IV, V, and VI injuries are all forms of dislocation of the acromioclavicular joint. These need to be reduced surgically and some form of reconstruction attempted. Early referral is indicated to minimize pain and dysfunction. Because the scapula is no longer suspended from the clavicle, the deltoid and trapezius muscles will become involved. These muscles may have been injured directly and therefore are ill-suited to take on the role of suspending the arm. The result is more significant pain and a greater chance for prolonged disability.

If the patient has sustained a fracture, surgery may be necessary, and referral to an orthopedist is appropriate. The severity of the injury will depend on whether the fracture is medial to the coracoclavicular ligaments or whether it involves the AC joint itself. Fractures medial to the ligaments can result in displacement of the clavicle and the patient therefore runs the risk of delayed union or non-union. The displacement can look like a type II or III sprain. Careful examination of the location and degree of pain should raise suspicions. Regardless, radiographs are indicated to assess the possibility of fracture.

Fractures in the joint will likely lead to arthrosis in the future. These patients may not need surgery initially—that will be decided by the patient and the orthopedist—but may require a protracted conservative course of symptomatic treatment.

Resection of the distal clavicle, tacking the acromion to the clavicle, re-creating the ligaments, and screw fixation of the AC joint or of the clavicle to the coracoid process have all been used to stabilize the joint. In chronic situations, the Weaver-Dunn procedure may be used. This includes resection of the distal clavicle, transfer of the coracoacromial ligament to the clavicle, and suture fixation of the clavicle to the coracoid.[3]

Potential Disease Complications

Patients may be left with a "bump" due to the depression of the acromion relative to the clavicle. This should be expected and is unavoidable without surgery. AC joint pain due to chronic instability is the most common complication.[3,10] Degenerative arthritis can occur because of the injury or due to instability. This can be treated symptomatically with modalities and injections. If the pain persists, surgery should be considered.

Potential Treatment Complications

Analgesics, NSAIDs, and COX-2 inhibitors have well-known side effects that most commonly affect the gastric, hepatic, and renal systems. COX-2 inhibitors may have fewer gastric side effects. Injecting the joint with too long a needle may result in injection into the subacromial space. This can cause diagnostic confusion, if not outright injury.[2] Injections can also be associated with infection in rare cases.

Direct complications of surgery can include infection, pain, wound or skin breakdown, and hypertrophic scar.[3,12] Following surgery, there can be a recurrence of the deformity,[12,13] hardware failure or migration,[4,12] or limitation of movement. Pain may persist due to insufficient resection, weakness, or joint instability.[2]

References

1. Stecco A, Sgambati E, Brizzi E, et al: Morphometric analysis of the acromioclavicular joint. Italian J Anat Embryol 1997;102(3):195–200.
2. Shaffer BS: Painful conditions of the acromioclavicular joint. J Am Acad Orth Surgeons 1999;7(3):176–188.
3. Turnbull JR: Acromioclavicular joint disorders. Med Sci Sports Exerc 1998;30:S26–S32.
4. Berg EE: An intra-articular fracture dislocation of the acromioclavicular joint. Am J Orthop 1998;7:555–559.
5. Gerber C, Galantay RV, Hersche O: The pattern of pain produced by irritation of the acromioclavicular joint and subacromial space. J Shoulder Elbow Surg 1998;7:352–355.
6. Buchberger DJ: Introduction of a new physical examination procedure for the differentiation of acromioclavicular joint lesions and subacromial impingement. J Manipulative Physiol Therapeutics 1999;22:316–321.
7. O'Brien SJ, Pagnani MJ, Fealy S, et al: The active compression test: A new and effective test for diagnosing labral tears and acromioclavicular joint abnormality. Am J Sports Med 1998;26:610–613.
8. Lemos M: Evaluation and treatment of the injured acromioclavicular joint in athletes. Am J of Sports Medicine 1998;26:137–144.
9. Yu JS, Dardani M, Fischer RA: MR observations of posttraumatic osteolysis of the distal clavicle after traumatic separation of the acromioclavicular joint. J Computer Assisted Tomography 2000;24(1):159–164.
10. Clarke HD, McCann PD: Acromioclavicular injuries. Orthop Clin North Am 2000;31:177–187.
11. McFarland EG, Blivin SJ, Doehring CB, et al: Treatment of grade III acromioclavicular separations in professional throwing athletes: Results of a survey. Am J Orthop 1997;26:771–774.
12. Phillips AM, Smart C, Groom AFG: Acromioclavicular dislocation. Conservative or surgical therapy. Clin Orthop Rel Res 1998;353:10–17.
13. Press J, Zuckerman JD, Gallagher M, Cuomo F: Treatment of grade III acromioclavicular separations. Bull Hosp Joint Dis 1997;56(2):77–83.

12 Adhesive Capsulitis

Robert P. Nirschl, MD, MS
Sharon Goldman Willett, PTA, STS

Synonyms

Frozen shoulder

Periarthritis of the shoulder

Stiff and painful shoulder

Periarticular adhesions

Humeroscapular fibrositis

ICD-9 Code

726.0
Adhesive capsulitis of shoulder

Definition

Primary frozen shoulder is a progressive soft tissue restriction of shoulder motion of uncertain etiology that is usually insidious in onset and often associated with pain. Accompanying diagnostic factors of secondary frozen shoulder may include rotator cuff tendinitis/tendinosis and extrinsic factors and maladies such as immobilization following wrist fracture, cervical radiculopathy, or intrathoracic conditions and systemic disorders such as diabetes and hypothyroidism. Women ages 40 to 65 years are most commonly affected. Individuals with depression or prolonged immobilization due to an injury are also at increased risk.

The key histopathological abnormality of primary frozen shoulder is an acute reddened angry synovial pannus in the inflammatory phase, followed by fibrosis, hyalination, and fibrinoid degeneration with contraction of the synovial and sub-synovial tissue in the maturing phase of the malady.

Symptoms

In the early stages, there is pain in the shoulder with active and passive movement. In late stages, complaints of stiffness, both actively and passively, at shoulder end ranges are common, with loss of motion localized to the glenohumeral joint. The history is usually devoid of specific injury to the shoulder. A full medical history must be taken to check for any predisposing factors such as autoimmune disease, diabetes, or myofascial pain syndrome.

Physical Examination

Adhesive capsulitis is noted with a measurable restriction in *both* passive and active shoulder range of motion. This is in contrast to a rotator cuff tear, in which active range of motion is restricted but passive range of motion is normal. Motion is painful especially at the extremes of range. A decrease or stiffness in the glenohumeral glide is noted, especially inferior translation. The relationship of the glenohumeral joint movement independent of scapularthoracic motion should also be addressed. Patients with adhesive capsulitis typically cannot put their palms together in a prayer position. The shoulder is usually painful to palpation around the rotator cuff.

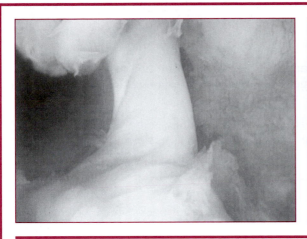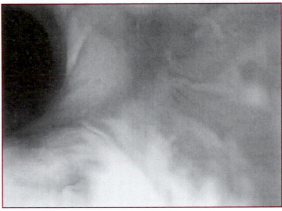

FIGURE 1. Arthroscopic view of acute adhesive capsulitis synovitis.

Manual muscle testing done in the available range may detect weakness, suggesting a rotator cuff component.

Cervical range of motion should also be evaluated to rule out the neck as a possible source of pain. Sensation and deep tendon reflexes are normal.

Functional Limitations

Patients may experience sleep disruption due to pain and/or inability to sleep on the affected side. Inability to perform activities of daily living is common (e.g., fastening a bra in the back, putting on a belt, reaching for a wallet in the back pocket, reaching for a seatbelt, combing the hair, etc.). Work activities may be limited—particularly those that require reaching (e.g., filing above waist level, stocking shelves, lifting boards or other items, etc.). Recreational activities may also be affected (e.g., difficulty serving or throwing a ball, inability to do the crawl stroke in swimming, etc.).

Diagnostic Studies

X-rays are typically done to rule out an underlying arthritis, tumor, or calcium deposit. In adhesive capsulitis, they are generally normal. MRI or arthrogram (if MRI is not available) is generally done in patients who don't improve after a trial of conservative treatment (at least 6 to 12 weeks). Arthrography will typically show decreased volume of contrast that can be injected into the joint (less than 5 ml). Diagnostic arthroscopy (Fig. 1) may also be utilized. Routine blood work should be done to rule out diabetes, thyroid disorders, and autoimmune diseases that may be causing secondary frozen shoulder.

Differential Diagnosis

Osteoarthritis	Biceps tendinitis	Humeral fracture
Avascular necrosis	Subacromial bursitis	Tumor
Rotator cuff disease	Thoracic outlet syndrome	Scapular muscle dyskinesia
Cervical radiculopathy	Brachial plexopathy	

Treatment

Initial

The initial treatment goals are to decrease pain and increase range of motion at the shoulder (including accessory glenohumeral glide and proper scapular rhythm). The patient should be given some basic shoulder exercises initially (Fig. 2).

Reducing any inflammation and pain using NSAIDs/COX-2 inhibitors is generally advocated. Occasionally, oral steroids are recommended. The use of cold/ice therapy is also a helpful adjunct to pain control (20 minutes 2 to 3 times daily).

Rehabilitation

Preparatory modalities to decrease pain, such as ultrasound, moist hot packs, and electrical stimulation, are helpful. Iontophoresis with topical steroids may offer opportunities for enhanced pain control. Passive manipulation of the glenohumeral joint, the restoration of glenohumeral glide, and stretching of the tissues are the most important aspects in restoring range of motion. Exercises initiated in a structured environment, for muscle re-education and strengthening to aid in functional improvement and enhancement of active stretching as well as to help prevent re-aggravation, are recommended. Follow-up home exercise programs to ensure progressive rehabilitation are helpful. Postexercise icing is beneficial in reducing pain and soreness. If there is any additional diagnosis such as rotator cuff tendinitis/tendinosis or bicipital tendinitis, ice can help decrease inflammation, edema, and pain. With less pain the patient may be more willing to move the extremity, thereby enhancing the rehabilitation process.

Once pain is managed and the patient begins to regain some shoulder range of motion, gentle strengthening exercises are initiated. Patients should be encouraged to continue their exercises once supervised physical therapy ends in order to maintain their range of motion.

Procedures

Procedural opportunities include injections and surgery. As an adjunct to pain control, subacromial injections may aid pain control from a companion rotator cuff tendinitis/tendinosis or inflammatory adhesive capsulitis/bursitis (see Chapters 16 and 17).

Surgery

If loss of motion and pain become recalcitrant, surgical intervention may be considered. Decision for surgery is usually based on lack of rehabilitation progress and unacceptable quality of life. The traditional approach of manipulation under anesthesia followed by immediate and aggressive physical therapy has had some success. Improved success with more rapid maximum benefit (weeks rather than months) occurs with the addition of arthroscopic debridement of the glenohumeral adhesive synovitis and coracoacromial arch bursitis.

Potential Disease Complications

Adhesive capsulitis may result in the persistence of signs and symptoms including permanent loss of motion and chronic pain. A patient with secondary capsulitis and systemic disease may suffer the complications of the underlying disease.

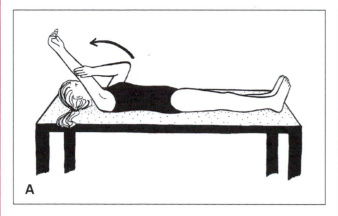

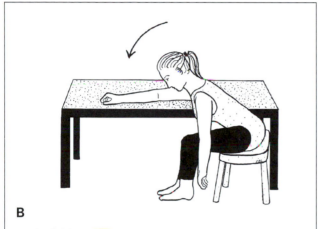

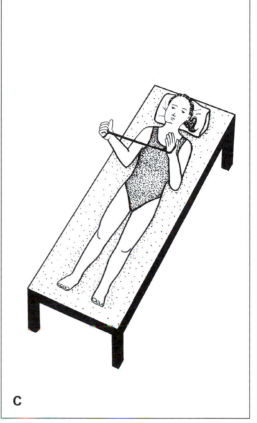

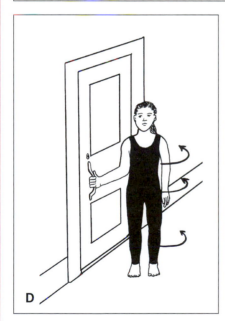

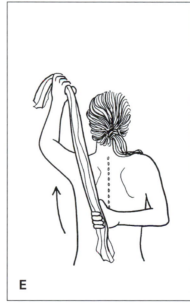

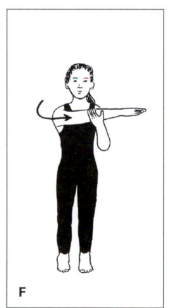

FIGURE 2.   University of Washington (Jackins) exercises for improving range of motion. *A,* Stretch in overhead reach using the opposite arm to push the affected arm. *B,* Gently lean forward to stretch the shoulder. *C,* Stretch in external rotation using the opposite hand to push a cane or other stick. *D,* Turn the body away from a fixed object to apply a gentle stretching force in external rotation. *E,* Use towel to apply a gentle stretching force in internal rotation. *F,* Stretch in cross-body reach using the opposite arm to pull the affected arm.

Potential Treatment Complications

Complications, other than medication issues are unusual. Analgesics, NSAIDs, and COX-2 inhibitors have well-known side effects that most commonly affect the gastric, hepatic, and renal systems. Surgical complications of standard nature can occur as well as focused musculoskeletal issues. Fracture of the humerus secondary to manipulation has been reported.

References
1. Owens-Burkhard H: Management of the frozen shoulder, 2nd ed. In Donatelli R (ed): Physical Therapy of the Shoulder. New York, Churchill Livingston, 1991, pp 91–113.
2. Coumo F: Diagnosis, classification, and management of the stiff shoulder. In Iannotti J, Williams G (eds): Disorders of the Shoulder: Diagnosis and Management. Philadelphia, Lippincott, Williams, & Wilkins, 1999.

13 Biceps Tendinitis

Jeffrey A. Strakowski, MD
Julie K. Silver, MD

Synonyms

Biceps tendinosis

Bicipital tendinitis

ICD-9 Codes

726.11
Calcifying tendinitis of shoulder

726.12
Bicipital tenosynovitis

Definition

Biceps tendinitis is a general term used to describe inflammation, pain, or tenderness in the region of the biceps tendon. The actual origin of the pain may be due to a degenerative process called tendinosis. This usually occurs in "watershed" areas of vascular supply of tendons.[1] Biceps tendinitis rarely occurs alone, but rather is typically associated with rotator cuff pathology and impingement. The precipitating forces in biceps tendinitis are multifactorial and include repetitive overuse, multidirectional instability, compressive forces from degenerative joint disease and spurring, calcifications into the tendon, and direct trauma.[2,3] The majority of shoulder movement occurs about the glenohumeral joint, which is a ball-and-socket joint. This joint has great mobility at the expense of stability, and dynamic effects of muscle strength and function are highly interdependent. Injury or compromise of a single muscle of the dynamic shoulder stabilizers can adversely affect other muscles and impair function of the entire joint.

Symptoms

Biceps tendinitis usually presents with complaints of anterior shoulder pain that is worse with activity. Often, pain will also occur with prolonged rest and subsequent immobility, particularly at night.[4] Attention should be given to onset, duration, and character of the pain. Some individuals will present only with complaints of fatigue with shoulder movement in the early stages of tendinitis. History of prior trauma, athletic and occupational endeavors, and systemic diseases should be considered when evaluating the shoulder. Patients with accompanying supraspinatus tendinitis or "impingement syndrome" often complain of a "pinching" sensation with overhead activities and a "toothache" sensation in the lateral proximal arm.[5] In bicipital tendinitis, anterior shoulder pain occurs with shoulder flexion and lifting activities that involve elbow flexion.[6]

Physical Examination

A physical examination should begin with adequate inspection of the shoulder and neck region. Attention is given to prior scars, structural deformities, posture, and muscle bulk. Determination of the exact location

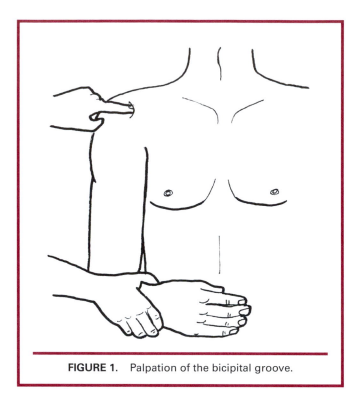

FIGURE 1. Palpation of the bicipital groove.

of pain can be helpful for diagnosis. Biceps tendinitis commonly presents with palpable tenderness over the bicipital groove (Fig. 1). Side-to-side comparisons should be made because the tendon is typically slightly tender to direct palpation. Tenderness over the lateral aspect of the shoulder suggests tendinitis or muscular strain of the deltoid or the underlying bursa. Range of motion may be limited if the rotator cuff is involved. Motion limitation is not seen in isolated tendonopathies but is often seen in concomitant degenerative joint diseases, impingement syndromes, tendon tears, or adhesive capsulitis. A neurologic examination should be normal, including sensation and deep tendon reflexes. Occasionally, strength is limited due to pain.

Special tests of the shoulder should be performed routinely. These include impingement tests[4] and supraspinatus tests[7] in rotator cuff tendinitis. Speed's and Yergason's tests (see Figs. 2 and 3) are considered specific for bicipital tendinitis.[8,9] Other maneuvers to assess for instability and arthritis should be performed.

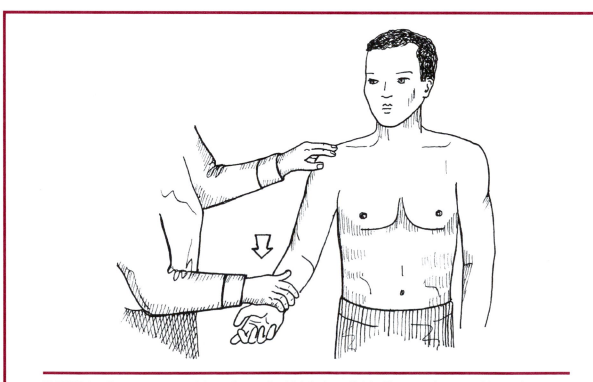

FIGURE 2. Demonstration of Speed's test for bicipital tendinitis. The examiner provides resistance to forward flexion of the shoulder with the elbow in extension and supination of the forearm. Pain is elicited in the intertubercular groove in a positive test.

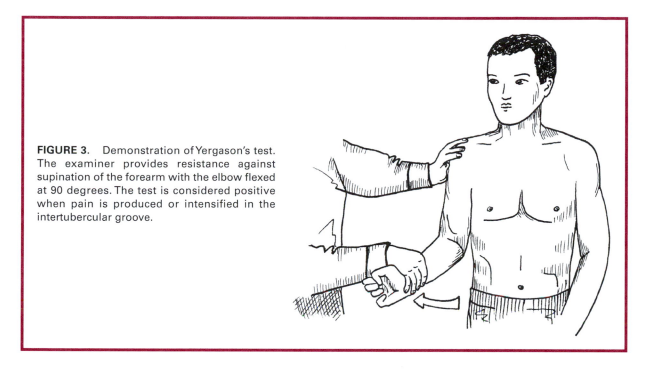

FIGURE 3. Demonstration of Yergason's test. The examiner provides resistance against supination of the forearm with the elbow flexed at 90 degrees. The test is considered positive when pain is produced or intensified in the intertubercular groove.

Functional Limitations

Biceps tendinitis may cause patients to limit their activities at home and at work. Limitations may include difficulty with lifting and carrying groceries, garbage bags, and brief cases. Athletics that involve the affected arm may be curtailed, such as swimming, tennis, and throwing sports. Pain may impair sleep.

Diagnostic Studies

Biceps tendinitis is generally diagnosed on a clinical basis, but imaging studies are helpful for excluding other pathology. Plain film x-rays can show calcifications in the tendon and degenerative disease of the joint. The Fisk view is utilized when evaluating bicipital tendinitis to assess the size of the intertubercular groove. This helps determine whether there is a relative risk of developing recurrent subluxation of the tendon, which is seen in individuals with short and narrow margins of the intertubercular groove.[10] Arthrograms have been used in the past for rotator cuff disease but are generally only helpful in full thickness tears and have lost favor to magnetic resonance imaging (MRI). MRI can detect partial thickness tendon tears; evaluate muscle substance, soft tissue abnormalities, and labral disease; and assess for masses. Ultrasound is used in some centers for dynamic assessment of tendon function but has not reached widespread acceptance.[11] Electrodiagnosis is utilized when concomitant peripheral neuropathies need assessment. Arthroscopy is a useful procedure for the evaluation of intraarticular pathology but does not play a role in isolated tendinitis.

Differential Diagnosis

Rotator cuff tendinitis and tears

Multidirectional instability

Biceps brachii rupture

Acromial clavicular joint sprain

Degenerative joint disease

Rheumatoid arthritis

Crystalline arthropathy

Adhesive capsulitis

Cervical spondylosis

Cervical radiculopathy

Brachial plexopathy

Peripheral entrapment neuropathy

Referral from visceral organs

Diaphragmatic referred pain

Treatment

Initial

The hallmark for treatment of biceps tendinitis involves activity modification, anti-inflammatory measures, heat and cold modalities, and a therapeutic exercise program for promoting strength and flexibility of the dynamic shoulder stabilizers.[9] Overhead activities and lifting are to be avoided initially. Workstation assessment and modification can be helpful for laborers. Evaluation of athletic technique and training adaptations are important in athletes. NSAIDs/COX-2 inhibitors can assist with decreasing the pain and inflammation. Shoulder stretching is helpful to maintain range of motion and flexibility and is emphasized in all parameters of abduction, adduction, and internal and external rotation.[12] Moist heat can be useful prior to activity. Ice is helpful after exercise for minimizing pain.

Rehabilitation

Rehabilitation for biceps tendinitis is similar to that of rotator cuff tendinitis (see Chapter 16). Moreover, since biceps tendinitis rarely occurs in isolation, it is important to rehabilitate the patient by accounting for all of the shoulder pathology that is present (e.g., instability, impingement) Modalities such as ultrasound can be applied easily to focal tendinitis as a deep heating modality using 1 to 2.5 watts/cm^2. Progressive resistance exercises are utilized to strengthen the dynamic shoulder stabilizers. Athletes are returned to play gradually when pain is minimal or absent.

Procedures

Steroid injections are a useful adjunct for biceps tendinitis (Fig. 4). Care is taken to avoid injection into the tendon substance itself. These serve as an adjunct to diminish pain and inflammation and

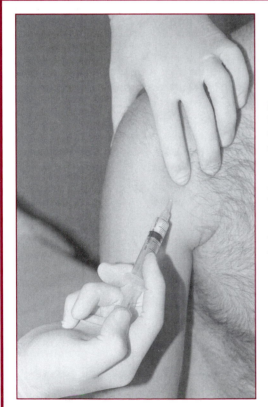

FIGURE 4. Injection technique for the long head of the biceps brachii. Under sterile conditions using a 25-gauge 1.5-inch disposable needle and a local anesthetic/corticosteroid combination, the area surrounding the biceps tendon is injected. It is important to bathe the tendon sheath in the preparation rather than to inject the tendon itself. Typically a 1–3 cc aliquot of the mixture is used (e.g., 1 cc of 1% lidocaine mixed with 1 cc of betamethasone). Immediate post-injection care includes icing for 5–10 minutes, and the patient may continue to ice at home for 15–20 minutes, 2–3 times daily for several days. The patient should be instructed to avoid heavy lifting or vigorous exercise for 48–72 hours post-injection. It is advisable not to repeat the injection more than 2–3 times, owing to the possibility of weakening the tendon. (From Lennard TA (ed): Pain Procedures in Clinical Practice, 2nd ed. Philadelphia, Hanley & Belfus, 2000, p 150.)

facilitate the rehabilitation process. Injections must be used judiciously to avoid weakening tendon substance.[13] Depending on the shoulder pathology, other injections may also be useful (e.g., subacromial).

Surgery

Surgery is generally not indicated for biceps tendinitis.

Potential Disease Complications

Progressive biceps tendinitis and pain can lead to diminished activity and subsequent adhesive capsulitis. Compensatory problems with other tendons can develop due to their interdependence for proper shoulder movement. The development of myofascial pain of the surrounding shoulder girdle muscles is another common complication in shoulder tendinitis.

Potential Treatment Complications

The exercise program should be properly supervised initially to prevent aggravation of tendinitis of other muscle groups. Analgesics, NSAIDs, and COX-2 inhibitors have well-known side effects that most commonly affect the gastric, hepatic, and renal systems. Repeated steroid injections in or near tendons result in compromise of the tendon substance and should be avoided.

References

1. Brooks CH, Rewell WJ, Heaely FW: A quantitative histological study of the vascularity of the rotator cuff tendon. J Bone Joint Surg 1992;74B:151–153.
2. Codman EA: Rupture of the supraspinatus tendon and lesions in or about the subacromial bursa. In The Shoulder. Boston, Thomas Todd, 1934, pp 65–177.
3. Wolf WB: Shoulder tendinoses. Clin Sports Med 1992;11:871–890.
4. Neer CS, Foster CR: Impingement lesions. Clin Orthop 1983;173:70.
5. Hawkins RJ, Kennedy JC: Impingement syndrome in athletes. Am J Sports Med 1980;8:3.
6. Post M, Benca P: Primary tendinitis of the long head of the biceps. Clin Orthop 1989;246:117–125.
7. Jobe FW, Jobe CM: Painful athletic injuries of the shoulder. Clin Orthop 1983;173:117–124.
8. Nevlaser RJ: Lesions of the biceps and tendonitis of the shoulder. Orthop Clin N Am. 1980;11:334–340.
9. Jobe FW, Brodley JP: The diagnosis and nonoperative treatment of shoulder injuries in athletes. Clin Sports Med 1989;8:419–438.
10. Cone RO, Danzig L, Resnick D, Godman AB: The bicipital groove: Radiographic, anatomic and pathologic study. AJR 1983;141:781–788.
11. Middleton WD, Reinus WR, Totty WG: Ultrasonographic evaluation of the rotator cuff and biceps tendon. J Bone Joint Surg 1986;68(A);440–450.
12. Nevlaser RJ: Painful shoulder conditions. Clin Orthop 1983;173:63–69.
13. Fatal PD, Wigins ME: Corticosteriod injections: Their use and abuse. J Am Acad Orthop Surg 1994;2:133–140.

14 Biceps Tendon Rupture

Jeffrey A. Strakowski, MD

Synonyms

Biceps brachii rupture

Biceps tear

Bicipital strain

ICD-9 Codes

727.62
Rupture of tendon of biceps (long head), non-traumatic

840.8
Sprain/strain of other specified site of shoulder and upper arm

Definition

Biceps tendon rupture (either complete or partial) is a disruption of the tendon of the biceps brachii muscle, which can occur proximally or distally. The more common proximal ruptures are frequently seen in older individuals who have had chronic, often asymptomatic, tendinitis of the long head of the biceps tendon and have concomitant rotator cuff disease and degenerative joint disease of the shoulder[1] (Fig. 1). The vast majority of cases involve the long head of the biceps brachii and present as a partial or complete avulsion from the superior rim of the anterior glenoid labrum.[2]

The distal biceps rupture is relatively uncommon and typically occurs in middle-age males. This often develops suddenly with stressing of the flexor mechanism of the elbow. Distal biceps rupture usually occurs as a single traumatic event such as heavy lifting and is often an avulsion of the tendon from the radial tuberosity but can also occur as a midsubstance tendon rupture.[3]

Symptoms

Proximal ruptures are often asymptomatic and are commonly discovered with awareness of distal migration of the biceps brachii muscle mass or may occur suddenly by a seemingly trivial event. Often, individuals will note an acute "popping" sensation, and edema and ecchymosis can also be seen. The proximal ruptures are typically less painful but can be preceded by chronic shoulder discomfort.[4]

An acute distal rupture is often associated with pain at the antecubital fossa that is typically aggravated by resisted elbow flexion. The pain is usually sharp initially but improves with time and is often described as a dull ache.[5] Swelling, distal ecchymosis, and proximal migration of the biceps brachii muscle mass accompany this injury with a magnitude dependent on the degree of injury.

Physical Examination

Visual inspection of the biceps brachii, including comparison with the unaffected limb, is the critical element in the physical examination of this condition. Ludington's test[6] is a recommended position to observe differences in the contour and shape of the biceps (Fig. 2). Complete ruptures are relatively easy to diagnose, whereas partial ruptures can be more difficult. The clinician should also assess for the presence of ecchymosis or swelling as a sign of acute injury. Palpation for point tenderness will often reveal pain at the rupture site. Effort should also be made to determine whether the rupture is complete by palpation of the tendon. Thorough assessment of the shoulder and elbow should be made for range of motion and laxity. Yergason's[7] and Speed's tests[8] (see Chapter 13), which are utilized in the assessment of bicipital tendinitis, are also recommended. A thorough neurologic and vascular examination is performed and should be normal in the absence of concomitant problems. Caution should be used with strength testing to avoid worsening an incomplete tear.

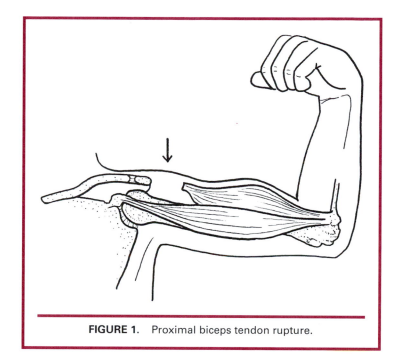

FIGURE 1. Proximal biceps tendon rupture.

Functional Limitations

The functional limitations are generally relatively minimal with proximal biceps rupture,[9] and patient concern is commonly centered around cosmetic considerations. More significant weakness of elbow flexion and supination is noted after a distal tendon disruption. Pain can be acutely limiting after both situations but is typically more problematic in distal rupture. The primary role of the biceps brachii is supination of the forearm. Elbow flexion is functional by the action of the brachialis and brachioradialis. A degree of residual weakness with supination and elbow flexion, particularly after distal tendon rupture, can cause functional impairment for individuals who perform heavy physical labor, such as moving boxes, wood boards, or heavy equipment.[10] Fatigue with repetitive work is also a common complaint with non-surgically treated distal tendon ruptures.[11] The long head of the biceps is believed to play a role in anterior stability of the shoulder[12,13] and is an issue for people who perform overhead activities, such as lifting, filing, painting, etc.

Diagnostic Studies

The diagnosis of biceps brachii rupture is often made on a clinical basis alone. Magnetic resonance imaging is helpful in

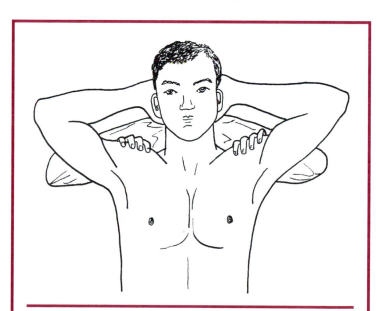

FIGURE 2. Ludington's test is performed by having the patient clasp both hands onto or behind the head, allowing the interlocking fingers to support the arms. This action allows maximum relaxation of the biceps tendon in its resting position. The patient then alternately contracts/relaxes the biceps while the clinician palpates the tendon and muscle. In a complete tear, contraction will not be felt on the affected side.

confirming the diagnosis and assessing the extent of the injury. It is particularly useful in partial ruptures.[14] MRI studies can also assess concomitant rotator cuff disease. Imaging of the entire insertion site as well as elbow structures should be performed in distal ruptures. Plain roentgenograms sometimes show hypertrophic bone formation related to chronic degenerative tendon abnormalities as a predisposition to rupture. X-rays are also performed in acute traumatic cases to rule out fractures. Electrodiagnostic testing (i.e., EMG and nerve conduction studies) to rule out peripheral nerve dysfunction is considered when appropriate.

Differential Diagnosis

Musculocutaneous neuropathy

Brachial plexopathy

Tumor

Dislocated biceps tendon

Glenohumeral arthritis

Rotator cuff pathology

Pectoralis major muscle rupture

Hematoma

Cervical radiculopathy

Treatment

Initial

For most patients, treatment for proximal biceps tears is conservative. Surgery is rarely necessary, since there is little loss of function, and the cosmetic deformity is generally acceptable without surgical repair.[15]

Young athletes or heavy laborers may be the exception since they typically need the lost strength that occurs with loss of the continuity of the biceps tendon. Distal tears are more commonly referred to surgery acutely. However, initial treatment of partial distal ruptures consists of splint immobilization in flexion, which should be continued for 3 weeks. This is followed by a gradual return to normal activities. Analgesics, NSAIDs/COX-2 inhibitors, and ice assist with the discomfort and swelling in both proximal and distal ruptures.

Rehabilitation

Non-surgical treatment includes range of motion of the elbow and shoulder for contracture prevention. Modalities (e.g., ultrasound) can be used for pain control. Gentle strengthening can typically be done after the acute phase (i.e., when there is little swelling or pain) in complete tears that are not going to be repaired because there is little chance of further injury.

Postoperative rehabilitation for distal biceps rupture repairs consists of immobilization of the elbow in 90 degrees of flexion for 7 to 10 days, followed by the use of a hinged flexion-assist splint with a 30-degree extension block for 8 weeks after surgery. Gentle range-of-motion and progressive resistance exercises are started after that. Unlimited activity is not allowed until 5 months postoperatively.[16]

Procedures

No procedures are performed in biceps tendon rupture.

Surgery

Prompt assessment is necessary for complete distal biceps ruptures under consideration for surgical repair. The same is true for proximal ruptures in very active individuals who require maximal upper body strength for their vocation or sport. Optimal surgical outcomes are obtained if treatment occurs within the first 4 weeks after injury. Partial distal ruptures are generally followed non-operatively until a complete rupture occurs. The partial rupture can scar and remain in continuity.[4] The goal of surgical treatment is to restore strength of supination and flexion. For distal repairs, this is typically performed by a two-incision technique involving reinsertion of the biceps tendon to the radial tuberosity.[17]

Potential Disease Complications

Complications from isolated biceps rupture are relatively rare. Partial tears can become complete tears. Attention should be given to potential contracture formation. Median nerve compression has been reported to presumably be related to an enlarged synovial bursa associated with a partial distal biceps tendon rupture.[18] Compartment syndrome has also been reported in proximal biceps rupture in a patient receiving systemic anticoagulation.[19]

Potential Treatment Complications

Analgesics, NSAIDs, and COX-2 inhibitors have well-known side effects that most commonly affect the gastric, hepatic, and renal systems. Advancing the extent of the rupture can occur with overly aggressive strengthening measures and passive stretching. The potential for serious surgical complications is most significant with distal rupture because of the important neurovascular structures in that region, including the median and radial nerves and brachial artery and vein.[20] The complication rate increases with the length of time after rupture that the surgery is performed. Proximal radial ulnar synostosis and heterotopic ossification have also been reported as rare postsurgical complications.[16] Stiffness and contractures are possible with or without surgical intervention.

References
1. Neer CS: Impingement lesions. Clin Orthop 1983;173:70–77.
2. Gilcreest EL: The common syndrome of rupture, dislocation and elongation of the long head of the biceps brachii. An analysis of one hundred cases. Surg Gynecol. Obstet 1934;58:322.
3. Le Huec JC, Moinard M, Liquois F, Zipoli B: Distal rupture of the tendon of biceps brachii. Evaluation by MRI and the results of repair. J Bone Joint Surg Br 1996;78:767–770.
4. Waugh RI, Hathcock TA, Elliott JL: Ruptures of muscles and tendons: with particular reference of rupture (or elongation of the long tendon) of biceps brachii with report of fifty cases. Surgery 1949;25:370–392.
5. Bourne MH, Morrey BF: Partial rupture of the distal biceps tendon. Clin Orthop Rel Res 1991;271:143–148.
6. Ludington NA: Am J Surg 1923;77:358.
7. Yergason RM: Rupture of biceps. J Bone Joint Surg 1931;13:160.
8. Gilcreest EL, Albi P: Unusual lesions of muscles and tendons of the shoulder girdle and upper arm. Surg Gynecol Obstet 1939;68:903–917.
9. Phillips, BB, Canale ST, Sisk TD, et al: Ruptures of the proximal biceps tendon in middle-aged patients. Orthopedic Rev 1993;22:349–353.
10. Pearl ML, Bessos K, Wong K: Strength deficits related to distal biceps tendon rupture and repair. A case report. Amer J Sports Med 1998;26:295–296.
11. Davison BL, Engber WD, Tigert LJ: Long term evaluation of repaired distal biceps brachii tendon ruptures. Clin Orthop Rel Res 1996;333:188–191.
12. Rodosky MW, Harner CD, Fu FH: The role of the long head of the biceps muscle and superior glenoid labrum in anterior stability of the shoulder. Amer J Sports Med 1994;22:121–130.
13. Warner JJ, McMahon PJ: The role of the long head of the biceps brachii in superior stability of the glenohumeral joint. J Bone Joint Surg 1995;77:363–372.
14. Erickson SJ, Fitzgerald SW, Quinn SF, et al: Long bicipital tendon of the shoulder: Normal anatomy and pathologic findings on MR imaging. Am J Roent 1992;158:1091–1096.
15. Hawkins RJ, Kennedy JC: Impingement syndrome in athletes. Am J Sports Med 1980;8:151–158.
16. Ramsey, ML: Distal biceps tendon injuries: Diagnosis and management. J Am Acad Orthop Surg 1999;7:199–207.
17. Boyd HD, Anderson LD: A method for reinsertion of the distal biceps brachii tendon. J Bone Joint Surg 1961;43:1041–1043.
18. Foxworthy M, Kinninmonth AWG: Median nerve compression in the proximal forearm as a complication of partial rupture of the distal biceps brachii tendon. J Hand Surg [Br] 1992;17:515–517.
19. Richards AM, Moss AL: Biceps rupture in a patient on long-term anticoagulation leading to compartment syndrome and nerve palsies. J Hand Surg Br 1997;22:411–412.
20. Rantanen J, Orava S: Rupture of the distal biceps tendon. A report of 19 patients treated with anatomic reinsertion, and a meta-analysis of 147 cases found in the literature. Am J Sports Med 1999;27:128–132.

15 Glenohumeral Instability

William F. Micheo, MD
Edward Ramos, MD

Synonyms

Dislocation

Subluxation

Recurrent dislocation

Multidirectional instability

ICD-9 Codes

718.81
Instability of shoulder joint

831.00
Closed dislocation shoulder, unspecified

Definition

Shoulder instability represents a spectrum of disorders ranging from shoulder *subluxation*, in which the humeral head partially slips out of the glenoid fossa, to shoulder *dislocation*, which is a complete displacement out of the glenoid. It is classified as anterior, posterior, or multidirectional, and based on its frequency, etiology, direction, and degree.[1] Instability can result from macrotrauma, such as shoulder dislocation, or repetitive microtrauma associated with throwing, and it can occur without trauma in individuals with generalized ligamentous laxity.

The glenohumeral joint has a high degree of mobility at the expense of stability. Static and dynamic restraints maintain the shoulder in place with overhead activity. Muscle action, particularly that of the rotator cuff and scapular stabilizers, is important in maintaining joint congruity in midranges of motion. Static stabilizers such as the glenohumeral ligaments, joint capsule, and glenoid labrum are important for stability in the extremes of motion.[2]

Symptoms

In the case of traumatic instability the individual usually falls on the outstretched externally rotated, abducted arm with a resulting anterior dislocation. A blow to the posterior aspect of the externally rotated, abducted arm can also result in anterior dislocation. Posterior dislocation usually results from a fall on the forward flexed, adducted arm or by direct blow in the posterior direction when the arm is above the shoulder.[2]

With recurrent instability or subluxation, identifying an initial precipitating event may be difficult. Usually, symptoms result from repetitive activity, e.g., throwing, racquet sports, swimming, or work-related tasks. Repeated stresses place great demands on the dynamic and static stabilizers of the glenohumeral joint, leading to increased translation of the humeral head and pain associated with impingement of the rotator cuff. Patients may report that the shoulder slips out of the joint or the arm goes "dead," and they may report weakness associated with overhead activity. [3]

Physical Examination

The shoulder should be inspected for presence of deformity, atrophy of surrounding muscles, asymmetry, and scapular winging. Individuals should be observed from anterior, lateral, and posterior positions. Palpation of soft tissue and bone should be systematically addressed and include the rotator cuff, biceps tendon, and subacromial region.

Passive and active range of motion should be evaluated. Differences between passive and active motion may be secondary to pain, weakness, or neurologic damage. Repeated overhead activity may also lead to an increase in measured external rotation accompanied by a reduction in internal rotation. Manual strength testing should be performed to identify weakness of specific muscles of the rotator cuff and the scapular stabilizers. The supraspinatus muscle can be tested in the scapular plane with internal rotation or external rotation of the shoulder. The external rotators can be tested with the arm at the side of the body, and the subscapularis muscle can be tested by using the "lift-off test," in which the palm of the hand is lifted away from the lower back (Fig. 1). The scapular stabilizers, such as the serratus anterior and the rhomboid muscle, can be tested in isolation or by doing wall push-ups. Sensory and motor exam of the shoulder girdle and arm should be performed to rule out nerve injuries.

Testing the shoulder in 90 degrees of forward flexion with internal rotation can assess for rotator cuff impingement, and using extreme forward flexion with the forearm supinated may reproduce symptoms (Fig 2). Glenohumeral translation testing to determine laxity or instability should be documented. Apprehension testing can be performed with the patient sitting, standing, or in the supine position (Fig. 3); the shoulder joint is stressed in abduction and external rotation to assess for reproduction of the feeling of instability in the patient. A relocation maneuver that reduces the symptoms also aids in the diagnosis (Fig. 4). Other tests include the load-and-shift maneuver to document humeral head translation in anterior or posterior directions; the sulcus sign to document inferior humeral head laxity; and the active compression test, in which a downward force is applied to the

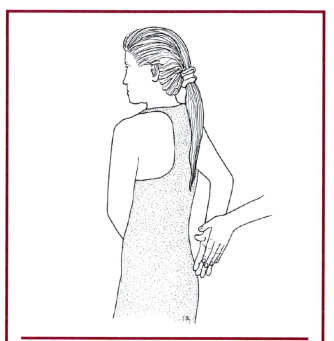

FIGURE 1. In the "lift-off test" of the subscapularis, the patient places the arm on the lower back area and attempts to forcefully internally rotate against the examiner's hand. It is important to document first that the patient has enough passive motion to allow the shoulder to be internally rotated away from the lower back area.

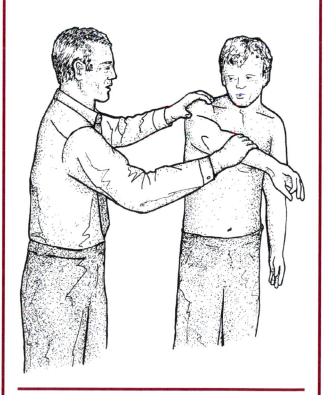

FIGURE 2. Impingement test. Testing for impingement against the coracoacromial arch.

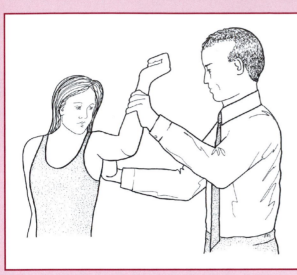

FIGURE 3. In the apprehension test, the arm is abducted to approximately 90° and progressively externally rotated while the patient's response is noted. A positive response is elicited by the patient having a sensation that the shoulder will slip out of joint.

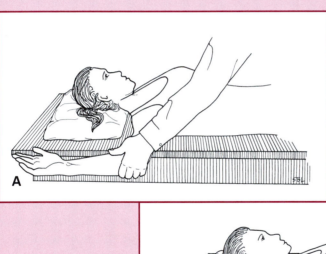

A

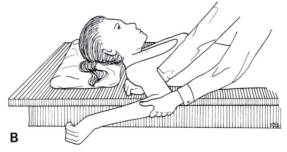

B

FIGURE 4. *A,* Apprehension relocation test in supine position with arm in 90° of abduction and maximal external rotation. *B,* Reduction of symptoms of apprehension with posteriorly directed force on proximal humerus. *C,* Increased symptoms of apprehension or pain with anterior force applied on proximal humerus.

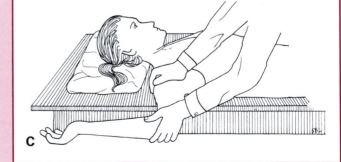

C

forward flexed, adducted, and internally rotated shoulder to reproduce pain associated with labral tears.[2-6]

Functional Limitations

Limitations include reduced motion, muscle weakness, and pain, which interfere with overhead activities, such as reaching into cupboards and brushing hair. Athletes, particularly those participating in throwing sports, may experience a decrease in the velocity; for instance, baseball or softball players may lose control of pitching, and tennis players may lose control of their serve. Recurrent instability often leads to avoidance of activities that require abduction and external rotation because of reproduction of symptoms.

Diagnostic Studies

The standard radiographs that are obtained to evaluate the patient with shoulder symptoms include anteroposterior views in external and internal rotation and outlet, axillary lateral, and stryker notch views. These will allow an assessment of the greater tuberosity and the shape of the acromion and will reveal irregularity of the glenoid or posterior humeral head. Special tests that also can be ordered include arthrography, CT arthrography, and magnetic resonance imaging (MRI). These should be ordered when looking for rotator cuff or labral abnormalities in the patient who has not responded to treatment. MRI has become the current standard technique for evaluation of rotator cuff and labral pathology. The use of gadolinium contrast enhancement appears to increase the sensitivity of MRI in identifying labral pathology.[7] Diagnostic arthroscopy can be utilized in some cases but is generally not necessary.

Differential Diagnosis

Rotator cuff tendinitis/tendinosis

Rotator cuff tear

Glenoid labral tear

Suprascapular neuropathy

Treatment

Initial

Acute management of glenohumeral instability is non-operative in the majority of cases. This includes relative rest, ice, and analgesic or anti-inflammatory medication. Goals at this stage include pain reduction, protection from further injury, and starting an early rehabilitation program.

If the injury was observed (as often occurs in athletes) and no evidence of neurologic or vascular damage is evident on clinical exam, reduction may be attempted with traction in forward flexion and slight abduction and followed by gentle internal rotation. If this fails, the patient should be transported from the playing area, and reduction may be attempted by placing the patient prone, sedating the individual, and allowing the injured arm to hang from the bed with a 5 to 10 pound weight attached to the wrist.[2]

If there is suspicion of fracture or posterior dislocation, the patient should undergo radiologic evaluation before a reduction is attempted. After the reduction, radiologic studies should be repeated.

TABLE 1. Glenohumeral Instability Rehabilitation

	Acute Phase	Recovery Phase	Functional Phase
Therapeutic intervention	Active rest Cryotherapy Electrical stimulation Protected motion Isometric exercise to shoulder and scapular muscles General conditioning NSAIDs	Modalities: superficial heat ultra-, sound, electrical stimulation Range-of-motion exercises, flexibility exercises for posterior capsule Scapular control: closed chain exercises, proprioceptive neuro-muscular facilitation patterns Dynamic upper extremity strengthening exercise: isolated rotator cuff exercises Sports-specific exercises: surgical tubing, multiplanar joint exercises, trunk and lower extremity General conditioning Gradual return to training	Power and endurance in upper extremities: diagonal and multiplanar motions with tubing, light weight, medi-cine balls; plyometrics Increase multiple-plane neuromuscular control Maintenance: general flexibil-ity training, strengthening, power and endurance exercise program Sports-specific progression
Criteria for advancement	Pain reduction Recovery of pain-free motion Strength of the shoulder muscles to 4/5	Full-non-painful motion Normal scapular stabilizers and rotator cuff strength Correction of posterior capsule inflexibility Symptom-free progression in a sports-specific program	Normal clinical examination Normal shoulder mechanics Normal kinematic chain integration Completed sports-specific program Normal throwing motion

Rehabilitation

The rehabilitation of glenohumeral instability should begin as soon as the injury occurs. The goals of non-surgical management include reducing pain, restoring full motion, correcting muscle strength deficits, achieving muscle balance, and returning to full activity free of symptoms. The rehabilitation program consists of acute, recovery, and functional phases (Table 1).[8–10]

Acute phase (1 to 2 weeks): This phase should focus on treating tissue injury and clinical signs and symptoms. The goal in this stage should be to allow for tissue healing while reducing pain and inflammation. Re-establishment of non-painful range of motion, prevention of muscle atrophy, and maintenance of general fitness should also be addressed.

Recovery phase (2 to 6 weeks): This phase should focus on obtaining normal passive and active glenohumeral range of motion, improving scapular muscle control, and achieving normal muscle strength and balance. Biomechanical and functional deficits, including abnormalities in the throwing motion, should also be addressed.

Functional phase (6 weeks to 6 months): This phase should focus on increasing the power and endurance of the upper extremities while improving neuromuscular control. Rehabilitation at this stage should work on the entire kinematic chain, addressing specific functional deficit. This program should be continuous with the ultimate goal of prevention of recurrent injury.

Procedures

If the individual persists with some symptoms of pain secondary to rotator cuff irritation, despite an appropriate rehabilitation program, a subacromial injection could be considered (Figs. 5 and 6). The patient at that time should be re-evaluated for identification of residual functional and biomechanical deficits that need to be addressed in combination with the injection. Under sterile conditions, using a 25-gauge, 1.5-inch disposable needle, inject an anesthetic/corticosteroid preparation using an anterior, posterior, or lateral approach. Typically 4–8 cc is injected (e.g., 4 cc of 1% lidocaine and 2 cc of 40 mg/cc betamethasone). Alternately, the lidocaine may be injected

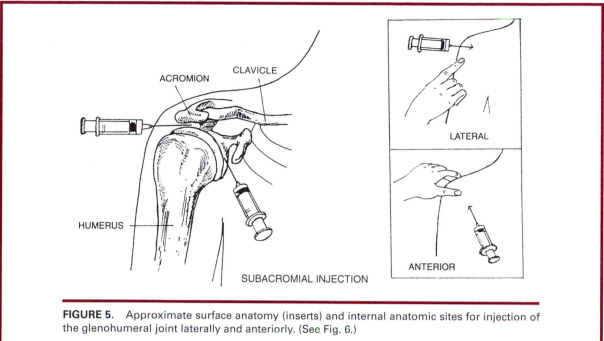

FIGURE 5. Approximate surface anatomy (inserts) and internal anatomic sites for injection of the glenohumeral joint laterally and anteriorly. (See Fig. 6.)

first followed by the corticosteroid. Post-injection care includes local ice for 5–10 minutes. The patient should be instructed to ice the shoulder for 15–20 minutes 3–4 times daily for the next few days and to avoid aggressive overhead activities.

Surgery

Traditionally the treatment of an acute initial shoulder dislocation has consisted of a period of immobilization followed by rehabilitation and a gradual return to full activity. However, because of

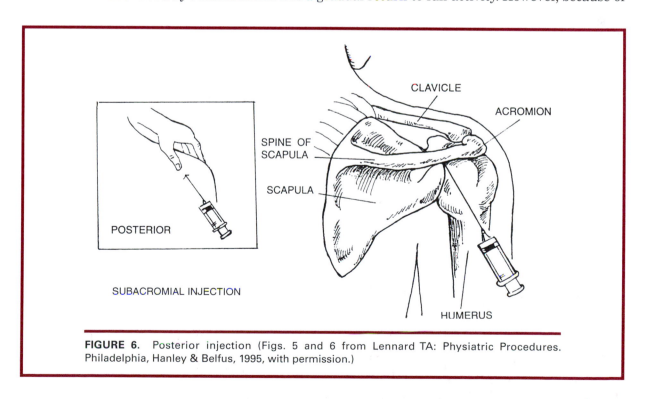

FIGURE 6. Posterior injection (Figs. 5 and 6 from Lennard TA: Physiatric Procedures. Philadelphia, Hanley & Belfus, 1995, with permission.)

high rates of recurrent instability after conservative treatment in the active athletic population, and in particular throwers, early surgical intervention is gaining acceptance.[7,11] Early arthroscopic repair of the inferior labral defect associated with acute shoulder dislocation is becoming widespread because of an apparent reduction in postoperative morbidity, which may allow the athlete an early return to function.

In the individual with recurrent instability, surgical treatment may need to address abnormalities in the shoulder capsule, glenoid labrum, and rotator cuff. Surgical interventions include capsular procedures, such as the capsular shift, and thermal capsulorrhaphy, labral, and rotator cuff procedures, such as debridement or repair.[11–13]

In many instances these procedures need to be combined for optimal results in the patient, followed by an appropriate rehabilitation program with guidelines similar to those for the patient treated non-operatively.

Potential Disease Complications

Complications include recurrent instability with overhead activity, pain of the shoulder region, nerve damage, and weakness of the rotator cuff and scapular muscles. These tend to occur more commonly in patients with multidirectional atraumatic instability. Loss of function may include inability to lift overhead and loss of throwing velocity and accuracy.

Potential Treatment Complications

Complications of treatment include loss of motion, failure of surgical repair with recurrent instability, and inability to return to previous level of function. Analgesics, NSAIDs, and COX-2 inhibitors have well-known side effects that most commonly affect the gastric, hepatic, and renal systems.

References
1. Speer KP: Anatomy and pathomechanics of shoulder instability. Clin Sports Med 1995;14:751–760.
2. Bahr R, Craig E, Engerbretsen L: The clinical presentation of shoulder instability including on-field management. Clin Sports Med 1995;14:761–776.
3. Laurencin CT, O'Brien SJ: Anterior shoulder instability: Anatomy, pathophysiology, and conservative management. In Andrews JR, Zarims B, Wilk K (eds): Injuries in Baseball. Philadelphia, Lippincott-Raven, 1998, pp 189–197.
4. Clarnette RC, Miniaci A: Clinical exam of the shoulder. Med Sci Sports Exerc 1998;30(S):1–6.
5. Meister K: Current concepts. Injuries to the throwing athlete. Part One: Biomechanics/pathophysiology/classification of injury. Am J Sports Med 2000;28:265–275.
6. O'Brien SJ, Pagnani MJ, Fealy S, et al: The active compression test: A new and effective test for diagnosing labral tear and acromioclavicular joint abnormality. Am J Sports Med 1998;26:610–613.
7. Meister K: Current concepts. Injuries to the throwing athlete. Part Two: Evaluation/treatment. Am J Sports Med 2000;28:587–601.
8. Cavallo RJ, Speer KP: Shoulder: Instability and impingement in throwing athletes. Med Sci Sports Exerc 1998;30(S):18–25.
9. Kibler WB, Livingston B, Bruce R: Current concepts in shoulder rehabilitation. Adv Oper Orthop 1995;3:249–300.
10. Ellen M, Smith J: Musculoskeletal rehabilitation and sports medicine: Shoulder and upper extremity injuries. Arch Phys Med Rehabil 1999;80(S):50–58.
11. Nelson BJ, Arciero RA: Arthroscopic management of glenohumeral instability. Am J Sports Med 2000;28:602–614.
12. Ticker JB, Warner JJP: Selective capsular shift technique for anterior and anterior-inferior glenohumeral instability. Clin Sports Med 2000;19:1–17.
13. Burkhart SS, Morgan CD, Kibler WB: Shoulder injuries in overhead athletes: The "dead arm" revisited. Clin Sports Med 2000;19:125–158.

16 | Rotator Cuff Tendinitis

Jay E. Bowen, DO
Gerard A. Malanga, MD

Synonyms

Impingement syndrome
Rotator cuff tendinosis

ICD-9 Code

726.10
Rotator cuff syndrome

Definition

Rotator cuff tendinitis is a common phenomenon affecting both athletes and non-athletes. The muscles that comprise the rotator cuff (RTC)—the supraspinatus, infraspinatus, subscapularis, and teres minor (the SITS muscles)—may become inflamed or impinged by the acromion, coracoacromial ligament, acromioclavicular joint, and the coracoid process. Recent evidence suggests that fibroblastic hyperplasia (tendinosis) may play a role as well. The supraspinatus tendon is the most commonly involved.

Rotator cuff tendinitis may result from a variety of factors including the muscle—usually the tendon or its musculotendinous junction can be "squeezed" along its course from a relatively narrowed space, as a result of degeneration from the aging process, or from underlying subtle instability of the humeral head.

In chronic RTC tendinitis, the muscles of the RTC and surrounding scapulothoracic stabilizers may become weak. These muscles can become weak from disuse or overtraining. Use beyond the endurance of the muscles can fatigue the stabilizing musculature, resulting in altered biomechanics. The humeral head moves excessively off the center of the glenoid, usually superiorly. From this abnormal motion, impingement of the rotator cuff occurs, causing inflammation of the tendon. Over time and/or with aging modifications of the acromion occur, resulting in osteophyte formation or "hooking" of the acromium (Fig. 1). With repeated

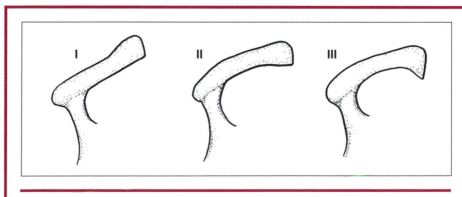

FIGURE 1. Types of acromial morphology (lateral view).

superior migration and acromial changes, degeneration of the musculotendinous junction can lead to tearing of the RTC (see Chapter 17). This is what many refer to as impingement or impingement syndrome.

With prolonged pain, patients can develop adhesive capsulitis from the lack of active motion. (See Chapter 12.)

Symptoms

Patients normally present with pain in the posterolateral shoulder region and, often, deltoid muscle pain, which is referred from the shoulder. The pain is described as dull and achy. Complaints occur with activities above the shoulder level, usually when the arm is abducted greater than 90 degrees. Symptoms are also noted in movements involving eccentric contractions and from sleeping on the affected side. RTC tendinitis is common in persons with overhead activity requirements (e.g., swimmers, painters).

Physical Examination

The shoulder examination should be approached systematically in every patient and should include inspection, palpation, range of motion, muscle strength, and performance of special tests of the shoulder as clinically indicated.

The examination begins with observation of the patient during the history portion of the evaluation. The shoulder should be carefully inspected from the anterior, lateral, and posterior positions. Atrophy of the supraspinatus and infraspinatus muscles can be seen in massive rotator cuff tears, as well as in entrapments of the suprascapular nerve. Scapular winging is rare in rotator cuff injuries; however, abnormalities of scapulothoracic motion are often present and should be addressed as part of the treatment plan.

Tenderness is often localized to the greater tuberosity, subacromial bursa, or long head of the biceps.

Total active and passive range of motion in all planes, and scapulohumeral rhythm should be evaluated. Maximal total elevation occurs in the plane of the scapula, which lies approximately 30 degrees forward of the coronal plane. Patients with rotator cuff tears tend to have altered scapulothoracic motion during active shoulder elevation. Decreased active elevation with normal passive range of motion is usually seen in rotator cuff tears secondary to pain and weakness. When both active and passive range of motion are similarly decreased, this usually suggests the onset of adhesive capsulitis. Glenohumeral internal rotation is assessed most accurately by abducting the shoulder to 90 degrees and manually fixing the scapula. From this point, the elbow is flexed to 90 degrees and the humerus is internally rotated. The impingement syndrome associated with rotator cuff injuries tends to cause pain with elevation between 60 to 120 degrees (painful arc), when the rotator cuff tendons are compressed against the anterior acromion and coracoacromial ligament.

Strength testing should be done to isolate the relevant muscles individually. The anterior cuff (subscapularis) can be assessed using the lift-off test (see page 177), which is performed with the arm internally rotated behind the back. Lifting the hand away from the back against resistance tests the strength of the subscapularis muscle. The posterior cuff (infraspinatus and teres minor) can be tested with the arm at the side and elbow flexed to 90 degrees. Significant weakness in external rotation will be seen in large tears of the rotator cuff. The supraspinatus muscle is specifically tested by abducting the patient's arm to 90 degrees, horizontally adduct to 20 to 30 degrees, and internally rotating the arm to the thumb's-down position. Testing of the scapula rotators, the trapezius and the serratus anterior, is also important. The serratus anterior can be tested by having the patient lean against a wall, winging of the scapula as the patient pushes against the wall indicates weakness.

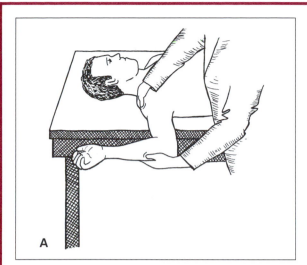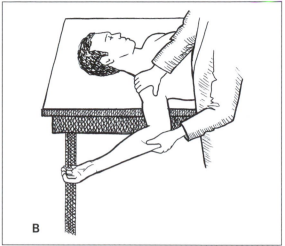

FIGURE 2. Relocation test. *A*, Abduction, maximum external rotation is limited by pain in certain shoulders. *B*, By applying pressure on the anterior shoulder, the discomfort is eliminated and greater external rotation is noted.

Drop-Arm Test

The clinician abducts the patient's shoulder to 90 degrees and then asks the patient to slowly lower the arm to the side in the same arc of movement. A positive test is indicated if the patient is unable to return the arm to the side slowly, or has severe pain when attempting to do so. A positive result indicates a tear of the rotator cuff.

Impingement Sign

The shoulder is forcibly forward flexed with the humerus internally rotated, causing a jamming of the greater tuberosity against the anterior-inferior surface of the acromion. Pain with this maneuver reflects a positive test and indicates an overuse injury to the supraspinatus muscle and possibly to the biceps tendon. (See page 77.)

Apprehension Test

The arm is abducted 90 degrees and then fully externally rotated while an anteriorly directed force is placed on the posterior humeral head from behind. The patient will become apprehensive and resist further motion if chronic anterior instability is present. (See page 78).

Relocation Test

Perform the apprehension test with the patient supine and the shoulder at the edge of the table (Fig. 2). A posteriorly directed force on the proximal humerus will cause resolution of the patient's symptoms of apprehension, which is another indicator of anterior instability (see page 78).

Functional Limitations

Patients with rotator cuff tendinitis complain of pain with overhead activities (e.g., throwing a baseball, painting a ceiling), greatest above 90 degrees of abduction secondary to pain. Pain may also occur with internal and external rotation and may affect daily self-care activities. Women typically have difficulty hooking their bras in back. Work activities such as filing, hammering overhead, and lifting can be affected. The patient can be awoken by pain in the shoulder, which impairs their sleep.

Diagnostic Studies

In the event of trauma to the shoulder and complaints consistent with rotator cuff tendinitis, the clinician should obtain x-rays to avoid missing an occult fracture. AP view with internal and external rotation is sufficient for screening. If dislocation is suspected, further views should be obtained, including West Point axillary, true AP, and Y views.

MRIs are the study of choice when a patient is not progressing with conservative management or to rule out alternative pathology (e.g., rotator cuff tear). In tendinitis, the films will demonstrate an increased signal within the substance of the tendon. Diagnostic arthroscopy is utilized in some cases but is generally not necessary.

Electrodiagnostic studies can be ordered to exclude alternative diagnoses as well (e.g., cervical radiculopathy).

Subacromial anesthetic injections (see page 81) have been discussed as diagnostic tools to assist in confirming the diagnosis of rotator cuff tendinitis. This procedure is not as important for diagnosing tendinitis but rather for helping to rule out a tear. If the patient cannot provide good effort to abduction during the physical examination, the clinician can inject the anesthetic into the subacromial space. After the injection, if there is significant reduction in the pain level and the patient can provide adequate and near maximal abduction, the diagnosis of tendinitis is more likely than a rotator cuff tear.

Differential Diagnosis

Rotator cuff tear

Glenolabral tear

Muscular strain

Subacromial bursitis

Bicipital tendinitis

Myofascial pain

Fracture

Acromioclavicular sprain

Tumor

Myofascial/vascular thoracic outlet syndrome

Cervical radiculopathy

Traumatic or atraumatic brachial plexus pathology (e.g., Parsonage–Turner [acute brachial neuritis])

Suprascapular neuropathy

Thoracic outlet syndrome

Treatment

There are five basic phases of treatment (Table 1).

TABLE 1. Treatment Phases for Rotator Cuff Tendinitis

I. Pain control and reduction of inflammation.

II. Restoration of normal shoulder motion; both scapulothoracic and glenohumeral.

III. Normalization of strength and dynamic muscle control.

IV. Proprioception and dynamic joint stabilization.

V. Sport- or task-specific training.

Initial

Initially, pain control and inflammation reduction are required to allow progression of healing and the initiation of an active rehabilitation program. This can be accomplished with a combination of relative rest from aggravating activities, icing (20 minutes 3 to 4 times a day), and electrical stimulation. Acetaminophen may help with pain control. NSAIDs/COX-2 inhibitors may be used to help control pain and inflammation.

Having the patient sleep with a pillow between the trunk and arm will decrease the tension on the supraspinatus tendon and prevent compromise of blood flow in its watershed region.

Rehabilitation

Restoration of Shoulder Range of Motion

Physical therapy may also help with pain management. Initially, ultrasound to the posterior capsule followed by gentle, passive, prolonged stretch may be needed. The use of ultrasound should be closely monitored to avoid heating an inflamed tendon, which will worsen the situation.

After the pain has been managed, restoration of shoulder motion can be initiated. The use of Codman's pendulum exercises, wall walking, stick or towel exercises, and/or a physical therapy program are useful in attaining full pain-free range. It is important to address any posterior capsular tightness because it can result in anterior and superior humeral head migration, resulting in impingement. A tight posterior capsule and the imbalance it causes force the humeral head anterior, producing shearing of the anterior labrum and causing additional injury. Stretching of the posterior capsule is a difficult task to isolate. The horizontal adduction that is usually performed tends to stretch the scapular stabilizers, not the posterior capsule. However, stretching of the posterior capsule is possible if care is taken to fix and stabilize the scapula, preventing stretching of the scapulothoracic stabilizers. The focus of treatment in this early stage should be on improving range, flexibility of the posterior capsular, and postural biomechanics and restoring normal scapular motion.

Postural biomechanics are important because with poor posture (e.g. excessive thoracic kyphosis and protracted shoulders), there is increased outlet narrowing, resulting in greater risk for rotator cuff impingement. Restoring normal scapular motion is also essential because the scapula is the platform upon which the glenohumeral joint rotates.[1,2] Thus, an unstable scapula can secondarily cause glenohumeral joint instability and resultant impingement. Scapular stabilization includes exercises such as wall push-ups and biofeedback (visual and tactile).

Strengthening

The third phase of treatment is strengthening, which should be performed in a pain-free range. Strengthening should begin with the scapulothoracic stabilizers and the use of shoulder shrugs, rowing, and push-ups, which will isolate these muscles and help return smooth motion, allowing normal rhythm between the scapula and the glenohumeral joint. This will also provide a firm base of support upon which the arm can move. Attention should then be turned toward strengthening the rotator cuff muscles. Positioning of the arm at 45 and 90 degrees of abduction for exercises prevents the "wringing out" phenomenon that hyperadduction can cause by stressing the tenuous blood supply to the tendon of the exercising muscle. The "thumbs-down" position with the arm in greater than 90 degrees of abduction and internal rotation should also be avoided to minimize subacromial impingement. After the scapular stabilizers and rotator cuff muscles are rehabilitated, the prime movers should be addressed to prevent further injury and facilitate return to prior function.

There are many ways to strengthen muscles. The rehabilitation program should start with static and co-contractions, progress to concentric exercises, and be completed with eccentric exercises and endurance training. There are many techniques to strengthen muscles, including static and dynamic exercises. A therapy prescription should include the number of repetitions, number of sets, and the intensity at which the specific exercise should be performed. When strength is restored, a maintenance program should be continued for fitness and prevention of re-injury.

Proprioception

The fourth phase is proprioceptive training. This is important to retrain the neurologic control of the strengthened muscles, providing improved dynamic interaction and coupled execution of tasks for harmonious movement of the shoulder and arm. Tasks should begin with closed kinetic chain exercises to provide joint stabilizing forces. As the muscles are re-educated, exercises can progress to open chain activities, which may be used in specific sports or tasks. In addition, proprioceptive neuromuscular facilitation (commonly called PNF) is designed to stimulate muscle/tendon stretch receptors for re-education.

Task- or Sport-Specific

The last phase of rehabilitation is to return to task- or sport-specific activities. This is an advanced form of training for the muscles to relearn prior activities. This is important and should be supervised so the task is performed correctly, and to eliminate the possibility of re-injury or injury in another part of the kinetic chain from improper technique. The rehabilitation begins at a cognitive level but must be repeated so that it transitions to unconscious motor programming.

The aforementioned phases may overlap and can be progressed as rapidly as tolerated, but each should be performed to speed recovery and prevent re-injury.

Procedures

A subacromial injection of anesthetic (impingement test) can be beneficial in diagnosing a rotator cuff tear from tendinitis. Patients with pain that limits the validity of their strength testing may be able to provide almost full resistance to abduction and external rotation after the injection, suggesting rotator cuff tendinitis. On the other hand, if there is continued weakness, one must consider a rotator cuff tear.

Many clinicians include a corticosteroid with the anesthetic to avoid the need for a second injection. This procedure can be both diagnostic and therapeutic. If one makes the diagnosis of rotator cuff tendinitis, the corticosteroid injection will decrease the inflammation and allow accelerated rehabilitation.

Refer to the injection procedure on page 81.

Surgery

Surgery should be considered if the patient fails to improve with a progressive non-operative therapy program of 3 to 6 months. Surgical procedures may include subacromial decompression arthroscopically or, less commonly, open. At that time, the surgeon may debride the tendon and explore for other pathology.

Potential Disease Complications

The greatest risks for not treating rotator cuff tendinitis is rupture or tear of a tendon or the development of a labral tear. As previously discussed, with prolonged impairment in motion and strength and subtle instability, hooking of the acromion can develop. Adhesive capsulitis may develop with chronic pain and decreased shoulder movement as well.

Potential Treatment Complications

There are minimal possible complications from non-operative treatment of rotator cuff tendinitis. Since NSAIDs are used frequently, one must remain vigilant to their potential side effects (e.g., gastritis, ulcers, renal impairment, bronchospasm). COX-2 inhibitors may have fewer gastric side effects. Injections may cause rupture of the diseased tendon.

References
1. Gross J, Fetto J, Rosen E: Musculoskeletal Examination. Massachusetts, Blackwell Science, 1996.
2. Smith L, Weiss E, Lehmkuh L: Brunnstrom's Clinical Kinesiology, 5th ed. Philadelphia, F.A. Davis, 1996.
3. Cailliet R: Shoulder Pain, 3rd ed. Philadelphia, F.A. Davis, 1991, pp 42–46.
4. Malanga GA, Bowen JE, Nadler SF, Lee A: Non-operative management of shoulder injuries. J Back Musculolskeletal Rehab 1999;12(12):179–189.
5. Hawkins RJ: Basic science and clinical application in the athlete's shoulder. Clin Sports Med 1991;10(4):693–971.
6. Poppen NK, Walker PS: Normal and abnormal motion of the shoulder. J Bone Joint Surg 1976;58A:195–201.

7. Kibler WB: Role of the scapula in the overhead throwing motion. Contemporary Orthop 1991;22(5): 525–532.
8. DeLateur BI: Exercise for strength and endurance. In Basmajian JV (ed): Theraputic Exercise, 4th ed. Baltimore, Williams & Wilkins, 1984.
9. Steindler A: Kinesiology of Human Body under Normal and Pathological Conditions. Springfield, IL, Carles C. Thomas, 1995.
10. Howell SM, Galinat BJ: The glenoid-labral socket—a constrained articular surface. Clin Orthop 1989;243:122–125.
11. Steinbeck J, Liljenqvist U, Jerosch J: The anatomy of the glenohumeral ligamentous complex and its contribution to anterior shoulder stability. J Should Elbow Surg 1998;7:122–126.
12. Inman VT, Saunders JBCM, Abbott LC: Observations of the function of the shoulder. J Bone J Surg 1944;26:1–30.
13. Saha AK: Dynamic stability of the glenohumeral joint. Acta Orthop Scand 1971;42:491.
14. Wuelker N, Korell M, Thren K: Dynamic glenohumeral joint stability. J Should Elbow Surg 1998;7:43–52.
15. Ozaki J, Fujimoto S, et al: Tears of the rotator cuff of the shoulder associated with pathologic changes in the acromium: A study in cadavers. J Bone Joint Surg 1988;(70B):1224–1230.
16. Codman EA: The Shoulder: Rupture of The Supraspinatus Tendon and Other Lesions in or About the Subacromial Bursa. Boston, Thomas Todd, 1934.
17. Rathburn JB, Macnab I: The microvascular pattern of the rotator cuff of the shoulder. J Bone Joint Surg 1970;52B:540.
18. Lohr JF, Uhthoff HK: The microvascular pattern of the supraspinatus tendon. Clin Orthop 1990;254:35–38.
19. Swiontkowski M, Iannotti JP, Esterhai JL, et al: Intraoperative assessment of rotator cuff vascularity using laser Doppler flowmetry. Presented at 56th Annual Meeting of AAOS, Las Vegas, Feb 10, 1989
20. Biglianni LU, Morrison D, April EW: The morphology of the acromium and its relationship to rotator cuff tears. Orthop Trans 1986;10:228.
21. Neer CS: Anterior acromioplasty for the chronic impingement syndrome in the shoulder. A preliminary report. J Bone Joint Surg 1972;54A(1):41–50.
22. Flatlow E, Soslowshy L, Ticker J, et al: Excursion of the rotator cuff under the acromium: patterns of subacromial contact. Am J Sports Med 1994;22:779–787.
23. Brems JJ: Management of atraumatic instability techniques and results. Instructional Course lecture 179. AAOS Annual Meeting, Atlanta, Feb 26, 1996.
24. Yoneda B, Welsh R: Conservative treatment of shoulder dislocation in young males. J Bone Joint Surg 1982;64B(2):254–255.
25. Burkhead WZ Jr, Rockwood CA Jr: Treatment of instability of the shoulder with an exercise program. J Bone Joint Surg (Am) 1992;74(6):890–896.
26. Rockwood CA, Matsen FA: The Shoulder. Philadelphia, W.B. Saunders, 1990.
27. Nicholas JA, Hershman EB: The Upper Extremity in Sports Medicine. St Louis, Mosby, 1990.
28. Reid DC: Sports Injury Assessment and Rehabilitation. New York, Churchill Livingstone, 1992.
29. Simonet WT, Cofield RH: Prognosis in anterior shoulder dislocation. Am J Sports Med 1984;12:19–24.
30. Plancher KD, Litchfield R, Hawkins RJ: Rehabilitation of the shoulder in tennis players. Clin Sports Med 1995;14(1):116–118.
31. Dines DM, Levinson M: The conservative management of the unstable shoulder including rehabilitation. Clin Sports Med 1995;14(4):799–813.
32. Harryman DT, Sidles JA, Clark JM, et al: Translation of the humeral head on the glenoid with passive glenohumeral motion. J Bone Joint Surg 1990;72A:1334–1343.
33. Kibler WB, Chandler TJ: Functional scapular instability in throwing athletes. AAOS Society for Sports Medicine's 15th Annual Meeting, Traverse City, June 19–22, 1989.
34. Borsa PA, Lephart SM, Kocher MS, Lephart SP: Functional assessment and rehabilitation of shoulder proprioception for the glenohumeral instability. J Sports Rehab 1994;3(1):84–104.
35. Janda DH, Loubert P: A preventive program focusing on the glenohumeral joint. Clin Sports Med 1991;10:955–971.
36. Kabat H: Proprioception facilitation in theraputic exercise. In Kendall HD (ed): Theraputic Exercises. Baltimore, Waverly Press, 1965, pp 327–343.
37. Malanga GA, Jenp Y, Growney E, An K: EMG analysis of shoulder positioning in testing and strengthening the supraspinatus. Med Sci Sports Exerc 1996;28(6):661–664, 1996.
38. Jenp Y, Malanga GA, Growney E, An K: Activation of the rotator cuff in generating isometric shoulder rotation torque. Am J Sports Med 1996;24(4):477–485.
39. Wang JC, Shapiro MS: Changes in acromial morphology with age. J Should Elbow Surg 1997;6:55–59.
40. Cordasco FA, Wolfe IN, et al: An electromyographic analysis of the shoulder during a medicine ball rehabilitation program. Am J Sports Med 1996;24(3):386–392, 1996.
42. Blasier RB, Carpenter JE, Huston LJ: Shoulder proprioception: Effect of joint laxity, joint position, and direction of motion. Orthop Review 1994;23(1):45–50.
43. Basmajian J: Muscles Alive: Their functions Revealed by Electromyography, 5th ed. Philadelphia, Williams & Wilkins, 1985.

17 Rotator Cuff Tear

Gerard A. Malanga, MD
Jay E. Bowen, DO

Synonyms

Shoulder tear

Torn shoulder

ICD-9 Codes

726.10
Rotator cuff syndrome

727.61
Nontraumatic complete rupture of rotator cuff

840.4
Rotator cuff sprain

Definition

Three types of tears can occur to the rotator cuff (RTC). A full-thickness tear can be massive and cause immediate functional impairments. Another type of tear, a partial-thickness tear, can be broken down into a tear on the superior surface into the subacromial space or inferior surface on the articular side. These tears can be either traumatic or degenerative.[1-7] (See Figs. 1 to 3.)

Traumatic tears occur in the younger population of athletes and laborers, whereas degenerative tears occur in older individuals. Because there are more male heavy laborers, RTC tears are more common in men. The incidence of degenerative tears is increased for both sexes older than 35 years.[4,6,8]

Symptoms

Symptoms are similar to RTC tendinitis. Pain is referred to the lateral triceps and sometimes more globally in the shoulder. Often, there is co-existing inflammation and the pain quality is dull and achy. Weakness occurs because of the pain, which is caused by the impaired motion or from the tear itself. Persons have difficulty with overhead activities.

Physical Examination

Examination is essentially the same as for RTC tendinitis. The arm drop test may demonstrate greater weakness than expected from an inflamed, intact tendon, although one can be easily fooled. As with RTC tendinitis, an anesthetic injection into the subacromial space may help discern tear. Even though the pain may be improved or resolved from the injection, resisted abduction will be just as weak since the torn tendon cannot withstand the stress.[9]

Remember to examine the cervical spine to avoid missing underlying pathology. Some individuals develop a RTC tear as a result of a radiculopathy or other nerve impairment. The dysfunction of the shoulder from a radiculopathy or suprascapular neuropathy results in weakness of the rotator cuff and/or the scapular stabilizers. This dysrhythmia causes impingement of the tendons with other structures and eventually leads to fraying and tearing.[10-12]

Functional Limitations

The greatest limitation that patients complain of is performing overhead activities.[2,7,13–15]

Diagnostic Studies

The diagnosis of a RTC tear depends mostly on the history and physical examination. However, imaging studies may be used to confirm the clinician's diagnosis and to eliminate other possible pathologies.

MRI of the shoulder is the "gold standard." Computerized tomography (CT) scans show osseous structures better but are less effective at demonstrating a soft tissue injury.

Roentgenograms are often obtained to rule out any osseous problem. A suggestion of a tear can be inferred if there is evidence of humeral head upward migration or sclerotic changes at the greater tuberosity where the tendons insert.

Similar to the evaluation of a person with RTC tendinitis, an anesthetic injection can be performed to differentiate a tear from tendinitis.

Shoulder arthrograms are performed less often since the advent of MRI. An arthrogram includes injection of contrast material into the glenohumeral joint followed by plain film x-rays. Dye should remain

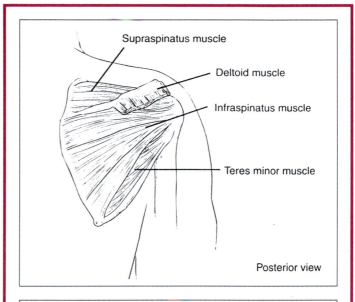

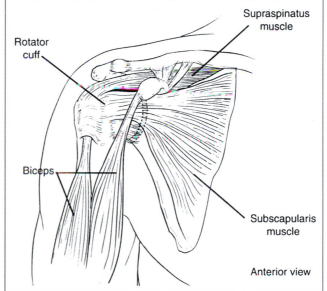

FIGURE 1. Muscles of the rotator cuff, posterior view (*top*), anterior view (*bottom*). (From Snider RKI: Essentials of Musculoskeletal Care. Rosemont, II, American Academy of Orthopaedic Surgeons, 1997, with permission.)

contained in the joint space. If it extravasates, this signifies a tear. Partial-thickness RTC tears can be missed, especially tears on the superior surface. Some centers have been combining gadolinium dye injections followed by an MRI. This is used mostly to identify a labral tear, not a RTC tear.

Ultrasound imaging can also be used in the diagnosis of full-thickness rotator cuff tears. Ultrasound is less commonly used than MRI in the United States; however, it can be a very helpful study when performed in centers with clinicians who have experience in musculoskeletal ultrasound imaging. It is generally believed that ultrasound is less sensitive than MRI in the diagnosis of partial-thickness rotator cuff tears.[4,6,8,9,12,13,16,17]

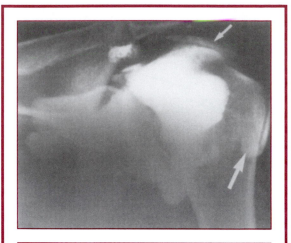

FIGURE 2. Rotator cuff tear with contrast extending into the subacromial (*short arrow*) and subdeltoid (*long arrow*) bursae. (From West SG (ed): Rheumatology Secrets. Philadelphia, Hanley & Belfus, 1997, p 373, with permission.)

Diagnostic arthroscopy is done in some instances but is not generally necessary.

Differential Diagnosis

Non-neurologic
    Rotator cuff tendinitis
    Glenolabral tear
    Acromioclavicular sprain
    Occult fracture
    Osteoarthritis
    Rheumatoid arthritis
    Adhesive capsulitis
    Myofascial pain syndrome
    Myofascial thoracic outlet syndrome
Neurologic
    Cervical radiculopathy
    Brachial plexopathy
    Suprascapular neuropathy
    Neurogenic (true) thoracic outlet syndrome

Treatment

Initial

Initial treatment of a RTC tear is similar to that for RTC tendinitis as previously discussed (see Chapter 16); however, if the symptoms do not respond to a rehabilitation program, the clinician should consider surgical consultation earlier in the course of injury.

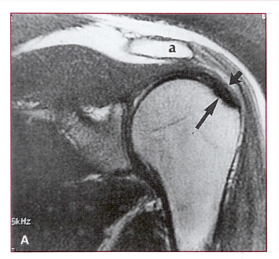
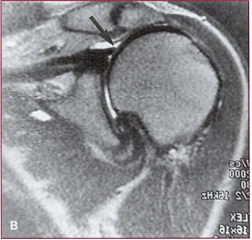

FIGURE 3. **A**, Normal shoulder MRI. The supraspinatus tendon is uniformly low signal and continuous (*arrows*). The space between the humeral head and the acromion (*a*) is maintained. **B**, Chronic rotator cuff tear. The supraspinatus tendon is completely torn and retracted to the level of the glenohumeral joint (*arrow*), where it is surrounded by fluid. Note the high-riding humeral head, in close proximity to the acromion. This is due to the atrophy of the cuff muscles associated with chronic tendon tears.

The basic phases of rehabilitation include the following[12]
1. Pain control and reduction of inflammation
2. Restoration of normal shoulder motion—both scapulothoracic and glenohumeral
3. Normalization of strength and dynamic joint stabilization
4. Proprioception and dynamic joint stabilization
5. Sport-specific training

Initially, pain control and inflammation reduction are required to allow progression of healing and the initiation of an active rehabilitation program. These can be accomplished with a combination of relative rest, icing (20 minutes 3 to 4 times a day), electrical stimulation, and acetaminophen or a nonsteroidal anti-inflammatory drug. The following program's progression can be added as tolerated by the patient. Having the patient sleep with a pillow between his or her trunk and arm will decrease the tension on the supraspinatus tendon and prevent compromise of blood flow in its watershed region.

Rehabilitation

Due to the interrelationship of instability and impingement previously discussed, there is a great deal of overlap in the rehabilitation of these shoulder problems. Treatment must be individualized and based on the restoration of optimal *function* and not merely based on surgical correction of anatomic changes. Supervised physical therapy is the mainstay of treatment and is successful in the vast majority of patients.

Restoration of Shoulder Range of Motion

As with all musculoskeletal disorders, the entire body must be taken into consideration. Abnormalities in the kinetic chain can also affect the shoulder. If there are restrictions or limitations in range of motion or strength, the forces will be transmitted to other portions of the kinetic chain, resulting in an overload of those tissues and possibly injury.

After the pain has been managed, restoration of motion can be initiated. The use of Codman's pendulum exercises, wall walking, stick or towel exercises, and/or a physical therapy program is beneficial in attaining full pain-free range. It is important to address any posterior capsular tightness because this can cause anterior and superior humeral head migration, resulting in impingement. A tight posterior capsule and the imbalance it causes forces the humeral head anteriorly, producing shearing of the anterior labrum and causing an additional injury. Stretching of the posterior capsule is a difficult task. The horizontal adduction that is usually performed tends to stretch the scapular stabilizers rather than the posterior capsule. If care is taken to fix and stabilize the scapula and therefore prevent the stretching of the scapulothoracic stabilizers, stretching of the posterior capsule can be achieved. The focus of treatment in this early stage should be on improving range and flexibility of the posterior capsular, improving postural biomechanics, and restoring normal scapular motion.

Initially, ultrasound to the posterior capsule followed by gentle, passive prolonged stretch may be needed. The use of ultrasound should be closely monitored to prevent heating an inflamed tendon, which will worsen the injury.

Postural biomechanics are important because with poor posture (e.g., excessive thoracic kyphosis and protracted shoulders), there is increased outlet narrowing, resulting in greater risk for rotator cuff impingement. Restoring normal scapular motion is also essential because the scapula is the platform upon which the glenohumeral joint rotates.[18,19] Thus, an unstable scapula can secondarily cause glenohumeral joint instability and resultant impingement. Scapular stabilization includes exercises such as wall push-ups and biofeedback (visual and tactile).

Strengthening

The third phase of treatment is strengthening and should be performed in a pain-free range. Strengthening should begin with the scapulothoracic stabilizers and the use of shoulder shrugs, rowing, and push-ups, which will isolate these muscles and help return smooth motion, allowing normal rhythm between the scapula and the glenohumeral joint. This will also provide a firm base of support on which the arm can move. Attention should then be turned toward strengthening of the rotator cuff muscles. Positioning of the arm at 45 and 90 degrees of abduction for exercises prevents the "wringing out" phenomenon that hyperadduction can cause by stressing the tenuous blood supply to the tendon of the exercising muscle. The "thumbs-down" position with the arm in greater than 90 degrees of abduction and internal rotation should also be avoided to minimize subacromial impingement. After the scapular stabilizers and rotator cuff muscles are rehabilitated, the prime movers should be addressed to prevent further injury and facilitate return to prior function.

There are many ways to strengthen muscles. The rehabilitation program should start with static and co-contractions, progress to concentric exercises, and be completed with eccentric exercises and endurance training. The Body Blade can be used for co-contraction in multiple planes and positions for rhythmic stabilization. There are many techniques to strengthen muscles, including static and dynamic exercises. A therapy prescription should include the number of repetitions, number of sets of repetitions, and the intensity at which the specific exercise should be performed. When strength is restored, a maintenance program should be continued for fitness and prevention of re-injury.

Proprioception

The fourth phase is proprioceptive training. This is important to retrain the neurologic control of the strengthened muscles in providing improved dynamic interaction and coupled execution of tasks for harmonious movement of the shoulder and arm. Tasks should begin with closed kinetic chain exercises to provide joint stabilizing forces. As the muscles are re-educated, exercises can progress to open chain activities that may be used in specific sports or tasks. Exercises such as those using the Body Blade or pliometrics will also address proprioception. In addition, proprioceptive neuromuscular facilitation (PNF) is designed to stimulate muscle/tendon stretch receptors for re-education. Kabat has described shoulder PNF techniques in detail.[20]

Task- or Sport-Specific

The last phase of rehabilitation is to return to task- or sport-specific activities. This is an advanced form of training for the muscles to relearn prior activities. This is important and should be supervised so that the task performed is correct and to eliminate the possibility of re-injury or injury in another part of the kinetic chain from improper technique. The rehabilitation begins at a cognitive level but must be practiced so that it ultimately becomes part of unconscious motor programming.

The previously described phases may overlap and can be progressed as rapidly as tolerated, but all should be performed to speed recovery and prevent re-injury.

Procedures

Subacromial injections of anesthetic and corticosteroid may be both diagnostic and therapeutic (see page 81).

Surgery

If the patient's condition has not progressed with a conservative rehabilitation after 2 to 3 months, a surgical consultation should be considered. If the patient is unable to perform all the activities he or she demands (vocationally and avocationally) after 6 months of treatment and independent exercise performance, a surgical consultation should be obtained. If the patient is a high level athlete or worker, earlier consultation may be appropriate. The younger patient population is more amenable to surgical intervention.[6,8]

If surgery is contemplated, repair, debridement, decompression, or a combination of these may be considered. A concomitant injury should be considered, such as a labral tear. The detail of these surgical procedures is beyond the scope of this text.

Potential Disease Complications

Partial rotator cuff tears can progress to full-thickness tears, especially if untreated. Rehabilitation attempts to restore biomechanics as close to normal to prevent excessive wear on the tendon, which can cause further degeneration. Chronic untreated rotator cuff tears can lead to shoulder arthropathy.[6,11]

Potential Treatment Complications

Analgesics, NSAIDs, and COX-2 inhibitors have well-known side effects that most commonly affect the gastric, hepatic, and renal systems. There are minimal disadvantages to coordinating a rehabilitation program that may improve the patient's symptoms to a level at which the patient is satisfied and functional. However, an overly aggressive program can progress a partial tear to a complete tear. As for surgery, in general, the potential problems include bleeding, infection, worsening of the complaints, and nerve injury.

References
1. Biglianni LU, Morrison D, April EW: The morphology of the acromium and its relationship to rotator cuff tears. Orthop Trans 1986;10:228.
2. Codman EA: The Shoulder: Rupture of the Supraspinatus Tendon and Other Lesions in or About the Subacromial Bursa. Boston, Thomas Todd, 1934.
3. Flatlow E, Soslowshy L, Ticker J, et al: Excursion of the rotator cuff under the acromium: Patterns of subacromial contact. Am J Sports Med 1994;22:779–787.
4. Hawkins RJ: Basic science and clinical application in the athlete's shoulder. Clin Sports Med 1991;10(4):693–971.
5. Neer CS: Anterior acromioplasty for the chronic impingement syndrome in the shoulder. A preliminary report. J Bone Joint Surg 1972;54A(1):41–50.
6. Rockwood CA, Matsen FA: The Shoulder. Philadelphia, W.B. Saunders, 1990.
7. Ozaki J, Fujimoto S, et al: Tears of the rotator cuff of the shoulder associated with pathologic changes in the acromium: A study in cadavers. J Bone Joint Surg 1988;70(8):1224–1230.
8. Reid DC: Sports Injury Assessment and Rehabilitation. New York, Churchill Livingstone, 1992.
9. Gross J, Fetto J, Rosen E: Musculoskeletal Examination. Blackwell Science, 1996.
10. Basmajian J: Muscles Alive: Their Functions Revealed by Electromyography, 5th ed. Philadelphia, Williams & Wilkins, 1985.
11. Kibler WB: Role of the scapula in the overhead throwing motion. Contemp Orthop 1991;22(5):525–532.
12. Malanga GA, Bowen JE, Nadler SF, Lee A: Non-operative management of shoulder injuries. J Back Musculoskeletal Rehab 1999;12(12):179–189.
13. Dines DM, Levinson M: The conservative management of the unstable shoulder including rehabilitation. Clin Sports Med 1995;14(4):799–813.
14. Harryman DT, Sidles JA, Clark JM, et al: Translation of the humeral head on the glenoid with passive glenohumeral motion. J Bone Joint Surg 1990;72A:1334–1343.
15. Steinbeck J, Liljenqvist U, Jerosch J: The anatomy of the glenohumeral ligamentous complex and its contribution to anterior shoulder stability. J Shoulder Elbow Surg 1998;7:122–126.
16. Cailliet R: Shoulder Pain, 3rd ed. Philadelphia, F.A. Davis, 1991, pp 42–46.
17. Nicholas JA, Hershman EB: The Upper Extremity in Sports Medicine. St Louis, Mosby, 1990.
18. Kibler WB, Chandler TJ: Functional scapular instability in throwing athletes. AAOS Society for Sports Medicine's 15th Annual Meeting, Traverse City, MI, June 19–22, 1989.
19. Nuber GW, Jobe FW, Perry J, et al: Fine wire electromyography analysis of the shoulder during swimming. AJSM 1985;13(4):216–222.
20. Kabat H: Proprioception facilitation in therapeutic exercise. In Kendall HD (ed): Therapeutic Exercises. Baltimore, Waverly Press, 1965, pp 327–343.

18 Scapular Winging

Tamara D. Lauder, MD

Synonyms

Rug sac palsy

Long thoracic nerve palsy

Scapulothoracic winging

ICD-9 Codes

352.4
Disorders of accessory (11th) nerve

353.5
Neuralgic amyotrophy (Parsonage-Aldren-Turner syndrome)

354.9
Mononeuritis of upper limb, unspecified

Definition

Scapular winging is a condition in which the scapula (usually the medial and inferior borders) is displaced away from the body. Winging of the scapula may be present at rest but is usually accentuated with movement of the shoulder. Scapular winging can occur from neuromuscular, musculoskeletal, or structural causes (Table 1).

Symptoms

Patients typically report pain in the shoulder, scapula, or cervical region(s). Range of motion of the shoulder is usually difficult and painful, and the patient may experience clicking and popping with use of the shoulder. The specific symptoms that a patient manifests often depend on the cause of the scapular winging. Patients with scapular winging may have symptoms suggestive of other clinical conditions and, therefore, it is essential that an examination of the scapula always be performed for any shoulder, neck, or upper extremity symptoms to avoid misdiagnosis.

Patients with scapular winging due to a *spinal accessory nerve* lesion may complain of drooping of the affected shoulder and pain in the shoulder, upper trapezius, and posterolateral cervical regions, exacerbated with shoulder abduction. Abduction of the shoulder of more than 70 to 90 degrees is usually difficult.[1]

Patients who have lesions of the *long thoracic nerve* present predominantly with shoulder and scapular pain, although patients may experience pain radiating into the upper arm and lateral cervical region, as well. Forward flexion of the arm is difficult and painful. Patients may report that they have been told by others that their "shoulder blade sticks out" or may complain of their shoulder blade hooking over the back or side of a chair when seated.[1]

Other causes of scapular winging may give a constellation of the symptoms previously described. Patients also often complain of weakness in the upper extremity, muscle fatigue with use of the shoulder, and morning stiffness in the shoulder region.[1,2]

Several critical historic components are necessary for an accurate diagnosis. The timing and severity are especially important, because patients with *Parsonage-Turner syndrome* (amyotrophic brachial neuralgia) usually have sudden severe pain followed several days later by upper extremity weakness. This entity commonly involves the *long thoracic nerve*, and patients may present with scapular winging and shoulder symptoms. A history of recent trauma, illness, immunizations, or surgeries (especially to the neck, shoulder, axilla, or thorax), or carrying heavy loads across the shoulder(s) should also be elicited.

Physical Examination

Although scapular winging may not be due to primary shoulder pathology, the synergistic role of the scapula in regard to proper functioning and motion of the shoulder makes it difficult for patients to distinguish between pain originating from the shoulder and the scapula. A careful clinical examination of all components of the musculoskeletal system contributing to the biomechanics of the upper limb is essential in patients with upper limb and shoulder symptoms. Knowledge of the anatomy of the muscles attaching to the scapula allows the clinician to better understand the examination abnormalities.

Anatomy

Although several muscles contribute to proper glenohumeral and scapulothoracic biomechanics, there are a few key muscles that work to prevent movement of the scapula away from the chest wall with upper limb movement.[3] The muscular attachments of the serratus anterior muscle allow it to rotate the scapula forward and the glenoid upward during forward flexion of the shoulder. It also holds the medial (vertebral) border of the scapula against the chest wall. The serratus anterior is innervated by the long thoracic nerve (C5, C6, C7), of which C7 may make a major contribution, especially to the lower most powerful muscles fibers.[4,5]

TABLE 1.   Causes of Scapular Winging*

Primary
  Neurogenic
    Serratus anterior involvement
      Long thoracic nerve
      C6–C7 nerve root lesion[5]
    Trapezius involvement
      Spinal accessory nerve lesion
    Rhomboid involvement
      C5 nerve root
      Dorsal scapular nerve
    Brachial plexus lesion (e.g., Parsonage-Turner syndrome, stretch injury, local compression)
  Structural
    Bony
      Osteochondroma (e.g., scapular, rib)
      Scapular fracture nonunions
      General static skeletal deformity (e.g., scoliosis, cleidocranial dysostosis)[10]
    Muscular
      Direct muscle injury—serratus anterior, trapezius, rhomboid (e.g., trauma, surgical)
      Congenital absence of periscapular muscles (e.g., serratus anterior, trapezius, rhomboid major)
      Muscular dystrophies (e.g., fascioscapulohumeral dystrophy)
    Bursal
      Scapulothoracic bursae
      Exostosis bursata[11]

Secondary
  Contractural winging
    Unbalanced muscle contractures (e.g., brachial plexus injuries)
    Fibrosis of deltoid muscle (e.g., injections)
  Primary glenohumeral or subacromial pathology
    Rotator cuff pathology (subacromial impingement, rotator cuff tear)
    Shoulder instability
    Acromioclavicular joint disorders
    Nonunion or malunion of acromion or clavicular fractures
    Glenoid fracture
    Avascular necrosis of the humeral head
    Acromegalic arthropathy of the shoulder
    Voluntary posterior shoulder subluxation

Voluntary Scapular Winging

* Modified from Kuhn, 1997.

The trapezius is composed of three groups of fibers known as the upper, middle, and lower trapezius. Together, they rotate the glenoid upward and depress the superior border of the scapula with shoulder abduction. They also retract (pull back) the shoulders. The trapezius is innervated by the spinal portion of the *spinal accessory nerve* (cranial nerve XI) and receives some fibers from the cervical plexus (C2, C3, C4).

The rhomboids (rhomboid major and minor) rotate the scapula, turning the glenoid downward. They prevent winging of the inferior angle of the scapula when the upper extremity is pushing forward against resistance by holding the lower angle of the scapula close to the ribs. The rhomboids are innervated by the *dorsal scapular nerve* (C5).

The levator scapulae has a small attachment on the vertebral border of the scapula. It assists the rhomboids and latissimus dorsi in rotating the glenoid fossa downward and elevating the scapula when a person shrugs the shoulder. The levator scapulae is innervated by the *cervical plexus* (C3, C4) and occasionally by fibers of the dorsal scapular nerve (C5).

Examination

When examining a patient for evidence of scapular winging, the patient must be inspected both at rest and with range-of-motion activities of the shoulders. The patient should remove enough clothing to provide the clinician an unobstructed assessment of the scapula.

At Rest

Inspect the patient's thorax and shoulders both anteriorly and posteriorly, looking for any evidence of muscle atrophy, asymmetry, or scapular winging. Also observe the patient's overall posture. Patients with neurogenic or primary muscular causes of scapular winging may have atrophy of the trapezius or rhomboid or a deeper suprascapular fossa than on the unaffected side.[2] With a *spinal accessory nerve* injury, the superomedial border of the scapula is displaced upward. With a *long thoracic nerve* lesion, the scapula may look normal or the inferior angle may be rotated toward the midline with mild winging away from the thorax.[1,2] Muscle spasm may be seen or palpated in various muscles secondary to unopposed contractions of the unaffected muscles.[6]

The clinician should then observe the patient from behind while the patient performs several range-of-motion activities.

During Active Shoulder Forward Flexion (Fig. 1)

Winging and medial displacement of the medial border of the scapula when the arm is forward flexed is more pronounced with dysfunction of the serratus anterior muscle or its innervation (*long thoracic nerve*). Having the patient resist while the arm is in the outstretched, forward flexed position both at shoulder and waist levels (e.g., wall push-up) can accentuate winging of the medial border of the scapula with *long thoracic nerve* lesions. In partial *long thoracic nerve* lesions, putting the serratus anterior at a mechanical disadvantage by lowering the arms to waist level when pushing forward may accentuate the winging more dramatically than at shoulder level.[5] One may also see slight elevation of the superior border of the scapula with a *long thoracic nerve* lesion, although this is not nearly as pronounced as is seen with shoulder abduction with a *spinal accessory nerve* lesion.

If there is weakness of the rhomboid muscles, displacement of the scapula downward and laterally occurs with forward flexion secondary to the unopposed serratus anterior.[7] Displacement of the scapula laterally and dorsally, especially the lower portion, can be seen by slowly lowering the arms from the forward flexed position.[2]

During Active Shoulder Abduction (Fig. 2)

Winging of the scapula with shoulder abduction is more pronounced with dysfunction of the trapezius muscle or its innervation (*spinal accessory nerve*). Elevation of the scapula and lateral displacement are seen within the first 90 degrees of shoulder abduction.[1,2] In *spinal accessory nerve* lesions, these findings become less pronounced with abduction past 90 degrees, whereas patients with *long thoracic nerve* lesions may have a more difficult time elevating the arm above 90 degrees.[1,7]

The *scapular stabilization test* can also be useful in confirming that pain and limitation of shoulder elevation are caused by loss of scapular stabilization. This involves the clinician

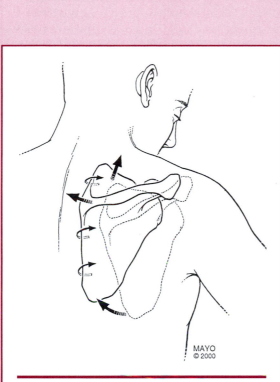

FIGURE 1. Position of the scapula with a *long thoracic nerve* lesion or serratus anterior weakness during shoulder forward flexion. Note pronounced winging of the medial border of the scapula, medial displacement, mild medial rotation of the inferior angle, and slight elevation of the superior border.

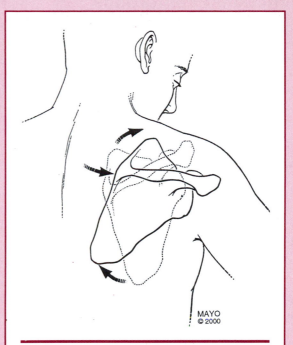

FIGURE 2. Position of the scapula with a *spinal accessory nerve* lesion or trapezius weakness during shoulder abduction. Note pronounced elevation of the superomedial border of the scapula, lateral displacement, and medial rotation of the inferior angle.

compressing the scapula against the patient's back. This maneuver should relieve pain and allow shoulder elevation above the horizontal.[8]

Although dysfunctions of the serratus anterior, trapezius, and rhomboid muscles are three of the more recognized causes of scapular winging and result in well-described patterns of abnormality, there are other causes of winging of the scapula (see Table 1). Scapular winging secondary to structural causes may not vary with arm position and may be associated with scapular crepitation, especially those secondary to bony or bursal abnormalities.[7] Primary glenohumeral or subacromial pathology may also result in secondary scapular winging due to increased compensatory scapulothoracic motion.

A careful neurologic examination that includes cranial nerve testing (especially cranial nerve XI testing with shoulder shrug); manual muscle testing of all other upper and lower extremity muscles, neck and facial muscles; reflexes; and sensory testing is essential to rule out evidence of additional neuromuscular abnormalities. Also, a thorough musculoskeletal examination of the shoulder and neck that includes active and passive range-of-motion and provocative maneuvers is essential in ruling out other primary causes or secondary manifestations of scapular winging.[9]

Functional Limitations

Functional limitations include difficulty with elevating the arm above the horizontal secondary to pain, weakness, and disturbed biomechanical movements of the shoulder. Such a limitation interferes with many activities of daily living (e.g., brushing hair, reaching in a cupboard), as well as recreational and sporting activities that require upper extremity use (e.g., volleyball, tennis). Patients may also have difficulty sleeping secondary to pain, which can lead to fatigue, stress, and anxiety. The degree of dysfunction or pain that a patient experiences depends on the source of the winging.

Diagnostic Studies

The presence of scapular winging is a clinical diagnosis; however, further diagnostic testing is warranted to determine the cause. Electrodiagnostic studies that consist of electromyography (EMG) and nerve conduction studies (NCS) are the most helpful and can confirm the presence of neuromuscular causes.

Although radiographs are rarely diagnostic, they may reveal evidence of primary bony etiologies, such as scapular osteochondromas, or secondary causes of the scapular winging, such as primary shoulder pathology, mass lesions, or cervical spondylosis contributing to nerve root pathology. Radiographs of the scapula, shoulder, cervical spine, or chest therefore should be considered.

CT or MRI of the neck, shoulder, scapula, or brachial plexus may be indicated as well, depending on the clinical suspicion of the cause.

Differential Diagnosis

Rotator cuff pathology

Cervical radiculopathy (especially C6 and C7)

Adhesive capsulitis

Myofascial pain syndrome

Tumors of the shoulder girdle, lung, upper extremity, spine

Shoulder arthritis

Treatment

Initial

Pain control may be necessary early on and can usually be achieved with analgesic or anti-inflammatory medications. The use of superficial heat and ice can also be used to help relieve associated muscle spasm and pain. Depending on the patient's vocation or recreational hobbies, activity modifications or restrictions may also be necessary (e.g., lifting restrictions). While the use of a sling is not advocated in most cases, it may offer the patient some pain relief when used within the first week of acute primary shoulder pathology causing secondary scapular winging.

Rehabilitation

Although specific treatment measures may vary slightly depending on the exact cause of the winging, the following general principles apply. Range-of-motion exercises of the shoulder must be started early to prevent contracture. A physical or occupational therapist should initiate these exercises because passive range of motion of the shoulder while stabilizing the scapula is usually necessary. It is also important to have the patient work with a therapist early on to avoid having the patient learn unwanted muscle substitution patterns, which may be hard to break later. Scapular stabilization exercises and a progressive strengthening program of the remaining functional periscapular and shoulder muscles should be instituted as the patient's pain permits.

Functional retraining of muscle substitution patterns may be necessary. Patients should progress to a home program only when they can perform the exercises properly. Scapular stabilizing braces have been used, but results have been equivocal.[12]

Procedures

Procedures, such as local steroid injections, are generally not necessary but should be considered if the patient has or develops associated musculoskeletal conditions (e.g., rotator cuff tendonopathy secondary to the altered shoulder biomechanics, or as the primary pathology).

Surgery

Chronic, painful, and refractory scapular winging can be treated with surgical techniques. If the patient's scapular winging is secondary to a single nerve injury, surgical procedures are usually only considered after an adequate time for recovery of nerve function (at least 1 to 2 years).

Surgical interventions can be separated into three categories: scapulothoracic fusion, static scapular stabilization, and dynamic scapular stabilization.[6]

Scapulothoracic fusion involves fusing the scapula to the thorax and is used in cases of generalized muscle weakness, such as fascioscapulohumeral dystrophy, or as a salvage procedure after other surgical failures.

Static scapular stabilization involves tethering the scapula to a fixed anatomic structure such as vertebral spinous processes or ribs.

Dynamic scapular stabilization offers not only stabilization of the scapula but also better restoration of function than the other methods. Transfer of the sternal portion of the pectoralis major muscle to the inferior angle of the scapula is currently the preferred method to restore scapular stabilization and shoulder function, although different dynamic muscle transfer techniques have been described.[6–8]

In the case of scapular winging secondary to a known single nerve injury (e.g., spinal accessory nerve injury from direct trauma), one must also consider the option of nerve exploration and nerve repair.[7]

Potential Disease Complications

Complications include loss of shoulder function or range of motion, shoulder adhesive capsulitis, chronic muscle atrophy, chronic shoulder pain, and cosmetic deformity.

Potential Treatment Complications

Analgesics, NSAIDs, and COX-2 inhibitors have well-known side effects that most commonly affect the gastric, hepatic, and renal systems. Potential complications of local steroid injections, if needed, include but are not limited to infection, bleeding, allergic reaction to the medication, skin depigmentation, and tendon rupture.

Inappropriate or overly aggressive exercises that do not attempt to stabilize the scapula or correct muscle substitution patterns may lead to further pain and unnecessary stretching of the affected muscles, making improvement of the scapular winging, upper extremity function, and cosmetic deformity difficult.

There are many potential treatment complications associated with the surgical options previously mentioned. Surgical complication may include cosmetic deformity from the surgical procedure, wound infection, failure of the graft, graft site morbidity, pneumothorax, pseudarthrosis and loss of scapulothoracic motion with scapulothoracic fusion, stretch of the scapular attachment site, and recurrent winging with a static stabilization.[6,8]

References

1. Hammond SR, Danta G: A clinical and electrophysiological study of neurogenically induced winging of the scapula. Clin Exper Neurol 1981;17:153–166.
2. Saeed MA, Gatens PF, Singh S: Winging of the scapula. Am Fam Physician 1981;24:139–143.
3. Travell JG, Simons DG: Myofascial Pain and Dysfunction: The Trigger Point Manual. Baltimore, Williams & Wilkins, 1983, pp 185–186, 334–335, 425–426, 622–625.
4. Horwitz MT, Tocantins LM: An anatomical study of the role of the long thoracic nerve and the related scapular bursae in the pathogenesis of local paralysis of the serratus anterior muscle. Anat Rec 1938;71:375–385.
5. Makin GJV, Brown WF, Ebers GC: C7 radiculopathy: Importance of scapular winging in clinical diagnosis. J Neur Neurosurg Psychiatry 1986;49:640–644.
6. Wiater MJ, Flatow EL. Long thoracic nerve injury. Clin Ortho Rel Research 1999;368:17–27.
7. Kuhn JE, Hawkins RJ. Evaluation and treatment of scapular disorders. In Warner JJP, Iannotti JP, Gerber C (eds): Complex and Revision Problems in Shoulder Surgery. Philadelphia, Lippincott-Raven, 1997, pp 357–375.
8. Warner JJP, Navarro RA: Serratus anterior dysfunction: Recognition and treatment. Clin Ortho Rel Research 1998;349:139–148.
9. Magee DJ. Cervical Spine and Shoulder in Orthopedic Physical Assessment. Philadelphia, W.B. Saunders, 1992 pp 34–70, 90–142.
10. Duralde XA: Evaluation and treatment of the winged scapula. J South Orthop Assoc 1995;4(1):38–52.
11. Cuomo F, Blank K, Zuckerman JD, Present DA: Scapular osteochondroma presenting with exostosis bursata. Bul Hospital Joint Diseases 1993;52:55–58.
12. Marin R: Scapula winger's brace: A case series on the management of long thoracic nerve palsy. Arch Phys Med Rehabil 1998;79:1226–1230.

19 | Shoulder Arthritis

Robert P. Nirschl, MD, MS

Synonyms

Glenohumeral arthritis

Osteoarthritis

Arthritic frozen shoulder

ICD-9 Codes

715.11
Primary osteoarthritis, shoulder

715.21
Secondary osteoarthritis, shoulder (rotator cuff arthropathy)

716.11
Traumatic arthropathy, shoulder

716.91
Arthropathy, unspecified, shoulder

Definition

Osteoarthritis of the shoulder occurs when there is loss of articular cartilage that results in narrowing of the joint space (Fig. 1). Synovitis and osteocartilaginous loose bodies are commonly associated with shoulder arthritis. Pathologic distortion of the articular surfaces of the humeral head and glenoid can occur due to increasing age, overuse, heredity, or trauma. This condition is most commonly seen in people older than 50. Longstanding complete rotator cuff tears can predispose one to shoulder arthritis. The medical history should include any history of fracture, dislocation, or rotator cuff tear, suggesting a posttraumatic etiology.

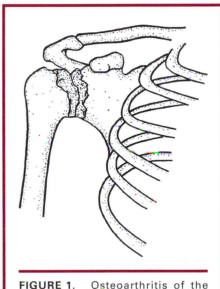

FIGURE 1. Osteoarthritis of the shoulder.

Symptoms

Symptoms include constant shoulder pain intensified by activity and usually partially relieved with rest. Pain is usually noted in all shoulder movements. Major restriction of shoulder motion and disuse weakness are common and progressive. The pain is typically restricted to the area of the shoulder but may be felt around the deltoid region or even into the forearm. The pain is generally characterized as dull and aching but may become sharp at the extremes of range of motion. Neurologic symptoms such as numbness and paresthesias should be absent. Pain may interfere with sleep and may be worse in the morning.

Physical Examination

Restriction of shoulder motion is a major clinical component, especially loss of external rotation and abduction. Both active and passive range of

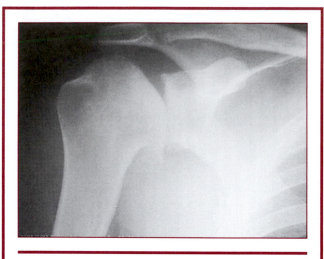

FIGURE 2. X-ray typical of glenohumeral osteoarthritis.

motion are affected in shoulder arthritis, as compared to only active motion being affected in rotator cuff tears (passive range is normal in rotator cuff injuries unless adhesive capsulitis is present). Pain increases when the extremes of the restricted motion are reached, and crepitus is common with movement. Tenderness may be present over the anterior rotator cuff and over the posterior joint line. If acromioclavicular (AC) joint osteoarthritis is an accompanying problem, the AC joint will be tender as well. There may be wasting of the muscles surrounding the shoulder due to disuse atrophy. Sensation and deep tendon reflexes should be normal.

Functional Limitations

All activities that require upper extremity strength, endurance, and flexibility can be affected. Most commonly, activities that require reaching overhead in external rotation are limited. These include brushing hair, putting on a shirt, throwing a baseball, reaching for groceries on high shelves, etc. If pain is severe and constant, sleep may be interrupted, and the patient may experience depressive symptoms.

Diagnostic Studies

Routine shoulder x-rays with four views (A-P internal and external rotation, axillary, and scapular Y view) are generally sufficient for evaluating loss of articular cartilage and glenohumeral joint space narrowing (Fig. 2). Other findings on plain x-rays that suggest shoulder arthritis include flattening of the humeral head, marginal osteophytes, and the presence of subchondral cysts in the humeral head and glenoid. If there is a chronic rotator cuff tear that is contributing to the destruction of the articular cartilage, the humeral head will be seen pressing against the undersurface of the acromion. Associated AC joint arthritis can be seen on the AP view. CT scan for more unique skeletal architecture and MRI to assess the rotator cuff may be occasionally indicated.

Differential Diagnosis

Rotator cuff pathology	Synovitis	Cervical osteoarthritis
Shoulder instability	Rheumatoid arthritis	Cervical radiculopathy
Labral degeneration and tear	Pseudogout	Charcot's joint
Biceps tendon abnormalities	Infection	Fracture of the humerus
Adhesive capsulitis	Neoplasms	Avascular necrosis

Treatment

Initial

Shoulder arthritis is a chronic issue, but acute exacerbations in pain can be treated with NSAIDs/COX-2 inhibitors. Occasionally these are used on a long-term basis, but the risk of side effects increases substantially. Non-narcotic analgesic medications can also help with pain. Capsaicin cream may be used topically on a prn basis. The use of ice and heat may relieve pain as well. Gentle stretching exercises help to keep the range of motion and prevent secondary adhesive capsulitis.

Rehabilitation

The rehabilitative efforts are dedicated to the restoration of strength, endurance, and flexibility. Supervised physical or occupational therapy will focus on the upper back; neck; and scapular muscle groups; and the entire upper extremity, including the rotator cuff, arm, forearm, wrist, and hand. Many patients benefit from aquatic therapy and can easily be taught exercises and then transitioned to an independent pool exercise program that they can continue long term.

The success of flexibility return will be determined by the extent of mechanical bony blockade, which in turn is determined by the magnitude of glenohumeral incongruous distortion, loose bodies, and osteophyte formation.

Pain control can be assisted with the use of modalities such as ultrasound, iontophoresis, and electrical stimulation.

Procedures

If rehabilitation fails, the patient has several treatment options. First, periarticular injections may offer some help to control pain of associated problems, such as subacromial bursitis and rotator cuff tendinitis/tendinosis. Second, intra-articular injections may also afford some pain relief—particularly in the early stages. However, injections have not been shown to alter the underlying arthritis pathoanatomy (Fig. 3). The final treatment option is surgery.

With the patient seated with the arm either in the lap or hanging down by the side, the internal rotation and gravity pull of the arm will open the space, leading to the glenohumeral joint. Then, under sterile conditions, using a 25-gauge, 1.5-inch disposable needle, inject a 3 to 4 cc mixture of a local anesthetic/corticosteroid combination (e.g., 1 cc 1% lidocaine mixed with 3 cc

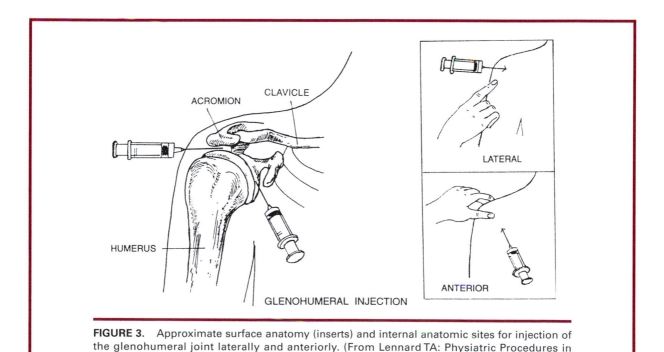

FIGURE 3. Approximate surface anatomy (inserts) and internal anatomic sites for injection of the glenohumeral joint laterally and anteriorly. (From Lennard TA: Physiatric Procedures in Clinical Practice. Philadelphia, Hanley & Belfus, 1995, p 17.)

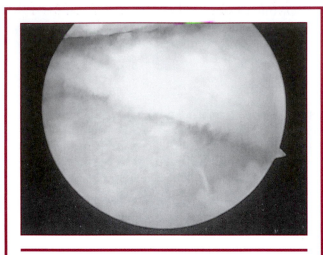

FIGURE 4.   Arthroscopic surgical view of osteoarthritis.

betamethasone [Celestone] 6 mg/cc). Alternately, the anesthetic may be injected first.

Postinjection care should include icing the shoulder for 5 to 10 minutes immediately and then for 15–20 minutes 2 to 3 times a day over the next 24 to 48 hours. Patients should be cautioned to avoid aggressive activities for the first few days following the injection.

Surgery

If unacceptable symptoms persist despite conservative treatment, the patient may decide to reduce his or her activity level to minimize pain or proceed with surgical intervention. It is important to inform the patient that regardless of the treatment approach, with osteoarthritis, a return to normal shoulder function, either by rehabilitation or surgery, is not possible. Pain control and some increased function are, however, usually achievable.

Surgical options include debridement of the glenohumeral joint by either open or arthroscopic techniques or joint replacement. If reasonable congruity between the humeral head and glenoid is present, good improvement in pain control and some functional improvement can be anticipated with debridement, even in the presence of severe chondromalacia. Arthroscopic techniques are quite successful provided that mechanical blockading osteophytes and loose bodies are removed (Fig. 4).[2] If major incongruity is present between the humeral head and glenoid, total joint arthroplasty may be indicated.[3] Most shoulders, however, can be aided arthroscopically with appropriate technique, which often necessitates a second posterior portal and a highly experienced shoulder arthroscopist.[2]

Potential Disease Complications

Disease complications include chronic intractable pain and loss of shoulder range of motion resulting in diminished functional ability to use the arm, disuse weakness, difficulty with sleep, inability to perform work and recreational activities, and sometimes, depression.

Potential Treatment Complications

Analgesics, NSAIDs, and COX-2 inhibitors have well-known side effects that most commonly affect the gastric, hepatic, and renal systems. Infection or an allergic reaction to the medications used are rare side effects of injections. Surgical complications also are not common, but the usual possibilities, including neurovascular issues, have been reported.

References
1. Williams GR, Iannotti JP: Biomechanics of the glenohumeral joint: Influence on shoulder arthroplasty. In Iannotti J, Williams G (eds): Disorders of the Shoulder: Diagnosis and Management. Philadelphia, Lippincott, Williams, and Wilkins, 1999.
2. Nirschl RP: Arthroscopy in the treatment of glenohumeral osteoarthritis. Presented to the Brazilian Congress of Upper Extremity Surgeons. Belo Horizonte, Brazil, Sept 29, 2000.
3. Schenk T, Iannotti JP: Prosthetic arthroplasty for glenohumeral arthritis with an intact of repairable rotator cuff: Indications, techniques, and results. In Iannotti J, Williams G (eds): Disorders of the Shoulder: Diagnosis and Management. Philadelphia, Lippincott, Williams, and Wilkins, 1999.

20 | Elbow Arthritis

Paul R. Greenlaw, MD
Charles Cassidy, MD

Synonyms

Rheumatoid elbow

Primary degenerative arthritis

Osteoarthritis of the elbow

ICD-9 Codes

714.12
Rheumatoid arthritis of the elbow

715.12.1
Osteoarthritis, primary, of the elbow

715.22
Osteoarthritis, secondary, of the elbow

716.12
Traumatic arthritis of the elbow

Definition

In the simplest of terms, arthritis of the elbow reflects a loss of articular cartilage in the ulnotrochlear and radiocapitellar articulations. Destruction of the articulating surfaces and bone loss or, alternatively, excess bone formation in the form of osteophytes can be present. Joint contractures are common. Joint instability can result from inflammatory or traumatic injury to the bony architecture, capsule, and ligaments. The spectrum of disease ranges from intermittent pain or loss of motion with minimal changes detectable on x-rays to the more advanced stages of arthritis showing complete loss of joint space, osteophyte formation, severe loss of motion, and constant pain. Both complete ankylosis and total instability of the elbow are potential final outcomes of the destructive process.

The major causes of elbow arthritis are the inflammatory arthropathies, of which rheumatoid arthritis is the predominant disease. Approximately 20% to 50% of rheumatoid patients eventually develop arthritis of the elbow.[1] Involvement of the elbow in juvenile rheumatoid arthritis is not uncommon. Other inflammatory conditions affecting the elbow joint include systemic lupus erythematosus, the seronegative spondyloarthropathies (ankylosing spondylitis, psoriatic arthritis, Reiter's syndrome, and enteropathic arthritis), and crystalline arthritis (gout and pseudogout). Post-traumatic arthritis can result from intra-articular fractures of the elbow. Osteonecrosis of the capitellum or trochlea, leading to arthritis, has also been described.[2] Primary osteoarthritis of the elbow is a rare condition, responsible for less than 5% of elbow arthritis.[3] Interestingly, the incidence is significantly higher in the Alaskan Eskimo and Japanese populations.[4] Primary elbow arthritis usually affects the dominant arm of men in their 50s. Repetitive, strenuous arm use appears to be a factor, as the condition has been reported in heavy laborers, throwing athletes, and weight lifters.

Symptoms

The symptoms of elbow arthritis reflect, in part, the underlying etiology and severity of the disease process. Regardless of the etiology, however, the inability to fully straighten (extend) the elbow is a nearly universal complaint of patients with elbow arthritis. Associated symptoms of cubital tunnel syndrome (ulnar neuropathy at the elbow) include numbness in the ring and small fingers, loss of hand dexterity, and an aching pain along the ulnar aspect of the forearm. Cubital tunnel syndrome is neither uncommon nor unexpected, given the proximity of the ulnar nerve to the elbow joint. (See Chapter 25.)

Patients with early rheumatoid involvement complain of a swollen, painful joint with morning stiffness. Progressive loss of motion and/or instability is seen in later stages. Compression of the posterior interosseous nerve by rheumatoid synovitis can occasionally produce the inability to extend the fingers.

Patients with crystalline arthritis of the elbow may complain of severe pain, swelling, and limited motion; an expedient evaluation is warranted to rule out a septic elbow in such cases.

Post-traumatic or idiopathic arthritis of the elbow, in contrast, usually manifests with painful loss of motion without significant effusions, warmth, or the constant pain associated with an inflamed synovium. These patients usually complain of pain at the extremes of motion, and they have more trouble extending the elbow than flexing it. Pain throughout the arc of motion implies advanced arthritis.

The final stages of arthritis, irrespective of cause, can include complaints of severe pain and decreased motion that hinders activities of daily living, as well as the cosmetic deformity of the flexed elbow posture.

Physical Examination

Physical examination findings depend on the cause, as well as the stage, of the elbow arthritis. As mentioned, however, a flexion contracture is almost always present. The range of motion should be monitored at the initial examination and at subsequent follow-up exams.

Normal elbow range of motion in extension-flexion is from 0 to about 150 degrees, with pronation averaging 75 degrees and supination averaging 85 degrees. A functional range of motion is considered to be from –30 to 130 degrees, with 50 degrees each of pronation and supination.[5]

All other joints should be assessed as well. Strength should be normal, but may be impaired in longstanding elbow arthritis due to disuse or in more acute cases due to pain. Weakness may also be noted in the presence of associated neuropathies. In the absence of associated neuropathies, deep tendon reflexes and sensation should also be normal.

Associated ulnar nerve irritation can produce a sensitive nerve with a positive Tinel's sign over the medial elbow (cubital tunnel), diminished sensation in the small finger and ulnar half of the ring finger, and weakness of the intrinsic muscles (see Chapter 25). Numbness provoked by acute flexion of the elbow for 30 to 60 seconds is termed a positive elbow flexion test.

Effusions, synovial thickenings, and erythema are commonly noted in the inflammatory arthropathies during acute flares. Loss of motion in flexion and extension, as well as pronation and supination, can be present as the synovitis affects all articulating surfaces in the elbow. Pain, limited motion, and crepitus worsen as the disease progresses. Occasionally, rheumatoid destruction of the elbow will produce instability, which may be perceived by the patient as weakness. Examination of such elbows will demonstrate laxity to varus and valgus stress; anteroposterior instability may also be seen.

In contrast, progressive idiopathic or post-traumatic arthritis of the elbow results in stiffness. The loss of extension is usually worse than the loss of flexion. Pain is present with forced extension or flexion. Crepitus is palpable with flexion/extension and forearm rotation.

Functional Limitations

The elbow functions to position the hand in space. Significant loss of extension can hinder an individual's ability to interact with the environment, whereas significant loss of flexion can interfere with essential tasks such as eating, shaving, and washing. Activities such as carrying groceries or briefcases that require full extension of the elbow are painful.

A normal shoulder can compensate well for a lack of pronation, whereas a normal shoulder, wrist, and cervical spine can compensate, albeit awkwardly, for a lack of elbow flexion. There is no simple solution for a significant lack of elbow extension; the body must be moved closer to the desired object. Compensatory mechanisms are often impaired in patients with rheumatoid arthritis, magnifying the impact of the elbow arthritis on function.

TABLE 1. Radiographic Classification of Rheumatoid Arthritis[6]

I	Synovitis with a normal appearing joint
II	Loss of joint space but maintenance of the subchondral architecture
IIIa	Alteration of the subchondral architecture
IIIb	Alteration of the architecture with deformity
IV	Gross deformity

Diagnostic Studies

Plain x-rays are usually sufficient to diagnose elbow arthritis. Joint space narrowing, osteophyte formation, bone destruction, and cyst formation can all be easily identified by quality AP and lateral x-rays of the elbow. For the rheumatoid patient, the Mayo clinic radiographic classification of rheumatoid involvement is useful (Table 1).[6] Dramatic loss of bone is evident as the disease progresses (Fig. 1). This pattern of destruction is not seen, however, in the post-traumatic or

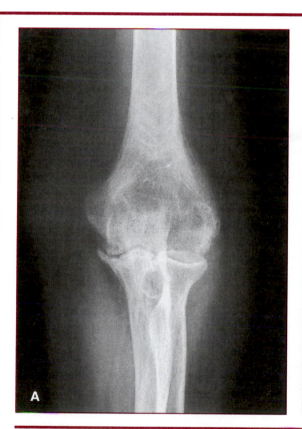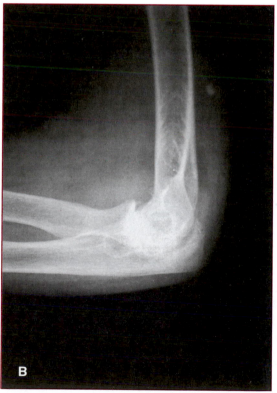

FIGURE 1. Rheumatoid arthritis. AP (*A*) and lateral (*B*) elbow radiographs of a 40-year-old female with longstanding elbow pain. Osteopenia and symmetric joint space narrowing are present. The lateral radiograph demonstrates early bone loss in the ulna. This would be categorized as stage IIIa.

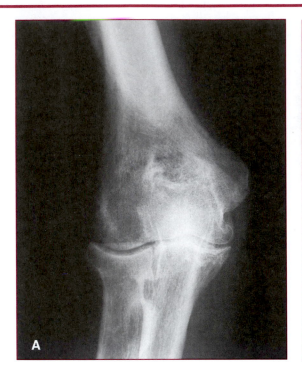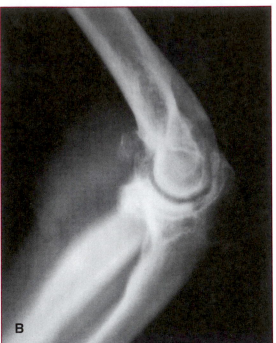

FIGURE 2. Primary degenerative elbow arthritis. AP (*A*) and lateral (*B*) elbow radiographs of a 52-year-old male with dominant right elbow pain at the extremes of motion. *A*, Joint space narrowing and obliteration of the coronoid fossa. *B*, Coronoid and olecranon spurs and a large anterior loose body are evident.

idiopathic patient. Radiographic features in these patients include spurs or osteophytes on the coronoid and olecranon, loose bodies, and narrowing of the coronoid and olecranon fossae (Fig. 2).

Lateral tomograms or a CT arthrogram may be helpful to localize suspected loose bodies. MRI is most valuable to confirm suspected osteonecrosis.

The diagnosis of rheumatoid arthritis will have already been made in the majority of patients who present with rheumatoid elbow involvement. When isolated inflammatory arthritis of the elbow is suspected, appropriate serologic studies may include a rheumatoid factor, ANA, HLA B-27, as well as an erythrocyte sedimentation rate. Elbow aspiration may be needed to rule out a crystalline or infectious etiology in patients who present with a warm, stiff, swollen, and painful joint and no history of trauma or inflammatory arthritis.

Differential Diagnosis

Medial or lateral epicondylitis

Elbow instability

Septic arthritis

Acute fracture

Cubital tunnel syndrome

Median nerve compression

Radial tunnel syndrome

Cervical radiculopathy

Elbow contracture

Treatment

Initial

Treatment of elbow arthritis depends on the diagnosis, degree of involvement, functional limitations, and pain. When the elbow is one of a number of joints actively involved with inflammatory arthritis, the obvious treatment is systemic. Disease modifying agents have had a dramatic effect in relieving symptoms and retarding the progression of arthritis for many of these patients. For systemic disease, a rheumatology consult can be beneficial.

The initial local treatment for an acutely inflamed elbow joint includes rest. A simple sling places the elbow in a relatively comfortable position. The patient should be encouraged to remove the sling for gentle range of motion exercises of the elbow and shoulder several times daily. Icing the elbow for 15 minutes several times a day for the first few days may be beneficial.

Non-operative treatment for primary osteoarthritis of the elbow primarily consists of activity modification and NSAIDs/COX-2 inhibitors. Oral analgesics may help with pain control. Topical treatments such as capsaicin can be tried as well.

Patients who have associated cubital tunnel symptoms are instructed to avoid direct pressure over the elbow and to avoid prolonged elbow flexion. A static night splint maintaining the elbow in about 30 degrees of flexion may help to alleviate the cubital tunnel symptoms (see Chapter 25).

Rehabilitation

Once the acute inflammation has subsided, physical or occupational therapy is instituted to regain elbow motion and strength and to educate the patient on activity modification and pain-control measures.

Therapy should focus on improving range of motion and strength throughout the upper body because this will improve function regardless of the degree of elbow arthritis. Adaptive equipment such as reachers can be recommended. Ergonomic workstation equipment may also be useful (e.g., voice-activated computer software, forearm rests).

Modalities such as ultrasound and iontophoresis may help with pain control.

Night-time static, static-progressive, or dynamic extension splinting may be indicated to relieve significant elbow contractures. Braces may be effective in the setting of instability. It is important to remember that *functional* rather than full elbow motion is the goal of therapy.

In primary osteoarthritis of the elbow, corrective splinting is not indicated since bony impingement is usually present. Similarly, therapy may actually aggravate the symptoms and should be ordered judiciously.

Rehabilitation is critical to the success of surgical procedures about the elbow. The rheumatoid patient commonly has multiple joint problems, which must not be neglected during treatment of the elbow. The shoulder is at particular risk for stiffness. A good operation, a motivated patient, and a knowledgeable and skillful therapist are necessary to optimize postoperative results. Postoperative rehabilitation depends on the procedure and the surgeon's preference. However, in general, physical or occupational therapy should be recommended to restore range of motion and strength.

Procedures

For recalcitrant symptoms, intra-articular steroid injections are quite effective in relieving the pain associated with synovitis (Fig. 3).

The elbow joint is best accessed through the "soft spot"—the center of the triangle formed by the lateral epicondyle, the tip of the olecranon, and the radial head. The patient is placed with the elbow between 50 to 90 degrees of flexion. For the posterolateral approach, the lateral epicondyle

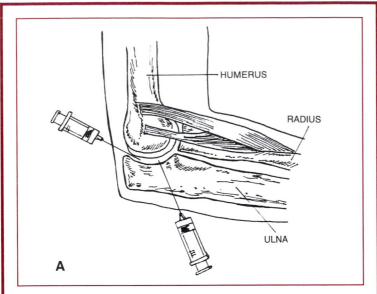

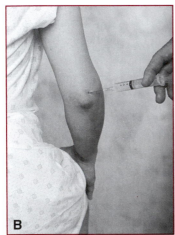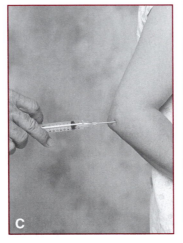

FIGURE 3. Internal anatomic (*A*) and approximate surface anatomic (*B*, lateral; *C*, posterior) sites for injection of the elbow laterally and posteriorly. (From Lennard TA: Pain Procedures in Clinical Practice, 2nd ed. Philadelphia, Hanley & Belfus, 2000, with permission.)

and the posterior olecranon are palpated. Under sterile conditions, using a 25 gauge 1½ inch needle, inject 3–4 cc of an anesthetic corticosteroid mixture (e.g., 1 cc [80 mg] of methylprednisolone and 3 cc of 1% lidocaine). The needle is directed proximally toward the head of the radius and medially into the elbow joint (*A* and *C*). No resistance should be noted as the needle enters the joint. If an effusion is present, aspiration may be done prior to injecting the anesthetic/corticosteroid mixture.

For the posterior approach, the olecranon is palpated with the lateral olecranon groove located just posterior to the lateral epicondyle. The needle is then inserted above the superior aspect of and lateral to the olecranon. Again, it should enter the joint without resistance (*A* and *B*).

Postinjection care may include icing the elbow for 10 to 20 minutes following the injection and then 2 to 3 times daily thereafter. The patient should be informed that the pain may worsen for the first 24 to 36 hours and that the medication may take 1 week to work.

In general, repeat injections are not recommended. Although the intra-articular steroids are effective in treating the synovitis, they also temporarily inhibit chondrocyte synthesis, an effect that could potentially accelerate the arthritis.

Surgery

Patients whose treatment has failed after 3 to 6 months of adequate medical therapy are potential candidates for surgery. Refractory pain is the best indication for surgery. When assessing the surgical candidate with primary elbow arthritis, it is important to listen carefully to the complaints. Many patients are dissatisfied with the simple fact that they cannot fully straighten the elbow. Such patients will usually be less than satisfied with surgery.

Intermittent locking or catching suggestive of a loose body is often best treated with arthroscopy. Pain at the extremes of motion is consistent with impingement. An ulnohumeral arthroplasty, or surgical debridement of the elbow joint, may be recommended. Arthroscopic as well as open surgical techniques can be used to remove the impinging olecranon and coronoid osteophytes.

Ulnohumeral arthroplasty is successful at achieving its principal goal—pain relief at the extremes of motion. However, it is only marginally successful at actually improving motion, with an average improvement in extension of 12 degrees and an average improvement in flexion of 8 degrees. Overall, 86% of patients in one series were satisfied with the results.[3] As expected, the results deteriorate with time.

Less commonly, patients with primary arthritis complain of pain throughout the arc of motion. Their radiographs will likely demonstrate advanced arthritis with severe joint space narrowing. Simply removing the osteophytes will not likely be successful. Total elbow arthroplasty would seem to be a reasonable option. However, unlike their rheumatoid counterparts, the vast majority of these patients are otherwise healthy, vigorous people who would regularly stress their joint replacement. For this reason, total elbow arthroplasty in this setting is best reserved for the older (age greater than 65), sedentary patient.[12]

For the younger patient with advanced primary arthritis, an interposition arthroplasty is recommended.[13] This procedure involves a radical debridement of the joint followed by a resurfacing of the joint surfaces with an interposition material, such as autologous fascia lata or allograft Achilles tendon. A hinged external fixator is then applied, which will protect the healing interposition material while simultaneously maintaining elbow stability and permitting motion. This procedure certainly does not produce a normal elbow.[14] Other surgical options include elbow arthrodesis and resection arthroplasty. There is no ideal position for an elbow fusion. The elbow looks better when it is relatively straight. However, this position is relatively useless. Consequently, elbow arthrodesis is performed rarely, usually in the setting of intractable infection. Resection arthroplasty is an option for a failed total elbow arthroplasty. This procedure permits some elbow motion, although the elbow tends to be very unstable.

Elbow synovectomy and debridement provide predictable short-term pain relief in the majority of rheumatoid patients.[7] Interestingly, the results do not necessarily correlate with the severity of the arthritis. The results do, however, deteriorate somewhat over time, drifting down from 90% success at 3 years to 70% success by 10 years as the synovitis recurs.[8] Elbow motion is not necessarily improved by synovectomy; only 40% of patients obtain better motion.

Total elbow arthroplasty is a reliable procedure for the rheumatoid patient with advanced elbow arthritis.[9,10] The Mayo clinic has reported excellent results using a semi-constrained prosthesis,[11] with pain relief in 92% of patients, and an average arc of motion of 26 to 130 degrees, with 64 degrees pronation and 62 degrees supination. However, the complication rate is significantly higher than for the more conventional hip and knee replacements.

Potential Disease Complications

End-stage rheumatoid arthritis of the elbow can produce either severe stiffness or instability. Advanced primary arthritis invariably produces stiffness. Either outcome results in pain and limited function of the involved extremity. In addition, entrapment or traction neuritis of the ulnar nerve is not uncommon. Compressive injury to the posterior interosseous nerve from rheumatoid synovial hyperplasia has been reported.

Potential Treatment Complications

The systemic complications of the disease modifying agents used in treating rheumatoid arthritis are numerous and are beyond the scope of this chapter (see Chapters 32 and 39). Analgesics, NSAIDs, and COX-2 inhibitors have well-known side effects that most commonly affect the gastric, hepatic, and renal systems. COX-2 inhibitors may have fewer gastric side effects. Intra-articular steroid injections introduce the risk of iatrogenic infection and may produce transient chondrocyte damage.

Surgical complications include infection, wound problems, neurovascular injury, stiffness, recurrent synovitis, and iatrogenic instability. With total elbow arthroplasty, wound healing problems, infection, and loosening are the principal complications, each occurring in approximately 5% to 7% of patients. In addition, most surgeons place lifelong restrictions on high-impact loading to minimize the need for revision surgery.

References

1. Porter BB, Park N, Richardson C, Vainio K: Rheumatoid arthritis of the elbow: The results of synovectomy. J Bone Joint Surg 1974;56B:427–437.
2. Le TB, Mont MA, Jones LC, et al: Atraumatic osteonecrosis of the adult elbow. Clin Orthop 2000;373:141–145.
3. Morrey BF: Primary degenerative arthritis of the elbow: Treatment by ulnohumeral arthroplasty. J Bone Joint Surg 1992;74B:409–413.
4. Ortner DJ. Description and classification of degenerative bone changes in the distal joint surface of the humerus. Am J Phys Anthrop 1968;28:139–155.
5. Morrey BF, Askew L, An KN, et al: A biomechanical study of normal functional elbow motion. J Bone Joint Surg 1981;63A:872–877.
6. Morrey BF, Adams RA: Semi-constrained arthroplasty for the treatment of rheumatoid arthritis of the elbow. J Bone Joint Surg 1992;74A:479–490.
7. Ferlic DC, Patchett CE, Clayton ML, Freeman AC: Elbow synovectomy in rheumatoid arthritis. Clin Orthop 1987;220:119–125.
8. Alexiades MM, Stanwyck TS, Figgie MP, Inglis AE: Minimum ten-year follow-up of elbow synovectomy for rheumatoid arthritis.Orthop Trans 1990;14:255.
9. Hargreaves D, Emery R: Total elbow replacement in the treatment of rheumatoid disease. Clin Orthop 1999;366:61–71.
10. Ferlic DC: Total elbow arthroplasty for treatment of elbow arthritis." J Shoulder Elbow Surg 1999;8:367–378.
11. Gill DRJ, Morrey BF: The Coonrad-Morrey total elbow arthroplasty in patients with rheumatoid arthritis: A 10–15 year follow-up study. J Bone Joint Surg 1998;80A:1327–1335.
12. Moro JK, King GJ: Total elbow arthroplasty in the treatment of posttraumatic conditions of the elbow. Clin Orthop 2000;370:102–114.
13. Wright PE, Froimson AI, Morrey BF: Interposition arthroplasty of the elbow. In Morrey BF (ed): The Elbow and its Disorders, 3rd ed. Philadelphia, W.B. Saunders, 2000, pp 718–730.
14. Cheng SL, Morrey BF: Treatment of the mobile, painful, arthritic elbow by distraction interposition arthroplasty. J Bone Joint Surg 2000;82B:223–228.

21 Epicondylitis

Lyn D. Weiss, MD
Jay M. Weiss, MD

Synonyms

Tendinosis[1]
Lateral epicondylitis
Medial epicondylitis
Tennis elbow
Pitcher's elbow
Golfer's elbow

ICD-9 Codes

726.31
Medial epicondylitis
726.32
Lateral epicondylitis

Definition

Epicondylitis is a general term used to describe inflammation, pain, or tenderness in the region of the medial or lateral epicondyle. The actual nidus of pain and pathology has been debated. Lateral epicondylitis implies an inflammatory lesion with degeneration at the origin of the extensor muscles (the lateral epicondyle of the humerus). The extensor carpi radialis brevis (ECRB) is the muscle primarily affected. Other muscles that can contribute to the condition are the extensor carpi radialis longus and the extensor digitorum communis. In medial epicondylitis, the flexor muscle group is affected.

Although the term epicondylitis refers to an inflammatory process, inflammatory cells are not identified histologically. Instead, the condition may be secondary to failure of the musculotendinous attachment with resultant fibroplasia,[2] termed tendinosis. Other postulated primary lesions include angiofibroblastic tendinosis, periostitis, and enthesitis.[3] Overall, the focus of injury appears to be the muscle origin. Symptoms may be related to the failure of an appropriate repair process.[4]

Repetitive stress has been implicated as a factor in this condition.[5]

Symptoms

Patients usually report pain in the area just distal to the lateral epicondyle (lateral epicondylitis) or the medial epicondyle (medial epicondylitis). The patient may complain of pain radiating proximally or distally. Patients may also complain of pain with wrist/hand movement, such as gripping a doorknob or carrying a briefcase. Patients occasionally report swelling, as well.

Physical Examination

On examination, the hallmark of epicondylitis is tenderness over the extensor muscle origin (lateral epicondylitis) or flexor muscle origin (medial epicondylitis). The origin of the extensor or flexor muscles can be located one fingerbreadth below the lateral or medial epicondyle, respectively. With lateral epicondylitis, pain is increased with resisted wrist extension, especially with the elbow extended, the forearm pronated, the wrist radially deviated, and the hand in a fist. The middle finger test can also be used to assess for lateral epicondylitis. Here, the proximal interphalangeal joint of the long finger is resisted in extension, and pain is elicited over the lateral epicondyle. Swelling is occasionally present. With medial epicondylitis, pain is increased with resisted wrist flexion.

Functional Limitations

The patient may complain of an inability to lift or carry objects on the affected side, secondary to increased pain. Typing, using a computer mouse, or working on a keyboard may re-create the pain. Even handshaking or squeezing may be painful in both lateral and medial epicondylitis. Athletic activities may cause pain; hence the names tennis elbow for lateral epicondylitis and pitcher's/golfer's elbow for medial epidondylitis.

Diagnostic Studies

The diagnosis is usually made on clinical grounds. MRI, which is particularly useful for soft tissue definition, can be used to assess for tendinitis, tendinosis/degeneration, partial tears, or complete tears/detachment of the common flexor or common extensor tendons at the medial and lateral epicondyles, respectively.[6] MRI, however, is rarely needed, except in recalcitrant epicondylitis, and in the early stages will not alter the treatment significantly. The medial and lateral collateral ligament complexes can be evaluated for tears, as well as for chronic degeneration and scarring. Arthrography may be beneficial if capsular defects and associated ligament injuries are suspected. Radiographs are of little use in this condition but may be useful in cases of resistant tendinitis and for ruling out occult fractures, arthritis, or an osteochondral loose body.

Differential Diagnosis

Posterior interosseous nerve syndrome

Median or ulnar neuropathy about the elbow

Acute calcification about the lateral epicondyle[7]

Anconeus compartment syndrome[8]

Degenerative arthrosis[9]

Lateral ligament instability[10]

Bursitis

Bone infection or tumors

Osteoarthritis

Osteochondral loose body

Triceps tendinitis

Elbow synovitis

Radial head fracture

Collateral ligament tears

Treatment

Initial

Initial treatment consists of relative rest, avoidance of repetitive motions involving the wrist, activity modification to avoid stress on the epicondyles, anti-inflammatory medication, heat modalities, or ice for acute pain. Patients who develop lateral epicondylitis from tennis should modify their stroke (especially improving the backhand stroke to ensure that the forearm is in midpronation and the trunk is leaning forward) and modify their equipment, usually by reducing string tension and enlarging the handle size.[5] Frequently, a two-handed backhand will relieve the stress sufficiently. Patients who develop medial epicondylitis from golf should consider modifying their swing to avoid excessive force on wrist flexor muscles.

In addition, a forearm band (counterforce brace) worn distal to the flexor or extensor muscle group origin can be beneficial. The theory is to dissipate the forces over a larger area of tissue than only the medial or lateral attachment site. Alternatively, the use of a wrist immobilization splint, set in neutral (for either medial or lateral epicondylitis) or in 30 to 40 degrees of wrist extension (for lateral epicondylitis only), will relieve the tension on the extensor carpi radialis brevis muscle, as well as other wrist and finger extensors.[11]

Rehabilitation

Rehabilitation may include physical or occupational therapy. Therapy should include two phases. The first phase should be directed at decreasing pain (ultrasound, electrical stimulation, phonophoresis, heat, ice, massage) and decreasing disability (education, decreasing repetitive stress, and preservation of motion). When the patient is pain

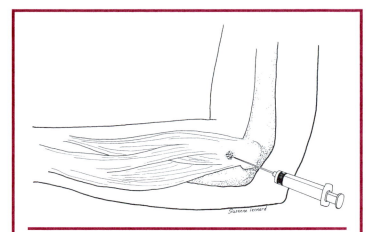

FIGURE 1. Under sterile conditions, using a 27-gauge needle and 1 to 2 cc of a local anesthetic combined with 1 to-2 cc of a corticosteroid preparation, inject the solution approximately 1 to 5 cm distal to the lateral epicondyle. The injected materials should flow smoothly—resistance generally indicates that the solution is being injected directly into the tendon, and this should be avoided.

free, a gradual program to improve strength and endurance of wrist extensors (for lateral epicondylitis) or wrist flexors (for medial epicondylitis) should be implemented. This program must be carefully monitored to permit strengthening of the muscles and work hardening of the tissues, without itself causing an overuse situation. The patient should start with static exercises and advance to progressive resistive exercises. Theraband, light weights, or manual (self) resistance exercises can all be used.

Work or activity restrictions or modifications may be required for a period of time.

Procedures

Injection of corticosteroid, usually with a local anesthetic into the area of maximum tenderness (approximately 1 to 5 cm distal to the lateral epicondyle), has been shown to be effective in treating lateral epicondylitis (Fig. 1).[12] To confirm the diagnosis, a trial of lidocaine alone may be given. An immediate improvement in grip strength should be noted postinjection. Postinjection treatment should include icing the affected area both immediately (for 5 to 10 minutes) and thereafter (a reasonable regimen is 20 minutes 2-3 times per day for 2 weeks), wearing a wrist splint (particularly for activities that involve wrist movement) for at least 2 to 3 days, and avoiding exacerbating activities.

Injection of botulinum toxin into the extensor digitorum communis III and IV has been reported to be beneficial in treating chronic treatment-resistant lateral epicondylitis.[13]

Injections for medial epicondylitis are generally not recommended because of the risk of injury to the ulnar nerve (either by direct injection or by tissue changes that may promote nerve injury).

Surgery

Surgery may be indicated in those patients with continued severe symptoms who do not respond to conservative management. For lateral epicondylitis, surgery is aimed at excision and revitalization of the pathologic tissue in the extensor carpi radialis brevis and release of the muscle origin.[14]

Potential Disease Complications

Possible long-term complications of untreated epicondylitis include chronic pain, loss of function, and possible elbow contracture. Medial epicondylitis may lead to reversible impairment (neurapraxia) of the ulnar nerve.[15] Generally, epicondylitis is more easily and successfully treated in the acute phase.

Potential Treatment Complications

Analgesics, NSAIDs, and COX-2 inhibitors have well-known side effects that most commonly affect the gastric, hepatic, and renal systems. Local steroid injections may increase the risk of disrupting tissue planes, create high-pressure tissue necrosis, rupture tendons,[1] damage nerves, promote skin depigmentation or atrophy, or cause infection.

References

1. Kraushaar BS, Nirschl RP: Tendinosis of the elbow (tennis elbow). Clinical features and findings of histological, immunohistochemical, and electron microscopy studies. J Bone Joint Surg 1999;81(2):259–278.
2. Nirschl RP, Petrone FA: Tennis elbow. J Bone Joint Surg 1070;61-A:832–839.
3. Nirschl RP: Elbow tendinosis/tennis elbow. Clin Sports Med 1992;11:851.
4. Putnam MD, Cohen M: Painful conditions around the elbow. Orthop Clin North Am 1999;30(1):109–118.
5. Cassvan A, Weiss LD, Weiss JM, et al: Cumulative trauma disorders. Boston, Butterworth-Heinemann, 1997.
6. Braddom RL: Physical Medicine and Rehabilitation. Philadelphia, W.B. Saunders, 1996, p 222.
7. Hughes E: Acute deposition of calcium near the elbow. J Bone Joint Surg Br 1950;32:30–34.
8. Abrahamsson S, Sollerman C, Soderberg T, et al: Lateral elbow pain caused anconeus compartment syndrome. Acta Orthop Scand 1987;58:589–591.
9. Brems JJ: Degenerative joint disease of the elbow. In Nicholas JA, Hershman EB (eds): The Upper Extremity in Sports Medicine. St Louis, Mosby, 1995, pp 331–335.
10. Morrey BF: Anatomy of the elbow joint. In Morrey BF (ed): The Elbow and Its Disorders, 2nd ed. Philadelphia, W.B. Saunders, 1993, p 16.
11. Plancher KD: Clinics in Sports Medicine: The Athletic Elbow and Wrist, Part I. Diagnosis and Conservative Treatment, vol 14. Philadelphia, W.B. Saunders, 1995, pp 433–435.
12. Hay EH, Paterson SM, Lewis M, et al: Pragmatic randomized controlled trial of local corticosteroid injection and naproxen for treatment of lateral epicondylitis of elbow in primary care. BMJ 1999;319:964–968.
13. Morre HH, Keizer SB, van Os JJ: Treatment of chronic tennis elbow with botulinum toxin. Lancet 1997;349(9067):1746.
14. Organ SW, Nirschl RP, Kraushaar BS, Guidi EJ: Salvage surgery for lateral tennis elbow. Am. J. Sports Med 1997;25:746–750.
15. Barry NN, McGuire JL: Overuse syndromes in adult athletes. Rheumatic Dis Clin North Am 1996;22(3):515–530.

22 Median Neuropathy

Francisco H. Santiago, MD
Ramon Vallarino Jr., MD

Synonyms

Pronator Teres Syndrome
Pronator Syndrome

Anterior Interosseous Syndrome
Kiloh-Nevin Syndrome

ICD-9 Code

354.1
Other lesion of median
nerve (median nerve
neuritis)

Definition

There are three general areas in which the median nerve can become entrapped around the elbow and forearm. Since this chapter mainly deals with entrapment below the elbow, the most proximal and least frequent entrapment will not be discussed, but merely mentioned. Forearm median nerve entrapment is the compression by a dense band of connective tissue called the ligament of Struthers, an aberrant ligament found immediately above the elbow.

The topics discussed in this chapter include (1) compression of the median nerve at or immediately below the elbow, where the pronator teres muscle usually compresses it, and (2) compression distally of a branch of the median nerve-the anterior interosseous nerve.

Pronator Teres Syndrome

Pronator teres syndrome[1] is a symptom complex that is produced as the median nerve crosses the elbow and becomes entrapped as it passes first beneath the lacertus fibrosus—a thick fascial band extending from the biceps tendon to the forearm fascia—then between the two heads (superficial and deep) of the pronator teres muscle and under the edge of the flexor digitorum sublimis (Fig. 1). Compression may be related to a local process such as pronator teres hypertrophy, tenosynovitis, muscle hemorrhage, fascial tear, postoperative scarring, or an anomalous median artery. It may also be injured by occupational pressure, such as carrying a grocery bag.

Anterior Interosseous Syndrome

The anterior interosseous nerve arises from the median nerve 5 to 8 cm distal to the lateral epicondyle.[1,2] Slightly distal to its course through the pronator teres muscle, the median nerve gives off the anterior interosseous nerve—a purely motor branch (Fig. 2). It contains no fibers of superficial sensation but does supply deep pain and proprioception to some deep tissues, including the wrist joint. This nerve may be damaged by direct trauma, forearm fractures, humeral fracture, injection into or blood-drawing from the cubital vein, supracondylar fracture, fibrous bands related to the flexor digitorum sublimis, and flexor digitorum profundus. In some patients, it is a component of brachial amyotrophy of the shoulder

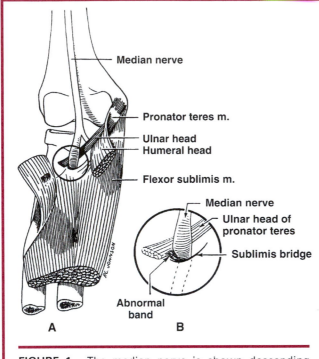

FIGURE 1. The median nerve is shown descending beneath the sublimis bridge after traversing the space between the two heads of the pronator teres. The nerve is compressed at the sublimis bridge. (From Kopell HP, Thompson WAL: Pronator syndrome: A confirmed case and its diagnosis. N Engl J Med 1958;259:713–715, with permission.)

girdle or related to cytomegalovirus infection or a bronchogenic carcinoma metastasis. The nerve maybe partially involved, but in a fully established syndrome, three muscles are weak: (1) flexor pollicis longus, (2) flexor digitorum profundus to the second and sometimes the third digits, and (3) pronator quadratus.

Symptoms

Pronator Teres Syndrome

In an acute compression, with unmistakable symptoms, the diagnosis is easy to establish.[2] In many cases of intermittent, mild, or partial compression, the signs and symptoms are vague and non-descript. The most common symptom is mild to moderate aching pain in the proximal forearm, sometimes described as tiredness and heaviness. Use of the arm may cause a mild or dull aching pain to become deep or sharp. Repetitive elbow motions are likely to provoke symptoms. As the pain intensifies, it may radiate proximally to the elbow or even to the shoulder. Paresthesias in the median nerve distribution may be reported, but they are generally not as severe or well localized as the complaints in carpal tunnel syndrome. When numbness is a prominent symptom, the complaints may mimic carpal tunnel syndrome. However, unlike carpal tunnel syndrome, pronator teres syndrome rarely has nocturnal exacerbation and the symptoms are not exacerbated by a change of wrist position.

Anterior Interosseous Syndrome

The onset of anterior interosseous syndrome can be related to exertion, or it may be spontaneous. In classic cases of spontaneous anterior interosseous nerve paralysis, there is acute pain in the proximal forearm or arm, lasting hours or days. There may be a history of local trauma or heavy muscular exertion at the time of onset of pain. As mentioned, the patient may complain of weakness of the forearm muscles innervated by the anterior interosseous nerve. Theoretically, there should be no sensory complaints.

Physical Examination

Pronator Teres Syndrome

Findings maybe ill defined and difficult to substantiate in pronator teres syndrome.[2] The most important physical finding is tenderness over the proximal forearm. Pressure over the pronator teres muscle produces discomfort and may produce a radiating pain and digital numbness. The symptomatic pronator teres muscle may be firm to palpation as compared with the other side. The contour of the forearm may be depressed, caused by the thickening of the lacertus fibrosus. Distinctive findings are (1) weakness of both the intrinsic muscles of the hands and muscles proximal to the wrist and in the forearm with tenderness, (2) Tinel's sign over the point of entrapment, and (3) absence of Phalen's sign. Pain may be elicited by pronation of the forearm, elbow flexion, or even by contraction of the superficial flexor of the second digit. Sensory examination findings are usually poorly defined but may involve not only the median nerve distribution of the digits but also the thenar region of the palm due to involvement of the palmar cutaneous branch of the median nerve. Deep tendon reflexes and cervical examination should be normal.

Anterior Interosseous Syndrome

To test the muscles that the anterior interosseous nerve innervates,[2] the clinician braces the metacarpophalangeal joint of the index finger and the patient is asked to flex only the distal phalanx. This isolates the action of the flexor digitorum profundus on the terminal phalanx and eliminates the action of the flexor digitorum superficialis. There is no terminal phalanx flexion if the anterior interosseous nerve is injured.

Another useful test is to ask the patient to make the "OK" sign.[3] In anterior interosseous syndrome, the distal interphalangeal joint cannot be flexed and this results in the index finger remaining relatively straight during this test (Fig. 3). The patient is asked to approximate forcefully the finger pulps of the first and second digits. The patient with weakness of the flexor pollicis longus and digitorum profundus muscles cannot touch with the pulp of the fingers, but rather the entire volar surfaces of the digits are in contact. This is due to the paralysis of the flexor pollicis longus and flexor digitorum profundus of the second digit. The pronator quadratus is difficult to isolate clinically, but an attempt can be made by flexing the forearm and asking the patient to resist supination. Sensation and deep tendon reflexes should be normal.

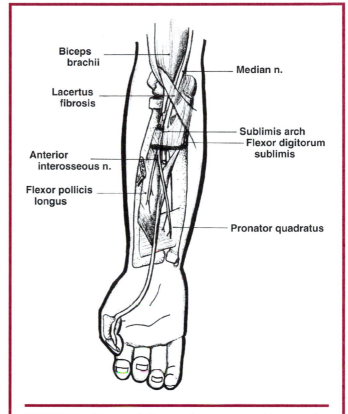

FIGURE 2. Course of the median nerve and its anterior interosseous branch.

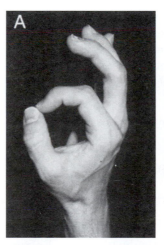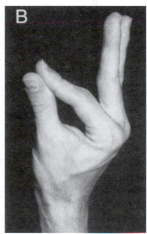

FIGURE 3. The anterior interosseous nerve innervates the flexor pollicis longus, as well as the flexor digitorum profundus to the index and long fingers. *A,* It is responsible for flexion on the thumb interphalangeal (IP) joint and the index finger distal IP joint. *B,* An injury to the median nerve high in the forearm or to the anterior interosseous branch of the median nerve results in inability to forcefully flex these joint. (From Concannon MJ: Common Hand Problems in Primary Care. Philadelphia, Hanley & Belfus, 1999, p 137, with permission.)

Functional Limitations

Pronator Teres Syndrome

In pronator teres syndrome, there is clumsiness, loss of dexterity, and a feeling of weakness in the hand. This may lead to functional limitations both at home and work. Repetitive elbow motions such as hammering, cleaning fish, serving tennis balls, and rowing are most likely to provoke symptoms.

Anterior Interosseous Syndrome

As weakness develops in anterior interosseous syndrome, there is loss of dexterity and pinching motion with difficulty picking up small objects with the first two digits. Activities of daily living, such as buttoning shirts and tying shoelaces, can be impaired. Patients may have difficulty with typing, handwriting, cooking, and so on.

Diagnostic Studies

Pronator Teres Syndrome

Electrodiagnostic testing (nerve conduction studies and EMG) is the "gold standard" for confirming pronator teres syndrome.[1] Nerve conduction studies may be abnormal in the median nerve distribution; however, the diagnosis may be best established by EMG studies demonstrating membrane instability (including increased insertional activity, fibrillation and positive sharp waves at rest, wide and high amplitude polyphasics on minimal contraction, and decreased recruitment pattern on maximal contraction) of the median nerve muscles below and above the wrist in the forearm, but with *sparing of the pronator teres*.

Imaging studies (e.g., x-ray, CT, and MRI) are used to exclude alternative diagnoses.

Anterior Interosseous Syndrome

Electrodiagnostic studies may also help establish the diagnosis of anterior interosseous syndrome.[3] Generally, routine motor and sensory studies are normal. The most appropriate technique is surface electrode recording from the pronator quadratus muscle with median nerve stimulation at the antecubital fossa. On EMG, findings of membrane instability are restricted to the flexor pollicis longus, flexor digitorum profundus (of the second and third digits), and pronator quadratus.

Again, imaging studies exclude other diagnoses.

Differential Diagnosis

Pronator Teres Syndrome

Carpal tunnel syndrome.

Cervical radiculopathy, particularly lesions affecting C6 or C7

Thoracic outlet syndrome with involvement of the medial cord

Elbow arthritis

Epicondylitis

Anterior Interosseous Syndrome

Paralytic brachial plexus neuritis

Entrapment or rupture of the tendon of the flexor pollicis longus

Rupture of the flexor pollicis longus and flexor digitorum profundus

Treatment

Initial

Pronator Teres Syndrome

Treatment is initially conservative, with rest and avoidance of the offending repetitive trauma.[2] NSAIDs/COX-2 inhibitors may help with pain and inflammation. Analgesics may be used for pain. Low-dose tricyclic anti-depressants may be used for pain and to help with sleep. Anti-seizure medications are also often used for neuropathic pain (e.g., carbamazepine, gabapentin, etc.).

Anterior Interosseous Syndrome

Treatment of the anterior interosseous syndrome depends on the cause.[2] Penetrating wounds require immediate exploration and repair. Impending Volkmann's contracture demands immediate decompression. In spontaneous cases associated with specific occupations, a trial of non-operative therapy is indicated. If spontaneous improvement does not occur by 6 to 8 weeks, consideration should be given to surgical exploration.

Conservative management includes avoiding the activity that exacerbates the symptoms. Pharmacologic treatment is similar to pronator teres syndrome.

Rehabilitation

Pronator Teres Syndrome

A splint that can put the thumb in an abducted, opposed position, such as a C bar, or a thumb poststatic orthosis can be utilized (Fig. 4),[4,5,8] and taping the index and middle fingers in a buddy splint to stabilize the lack of distal interphalangeal flexion may be helpful.

Rehabilitation may include modalities such as ultrasound, electrical stimulation, iontophoresis, and phonophoresis. The patient can be instructed in ice massage, as well. Once the acute symptoms have subsided, physical or occupational therapy can focus on exercises to improve forearm flexibility, muscle strength responsible for thumb abduction, opposition, and wrist radial flexion.

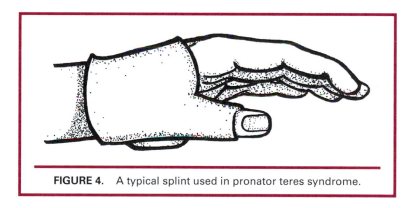

FIGURE 4. A typical splint used in pronator teres syndrome.

Anterior Interosseous Syndrome

Resting the arm by immobilizing the arm in a splint may be tried (Fig. 5).[7] If the symptoms subside, conservative physical or occupational therapy, including physical modalities as previously described and exercises to improve strength and function of the pronator quadratus, flexor digitorum profundus, and flexor pollicis longus, can be initiated.

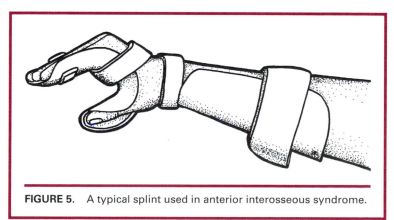

FIGURE 5. A typical splint used in anterior interosseous syndrome.

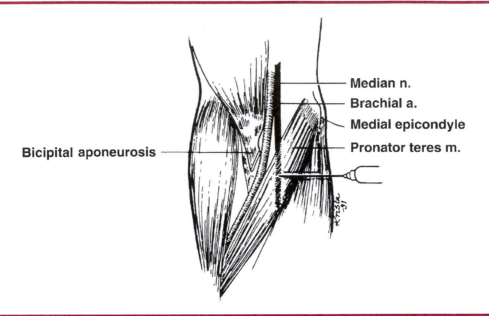

FIGURE 6. Pronator teres syndrome nerve block. At the elbow crease, make a mark at the midpoint between the medial epicondyle and the biceps tendon. Then, under sterile conditions insert a 25-gauge, 1.5-inch disposable needle into the pronator teres muscle approximately 2 cm below the mark or at the point of maximal tenderness in the muscle. Confirmation of needle placement can be done using a nerve stimulator. Then, inject 3–5 ml cortico-steroid/anestheic solution (e.g., 2 ml of methylprednisolone [40 mg/cc] combined with 2 ml of 1% licocaine). Post-injection care may include icing for 10–15 minutes and splinting the wrist and forearm in a functional position for a few days. Also, the patient should be cautioned to avoid aggressive use of the arm for at least 1–2 weeks. (From Lennard TA: Pain Procedures in Clinical Practice, 2nd ed. Philadelphia, Hanley & Belfus, 2000, p 98, with permission.)

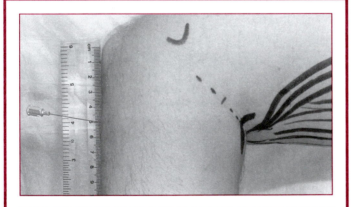

FIGURE 7. Anterior interosseous nerve block. The anterior interosseous nerve can be blocked using either an anterior or posterior approach. For the posterior approach, the posterior elbow is exposed and the forearm is placed in neutral. Under sterile conditions using a 2-inch, 25-gauge disposable needle, inject 3–5 ml of a corticosteroid/anesthetic solution (e.g., 2 ml of methylprednisolone [40 mg/cc]) approximately 5 cm distal to the tip of the olecranon. The needle should penetrate about 3.5–5 cm toward the biceps tendon insertion at the radius. A nerve stimulator is necessary to ensure proper placement. Post-injection care is similar to that of the pronator teres nerve block. (From Lennard TA: Pain Procedures in Clinical Practice, 2nd ed. Philadelphia, Hanley & Belfus, 2000, p 99, with permission.)

Procedures

In both anterior interosseous and pronator teres syndromes, a median nerve block may be attempted (Figs. 6 and 7).

Surgery

Pronator Teres Syndrome

If symptoms fail to resolve, surgical release of the pronator teres muscle and any constricting bands (ligament of Struthers and lacertus fibrosis) should be considered with direct exploration of the area. An S-shaped incision is typically utilized to extensively expose the entire median nerve from the forearm to the hand.

Anterior Interosseous Syndrome

If spontaneous improvement does not occur by 6 to 8 weeks, consideration should be given to surgical exploration. The surgical technique for exploration is exposure of the median nerve directly beneath the pronator teres or separating this muscle from the flexor carpi radialis, identifying the anterior interosseous nerve, and releasing the offending structures.

If surgical decompression was performed and failed to resolve the weakness, tendon transfers may be considered.

Potential Disease Complications

Pronator Teres Syndrome

Disease-related complications, if the condition is left unresolved, include permanent loss of the use of the pinch grasp, lack of wrist flexion, and incessant pain.

Anterior Interosseous Syndrome

If allowed to persist, this syndrome will result in an inability to perform the pinch grasp.

Potential Treatment Complications

Use of anti-inflammatory medications such as NSAIDs can induce gastric, renal, and hepatic side effects. COX-2 inhibitors may have fewer gastric side effects. Local steroid injections can induce skin depigmentation, local atrophy, or infection. Surgical complications include infection, bleeding, and injury to surrounding structures.

References
1. Liveson J: Peripheral Neurology—Case Studies in Electrodiagnosis, 2nd ed. Philadelphia, FA Davis, 1991, p 23–26.
2. DawsonD, Hallett M, Millender L: Entrapment Neuropathies, 2nd ed. Boston, Little, Brown, 1990, pp. 97–123.
3. Dumitru D: Electrodiagnostic Medicine. Philadelphia, Hanley & Belfus, 1994, pp 864–867.
4. Braddom, R: Physical Medicine and Rehabilitation. Philadelphia, W.B. Saunders, 1996, pp 328–329.
5. Hunter J, Mackin E, Callahan A (eds): Rehabilitation of the Hand: Surgery and Therapy, 4th ed. St. Louis, Mosby–Year Book, 1995, pp 686–690.
6. Boscheinen-Morrin, Judith, The Hand Fundamentals of Therapy, 2nd ed. Wobrun, Butterman-Heinemann, 1999, pp 87–93.
7. Trombly C (ed): Occupational Therapy for Physical Dysfunction, 4th ed. Philadelphia, Lippincott Williams & Wilkins, 1997, pp 556–558.
8. Lennard T: Physiatric Procedures in Clinical Practice. Philadelphia, Hanley & Belfus, 1995, pp 140–142.

23 Olecranon Bursitis

Sarah Shubert, MD
Charles Cassidy, MD

Synonyms

Miner's elbow
Student's elbow
Draftsman's elbow
Dialysis elbow
Elbow bursitis

ICD-9 Code

726.23
Olecranon bursitis

Definition

Olecranon bursitis is a swelling of the subcutaneous, synovial lined sac that overlies the olecranon process. The bursa functions to cushion the tip of the olecranon and reduce friction between the olecranon and the overlying skin during elbow motion. Because of the paucity of soft tissue covering the elbow, the olecranon bursa is susceptible to injury.

The causes of olecranon bursitis can be classified as traumatic, inflammatory, septic, and idiopathic.[1] Traumatic bursitis may result from a single, direct blow to the elbow or from repetitive stress. Football players, particularly those who play on artificial turf, are at risk for developing acute bursitis. More commonly, repeated minor trauma from direct pressure on the elbow or elbow motion is responsible for the problem. Trauma is thought to stimulate increased vascularity, resulting in bursal fluid production and fibrin coating of the bursal wall.[2] Persons engaged in certain occupations or certain activities are susceptible to olecranon bursitis, including auto mechanics, gardeners, plumbers, carpet-layers, students, gymnasts, wrestlers, and dart-throwers. Interestingly, approximately 7% of hemodialysis patients develop olecranon bursitis.[3] Repeated, prolonged positioning of the elbow and anticoagulation appear to be contributing factors.

Inflammatory causes include diseases that affect the bursa primarily, such as rheumatoid arthritis, gout, and chondrocalcinosis. Olecranon bursitis is commonly seen in rheumatoid patients, in whom the bursa may actually communicate with the affected elbow joint. Crystal-induced olecranon bursitis may be difficult to differentiate from septic bursitis.

Septic olecranon bursitis comprises 20% of olecranon bursitis.[4] The source is most often transcutaneous, and about half have identifiable breaks in the skin. When positive, cultures of the bursal fluid usually contain *Staphylococcus aureus*.[5] Sepsis is unusual. Both underlying bursal disease (gout, rheumatoid arthritis, chondrocalcinosis) and systemic conditions such as diabetes mellitus, uremia, alcoholism, intravenous drug use, and steroid therapy are considered predisposing factors.

In approximately 25% of cases, no identifiable cause of the olecranon bursitis is found. Presumably, repetitive, minor irritation is responsible for the bursal swelling.

Symptoms

Painless swelling is the chief complaint in non-inflammatory, aseptic olecranon bursitis. When symptomatic, patients usually have discomfort when the elbow is flexed beyond 90 degrees and have trouble resting on the elbow. Moderate to severe pain is the predominant complaint of patients with septic or crystal-induced olecranon bursitis. These patients may also have fever, malaise, and limited elbow motion.

Physical Examination

The physical examination varies somewhat depending on the underlying condition. With non-inflammatory aseptic bursitis, a non-tender fluctuant mass is present over the tip of the elbow (Fig. 1). Elbow motion is usually full and painless. With chronic bursitis, the fluctuance may be replaced with a thickened bursa (Fig. 2).

The distinction between crystal-induced and septic bursitis may be subtle. Both conditions may produce tender fluctuance, induration, swelling, warmth, and local erythema. Elbow flexion may be somewhat limited, though not as limited as with septic arthritis of the elbow joint. Fever or a break in the skin over the elbow are important clues to an underlying septic process (Fig. 3). Cellulitis extending distally along the forearm is also more likely to be due to an infection.

In inflammatory cases, pain inhibition may produce mild weakness of elbow flexion and extension. Sensation and distal pulses are unaffected. Examination of other joints should also be normal.

Functional Limitations

Functional limitations vary depending on the underlying diagnosis. Traumatic olecranon bursitis usually causes minimal functional limitation. Patients may note some mild discomfort with direct pressure over the tip of the elbow (e.g., when sitting

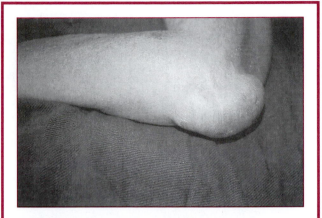

FIGURE 1. Atraumatic olecranon bursitis in a 55-year-old female. A large fluctuant mass is present.

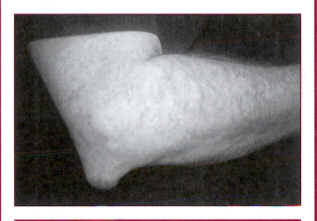

FIGURE 2. Chronic gouty olecranon bursitis. The prominence at the tip of the elbow is firm with thinning of the overlying skin.

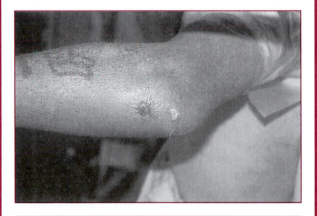

FIGURE 3. Septic olecranon bursitis. Cellulitis is present over a wide area. The white scab at the tip of the elbow represents the site of the penetrating injury. Distally, the draining area of granulation tissue developed at the site of needle aspiration. Aspiration of the bursa should be done by using a long needle inserted well away from the fluctuant area.

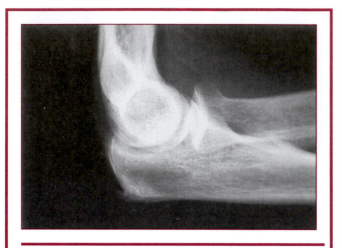

FIGURE 4. Lateral radiograph of the elbow in a patient with chronic olecranon bursitis. Note the olecranon spur.

at a desk or resting their arm on the armrest of a chair or in the car). With crystal-induced and septic bursitis, pain is the predominant issue. Patients may have trouble sleeping and have difficulty with most activities of daily living that involve the affected extremity (e.g., dressing, grooming, cleaning, shopping, and carrying packages).

Diagnostic Studies

The diagnosis of aseptic, non-inflammatory olecranon bursitis is usually straightforward, based on a characteristic appearance on physical examination. In this setting, additional studies are not usually necessary. However, plain radiographs may demonstrate an olecranon spur in about one third of cases (Fig. 4). Because this is an extra-articular process, a joint effusion is not present.

If crystal-induced or septic bursitis is suspected, aspiration of the bursal fluid is usually indicated. The fluid should be sent for cell count, gram stain and culture, and crystal analysis. Acute, traumatic bursal fluid typically has a serosanguineous appearance, containing fewer than 1000 white blood cells (WBCs) per high-power field, with a predominance of monocytes. Infected bursal fluid usually contains an increased WBC count, with a high percentage of polymorphonuclear cells. The gram stain is positive in only 50% of septic cases. Even in the setting of infection, the fluid should be examined under a polarizing microscope, since simultaneous infectious and crystal-induced arthritis can occur.[6]

A complete blood cell count and serum uric acid level may provide supportive information in confusing cases, although a normal serum WBC count does not preclude septic bursitis.

MRI may be of some value to rule out osteomyelitis of the olecranon in longstanding cases of septic bursitis. The use of MRI may also help to clarify the diagnosis for unusual masses about the elbow.

Differential Diagnosis

Rheumatoid nodule   Lipoma
Tophus   Elbow synovitis
Olecranon spur

Treatment

Initial

Treatment of traumatic olecranon bursitis begins with prevention of further injury to the involved elbow. An elastic elbow pad provides compression and protects the bursa. The patient should be counseled on ways of protecting the elbow at work and during recreation. NSAIDs/COX-2 inhibitors are usually prescribed. Traumatic, non-inflammatory bursitis usually resolves with this treatment.[7] Occasionally, when the bursa is very large, aspiration of the bloody fluid will be a first-line treatment. This is followed by applying a compressive wrap and splint for several days.

In suspected cases of septic olecranon bursitis, it is important to palpate for fluctuance. If a fluid collection is appreciated, the bursa should be aspirated (see the *Procedures* Section). When cellulitis over the tip of the elbow is present without an obvious collection, empiric treatment with antibiotic therapy to cover penicillin-resistant *Staphylococcus aureus*, the most common offender, is recommended. (Less common offenders are are Group A *Streptococcus* and *S. epidermidis*.) The decision whether to use oral or intravenous antibiotics depends on the appearance of the elbow, signs of systemic illness, and the general health of the patient. The elbow should be splinted in a semi-flexed position (~60 degrees) without pressure on the olecranon. NSAIDs/COX-2 inhibitors may be prescribed unless contraindicated as empiric treatment for gout and pseudogout. When final culture results return, the antibiotic therapy should be adjusted appropriately. Outpatient cases should be followed very closely, with any changes in the size of the bursa and the quality of the overlying skin noted; oral antibiotic therapy should continue for at least 10 days.

Patients with extensive infection or underlying bursal disease, systemic disease, or immunosuppression and outpatients refractory to oral treatment should be hospitalized for treatment with an intravenous cephalosporin. In one study, the average duration of intravenous therapy was 4.4 days if symptoms had been present for less than 1 week and 9.2 days if longer than 1 week.[8] The conversion to oral antibiotics should occur only after consistent improvement is seen in the appearance of the patient and the elbow. Serial aspirations may also constitute part of the therapy, or alternatively, some clinicians use a suction irrigation system placed into the bursa. Surgical consultation is recommended by the authors if the bursitis has failed to improve within several days of appropriate management.

Rehabilitation

Since the process is extra-articular, permanent elbow stiffness is not usually a problem. Physical or occupational therapy for gentle range of motion may be indicated once the olecranon wound has clearly healed. Extreme flexion should be avoided early on because this position puts tension on the already compromised skin. If prolonged immobilization is necessary to permit the soft tissues to heal, therapy may include range of motion and strengthening of the arm and forearm.

Patients who have traumatic or recurrent olecranon bursitis should be counseled on ways to modify their home and work activities to eliminate irritation to the bursa. This might include the use of ergonomic equipment such as forearm rests (also called data arms) that do not contact the elbow. In some instances, vocational retraining may be indicated.

Procedures

Needle aspiration is therapeutic as well as diagnostic and usually reduces symptoms (Fig. 5). It can be performed for traumatic bursitis patients if they have symptoms compromising their regular activities and should be done (as previously described) for patients in whom inflammatory or septic causes are suspected.

The elbow should be prepared in a sterile fashion. The skin is infiltrated locally with 1% lidocaine (Xylocaine). To minimize the risk of persistent drainage following aspiration, it is recommended to insert a long 18-gauge needle at a point well proximal to the tip of the elbow. The bursa should be

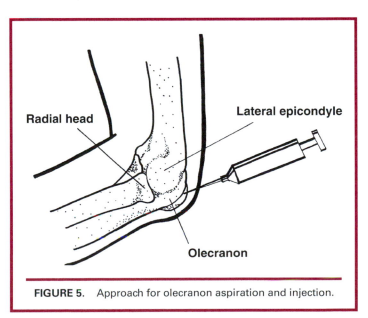

FIGURE 5. Approach for olecranon aspiration and injection.

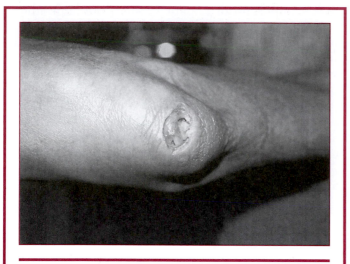

FIGURE 6. Untreated septic bursitis with a large olecranon ulcer. The periosteum of the olecranon is visible in the wound. This problem is very difficult to manage, and often requires flap coverage.

drained as completely as possible. The fluid should be sent for gram stain, culture and sensitivity, cell count, and crystal analysis.

Post-injection care should include local icing for 10 to 20 minutes. A sterile compressive dressing is then applied, followed by an anterior plaster splint that maintains the elbow in 60 degrees flexion.

Corticosteroid injections into the bursa have been proven to hasten the resolution of traumatic and crystal-induced olecranon bursitis.[9] However, the risk of complications is high, including infection, skin atrophy, and chronic local pain. Consequently, the routine use of steroid injections for olecranon bursitis is not recommended.

Surgery

Surgery is rarely indicated for traumatic olecranon bursitis. Chronic drainage of bursal fluid is the most common indication for surgery.[1] Bursectomy is conventionally done through an open technique, although a recently developed arthroscopic method has shown some promise. Surgery is usually curative for both traumatic and septic bursitis. However, the success rates are very different for patients with rheumatoid arthritis—surgery provides successful relief for 5 years in only 40% of rheumatoid arthritis patients versus 94% of non-rheumatoid patients.[10]

After surgery, suction drains are often placed for several days. Splinting of the elbow at 60 degrees of flexion or greater for 2 weeks is thought to help prevent recurrence.

Potential Disease Complications

Septic bursitis poses the greatest threat with regard to disease complications. If neglected, the infection may thin the overlying skin and eventually erode through it (Fig. 6). This complication is quite difficult to manage, often requiring extensive debridement and flap coverage. Persistent infection can also result in osteomyelitis of the olecranon process. Immunocompromised patients are at risk of sepsis from olecranon bursitis. Necrotizing fasciitis originating from a septic olecranon bursitis, although rare, may prove to be fatal.

Potential Treatment Complications

Analgesics, NSAIDs, and COX-2 inhibitors have well-known side effects that most commonly affect the gastric, hepatic, and renal systems. Persistent drainage from a synovial fistula is an uncommon complication of aspiration of the olecranon bursa; however, this problem is serious enough to discourage the routine aspiration of olecranon bursal fluid in non-inflammatory conditions. Complications of steroid injection, as described earlier, can be serious. In addition, wound problems are the major complication associated with surgical treatment of olecranon bursitis. Because of the superficial location of the olecranon and the tenuous blood supply of the overlying skin, wound healing can be difficult. Malnourished and chronically ill patients are especially at risk for surgical complications.

References

1. Morrey BF: Bursitis. In Morrey BF (ed): The Elbow and its Disorders, 3rd ed. Philadelphia, W.B. Saunders, 2000, pp 901–908.
2. Canoso JJ: Idiopathic or traumatic olecranon bursitis. Clinical features and bursal fluid analysis. Arthritis Rheum 1977;20:1213–1216.
3. Irby R, Edwards WM, Gatter RJ: Articular complications of hemotransplantation and chronic renal hemodialysis. Rheumatology 1975;2:91–99.
4. Jaffe L, Fetto JF: Olecranon bursitis. Contemp Orthop 1984;8:51–56.
5. Zimmerman B III, Mikolich DJ, Ho G Jr: Septic bursitis. Semin Arthritis Rheum 1995;24:391–410.
6. Gerster JC, Lagier R, Boivin G: Olecranon bursitis related to calcium pyrophosphate dihydrate deposition disease. Arthritis Rheum 1982;25:989–996.
7. Smith DL, McAfee JH, et al: Treatment of nonseptic olecranon bursitis. A controlled, blinded prospective trial. Arch Intern Med 1989;149:2527–2530.
8. Ho G, Su EY: Antibiotic therapy of septic bursitis. Arthritis Rheum 1981;24:905–911.
9. Weinstein PS, Canso JJ, Wohlgethan JR: Long-term follow-up of corticosteroid injection for traumatic olecranon bursitis. Ann Rheum Dis 1984;43:44–46.
10. Stewart NJ, Manzanares JB, Morrey BF: Surgical treatment of aseptic olecranon bursitis. J Shoulder Elbow Surg 1997;6:49–54.

24 Radial Neuropathy

Faren H. Williams, MD

Faren H. Williams, MD

Synonyms

Radial nerve palsy

Radial nerve compression

Wrist drop neuropathy

Finger/thumb extensor paralysis

Saturday night palsy

Supinator syndrome

Radial tunnel syndrome

ICD-9 Code

354.3
Lesion of the radial nerve

Definition

Lesions can occur anywhere along the radial nerve, which is the terminal branch off the posterior cord of the brachial plexus (Fig. 1). The radial nerve is primarily motor, although sensation can be affected with more proximal lesions if the posterior antebrachial cutaneous nerve, which branches off from the main nerve at the distal end of the spiral groove, is involved. With more distal nerve injury, the superficial radial sensory nerve may be affected and sensation on the radial innervated dorsum of the hand will be altered.[1,2] Traumatic events such as humerus fractures account for the more significant radial nerve lesions, and extrinsic compression on the radial nerve is one of the most common causes of radial nerve palsy. For example, the so-called Saturday night palsy occurs when an individual lies with the arm in an awkward position, such as over a sharp ledge or backrest of a chair, due to extreme fatigue or drug or alcohol intoxication.

With high axillary lesions, the triceps function is affected. The branches that innervate the triceps leave the radial nerve near the origin of the long head of the triceps above the spiral groove; the brachioradialis may also be affected by a proximal lesion because its innervation is at or just distal to the spiral groove of the humerus. In the spiral groove, the nerve and deep brachial artery lie on bare bone, which is why it is more susceptible to trauma or compression at that point.

Symptoms

The primary complaint is that of weakness in the affected arm. Patients may not report any pain initially, except as related to other problems, such as a humerus fracture.[3–5]

If the superficial radial sensory nerve is severed, as with a wrist laceration, the patient will have complete anesthesia over the distal radial nerve sensory distribution. If instead, the nerve is entrapped, the patient may complain of numbness and tingling (paresthesias) or burning and pain (dysesthesias) over the dorsoradial aspect of the forearm, wrist and dorsal hand, thumb, first web space, and index finger on the dorsum (Fig. 1). As the wrist flexes and extends, the radial sensory nerve stretches, and entrapment of the nerve may cause sharp, shooting pains. This wrist pain in general may be similar to that from a tenosynovitis. If this pain is significant, it may affect pinch and grip strength. The patient may also experience pain with pronation and supination of the forearm since these movements increase pressure on the radial sensory nerve as it exits between the brachioradialis and the extensor carpi radialis longus tendons.[1]

There are some spontaneous idiopathic radial neuropathies that present with attacks of pain along the course of the nerve, which are usually worse with exertion. Some patients do not develop muscle weakness, whereas others experience weakness of the radial innervated muscles after several months.

Physical Examination

With high axillary lesions, triceps (elbow extension) is weak. To evaluate triceps function, support the arm in the horizontal plane, and ask the patient to extend at the elbow. If the arm is at the patient's side, it may appear that some triceps are contracting, even though the only muscle working is the biceps. To determine whether patients have antigravity triceps strength, ask them to extend their arm up to the ceiling. It is important to test the extent of weakness because many radial nerve injuries may be incomplete. Elbow flexion and supination should be tested and strength compared with the opposite side since the radial nerve innervates the brachioradialis and a portion of

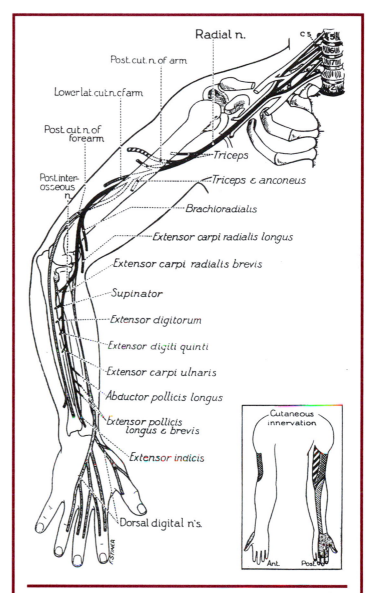

FIGURE 1. Neural branching of the radial nerve. Its origin in the axilla to the termination of its motor and sensory branches is shown. The inset demonstrates the cutaneous distribution of the various sensory branches of the radial nerve. (From Haymaker W, Woodhall B: Peripheral Nerve Injuries. Philadelphia, W.B. Saunders, 1953, with permission.)

the brachialis, which are elbow flexors. This weakness may be more subtle since the primary elbow flexors are supplied by the musculocutaneous nerve. Weakness of the triceps places the radial nerve lesion above the spiral groove, and decreased elbow flexion strength suggests a nerve injury at or near the spiral groove. The more proximal radial nerve problems may be caused by axillary crutches with compression on the nerve or an injury secondary to humeral artery catheterization. In the latter case, a hematoma may be responsible for the compression. One also needs to look for other causes, such as a tumor. Sensory loss is usually incomplete.[3,5]

Compression of the radial nerve in the spiral groove will produce findings of strong elbow extension combined with weak wrist and finger extension. The patient may also have sensory loss in the distribution of the radial nerve, including the dorsolateral aspect of the forearm, which is

TABLE 1. Extensor Tendon Compartments—Wrist*

Muscles	Insertion	Evaluation
1. Abductor pollicis longus Extensor pollicis brevis	Dorsal—base of thumb metacarpal Proximal phalanx—thumb	Bring thumb out to side
2. Extensor carpi radialis longus Extensor carpi radialis brevis	Dorsal base of index and middle metacarpals	Dorsiflex the wrist with the hand in a fist and apply resistance radially
3. Extensor pollicis longus	Distal phalanx of the thumb	Hand flat on table Lift only thumb
4. Extensor digitorum communis Extensor indicis proprius	Extensor hood and base of proximal phalanges of the ulnar four digits	Extend fingers with wrist in neutral Extend index finger
5. Extensor digiti minimi	Proximal phalanx of the little finger	Straighten little fingers with other fingers in fist
6. Extensor carpi ulnaris	Dorsal base of the fifth metacarpal	Wrist extension with ulnar deviation

* From American Society for Surgery of the Hand: The Hand: Examination and Diagnosis. New York, Churchill Livingstone, 1983.

innervated by the posterior antebrachial cutaneous nerve, which branches off from the radial nerve at the distal end of the spiral groove. With idiopathic radial neuropathies, patients may have painful trigger points focally along the course of the radial nerve, or they may have pain and tenderness along the entire nerve. Patients with this problem may have strangulation of the nerve within the spiral groove, which is identified during surgery. With a more proximal nerve injury, the triceps reflex may be decreased. With injuries around the spiral groove, the brachioradialis reflex may be decreased or absent.[3,6]

At the elbow, the radial nerve divides into two terminal branches: (1) the superficial branch—the superficial radial sensory nerve and (2) the deep branch—the posterior interosseous nerve. More distal lesions cause lack of wrist and/or finger and thumb extension. If only the posterior interosseous branch is affected, then the patient will have weakness of finger extension.

Posterior interosseous nerve or *supinator syndrome* is due to compression that is distal and may be caused by cysts, bursae, ganglia, or synovitis within the elbow joint or trauma to the elbow and/or radial head. The patient will have intact elbow extension and flexion and wrist extension with radial deviation since the extensor carpi radialis longus and brevis muscles are spared, but the extensor carpi ulnaris muscle is not working. Sensation to the posterior lateral hand will be intact. The patient may experience lateral elbow pain with elbow, wrist, and middle finger extension against resistance. The point of maximum tenderness to palpation will be over the mobile extensor muscle mass, 1 to 2 cm distal to the lateral epicondyle, unlike tennis elbow, which is generally more tender directly over the epicondyle. Resisted supination is also painful with a posterior interosseous nerve palsy. In a partial posterior interosseous palsy, the index finger may have some preserved extension compared with the other finger extensors and will stick out straight.[2,6]

Depending on the extent of nerve injury, there may be some visible autonomic changes in the distribution of the radial nerve. These include a decrease in sweating and some skin color changes, compared with skin innervated by other upper extremity nerves.

Finkelstein's test, in which the thumb is enclosed in a clenched fist and the wrist passively stretched, may cause pain with a radial sensory neuropathy, as well as with de Quervain's tenosynovitis.

Functional Limitations

The patient will have decreased wrist range of motion, decreased hand grip, and less pinch strength. Depending on the loss of range, some patients may have difficulty with functional activities, such as buttoning and writing, especially if their dominant hand is affected. Patients who do more physical work will have problems with using tools such as wrenches, screwdrivers, and hammers, all of which require some torque about the wrist, good grip strength, and hand motion.[6]

Diagnostic Studies

Electrodiagnostic studies (EMG and nerve conduction studies) are the "gold standard" in evaluating radial nerve injuries, since they can help to differentiate between partial and complete lesions and provide information regarding the extent of axonal loss and/or demyelination. Complete axonotmesis lesions lead to total lack of motor conduction and total loss of the sensory action potential. Therefore, it is important to study both the motor and sensory components of the radial nerve.[1,6] EMG will provide more information about acute denervation if the study is done 3 to 4 weeks after the injury since it takes that long for membrane instability to evolve, although membrane instability in muscles closer to the site of the lesion may be detected after 10 to 14 days.

Electrodiagnostic studies can help to establish both the diagnosis and the prognosis for radial nerve injuries. Additionally they can help to rule out other nerve injuries (e.g., cervical radiculopathies, brachial plexopathies, carpal tunnel syndrome). It may be worthwhile to repeat these studies 2 to 3 months after the initial study in order to monitor the healing process.[7]

Imaging studies such as x-rays and MRIs are used to rule out other diagnoses or to assess whether a radial nerve injury is being caused by a mass (e.g., ganglion, tumor).

Differential Diagnosis

Cervical radiculopathy (C5 to C8)

Lesion of the posterior cord/brachial plexopathy

Brachial neuritis

Axillary nerve injury

Extensor tendon rupture

Epicondylitis

Tenosynovitis—extensor pollicus longus (de Quervain's)

Upper extremity extensor compartment syndrome

Hematoma

Tumor

Carpal tunnel syndrome

Ulnar neuropathy

Peripheral neuropathy

Treatment

Initial

Radial nerve injuries can take 6 to 12 months to heal. In some instances, only partial recovery will occur, regardless of treatment.

If there is swelling associated with the initial injury, then nonsteroidal anti-inflammatory drugs (NSAIDs, including cyclooxygenase-2 [COX-2] inhibitors) may be helpful. If there was significant traction on the nerve and possible muscle spasm, then muscle relaxants may be beneficial. Since some muscle relaxants are sedating, they may also help provide more restful sleep.

If there is pain associated with the nerve injury, then medications, such as some antidepressants or anticonvulsants, may be efficacious. If the pain is more of a hypersensitivity, then desensitization techniques may be helpful.

Transcutaneous electrical nerve stimulation (TENS) may help to decrease pain.[12]

Rehabilitation

Supervised physical therapy or occupational therapy on an ongoing basis is usually not necessary initially, except a therapist trained in hand therapy would need to be involved in making special splints. Aggressive activity should not be initiated too soon in the denervated muscle because newly reinnervated neuromuscular units may be damaged, especially if there are too few functioning motor units to support the increased level of activity.[9] Studies found that increasing the activity 4 weeks after nerve injury was more favorable for recovery than 3 weeks after injury.[8]

Splints may help to keep denervated extensor muscles from staying in an overstretched position and may prevent shortening of the finger flexor tendons. They can help to prevent joint contractures and allow for more functional usage of the hand as a helper in activities such as grooming or dressing. Splints also prevent the patient from overusing the hand. A splint that allows tenodesis will facilitate finger extension with wrist flexion, and wrist extension with finger flexion. A spring-loaded extensor brace may help improve function further; this is a static wrist extension splint with dynamic extension outriggers for the fingers and thumbs. Patient compliance and tolerance for a more bulky orthotic may be less, especially if the affected hand/arm is the non-dominant one, so this should be considered before prescribing such devices.

Later, if there has been significant loss of range of motion in the upper extremity from immobilization with capsular tightness, more intense therapy may be indicated. Certain modalities such as ultrasound, in conjunction with prolonged passive stretch for 20 to 30 minutes 4 times a day, may help to improve range of motion. Electrical stimulation may help to prevent muscle atrophy, but it has not been shown to enhance reinnervation, and it may hinder terminal sprouting of motor axons.[8] In addition, too much discomfort associated with the intensity, duration, and frequency (Hz) of current required to activate denervated muscle may be a problem.

If there is more limited range of motion, then serial, static splinting or casting or use of rubber bands on a dynamic splint may offer additional improvement. Patients who have been immobilized for a period of time also lose muscle strength, and exercises help regain some of the strength. If the patient has altered sensation that makes the arm or hand painful to touch, then desensitization techniques administered by a therapist may be helpful.[6,9]

Postoperative rehabilitation depends on the type of surgery done, decompression versus tendon transfer, and the extent of concomitant problems. Some immobilization after tendon transfers is indicated to allow for healing, but it should be kept at a safe minimum to prevent adhesions about the transferred tendon. After tendon transfer, prolonged tension on the tendon should be avoided to prevent gap formation, with subsequent potential for rupture with remobilization, at the site of tendon anastomosis.

It is important to begin passive range-of-motion exercises as soon as feasible after surgery, progressing to active assisted and active range-of-motion exercises to prevent further loss of function.

Postoperative prevention of edema is also important, along with neuromuscular re-education for using the transferred muscle for its new function. The latter begins approximately 3 weeks after the surgery. The patient should be asked to produce the motion originally done by the transferred muscle, not the one for which the tendon transfer was done. The therapist then blocks manually the original so that the transferred tendon can perform the new motion. The patient needs to first perceive the new kinesthetic sensations, and then with repetitious practice, develop the new motor skill. When these motions can be done consistently, functional training with light functional activities is started. Six weeks after surgery, some resistance which is used during normal activities, can be applied. Therapy needs to be consistent and regular to prevent deterioration of the new motor patterns. Range of motion throughout the therapy sessions can be increased over a 6-week period.[9,10]

Procedures

Anesthetic blocks into the most painful areas may help decrease pain. Likewise, focal trigger point injections may be effective if these points can be palpated and palpation of them reproduces the pain.[11]

Surgery

If there is some suspicion of involvement of the radial nerve with a humerus fracture or if the nerve is compressed by a tumor, etc., then surgery should be considered.[10] If the radial nerve appears completely severed on electrodiagnositc studies, then prompt surgical intervention to reanastomose the nerve may be indicated.

For most radial nerve injuries, one can consider surgery after a 3- to 6-month period of observation and conservative treatment. A variety of surgical approaches has been advocated in these instances; however, it is important to remember that recovery of the radial nerve can take up to 1 year or more without any surgical intervention.[10] Surgery is more appropriate for lesions closer to the spiral groove or in the more distal forearm. Response rates to surgery vary from 51% to more than 80%,[10] with the worst results being seen in patients with work-related injuries, longstanding epicondylar pain, and poor localization of symptoms on physical examination.

When patients have complete denervation of the radial nerve that does not improve over time and corresponding problems with functional activities of daily living, then tendon transfers to improve hand function should be considered.[9] Strength of the muscle to be transferred should at least be grade 4/5 since muscles may lose a grade of strength with the change in routing of the tendon. The goal is to improve function for the patient. There should be a preoperative program before a tendon transfer that aims to restore passive range of motion for the expected function of the transfer and includes maximal strengthening of the muscle to be transferred and training for conscious perception of kinesthetic sensations relating to neuromuscular re-education.

Potential Disease Complications

The radial nerve may not recover, and depending on the site of injury, the patient will have significant loss of upper extremity function, as previously described. Patients who do not continue to use the hand may be at risk for developing a reflex sympathetic dystrophy with more refractory pain and possibly swelling.[3]

Refractory neurogenic pain from the nerve injury itself and autonomic changes are always potential complications of peripheral nerve injury.

Potential Treatment Complications

Complications are related to the specific treatments. Any medications may cause side effects unique to that medication. With any injection or surgery, there is always the risk for infection, and the procedure may not lead to significant improvement in pain or function. With prolonged immobilization, the patient may develop a tight joint capsule at the wrist, elbow, or shoulder that is painful with motion, or the patient may develop a reflex sympathetic dystrophy with corresponding atrophic skin changes and pain. Both of these problems significantly limit the patient's ability to use that limb functionally and further impair the patient's independence with activities of daily living. The impairment is more limiting if it is in the patient's dominant hand and if the patient has a moderate-to-heavy duty physical job that involves forceful use of the hand and lifting. A patient who does not regain significant functional usage of the involved extremity may need to do a different type of work if the present job requires full arm movement and strength.

References

1. Dawson DM: Entrapment Neuropathies, 3rd ed. Philadelphia, Lippincott–Raven, 1999.
2. Oh J: Clinical Electromyography: Nerve Conduction Studies. Baltimore, University Park Press, 1984.
3. Cailliet R: Hand pain and impairment. Philadelphia, F.A. Davis, 1988.
3. Jenkins DB: Hollinshead's Functional Anatomy of the Limbs and Back. Philadelphia, W.B. Saunders, 1991.
5. Eaton CJ, Lister GD: Radial nerve compression. In Rayan GM (ed): Hand Clinics. Philadelphia, W.B. Saunders, 1992.
6. American Society for Surgery of the Hand: The Hand: Examination and Diagnosis. New York, Churchhill. Livingstone, 1983.
7. Delisa JA. Gans BM: Rehabilitation Medicine: Principles and Practice. Philadelphia, Lippincott-Raven, 1998.
8. Dumitru. Electrodiagnostic Medicine, 2nd ed. Philadelphia, Hanley & Belfus, 2002.
9. Herbison G: Treatment of peripheral neuropathies. Plenary session. Neuropathy: From genes to function. Philadelphia, American Association of Electrodiagnostic Medicine, 2000.
11. Hunter, J.M., Mackin, E.J., and Callahan, A.D. Rehabilitation of the hand: surgery and therapy. Mosby. Philadelphia, 1995.
10. Kottke FJ, Lehmann JF: Krusen's Handbook of Physical Medicine and Rehabilitation. Philadelphia, W.B. Saunders, 1990.
12. Wolf SL: Clinics in physical therapy. Electrotherapy. New York, Churchill Livingstone, 1981.

25 Ulnar Neuropathy (Elbow)

Wayne Stokes, MD

Synonyms

Cubital tunnel syndrome

Tardy ulnar palsy

Ulnar neuritis

Compression of the ulnar nerve

ICD-9 Code

354.2
Lesion of ulnar nerve

Definition

Compression, repetitive stretching, friction, or a direct blow to the ulnar nerve as it travels through the medial elbow may result in sensory and intrinsic motor changes in the hand and can be associated with elbow pain (Fig. 1). The superficial anatomic location and multiple potential sites of compression at the arcade of Struthers' ligament, cubital tunnel, and flexor carpi ulnaris aponeurosis (arcuate ligament) make the nerve vulnerable to injury with repetitive elbow flexion/extension or recurrent nerve subluxation at the elbow. Since the ulnar nerve lengthens with flexion, friction from a scarred ulnar collateral ligament, arthritis within the groove, traction at compression site, or valgus traction overload in a throwing athlete can contribute to the second most common neuropathy in the upper extremity.[1] Median neuropathy (carpal tunnel syndrome) at the wrist is the most common.

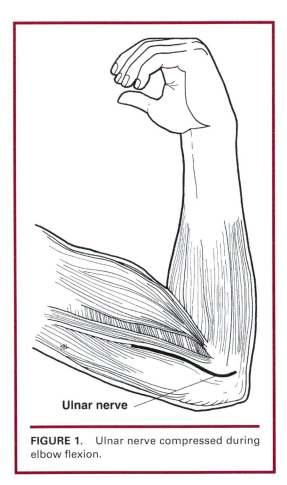

FIGURE 1. Ulnar nerve compressed during elbow flexion.

Symptoms

Patients report numbness and paresthesias in the little and ring fingers (Fig. 2). Hand clumsiness, decreased strength, and elbow pain with radiation down the forearm may be seen. The patient may report a

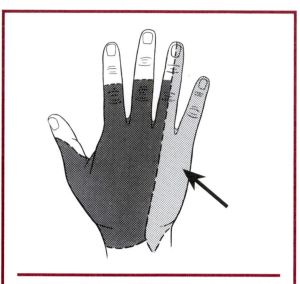

FIGURE 2. Patients with injury or pathology of the ulnar nerve complain of decreased sensation in the ulnar nerve distribution (*light grey area, arrow*). (From Concannon M: Common Hand Problems in Primary Care. Philadelphia, Hanley & Belfus, 1999, with permission.)

previous elbow trauma or surgery from years ago (tardy ulnar palsy).

Physical Examination

The medial elbow can be tender to palpation. Compression of the nerve in the ulnar groove behind the medial epicondyle may cause pain at the elbow and paresthesias in the ring and little fingers. The ulnar nerve may subluxate with flexion/extension of the elbow.[2] Sensory changes may occur in the ulnar distribution of the hand, although motor testing is usually normal. Subtle sensory changes can be highlighted through 2-point discrimination testing. The elbow flexion test involves holding both elbows in full flexion with full extension of the wrists. Onset of numbness and tingling in the ring and little fingers should be noted, compared with the other side, and the symptoms should resolve after release of full flexion. Intrinsic muscle weakness and muscle wasting may occur later (Fig. 3). Atrophy is best visualized at the web space between the thumb and index fingers (Fig. 4). Examination for ulnar collateral ligament laxity can be done in 30- to 40-degree flexion with valgus loading.

Functional Limitations

The patient may have a weak hand, clumsiness, or poor coordination. There can be medial elbow pain or ache with increase in activity. Resting the elbow on a hard surface or a prolonged flexion position may result in elbow pain and numbness in the ring and little fingers.

Differential Diagnosis

Medial epicondylitis
Carpal tunnel syndrome
Cervical radiculopathy
Thoracic outlet syndrome
Ulnar nerve entrapment at the wrist
Brachial plexopathy

Diagnostic Studies

X-rays of the elbow with cubital tunnel views should be obtained when symptoms persist 4 weeks or longer. These films may detect spurs, arthritic changes, and previous elbow trauma.

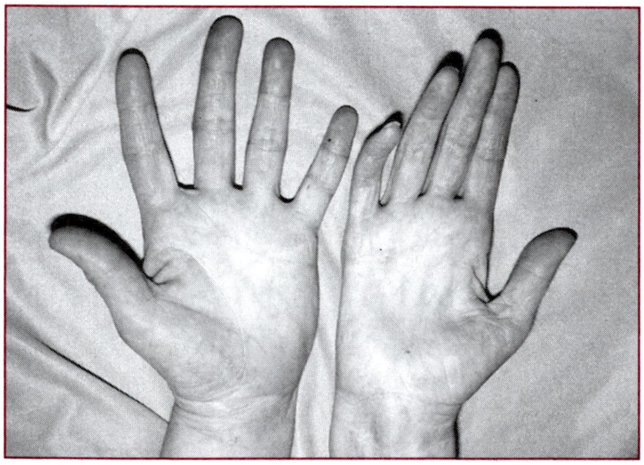

FIGURE 3. When evaluating hand musculature and possible atrophy, it is helpful to compare to the contralateral (uninjured) hand. In comparison, subtle differences may become quite obvious. Here, the atrophy is striking and dramatic. (From Concannon M: Common Hand Problems in Primary Care. Philadelphia, Hanley & Belfus, 1999, with permission.)

Electrodiagnostic testing (EMG and nerve conduction studies) can help locate and determine the extent of nerve compression across the elbow. They also can help localize and rule out alternative diagnoses (e.g., cervical root impingement, brachial plexopathy). Electrodiagnostic testing is most valuable when done at least 3 weeks after symptoms begin.

MRI with arthrogram may highlight tears of ulnar collateral ligament[3] and document more subtle soft tissue and bony pathology but is rarely necessary.

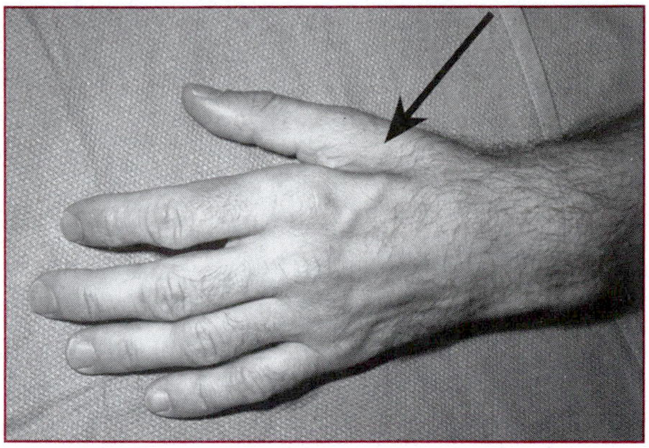

Treatment

Initial

Treatment initially involves rest and avoidance of prolonged or repetitive flexion at work (computer keyboard/mouse) and the athlete should refrain from repetitive valgus stress in throwing. Direct contact to the nerve should be decreased, which may be accomplished by avoiding resting the elbows on hard surfaces, such as desktops and counters. Elbow pads may be beneficial. Splinting at night in mild flexion can be accomplished with a towel wrapped around the elbow or with plastic splints. NSAIDs may be helpful.

FIGURE 4. It is not unusual for patients with cubital tunnel syndrome to present with signs of muscle atrophy. It is most noticeable at the first web space, where atrophy of the first dorsal interosseous muscle leaves a hollow between the thumb and the index rays (*arrow*). (From Concannon M: Common Hand Problems in Primary Care. Philadelphia, Hanley & Belfus, 1999, with permission.)

Rehabilitation

A rehabilitation program to increase strength of the forearm pronator and flexor muscles can be instituted. Flexibility exercises maintain range of motion and prevent muscle tightness. Advanced strengthening including eccentric and dynamic joint stabilization exercises may be added as tolerated.[4] Workstation modifications may be very helpful. Repositioning the desk chair, lowering the keyboard, moving the computer mouse to the unaffected hand, and substituting headphones for telephone handset may decrease prolonged/repetitive elbow flexion. Forearm rests that support the arms during typing are also helpful. Ideally, these armrests should not place any pressure at the elbow but should just give support at the forearm level. In athletes, altering throwing mechanics may decrease abnormal forces at the elbow.

Procedures

Procedures are not typically performed in ulnar neuropathy at the elbow.

Surgery

Failure of conservative care, including rest, splinting, therapy, and avoidance of provocative activities, may lead to surgery. The extent of pain, motor loss, and sensory abnormalities will also affect surgical planning. Surgery may include release of compression from the arcade of Struthers' ligaments to the aponeurosis of the flexor carpi ulnaris. The nerve usually is transposed anteriorly, either submuscularly or subcutaneously.[5] If the ulnar collateral ligament is damaged, its repair will also need to be addressed.[6]

Potential Disease Complications

Chronic pressure or repetitive traction on the ulnar nerve may lead to motor deficits, including hand weakness, poor coordination, intrinsic muscle atrophy, and sensory loss. Flexion contracture, valgus deformity, and chronic pain may develop at the elbow.

Potential Treatment Complications

The results of surgery are based on the extent of ulnar nerve compression, thoroughness of release of compression sites, and the degree of prior intrinsic muscle loss and previous sensory loss.[5,7] NSAIDs may cause gastric, hepatic, or renal complications.

References

1. Butters K, Singer K: Nerve lesions of the arm and elbow. In DeLee J, Drez D (ed): Orthopaedic Sports Medicine, Principles and Practice. Philadelphia, W.B. Saunders, 1994, pp 802–811.
2. Childress H: Recurrent ulnar nerve dislocation at the elbow. Clin Orthop 1975;180:168–173.
3. Timmerman L, Schwartz M, Andrews J: Preoperative evaluation of the ulnar collateral ligament by magnetic resonance imaging and computed tomography arthrography: Evaluation of 25 baseball players with surgical confirmation. Am J Sports Med 1994;22:26–32.
4. Wilk K, Chmielewski T: Rehabilitation of the elbow. In Canavan P (ed): Rehabilitation in Sports Medicine. Stamford, CT, Appleton & Lange, 1998, pp 237–256.
5. Dellon A: Review of treatment for ulnar nerve entrapment at the elbow. J Hand Surg 1989;14A:688–700.
6. Azar F, Andrews J, Wilk K, Groh D: Operative treatment of ulnar collateral ligament injuries of the elbow in athletes. Am J Sports Med 2000;28:16–23.
7. Jobe F, Fanton G: Nerve injuries. In Morrey B (ed): The Elbow and Its Disorders. Philadelphia, W.B. Saunders, 1985, p 497.

26 | de Quervain's Tenosynovitis

Alan F. Doyle, DO

Synonyms

Washerwomen's sprain

Stenosing tenosynovitis

Tenovaginitis

Tendinosis

ICD-9 Code

727.04
de Quervain tenosynovitis

Definition

Tenosynovitis of the first dorsal compartment of the wrist (Fig. 1) is a chronic inflammation of the extensor pollicis brevis (EPB) and abductor pollicis longus (APL) tendons. The condition was initially described by Fritz de Quervain in 1895.[1]

Symptoms

Patients complain of pain when using their thumb in either extension or grasping motions. Swelling is often present over the tendons on the thumb side of the wrist.[2] If persistent, the tendon sheath may thicken and constrict the tendon when the thumb is used. This may result in a triggering or locking phenomenon with thumb abduction or extension and can imply a more recalcitrant course.[3] Symptoms of paresthesias or numbness should alert the clinician that an alternative diagnosis is more likely (e.g., carpal tunnel syndrome, cervical radiculopathy).

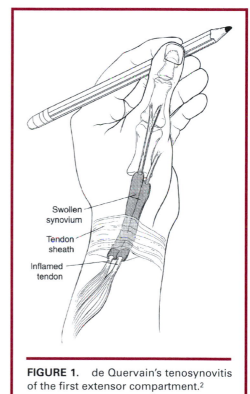

Swollen synovium

Tendon sheath

Inflamed tendon

FIGURE 1. de Quervain's tenosynovitis of the first extensor compartment.[2]

Physical Examination

On exam, pain, swelling, erythema, and tenderness are often present on the radial side of the wrist. The diagnosis is confirmed by pain that is exacerbated by passive wrist ulnar deviation while the thumb is flexed and the fingers curled around it (Finkelstein's test).[4] Strength, particularly grip and pinch strength, may be decreased due to pain or disuse secondary to pain. Sensation and deep tendon reflexes are normal.

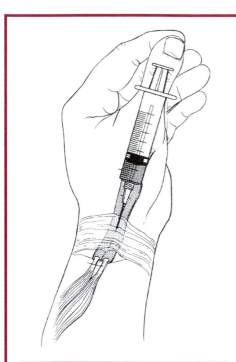

FIGURE 2. Under sterile conditions, using a 27-gauge, ⅝-inch needle, inject a mixture of 0.5 to 1 cc local anesthetic with 1 to 2 cc corticosteroid. The needle should be held at a 45-degree angle and in line with the two tendons. Advance the needle until it strikes the tendon, and then withdraw just slightly. The injected material should flow freely; if not, the needle is probably within the tendon and this should be avoided. After the injection, icing for 5 to 10 minutes is helpful. Thereafter, instruct the patient to ice the injected area for 20 minutes (2 to 3 times daily) for 1 to 2 weeks. It is advisable to give the patient a thumb spica splint to be worn most of the time for the first week postinjection and then intermittently during the next 2 to 3 weeks. An increase in pain for the first few days after the injection is typical.[2]

Functional Limitations

Limitations are associated with activities that require forceful grasp coupled with ulnar deviation or repetitive use of the thumb.[5] Some examples include griping a golf club or a tennis racket, as well as using a keyboard. In patients who are very symptomatic, even less strenuous activities, such as gripping a steering wheel while driving or turning a door knob, may be difficult due to pain.

Diagnostic Studies

Tenosynovitis of the wrist is a clinical diagnosis, but some authors recommend obtaining a wrist radiograph to rule out other potential causes of wrist pain.[2,4] Recently, ultrasonography is being used in the diagnosis of tendinitis because it is more sensitive than MRI in the detection of synovitis and tenosynovitis.[6]

Differential Diagnosis

Carpal joint arthritis	Triscaphoid arthritis
Rheumatoid arthritis	Intersection syndrome
Radial nerve injury	Ganglion cyst
Cervical radiculopathy	Scaphoid fracture
Carpal tunnel syndrome	Radioscaphoid arthritis
Kienbock's disease	

Treatment

Initial

Relative rest by avoiding activities that exacerbate pain in the wrist is the mainstay of treatment and should be prescribed for 1 to 2 weeks initially. In some cases a much longer period of time is necessary. In addition to rest, ice, elevation, and nonsteroidal anti-inflammatory drugs (NSAIDs), including cyclooxygenase-2 (COX-2) inhibitors, can decrease pain and inflammation.[5] Some clinicians prescribe a hand-based thumb spica splint to immobilize the metacarpophalangeal (MP) joint of the thumb. Inflammation may be reduced when the thumb MP joint is immobilized.[7]

Rehabilitation

For effective treatment results, the goal is to decrease inflammation and pain initially and then to strengthen the surrounding muscles so that symptoms do not return. A comprehensive physical or occupational therapy approach is helpful and should include pain relief modalities (e.g., ultrasound, iontophoresis), soft-tissue manipulation, worksite evaluation, and a home exercise program.[7]

Friction massage perpendicular to the tendon direction can also be beneficial. The return to full activity needs to occur slowly over time. Rehabilitation could follow the 10% rule (i.e., an increase in weight or repetitions by no more than 10% each week).[5]

The home exercise program should include gentle range-of-motion exercises, combined with a stretching program. The worksite evaluation can be done at the worksite or by having the patient bring in photos of the worksite. Typical recommendations for an office worker might include switching the computer mouse and phone to the unaffected side, using a track ball or foot computer mouse, and alternating thumbs that strike the space bar on the computer keyboard.

Procedure

A mixture of local anesthetic combined with an aqueous steroid preparation injected into the first dorsal compartment can provide significant relief of symptoms (Fig. 2). In one study, 60% of patients were treated successfully with one injection, and an additional 24% were pain free after two injections.[1] In general, two to three injections are standard for cases that don't completely resolve after the first injection. Failure to respond to conservative treatment or recurrent disease is an indication for surgical release.[4]

Surgery

The role for surgery in the treatment of de Quervain's tenosynovitis has changed in the past 15–20 years. Prior to 1985 nearly every writer on the topic supported surgery as the initial treatment for this condition.[8] However, given the popularity of local steroid therapy combined with its safety, cost-effectiveness, and absence of complications, surgery is now considered a second-line treatment.[9]

Potential Disease Complications

Patients who continue to "work through their pain," are at risk for developing an overuse syndrome. Fibrosis may eventually result from continued or repeated release of inflammatory products, leading to thick, unyielding, restrictive tendon sheaths or retinacular tunnels.[5] In a study of patients with de Quervain's tenosynovitis, the tendon sheaths were up to five times thicker than in controls from the deposition of dense fibrous tissue.[10]

Potential Treatment Complications

Analgesics, NSAIDs, and COX-2 inhibitors have well-known side effects that most commonly affect the gastric, hepatic, and renal systems. With any type of steroid injection there is a risk of bleeding, infection, and skin depigmentation. Repeated steroid injections have the potential to weaken the tendon and may cause a tendon rupture. Surgical treatment complications include radial nerve injury, incomplete retinacular release, and tendon subluxation.[9]

References
1. Rankin ME, Rankin EA: Injection therapy for management of stenosing tenosynovitis (de Quervain's disease). J Nat Med Assoc 1998;90:474–476.
2. Snider RK: Essentials of Musculoskeletal Care, 1st ed. Rosemont, IL, American Academy of Orthopedic Surgeons, 1997.
3. Alberton GM, High WA, Shin AY, Bishop AT: Extensor triggering in de Quervian's stenosing tenosynovitis. J Hand Surg 1999;24A(6):1311–1314.
4. Cooney WP, Linscheid RL, Dobyns JH: The wrist diagnosis and operative treatment, 1st ed. St Louis, Mosby, 1998.
5. Verdon ME: Overuse syndromes of the hand and wrist. Primary care. ClinOffice Practice 1996;23(2):306–310.
6. Grassi W, Filippucci E, Farina A, Cervini C: Sonographic imaging of tendons. Arthritis Rheum 2000;43(5):969–976.
7. Bensich S, Melicher S: De Quervain's management starts with differential diagnosis. Biomechanics 2000;7(5):63–70.
8. Kay NRM: De Quervain's disease changing pathology of changing perception. J Hand Surg Br, 2000;25B(1):65–69.
9. Kent TT, Eidelman D, Thomson JG: Patient satisfaction and outcome of surgery for de Quervain's tenosynovitis. J Hand Surg 1999;24A(5):1071–1077.
10. Clark MT, Lyall HA, Grant JW, et al: The histopathology of de Quervain's disease. J Hand Surg Br 1998;23B:732–734.

27 Dupuytren's Contracture

Jeffrey A. Strakowski, MD

Synonyms

Dupuytren's disease

ICD-9 Code

728.6
Dupuytren's contracture

Definition

Dupuytren's disease is characterized by shortening of the palmar fascia, leading to progressive flexion deformity of the palm and digits (Fig. 1). The nodule in the palm is the primary lesion in Dupuytren's contracture. It is a firm, soft tissue mass that is fixed to both the skin and the deeper fascia. It is characterized histologically by dense, non-inflammatory, chaotic cellular tissue and appears on the anterior aspect of the palmar aponeurosis. The myofibroblast is felt to be the key cell for tissue contraction in Dupuytren's disease.[1] As the nodule extends slowly, it induces shortening and tension on the longitudinal fascial bands of the palmar aponeurosis, resulting in cords of hypertrophied tissue. Dupuytren's disease is believed to begin in the overlying dermis.[2] Unlike the nodule, the chord is strikingly different histologically as it contains few to no myofibroblasts and few fibroblasts in a dense collagen matrix with less vascularity. Skin changes can be the earliest signs of Dupuytren's disease, which is characterized by thickening of the palmar skin and underlying subcutaneous tissue. Rippling of the skin can occur prior to the development of a digital flexion deformity.[3]

It has been suggested, in controversy, that Dupuytren's disease is related to manual labor and repetitive "microtrauma."[4] This suggestion has not held up under scrutiny, and it is now believed that microruptures are related to the contracture rather than a primary cause of it.[5] Cessation of manual labor can lead to acceleration of the disease, which has been noted in laborers after retirement.[6] Dupuytren's disease is known to have a genetic predisposition and is believed to be inherited as an autosomal dominant trait with variable penetrance.[7] Family history is often unreliable, as many individuals are unaware they have family members who have the condition. Dupuytren's disease has been termed "Viking's disease"[8] because it has a high prevalence in areas that were populated by the Vikings, including Scandinavia, Canada, and Western Europe, and in Australia, where the Vikings eventually migrated. It is very rare in non-Caucasian races. Dupuytren's disease occurs more commonly in the elderly but tends to be expressed more severely when it develops in younger patients. Women are affected half as often or less as men.[9] It has been associated with multiple other factors. There is no relationship to handedness; however, affected individuals tend to complain more frequently about the dominant hand. Other associations with the condition include increasing age, diabetes mellitus,[10] epilepsy,[11] alcohol consumption,[12] cigarette smoking,[13] HIV infection,[14] and Colles' fracture.

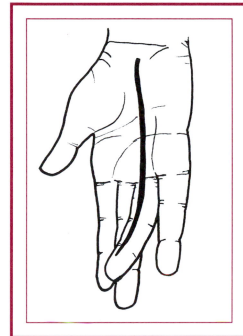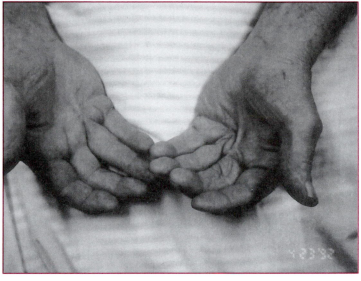

FIGURE 1. Dupuytren contracture of the ring finger.

There are secondary findings in Dupuytren's disease that are rarely seen, but when present suggest a strong Dupuytren's diathesis (genetic penetrance of the disease). These findings include knuckle pads (Garrod's nodes), plantar fascial disease (Lederhose's disease), and contracture of the penile fascial envelope (Peyronie's disease). The contractile tissue in all of these conditions resemble the pathologic findings of Dupuytren's in the palm.[15] These associated conditions are found in an estimated 1% or fewer of patients with Dupuytren's disease.[16] All patients with the disease have a diathesis; however, the association with these conditions, as well as onset at an early age and family history, suggests the diathesis is strong. Their association to a strong Dupuytren's diathesis makes recognition important for awareness of possible poor prognosis and likelihood of recurrence with surgical treatment.

Symptoms

Dupuytren's disease typically has a painless onset and progression. Pain can be a result of concomitant injuries to the hand that can precede the development or worsening of Dupuytren's. The progression of the condition is generally considered to be a result of immobility after an injury in a predisposed individual, rather than from the injury itself.

Physical Examination

The most common first sign of Dupuytren's disease is a lump in the palm in close proximity to the distal palmar crease and in the axis of the ray of digit IV (Fig. 1). It can also present in the digit, generally over the proximal phalanx. The thumb and index finger are the least affected of the five digits. The nodule can be tender to palpation. In most cases, the skin is closely adherent to the nodule, and movement with tendon excursion often suggests other conditions, such as stenosing tenosynovitis. The condition is more readily apparent when it presents in a more advanced stage with palmar nodule, cord, and digital flexion contracture. Associated conditions with this disease include fat pads at the knuckles as well as evidence of the disease in the plantar fascia.

Functional Limitations

The majority of individuals seen with this condition have little functional limitation. With more advanced contracture, properly opening the palm while grasping can become difficult, making gripping activities troublesome.

Diagnostic Studies

The diagnosis of Dupuytren's disease is generally made on a clinical basis. Biopsy is considered when a palmar soft tissue mass cannot be reliably differentiated from sarcoma. The suspicion for this is higher in a younger individual with no strong evidence of Dupuytren's disease because sarcoma is more likely in younger age groups. Unfortunately, histologic differentiation is not always easy since a Dupuytren's nodule can appear very cellular with mitotic figures and closely resemble an aggressive sarcoma.

Differential Diagnosis

Fibromas	Lipomas	Sarcomas
Giant cell tumors	Neurofibromas	Tendon nodules of stenosing tenosynovitis
Inclusion cysts	Retinacular ganglions at the A1 pulley	Tophi

Treatment

Initial

Appropriate identification of the purpose of the encounter with the patient is important. Dupuytren's disease is typically not painful and commonly not functionally limiting. Many patients who seek consultation for Dupuytren's disease are merely looking for reassurance that they do not have malignancy and are satisfied to learn that the contracture is not a sign of serious disease.

Conventional non-invasive treatment has generally been of little or no value in the prevention of contracture or recurrence in Dupuytren's disease. This includes the use of steroid injections, splinting, ultrasound, and nonsteroidal anti-inflammatory medications (NSAIDs). Radiotherapy, topical DMSO, colchicine, and interferon have also been proposed but lack data demonstrating long-term efficacy. Traumatic rupture has never gained acceptance as a method of correcting flexion contracture; however, anecdotal reports of individuals correcting their deformity in such a fashion exist.[17]

Continuous passive traction has been proposed by some for severely flexed digit contractures;[19] however, this is utilized as a pre-operative adjunctive procedure and not done in isolation.

Ergonomic assessment and equipment modification can be of use in some instances with laborers who are functionally limited by contracture.

Rehabilitation

Rehabilitation efforts are minimal preoperatively and focus on adaptive equipment recommendations for work and home (large-handled tools for gripping, etc.). Splinting may be done by therapists with pre-fabricated or custom designs. Continuous passive traction of Messina has been proposed by some for severely flexed digit contractures[18]; however, this is utilized as a preoperative adjunctive procedure and not done in isolation.

Postoperative rehabilitation is needed to facilitate satisfactory outcome. The length of the rehabilitation generally reflects the invasiveness of the surgical procedure, with limited fasciotomies often involving a period of 4 to 6 weeks, whereas more extensive surgery may necessitate a formal rehabilitation process of up to 3 to 6 months. Stretching, splinting in palmar extension, and continuous passive traction in some individuals are used early postoperatively. Strengthening and functional activities are added later after incision healing. Again, splinting may be an option to prevent recurrence and adaptive equipment recommendations can help with resuming functions that involve gripping or repetitive hand use.

Procedures

Closed needle fasciotomy has been utilized by some[18] but is prone to complications, including infection, nerve injury, and skin breakdown as well as recurrence.

Enzymatic fasciotomy with collagenase has more recently shown promise for non-surgical relief of contracture. Purified collagenase is derived from *Clostridium histolyticum*. This treatment has been used in the past for debridement of burns and skin ulcers as well as Peyronie's disease.[20] In vitro studies have shown efficacy,[21] and current clinical studies are ongoing.

Steroid injection into the palmar nodule can be a useful adjunct to flatten the nodule. Concern for potential adverse effect on the underlying flexor tendons has prevented widespread use. Injection of collagenase into the central cord is gaining popularity. Care must be taken to avoid injection into the underlying flexor tendons.[22]

Surgery

Appropriate selection is critical for patients considering surgical treatment. The potential for recurrence and worsening after surgery is high in patients with a strong diathesis. Recurrence is defined as the development of nodules and contracture in the area of previous surgery. Extension is the development of lesions outside of the surgical area where there had previously been no disease. All patients should be made aware that surgery is not curative for this disease and that recurrence and extension are likely at some time. Extensive recurrence is more likely if surgery is performed during the proliferative phase of the condition.

Nevertheless, many individuals have improved hand function after surgical treatment, compared with their pre-operative status for years upon followup.[23] The goal of surgical treatment, when indicated, is to improve function, reduce deformity, and prevent recurrence. Surgical indication is generally felt to include digital flexion contracture of the proximal interphalangeal (PIP) and metacarpophalangeal (MCP) joints and web space contracture. MCP joint contractures are often fully correctable; however, PIP joint contractures often have residual deformity.[24]

There have been multiple surgical procedures described for the treatment of Dupuytren's contracture. These include variations of subcutaneous fasciotomy, fasciectomy, and skin grafting. Fewer complications are seen with limited fasciectomy, and this is often the procedure of choice in for higher risk patients in which temporary relief is favored over long-term results. Full thickness skin grafting has been shown to prevent recurrence and is considered in patients with a strong diathesis who have functionally limiting contracture.

Potential Disease Complications

In some individuals, the condition can become functionally limiting due to severe contracture. The thumb and index finger tend to be less affected than the other digits. Secondary contracture of the PIP joints can also develop in longstanding deformity.

Potential Treatment Complications

Recurrence of the disease is common in many individuals after surgical treatment. Loss of flexion into the palm is particularly disturbing to patients. The presence of thickly calloused hands can result in increased postoperative swelling, leading to longer periods of postoperative supervision and swelling. The term "flare reaction"[25] is a postoperative complication that occurs 3 to 4 weeks after surgery and is characterized by redness, swelling, pain, and stiffness. This occurs in 5% to 10% of patients.[26] Although women with the disease less frequently meet operative criteria, they are thought to have a higher incidence of reflex sympathetic dystrophy (i.e., complex regional pain syndrome) postoperatively.[27] Other potential surgical complications include hematoma, granulation, inadvertent division of a digital nerve or artery, infection, and graft failure in full thickness grafting procedures. Potential complications of injection therapy include injury to nearby structure, including the digital artery, nerve, and flexor tendons.

References

1. Tomasek JJ, Schultz RJ, Haaksma CJ: Extracellular matrix-cytoskeletal connections at the surface of the specialized contractile fibroblast (myofibroblast) in Dupuytren's disease. J Bone Joint Surg Am 1987;69:1400.
2. Hueston JT: Digital Wolfe grafts in recurrent Dupuytren's contracture. Plast Reconstr Surg 1962;29:342.
3. McFarlane RM: Patterns of the diseased fascia in the fingers in Dupuytren's contracture. Plast Reconstr Surg 1974;54:31–44.
4. Skoog T: The pathogenesis and etiology of Dupuytren's contracture. Plast Reconstr Surg 1963;31:258.
5. Early P: Population studies in Dupuytren's dontracture. J Bone Joint Surg 1962;44B:602–613.
6. Liss GM, Stock SR: Can Dupuytren's contracture be work-related? Review of the literature. Am J Indust Med 1996;29:521–532.
7. Ling RSM: The genetic factors in Dupuytren's disease. J Bone Joint Surg Br 1963;45:709.
8. Hueston J: Dupuytren's contracture and occupation. J Hand Surg Am 1987;12:657.
9. Yost J, Winters T, Fett HC: Dupuytren's contracture: A statistical study. Am J Surg 1955;90:568–572.
10. Noble J, Heathcote JG, Cohen H: Diabetes mellitus in the aetiology of Dupuytren's disease. J Bone Joint Surg Br 1984;66:322.
11. Lund M: Dupuytren's contracture and epilepsy. Acta Psychiatr Neurol 1941;16:465–492.
12. Noble J, Arafa M, Royle G, et al: The association between alcohol, hepatic pathology and Dupuytren's disease. J Hand Surg Br 1992;17:71.
13. An JS, Southworth SR, Jackson T, et al: Cigarette smoking and Dupuytren's contracture of the hand. J Hand Surg Am 1994;19:442.
14. Bower M, Nelson M, Gazzard BG: Dupuytren's contractures in patients infected with HIV. Br Med J 1990;300:165.
15. Hueston JT: Some observations on knuckle pads. J Hand Surg 1984;9B:75.
16. Cavolo DJ, Sherwood GF: Dupuytren's disease of the plantar fascia. J Foot 1982;21(1): 12.
17. Sirotakova M, Elliot D: A historical record of traumatic rupture of Dupuytren's contracture. J Hand Surg Br 1997;22:198–201.
18. Badois F, Lermusiaux J, Masse C, et al: Nonsurgical treatment of Dupuytren's disease using needle fasciotomy. Rev Rhum Engl Ed 1993;60:692–697.
19. Citron N, Mesina J: The use of skeletal traction in the treatment of severe primary Dupuytren's disease. J Bone Joint Surg Br 1998;80:126–129.
20. Gelbard M, James K, Riach P, et al: Collagenase versus placebo in the treatment of Peyronie's disease: A double-blind study. J Urol 1993;149:56–58.
21. Starkwether KD, Lattuga S, Hurst LC, et al: Collagenase in the treatment of Dupuytren's disease: An in vitro study. J Hand Surg 1996;21:490–495.
22. Badalamente M, Hurst L: Enzyme injection as a non-operative treatment for Dupuytren's disease. Drug Delivery 1996;3:33–40.
23. Forgon M, Farkas G: Results of surgical treatment of Dupuytren's contracture. Handchir Mikrochir Plast Chir. 1988;20:279–284.
24. Riolo J, Young L, Ueda K, Pidgeon L: Dupuytren's contracture. So Med J 1991;84:983–996.
25. Howard LD Jr: Dupuytren's contracture: A guide for management. Clin Orthop 1959;15:118.
26. McFarlane RM: The current status of Dupuytren's disease. J Hand Surg 1983;8:703.
27. Zemel NP, Balcomb TV, Stark HH, et al: Dupuytren's disease in women: Evaluation of long-term results after operation. J Hand Surg 1987;12(6):1012.

28 Extensor Tendon Injuries

Jeffrey S. Brault, DO, PT

Synonyms

Mallet finger
Extensor hood injury
Central slip injury
Extensor sheath injury
Boutonnière deformity
Buttonhole deformity

ICD-9 Codes

727.63
Hand extensor injury
736.1
Mallet finger
736.21
Boutonnière deformity

Definition

Extensor tendon injuries are more common than flexor tendon injuries. Because of their superficial position, extensor tendons are prone to laceration, abrasion, crushing, burns, and bites.[1] These injuries result in the inability to extend the finger due to extensor lag, joint stiffness, and poor tendon excursion if treatment is suboptimal.[2,3] There are seven zones to the extensor mechanism where injury can result in differing pathomechanics[4] (Fig. 1).

Symptoms

Patients typically lose the ability to fully extend the involved finger (Fig. 2). This lack of motion may be confined to a single joint or the entire digit. Pain often accompanies the loss of motion and can be in surrounding regions because of abnormal tissue stresses. Diminished sensation may be present if there is concomitant injury to digital nerves.

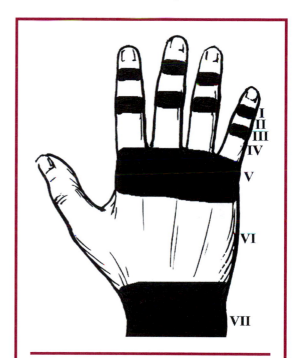

FIGURE 1. Zones of extensor tensons. Roman numerals are used to identify the zones: odd numbers overlie the respective joints, and even numbers overlie areas of intermediate tendon regions.

Physical Examination

Physical exam begins with observation of the resting hand position. If the extensor tendon is completely disrupted, the unsupported finger will assume a flexed posture.

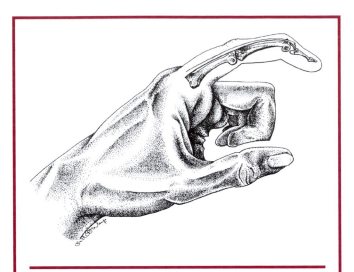

FIGURE 2. Mallet finger. The extensor tendon is usually torn near its insertion. Occasionally a small fragment of the distal phalanx is avulsed by the tendon. The DIP joint cannot be actively extended. (From Mellion MB: Office Sports Medicine, 2nd ed. Philadelphia, Hanley & Belfus, 1996, with permission.)

Range of motion, both active and passive, is evaluated for each finger joint. Grip strength is commonly measured by use of a handheld dynamometer. Individual finger extension strength can be recorded via manual muscle testing or finger dynamometry.

Sensation should be checked because of the close proximity of the extensor mechanism to the digital nerves.

Functional Limitations

Functional limitations manifest as the inability to produce finger extension in preparation for grip or pinch. Writing and manipulation of small objects can be problematic. Patients have difficulty reaching into confined areas (e.g., pockets) without the finger getting in the way.

Diagnostic Studies

A lateral radiograph of the finger shows whether the extensor injury is the result of a fracture. Anterior/posterior finger x-rays demonstrate joint malalignment. MRI and ultrasound are generally not necessary.

Differential Diagnosis

Fracture dislocation   Osteoarthritis
Joint dislocation   Rheumatoid arthritis
Peripheral nerve injury   Trigger finger (stenosing tenosynovitis)

Treatment

Initial

Treatment protocols for extensor tendon injuries vary by zone, mechanism, and time elapsed since the injury. If the disruption of the extensor mechanism is due to a laceration, crush injury, burn, or bite, then surgical review is warranted. Wound care to reduce the chance of infection and splinting of the finger in a protective position are required before surgery. In closed injuries, conservative splinting can be attempted for zone I and II injuries.

NSAIDs, including COX-2 inhibitors, and analgesics may be used for pain control.

Rehabilitation

Preoperative

Conservative treatment and splinting have been recommended for zone I and II injuries. Zone III through IV injuries usually require surgical repair.

TABLE 1 Zone I and II Injuries

Acute DIP injuries, mallet deformity (less than 3 weeks)

Weeks	Splint	Exercises	Wound and Skin Care
0–5	Continuous DIP extension (stack)	Active flexion and extension of PIP and MCP (hourly)	Remove splint daily to check for skin integrity and hygiene (maintain DIP in extension)
6	Worn between exercises and at night	Active flexion and extension of of DIP (hourly)	↓
7	Worn between exercises and at night	Passive flexion and extension of DIP (hourly)	↓
8	If no extensor lag may gradually wean splint	Continue with active and passive DIP exercises	↓

Chronic DIP injuries, mallet deformity (greater than 3 weeks)

Weeks	Splint	Exercises	Wound and Skin Care
0–7	Continuous DIP joint extension (stack)	Active flexion and extension of PIP and MCP (hourly)	Remove splint daily to check for skin integrity and hygiene (maintain DIP in extension)
8	Worn between exercises and at night	Active flexion and extension of of DIP (hourly)	↓
9	Worn between exercises and at night	Passive flexion and extension of DIP (hourly)	↓
10	If no extensor lag may gradually wean splint	Continue with active and passive DIP exercises	↓

From Brault J: OperTech Plast Reconstr Surg 2000;7:25–30.

Zone I (mallet deformity). Injury in this region is the result of forced hyperflexion of the distal interphalangeal (DIP) joint with tendinous disruption or avulsion fracture of the insertion. In closed injury the most common treatment is 6 weeks of continuous immobilization in slight hyperextension (0 to 15 degrees).[5,6] Although many types of splints are available, stack splints are the most commonly utilized. The splint should be worn continuously except during hygiene. When the splint is removed, the DIP joint should be maintained in extension. At 7 weeks, if no extensor lag is identified, passive, pain-free, DIP range of motion can be initiated, 10 repetitions hourly. The splint should be worn during exercise and at night. At 8 weeks, exercises are progressed to active extension, and splinting may be discontinued. In chronic mallet deformities, in which no treatment is initiated for 3 weeks following injury, splinting is recommended for 8 weeks before beginning exercises (Table 1).[6]

Zone II. Zone II injuries are often due to hyperflexion of the DIP joint. Laceration of the terminal extensor slip can occur and requires surgical repair. These injuries are treated similar to zone I injuries (see Table 1).[6,7]

Postoperative

Conservative treatment of zone III through VII injuries has limited success in restoring normal range of motion and function. Acute injuries in these zones are usually surgically corrected, and chronic injuries often require surgical review.

Zone III (boutonnière deformity). Injuries in this zone usually result from direct forceful flexion of an extended proximal interphalangeal (PIP) joint, laceration, or bite. If the lateral bands slip volarly, a boutonnière deformity results. Acute open injuries require primary surgical repair. Postoperative rehabilitation has changed in recent years with the implementation of early protected motion.[5,6,8] Postoperatively, the finger is immobilized in a PIP gutter splint. This splint is removed hourly to perform guarded active motion exercises. Therapy may consist of using two exercise braces that provide optimal gliding of the extensor mechanism (Table 2).

TABLE 2. Zone III and IV Injuries (Immediate Motion)

Weeks	Splint	Exercises	Wound and Skin Care
Start 24–48 hrs 0–2 weeks	DIP and PIP neutral splint	Exercise hourly with two splints Splint 1—allows 30 degrees of PIP and 25 degrees of DIP ROM Splint 2—PIP in neutral, DIP joint	Daily removal of splint for wound cleaning Edema control with compressive wrap
2–3	If no extensor lag noted	Splint 1—increase PIP flexion to 40 degrees Splint 2—continue	↓
4–5	If no extensor lag noted	Splint 1—increase PIP flexion to 40 degrees Splint 2—continue	↓
6	If no extensor lag noted, discontinue use of splints	Allow full active PIP and DIP flexion	↓

From Brault J: Oper Tech Plast Reconstr Surg 2000;7:25–30.

Zone IV. In this region, tendon injuries usually spare the lateral bands.[9] Because of the intricate relationship of the tendon and bone in this area, there are often considerable adhesions and loss of motion. Rehabilitation and splinting techniques are similar to that in zone III (see Table 2).

Zone V. Zone V is located over the metacarpophalangeal (MCP) joints. This is the most common area of extensor tendon injuries resulting from laceration, bites, or joint dislocation.[1] Acute open injuries are surgically repaired if not the result of a human bite, fist to mouth. Many authors have recently recommended that dynamic splinting be initiated in the first week.[5,6,9,10] This is accomplished with a dorsal dynamic extension splint that has stop beads on the suspension line, which limits flexion (Fig. 3A). Patients are instructed to perform active flexion of the fingers hourly (Fig. 3B). The rubber band suspension provides passive extension. Therapy is initiated early by a skilled therapist by positioning the wrist in 20 degrees of flexion and passively flexing the MCP joint to 30 degrees. This provides for safe protected gliding of the extensor mechanism. At postoperative week 7, progressive strengthening exercises can be initiated. At week 9, all bracing may be discontinued if no extensor lag is present (Table 3).

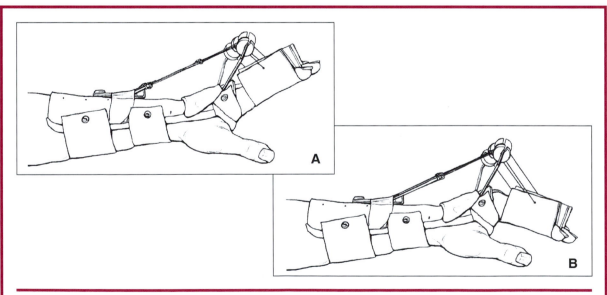

FIGURE 3. *A,* Splint allows for 30 to 40 degrees of active MP flexion with passive return to neutral. *B,* Flexion is limited by "stop beads" on the outrigger strings.

TABLE 3. Zone V, VI, and VII Injuries

Weeks	Splint	Exercises	Wound and Skin Care
Start 24–48 hrs	Dorsal dynamic extension splint (see Fig. 3A–3B) Night splint—MCP block	Exercise hourly in extension splint—allows 30–40 degrees of MCP flexion With skilled therapist—wrist at 20 degrees, passive MCP flexion to 30 degrees—patient performs active extension (daily to 3 × week)	Daily removal of splint for wound cleaning Edema control with 0–3 compressive wrap
4	Continue with dynamic day splint, static night splint	Increase active ROM to 50–60 degrees	↓
5	Discontinue dynamic extension splint MCP block splint worn at night and between exercises	Increase active ROM exercises to full motion	↓
6	MCP block splint	Passive flexion exercises of MCP and IP joints (buddy tape)	↓
7	↓	Progressive extension exercises, with mild resistance	↓
9	If no extensor lag, discontinue all splints	Continue with active and passive DIP exercises	↓

From Brault J: OperTech Plast Reconstr Surg 2000;7:25–30.

Zone VI. This area lies over the metacarpals. Injuries in this area present with similar clinical pictures to zone V injuries and are treated as such (see Table 3).[6,9,10]

Zone VII. Zone VII is at the level of the wrist. Tendons in this region run through a fibro-osseous tunnel and are covered by the extensor retinaculum. Complete lacerations of the tendons in this region are rare. Tendon retraction is a significant problem in this region and primary repair is warranted. Rehabilitation is similar to that in zone V (see Table 3).[6,9,10]

Procedures

Procedures other than surgical repair are rarely performed on extensor tendon injuries.

Surgery

Surgical correction of injuries in zones I and II results from failed conservative bracing, usually in a younger patient. For cosmetic reasons, patients may elect to have either the terminal extensor tendon repaired or the DIP joint fused. In older individuals with fixed deformities and painful degenerative joints, management is through arthrodesis.

Surgical intervention in zones III to VII is usually primary repair of the injured extensor tendon mechanism. If primary repair is not possible, tendon grafting has been described.[4]

Potential Disease Complications

Extensor tendon injury can result in permanent loss of finger extension, primarily due to adhesion formation or joint contracture. Painful degeneration of the affected joints can occur if normal motion is not restored.

Potential Treatment Complications

Analgesics, NSAIDs, and COX-2 inhibitors have well-known side effects that most commonly affect the gastric, hepatic, and renal systems. Acute tendon ruptures as a result of aggressive therapy necessitate reoperation and, potentially, tendon grafting. Therapy programs that are not aggressive enough often result in reduced range of motion and strength. Surgical complications include infection, adhesion formation, and advanced joint degeneration.

References

1. Hart R, Uehara D, Kutz J: Extensor tendon injuries of the hand. Emerg Med Clin North Am 1993;11:637.
2. Evans R, Burkhalter W: A study of the dynamic anatomy of extensor tendons and implications for treatment. J Hand Surg 1986;11A:774–779.
3. Newport M, Blair W, Steyers C: Long-term results of extensor tendon repair. J Hand Surg 1990;15A:961–966.
4. Kleinert H, Verdan C: Report of the committee on tendon injuries. J Hand Surg 1983;8:795.
5. Evans R: An update on extensor tendon management. In Hunter J, Mackin E, Callahan A (eds): Rehabilitation of the Hand: Surgery and Therapy, vol 1, 4th ed. St. Louis, MO, Mosby, 1995, pp 565–606.
6. Minamikawa Y: Extensor repair and rehabilitation. In Peimer C (ed): Surgery of the Hand and Upper Extremity, vol 1. New York, NY, McGraw-Hill, 1996, pp 1163–1188.
7. Evans RB: Early short arc motion for the repaired central slip. J Hand Surg 1994;19A:991–997.
8. Rosenthal E: The extensor tendon: Anatomy and management. In Hunter J, Mackin E, Callahan A (eds): Rehabilitation of the Hand: Surgery and Therapy, vol 1, 4th ed. St. Louis, MO, Mosby, 1995, pp 519–564.
9. Brault J: Rehabilitation of extensor tendon injuries. Oper Tech Plast Reconstr Surg 2000;7:25–30.
10. Thomas D: Postoperative management of extensor tendon repairs in zones V, VI, VII. J Hand Ther 1996;9:309–314.

29 Flexor Tendon Injuries

Jeffrey S. Brault, DO, PT

Definition

The flexor tendons of the hand are vulnerable to laceration and rupture. These injuries are most commonly seen in manual laborers who work around moving equipment, people with rheumatoid arthritis, and athletes (jersey finger). The flexor digitorum profundus (FDP) of the ring finger is the most commonly involved.[1] Incomplete injuries to the flexor tendon are easily missed on physical examination and can progress to full ruptures.

Regions of potential tendon injury are divided into five zones (Fig. 1).[2] Zone I is from the tendon insertion at the base of the distal phalanx to the midportion of the middle phalanx. Laceration or injury in this zone results in disruption of the FDP tendon and the inability to flex the distal interphalangeal (DIP) joint. Zone II extends from the midportion of the middle phalanx to the distal palmar crease. This zone is known as *no man's land* due to the poor functional results after tendon repair.[3] Tendon injury in this zone usually involves both FDP and flexor digitorum superficialis (FDS) tendons and results in inability to flex the DIP and proximal interphalangeal (PIP) joints. Zone III is located from the distal palmar crease to the distal portion of the transverse carpal ligament. This zone includes the intrinsic hand muscles and vascular arches. Zone IV overlies the transverse carpal ligament in the area of the carpal tunnel. In this zone, injuries usually involve multiple FDP and FDS tendons. Zone V extends from the wrist

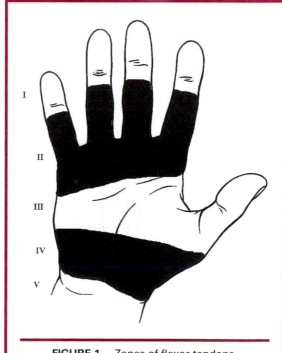

FIGURE 1. Zones of flexor tendons.

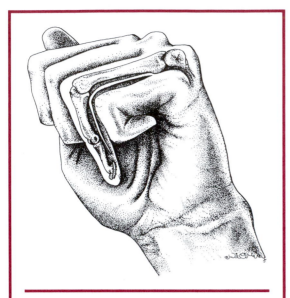

FIGURE 2. Jersey finger. The flexor profundus tendon is detached by a forced hyperextension of the DIP joint. (From Mellion MB: Office Sports Medicine, 2nd ed. Philadelphia, Hanley & Belfus, 1996, with permission.)

crease to the level of the musculotendinous junction of the flexor tendons. Injuries in this region most often result from self-inflicted laceration (suicide attempts).

Symptoms

Inability to flex the affected joint may be the presenting complaint.

Sensation of the involved finger is often affected due to the close proximity of the flexor tendons with the neurovascular bundle. It is important to include a detailed history to outline the mechanism of injury.

Physical Examination

Evaluation begins with observation of the resting hand position. If the flexor tendon is completely severed, the unsupported finger will assume an extended position (Fig. 2).[4] Active flexion of all finger joints needs to be assessed. Flexion strength of each digit should be evaluated by manual muscle testing or finger dynamometry. Strength is evaluated by having the patient individually flex both the DIP and then the PIP joints against applied resistance. It is possible to have a complete laceration of the flexor tendons with preservation of peritendinous structures and active motion. In these cases, however, flexion will be weak.[5]

To check individual function of the FDP, the patient is asked to flex the fingertip at the DIP joint while the PIP joint is maintained in extension. If there is injury to the FDP, the patient will be unable to flex the DIP joint.

It is difficult to diagnose solitary injuries of the FDS due to the FDP's ability to perform flexion of all finger joints via intertendinous connections. To isolate the integrity of the FDS, all the fingers are held straight, placing the FDP in a biomechanical disadvantaged position. The patient actively attempts to flex the finger to be tested while the other fingers are held in relative extension. If the patient is unable to move the finger, injury most likely has occurred to the FDS tendon. This test is only reliable for the middle, ring, and small fingers.

Sensation of the finger should be evaluated since open tendon injuries often are accompanied by injuries of the nearby digital nerves.

Functional Limitations

Functional limitations include difficulty with power grasp if the ulnarly sided tendons are involved and precision grasp problems if the radially sided tendons are involved. The patient may present with inability to button shirts, pinch small objects, or firmly grasp objects.

Diagnostic Studies

Radiographic evaluation should include anterior/posterior and lateral views of the involved finger(s). These assist in identification of joint dislocation, articular disruption, avulsion, and long bone fractures. Ultrasound and MRI are utilized to identify partially lacerated or ruptured tendons.

Differential Diagnosis

Partial tendon laceration

Trigger finger (stenosing tenosynovitis)

Anterior interosseous nerve injury

Median nerve injury

Treatment

Initial

Surgical intervention is almost always required for flexor tendon injuries. Protection of the affected finger in a bulky dressing and meticulous wound care are recommended prior to surgical correction.

Cleaning and repair of superficial wounds should be performed if surgical referral is delayed. Optimally, surgical correction of the flexor tendon injury occurs within the first 12 to 24 hours. Delayed primary repair is performed in the first 10 days. If primary repair is not performed secondary to infection, secondary repair can be performed up to 4 weeks. If repair is not performed within 4 weeks, the tendon usually is retracted within the sheath, making surgical repair difficult.[5]

Analgesics and NSAIDs, including COX-2 inhibitors, may be used for pain control.

Rehabilitation

Postoperative rehabilitation of repaired tendons has changed greatly in the past 10 years through initiation of early protected motion.[6–8] Historically, the repaired fingers were placed in an immobilization splint for up to 2 months. This often led to adhesion formation and ultimately the loss of motion and function.

The new rehabilitation scheme for repaired flexor tendons is essentially the same for all zones. Immediately postoperatively the hand is placed in a protective dorsal splint with 30 to 40 degrees of wrist flexion. All metacarpophalangeal (MCP) joints are placed in 45 degrees of flexion. A dorsal hood extends to the fingertip level, allowing PIP and DIP joint extension to 0 degrees. All of the fingers are held in flexion by dynamic traction applied by rubberbands originating from the proximal forearm with pulley at the palm and attachment to the fingernails.(Fig. 3A)

The patient is instructed to actively extend the fingers against the rubberband traction to the dorsal block, 10 repetitions hourly (Fig. 3B). The rubberband traction passively returns the fingers

TABLE 1.   Flexor Tendon Injuries (Immediate Motion)

Days	Splint	Exercises	Wound and Skin Care
Postop— day 21	Postop dynamic flexion splint with dorsal hood (Fig. 3) Wrist flex at 30–40° MCP 45°, PIP and DIP 0° of extension	Patient actively extends each finger 10 times hourly Under the direction of a hand therapist, wrist flexion is used to produce less tension on the flexor tendon during active exercises	Daily removal of splint for wound cleaning Edema control with compressive wrap
21–28	Progressive reduction in use of splint	Patient may begin to perform active flexion exercises without therapist	↓
28	Discontinue splint	Progress to increased active and passive flexion exercises. Grip strengthening	↓

From Lund A: Oper Tech Plast Reconstruc Surg 2000;7:20–24.

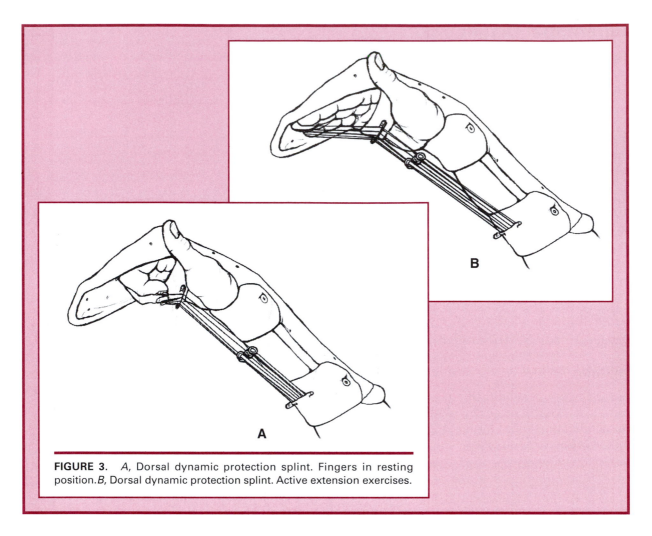

FIGURE 3. *A*, Dorsal dynamic protection splint. Fingers in resting position. *B*, Dorsal dynamic protection splint. Active extension exercises.

to a flexed position. At night the traction is removed and the fingers are strapped to the dorsal hood with the PIP and DIP joints in extension.

The rehabilitation program may involve immediate short arc motion (SAM).[6] Under the supervision of a skilled therapist, the injured digit is placed in moderate flexion with the wrist in 30-40° of extension, MCP joints 80° of flexion, PIP joints 75° of flexion and DIP joints in 30 to 40 degrees of flexion. The patient is then instructed to actively hold this position for 10 seconds. On completion of the static contraction, the therapist passively flexes the wrist. This allows for natural tenodesis to extend the fingers. At day 21 the patient can initiate unsupervised active flexion exercises. At 28 days the dorsal digital splint is removed and active tendon gliding exercises are initiated.[9]

Modalities such as paraffin baths, ultrasound, etc., may be used to promote range of motion.

Procedures

Procedures are generally not indicated in flexor tendon injuries.

Surgery

Optimally, repair of the flexion tendon should occur within the first 48 hours after injury. Improper handling of tissues during repair can result in hematoma, damage to the pulley integrity, and damage to the vincula—the vascular supply of the tendons.

Potential Disease Complications

Injury to the flexor tendon mechanism can result in permanent loss of finger flexion. Partial tendon damage can easily be missed and result in either weakness or complete rupture.

Potential Treatment Complications

Analgesics, NSAIDs, and COX-2 inhibitors have well-known side effects that most commonly affect the gastric, hepatic, and renal systems. Postsurgical complications include adhesion formation and tendon rupture. Postsurgical tendon rupture is usually the result of aggressive motion, either by the patient or therapist that results in failure of the repair. Re-operation is often required, which results in the greater propensity for adhesion formation. Adhesion formation and the loss of motion and strength complicate surgical repair, particularly in zone II.[3]

Many other factors affect healing of the tendon and postoperative rehabilitation. Factors such as advanced age, poor circulation, tobacco, and caffeine use, and generalized poor health can contribute to impaired healing. Scar formation can result in adhesion formation and decreased movement. Poor motivation and compliance with the therapy program result in less-than-optimal recovery.

References
1. Amadio P: Epidemiology of hand and wrist injuries in sports. Hand Clinic 1990;6:429–453.
2. Kleinert H, Schepel S, Gill T: Flexor tendon injuries. Surg Clin North Am 1981;61:267–286.
3. Chow J, Thomas L, Dovell S, et al: A combined regimen of controlled motion following flexor tendon repair in "No Man's Land". Plastic Rec Surg 1987;79:447–453.
4. Idler R, Manktelow R, Lucus G, et al: The Hand: Examination and Diagnosis, 3rd ed. New York, Churchill, Livingstone, 1990, pp 59–62.
5. Strickland J: Flexor tendons—acute injuries, In Green D, Hochkis R, Peterson W (eds): Green's Operative Hand Surgery, 4th ed. Philadelphia, Churchill Livingstone, 1999, pp 1851–1897.
6. Evans R: Immediate active short arc motion following tendon repair. In Hunter J, Schneider L, Mackin E (eds): Tendon and Nerve Surgery in The Hand—A Third Decade. St Louis, Mosby, 1997, pp 362–393.
7. Lund A: Flexor tendon rehabilitation: A basic guide. Oper Tech Plastic Reconstruc Surg 2000;7:20–24.
8. Strickland J: Biologic rationale, clinical application and result of early motion following flexor tendon repair. J Hand Ther 1989;2:71–83.
9. Werntz J, Chesher S, Breiderbach W, et al: A new dynamic splint and postoperative treatment of flexor tendon injury. J Hand Surg 1989;14A:559–566.

30 Hand and Wrist Ganglia

Charles Cassidy, MD
Sarah Shubert, MD

Synonyms

Carpal cyst

Synovial cyst

Mucous cyst

Intraosseous cyst

ICD-9 Codes

727.41
Ganglion of joint

727.42
Ganglion of tendon
sheath

Definition

Hand and wrist ganglia account for 50% to 70% of all hand masses. The ganglion is a benign, mucin-filled cyst found in relation to a joint, ligament, or tendon. It is typically filled from the joint via a tortuous duct, or "stalk," which functions as a valve directing the flow of fluid. The mucin itself contains high concentrations of hyaluronic acid, as well as glucosamine, albumin, and globulin.[1] When used to describe ganglia, the term "synovial cyst" is actually a misnomer since ganglion cysts do not contain synovial fluid and are not true cysts lined by epithelium, but rather by flat cells. The etiology of ganglia remains a mystery, although many believe that ligamentous degeneration or trauma plays an important role.[1,2]

By far, the most common location for a ganglion is the dorsal wrist (Fig. 1), with the pedicle arising from the scapholunate ligament in virtually all cases. Only 20% of ganglia are found on the volar wrist (Fig. 2) This type may originate from either the radioscaphoid or scaphotrapezial joint. Alternatively, ganglia can occur near the joints of the finger. One subtype of hand/wrist ganglia is the "occult" cyst, which is not palpable on physical exam.

Ganglion cysts occur more commonly in women, usually between the ages of 20 and 30 years. However, they can develop in either sex at any age. Ganglia of childhood usually resolve spontaneously over the course of several months. The most commonly

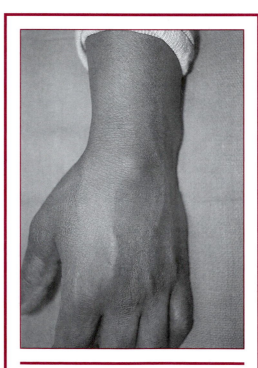

FIGURE 1. Dorsal wrist ganglion. The mass is typically found overlying the scapholunate area in the center of the wrist.

seen ganglion of the elderly, the mucous cyst, arises from an arthritic distal interphalangeal joint (DIP) (Fig. 3).

Other common types of ganglia in the hand include the retinacular cyst (flexor tendon sheath ganglion) (Fig. 4), proximal interphalangeal joint (PIP) ganglion, and first extensor compartment cysts associated with de Quervain's tenosynovitis. Less common ganglia include cysts within the extensor tendons or carpal bones (intraosseous) and those associated with a second or third carpometacarpal boss (arthritic spur). Rarely, ganglia located within the carpal tunnel or Guyon's canal can produce carpal tunnel syndrome or ulnar neuropathy.

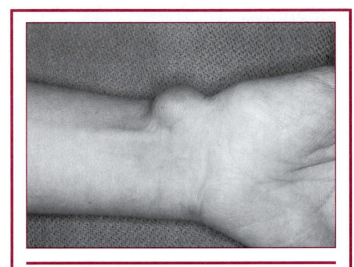

FIGURE 2. Clinical appearance of a volar wrist ganglion.

As noted, the cause of ganglion cyst formation is not known, but there may be a link to light, repetitive activity, demonstrated by an increased incidence in typists, musicians, and draftsmen. Interestingly, there is no increased risk in heavy laborers, who bear a greater load on their wrists. Wrist instability has also been discussed as both a possible cause and effect of the disease. Overall, there is a history of trauma in 10% to 30% of people presenting with the disease.[2]

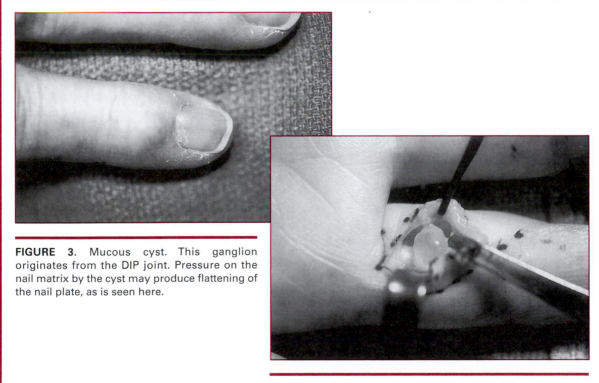

FIGURE 3. Mucous cyst. This ganglion originates from the DIP joint. Pressure on the nail matrix by the cyst may produce flattening of the nail plate, as is seen here.

FIGURE 4. Retinacular cyst. This ganglion originates from the flexor tendon sheath.

Symptoms

Patients with a wrist ganglion usually present with a painless wrist or hand mass of variable duration. The cyst may fluctuate in size or disappear altogether for a period of time. Pain and weakness of grip are occasional presenting symptoms; however, an underlying concern about the appearance and/or seriousness of the problem is usually the reason for seeking medical attention. The pain, when present, is most often described as aching and aggravated by certain motions. With dorsal wrist ganglia, patients often complain of discomfort as the wrist is forcefully extended (e.g., when pushing up from a chair). Interestingly, dorsal wrist pain may be the principal complaint of patients with an "occult" dorsal wrist ganglion, which is not readily visible. The wrist pain usually subsides as the mass enlarges.

With a retinacular cyst, patients usually complain of slight discomfort when gripping, for example, a racquet handle or shopping cart. Patients whose complaints of pain are primarily related to de Quervain's tenosynovitis (see Chapter 26) may notice a bump over the radial styloid area. Pain with grip is also a complaint of patients with a carpometacarpal boss. Mucous cysts can drain spontaneously and can also produce nail deformity, either of which may be presenting complaints. Symptoms identical to carpal tunnel syndrome will be noted by patients with a carpal tunnel ganglion. A ganglion in Guyon's canal will produce hand weakness (due to loss of intrinsic function) and may produce numbness in the ring and small fingers.

Physical Examination

Ganglia are typically solitary cysts, although they are often found to be multi-loculated on surgical exploration. They are usually mobile a few millimeters in all directions on physical examination. The mass may be slightly tender. When the cyst is large, transillumination (placing a penlight directly onto the skin overlying the mass) will help to differentiate it from a solid tumor.

The classic location for a dorsal wrist ganglion is ulnar to the extensor pollicus longus, between the third and fourth tendon compartments, or directly over the scapholunate ligament.[1] However, these ganglia may have a long pedicle that courses through various tendon compartments and exits at different locations on the dorsal wrist, or even the volar wrist. When the ganglion is small, it may be apparent only with wrist flexion. Wrist extension and grip strength may be slightly diminished. Dorsal wrist pain and tenderness with no obvious mass or instability should arouse suspicion for an occult ganglion.

Volar ganglia occur most commonly at the wrist flexion crease on the radial side of the flexor carpi radialis tendon but may extend into the palm or proximally, or even dorsally, into the carpal tunnel. They can involve the radial artery, complicating their surgical removal. They may seem to be pulsatile, although careful inspection will demonstrate that the radial artery is draped over the mass.

Retinacular cysts are usually not visible but are palpable as pea-sized masses, typically located at the volar aspect of the digit at the palmar digital crease. They are adherent to the flexor tendon sheath and do not move with finger flexion. Alternatively, intratendinous ganglia are distinguished by the fact that they move with finger motion.

Mucous cysts are located over the DIP joint, and the overlying skin may be quite thin. They are occasionally mistaken for warts. Spontaneous drainage and even septic DIP arthritis are not uncommon. Nail plate deformity is an associated finding. PIP joint ganglia are located on the dorsum of the digit, slightly off midline. Ganglia associated with carpometacarpal bosses produce tender prominences on the dorsum of the hand distal to the typical location for a wrist ganglion.

Important signs to look for on physical exam, especially when planning for surgery, are compression of the median or ulnar nerves or of the radial artery. An Allen's test should be performed prior to surgery to evaluate radial and ulnar artery patency, particularly in the case of a volar cyst (Fig. 5).

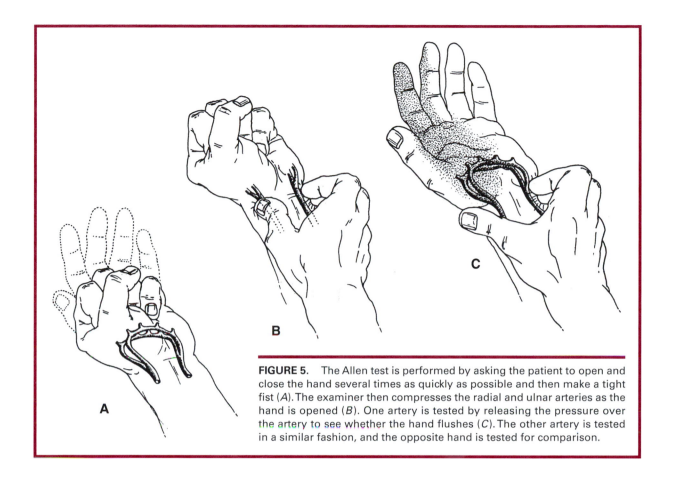

FIGURE 5. The Allen test is performed by asking the patient to open and close the hand several times as quickly as possible and then make a tight fist (*A*). The examiner then compresses the radial and ulnar arteries as the hand is opened (*B*). One artery is tested by releasing the pressure over the artery to see whether the hand flushes (*C*). The other artery is tested in a similar fashion, and the opposite hand is tested for comparison.

Functional Limitations

Physical limitations due to ganglion cysts are rare. With dorsal wrist ganglia, fatigue and weakness are occasional findings. Patients may have difficulty with weight bearing on the affected extremity with the wrist extended (e.g., when pushing up from a chair).

Diagnostic Studies

The diagnosis of a ganglion cyst is usually straightforward, and ancillary studies are often unnecessary. With wrist ganglia, plain radiographs of the wrist are usually obtained preoperatively to evaluate the carpal relationships and to exclude the possibility of an intraosseous ganglion. With a mucous cyst, radiographs of the affected digit will usually demonstrate a DIP joint osteophyte. Ultrasound or MRI may be useful in identifying deep cysts or cases of vague dorsal wrist pain. Specifically, MRI is indicated to rule out Kienbock's disease in patients with dorsal wrist pain and no obvious ganglion or wrist instability. Cyst aspiration is the single best confirmatory study. Aspiration characteristically yields a viscous, clear/yellowish fluid with the appearance and consistency of apple jelly. Occasionally the fluid will be blood-tinged.

Differential Diagnosis

Lipoma

Extensor tenosynovitis

Giant cell tumor of tendon sheath

Carpal boss

Scapholunate ligament injury/sprain

Kienböck's disease (avascular necrosis of the lunate)

Treatment

Initial

Reassurance is the single most important initial treatment. Many patients are satisfied to know that they do not have a serious illness. It is important to tell patients that the cyst(s) often fluctuates in size and occasionally disappears on its own. Undoubtedly, observation is the most appropriate treatment for ganglia in children, as long as the diagnosis is certain. In adults, splinting is an appropriate initial treatment for cysts associated with discomfort. A cock-up wrist splint is prescribed for carpometacarpal and dorsal/volar wrist ganglia, whereas a radial gutter splint is prescribed for ganglia associated with de Quervain's tenosynovitis. Traditional methods of crushing the cyst with a coin or a Bible, even though occasionally successful, are not recommended. Anecdotally, daily massage of mucous cysts by patients may be successful in resolving them as long as the overlying skin is healthy. Analgesics or NSAIDs/COX-2 inhibitors may be used on a limited basis for discomfort but do little to treat the disorder.

Rehabilitation

Rehabilitation has a role primarily in the postsurgical setting. The usual course of treatment following dorsal ganglion excision involves 7 to 14 days of immobilization in slight wrist flexion to minimize loss of wrist *flexion* secondary to scarring. Frequent, active range of motion of the wrist should be started after splint removal, and the patient should be able to return to relatively normal activity approximately 3 weeks after surgery.[1] Most patients are able to carry out their own rehabilitation at home. Formal therapy can be ordered if patients have difficulty returning to normal functioning. Therapy may include modalities for pain control, active assisted and passive range-of-motion exercises, and strengthening exercises. Therapists may also evaluate return to work issues including adaptive equipment that may assist patients in their daily work functions.

Procedures

Aspiration of the cyst serves two purposes: it confirms the diagnosis, and it may be therapeutic. Unfortunately, the recurrence rate following ganglion aspiration is quite high. One study[3] demonstrated long-term success rates of 27% and 43% for dorsal and volar wrist ganglia, respectively, treated with aspiration, multiple puncture, and 3 weeks of immobilization. Importantly, cysts present for longer than 6 months almost uniformly recurred. The results for aspiration of retinacular cysts were somewhat better, averaging 69% successful.

However, a significant number of patients may elect to proceed with cyst aspiration despite of the high likelihood of recurrence. It is important to note that aspirating volar wrist ganglia may cause displacement of the cyst and envelop the radial artery. Aspiration of mucous cysts is not recommended.

Steroids have *not* been shown to add any therapeutic benefit to ganglia aspiration.

Surgery

Many patients opt for surgical excision of the cyst, often for primarily cosmetic reasons. Surgery should be advised when the diagnosis is unclear. To minimize the likelihood of recurrence, the surgeon should not only remove the cyst, but should trace the stalk to its origin within the joint. For wrist ganglia, the surgeon often finds that the visible mass grossly underestimates its actual size and extent. Because these procedures require opening the wrist joint, they cannot be performed with the use of local anesthesia. With proper technique, recurrence rates should be less than 5%. Volar ganglia are more difficult to access and more often variable in their shape and location, making for more complicated surgery. It is important that the risks and benefits of surgical treatment for ganglion cysts be carefully discussed with the patient.

The surgical management of mucous cysts must include excision of the cyst stalk as well as the offending osteophyte, which originates either from the dorsal base of the distal phalanx or the head of the middle phalanx. The nail deformity should resolve over several months.[4]

Potential Disease Complications

Chronic wrist pain as the result of an untreated wrist ganglion is rare. The cosmetic deformity, however, is obvious. The most important complication associated with a neglected cyst is septic DIP joint arthritis resulting from spontaneous drainage of a mucous cyst. For that reason, the authors recommend mucous cyst excision when the overlying skin is thin or spontaneous drainage has occurred.

Potential Treatment Complications

Analgesics, NSAIDs, and COX-2 inhibitors have well-known side effects that most commonly affect the gastric, hepatic, and renal systems. The patient must understand that surgery will replace a bump with a scar. Slight limitation of wrist flexion following dorsal ganglion excision is not uncommon. Other risks include injury to the iatrogenic scapholunate ligament, extensor tendon, and cutaneous nerve. Recurrence is another possibility.

Surgery performed on the *volar* wrist carries a greater risk of injury to artery and nerve. The structures most at risk are the palmar cutaneous branch of the median nerve and the terminal branches of the lateral antebrachial cutaneous nerve, as well as the radial artery, which is often intertwined with the cyst. Perhaps because of the more intricate nature of its surgical removal, the volar cyst is associated with a higher rate of recurrence after surgery.

References
1. Angelides AC: Ganglions of the hand and wrist. In Green DP et al (eds): Green's Operative Hand Surgery, 4th ed. Philadelphia, Churchill Livingstone, 1999.
2. Peimer C (ed): Surgery of the Hand and Upper Extremity, vol 1. New York, McGraw Hill, 1996, p 837–852.
3. Richman JA, Gelberman RH, Engber WD, et al: Ganglions of the wrist and digits: Results of treatment by aspiration and cyst wall puncture. J Hand Surg 1987;12A:1041–1043.
4. Kasdan ML, Stallings SP, Leis VM, Wolens D: Outcome of surgically treated mucous cysts of the hand. J Hand Surg 1994;19A:504–507.

31 Hand Osteoarthritis

Leo M. Rozmaryn, MD

Synonyms

Arthritis

Degenerative arthritis

Osteoarthritis

Degenerative joint disease

Joint destruction

ICD-9 Codes

715.14
Osteoarthritis, primary, localized to the hand

715.24
Osteoarthritis, secondary, localized to the hand

716.14
Traumatic arthropathy of the hand

Definition

Osteoarthritis of the hand is a degenerative condition in which the hyaline cartilage disorder develops in the diarthrodial joints of the hand. It is distinct from inflammmatory arthropathies such as rheumatoid arthritis in which the primary component is an inflammatory or systemic pathophysiology. Primary idiopathic osteoarthritis is reserved to describe situations in which articular cartilage degeneration occurs without clear etiology. Idiopathic osteoarthritis excludes post-traumatic arthritis or arthritic conditions resulting from pyrophosphate deposition disease, infection, or other known causes. The prevalence of osteoarthritis of the hand increases with age and is more common in men than women until menopause. In individuals older than 65 years, osteoarthritis of the hand has been estimated to be as high as 78% in men and 99% in women.[1] The distal interphalangeal and proximal interphalangeal joints and the base of the thumb are the most affected joints.

Symptoms

Patients typically report pain, stiffness, episodic swelling, erythema, and induration of the affected joints. Initially, the pain and the stiffness may be mild, but over time, symptoms progress steadily. Pain is commonly worse at night and may affect one or more digits or one or more joints in the same digit. Stiffness and pain are also common first thing in the morning. A certain percentage of patients feel no pain but experience a steadily progressive enlargement of the affected joints with stiffness and a loss of function. It is not understood at this time why some patients have pain and some do not.

Physical Examination

Distal Interphalangeal Joint

Osteoarthritis of the distal interphalangeal joint is characterized by primary enlargement of the distal joint with formation of so-called Heberden's nodes (Fig. 1). It is often painless and unnoticeable, primarily because of the deformity near the joint. After loss of joint space and formation of Heberden's nodes, angulatory and rotatory deformities of the terminal phalanx can develop (Fig. 2). Modular involvement of the joint

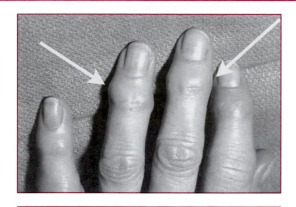

FIGURE 1. Patients with degenerative joint disease of the hands can present with Heberden's nodes (arrows). These nodules represent osteophytes at the DIP joint. (From Concannon MJ: Common Hand Problems in Primary Care. Philadelphia, Hanley & Belfus, 1999, with permission.)

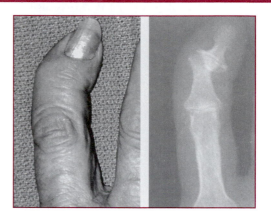

FIGURE 2. Severe osteoarthritis at the DIP joint of the fifth finger. Osteophyte formation, joint destruction, and angulation are demonstrated. (From Concannon MJ: Common Hand Problems in Primary Care. Philadelphia, Hanley & Belfus, 1999, with permission.)

combined with bone spurs can lead to the formation of ganglion cysts or mucous cysts on the dorsal aspect of the distal interphalangeal joint. There may be secondary deformity of the nail plate, with grooving and splitting of the nail plate. The proximal interphalangeal joint is less commonly involved with osteoarthritis than the distal joint. Again, the development of progressive pain, stiffness, and enlargement of the joint with periodic flares of erythema and increased pain may occur. The development of a progressive flexion deformity and contracture of the joint or an angulatory or rotatory deformity such as ulnar deviation of the finger as the joint space collapses are also possible. Some patients may have severe deformities of the proximal interphalangeal joints with no pain.

Metacarpophalangeal Joint

Osteoarthritis in the metacarpophalangeal joint usually results in pain, swelling, grinding, and loss of movement of the joint. Digital deformity in the radial ulnar plane is rare, although flexion deformities are common. These may involve one or several metacarpophalangeal joints at the same time.

Trapeziometacarpal Joint

The trapeziometacarpal joint is a very common site for the development of osteoarthritis. This complex saddle joint that allows thumb flexion, extension, abduction, adduction, and circumduction may fail as the articular cartilage degenerates and there is loosening of the complex primary ligamentous and secondary muscular restraints around the carpometacarpal joint. This condition may be accompanied by joint subluxation at the metacarpal base.[2] Onset of pain may be vague and can take months or even years to become clinically evident. Osteoarthritis presents with pain and crepitance and the characteristic deformity on the radial aspect of the base of the metacarpophalangeal joint. Any compressive or rotatory movement becomes very painful. Curiously, there is poor correlation between the radiographic appearance of the joint and the degree of symptoms. Patients gradually become unable to perform even the simplest tasks of daily living.

Examination of any of these joints will include documenting the active and passive range of motion of these joints. The presence of peri-articular bone spurs or osteophytes should be noted. The condition of the skin, whether it is erythematous and the pain exhibited by the patient when passive movement to the joint is attempted should be noted. The arc of active and passive movement should be documented as well. Grip and pinch strength are usually diminished. The digits and the thumb need to be evaluated for dynamic or static deformities, and the degree of deformity should be noted. Neurologic examination including sensation and deep tendon reflexes should be normal.

Functional Limitations

Functional limitations include weak grasp, pain, and stiffness with finger movement, impeding manual exertion. This may limit opening jars and doors, or gripping a steering wheel or tools. Fine motor tasks become increasingly difficult as the pain, stiffness, and deformity progress. Patients may have difficulty typing at work, opening mail, chopping vegetables, buttoning clothes, tying shoelaces, etc.

Diagnostic Studies

The imaging modality of choice is the plain x-ray. Characteristic findings include joint space narrowing, subchondral sclerosis, osteophyte formation, and degenerative cyst formation in the subchondral bone. As the joint space collapses, there may be shortening of the involved digit or ulna deviation of the digits. Four radiographic changes are characteristic of basal joint arthritis of the thumb.[3] In stage I the articular contours are normal with no subluxation or joint debris. The joint space may be widened if an effusion is present. In stage II there is slight narrowing of the thumb trapezial metacarpal joint, but the joint space and articular contours are preserved. Joint debris is less than 2 mm and may be present. In stage III there is significant trapezial metacarpal joint destruction with sclerotic resistive changes and subchondral bone with osteophytes greater than 2 mm . Stage IV is characterized by pantrapezial arthritis in which both the trapezial metacarpal and scaphoid trapezial joints are affected. The base of the thumb metacarpal may be radially subluxed early in the disease.

Differential Diagnosis

Inflammatory arthritis (e.g., lyme disease, gout, rheumatoid arthritis, psoriatic arthritis)
Calcium pyrophosphate deposition disease
Septic arthritis
Systemic lupus erythematosus
Scleroderma

Treatment

Initial

Initial treatment of osteoarthritis of the hand and wrist is directed from mechanical and biologic aspects of the disease. To decrease mechanical stresses in the affected joints, activity modification, rest, and judicious splinting are appropriate. For the interphalangeal joint, finger splints for night use and selective day use can be considered. For the basilar thumb joint, an opponens splint, either hand-based or across the wrist, can be beneficial. Similarly, a cock-up brace can be used for intercarpal and radial carpal osteoarthritis. The medical treatment of osteoarthritis includes NSAIDs/COX-2 inhibitors. Although there is a myriad of these medications available, no single compound has been found to be singularly effective in the treatment of osteoarthritis. Recently the use of chondroitin sulfate,[3] glucosamine,[4] and the intra-articular injection of Hyalgan[5] have been advocated. Capsaicin cream can also be tried.

Rehabilitation

Therapeutic intervention for conservative, non-operative treatment of osteoarthritis begins with resting the involved joints. Activities that stress the joint should be identified and modified or discontinued. Instruction in joint protection (Table 1) and work simplification techniques is helpful, as well as encouraging the patient to perform routine tasks more proficiently and with less stress to the joints.

For the arthritic patient, hand splints are used to rest inflamed joints, maintain proper joint alignment, improve functional control, and support weak structures. The most commonly used splints include a resting hand splint, ulnar deviation splint, tri-point proximal interphalangeal joint splint, and thumb spica splint. Each splint should be fabricated to minimize interference with the uninvolved joint function and maximize independence and activities of daily living. Patients should be supplied with instructions on the splint wear time, care procedures, donning and doffing procedures and skin care. Therapeutic modalities such as warm water soaks and paraffin baths are used in the treatment of the non-acute arthritic hand. Contraindications for using heat on an arthritic hand include acute exacerbation of joint inflammation, peripheral neuropathies, auto sensory disturbances, and skin irritations or open wounds. Gentle range-of-motion exercise of all digits is helpful, preceded by application of moist heat.

Procedures

Injections can be used for painful arthritic joints. These are typically done no more than 2 to 3 times annually using a corticosteroid/anesthetic preparation (Fig. 3).

Under sterile conditions, using a 25- to 27-gauge needle and a mixture of local anesthetic (e.g., 0.5 to 1 cc 1% lidocaine) and corticosteroid (e.g., 0.5 to 1 cc triamcinolone), the joint is injected. It is

---

TABLE 1   Basic Principles of Joint Protection

1. Respect pain: The patient must learn to distinguish between a debilitating pain that can exacerbate symptoms versus an uncomfortable pain associated with a particular activity. Activities ought to be modified on that basis.

2. Balance activity and rest: The patient's daily activity schedule must be outlined and modified to ensure proper planning, pacing, and prioritization of activities. Daily routines must incorporate adequate time for rest that involves joints.

3. Employ work simplification techniques: Patients are encouraged to use proper body mechanics and to arrange their living quarters and daily routines to minimize unnecessary use of energy and unnecessary stress on the joints.

4. Maintain strength and range of motion: Patients are encouraged to maintain at least minimal involvement in the majority of self-care tasks to preserve active range of motion. Daily activities may be supplemented with active range-of-motion exercises targeted for specific joints.

5. Avoid positions of deformity: Positions or motions that stress the joint toward positions of deformity are to be avoided or eliminated. Ulnar stress and twisting motions are to be avoided.

6. Use stronger muscles and larger joints: The patient is taught adaptive techniques in which less stress is placed on the smaller joints and weaker muscles of the hand. In addition, the patient should be taught to carry items close to the body or cradle them in the entire arm to distribute loads, rather than relying on smaller muscles and joints of the hand to bear the entire load.

7. Use adaptive equipment or splints: The patient is provided with information on specific adaptive devices that are helpful in reducing or eliminating positions of deformity or unnecessary stress on the smaller joints. Splints are fabricated as indicated to preserve joint integrity and to avoid positions of deformity.

8. Avoid activities that cannot be interrupted or stopped: Strenuous activities that may cause severe pain or joint stress should be avoided. Activities such as lifting a small child or carrying a hot pan should be discouraged because the patient is not only at risk for joint stress, but also for injury to others and further injury to himself or herself if the hand cannot withstand the joint forces.

9. Avoid sustained positions: Sustained gripping should be eliminated. The patient is encouraged to use frequent rests or adaptive equipment to avoid static positions that facilitate joint stress and muscle fatigue.[6]

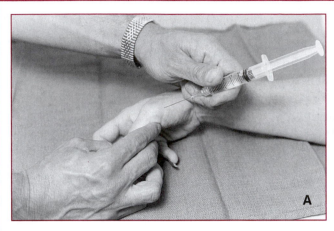

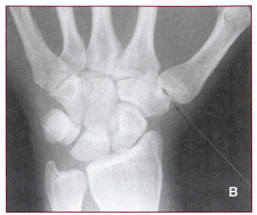

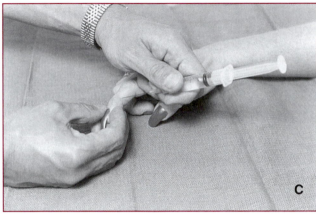

FIGURE 3. *A*, Needle placement into the carpo-metacarpal joint. *B*, Anteroposterior x-ray of the hand demonstrating needle placement into the first carpometacarpal joint. *C*, Needle placement into the interphalangeal joint. (From Lennard TA: Pain Procedures in Clinical Practice, 2nd ed. Philadelphia, Hanley & Belfus, 2000, with permission.)

important to note that small joints of the hand will not accommodate large volumes, so the total amount of fluid injected should typically be in the range of 1 to 2 cc.

Post injection care may include icing for 5 to 10 minutes and splinting the injected joint for up to 1 week after the procedure.

Surgery

Distal Interphalangeal Joint

For the mucous cyst and painful Heberden's nodes, the main surgical treatment has consisted of debridement of the Heberden's nodes and removal of the mucous cyst. In rare circumstances, when joint destruction is severe and maintenance of a distal interphalangeal joint is acceptable and alignment is difficult to achieve by other means, arthrodesis is considered, especially to correct severe angulatory or rotatory deformities that are functionally or cosmetically unacceptable to the patient.

Silicone interpositional arthroplasties have been described at the distal interphalangeal joint but have limited applications in this setting.

Proximal Interphalangeal Joint

The main indications for surgery are pain refractory to medical treatment, deformity that interferes with function, and contractures secondary to osteophyte formation and soft tissue fibrosis. Because proximal interphalangeal joint motion is so critical to normal hand functions, surgery should be avoided when an acceptable arc of motion is present. Infrequently, significant instability associated with joint destruction, joint deformity, and pain is an indication for surgical reconstruction by arthrodesis or arthroplasty .

Total collateral ligamentous incision for fibrosis of the soft tissues in a contracted proximal interphalangeal joint has been demonstrated to be effective in relieving the contracture. This can be coupled with flexor tendon sheath release, volar plate contracture release, and modest, marginal osteophyte excision.

Arthrodesis is favored over arthroplasty in cases of gross instability, prior history of sepsis, deficient bone stock, and inadequate soft tissue coverage. There are multiple techniques for achieving arthrodesis.

Silicone implant arthroplasty remains a viable and appropriate treatment option for severe osteoarthritis of the proximal interphalangeal joints, and retrospective reviews of patients with proximal interphalangeal joint arthroplasties revealed excellent clinical results.[7]

Trapeziometacarpal Joint

The trapeziometacarpal joint is the most common upper extremity site of surgical reconstruction for osteoarthritis. The indications for surgery are primarily pain and secondary deformity that interferes with activities of daily living. The decision to treat basal joint disease and ultimately to perform surgery should be independent of x-ray staging. Patients may have severe disease on x-ray but not exhibit any pain. Ligamentous reconstruction using the slip of flexor carpi radialis tendon may be very effective in preventing further degeneration in early disease if joint surfaces are free of degeneration or chondromalacia but exhibit instability in subluxation.[8]

In more advanced disease, reconstructive efforts are directed at eliminating the painful arthritic joints about the trapezium to decrease pain and preserve function. Occasionally, trapeziometacarpal joint arthrodesis has been used, especially in young laborers; however, this results in the scaphoid trapezial joint bearing the brunt of all thumb motion after surgery and can result in arthrosis of that articulation.[9]

A more popular method of basal joint reconstruction is arthroplasty. This may vary from simple excisional arthroplasty in which the trapezium is removed, the metacarpal is held out to length using wires or external fixation, or a tendon is placed into positional material such as an "anchovy spacer" using a tendon graft. Other materials such as fascia, gel foam, and silicone have been used to treat and to fill the space left by the excision of the trapezium.[10] Silicone implant usage has now fallen into disfavor because of the high incidence of resultant silicone synovitis and progressive joint destruction. Metal and plastic prostheses have been used with some success but have been found to loosen over time, necessitating further surgery. Spherical implants have recently been advocated, but it is too soon to evaluate their long-term effectiveness.[11] Most recently the Burton ligament reconstruction tendon interposition (LRTI) has been used as a modification of the original anchovy procedure. Long-term results have demonstrated that these ligament reconstructions have excellent long-term durability with pain relief and even late increases in strength.[12] There are some newer techniques for arthroscopic partial resection of the trapezium and interpositional arthroplasty, but again, it is too soon to assess their long-term effectiveness.

Potential Disease Complications

If left untreated this disease produces steadily increasing deformity, pain, and stiffness in the digits and the thumb with diminished strength, range of motion, and ability to carry on activities of daily living.

Potential Treatment Complications

Analgesics, NSAIDs, and COX-2 inhibitors have well-known side effects that most commonly affect the gastric, hepatic, and renal systems. The primary risks associated with injections include infection and an allergic reaction to the medication used. Potential surgical complications include wound infection, silicone implant synovitis, dissolution or extrusion of tendon interpositional spacers with proximal migration and impingement of the base of the thumb metacarpal, and loosening of trapeziometacarpal implantation with breakage of the implant.

Complications of arthrodeses procedures include non-union, infection, implant breakage, or extrusion. For digital silicone implants, breakage of the implants and synovitis have been reported.[14]

References

1. Chaisson CE, Zhang Y, McAlindon TE, et. al: Radiographic hand osteoarthritis incidents, patterns, and influence of pre-existing disease in a population base sample. J Rheumatol 1997;24:1337–1343.
2. Burton RI: Basal joint arthrosis of the thumb. Orthop Clin North Am 1973;4(2):331–348.
3. Eaton RG, Littler JW: A study of the basal joint of the thumb. Treatment of its disabilities by fusion. J Bone Joint Surg 1969;51A:661–668.
4. Ronca F, Palmierri L, Panicucci T, Ronca G: Anti-inflammatory activity of chondroitin sulfate. Osteoarthritis Cartilage 1998;6(Suppl A):14–21.
5. Towheed TE, Anastassiades TP: Glucosamine therapy for osteoarthritis. J Rheumatol 1999;26:2294–2297.
6. Corrado EM, Peluso GF, Giglioiti S, et. al: The effects of intra articular administration of highly uronic acid on osteoarthritis of the knee: A clinical study with the immunologic and biochemical evaluations. Eur J Rheumatol Inflamm 1995;15(1).
7. Dovelle S, Heeter PK: Hand Injuries: A Rehabilitation Perspective in Orthopedic Assessment and Treatment of the Geriatric Patient. St Louis, Mosby, 1993, p 205.
8. Lynn HH, Wyrick JD, Stern PJ: Proximal interphalangeal joint silicone replacement arthroplasty: Clinical results using an interior approach. J Hand Surg 1995;20A:123–132.
9. Burton RI, Pellegrini VD Jr: Surgical management of basal joint arthritis of the thumb. Part 2: Ligament reconstruction with tendon interposition arthroplasty. J Hand Surg 1986;11A:324–332.
10. Eaton RG, Littler JW: A study of the basal joint of the thumb. J of Bone and Joint Surg 1969;51A:661–668.
11. Thompson JS: Complications and salvage of trapezial metacarpal arthroplasties. In Barr JS Jr (ed): Instructional course lectures XXXVIII. Park Ridge, IL, American Academy of Orthopedic Surgeons, 1989, pp 3–13.
12. Calandruccio JH, Jobe MT: Arthroplasty of the thumb carpometacarpal joint. Semin Arthroplasty 1997;8(2):135–147.
13. Tomiano MM, Pellegrini VD Jr, Burton RI: Arthroplasty of the basal joint of the thumb: Long-term follow-up after ligament reconstruction with tendon interposition. J Bone Joint Surg 1995;77A:346–355.
14. Foliart EE: Swanson silicone finger joint implants. A review of the literature regarding long-term complications. J Hand Surg 1995;20A:445–449.

32 Hand Rheumatoid Arthritis

Leo M. Rozmaryn, MD

Synonyms

Rheumatoid arthritis

Rheumatism

Inflammatory arthritis

ICD-9 Code

714.0
Rheumatoid arthritis

Definition

Rheumatoid arthritis is a systemic autoimmune disorder of unknown etiology. It is a slowly progressive disorder that affects virtually any joint in the body and can have a profound effect on the hand. Rheumatoid synovitis in the hand releases lytic substances that destroy articular cartilage as well as joint capsule, bone, or tendon sheath. Understanding these patterns will dictate the timing and indication for surgical and non-surgical treatment. The disease can take three forms: *monocyclic, polycyclic*, and *progressive*, and it is often difficult to predict which pattern the patient will follow. Although primary treatment for the condition is medical, surgery is reserved for cases of progressive deformity and failure of medical treatment to stem the synovitis or impending tendon rupture.

Symptoms

The chief complaints are finger joint pain, stiffness, swelling, erythema, and progressive deformity. Pain is usually worse at night, and morning stiffness is common. The swelling may either be localized and modular or diffuse.

Physical Examination

The evaluation of a rheumatoid arthritic hand should include the following:

1. Joint pathology and joint stability
2. Joint pain and inflammation
3. Limitations in active and passive range of motion for grip and pinch strength deficits
4. Limitations in hand dexterity
5. The degree of disability with respect to self-care, and vocational and recreational activities

The examination of a rheumatoid hand is complex and varies with the stage of the disease. Early in the process, joints are usually stiff, painful, swollen, and red as a tense synovitis predominates. There may be large tenosynovitis on the dorsum of the hand and wrist. There also may be triggering of the digits secondary to flexor tenosynovitis, but the swelling on the volar side is less apparent than on the dorsum. As the disease progresses, the joints may become very loose and frail as they are destroyed. This is common in the

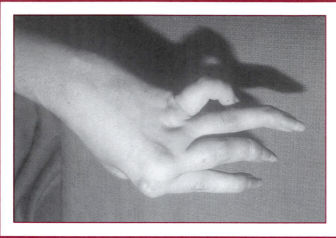

FIGURE 1. Rheumatoid hand. Note the multiple presentations in one hand.
1. Ulnar drift at the metacarpophalangeal joints.
2. Swan neck deformities of the third and fourth fingers.
3. Boutonnière deformity of the fifth finger.
4. Volar subluxation at the metacarpophalangeal joint.
5. Radial rotation of the metacarpals.

interphalangeal joints of the fingers and the thumb and is due to complete destruction of the articular surface of the joint and destruction of the collateral ligaments. Either boutonnière deformities (with flexion deformities of the proximal interphalangeal joint and extension deformities of the distal interphalangeal joint of the digits) or swan neck deformities (with hyperextension of the proximal interphalangeal joint with flexion of the distal interphalangeal joint) may predominate, and one can see varying patterns on the fingers of one hand (Fig. 1).

The thumb undergoes similar deformity. The metacarpal phalangeal joints may exhibit full or partial subluxation of the proximal phalanges on the metacarpal heads with the decided ulnar drift. Later in the disease, there may not be any synovitis because it may have burned itself out, and left joint destruction in its wake. In the thumb, typically the carpal metacarpal joint is dislocated with an abduction deformity of the metacarpal, causing a swan neck deformity. There may be an inability to extend one or more digits or the thumb secondary to rupture of the extensor tendons from dorsal tenosynovitis or inability to flex the fingers secondary to attritional rupture of a flexor tendon or locking of a tight trigger digit. With subluxation of the extensor tendons, the metacarpal phalangeal joints may appear in a flexion deformity without rupture of the extensor tendons.

Functional Limitations

Functional limitations in these patients may progress very slowly, and because of this, patients may remain fully functional for an extended period of time and may be able to continue activities of daily living, fine motor coordination, and gross grasping and gripping functions until severe deformities predominate. However, during acute exacerbations, activities of daily living and the ability to grip grossly and perform fine manipulations may be severely curtailed.

Diagnostic Studies

The plain x-ray remains the "gold standard" for diagnostic imaging. A diffuse osteopenia, especially in the periarticular regions, and joint space narrowing may predominate early, before deformities develop. A zigzag deformity with radial deviation of the metacarpals and ulnar deviation of the proximal phalanges at the metacarpophalangeal joint is typical. As lysosomal enzymatic degradation of the articular surfaces and the subchondral bone progresses, all architecture of the fine interphalangeal and metacarpophalangeal joints and the basal joints of the thumb may be destroyed. One can easily see the presence of boutonnière's and swan neck deformities on x-rays.

Laboratory tests include testing for rheumatoid factor.

Differential Diagnosis

Septic arthritis

Lyme's disease

Systemic lupus erythematosus

Psoriatic arthritis

Gout

Pyrophosphate deposition disease

Treatment

Initial

Nonsteroidal anti-inflammatory drugs (NSAIDs), including cyclooxygenase-2 (COX-2) inhibitors, may decrease pain and inflammation but will not inhibit synovial proliferation. The effectiveness of NSAIDs is related to the prevention of prostaglandin synthesis. Low dose corticosteroids are often beneficial in treating symptoms of inflammatory joints. Remittive agents, including antimalarial drugs, sulfasalazine, methotrexate, gold, D-penicillamine, immunosuppressive agents (azathioprine and cyclophosphamide) and cyclosporine, are used regularly.

Rehabilitation

Rehabilitation of the rheumatoid hand involves resting the involved joints, modification of activities that stress the joints, joint protection and work simplification instructions (refer to Table 1 on page 171), splinting regimens, heat modalities followed by gentle active range-of-motion exercise, and resistive exercise (see also Chapters 28 and 29).

Extensor Tendon Postoperative Rehabilitation

Within 5 days after surgical reconstruction of the extensor tendons, patients are placed into dynamic extension-assist orthotics for a program of flexion and passive extension exercises, under rubber band protection that allows for movement of the extensor mechanism without undue tension across the suture sites. After 6 weeks, the splints are discontinued and full active and passive range-of-motion exercises are commenced with a strengthening program.

Flexor Tendon Postoperative Rehabilitation

Within 5 days after operative repair of flexor tendons, the patient is placed in a flexion-assist orthotic, allowing active extension and passive flexion, under rubber band control that allows full gliding of flexor tendons without undue tension across the suture sites. Then under the supervision of a hand therapist, after 6 weeks, all splinting is discontinued, and full active and passive range-of-motion exercises are commenced, and a slow, progressive strengthening program is begun.

Metacarpophalangeal Postoperative Rehabilitation

After introduction of metacarpophalangeal silastic implants, several methods of postoperative rehabilitation can be used; however, the classic method is to immobilize for a period of 10 to 14 days and then begin gentle, slow active and passive range-of-motion exercise.

A more recently advocated treatment protocol is either immediate use of a passive motion machine, allowing full range of motion at the metacarpophalangeal joint, or early intervention with a hand therapist utilizing extension-assist orthotics under light tension of all four palmar digital metacarpophalangeal joints, allowing full flexion of the metacarpophalangeal joints in the extension-assist device. Full range of motion of the metacarpophalangeal joints and the interphalangeal joints is achieved with the help of a hand therapist. In about $4\frac{1}{2}$ weeks, all splinting is discontinued and a full strengthening program of the metacarpophalangeal joints is commenced.

Interphalangeal Joint Postoperative Rehabilitation

After an interphalangeal joint arthrodesis, pins are kept in place for 8 weeks, and the splint is protected in a Therma plast orthosis to obtain the position of the arthrodesis, at the same time mobilizing the adjacent joints to prevent contractures. After 8 weeks, the pins are removed, and once it has been ascertained that fusion has taken place, strengthening exercises can begin.

After an implant arthroplasty, gentle active and passive full range of motion of the proximal interphalangeal joint is begun under supervision of a hand therapist. Flexion is achieved utilizing active, active assist, passive, and joint blocking techniques. At 5 weeks, formal strengthening is begun.

Procedures

Injection of intra-articular steroids may halt progression of the synovitis in a given joint. A good rule of thumb is no more than three injections spaced at least 3 months apart (refer to page 172 for procedure details).

Surgery

Priorities for managing patients with rheumatoid disease of the hand are pain relief, restoration or improvement of function, prevention of deformities, and lastly, the appearance of the hand. The presence of a deformity is not in of itself an indication for surgery. If similar deformities exist in both hands and present a functional problem, one hand should be corrected to facilitate large object grasp; the contralateral hand may be left undisturbed to provide small object grasp and power. It is important to evaluate the stage of the disease of any particular deformity because the management of deformities vary from stage to stage. In general, stage II deformity is usually flexible, stage III exhibits limited movement, and stage IV present with a formation of fixed joint contractures.

Frequently the wrist needs to be addressed before finger deformities are addressed so that hand rehabilitation can proceed in an orderly fashion. In general, proximal joints such as the shoulder and elbow should be operated on before the distal ones (hand and wrist). Metacarpophalangeal joints should be reconstructed before proximal interphalangeal joints. Arthrodesis of the wrist and thumb metacarpophalangeal joint arthrodesis can be accomplished simultaneously; however, combining these with metacarpophalangeal implant arthroplasties that require prompt remobilization may compromise the end result.[1]

Extensor Tendon Surgery (see also Chapter 28)

Extensor tenosynovitis presents with a painless dorsal wrist mass distal to the retinaculum of the wrist. A tenosynovectomy is indicated for persistent tenosynovitis unresponsive to medical treatment, a tenosynovial mass increasing in size, or rupture of an extensor tendon.

The most serious complication of untreated dorsal tenosynovitis is tendon rupture. Patients present with a sudden loss of finger extension. Treatment usually involves transfer of the distal end of the ruptured tendon to an adjacent tendon. In the event of multiple tendon ruptures, tendon transfer from the volar side may be indicated. When both wrist extensor tendons are ruptured on the radial side, arthrodesis is required.[2]

Flexor Tendon Surgery (see also Chapter 29)

Flexor tenosynovitis can contribute to a rheumatoid patient's complaints of weak grasp, morning stiffness, volar swelling, and median nerve compression. A tenosynovitis may be diffuse or create discreet nodules that can limit tendon excursion. At the wrist, tenosynovial biopsy is indicated for median nerve compression, a painful tenosynovial mass, or tendon rupture. The tendon most commonly ruptured is the flexor pollicis longus. A tendon bridge graft, a two-stage flexor graft, or a tendon transfer can be performed to reconstruct the rupture. A ruptured profundus tendon is sutured to an adjacent intact tendon. The presence of one tendon rupture is an indication to promptly perform surgery to prevent further tendon damage.[3]

The palm is the most common location of flexor tenosynovitis. Indications for flexor tenosynovectomy in the palm include pain with use, triggering, tendon rupture, and passive flexion of the fingers that is greater than active flexion. For tendon rupture within a digit, a distal interphalangeal joint fusion should be considered. When both tendons are ruptured in the digit, consideration should be given to a stage tendon graft or fusion of both the PIP and the distal interphalangeal (DIP) joints.

Metacarpophalangeal Joint Surgery

The most common deformities of the metacarpophalangeal joint are palmar dislocation of the proximal phalanx and ulnar deviation of the fingers. As the inflammatory process disrupts the digit stabilizers, anatomic forces during use of the hand propel the digits into ulnar deviation. Metacarpophalangeal synovectomy is indicated for the painful, persistent metacarpophalangeal joint synovitis that has not responded to medical treatment and demonstrates minimal cartilage destruction on inspection or radiographically. Silicone implant arthroplasty is indicated in patients with diminished range of motion, marked flexion contractures, poor functional position, severe ulnar drift, and loss of function. Long-term studies have shown mild loss of motion over time and some recurrent deformity in patients whose disease course is progressive, but in general, the results are excellent.

Interphalangeal Joint Surgery

There are two types of proximal interphalangeal joint deformities, the boutonnière deformity and the swan neck deformity. Surgical intervention, such as flexor sublimis tenodesis or oblique retinacular ligament reconstruction, is designed to prevent hyperextension. Occasionally there is a mallet of the distal interphalangeal joint that can be corrected by partial extension.[4] In later disease, intrinsic tightness requires release. In late swan neck deformity with loss of PIP movement, PIP implant arthroplasty is required, as well as sufficient soft tissue immobilization and release to achieve movement in flexion once again.[5] In late deformities, especially in the index and middle fingers, arthrodesis may be required. Implant arthroplasties are recommended for the PIP joints of the ring and small finger joints.

In early boutonnière deformity, proximal interphalangeal (PIP) synovectomy may be performed, accompanied by postoperative splinting or joint injection. In distal extensor, tenotomy can gain distal interphalangeal joint flexion. In late disease, fixed flexion contracture with inability to passively extend the PIP joint may be present. Restoration of the extensor tendon function by itself will be unsuccessful. Treatment options are PIP arthrodesis or arthroplasty with a silastic implant. Long-term results reveal significant loss of range of motion of the PIP joint, but the deformity and pain level are markedly improved.

The thumb presents with two types of deformities. One is the boutonnière deformity with flexion of the MP joint and the extension of the interphalangeal joint. The other is the swan neck deformity with abduction subluxation of the base of the thumb metacarpal, hyperextension of the metacarpophalangeal joint, and flexion deformity of the interphalangeal joint of the thumb. This once again is caused by synovitis, and synovectomy and tendon reconstruction in early deformity may be quite helpful. For more severe swan neck deformity, carpometacarpal arthrodesis or arthroplasty may be necessary. There are many more complex deformities that can be discussed, but they are beyond the scope of this chapter.

Potential Disease Complications

Complications of rheumatoid disease in the hand include severe loss of function with complete joint destruction, severe flexion and ulnar deviation deformities of the digits, and severe swan neck and boutonnière deformities. Chronic intractable pain is also a common complication of the disease.

Potential Treatment Complications

Complications of treatment include infection, hardware breakage, non-union, silastic implant breakage, silicone synovitis, and progression of deformity. All of these would eventually lead to loss of function of the hand. Analgesics, NSAIDs, and COX-2 inhibitors have well-known side effects that most commonly affect the gastric, hepatic, and renal systems.

References

1. Millender LH, Phillips C: Combined wrist arthrodesis and metacarpophalangeal joint arthroplasty in rheumatoid arthritis. Orthop 1978;1:43–48.
2. Millender LH, Nalebuff EA: Arthrodesis of the rheumatoid wrist. An evaluation of 60 patients and a description of a different surgical technique. J Bone Joint Surg 1973;55A:1026–1034.
3. Ertel AN: Flexor tendon ruptures in rheumatoid arthritis. Hand Clin 1989;5:177–190.
4. Littler JW: Principles of reconstructive surgery of the hand. In Littler JW, Converse JM (eds): Reconstructive plastic surgery. Philadelphia, W.B. Saunders, 1977, pp 3103–3153.
5. Littler JW, Eaton RG: Reduced redistribution of forces in the correction of the boutonniere deformity. J Bone Joint Surg Am1967;49A:1267.

33 Kienbock's Disease

Sarah Shubert, MD
Charles Cassidy, MD

Synonyms

Lunatomalacia

Osteonecrosis of the lunate

Avascular necrosis of the lunate

ICD-9 Codes

715.23
Osteoarthrosis of the wrist, secondary

732.3
Kienbock's disease

Definition

Kienbock's disease is defined as avascular necrosis of the lunate, unrelated to acute fracture, often leading to fragmentation and collapse. While the precise etiology and natural history of this disorder remain unknown, interruption of the blood supply to the lunate is undoubtedly a part of the process. Trauma has been implicated as a cause.[1–3] The disease occurs most often in the dominant hand of men in the age group of 20 to 40 years. Many of these patients are manual laborers who report a history of a major or repetitive minor injury. Associations have also been made between Kienbock's disease and corticosteroid use, cerebral palsy, systemic lupus erythematosus, and streptococcal infection.

An important radiographic observation has been made regarding the radius-ulna relationship at the wrist and the development of Kienbock's disease.[4] In these patients, the ulna is generally shorter than the radius, a finding termed ulnar negative variant. Normally, the lunate rests on both the radius and the triangular fibrocartilage complex covering the ulnar head. It has been speculated that when the ulna is significantly shorter than the radius, a shearing effect occurs in the lunate, which can make it more susceptible to injury.

Symptoms

Presenting symptoms include chronic wrist pain, decreased motion, and weakness.[5] The pain is usually deep within the wrist, although the patient often points to the dorsum of the wrist, and is aggravated by activity. Some patients complain of a pressure-like pain that may awaken them. A history of recent trauma is often provided; however, many patients report having had longstanding mild wrist pain preceding the recent injury.

Physical Examination

Mild dorsal wrist swelling and tenderness in the middorsal aspect of the wrist may be present. Wrist flexion and extension are limited. Forearm rotation is usually preserved. Grip strength is often considerably less on the affected side.

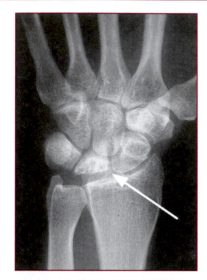

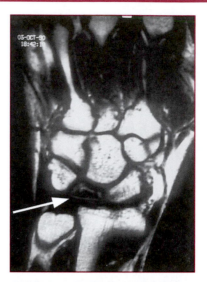

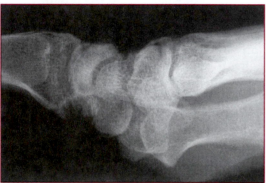

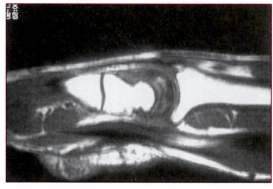

FIGURE 1. Advanced Kienbock's disease. Cystic and sclerotic changes are present within the collapsed lunate.

FIGURE 2. MRI in Kienbock's disease. T1-weighted images demonstrate diffuse low signal within the lunate.

Functional Limitations

Functional limitations include difficulty with heavy lifting, gripping, and activities involving the extremes of wrist motion. Many heavy laborers are unable to perform the essential tasks required of their occupation.

Diagnostic Studies

The initial diagnostic imaging for suspected Kienbock's disease includes standard wrist radiographs. Early in the disease process, the x-rays may be normal. With time, a characteristic pattern of deterioration occurs, beginning with sclerosis of the lunate, followed by fragmentation, collapse, and finally arthritis (Fig. 1).[6,7]

For clinical suspicion of Kienbock's disease with normal radiographs, a technetium bone scan or magnetic resonance imaging (MRI) may be helpful. In fact, MRI has probably supplanted plain x-ray for the detection and evaluation of Kienbock's disease. Characteristic signal changes include decreased signal on T1-weighted and increased signal on T2-weighted images (Fig. 2). Computed tomography (CT) is more effective than MRI at assessing for fracture of the lunate, but provides limited information regarding its vascularity. (See also Figs. 3 and 4.)

Differential Diagnosis

Wrist sprain

Osteoarthritis

Inflammatory arthritis (e.g., rheumatoid arthritis)

Scaphoid fracture

Scapholunate ligament tear

Ganglion

Preiser's disease (avascular necrosis of the scaphoid)

Tendinitis

Treatment

Initial

Given the limited information regarding the etiology and natural history of this uncommon disease, it is not surprising that the treatment has not been standardized. Without surgery, progressive radiographic collapse and radiographic arthritis almost invariably occur.[5] However, symptoms correlate only weakly with the radiographic appearance, and many patients maintain good long-term function.[8] The goals of surgery ideally would be to relieve the pain and halt the progression of the disease. Surgical interventions appear to be relatively effective in achieving the first goal but have not, as yet, reliably altered the radiographic deterioration of the lunate. Consequently, treatment options range from simple splints to external fixation and from radial shortening to vascularized grafts to fusions. Factors taken into consideration when assigning treatment include stage of the disease; ulnar variance; and patient age, occupation, pain, and functional impairment.[9] In general, young, active patients should be treated more conservatively before moving to major procedures that compromise wrist function and range of motion.

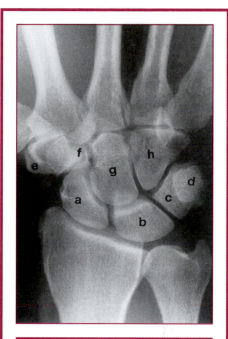

FIGURE 3. PA view of the wrist demonstrating the proximal and distal carpal rows. *A,* scaphoid; *B,* lunate; *C,* triquetrum; *D,* pisiform; *E,* trapezium; *F,* trapezoid; *G,* capitate; and *H,* hamate. (From Jebson PJL, Kasdan ML (eds): Hand Secrets. Philadelphia, Hanley & Belfus, 1998, p 220, with permission.)

Many clinicians prefer to begin with symptomatic treatment. Depending on the situation, this may involve a splint and activity modification or a short arm cast. However, an appropriate length of immobilization has not been established. Some clinicians have attempted this treatment for as long as 1 year, but most clinicians prescribe a cast for 6 to 12 weeks. The immobilization probably helps the pain associated with synovitis and wrist activity and motion; however, it does nothing to alter the vascularity of the bone or the shear stresses across the lunate. The patient should be informed that the x-rays will, in all likelihood, demonstrate worsening of the disease over time.

Pain can be treated with analgesics, NSAIDs, including COX-2 inhibitors. Narcotic medications are generally not recommended because of the chronicity of this condition.

Rehabilitation

Rehabilitation does not play a major role early in conservative treatment. Once the pain has subsided, gentle range of motion and strengthening may be initiated. Therapy is important for the postoperative patient, particularly if an intra-articular procedure has been performed or an external fixator has been applied. Typically the wrist is immobilized postoperatively until the vascularized graft or fusion has healed (about 6 weeks). At that point, occupational or physical therapy can effectively begin with gentle range of motion exercises, gradually progressing to strengthening exercises.

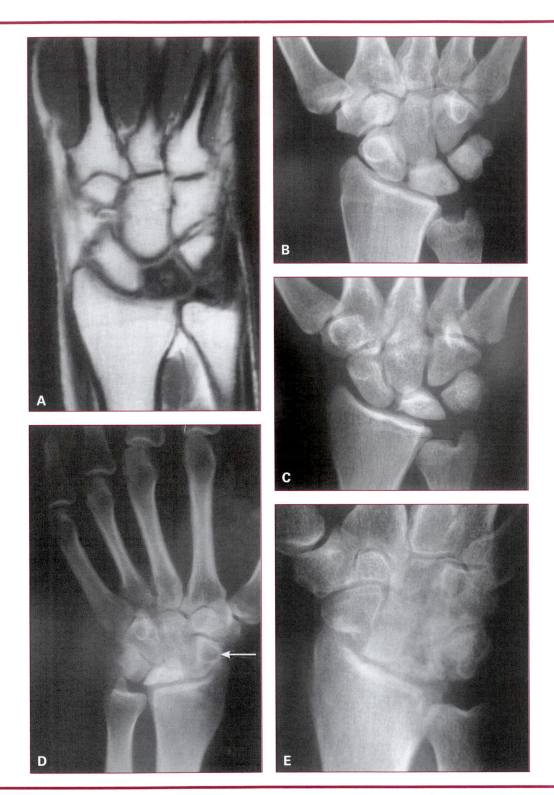

FIGURE 4.   The stages of Kienbock's disease. *A*, Stage I. T1-weighted MRI shows marked signal reduction in the lunate, compatible with loss of blood supply. *B*, Stage II. Density changes in the lunate as indicated by sclerosis. Note the ulnar-minus variance. *C*, Stage IIIA. Collapse of the lunate. There are no fixed carpal derangements. *D*, Stage IIIB. Decreased carpal height and proximal migration of the capitate. Note the scaphoid cortical ring sign (arrow). *E*, Stage IV. Generalized degenerative changes in the carpus. (From Weinzweig J (ed): Plastic Surgery Secrets. Philadelphia, Hanley & Belfus, 1999, pp 605–606, with permission.)

Procedures

Intra-articular steroids are of no proven benefit in the management of Kienbock's disease.

Surgery

Some authors feel that the majority of patients treated non-operatively do well,[6] whereas others believe that surgery is indicated for the majority of patients with Kienbock's disease.[11,13,14] The surgical treatment options for this disease may be divided into stress reduction (unloading), revascularization, lunate replacement, and salvage procedures.[9] Radial shortening of 2 to 3 mm is currently the most popular procedure for early stage Kienbock's in the setting of ulnar minus variant.[10,11] The goal is to make the radius and ulna lengths the same. Other unloading procedures include limited wrist fusion and external fixation.[12] Revascularization procedures have shown promise in the management of avascular necrosis of the hip; analogous techniques are being used in the wrist with encouraging early results. Lunate replacement has fallen out of favor due to reports of silicone synovitis and implant dislocation. When the lunate has collapsed to the point that it is not reconstructable, salvage procedures such as proximal row carpectomy or partial or total wrist arthrodesis are considered. Obviously, these procedures sacrifice motion in an effort to provide pain relief. The results of the various procedures are dependent on the stage of the disease. Nevertheless, most authors report 70% to 100% patient satisfaction.

Potential Disease Complications

Without surgery, progressive radiographic collapse of the lunate and arthritis of the wrist invariably occur.

Potential Treatment Complications

Analgesics, NSAIDs, and COX-2 inhibitors have well-known side effects that most commonly affect the gastric, hepatic, and renal systems. Infection is uncommon following hand surgery. Complications such as nerve injury, painful hardware, and stiffness of the wrist and digits are inherent in hand surgery. A radial shortening osteotomy or partial wrist fusion may fail to heal (non-union). Secondary wrist arthritis can develop following partial wrist fusions or proximal row carpectomy. Grip strength virtually never returns to normal. Finally—and most importantly—whether surgery favorably alters the natural history of this rare condition remains unproven.

References

1. Fredericks TK, Fernandez JE, Pirela-Cruz MA: Kienbock's disease. I. Anatomy and etiology. Int J Occup Med Environ Health 1997;10:11–17.
2. Fredericks TK, Fernandez JE, Pirela-Cruz MA: Kienbock's disease. II. Risk factors, diagnosis, and ergonomic interventions. Int J Occup Med Environ Health 1997;10:147–157.
3. Watson HK, Guidera PM: Aetiology of Kienbock's disease. J Hand Surg 1997;22B:5–7.
4. Hulten O: Uber anatomische variationen der handgelenkknochen. Acta Radiol 1928;9:155–168.
5. Beckenbaugh RD, Shives TS, Dobyns JH, Linscheid RL: Kienbock's disease: The natural history of Kienbock's disease and considerations of lunate fractures. Clin Orthop 1980;149:98–106.
6. Stahl F: On lunatomalacia (Kienbock's disease): Clinical and roentgenological study, especially on its pathogenesis and late results of immobilization treatment. Acta Chir Scand Suppl 1947;126:1–133.
7. Lichtman DM, Mack GR, MacDonald RI, et al: Kienbock's disease: The role of silicon replacement arthroplasty. J Bone Joint Surg 1977;59A:899–908.
8. Mirabello SC, Rosenthal DI, Smith RJ: Correlation of clinical and radiographic findings in Kienbock's disease. J Hand Surg 1987;12A:1049–1054.
9. Ruby LK, Cassidy C: Fractures and dislocations of the carpus. In Browner BD, et al (eds.): Skeletal Trauma: Fractures, Dislocations, and Ligamentous Injuries, 3rd ed. Philadelphia, W.B. Saunders, in press.
10. Almquist EE. Kienbock's disease. Hand Clin North Am 1987;3:141–148.
11. Salmon J, Stanley JK, Trail IA: Kienbock's disease: Conservative management versus radial shortening. J Bone Joint Surg 2000;82B:820–823.
12. Zelouf DS, Ruby LK: External fixation and cancellous bone grafting for Kienbock's disease. J Hand Surg 1996;21A:743–753.
13. Mikkelsen SS, Gelineck J: Poor function after nonoperative treatment of Kienbock's disease. Acta Orthop Scand 1987;58:241–243.
14. Delaere O, Dury M, Molderez A, Foucher G: Conservative versus operative treatment for Kienbock's Disease. J Hand Surg 1998;23B:1:33–36.

34 Median Neuropathy
(Carpal Tunnel Syndrome)

David Burke, MD

Synonyms

Median nerve
entrapment at the wrist
or carpal tunnel

Median nerve
compression

ICD-9 Code

354.0
Carpal tunnel syndrome

Definition

Carpal tunnel syndrome (entrapment of the median nerve at the wrist) is the most common compression neuropathy in the upper extremity and produces paresthesias, pain, and sometimes paralysis.

Carpal tunnel syndrome (CTS) is defined by a constellation of symptoms and presentations. While there is some variation as to what should be included in this definition, CTS is most often thought to include sensory changes in the lateral 3.5 digits of the hand, including a burning sensation or paresthesia. This condition is commonly nocturnal and often includes, in the latter stages, motor weakness in the thenar eminence. CTS is thought to result from impingement of the median nerve as it passes through the carpal tunnel.

It is helpful to think of the carpal tunnel as a structure with four sides, three of which are defined by the carpal bones and the carpal ligament "top" of the tunnel (Figs. 1 and 2). None of the sides of the tunnel yield well to

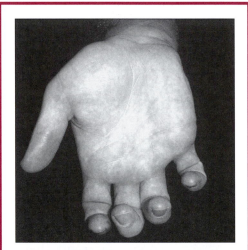
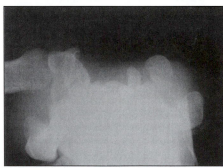

FIGURE 1.   Radiographic demonstration of the carpal tunnel (for orientation, the hand is in the same position as the x-ray). The carpal tunnel is formed radially, ulnarly, and dorsally by the carpal bones. (From Concannon M: Common Hand Problems in Primary Care. Philadelphia, Hanley & Belfus, 1999, with permission.)

expansion, so if there is swelling or increased pressure inside the tunnel, the median nerve may become compressed.

Symptoms

CTS symptoms include paresthesias in the lateral 3.5 digits of the hand and/or a burning sensation in the same distribution (Fig. 3). The sensation often includes the wrist, with sensory disturbances noted to be most often at night. The patient may describe the symptoms as being positional, with pain relieved by the shaking of a hand, often referred to as the "Flick" sign. Patients may complain of a subjective sense of swelling in the hands, often noting that they have difficulty wearing jewelry and/or watches, with this sensation fluctuating throughout the day and/or week.[1] In the latter stages of carpal tunnel syndrome, motor disturbances become apparent, with the patient complaining of subjective weakness manifested by decreased strength or frequent dropping of objects.

Physical Examination

Careful observation of the hands, comparing the affected side with the unaffected side, may demonstrate wasting of the thenar eminence. This may be apparent when comparing side-to-side on opposite hands or when comparing the thenar and hypothenar eminences of the same hand. A two-point discrimination task is often thought to be the most sensitive of the bedside examination techniques. This involves a side-to-side comparison of the two-point discriminating sensory ability of the median and ulnar nerve distribution of the hand. The more common examinations include Phalen's maneuver,

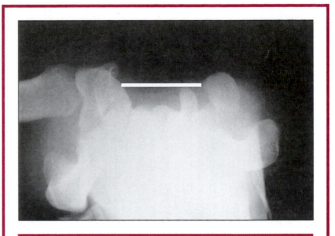

FIGURE 2. The volar carpal ligament (*line*) forms the roof of the carpal tunnel. This thick, fibrous structure does not yield to expansion, and increased pressure within the carpal tunnel can cause impingement of the median nerve. (From Concannon M: Common Hand Problems in Primary Care. Philadelphia, Hanley & Belfus, 1999, with permission.)

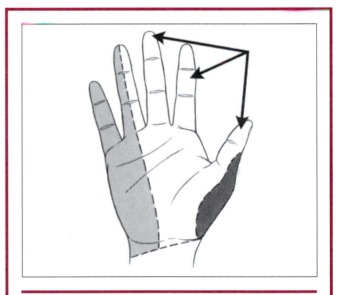

FIGURE 3. Patients with carpal tunnel syndrome complain of numbness or paresthesia within the median nerve distribution (*white area, arrows*). (From Concannon M: Common Hand Problems in Primary Care. Philadelphia, Hanley & Belfus, 1999, with permission.)

with a forced flexion at the wrist. This flexion is to 90 degrees and should last for a period of 1–2 minutes, reproducing the symptoms of CTS (Fig. 4). The reverse Phalen's maneuver is done with forced extension for a similar discovery. The second test, Tinel's, requires that the clinician tap sharply over the volar wrist; the sign is positive if symptoms radiate down the region of the distribution of the median nerve. A third test, the nerve compression test, involves placing two thumbs over the roof of the carpal tunnel, with pressure maintained for 1 minute. The sign is positive if symptoms are reproduced in the area of the distribution of the median nerve.

Functional Limitations

Functional limitations of CTS often include difficulty with sleep, with frequent awakening during the night, secondary to paresthesias and/or burning sensation. Some wrist positions during the day and some activities may become increasingly difficult, including driving for prolonged distances. Finally, weakness in the thenar eminence results in difficulty maintaining grip. Profound CTS results in functional limitations such as inability to tie one's shoes, button shirts, and put a key in a lock.

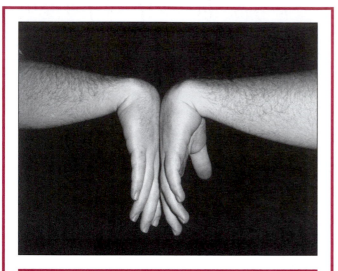

FIGURE 4. Phalen's test. Patients maximally flex both wrists and hold the position for 1–2 minutes. If symptoms of numbness or paresthesia within the median nerve distribution are reproduced, the test is positive. (From Concannon M: Common Hand Problems in Primary Care. Philadelphia, Hanley & Belfus, 1999, with permission.)

Diagnostic Studies

While CTS is a syndrome rather than a singular finding, it is often suggested that the definitive study of CTS is electrodiagnostic testing.

Others have advocated the injection of steroids into the carpal tunnel accompanied by relief of symptoms after several days as a reasonable means of diagnosing carpal tunnel syndrome.[2]

Differential Diagnosis

Medial or lateral epicondylitis

Radiculopathy involving the C5 to T1 nerve distribution

Rheumatoid arthritis or osteoarthritis at the wrist or digits

Hand/arm vibration syndrome

Arthritis of the carpal/metacarpal joint of the thumb

Tenosynovitis of the flexor carpi-radialis

Kienböck's disease

Median nerve compression at the elbow

Ulnar neuropathy at the elbow

Treatment

Initial

Since CTS is often thought to be secondary to overuse, relative rest at the affected wrist joint may prove effective. The wrist can be immobilized initially during the night, and if need be, as long as possible during the day with the use of a wrist splint placed at neutral. The optimal length of splinting before proceeding with more invasive techniques is not completely clear.[3] The vast majority of patients achieve their maximum level of symptom recovery within 2 weeks of the initial placement of the wrist splint. The use of oral anti-inflammatory medications or oral steroids has proven to be of some benefit, though not as impressive as those noted through injection.[4]

Long-term relief in CTS may be dependent on the general conditioning of the individual. Previous studies have suggested that the general conditioning of patients and their lifestyles account for approximately 32% of the variance for the development of CTS, whereas vocational tasks account for only 7% of the variance.[4]

Rehabilitation

Rehabilitation must address the issues of overuse, which exacerbates the symptoms of CTS in many individuals. As with all overuse syndromes, occupational or physical therapists can be helpful in instructing patients on relative rest throughout the day when patients are engaged in repetitive hand motion. During these periods of rest, flexion and extension stretching can be done, with the patient using the unaffected hand. Although many therapists advocate strengthening as part of a treatment program, aggressive strengthening exercises for hands weakened by carpal tunnel syndrome should be avoided until symptom relief is nearly complete. Since overuse syndromes involve a degree of inflammation, icing after long periods of use can be advocated to reduce the swelling within the carpal tunnel. Additionally, patients should be instructed on a program of general conditioning, since it is apparent that deconditioning exacerbates the symptoms of CTS.

Procedures

The patient can also be treated with steroid injections placed through the roof of the carpal tunnel, with one to three injections over the course of 1 to 2 months. A number of authors have suggested different injection techniques to prevent injury to the median nerve.[5–7]

For injections into the ulnar bursa (Fig. 5), under sterile conditions, using a ⅝-inch 27-gauge needle, place the needle proximal to the distal wrist crease and ulnar to the palmaris longus tendon. Direct the needle dorsally and angle it 30 degrees to a depth of about ⅝ inches (the length of the needle) or upon contact with a tendon. Slowly inject 1 to 2 ml of local corticosteroid. Anesthetics are not typically used in this injection. In individuals lacking a palmaris longus tendon (about 2% to 20% of the population), the needle can be placed midpoint between the ulna and radial styloid process.

Surgery

Surgery may be a reasonable alternative if conservative measures have failed. While the overall efficacy of this procedure seems good, the data are difficult to assess, given that much of the surgical literature has been presented with patients reporting subjective improvement of their symptoms but without a quantification of the improvement.[8,9]

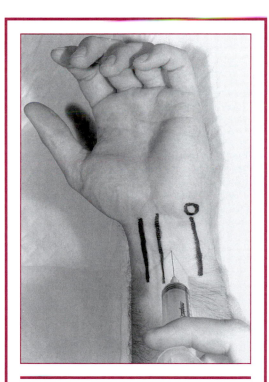

FIGURE 5. Preferred method for ulna bursa injection. Needle puncture is just ulnar to the palmaris longus tendon. The circle is over the pisiform bone. (From Lennard TA: Pain Procedures in Clinical Practice, 2nd ed. Philadelphia, Hanley & Belfus, 2000, p 100, with permission.)

Potential Disease Complications

As with any assault on a distal nerve, untreated carpal tunnel syndrome may result in permanent sensory disturbance and/or motor impairment in the area serviced by the median nerve. It is important that the clinician be wary of this and not allow the nerve disturbance to progress to permanent nerve damage.

Potential Treatment Complications

While oral analgesics may be important for symptomatic relief early in the stages of CTS, gastric, renal, and hepatic complications of nonsteroidal anti-inflammatory drugs should be monitored. Complications from local steroid injections include skin depigmentation, skin atrophy, a potential for tendon rupture, and the potential for injury to the median nerve at the time of injection.

Surgical complications have been noted to be rather few in the literature. These include accidental trans-section of the median nerve, with permanent loss of function distal to that trans-section. In addition, some have suggested that arthroscopic surgery might result in damage to the Berrettini branch of the median nerve, resulting in damage to this sensory branch of the median nerve.[10] While complications of surgical intervention are thought to be relatively infrequent, a number have been reported. The most common complication of surgical intervention is the incomplete sectioning of the transverse carpal ligament. Other potential complications include injury to the median nerve, palmar cutaneous branch recurrent motor branch, and superficial palmar arch; hypertrophied or thickened scar due to inappropriate incision; tendon adhesions because of wound hematoma; recurrence because of repair of the ligament; bowstringing of flexor tendons; malposition of the median nerve; inappropriate internal neurolysis resulting in scar compression; and reflex sympathetic dystrophy.[11–13]

References

1. Burke DT, Burke MAM, Bell R, et al: Subjective swelling: A new sign for carpal tunnel syndrome. Am J Phys Med Rehabil 1999;78(6):504–508.
2. Phalen GS. The carpal tunnel syndrome—clinical evaluation of 598 hands. Clin Orthop 1972;83:29–40.
3. Burke DT, Burke MM, Stewart GW, Cambre A: Splinting for carpal tunnel syndrome: In search of the optimal angle. Arch Phys Med Rehabil 1994;75(11):1241–1244.
4. Nathan PA, Keniston RC: Carpal tunnel syndrome and its relation to general physical condition. Hand Clin 1993;9(2):253–261.
5. Cyriax JH: The wrist and hand. In Illustrated Manual of Orthopaedic Medicine. Oxford, Oxford University Press, 1975, p 69.
6. Frederick HA, Carter PR, Littler T: Injection injuries to the median and ulnar nerves at the wrist. J Hand Surg Am 1992;17:645–647.
7. Kay NR, Marshall PD: A safe, reliable method of carpal tunnel injection. J Hand Surg Am 1992;17(6):1160–1161.
8. Chang B, Dellon AL: Surgical management of recurrent carpal tunnel syndrome. J Hand Surg Br 1993;18B:467–470.
9. Haupt WF, Wintzerg, Schop A: Long term results of carpal tunnel decompression: Assessment of 60 cases. J Hand Surg Br 1993;18:471–474.
10. Stancic MF, Micovic V, Potocnjak M: The anatomy of the Berrettini branch: Implications for carpal tunnel release. J Neurosurg 1999;91(6):1027–1030.
11. Langloh ND, Linscheid RL: Recurrent and unrelieved carpal-tunnel syndrome. Clin Orthop Rel Res 1972;83:41–47.
12. McDonald RI, Lichtman VM, Hanlon JJ, Wilson JN: Complications of surgical release for carpal tunnel syndrome. J Hand Surg Am 1978;3(1):70–76.
13. Kessler FB: Complications of the management of carpal tunnel syndrome. Hand Clin 1986;2(2):401–406.

35 | Trigger Finger

Julie K. Silver, MD
Jie Cheng, MD, PhD

Synonyms

Stenosing tenosynovitis

Digital flexor tenosynovitis

Locked finger

Tendinitis

ICD-9 Code

727.03
Trigger finger

Definition

Trigger finger is an often painful snapping, triggering, or locking of the finger as it is flexed and extended. This is due to a localized inflammation or a nodular swelling of the flexor tendon sheath that doesn't allow the tendon to normally glide back and forth under a pulley. *It occurs in the superficial and deep flexor tendons adjacent to the A1 pulley at the metacarpal head* (Fig. 1). The thumb and the middle and the ring fingers of the dominant hand of middle-aged females are most commonly affected.[1] It is often encountered in patients with diabetes and rheumatoid arthritis.[2,3] The relationship of trigger finger to repetitive trauma has been frequently cited in the literature[4,5]; however, the exact mechanism of this correlation is still open for debate.[6]

Symptoms

Patients typically complain of pain in the proximal interphalangeal (PIP) joint of the finger, rather than in the true anatomic location of the problem—at the metacarpophalangeal (MCP) joint. Some individuals may report swelling and/or stiffness in the fingers, particularly in the morning. Patients may also have intermittent locking in flexion or extension of the digit, which is overcome with forceful voluntary effort or passive assistance. Multiple finger involvement can be seen in patients with rheumatoid arthritis or diabetes.[2,3]

Physical Examination

The essential element in the physical examination is the localization of the disorder at the level of the MCP joint. There is palpable tenderness, and sometimes a tender nodule, over the volar aspect of the metacarpal head. Swelling of the finger may also be noted. Opening and closing of the hand actively produces a painful clicking as the inflamed tendon passes through a constricted sheath. Passive extension of the DIP or PIP joint while keeping the MCP joint flexed may be painless and done without triggering.[1] With chronic triggering, patient may develop IP joint flexion contractures.[1] Therefore it is important to determine whether there is normal passive range of motion in the MCP and interphalangeal (IP) joints. Neurologic examination including strength, sensation, and reflexes

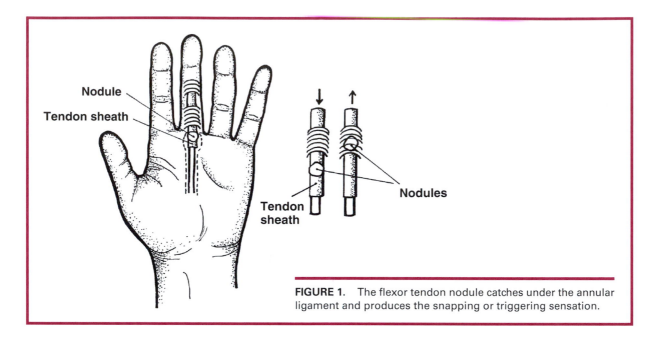

FIGURE 1. The flexor tendon nodule catches under the annular ligament and produces the snapping or triggering sensation.

Labels in figure: Nodule, Tendon sheath, Tendon sheath, Nodules

should be normal with the exception of severe cases that are associated with disuse weakness and/or atrophy. Co-morbidities can affect the neurologic exam as well (e.g., someone with diabetic neuropathy may have impaired sensation).

Functional Limitations

Functional limitations include difficulty with grasping and fine manipulation of objects due to pain, locking, or both. The patient may have problems with typing, buttoning a shirt, driving a car, using tools at work, etc.

Diagnostic Studies

This is a clinical diagnosis. Patients without a history of injury or inflammatory arthritis do not need routine radiographs.[7] MRI can confirm tenosynovitis of the flexor sheath, but this offers minimal advantage over clinical diagnosis.[8]

Differential Diagnosis

Anomalous muscle belly in the palm

Dupuytren's disease

Ganglion of the tendon sheath

Tumor of the tendon sheath

Rheumatoid arthritis

Treatment

Initial

The goal of treatment is to restore the normal gliding of the tendon through the pulley system. This can often be achieved with conservative treatment. However, typically the first line of treatment is a local steroid injection. The determination whether to inject first or try non-invasive measures is often based on the severity of the patient's symptoms (more severe symptoms generally respond better to injections), the level of activity of the patient (e.g., someone who needs to get back to work as quickly as possible) and the patient's and clinician's preferences.

Non-invasive measures generally involve splinting the MCP joint at 10 to 15 degrees for up to 2 weeks. This has been reported to be quite effective, although less so in the thumbs.[9] Also, DIP splinting provides a reliable and functional means of treating work-related trigger finger without lost time from work.[10] Additional conservative treatment includes icing the palm (20 minutes 2 to 3 times per day in the absence of vascular disease), NSAIDs/COX-2 inhibitors, and avoidance of exacerbating activities. Wearing padded gloves provides protection and may help to decrease inflammation by avoiding direct trauma.

Rehabilitation

Rehabilitation may include treatment with an occupational or physical therapist experienced in the treatment of hand problems. Supervised therapy is generally not necessary but may be useful in the following scenarios: (1) when a patient has lost significant strength, range of motion, and/or function from either not using the hand, from prolonged splinting, or post-operatively; (2) when modalities such as ultrasound or iontophoresis are recommended to reduce inflammation; and (3) when a customized splint is deemed to be necessary.

Therapy should focus on increasing function and decreasing inflammation and pain. This can be done by utilizing techniques such as ice massage, contrast baths, ultrasound, and iontophoresis with local steroid use. For someone with a very large or small hand or other anatomic variations (e.g., arthritic joints), a custom splint may fit better and allow him or her to function at work more easily than a pre-fabricated splint. Improving range of motion and strength can be done via supervised therapy either prior to surgery or postoperatively.

Procedures

A local steroid injection (Fig. 2) can be used as an alternative or in addition to other management.[11,12] The steroid injections are usually beneficial and frequently curative.[13,14] However, they may need to be repeated up to 3 times. This procedure is less effective with multiple digits involvement (such as in patients with diabetes or rheumatoid arthritis) or when the condition has persisted greater than 4 months.[14]

Surgery

Although steroid injections should be tried for most trigger finger cases prior to considering surgery, surgical intervention is highly successful for conservative treatment failures and should be considered for patients desiring quick and definitive relief from this disability.[15] Individuals with diabetes and rheumatoid arthritis are more likely to require surgery.[2,16] There

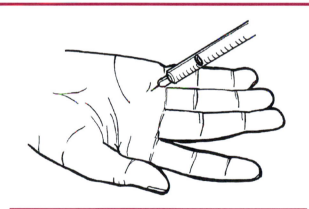

FIGURE 2. Under sterile conditions using a 27-gauge ⅝ inch needle, a 2–3 cc aliquot of a local anesthetic and steroid mixture (e.g., 2 cc of 1% lidocaine mixed with 1 cc [40 mg] of Depo-Medrol) is injected into the palm at the level of the distal palmar crease which directly overlies the tendon. Prior to cleaning the area to be injected, palpate for the nodule to exactly localize where the injection should be placed.

Post-injection care should include immediately icing the palm for 5–10 minutes and then 2–3 times a day for 15–20 minutes for the next few days. A splint can be worn post-injection for a few days, as it will help protect the injected area and allow the medication to take effect. The patient should be cautioned that it is normal to experience some post-injection pain for the first 24–48 hours. Additionally, the patient should be advised to avoid activities with the affected hand as much as possible for 1 week following the injection.

are two general types of surgery for this condition: the standard operative release of A1 pulley and the percutaneous A1 pulley release procedure. Both surgical procedures are generally effective and carry a relatively low risk of complications.[15,17]

Potential Disease Complications

Disease-related complications include permanent loss of range of motion from a contracture developing in the affected finger—most commonly at the PIP joint.[1] In rare instances, chronic intractable pain may develop despite treatment.

Potential Treatment Complications

Treatment-related complications from NSAIDs are well known (gastric, renal, and hepatic). COX-2 inhibitors may have fewer gastric-associated side effects. Complications from local steroid injections include skin depigmentation, skin atrophy, tendon rupture, digital sensory nerve injury, or infection. Individuals with rheumatoid arthritis are more likely to have tendon rupture[18]; therefore, repeated injections are not recommended in these cases. Possible surgical complications include infection, nerve injury, and flexor tendon bowstringing.[19–21]

References
1. Lapidus PW: Stenosing tenovaginitis. Surg Clin North Am 1953;33:1317–1347.
2. Stahl S, Kanter Y, Karnielli E: Outcome of trigger finger treatment in diabetes. J Diabetes & its Complications. 11(5):287-90, 1997.
3. Gray RG, Gottlieb NL: Hand flexor tenosynovitis in rheumatoid arthritis. Prevalence, distribution, and associated rheumatic features. Arthritis Rheum 1977;20(4):1003–1008.
4. Bonnici AV, Spencer JD: A survey of "trigger finger" in adults. J Hand Surg Br 1988;13(2):202–203.
5. Verdon ME: Overuse syndromes of the hand and wrist. [Review] [44 refs] Primary Care; Clin in Office Practice 1996;23(2):305–319.
6. Trezies AJ, Lyons AR, Fielding, Davis TR: Is occupation an etiological factor in the development of trigger finger? J Hand Surg Br 1998;23(4):539–540.
7. Katzman BM, Steinberg DR, Bozentka DJ, et al: Utility of obtaining radiographs in patients with trigger finger. Am J Orthopedics 1999;28(12):703–705.
8. Gottlieb NL: Digital flexor tenosynovitis: Diagnosis and clinical significance. J Rheum. 1991;18(7):954–955.
9. Patel MR, Bassini L: Trigger fingers and thumb: When to splint, inject, or operate. J Hand Surg Am 1992;17(1):110–113.
10. Rodgers JA, McCarthy JA, Tiedeman JJ: Functional distal interphalangeal joint splinting for trigger finger in laborers: A review and cadaver investigation. Orthopedics 1998;21(3):305–309; discussion 309–310.
11. Lambert MA, Morton RJ, Sloan JP: Controlled study of the use of local steroid injection in the treatment of trigger finger and thumb. J Hand Surg Br 1992;17(1):69–70.
12. Benson LS, Ptaszek AJ: Injection versus surgery in the treatment of trigger finger. J Hand Surg Am 1997;22(1):138–144.
13. Anderson B, Kaye S: Treatment of flexor tenosynovitis of the hand ("trigger finger") with corticosteroids. A prospective study of the response to local injection. Arch Intern Med 1991;151(1):153–156.
14. Newport ML, Lane LB, Stuchin SA: Treatment of trigger finger by steroid injection. J Hand Surg Am 1990;15(5):748–750.
15. Turowski GA, Zdankiewicz PD, Thomson JG: The results of surgical treatment of trigger finger. J Hand Surg Am 1997;22(1):145–149.
16. Stirrat CR: Treatment of tenosynovitis in rheumatoid arthritis. [Review] [15 refs] Hand Clin 1989;5(2):169–175.
17. Luan TR, Chang MC, Lin CF, et al: Percutaneous A1 pulley release for trigger digits. Chung Hua i Hsueh Tsa Chih—Chinese Med J 1999;62(1):33–39.
18. Ertel AN: Flexor tendon ruptures in rheumatoid arthritis. [Review] [21 refs] Hand Clin 1989;5(2):177–190.
19. Thorpe AP: Results of surgery for trigger finger. J Hand Surg Br 1988;13(2):199–201.
20. Heithoff SJ, Millender LH, Helman J: Bowstringing as a complication of trigger finger release. J Hand Surg Am 1988;13(4):567–570.
21. Carrozzella J, Stern PJ, Von Kuster LC: Transection of radial digital nerve of the thumb during trigger release. J Hand Surg Am 1989;14(2 Pt 1):198–200.

36 Ulnar Collateral Ligament Sprain

Sheila Dugan, MD

Synonyms

Skier's thumb

Ulnar collateral ligament tear/rupture

Gamekeeper's thumb

Break-dancer's thumb

Stener's lesion[1] (ruptured, displaced ulnar collateral ligament with interposed adductor aponeurosis)

ICD-9 Code

842
Sprains and strains of hand and wrist

Definition

Commonly called skier's thumb, this is a lesion of the ulnar collateral ligament (UCL) complex of the first metacarpophalangeal (MCP) joint. Tears can occur if an abduction stress is placed on an extended first MCP joint.[2] For example, acute injuries can occur when the strap on a ski pole forcibly abducts the thumb. Chronic ligamentous laxity is more common in occupational conditions associated with repetitive abduction force of the thumb. UCL injuries may be accompanied by avulsion fractures.

Symptoms

Patients report pain and instability of the thumb joint. Very often, patients can recall the instant of injury. If the UCL is ruptured, patients report swelling and hematoma formation; pain may be minimal with complete tears.

Physical Examination

Laxity of the UCL is the key finding on examination. Ligament injuries are graded as follows: *grade 1* sprains include local injury without loss of integrity; *grade 2* sprains include local injury with partial loss of integrity but end feel present; and *grade 3* sprains include complete tear with loss of integrity and end feel (Fig. 1). Passive abduction can be painful, especially in acute grade 1 and 2 sprains. The UCL should be tested with the first MCP in extension and flexion to evaluate all bands. The excursion should be compared with the uninjured side. Some authors recommend performing conventional x-rays before stressing the UCL to determine whether a large undisplaced fracture is present since stress testing could cause displacement.[3] There may be swelling or discoloration on the ulnar side of the first MCP joint. The patient may be unable to pinch.

Functional Limitations

Individuals describe difficulty with pinching activities (e.g., turning a key in a lock). Injuries affecting the dominant hand can have an impact on many fine motor manipulations, such as buttoning or retrieving objects from one's pocket. Injuries affecting the non-dominant hand can impair bilateral hand activities requiring stabilization of small objects.

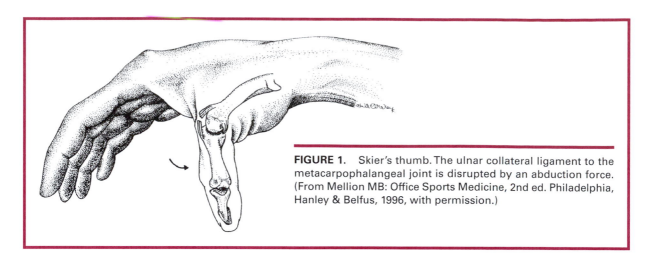

FIGURE 1. Skier's thumb. The ulnar collateral ligament to the metacarpophalangeal joint is disrupted by an abduction force. (From Mellion MB: Office Sports Medicine, 2nd ed. Philadelphia, Hanley & Belfus, 1996, with permission.)

Diagnostic Studies

Plain x-ray is essential to rule out an avulsion fracture of the base of the ulnar side of the proximal phalanx. A stress film with the thumb in abduction is occasionally useful and should be compared with the uninjured side. UCL rupture presents with an angle greater than 35 degrees.

Differential Diagnosis

Radial collateral ligament sprain/rupture

First MCP joint dislocation with and without volar plate injury

Thumb fracture/dislocation

Treatment

Initial

Pain and edema should be managed with ice, NSAIDs, including cyclooxygenase-2 (COX-2) inhibitors, and rest. Initial treatment for a first-degree (grade 1) UCL sprain includes taping for activity. Initial treatment for an incomplete (grade 2) UCL sprain involves immobilization in a thumb spica cast for 3 to 6 weeks with the thumb slightly abducted. Injuries involving non-displaced or small avulsion fractures when associated with an incomplete UCL tear can also be managed non-surgically and may require a longer course of immobilization. The cast can be extended to include the wrist for greater stability.[4] An alpine splint allows interphalangeal (IP) flexion while prohibiting abduction and extension of the first MCP joint.[5] Grade 3 injuries require surgical repair unless surgery is contraindicated for other reasons.

Rehabilitation

Physical or occupational therapy is important in the rehabilitation management of UCL sprains. Therapists who have completed special training and are certified hand therapists (often called CHTs) can be great resources. Range of motion of the unaffected joints of the arm, especially the interphalangeal joint of the thumb, must be maintained. In the setting of a grade 1 sprain, after a short course of modified rest and taping, therapy may be required to restore strength to the pre-injury level. In grade 2 sprains, a volar splint replaces the cast after 3 to 6 weeks. Splints may be custom molded by the therapist. They can be removed for daily active range-of-motion exercises. Passive range of motion and static strength training are initiated once pain at rest has resolved, and the patient is progressed to concentric exercise after about 8 weeks for non-surgical lesions and 10 to 12 weeks for postsurgical lesions. Prophylactic taping is appropriate for transitioning back to sports-specific activity (Fig. 2). Postsurgical rehabilitation is less aggressive, with avoidance of strengthening—especially a power pinch, for 8 to 12 weeks postoperatively.[6] Full activity after grade 2 tears with or without non-displaced avulsion fractures begins at 10 to 12 weeks compared with 12 to 16 weeks for surgically repaired injuries.[8]

Procedures

There are no specific non-surgical procedures performed for this injury.

Surgery

Early direct repair is required in the setting of a ruptured ligament (grade 3) injury. Grade 2 and 3 injuries resulting in severe instability, displaced fractures, or intra-articular fragments are also surgical candidates. Tension wiring is used to fixate avulsions; open reduction may be required for large displaced avulsion defects. Reconstruction may be necessary for a chronic tear.

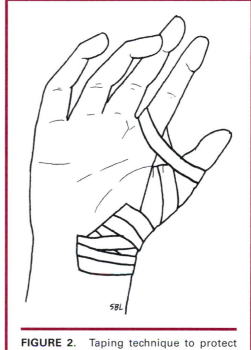

FIGURE 2. Taping technique to protect the ulnar collateral ligament.

Potential Disease Complications

Disease complications include chronic laxity with associated functional limitations, pain, and inability to pinch[7]; premature arthritis and persistent pain in the first MCP joint; and decreased range of motion of the thumb.

Potential Treatment Complications

Analgesics, NSAIDs, and COX-2 inhibitors have well-known side effects that most commonly affect the gastric, hepatic, and renal systems. Prolonged splinting can lead to loss of range of motion of the joint(s) and weakness and atrophy of muscles of the surrounding joints, depending on the extent of the injury and length of time spent in a splint. Surgical risks include non-union of avulsed fragments and the typical infrequent surgical complications such as infection and bleeding. Surgery can result in persistent numbness on the ulnar aspect of thumb.[8]

References
1. Stener B: Displacement of the ruptured ulnar collateral ligament of the metacarpophalangeal joint of the thumb. A clinical and anatomical study. J Bone Joint Surg 1962;44B:869–879.
2. McCue FC, Hussamy OD, Gieck JH: Hand and wrist injuries. In Zachazewski JE, Magee DJ, Quillen WS (eds): Athletic Injuries and Rehabilitation. Philedelphia, W.B. Saunders, 1996, p 589–599.
3. Kibler WB, Press JM: Rehabilitation of the wrist and hand. In Kibler WB, Herring SA, Press JM (eds): Functional Rehabilitation of Sports and Musculoskeletal Injuries. Gaithersburg, MD, Aspen Publications, 1998, pp 186–187.
4. Reid DC (ed): Sports Injury Assessment and Rehabilitation. New York, Churchill Livingstone, 1992, pp 1089–1092.
5. Moutet F, Guinard D, Corcella D: Ligament injuries of the first metacarpophalangeal joint. In Bruser P, Gilbert A (eds): Finger Bone and Joint Injuries. London, Martin Dunitz, 1999, pp 207–211.
6. Neviaser RJ: Collateral ligament injuries of the thumb metacarpophalangeal joint. In Strickland JW, Rettig AC (eds): Hand Injuries in Athletes. Philadelphia, W.B. Saunders, 1992, pp 95–105.
7. Smith RJ: Post-traumatic instability of the metacarpophalangeal joint of the thumb. J Bone Joint Surg 1977;59A:14.
8. Brown AP: Ulnar collateral ligament injury of the thumb. In Clark GL, Shaw Wilgis EF, et al (eds): Hand Rehabilitation: A Practical Guide, 2nd ed. New York, Churchill Livingstone, 1997, pp 369–375.

37 Ulnar Neuropathy (Wrist)

Ramon Vallarino Jr., MD
Francisco H. Santiago, MD

Synonyms

Guyon's canal entrapment

ICD-9 Code

354.2
Lesion of ulnar nerve

Definition

Entrapment neuropathy of the ulnar nerve occurs at the wrist in a canal formed by the hamate and its hook and the pisiform. These are connected by an aponeurosis that forms the roof of Guyon's canal (Fig. 1). This canal contains the ulnar nerve and the ulnar artery and vein. The following three types of lesions can be encountered:[1]

Type I: Affects the trunk of the ulnar nerve proximally in Guyon's canal and involves both the motor and sensory fibers. This is the most commonly seen lesion.

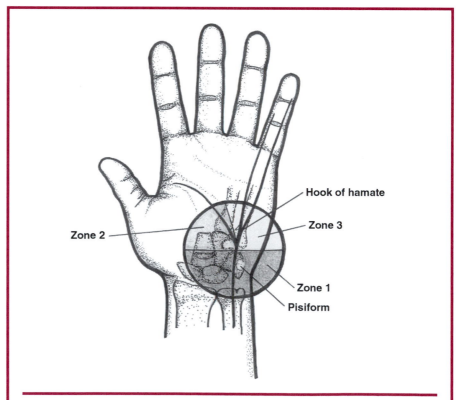

FIGURE 1. Distal ulnar tunnel showing the three zones of entrapment. Lesions in zone 1 give motor and sensory symptoms, lesions in zone 2 cause motor deficits; and lesions in zone 3 create sensory deficits.

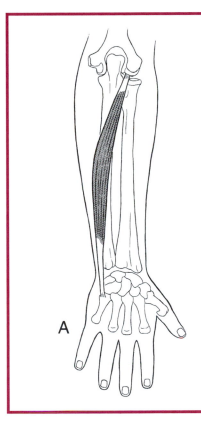

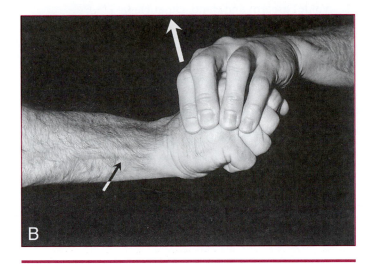

FIGURE 2. *A,* The extensor carpi ulnaris functions as a wrist extensor and an ulnar deviator. *B,* It can be tested by the patient forcefully extending (*large arrow*) and ulnarly deviating the wrist. The clinician should palpate the tendon (*small arrow*) while the patient performs this maneuver. (From Concannon MD: Common Hand Problems in Primary Care. Philadelphia, Hanley & Belfus, 1999, with permission.)

Type II: Affects only the deep (motor) branch distally in Guyon's canal and may spare the abductor digiti quinti depending on the location of its branching. A further classification is type IIa (still pure motor) in which all the hypothenar muscles are spared due to a lesion distal to their neurologic branching.

Type III: Affects only the superficial branch of the ulnar nerve, which provides sensation to the volar aspect of the fourth and fifth fingers and the hypothenar eminence. There is sparing of all motor function, although the palmaris brevis is affected in some cases. This is the least common lesion encountered.

Symptoms

Signs and symptoms can vary greatly and depend on which part of the ulnar nerve is affected and where along the extremity (Table 1). It is of great importance to be able to differentiate entrapment of the ulnar nerve at the wrist from the more common entrapment at the elbow. *The two clinical findings that confirm the diagnosis of Guyon's canal entrapment instead of ulnar entrapment at the elbow are (1) sparing of the dorsal ulnar cutaneous sensory distribution in the hand and (2) sparing of function of the flexor carpi ulnaris (FCU) and the two medial heads of the flexor digitorum profundus (FDP)* (Figs. 2 and 3). Otherwise, the symptoms in both conditions are similar and may include hand intrinsic muscle weakness and atrophy, numbness in the fourth and fifth fingers, hand pain, and sometimes, severely decreased function.

This injury is commonly seen in bicycle riders and people who use a cane, who place excessive weight on the proximal hypothenar area at the canal of Guyon and therefore are predisposed to distal ulnar nerve injury, especially affecting the deep ulnar motor branch (type II).[3] Entrapment at Guyon's canal has been associated with prolonged occupational use of tools, such as pliers and screwdrivers.[3]

TABLE 1. Volar Forearm and Hand: Ulnar Nerve

Muscle	Action
Flexor carpi ulnaris	Flex wrist, ulnarly deviate
Flexor digitorum profundus	Flex distal interphalangeal joint (4th and 5th)
Abductor digiti quinti*†	Analogous to dorsal interosseous
Flexor digiti quinti*†	Analogous to dorsal interosseous
Opponens digiti quinti*†	Flexes and supinates 5th metacarpal
Volar interossei*	Adduct fingers, weak flexion metacarpophalangeal
Dorsal interossei*†	Abduct fingers, weak flexion metacarpophalangeal
Lumbricals (ring and 5th)*†	Coordinate movement of fingers; extend interphalangeal joints; flex metacarpophalangel joints
Adductor pollicis*	Adduct thumb toward index finger
Lumbricals (ring, small)*	Coordinate movement of fingers; extend interphalangeal joints; flex metacarpophalangeal joints

* Hand intrinsic muscles.
† Hypothenar mass.

Physical Examination

Careful examination of the hand and a thorough knowledge of the anatomy of motor and sensory distribution of ulnar innervation are required to determine the location of the lesion. Except for the five muscles innervated by the median nerve (abductor pollicis brevis [APB], opponens pollicis, flexor pollicis brevis superficial head, and the first two lumbricals), the ulnar nerve supplies every other intrinsic muscle in the hand. Classically, there is notable atrophy of the first web space due to denervation of the first dorsal interosseous muscle (Fig. 4). In lesions involving the motor branches, there will be weakness and eventually atrophy of the interossei, the adductor pollicis, the fourth and fifth lumbricals, and the flexor pollicis brevis deep head. The palmaris brevis, abductor digitorum quinti (ADQ), opponens digitorum quinti, and flexor digitorum quinti may be involved or spared depending on

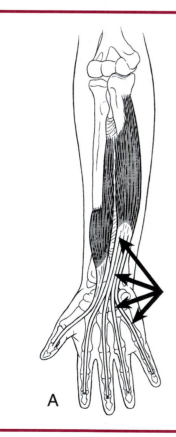
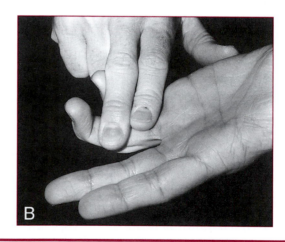

FIGURE 3. *A*, Flexor digitorum profundi (arrows). *B*, These tendons can be tested by the patient flexing the distal phalanx while the clinician blocks the middle phalanx from flexing. (From Concannon MD: Common Hand Problems in Primary Care. Philadelphia, Hanley & Belfus, 1999, with permission.)

the lesion. Sensory exam in all but type II reveals decreased sensation of the volar aspect of the hypothenar eminence and the fourth and fifth fingers (with splitting of the fourth in most). There is always sparing of the sensation of the dorsum of the hand medially as it is innervated by the dorsal ulnar cutaneous branch of the ulnar nerve, which branches off the forearm proximal to Guyon's canal.[1] The ulnar claw (hyperextension of the fourth and fifth metacarpophalangeal joints with flexion of the interphalangeal joints) seen in more proximal lesions may be more pronounced, presumably due to preserved function of the two medial heads of the FDP, which create a flexion moment that is unopposed by the weakened interossei and lumbricals.[1,4] The FCU has normal strength. All the signs of intrinsic hand muscle weakness that are seen in more proximal ulnar nerve lesions, such as Froment's paper sign, are also found in Guyon's canal entrapment, affecting the motor nerve fibers (Fig. 5).[5] Grip strength is invariably reduced in these patients.

Functional Limitations

Functional loss can vary from isolated decreased sensation in the affected region to severe weakness and pain with impaired hand movement. The patient may have trouble holding objects and performing many activities of daily living, such as occupation, daily household chores, grooming, and dressing. Vocationally, individuals may not be able to do the basic requirements of their jobs (e.g., operating a computer or cash register, carpentry work). This can be functionally devastating.

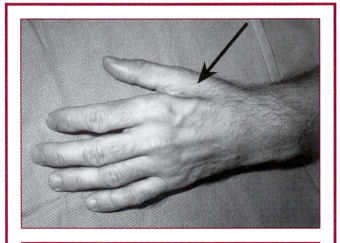

FIGURE 4. It is not unusual for patients with ulnar neuropathy to present with signs of muscle atrophy. It is most noticeable at the first web space, where atrophy of the first dorsal interosseous muscle leaves a hollow between the thumb and the index rays (*arrow*). (From Concannon MD: Common Hand Problems in Primary Care. Philadelphia, Hanley & Belfus, 1999, with permission.)

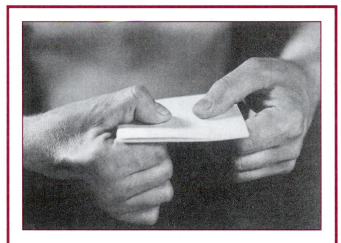

FIGURE 5. Ulnar nerve lesion. A patient with an ulnar nerve lesion is asked to pull a piece of paper apart with both hands. Note the affected side (right hand) uses the flexor pollicis longus muscle to prevent the paper from slipping out of the hand, thus substituting for the adductor pollicis muscle and generating Froment's sign. (From Haymaker W, Woodhall B: Peripheral Nerve Injuries. Philadelphia, W.B. Saunders, 1953, with permission.)

Diagnostic Studies

The cause of the clinical lesion suspected after careful history and physical examination can be investigated with the use of imaging techniques. Plain x-rays could reveal a fracture of the hamate or other carpal bones as well as the metacarpals and the distal radius, especially if there has been a traumatic injury. MRI and CT scan can be helpful if a fracture or a ganglion cyst is suspected.

Nerve conduction study and electromyography are helpful in confirming the diagnosis and the classification as well as in determining the severity of the lesion and the prognosis for functional recovery. As a rule, the dorsal ulnar cutaneous sensory nerve action potential (SNAP) is normal when compared with the unaffected side.[7] Abnormalities in both sensory and motor conduction studies are seen in type I. The ulnar SNAP recorded from the fifth finger is normal in type II, and an isolated abnormality is encountered in type III. The compound muscle action potential (CMAP) of the ADQ is normal in types IIa and III. For this reason, it is important to perform motor studies picking up from more distal muscles such as the first dorsal interosseous. Motor conduction studies should include stimulation across the elbow to rule out a lesion there, as it is far more common. Needle electromyography helps in documenting axonal loss, determining severity of the lesion to allow prognosis for recovery, and in more precisely localizing a lesion for an accurate classification. The FCU and the ulnar heads of the FDP should be completely spared in a lesion at Guyon's canal.[7]

Differential Diagnosis[8]

Ulnar neuropathy at the elbow (or elsewhere)

Cervical radiculopathy at C8-T1

Motor neuron disease

Thoracic outlet syndrome (generally lower trunk or medial cord)

Superior sulcus tumor (affecting the medial cord of the plexus)

Camptodactyly (an unusual developmental condition with a claw deformity)

Treatment

Initial

Initial treatment involves rest and avoidance of trauma (especially if occupational or repetitive causes are suspected). Ergonomic and postural adjustments can be very effective in these cases. The use of NSAIDs/COX-2 inhibitors in cases in which an inflammatory component is suspected can also be very beneficial. Analgesics may help control pain. Low-dose tricyclic anti-depressants may be used for both pain and to help with sleep. Prefabricated wrist splints may be beneficial and are often prescribed for night use. For individuals who continue their sport or work activities, padded shock absorbent gloves may be useful (e.g., for cyclists, jackhammer users).

Rehabilitation

A program of physical or occupational therapy performed by a skilled hand therapist can help to maintain normal range of motion and strength of the interossei and lumbrical muscles. Instructing the patient in a daily routine of home exercises should be done early in the diagnosis. Static splinting (often done as a custom orthosis) with an ulnar gutter will ensure rest of the affected area. In more severe cases, the use of static or dynamic orthotic devices may be considered to improve the patient's functional level. Weakness in the ulnar claw deformity can be corrected to improve grasp with the use of a dorsal metacarpophalangeal block (lumbrical bar) to the fourth and fifth fingers with a soft strap over the palmar aspect.[9]

A worksite evaluation may be beneficial as well. Ergonomic adaptations can prove very helpful to individuals with ulnar nerve entrapment at the wrist (e.g., switching to a foot computer mouse or voice activated computer software).

Procedures

Injections into Guyon's canal may be tried if a compressive entrapment neuropathy is suspected and generally provide symptomatic relief (Fig. 6).[3]

Under sterile conditions, using a 25-gauge, 2-inch disposable needle, a mixture of corticosteroid and 1% or 2% lidocaine totaling no more than 1 cc is injected into the distal wrist crease to the radial side of the pisiform bone and angled sharply distally so that its tip lies just ulnar to the palpable hook of the hamate.[3,10] Postinjection care includes ensuring hemostasis immediately after the procedure, local icing for 5–10 minutes, and instructions to the patient to rest the affected limb during the next 48 hours.

Surgery

Surgery is recommended when there is a fracture of the hook of the hamate or of the pisiform that causes neurologic compromise. Ganglion cyst and pisiohamate arthritis are also indications for surgical treatment. Surgery in general involves exploration, excision of the hook of hamate or pisiform (if fractured), decompression, and neurolysis of the ulnar nerve.[3]

Potential Disease Complications

As previously discussed, the severity and type of lesion of the ulnar nerve at the wrist will ultimately determine the complications. Severe motor axon loss will cause profound weakness and atrophy of ulnar innervated muscles in the hand and render the patient unable to perform even simple tasks due to lack of vital grip strength. Some patients also develop chronic pain in the affected hand, which can be severely debilitating, perhaps inciting a complex regional pain syndrome, and can predispose them to further problems such as depression and drug dependency.

Potential Treatment Complications

The use of NSAIDs should be carefully monitored because there are potential side effects, including gastrointestinal distress and cardiac, renal, and hepatic disease. COX-2 inhibitors may have fewer gastric side effects. Low-dose tricyclic anti-depressants are generally well tolerated but may cause fatigue, so they are usually prescribed for use in the evening. Injection complications include injury to a blood vessel or nerve, infection, and an allergic reaction to the medication used. Complications after surgery include infection, wound dehiscence, recurrence, and rarely, complex regional pain syndrome.

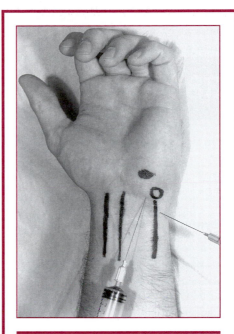

FIGURE 6. Approaches for two ulnar nerve blocks. The needle with syringe attached demonstrates the puncture for block at Guyon's canal. The circle is over the pisiform bone and the solid mark over the hook of the hamate. The second needle demonstrates the puncture site for an ulnar nerve block at the wrist, ulnar approach. (From Lennard TA: Pain Procedures in Clinical Practice, 2nd ed. Philadelphia, Hanley & Belfus, 2000, p 104, with permission.)

References
1. Dumitru D: Electrodiagnostic Medicine. Philadelphia, Hanley & Belfus, 1995, pp 887–891.
2. Concannon MD: Common Hand Problems in Primary Care. Philadelphia, Hanley & Belfus, 1999.
3. Dawson D, Hallet M, Millender L: Entrapment Neuropathies, 2nd ed. pp 193–195.
4. Liveson JA, Spielholz NI: Peripheral Neurology: Case Studies in Electrodiagnosis. Philadelphia, F.A. Davis, 1991.
5. Haymaker W, Woodhall B: Peripheral Nerve Injuries. Philadelphia, WB Saunders, 1953.
6. Snider RK: Essentials of Musculoskeletal Care. Rosemont, IL, American Academy of Orthopaedic Surgeons, 1997, pp 260–262.
7. Kim DJ, Kalantri A, Guha S, Wainapel SF: Dorsal cutaneous nerve conduction: Diagnostic aid in ulnar neuropathy. Arch Neurol 1981;38:321–322.
8. Patil JJP: Entrapment neuropathy. In O'Young BJ, et al (ed): PM&R Secrets, 2nd ed. Philadelphia, Hanley & Belfus, 2002, pp 144–150.
9. Irani KD: Upper limb orthoses. In Braddom RL (ed): Physical Medicine and Rehabilitation. Philadelphia, W.B. Saunders, 1996, pp 328–330.
10. Mauldin CC, Brooks DW: Arm, forearm, and hand blocks. In Lennard TA (ed): Physiatric Procedures. Philadelphia, Hanley & Belfus, 1995, pp 145–146.

38 Wrist Osteoarthritis

Leo M. Rozmaryn, MD

Definition

Degenerative arthritis in the wrist is a final common pathway to destruction, usually stemming from a previous injury. Such injuries include fractures of articular surfaces, ligamentous destruction, and articular cartilage destruction. There are two fundamental patterns:[1] (1) scapholunate advance collapse (SLAC) and (2) triscaphe arthritis. SLAC of the wrist usually occurs as a late sequela due to a scaphoid fracture malunion or scaphoid lunate dissociation. Triscaphe arthritis is located near the base of the thumb and can occur as a result of local trauma. The natural history of SLAC includes a pattern of progressive radial carpal and intercarpal arthritis.

Symptoms

Symptoms usually include radial-side wrist pain, localized swelling, progressive stiffness to wrist flexion/extension, and forearm pronation and supination. There may be weakness of grip. Symptoms are usually increased in the morning, with increased range of motion as the day progresses. The course may be indolent or rapidly progressive.

Physical Examination

There is usually radial-side wrist or distal radial ulna joint tenderness and pain with motion; swelling; and limitation of movement in flexion/extension, radial ulna deviation, and/or forearm pronation and supination. There is weakened grip and pinch strength, and there may be a joint effusion. The patient is more likely to report pain at the extremes of movement rather than throughout the entire range. The presence of limited flexion and extension depends on whether the radial carpal and midcarpal joints are involved. Greater involvement of the radial carpal joint produces decreased wrist flexion, whereas involvement of the midcarpal joint produces diminution in extension range of motion.

Functional Limitations

Functional limitations include a sense of stiffness, weak grasp, and pain with movement of the wrist, impeding the ability for manual exertion and positioning of the hand for fine motor coordination. There is a progressive limitation in activities of daily living.

Diagnostic Studies

The first and most common diagnostic modality is the plain x-ray. Characteristic findings include joint space narrowing; subchondral sclerosis; osteophyte formation; and degenerative cysts occurring in the SLAC pattern, triscaphe arthritis pattern, or isolated distal radial ulna joint pattern. In the first two patterns the radiolunate joint may be spared (Fig. 1). Radioscaphoid arthritis begins at the radial styloid and progresses proximally. In arthritis caused by scapholunate dissociation, the gap between the scaphoid and lunate widens and the capitate pushes down as a wedge between them, eventually reaching the radius. Triscaphe arthritis expresses itself as a localized narrowing between the scaphoid trapezium and trapezoid articulations.

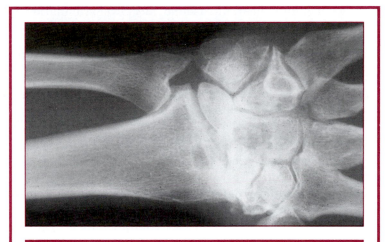

FIGURE 1. Osteoarthritis of the radial scaphoid articulation characteristic in SLAC wrists. Notice this near disappearance of the scaphoid, beaking of the radial styloid, subchondral sclerosis and cyst formation, relative sparing of the distal radial ulna joint, and the radiolunate articulation.

Differential Diagnosis

Inflammatory arthritis (e.g., Lyme disease)

Gout

Rheumatoid arthritis

Psoriatic arthritis

Calcium pyrophosphate deposition disease

Septic arthritis

Systemic lupus erythematosus

Scleroderma

Treatment

Initial

Initial treatment generally involves splinting the wrist in neutral or within 5 degrees of flexion or extension. This is usually accomplished with a light Therma plast splint that is worn during periods of heavy or strenuous use. The wrist sould be removed from the brace several times a day for gentle active and passive range-of-motion exercise, usually in hot water, alternating with cold water in a heat, stretch, ice sequence. The judicious use of nonsteroid anti-inflammatory drugs (NSAIDs), including cyclooxygenase-2 (COX-2) inhibitors, and the avoidance of heavy strenuous activity whenever possible are important. Recent use of oral chondroitinsulfate[2] and glucosamine has shown promise.

Rehabilitation

Rehabilitation by a therapist knowledgeable in treating hand disorders can be helpful. The following treatment is advocated: (1) active range-of-motion exercise; (2) passive stretching; (3) joint mobilization techniques through pain-free ranges of motion; (4) strengthening of wrist musculature and grip, beginning with static exercise and progressing to dynamic exercise with resisted movement; (5) functional activities in therapy and at home to facilitate range of motion, grip function, fine motor coordination; (6) the judicious use of modalities available in physical and/or occupational therapy settings, including heat, ultrasound, electrical stimulation, and ice to decrease pain, inflammation, edema, and increase mobility; and (7) the use of work hardening when appropriate.

Scaphoid Trapezium Trapezoid Postoperative Rehabilitation

The postoperative regimen includes 8 to 10 weeks of immobilization until fusion is complete, and then progressive active and passive range-of-motion exercises are initiated in a flexion extension plane radial ulna deviation and in pronation and supination planes.

Intercarpal and Radial Carpal Postoperative Rehabilitation

The postoperative regimen for wrist reconstruction depends entirely on the nature of the procedure performed. For soft tissue reconstructions that use pins to temporarily fix the radiocarpal or intercarpal joints while the soft tissue elements stabilize, the pins usually remain in place between 8 to 12 weeks. After removal of the pins, the wrist is mobilized by both active and passive range-of-motion exercises. Strengthening is begun almost immediately and continued for another 3 months. Functional and job retraining can begin at that time as well. Baseline function is not expected to return for at least 6 to 8 months.

For wrist arthrodesis with current plate technology, mobilization of the hand can begin immediately, and once the sutures are removed, full functional retraining and strengthening can commence. Additionally, wrist arthrodesis does not include the distal radio-ulnar joint, and full pronation and supination of the forearm can be expected.

Postoperative function remains a concern. While most patients can return to their original job, they need to modify their grips in order to do so. Perineal care and hand manipulation in tight spaces remain the most difficult tasks.

Procedures

The sparing use of intra-articular injected corticosteroid is a useful adjunct. A good rule of thumb is no more than three injections in a year and no more than one injection during a 3-month period. Intra-articular injection of Hyalgan also shows promise.

Surgery

Scaphoid Trapezium Trapezoid Surgery

The ideal treatment of symptomatic scaphoid trapezium trapezoid osteoarthritis is scaphoid trapezial trapezoid (STT) fusion.[3] These fusions are effective methods of maintaining overall carpal height and preventing carpal collapse. The disadvantage of intercarpal arthrodesis is that an alteration of normal wrist function occurs with a loss of approximately 50% of flexion and extension. With increased stress placed around adjacent joints, arthritis may progress in these other articulations; thus the overall rate of progressive radial carpal arthritis is 33%. Alternatives to STT fusion are trapezium excision and ligamentous reconstruction, or arthroplasty with trapezoid joint interposition.[4] This also prevents subsequent thumb metacarpal trapezial arthritis.

Intercarpal and Radial Carpal Surgery

In a SLAC wrist, there often is a normal radial lunate and midcarpal joint. In that case, excision of the scaphoid followed by capitolunate arthrodeses or a four-corner fusion (capitate lunate hamate triquetrum) addresses the radial scaphoid and possible capitolunate arthritis.[5] Most patients have a good to excellent result, with preservation of approximately 50% of motion in the flexion extension plane and 80% in the radial ulna deviation plane, as well as 80% of grip strength compared with the other side.[6]

Salvage procedures for symptomatic SLAC wrists and other osteoarthritic conditions that affect the radial carpal intercarpal joint include proximal row carpectomy and total wrist fusion. After this procedure, patients have excellent range of motion, ranging from 80 degrees to 94 degrees, with preservation of about 50% of grip strength.[7] In other studies, flexion extension arc averaged 61% of the other wrist, and grip strength averaged 80% of the other side.[8] The ultimate salvage for wrist osteoarthritis is total wrist arthrodesis.[9] This procedure has excellent reliability in terms of pain relief and durability and offers the patient upper strength that can be used for repetitive activities and heavy labor. The disadvantages of this fusion is that wrist flexion extension, radial and ulna deviation movements are eliminated. However, patients can pronate and supinate their forearms. Modern design of wrist fusion internal fixation plates have shortened the recovery and immobilization times. Usually, splints can be discontinued at 6 to 8 weeks. Finger and thumb movement normally can be begun immediately, and pronation and supination can start in 3 weeks, with the patient in a short arm cast.

Total Wrist Arthroplasty

During the past 15 years, much discussion has taken place about total wrist arthroplasty made of either a single silicone unit or a composite utilizing the same types of metal and plastic materials used in total knee replacement. Although the short-term results are excellent in terms of range of motion of the wrist and pain relief, there have been long-term problems with loosening of these prostheses.[10]

Potential Disease Complications

The history of this condition is the progression to joint ankylosis or autofusion, at which point movement differs from surgical arthrodesis in that the position of the joint may assume is predictable and may not be of functional use to the patient. By the time this stage is reached there is virtually no pain; however, pain can be protracted for a long period.

Potential Treatment Complications

Analgesics, NSAIDs, and COX-2 inhibitors have well-known side effects that most commonly affect the gastric, hepatic, and renal systems. Potential treatment complications include operative infection, hardware failure, nonunion of arthrodeses, and severe silicone synovitis. This form of synovitis can invade into surrounding bone structure, causing gross destruction of bone. Bilateral wrist arthrodesis can be quite disabling, and differing positions of arthrodesis may have to be used to allow the patient to address personal hygiene and activities of daily living.

References
1. Watson HK, Ryu J: Degenerative disorders of the carpus. Orthop Clin North Am 1984;15:337–353.
2. McAlandon TE, LaValley MP, Gulin JP, Felson DT: Glucosamine and chondroitin for treatment of osteoarthritis: A systemic quality assessment and metananalysis. JAMA 2000;283(11):1469–1484.
3. Fortin PT, Louis ES: Long-term follow-up of scaphoid trapezium trapezoid arthrodesis. J Hand Surg 1993;18A:675–681.
4. Tomaino MN, Tellegrini ED Jr, Burton RI: Arthroplasty of the basal joint of the thumb: Long-term follow-up after ligament reconstruction with tendon interposition. J Bone Joint Surg 1995;77A:346–355.
5. Ashmead D IV, Watson HK, Damon C, et al: Scapholunate advance collapse wrist salvage. J Hand Surg 1994;19A:741–750.
6. Krakauer JD, Bishop AT, Kooney WP: Surgical treatment of scapholunate advance collapse. J Hand Surg 1994;19A:751–759.
7. Tomaino MM, Delsignore J, Burton RI: Long-term results following proximal row carpectomy. J Hand Surg 1994;19A:694–703.
8. Tomaino MM, Miller RJ, Cole I, Burton RI: Scapholunate advance collapse wrist: Proximal row carpectomy or limited wrist arthrodesis with scaphoid excision. J Hand Surg 1994;19A:134–142.
9. Weiss AC, Wiedeman G Jr, Quenzer E, et al: Upper extremity function after wrist arthrodesis. J Hand Surg 1995;20A:813–817.
10. Meuli HC, Fernandez D VL: Uncemented total wrist arthroplasty. J Hand Surg 1995;20A:115–122.

39 | Wrist Rheumatoid Arthritis

Leo M. Rozmaryn, MD

Synonyms

Rheumatoid arthritis

Rheumatism

Inflammatory arthritis

ICD-9 Code

714.0
Rheumatoid arthritis

Definition

Rheumatoid arthritis is a systemic disease of the connective skeletal system as well as the lymphatic and circulatory systems. This is a slowly progressive disorder that affects virtually any joint in the body and can have a profound effect on the hand and wrist. Rheumatoid synovitis in the wrist releases lytic substances in clearly designed patterns that destroy articular cartilage as well as joint capsule, bone, or tendon sheath. The disease can take three different forms: monocyclic, polycyclic, and progressive, and it is difficult to predict which pattern the patient's condition will follow. Although the primary treatment for this condition is medical, surgery is an option for cases of progressive deformity and failure of medical treatment to stem the synovitis or impending tendon rupture.

Symptoms

The patient's chief complaints are generally joint pain, stiffness, and joint fatigue. During an exacerbation phase, the wrist may feel warm to the touch with the presence of either localized or diffuse edema. Morning stiffness is common. Patients may also complain of cosmetic issues, including joint swelling and deformity.

Physical Examination

The most common forms of wrist deformity observed are wrist flexion, deviation, and palmar subluxation (Fig. 1). Relative dorsal subluxation of the ulnar head occurs as the carpus supinates away from it, leading to the disruption of the distal radial ulna joint and displacement of the extensor carpi ulnaris tendon volarly, which in turn compromises ulna stability during wrist extension. Ankylosis of the intercarpal and carpal joints may occur as well, producing the inability to cup the hand. During an exacerbation phase, the wrist range of motion, particularly at the end range, is extremely painful with weakness on motor testing. There may be localized swelling about the extensor retinacular involving the fourth extensor compartment, occasionally involving the extensor pollicis longus. It begins beneath the extensor retinaculum and may extend distally over the dorsum of the hand and envelop the extensor tendons of the wrist and fingers. Lysosomal enzymes may digest and weaken the dorsal tendons and wrist ligaments and may directly invade the tendons themselves. If left unchecked the synovitis can cause tendon rupture and the palmar collapse deformity mentioned previously. Thus, patients may present with inability to extend the wrist or the fingers.

Strength may be limited by pain, disuse, or deformity (e.g., making grasping difficult); however, the remainder of the neurologic examination should be normal.

Functional Limitations

Functional limitations include inability to perform heavy lifting and gripping because of pain and inability to perform fine motor functions because of limitations of range of motion of the wrist. Patients may have difficulty with gripping a steering wheel or a grocery bag. They may have problems with cooking and cleaning due to difficulty with gripping tools. Activities of daily living such as shaving, shampooing the hair, etc., may be curtailed as well.

Diagnostic Studies

The "gold standard" for imaging remains the plain x-ray. Collapse of wrist architecture occurs in characteristic patterns in rheumatoid arthritis. These patterns are governed by the close proximity of synovial patches to supporting wrist ligaments. Collapse of the joint also results from articular cartilage and subchondral bone erosion. In the distal

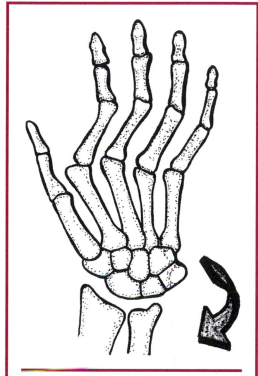

FIGURE 1. Characteristic Z-deformity of the hand and wrist in rheumatoid arthritis. The wrist translates ulnarly, the metacarpals angle radially, and the fingers deviate ulnarly at the metacarpophalangeal joints.

radial ulnar joint, synovitis can destroy the joint capsule and the triangular fibrocartilage complex. The head of the ulna becomes grossly deformed by destruction of the articular surfaces, and a relatively dorsal subluxation of the ulna occurs as the remaining carpus collapses volarly to the ulna head. This is known as the caput ulnae syndrome.[1] Other areas of involvement include the radial carpal joint, where intercarpal collapse patterns predominate. The destruction of the articular cartilage, the radial scaphoid, and radial lunar articulation will result in joint space narrowing. Insufficiency of the radial scaphoid lunate ligament may cause rotatory subluxation of the scaphoid and carpal malalignment, eventually leading to bony ankylosis. In addition, the distal carpal row rotates radially with the metacarpals giving rise to a zigzag deformity of the digits, radial deviation of the carpus, and ulnar deviation of the metacarpophalangeal joints. The subchondral collapse of the scaphoid fossa of the distal radius can cause proximal migration of the scaphoid into the radius (Fig. 2). The proximal migration of the capitate through a scaphoid lunate diastasis is a direct result of the weakening of the interosseus scaphoid lunate ligament.

Differential Diagnosis

Septic arthritis	Enteropathic arthritides
Lyme's disease	Osteoarthritis
Systemic lupus erythematosus	Gout
Psoriatic arthritis	Pyrophosphate deposition disease

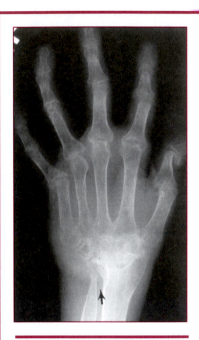

FIGURE 2. Advanced rheumatoid arthritis of the hand. Note the eroded distal ulna (arrow), loss of carpal height, erosions of the distal radius, loss of joint space, and periarticular erosions involving the metacarpophalangeal joints. (From Jebson PJL, Kasdan ML: Hand Secrets. Philadelphia, Hanley & Belfus, 1998, with permission.)

Treatment

Initial

The initial treatment of rheumatoid arthritis of the wrist may include the use of NSAIDs/COX-2 inhibitors, adjunctive antirheumatic agents, or oral steroids (see Chapter 134). Initial treatment may also include the use of intra-articular corticosteroid injections to cool down an acute synovitis.[2]

During the acute or postoperative phase the use of ice may be appropriate to decrease pain.

Patient education regarding the avoidance of exacerbating activities and the use of appropriate equipment at home and work to minimize pain and swelling and optimize function is important.

Rehabilitation

When initiating treatment of the rheumatoid wrist the clinician should be aware of the patient's clinical status since management in the acute and chronic stages are different.

Hot paraffin baths and whirlpool can be effective in increasing circulation and mobility. Splints such as wrist cock-up splints may improve deformity at the earliest stages of disease by providing relief from pain and swelling and thus maintaining proper alignment to the joints. During an exacerbation, general range-of-motion exercises are performed to prevent joint stiffness while avoiding the painful arc of movement. The therapist should be careful not to overstretch the joint because it can cause tissue damage. Active assisted range-of-motion exercises are appropriate, and strengthening should be limited to static exercise while the joint is inflamed. When inflammation subsides dynamic exercises may be initiated to promote movement and function. Strengthening of the wrist extensors will maintain hand function. Patients should be encouraged to perform as many functional activities as they can tolerate to prevent deformity and to take frequent rest periods during exercise and daily activity. When home exercises are prescribed, the patient should be instructed to perform short periods of exercise throughout the day rather than one long period of exercise.

The postoperative regimen for wrist reconstruction depends entirely on the nature of the procedures performed. For soft tissue reconstruction, if pins are used, they usually remain for 8 to 12 weeks. After removal of the pins, gentle passive and active range-of-motion exercises can mobilize the wrist. Strengthening exercises are typically done early in the course of treatment and often are progressed for up to 3 months after surgery. Functional and job retraining can be done after 8 to 12 weeks depending on the work demands. Baseline function may not resume until 6 to 8 months postoperatively.

Rehabilitative treatment must be dovetailed with sound medical management.

Procedures

The wrist may be injected to improve function and pain. Typically this can be done 2 to 3 times a year, but is not recommended repeatedly. Many of the small joints of the wrist have interconnecting synovial spaces, which make it possible to successfully inject the wrist via a

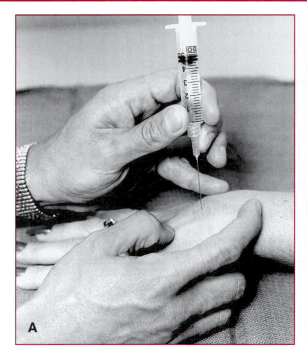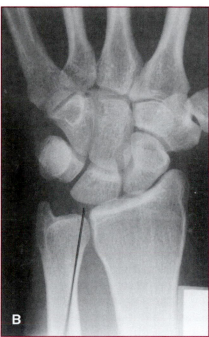

FIGURE 3. *A*, Dorsal wrist approach. The needle is inserted medial to the extensor pollicis longus tendon. *B*, Anteroposterior x-ray of the wrist demonstrating proper needle placement into the wrist using a dorsal approach. (From Lennard TA: Pain Procedures in Clinical Practice, 2nd ed. Philadelphia, Hanley & Belfus, 2000, with permission.)

number of approaches. The site of inflammation or desired anatomic area may determine the desired route.

The dorsal approach is often the preferred method for wrist injection (Fig. 3). This can be done best with the patient's wrist in slight flexion (over a rolled towel). Under sterile conditions, direct a 25- or 27-gauge needle just medial to the extensor pollicis longus tendon. Inject a mixture of local anesthetic (e.g., 1 cc 1% lidocaine) and corticosteroid (e.g., 1 cc triamcinolone).

Postinjection care may include local icing for 5 to 10 minutes and splinting for up to 1 week. Patients should avoid heavy lifting or carrying items after the injection.

Surgery

Tenosynovitis

Flexor and extensor tendons crossing the wrists are common sites of the relentless tenosynovitis that slowly destroys them. The tenosynovitis occurs as a result of direct invasion by rheumatoid pannus or lysosomal enzymes that digest the tendons. Sharp, bony prominences such as the ulnar head, Lister's tubercle, or the scaphoid tubercle form a mechanical shearing device that assists in this process. Digital extensor tendons that cross over the caput ulnar are affected most commonly. Ruptures usually affect the ulnar digits first and progress radially. Clinically, this could manifest suddenly and without pain. The extensor pollicis longus can be affected independently. Tenosynovitis can be cured and is of an urgent nature, especially if some of these tendons have begun to rupture. Flexor tendon ruptures must be distinguished from tendon subluxation and the possibility of radial nerve palsy secondary to rheumatoid tissue infiltration on the radial nerve. These can be evaluated by the "tenodesis" effect. If the digits cannot be extended at the metacarpophalangeal joint by flexing the wrist, the tendons likely have been ruptured. In the early stages of the disease the tendons can be repaired in a side-to-side fashion to intact extensor tendons. Direct end-to-end repair may work in very early stages but will become impossible later. If all the extensor tendons have been ruptured on the dorsum, reconstruction becomes increasingly difficult and will require tendon transfer from the volar side, usually a digital flexor. Flexor tendon rupture is much more difficult to treat. Tendon transfers or grafts are secondary and reconstruction may be necessary because direct repair is usually impossible. Fusions of the distal interphalangeal joint may be required when profundus tendon rupture becomes irreparable.[3]

Reconstruction of the Collapsed Wrist

Synovitis in the wrist characteristically starts on the ulnar aspect, and repair usually involves the distal radial ulnar and the radial carpal joint and spares the midcarpal joint. A dorsal wrist synovectomy is indicated for painful, poorly controlled synovitis and minimal articular damage. Following a synovectomy the dorsal retinaculum can be placed beneath the extensor tendons to reinforce the capsule and relocate the extensor carpi ulnaris dorsally. This is usually considered in patients in the early course of disease after about 6 months of medical therapy in which there is persistent pain, swelling, and loss of function as a result of inflammation.[4] Patients usually gain a strong sense of securing grip and do not mind the relative increase in stiffness after the procedure. Recently the arthroscope has been used to affect synovectomy of the wrist with minimal destruction of the soft tissue envelope. However, if the synovitis in the distal radioulnar joint progresses and instability results, a dorsally protuberant ulna can cause extensor tendon rupture. Shortening of the ulna; hemi-excision of the radial side of the ulna, leaving the ulna styloid intact; or excision of the distal 1 cm of the ulna head may be considered (Darrach procedure). The Darrach procedure has lost favor in the reconstruction of post-traumatic distal radial ulna joint problems in younger patients but affords older rheumatoid patients increased movement with less pain and removes the risk of extensor tendon rupture. There have been many attempts to reconstruct the ulna head with silastic prostheses to support the ulna carpus. This technique has had problems with implant fragmentation and silicone synovitis. In general, a well performed Darrach procedure is all that is necessary in this setting to achieve good results.[5]

Arthroplasty/Arthrodesis

As wrist disease progresses and pain and instability become more prominent, the clinician needs to consider arthroplasty or arthrodesis (Fig. 4). An arthrodesis will create a strong, painless wrist that is devoid of motion in the flexion extension and the radial ulnar plane. This can be problematic if the patient has another ankylosed joint in that extremity. To preserve wrist motion, numerous *arthroplasty* procedures have been described. These include synovectomy with stabilization, temporary pinning of the wrist, and creation of a fibrous ankylosis between the radius and the proximal carpal row. Silastic implants have been devised; however, although short-term results have been promising, these techniques over the long term have proven to be quite problematic. The elastic end of prostheses can fracture and can cause silicone synovitis.

A more permanent and stable solution is the wrist *arthrodesis*, either total or partial. Complete wrist radial carpal arthrodesis is indicated for severe wrist pain with deformity, bone loss, and ruptured extensor tendons. The best position for wrist fusion is neutral with slight flexion. The wrist joint is stabilized with pins (Fig. 4). This procedure has excellent long-term results with relief of pain and preservation of hand function.[6] This can also be performed in conjunction with a Darrach procedure.

Potential Disease Complications

Disease related complications include permanent loss of movement in the fingers, with collapse of the fingers secondary to tendon rupture; volar grip collapse with chronic pain; flexion deformity; and severe loss of activities of daily living.

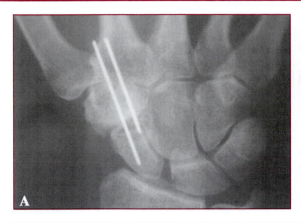
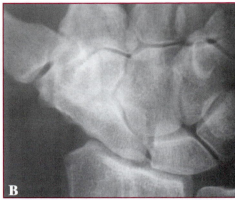

FIGURE 4. Triscaphe (STT) arthrodesis. A, Radiographic examination 6 weeks after triscaphe arthrodesis demonstrates typical pin placement and adequate bony consolidation. B, Three months after triscaphe fusion, the arthrodesis is radiographically solid. (From Weinzweig J: Plastic Surgery Secrets. Philadelphia, Hanley & Belfus, 1999, p 619, with permission.)

Potential Treatment Complications

Medical treatment complications are discussed in detail in Chapter 134. Surgical treatment complications include silicone synovitis from the use of silastic wrist; hardware loosening; and backing out, such as seen in wrist arthrodesis. These can secondarily puncture through the skin, creating infection. Non-union of the arthrodesis has been seen. The possibility of fracture about the wrist dramatically increases as the bones about the wrist become increasingly osteopenic.

Complications following total wrist replacement vary from 15% to 40%. In addition, bone resorption, component loosening, radial ulnar imbalance, and attritional tendon rupture have been seen.[7]

References
1. Millender H, Nalebuff EA: Preventive surgery-tenosynovectomy and synovectomy. Orthop Clin North Am 1975;6:765–792.
2. Massarotti EM: Medical aspects of rheumatoid arthritis: Diagnosis and treatment. Hand Clin 1996;12:463–475.
3. Wheen EJ, Tonkin MA, Green J, Bronkhorst N: Long-term results following digital flexor tenosynovectomy in rheumatoid arthritis. J Hand Surg 1995;20A:790–794.
4. Kulick RG, De Fiore JC, Straub LR, et al: Long-term results of dorsal stabilization in the rheumatoid wrist. J Hand Surg 1981:6:272–280.
5. Blank JE, Cassidy C: The distal radial ulna joint in rheumatoid arthritis. Hand Clin 1996;12:499–513.
6. American Academy of Orthopedic Surgeons: Orthopedic knowledge update III. Park Ridge, IL, American Academy of Orthopedic Surgeons, 1990, p 373.
7. Blair WF: An approach to complex rheumatoid hand and wrist problems. Hand Clin 1996;12:615–628.

40 Thoracic Compression Fracture

Toni J. Hanson, MD

Synonyms

Thoracic compression
fracture

Dorsal compression
fracture

Wedge compression

Vertebral crush fracture[1,2]

ICD-9 Code

805.2
Fracture of vertebral
column without mention
of spinal cord injury;
dorsal [thoracic], closed

Definition

A compression fracture is caused by forces transmitted along the vertebral body. The ligaments are intact, and compression fractures are usually stable.[3] Compression fractures in the thoracic vertebrae are commonly seen in osteoporosis with decreased bone mineral density. Such fractures may occur with trivial trauma and are usually stable. Pathologic vertebral fractures may occur with metastatic cancer (commonly in lung, breast, or prostate) as well as other processes affecting vertebrae. Trauma, such as a fall from a height or a motor vehicle accident, can also result in a thoracic compression fracture. Considerable force is required to fracture healthy vertebrae, which are resistant to compression. In such cases, the force required to produce a fracture may cause extension of fracture components into the spinal canal with neurologic findings. There may be evidence of additional trauma such as calcaneal fractures from a fall. Multiple thoracic compression fractures, as seen with osteoporosis, can produce a kyphotic deformity.[4–6] (See Fig. 1.)

Symptoms

Pain in the thoracic spine over the affected vertebrae is the usual hallmark of the presentation. It may be severe, sharp, exacerbated with movement, and decreased with rest. Severe pain may last 2 to 3 weeks and then decrease over 6 to 8 weeks; however, pain may persist for months. Typically, in osteoporotic fractures, the mid and lower thoracic vertebrae are affected. Acute fractures in osteoporosis, however, may result in little discomfort or poor localization.[7] Multiple fractures result in kyphosis (Dowager's hump). A good history and physical examination are essential since there may be indicators of a more ominous underlying pathology.[8,9]

Physical Examination

Tenderness with palpation or percussion over the affected region of the thoracic vertebrae is the primary finding on examination. Spinal movements also produce pain. Kyphotic deformity may be present in the patient who has had multiple prior compression fractures. Neurologic examination below the level of the fracture is recommended to assess for presence of reflex changes, Babinski's reflex, and sensory alteration. In an isolated compression fracture, the neurologic exam is normal. However, in some instances, the fracture may cause neurologic compromise. Sacral segments can be assessed through evaluation of rectal tone, volitional control, anal wink, and pinprick if there is concern about bowel and bladder function. The patient's height, weight, and chest expansion measurements are useful. Assessing the patient's gait for stability is also important. Co-morbid neurologic and orthopedic conditions may contribute to gait dysfunction and fall risk.[10,11]

Functional Limitations

Functional limitations in a patient with an acute painful compression fracture can be significant. The patient may experience loss of mobility and independence in activities of daily living, in addition to impact on social functioning. Hospitalization may be necessary for patients with severe symptoms.[12]

Diagnostic Studies

AP and lateral x-rays of the thoracic spine can confirm the clinical impression of a thoracic compression fracture. Radiographically in a thoracic compression fracture, the height of the

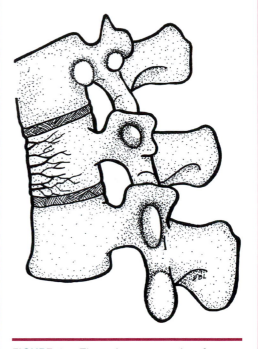

FIGURE 1. Thoracic compression fracture with reduction in anterior vertebral height and wedging of the vertebrae.

affected vertebrae is reduced, generally in a wedge-shaped fashion with anterior height less than posterior vertebral height. A bone scan may help localize (but not necessarily determine the etiology of) processes such as metastatic cancer, occult fracture, and infection. Percutaneous needle biopsy of the affected vertebral body can be helpful diagnostically in selected cases. Spinal imaging, such as CT or MRI, may also elucidate further detail.[13] Laboratory tests, including serum calcium, alkaline phosphatase, 24-hour urine collection, and bone mineral density testing,[14] may be helpful for metabolic processes. A CBC and sedimentation rate (which is a nonspecific, but sensitive indicator of an occult infection or inflammatory disease) may also be helpful. Diagnostic testing is directed, as appropriate, based on the entire clinical presentation.

Differential Diagnosis

Thoracic sprain

Thoracic radiculopathy

Thoracic disc herniation

Metastatic malignancy

Primary spine malignancy (uncommon, most frequently multiple myeloma)[15]

Benign spinal tumors

Infection, osteomyelitis (rare)[16]

Inflammatory arthritis

Referred pain (pancreatic cancer, abdominal aortic aneurysm)

Treatment

Initial

Initial treatment consists of activity modification, including limited bed rest. Cushioning with use of a mattress overlay (such as an egg crate) can also be helpful. Pharmacologic agents, including oral analgesics, muscle relaxants, and anti-inflammatory medications as appropriate for the patient are helpful. This includes agents such as tramadol 50 mg (1 or 2 q 4–6 hours, not exceeding 400 mg/day), propoxyphene napsylate 100 mg/acetaminophen 650 mg (1 q 4–6 hours), and acetaminophen 300 mg/codeine 30 mg (1 to 2 q 4–6 hours). If more severe or persistent pain is present, consideration can be given to an agent such as oxycodone CR (10 mg or 20 mg q 12 hours). Muscle relaxants, such as cyclobenzaprine 10 mg tid, may be helpful initially with muscle spasm. A variety of nonsteroidal anti-inflammatory drugs (NSAIDs), including the COX-2 inhibitors, can be considered, depending on the patient. Calcitonin (one spray daily, alternating nostrils providing 200 IU/0.09 ml per spray) has also been used for painful osteoporotic fractures. Stool softeners and laxatives may be necessary to reduce strain with bowel movements and constipation, particularly with narcotic analgesics.

Avoidance of spinal motion, especially flexion, via appropriate body mechanics (such as log rolling in bed) and spinal bracing is helpful. There are a variety of spinal orthoses that reduce spinal flexion. They must be properly fitted.[17,18] A lumbosacral orthosis (LSO) may be sufficient for a low thoracic fracture. A thoracolumbosacral orthoses (TLSO) is used frequently. If a greater degree of fracture immobilization is required, a custom-molded body jacket may be fit by an orthotist. Proper diagnosis and treatment of underlying contributors to the thoracic compression fracture are necessary. Most thoracic compression fractures will heal, but may produce permanent deformity.

Rehabilitation

Physical therapy is helpful to assist with gentle mobilization of the patient by employing proper body mechanics, optimizing transfer techniques, and training with gait aids to reduce biomechanical stresses on the spine and ensure gait safety. Pain-relieving modalities, such as therapeutic heat or cold, and transcutaneous electrical nerve stimulation may also be used. Exercise should not increase spinal symptoms. In addition to proper body mechanics and postural training (emphasizing spinal extension and avoidance of flexion), spinal extensor muscle strengthening, limb strengthening, stretching to muscle groups (such as the pectoral muscles, hips, and lower extremities), and deep breathing exercises may also be indicated. Weight-bearing exercises for bone health, balance, and fall prevention are also important. Proper footwear, with cushioning inserts, can also be helpful. Occupational therapy can help the patient with activities of daily living, reinforce proper spinal ergonomics, and address equipment needs and fall prevention. Successful rehabilitation is targeted at increasing the patient's comfort, decreasing deformity, decreasing resultant disability, and is individualized to address specific patient needs.[19–21]

Procedures

Invasive procedures are generally not indicated. Percutaneous vertebroplasty may be helpful to reduce pain and reinforce vertebral strength in selected cases.[21]

Surgery

Surgery is rarely necessary. Surgical stabilization can be considered in patients with continued severe pain after compression fracture as a result of non-union of the fracture or spinal instability or if neurologic complications occur. Referral to a spine surgeon is recommended in these cases for further assessment.[23]

Potential Disease Complications

Neurologic complications, including nerve or spinal cord compromise as well as orthopedic complications with continued pain, non-union, and instability, can occur. Underlying primary disease (e.g., metastatic thoracic compression) needs to be addressed. Patients with severe kyphosis may experience cardiopulmonary dysfunction. Severe thoracic pain accompanying a fracture may further limit deep breathing and increase the risk of pulmonary complications such as pneumonia. Progressive spinal deformity may produce secondary pain generators. The patient may have progressive levels of dependency as a result.

Potential Treatment Complications

Analgesics, NSAIDs, and COX-2 inhibitors have well-known side effects that most commonly affect the gastric, hepatic, and renal systems. It is important to select medications appropriately for individual patients. There may be difficulty with the use of spinal orthotics, such as intolerance in patients with gastroesophogeal reflux disease (GERD). Kyphotic patients frequently do not tolerate orthoses, and fitting is problematic. Surgery can result in many complications, not only from general anesthesia risks, but also from infection or bleeding difficulties such as hemorrhage or thromboembolism. Poor mechanical strength of bone, as in osteoporosis with paucity of dense lamellar and cortical bone, may result in suboptimal surgical outcome.

References

1. Benson LS: Orthopaedic PEARLS. Philadelphia: F. A. Davis, 1999, p 369.
2. Goldie B: Orthopaedic Diagnosis and Management—A Guide to the Care of Orthopaedic Patients. London, Blackwell Scientific, 1998, pp 183–209.
3. Benzel EC, Stillerman CB: The Thoracic Spine. St. Louis, Quality Medical Publishers, 1999, p 20.
4. Kesson M, Atkins E: The thoracic spine. In Kesson M, Atkins E: Orthopaedic Medicine—A Practical Approach. Butterworth/Heinemann, 1998, pp 262–281.
5. McRae R: The thoracic and lumbar spine. In Parkinson M (ed): Pocketbook of Orthopaedics and Fractures, vol 1. New York, Churchill Livingstone–Harcourt, 1999, pp 79–105.
6. Dandy D, Edwards D: Disorders of the spine. In Dandy D, Edwards D: Essential Orthopaedics and Trauma. New York, Churchill Livingstone, 1998, pp 431–451.
7. Bonner F, Chesnut C, Fitzsimmons A, Lindsay R: Osteoporosis. In DeLisa J, Gans BM (eds): Rehabilitation Medicine: Principles and Practice. Philadelphia, Lippincott-Raven, 1998, pp 1453–1475.
8. Van de Veld T: Disorders of the thoracic spine: Non-disc lesions. In Ombregt L (ed): A System of Orthopaedic Medicine. Philadelphia, W.B. Saunders, 1995, pp 455–469.
9. Errico T, Stecker S, Kostuik J: Thoracic Pain Syndromes. In Frymoyer J (ed): The Adult Spine: Principles and Practices. Philadelphia, Lippincott-Raven, 1997, pp 1623–1637.
10. Hu S, Carlson G, Tribus C: Disorders, diseases, and injuries of the spine. In Skinner H (ed): Current Diagnosis and Treatment in Orthopedics. New York, Lane Medical Books/McGraw-Hill, 2000, pp 177–246.
11. Pattavina C: Diagnostic imaging. In Hart R (ed): Handbook of Orthopaedic Emergencies. Philadelphia, Lippincott-Raven, 1999, pp 32–47, 116–126, 127–140.
12. Goldstein T: Treatment of common problems of the spine. In Goldstein T: Geriatric Orthopaedics—Rehabilitative Management of Common Problems. Gaithersburg, MD, Aspen Publications, 1999, pp 211–232.
13. Bisese J: Compression fracture secondary to underlying metastasis. In Bolger E, Ramos-Englis M (eds): Spinal MRI: A Teaching File Approach. New York, McGraw-Hill, 1992, pp 73–129.
14. Genant H, Lang P, Steiger P, et al: Osteoporosis: Assessment by bone densitometry. In Manelfe C (ed): Imaging of the Spine and Spinal Cord. New York, Raven Press, 1992, pp 221–242.
15. Heller JG, Pedlow FX Jr: Tumors of the Spine. In Garfin S, Vaccaro AR (eds): Orthopaedic Knowledge Update. Spine. Rosemont, IL, American Academy of Orthopaedic Surgeons, 1997, pp 235–256.
16. Levine MJ, Heller JG: Spinal Infections. In Garfin S, Vaccaro AR (eds): Orthopaedic Knowledge Update. Spine. Rosemont, IL, American Academy of Orthopaedic Surgeons, 1997, pp 257–271.
17. Saunders H: Spinal orthotics. In Saunders R (ed): Evaluation, Treatment and Prevention of Musculoskeletal Disorders, vol 1. Bloomington, MN, Educational Opportunities, 1993, pp 285–296.
18. Bussel M, Merritt J, Fenwick L: Spinal orthoses. In Redford J (ed): Orthotics Clinical Practice and Rehabilitation Technology. New York, Churchill Livingstone, 1995, pp 71–101.
19. Browngoehl L. Osteoporosis. In: Grabois M, Garrison, SJ, Hart, KA, Lehmkuhl, LD, ed. Physical Medicine & Rehabilitation The Complete Approach: Blackwell Science:1565-1577.
20. Eilbert W: Long-term care and rehabilitation of orthopaedic injuries. In Hart R, Rittenberry TJ, Uehara DT (eds): Handbook of Orthopaedic Emergencies. Philadelphia, Lippincott-Raven, 1999, 127–138.
21. Barr JD, Barr MS, Lemley TJ, McCann RM: Percutaneous vertebroplasty for pain relief and spinal stabilization. Spine 2000;25:923–928.
22. Kostuik J, Heggeness M: Surgery of the osteoporotic spine. In Frymoyer J (ed): The Adult Spine: Principles and Practice. Philadelphia, Lippincott-Raven, 1997, pp 1639–1664.
23. Snell E, Scarpone M: Orthopaedic issues in aging. In Baratz M, Watson AD, Imbriglia JE (eds): Orthopaedic Surgery: The Essentials. New York, Thieme Medicine Publishers, 1999, pp 865–870.

41 Thoracic Outlet Syndrome

Paul F. Pasquina, MD

Synonyms

Scalenus anticus syndrome

Cervical rib syndrome

First thoracic rib syndrome

Costoclavicular syndrome

Subcoracoid-pectoralis minor syndrome

Hyperabduction syndrome[1]

ICD-9 Code

353.0
Brachial plexus lesions (cervical rib syndrome, costoclavicular syndrome, scalenus anticus syndrome, thoracic outlet syndrome)

Definition

Thoracic outlet syndrome (TOS) remains a contentious area in medicine. The term is used to describe a number of conditions attributed to a compromise of the brachial plexus (typically the lower trunk), subclavian/axillary artery or vein, or both at one or more points between the base of the neck and the axilla. Because of the controversy and confusion surrounding this entity it is helpful to further subclassify the condition based on the neurovascular structure that is compromised: neurologic (axonal) TOS, vascular TOS, and disputed/symptomatic TOS.[2]

Vascular TOS refers to compromise of the subclavian/axillary artery or vein. Both are very rare and usually affect young to middle-aged persons. Vascular compromise may develop from trauma, thrombi, or congenital anomalies, such as a fully formed cervical rib or abnormal first thoracic rib. Traumatic causes such as midclavicular fractures may present acutely or as a late effect secondary to non-union or excessive callus formation. Repetitive trauma has also been implicated, such as that seen in throwing sports. Intimal damage to vascular structures may lead to thrombus or aneurysm formation.

Neurologic (axonal) TOS refers to true compression of the brachial plexus with resultant axonal damage, particularly to the lower trunk. This condition is also very rare, affecting young to middle-aged women more than men. Although many conditions may contribute to brachial plexus injuries (e.g., trauma, tumor, infections), the term "neurologic TOS" is used to describe a condition believed to be caused by the compression of the distal T1 and, to a lesser extent, the distal C8 anterior primary rami, by a taut band that extends from a rudimentary cervical rib or elongated C7 transverse process to the first thoracic rib.

"Disputed," or "symptomatic," TOS refers to a condition that occurs more commonly than both the vascular and true neurologic types. It is defined more as a symptom complex rather than a true anatomic pathologic process. Because of the difficulties in defining this condition, accurate etiologic data is not available, although it appears to affect women more than men. It is a diagnosis of exclusion, and therefore other conditions must be excluded prior to making the diagnosis. Physical examination should reveal normal neurologic and vascular findings.

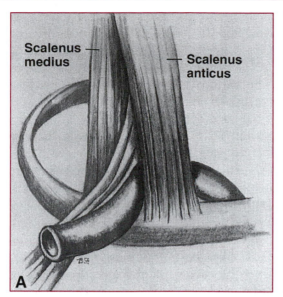
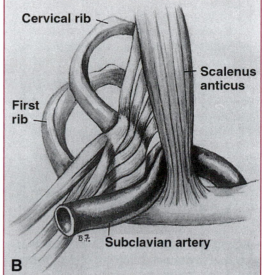
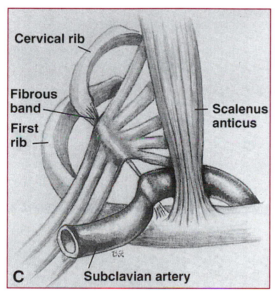
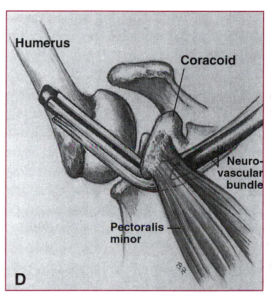

FIGURE 1. Areas of compression of the neurovascular bundle. A, Hypertrophy of scalene muscles. B, Presence of cervical rib. C, Presence of a fibrous band. D, Compression by pectoralis minor during hyperabduc tion. (From DePalma AF: Surgery of the Shoulder, 2nd ed. Philadelphia, J.B. Lippincott, 1973, pp 511–520, with permission.)

Symptoms

Patients typically report pain along the distal and ulnar aspects of their forearm and hand as well as sensory symptoms such as numbness, tingling, and burning. These symptoms are often aggravated by certain positions or activities, especially those involving overhead work. Subjective complaints of weakness or of dropping objects should be verified by physical examination. Those with vascular compromise may present with swelling, cyanosis, coldness, or even Raynaud's type symptoms.

Physical Examination

Physical examination should include an extensive evaluation of the patient's neck, shoulders, and upper extremities, with particular attention to the neurologic and vascular examinations. The patient should be undressed in order to assess any postural abnormalities or side-to-side atrophy.

Careful attention to the neck range of motion and a positive Spurling's test may reveal a cervical root lesion. Abnormal reflexes, weakness, and atrophy are consistent with a true neurologic deficit. Neurologic TOS, affecting primarily the lower trunk of the brachial plexus, may reveal atrophy of the thenar greater than hypothenar eminence in the hand, weakness of the hand intrinsic muscles, and sensory abnormalities of the medial forearm and hand.

Patients with vascular compromise to their upper extremity may have upper extremity swelling, discoloration, prominent dilated veins, subungual hemorrhages, and ulcerations of the fingertips.[3] These patients may also have a diminished radial pulse, especially after exercise.

Patients with disputed/symptomatic TOS, as discussed earlier, have normal neurologic and vascular examinations. This, however, may be difficult to establish, especially if a patient reports nonspecific decreased sensation or weakness associated with pain or "give-way" effort. These patients often present with a "droopy shoulder" posture, characterized by a long thin neck, and sloping, rounded, and often protracted shoulders, with horizontal clavicles.[4] Some patients may have tenderness in the supraclavicular fossa overlying the anterior/middle scalenes.

Careful palpation to the scalene, trapezius, levator scapulae, or supraspinatus muscles may reveal identifiable trigger points, reproducing the patient's symptoms. This finding would be more consistent with a diagnosis of myofascial pain syndrome.

Special tests, such as a Tinel's sign at the elbow or wrist and a positive Phalen's maneuver, may be helpful when considering the diagnosis of cubital or carpal tunnel syndrome. Other special tests advocated in evaluating TOS, such as Adson's, Allen's, hyperabduction, and costoclavicular tests, have disputed results.

Functional Limitations

Patients with all forms of TOS typically have difficulty with upper extremity function, particularly when their arms are in the overhead or abducted positions. In addition, the patient may report difficulty carrying heavy objects, such as groceries, when a downward load is applied to the upper extremities causing additional stretch to the plexus and vessels.

Patients with more advanced disease may have significant weakness and numbness of the hands, impairing their ability to perform fine motor activities such as writing, typing, buttoning a shirt, and working a cash register.

TOS has been reported in a subsection of patients who are instrumental musicians. Patients most affected were reported to play the violin or viola, followed by keyboard instrumentalists and flutists.[5]

Diagnostic Studies

Cervical spine x-rays are helpful to identify an elongated C7 transverse process or a rudimentary cervical rib. In addition, oblique films of the cervical spine are helpful to evaluate for significant neuroforaminal stenosis, which may be more consistent with a cervical radiculopathy. If the clinician has a high suspicion of cervical radiculopathy, even in the face of normal cervical spine x-rays, magnetic resonance imaging (MRI) should be performed to rule out a possible herniated nucleus pulposus.

Chest x-rays or clavicular films may reveal a possible pancoast tumor or an undiagnosed clavicular fracture.

Electrodiagnostic testing (e.g., EMG and nerve conduction studies) may be extremely helpful in determining the presence of true neurologic insult as well as localizing the injury to the root, plexus, or peripheral nerve (median or ulnar). Hallmark findings of neurologic (axonal) TOS include abnormal needle EMG activity in the C8/T1 myotomes as well as decreased amplitudes of the median greater than ulnar compound motor action potential (CMAP) and ulnar sensory nerve action potential (SNAP) with preservation of the median SNAP.[6] Abnormal ulnar motor conduction velocity studies across the "thoracic outlet" should be interpreted with skepticism, as these recordings have been shown to be of no use.[7] *Normal electrodiagnostic testing is expected in both vascular and disputed/symptomatic TOS.*

An MRI of the brachial plexus may be particularly helpful in identifying a possible soft tissue lesion, such as a tumor or hematoma, which may be compromising the plexus.

Arteriography and venography are indicated for further evaluation of possible vascular compromise; however, given the risk of potential complications from these more invasive procedures, they are typically done at the discretion of a vascular surgeon.

Differential Diagnosis

Cervical radiculopathy	Vasculitis	Mass lesion (tumor, hematoma)
Carpal tunnel syndrome	Myofascial pain syndrome	Arteriosclerosis
Traction plexopathy	Neuralgic amyotrophy	Multiple sclerosis
Thrombophlebitis	Ulnar neuropathy	Syringomyelia

Treatment

Initial

Initial treatment starts with an accurate diagnosis. Vascular compromises warrant immediate consultation with a vascular surgeon. True neurologic compromise to the brachial plexus, where structural lesions can be identified, warrant further evaluation by a neurosurgeon or a thoracic surgeon.

The vast majority of patients with disputed/symptomatic TOS, where no identifiable structural lesion can be identified, should be treated conservatively. Initial treatment involves activity modification and pain management. Medications that may be helpful include nonsteroidal anti-inflammatory drugs (NSAIDs), including cyclooxygenase-2 (COX-2) inhibitors, tricyclic antidepressants (e.g., amytryptiline, nortriptyline) as well as anticonvulsant medications (e.g., gabapentin, carbamezepine), especially when there is a large component of neuropathic pain.

Significant sleep disturbances should be addressed and treated appropriately. Patients may benefit by utilizing a cervical roll or wearing a soft cervical collar when sleeping. Symptoms of sleep apnea should be addressed. Poor sleep secondary to soft tissue pain or depression may greatly improve with the use of a low-dose antidepressant medication.

Rehabilitation

Rehabilitation regimens attempt to normalize the neck and upper trunk relationships, thereby helping to minimize any potential compression of the plexus or vascular structures at the various sites between the neck and the axilla, including the interscalene, costoclavicular, and subcoracoid areas. Some key components to this treatment program include postural training and awareness, correction of muscle imbalances through appropriate stretching and strengthening, weight reduction, and aerobic conditioning.[8,9] Some important points listed in Table 1.

TABLE 1. Rehabilitation Considerations

1. Postures that tend to exacerbate symptoms of TOS include when the head and cervical spine are anterior to the thorax and protraction of the scapulae. A figure-of-eight harness may be used to help correct this posture; however, it is typically poorly tolerated by most patients. Patients should be made aware of their posture, using visual aides such as mirrors, and should remind themselves during the day to avoid "slouching." In addition, an exercise program emphasizing stretching of the anterior muscles, such as the serratus anterior and pectoralis major and minor, coupled with strengthening of the lower scapular stabilizers and thoracic extensors may offer significant benefit.

2. Women with breast hypertrophy may benefit from a more supportive brassier with wider straps across the back.

3. Patients who perform most of their activities at a desk, especially those who use a keyboard, have a tendency to slide forward in their chair, thereby reducing lumbar lordosis, increasing thoracic kyphosis, and increasing cervical lordosis and head forward postures. Having the patient lower the keyboard may be an effective way to improve posture and decrease muscle effort in the upper extremity and minimize irritation of the cervicoscapular region.9 Further ergonomic assessments of patients' work or home environments may be warranted by an occupational therapist or other skilled provider.

4. Obesity may be a contributing factor to TOS symptoms; therefore, overweight patients should be referred to a nutritionist, who can assist with establishing an appropriate weight loss program.

5. Aerobic conditioning may be helpful in managing patients' chronic pain symptoms. In addition, patients with decreased respiratory efficiency tend to utilize their accessory respiratory muscles more, including the scalenes, upper trapezius, and sternocleidomastoid, which may contribute to TOS symptoms. Improving respiratory efficiency may be achieved by introducing aerobic conditioning and chest expansion exercises.

Procedures

Patients with neurologic symptoms attributed to other causes such as radiculopathy or peripheral nerve entrapment should be treated in the appropriate manner for such conditions.

Patients with identifiable trigger points, consistent with myofascial pain syndrome, may benefit greatly from local trigger point injections, spray and stretch treatments, or other myofascial release techniques.

Surgery

Prompt surgical evaluation and treatment is indicated for patients with vascular TOS. This may involve thrombolytic therapy, aneurysm repair, cervical rib removal, or bypass grafting, depending on the extent of damage.

Patients with true neurologic TOS often benefit from surgical sectioning of the congenital band between the tip of the cervical rib or elongated C7 transverse process and the first thoracic rib via a supraclavicular approach. Patients undergoing this procedure typically experience improved sensory symptoms and some improved hand strength, although one should not expect significant improvement of hand intrinsic muscle atrophy.[10]

Because of the potential risk of serious complications and inconsistent results, surgery should be considered as a last resort for patients in whom no structural lesion is identified on imaging and/or no objective abnormalities are noted on physical examination or electrodiagnostic testing.

Potential Disease Complications

Potential complications from unrecognized or undiagnosed vascular or neurologic TOS include progressive and irreversible loss of limb function by either ischemia or nerve damage. In cases of thrombus formation, proximal embolization into the carotids and brain is unlikely but has been reported.[11]

Potential Treatment Complications

Analgesics, NSAIDs, and COX-2 inhibitors have well-known side effects that most commonly affect the gasdtric, hepatic, and renal systems.

Occasionally the use of medications such as tricyclic antidepressants (TCAs) and anticonvulsants for neuropathic pain is limited by their side effects. Most common side effects include drowsiness, constipation, dry mouth, and urinary retention. Patients with known cardiac disease should not be prescribed TCAs without a cardiologist's approval. Patients who are prescribed carbamezipine should receive liver function and complete blood count tests, per Federal Drug Administration (FDA) recommendations.

Surgery should be reserved for patients with identifiable structural lesions or patients with intractable pain and/or significant functional impairment unimproved by conservative treatment. Great care must be advocated with any surgical intervention because of the potential for grave harm to the patient. Potential complications from TOS surgery include exsanguinations, phrenic nerve laceration, long thoracic nerve palsy, wound infection, pleural effusion, pneumothorax, and severe permanent brachial plexus injuries.[12,13]

References

1. Peet RM, Henriksen JD, Anderson TP, Martin GM: Thoracic-outlet syndrome: Evaluation of a therapeutic exercise program. Mayo Clin Proc 1956;31:281–287.
2. Dawson DM, Hallett M, Wilbourn AJ: Thoracic outlet syndromes. In Terrano AL, Dawson DM, Hallet M, et al (eds): Entrapment neuropathies, 3rd ed. Philadelphia, Lippincott-Raven, 1999, pp 227–250.
3. Judy KL, Heymann RI: Vascular complications of thoracic outlet syndrome. Am J Surg 1972;123:521–531.
4. Swift TR, Nichols FT: The droopy shoulder syndrome. Neurology 1984;34:212–215.
5. Lederman RJ: AAEM Minimonograph #43: Neruomuscular problems in the performing arts. Muscle Nerve 1994;17:569–577.
6. Cuetter AC, Bartoszek DM: The thoracic outlet syndrome: Controversies, overdiagnosis, overtreatment, and recommendations for management. Muscle Nerve 1989;12:410–419.
7. Wilbourn AJ, Lederman RJ: Evidence for conduction delay in thoracic outlet syndrome is challenged. N Engl J Med 1984;310:1052–1053.
8. Lindgren KA, Manninen H, Rytkonen H: Thoracic outlet syndrome—a functional disturbance of the thoracic upper aperture? Muscle Nerve 1995;18:526–530.
9. Novak CB, Mackinnnon SE: Thoracic outlet syndrome. Orthop Clin North Am 1996;27:747–762.
10. Wilbourn AJ: Thoracic outlet syndromes. Neurol Clin 1999;17:477–497.
11. Prior AL, Wilson LA, Gosling RG, et al: Retrograde cerebral embolism. Lancet 1979;2:1044–1047.
12. Moore WS, Machleder HI, Porter JM, Roos DB: Symposium: Thoracic outlet syndrome. Contemp Surg 1994;45:99–111.
13. Wilbourn AJ: Thoracic outlet surgery causing severe brachial plexopathy. Muscle Nerve 1988;11:66–74.

42 Thoracic Radiculopathy

Darryl L. Kaelin, MD

Synonyms

Thoracic radiculitis

Thoracic disc herniation

ICD-9 Code

724.4
Thoracic or lumbosacral
neuritis or radiculitis,
unspecified

Definition

Thoracic radiculopathy is generally a painful syndrome caused by mechanical compression, chemical irritation, or metabolic abnormalities of the thoracic spinal nerve root. Thoracic disc herniation accounts for less than 5% of all disc protrusions.[1,2] The majority of herniated thoracic discs (35%) occur between T8 and T12 with a peak (20%) at T11–12. Most patients (90%) present clinically between the fourth and seventh decades, with 33% presenting between the ages of 40 and 49 years. Approximately 33% of thoracic disc protrusions are lateral, preferentially encroaching on the spinal nerve root, whereas the remainder are central or central lateral, resulting primarily in various degrees of spinal cord compression. Natural degenerative forces and trauma are generally believed to be the most important factors in the etiology of mechanical thoracic radiculopathy. Perhaps one of the most common non-mechanical causes of thoracic radiculopathy is diabetes, often creating multi-level disease.[3]

Symptoms

The majority of patients (67%) present with complaints of "band-like" chest pain (Fig. 1). The second most common symptom (16%) is lower extremity pain.[4] Unlike thoracic radiculopathy, spinal cord compression produces upper motor neuron signs and symptoms consistent with myelopathy, whereas T11–12 lesions may damage the conus medullaris or cauda equina, creating bowel and bladder dysfunction and lower extremity symptoms. Thus, in a true thoracic radiculopathy, pain is the primary complaint. It is important to include in the history any trauma or risk factors for non-neurologic causes of chest wall or abdominal pain. Because thoracic radiculopathy is not common, it is important in non-traumatic cases to be suspicious of more serious pathology, such as malignancy. Therefore, a history of weight loss, decreased appetite, and previous malignancy should be elicited. Thoracic compression fractures that may mimic the symptoms of thoracic radiculopathy may be seen in young people with acute trauma, particularly falls—regardless of whether they land on their feet. In older people (particularly women with a history of osteopenia or osteoporosis) or in individuals who have prolonged history of steroid use, a compression fracture should be ruled out.

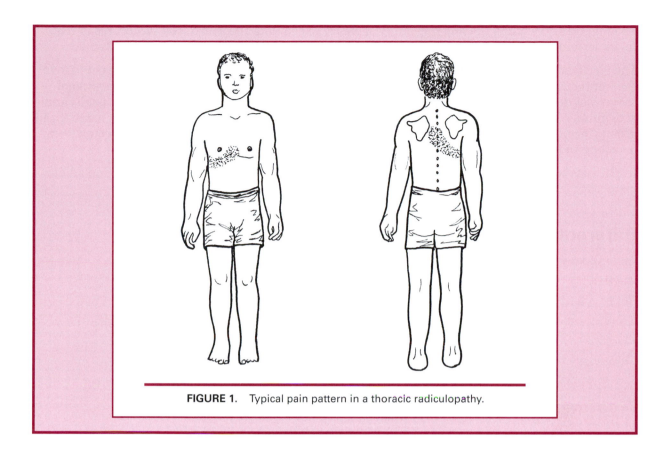

FIGURE 1. Typical pain pattern in a thoracic radiculopathy.

Physical Examination

The physical exam may only show limitations of range of motion generally due to pain—particularly trunk rotation, flexion, and extension. In traumatic cases, location of ecchymosis or abrasions should be noted. *Range of motion testing should not be done if a spinal fracture is suspected.* Pain with percussion over the vertebral bodies should alert the clinician to the possibility of vertebral fracture. Sensation may be abnormal in a dermatomal pattern. Any abnormalities of the spine should be noted, including the presence of scoliosis that is best detected when the patient flexes forward. Weakness or spasticity are seldom seen unless the spinal cord is compromised. Deep tendon reflexes should be normal. A thorough examination of the cardiopulmonary system, abdominal organs, and skin should be performed, particularly in individuals who have sustained trauma.

Functional Limitations

The pain produced by thoracic radiculopathy often limits an individual's movement and activity. Patients may complain of pain with dressing and bathing—particularly during activities that include trunk movements, such as putting on shoes. Work activities may be restricted, such as lifting, climbing, and stooping. Even sedentary workers may be so uncomfortable that they are not able to perform their jobs. Anorexia may result from pain in the abdominal region.

Diagnostic Studies

Because of the low incidence of thoracic radiculopathy and the possibility of serious pathology (e.g., tumor), the clinician should have a low threshold for ordering imaging studies in patients with persistent (more than 2 to 4 weeks) thoracic pain of unknown origin. Magnetic resonance imaging (MRI) remains the imaging study of choice to evaluate the soft tissue structures of the thoracic spine. CT scanning and CT myelography are alternatives if MRI cannot be obtained.

The electromyographic evaluation (EMG) of thoracic radiculopathy can be challenging because of the limited techniques available and lack of easily accessible muscles representing a myotomal nerve root distribution. The muscles most commonly tested are the paraspinals, intercostals, and abdominals. The clinician must investigate multiple levels of the thoracic spine to best localize the lesion. Techniques for intercostal somatosensory evoked potentials (SSEP) have also been shown to isolate individual nerve root levels.[5]

In patients who have sustained trauma, plain x-rays are advised to rule out fractures and spinal instability.

Differential Diagnosis

Intercostal neuralgia	Cholecystitis	Compression fracture
Angina	Peptic ulcer disease	Rib fracture
Aortic aneurysm	Pyelonephritis	Pott's disease
Esophageal disorders	Mastalgia	Malignancy (primary or metastatic)
Pleuritis	Postherpetic neuralgia	Adiposis dolorosa
Pulmonary embolism		

Treatment

Initial

Pain control is important early in the disease course. Patients should be advised to avoid activities that cause increased pain and to avoid heavy lifting. NSAIDs/COX-2 inhibitors are often the first line of treatment and help to control pain and inflammation. Oral steroids can be powerful anti-inflammatory medications and are typically used in the acute stages. This is generally done by starting at a moderate to high dose and tapering over several days. For example, a methylprednisolone [Medrol] dose pack is a prepackaged prescription that contains 24 pills. Each pill is 4 mg of Solu-Medrol. The pills are taken over the course of 6 days. On the first day, six tablets are taken, and then the dose is decreased by one pill each day. Care should be taken when using steroids in diabetic patients since they may elevate blood blood glucose levels. In patients with uncontrolled diabetes who present with thoracic radiculopathy, gaining glucose control should be attempted, although extremely elevated serum glucose levels have not been proven to cause the diabetic form of thoracic radiculopathy. Because of the risk of gastric ulceration, steroids are not typically used simultaneously with NSAIDs. Both non-narcotic and narcotic analgesics may be used to control pain. In subacute or chronic cases, other medications may be tried, such as tricyclic anti-depressants and anti-convulsants (e.g., gabapentin and carbamazepine), which have been effective in treating symptoms of neuropathic origin.

Moist heat or ice can be used, as tolerated, for pain. Transcutaneous electrical nerve stimulation (TENS) units may also help with pain.

Rehabilitation

Physical therapy can be used initially to assist with pain control. Modalities such as ultrasound and electrical stimulation may reduce pain and improve mobility. Physical therapy can then progress with spine stabilization exercises, back and abdominal strengthening, and a trial of mechanical spine traction. Some patients may benefit from a thoracolumbar brace to reduce segmental spine movement. Patients with significant spinal instability documented by imaging studies should be referred to a spine surgeon.

Additionally physical therapy should address postural retraining, particularly for individuals with habitually poor posture. Worksite evaluations can be done if indicated. All sedentary workers should be counseled on proper seating, including using a well-fitting adjustable chair with a lumbar support. More active workers should be advised on appropriate lifting techniques and avoidance of unnecessary trunk rotation.

Finally, physical therapy can focus on improving biomechanical factors that may play a role in abnormal loads on the thoracic spine. These include exercises for tight hamstring muscles and orthotics for pes planus (flat feet).

Procedures

Paravertebral spinal nerve root blocks have been shown to significantly reduce radiating pain.[6]

Surgery

Thoracoscopic microsurgical excision of herniated thoracic discs has been shown to create excellent outcomes with less surgical time, less blood loss, fewer postoperative complications, and shorter hospitalizations than more traditional and invasive surgical approaches.[7] Traditionally, mechanical causes of thoracic radiculopathy have been treated with posterior laminectomy, lateral costotransversectomy, or anterior discectomy via a transthoracic approach. In three series of 91 surgically treated cases, pain resolved or improved in 67% to 94% of patients, and myelopathy improved in 71% to 97% of patients.[8]

Potential Disease Complications

If left untreated, thoracic radiculopathy can result in chronic pain and its associated co-morbidities. If left unrecognized, progressive thoracic spinal cord compression can lead to paraparesis, neurogenic bowel and bladder, and spasticity.

Potential Treatment Complications

Analgesics, NSAIDs, and COX-2 inhibitors have well-known side effects that most commonly affect the gastric, hepatic, and renal systems. Rarely, short-term oral steroid use may produce avascular necrosis of the hip and, more commonly, glucose intolerance. Tricyclic anti-depressants may create dry mouth and urinary retention. Along with anti-convulsants, they may also cause sedation. Occasionally, physical therapy may exacerbate symptoms. The risks of invasive pain procedures and surgery, including bleeding, infection, and further neurologic compromise, are well documented.

References
1. Arce CA, Bohrmann GJ: Herniated thoracic discs. Neurol Clin 1985;3:382–392.
2. Brown CW, Deffer PA, Akmakjian J, et al: The natural history of thoracic disc herniation. Spine 1992;17(Suppl): S97–S102.
3. Dumitru D: Electrodiagnostic Medicine. Philadelphia, Hanley & Belfus, 1995, p 558.
4. Bicknell JM, Johnson SF: Widespread electromyographic abnormalities in spinal muscles in cancer, disc disease, and diabetes. Univ Mich Med Center J 1976;42:124–127.
5. Dreyfuss P, Dumitru D, Prewitt-Buchanan L: Intercostal somatosensory evoked potentials: A new technique. Am J Phys Med Rehabil 1993;72:144–150.
6. Richardson J, Jones J, Atkinson R: The effect of thoracic paravertebral blockade on intercostal somatosensory evoked potentials. Anesth Analg 1998;87(2):373–376.
7. Rosenthal D, Dickman CA: Thoracoscopic microsurgical excision of herniated thoracic discs. J Neurosurg 1998;89(2): 224–235.
8. Dretze DD Jr, Fessler RG: Thoracic disc herniations. Neurosurg Clin North Am 1993;4:75–90.

43 Thoracic Sprain/Strain

Darren Rosenberg, DO

Synonyms

Thoracic sprain
Pulled upper back
Benign thoracic pain

ICD-9 Code

847.1
Sprains and strains of other unspecified parts of back (thoracic)

Definition

Thoracic strain/sprain refers to the acute or subacute onset of pain in the region of the thoracic spine due to soft tissue injury of an otherwise normal back. This results in muscle spasm and limitation of thoracic range of motion and rib motion. Thoracic strain/strain injuries can occur in all age groups, but there is an increased prevalence among working-age patients.[1]

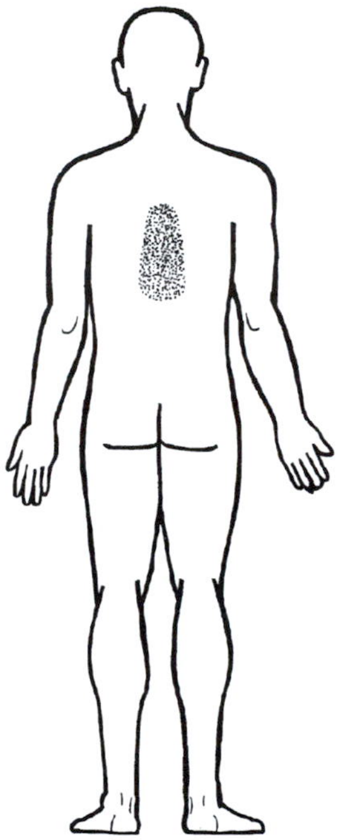

FIGURE 1. Typical pain diagram for a patient with a thoracic sprain/strain.

Symptoms

Patients typically report pain in their upper back (Fig. 1), which may be related to upper extremity movements and can be exacerbated by taking a deep breath or coughing. Pain may radiate locally. A history of trauma, cancer, recent infection, or bowel or bladder problems often warrants further investigation (Table 1).[2]

Physical Examination

The essential element in the physical examination is findings of thoracic muscle spasm, with a negative neurologic exam. Patients may exhibit pain when they lift their arms overhead, and they may have findings of rib motion restriction. Sensation, strength, and reflexes should be normal. A finding of lower extremity weakness, or neurological deficit in the lower extremity on physical examination suggests an alternative diagnosis and may warrant further investigation (see Table 1).[2]

Functional Limitations

Functional limitations include difficulty with bending, lifting, and overhead activities. These limitations affect both active and sedentary

TABLE 1. Red Flags for Potentially Serious Conditions

Possible fracture	**Possible cauda equina syndrome**
Findings from medical history:	*Findings from medical history:*
Major trauma, such as vehicle accident or fall from height	Saddle anesthesia
Minor trauma or even strenuous lifting (in older or potentially osteoporotic patients)	Recent onset of bladder dysfunction, such as urinary retention, increased frequency, or overflow incontinence
Possible tumor or infection	Severe or progressive neurologic deficit in the lower extremity
Findings from medical history:	*Findings from physical examination:*
Age over 50 years or under 20 years	Unexpected laxity of anal sphincter
History of cancer	Perianal/perineal sensory loss
Constitutional symptoms, such as recent fever or chills or unexplained weight loss	Major motor weakness: quadriceps (knee extension weakness), ankle plantar flexors, evertors, and dorsiflexors (foot drop)
Risk factors for spinal infection, recent bacterial infection (e.g., urinary tract infection), intravenous drug use, or immune suppression (from corticosteroid use, transplant, or HIV infection)	
Pain that is worse when in supine position, severe nighttime pain	

HIV = human immunodeficiency virus.
From American Family Physician: Acute low back problems in adults: Assessment and treatment. Am Family Physician 1995;470, with permission.

workers. Activities of daily living, such as upper extremity bathing and dressing, might be affected.

Diagnostic Studies

Thoracic sprain/strain injuries are typically diagnosed based on the history and physical examination. No tests are generally necessary during the first 4 weeks of symptoms, if the injury is non-traumatic. X-rays are indicated if the injury is associated with recent trauma or to rule out osteoporosis or malignancy. MRI is the study of choice when considering thoracic malignancy or in the patient with unilateral localized thoracic pain with sensorimotor deficits, to rule out thoracic disc herniations.[3]

It is important to note that MRI findings can be abnormal but unrelated to the patient's symptoms since many people who don't have pain have abnormal studies.[4]

Differential Diagnosis

Thoracic radiculopathy   Ankylosing spondylitis   Scoliosis/kyphosis

Spinal stenosis   Discitis   Extraspinal causes

Osteoarthritis   Vertebral fracture   (ulcer disease, pancreatitis,

Scheuermann's disease   Tumor   nephrolithiasis,)[5,6]

Treatment

Initial

The initial treatment for a thoracic sprain/strain injury generally involves the use of cold packs to decrease edema during the first 48 hours after strain and application of moist heat or cold to reduce pain and muscle spasm, thereafter. Bed rest for up to 48 hours may be beneficial, but prolonged bed rest is discouraged. Relative rest by avoiding activities that exacerbate pain is preferable to complete bed rest. Temporary use of a rib binder/ACE wrap may reduce pain and muscle spasm as well as increase activity tolerance. A short course of NSAIDs, including cyclooxygenase-2 (COX-2) inhibitors, acetaminophen, or muscle relaxants may be beneficial. Narcotics are generally not necessary.

Rehabilitation

Most acute thoracic sprain/strain injuries will heal spontaneously with rest and modalities used at home. However, if pain persists beyond a couple of weeks, physical therapy may be indicated and can include light massage (myofascial techniques) to reduce muscle spasm in the paraspinal musculature. Body mechanics and posture training are also important parts of the rehabilitation program for thoracic sprain/strain.[7,8] Focusing on correct posture at work and driving is also important. (Patients should be counseled to sit at their computers in an adjustable comfortable chair, etc.) Modalities for pain control should be used sparingly. Modalities that include use of superficial and deep heat/cold may help to increase range of motion and decrease pain.

Manual medicine (manipulation) may also be used for acute and subacute thoracic pain to help decrease muscle spasm, increase range of motion, and decrease pain.

Procedures

Trigger point injections (TPIs) may help restore range of motion, strength and balance to the dysfunctional segment.[9,10] (See page 81 for procedure.)

Surgery

Not indicated.

Potential Disease Complications

Thoracic sprain/strain injuries can occasionally develop into chronic intractable myofascial pain syndromes.

Potential Treatment Complications

Possible complications include GI side effects from NSAIDs. Other possible complications include somnolence/confusion from muscle relaxants; addiction from narcotics; bleeding, infection, and postinjection soreness from TPIs; and temporary post-treatment pain from manipulation.

References
1. Choi BC, Levitsky M, Lloyd RD, et al: Patterns and risk factors for sprains and strain in Ontario, Canada 1990. J Occup Environ Med 1996;38(4):379–389.
2. American Family Physician: Acute low back problems in adults: Assessment and treatment. Am Fam Physician 1995;51(2):469–484.
3. Dietze DD Jr, Fessler RG: Thoracic disc herniations. Neurosurg Clin N Am 1993;4(1):75–90.
4. Wood KB, Garvey TA, Gundry C, et al: Magnetic resonance imaging of the thoracic spine. Evaluation of asymptomatic individuals. J Bone Joint Surg AM 1995;77(11):1631–1638.
5. Snider RK: Essentials of Musculoskeletal Care. Rosemont, IL, American Academy of Orthopedic Surgeons, 1997.
6. Bruckner FE, Allard SA, Moussa NA: Benign thoracic pain. J R Soc Med 1987;80(5):286–289.
7. Guccione AA: Physical therapy for musculoskeletal syndromes. Rheum Dis Clin North Am 1996;22(3):551–562.
8. Turner JA: Educational and behavioral interventions for back pain in primary care. Spine 1996;21:2851–2859.
9. Rosen NB: The myofascial pain syndromes. Phys Med Rehabil Clin North Am 1993;4:41–63.
10. Travell JG, Simons DJ: Myofascial Pain and Dysfunction: The Trigger Point Manual, vols 1 and 2. Baltimore, Williams & Wilkins, 1983, 1991.

44 Lumbar Degenerative Disease

Michael K. Schaufele, MD
W. Alaric Van Dam, MD

Synonyms

Osteoarthritis of the spine

Spondylosis

Lumbar arthritis

Degenerative joint disease of the spine

Degenerative disc disease

ICD-9 Codes

721.3
Lumbosacral spondylosis without myelopathy

721.90
Spondylosis of unspecified site (spinal arthritis)

722.52
Degeneration of lumbar or lumbosacral intervertebral disc

724.2
Low back pain

Definition

Degeneration of the structures of the spine can occur as a result of normal aging. This process may be accelerated in patients with previous trauma or injury to the lumbar spine. L4 to L5 and L5 to S1 are the most commonly involved lumbar levels, given they undergo the greatest torsion and compressive loads. Degenerative processes may affect several anatomic structures, resulting in different clinical syndromes.

The *facet (zygapophyseal) joints and sacroiliac joints* may develop osteoarthritis similar to other synovial joints in the body.[1] The *intervertebral disc* experiences progressive disc dehydration as part of the normal aging process of the spinal structures. In certain patients, fissures in the annulus fibrosus may develop, causing an inflammatory response. Nociceptive pain fibers may grow into these fissures.[2] Further degeneration may result in progression of the disease or complete annular tears, which may be the source of discogenic low back pain, also referred to as internal disc disruption syndrome (IDD). Up to 39% of patients with chronic low back pain may suffer from IDD.[3] The loss of segmental integrity may lead to further degeneration of the disc, which results in narrowing of the intervertebral disc space. Because of increased loads on the posterior elements, facet degeneration may develop. Facet arthropathy may be an independent or concurrent source of low back pain. Further disc degeneration and subsequent loss of disc height may cause subluxation of the facet joints, resulting in degenerative spondylolisthesis, most commonly at the L4/L5 level.[4]

Other conditions seen with lumbar degeneration include spondylosis deformans and diffuse idiopathic skeletal hyperostosis (DISH). *Spondylosis deformans* is a degenerative condition marked by formation of anterolateral osteophytes and is mainly a radiologic diagnosis. In spondylosis deformans the intervertebral spaces are well preserved unlike in degenerative disc disease. The initiating factor in the development of this condition may be degeneration of the annulus fibrosus, primarily in the anterolateral disc space.[5] Spondylosis may become clinically symptomatic if excessive osteophyte formation leads to neural compression, such as in spinal stenosis. *DISH* involves ossification of the ligamentous attachments to the vertebral bones (entheses). Radiologic features consist of flowing, excessive anterior osteophyte formation. DISH affects 5% to 10% of patients older than 65 years.[6] This diagnosis is typically an incidental finding on radiologic studies.[7]

Other factors associated with lumbar degeneration include environmental, occupational, and psychosocial influences. Environmental influences include cigarette smoking and occupational activities that involve repetitive bending and prolonged exposures to stooping, sitting, or vibrational stresses. These repetitive actions may result in degeneration of the lumbosacral motion segments.[6] Psychosocial factors are well known to contribute to significant disability in low back pain, often in patients with only minimal structural impairment.[8]

Symptoms

Lumbar degenerative symptoms range from minor to debilitating. Common complaints include chronic back pain and stiffness. Patients may also report limited range of motion, especially with extension in the case of facet arthropathy or spinal stenosis. Symptoms of pain associated with lumbar flexion, coughing, sneezing, or Valsalva's maneuver are often associated with disc disease.

Lumbar degenerative disease is probably entirely asymptomatic in the majority of cases. Approximately one third of subjects have substantial abnormalities on MRI despite being clinically asymptomatic.[9] Because of factors not well understood, such as leakage of inflammatory factors from the disc, a chronic pain syndrome may develop in some patients, possibly from repetitive sensitization of nociceptive fibers in the annulus fibrosus.[10]

Clinicians should inquire about atypical symptoms of back pain, including night pain, fever, and recent weight loss. These may lead to the diagnosis of malignancy or infection.

Symptoms of chronic pain, including sleep disturbances and depression, should be sought.

Physical Examination

The purpose of the physical examination is to direct further evaluation and therapy toward one of the five most common sources of low back pain: (1) discogenic, (2) facet arthropathy/instability, (3) radiculopathy/ neural compression, (4) myofascial/soft tissue, or (5) psychogenic. Combinations of these sources of back pain often exist. This distinction will allow the use of advanced diagnostic tests and therapeutic options in the most cost-effective approach.

A standardized low back examination should include assessment of flexibility (lumbosacral flexion/extension, trunk rotation, finger-floor distance, hamstring and iliopsoas range-of-motion, and hip range-of-motion). An inclinometer may assist in standardizing lumbar range-of-motion measurements.[11] A complete examination should include inspection of lower extremities for atrophy and vascular insufficiency, muscle strength testing, and assessment for sensory abnormalities and their distribution. Asymmetries in deep tendon reflexes (patellar tendon [L4], hamstring tendon [L5], and Achilles tendon [S1]) are important to note and may be the most objective finding. Upper motor neuron signs such as Babinski's and Hoffmann's should also be tested. Functional strength testing should include heel-to-toe-walking, calf and toe raises, single leg knee bends, and a complete gait evaluation. Specific testing for lower back syndromes include straight-leg raising, femoral stretch sign, dural tension signs, sacroiliac joint provocative maneuvers (e.g., Faber's, Gillet's, Yeoman's, and Gaenslen's tests), as well as specific evaluation techniques such as the McKenzie technique. Assessing the patient for non-organic signs of back pain (Waddell's signs, Table 1) will help the clinician to recognize patients in which psychologic factors may contribute to their pain syndrome.[12]

Functional Limitations

Functional limitations in degenerative diseases of the lumbar spine depend on the anatomic structures involved.

All aspects of daily living, including self-care, work, and recreation, may be affected.

TABLE 1. Waddell's Signs

Five non-organic physical signs are described by Waddell:

1. Tenderness—non-organic tenderness may be either superficial or non-anatomic. Superficial tenderness can be elicited by lightly pinching over a wide area of lumbar skin. Non-anatomic pain is described as deep tenderness felt over a wide area rather than localized to one structure.

2. Simulation test—usually based on movement producing pain. Two examples include axial loading, in which low back pain is reported on vertical loading over the standing patient's skull by the clinician's hands, and rotation, in which back pain is reported when the shoulder and pelvis are passively rotated in the same plane as the patient stands relaxed with feet together.

3. Distraction test—if a positive physical finding is demonstrated in a routine manner, this finding is checked while the patient's attention is distracted. Straight-leg raising is the most useful distraction test. There are several variations to this test; most commonly, however, straight-leg raise is done in the supine position and then, while distracting the patient, in the sitting position. This is commonly referred to as the "flip test." However, one should keep in mind that biomechanically the two positions are very different.

4. Regional disturbances—regional disturbances involve a widespread area, such as an entire quarter or half of the body. The essential feature of this non-organic physical sign is divergence of the pain beyond the accepted neuroanatomy. Examples include give-away weakness in many muscle groups manually tested and sensory disturbances, such as diminished sensation to light touch. pinprick, or vibration, that do not follow a dermatomal pattern. Again, care must be taken not to mistake multiple root involvement for regional disturbance.

5. Overreaction—Waddell reports that overreaction during the examination may take the form of disproportionate verbalization, facial expression, muscle tension, tremor, collapsing, and even profuse sweating. Analysis of multiple non-organic signs showed that overreaction was the single most important non-organic physical sign. However, this sign is also the most influenced by the subjectivity of the observer.

Adapted from Geraci MC Jr, Alleva JT: Physical examination of the spine and its functional kinetic chain. In Cole AJ, Herring SA (eds): The Low Back Pain Handbook. Philadelphia, Hanley & Belfus, 1997, pp 58–59.

Patients with primary discogenic pain typically exacerbate symptoms during bending, twisting, stooping, and forward flexion. Patients with facet arthropathy/instability report increased pain with extension-based activity, including standing and walking. Pain is often relieved with sitting and other similar forward flexed positions. Patients with myofascial/soft tissue syndromes report pain that is worsened with static and prolonged physical activity. Symptomatic improvement may be associated with rest and modalities including heat, cold, and pressure. Patients with contributing psychologic factors, such as depression or somatization disorders, typically report pain out of proportion to their underlying pathology, poor sleep, and significant disability in their daily activities.

Diagnostic Studies

Diagnostic testing should be directed by the history and physical examination and should only be ordered if the therapeutic plan will be significantly influenced by the results. AP and lateral lumbar spine x-rays are helpful for identifying loss of disc height as a result of disc degeneration, spondylosis/osteophyte formation, and facet arthropathy (Fig. 1, A and B). Oblique views are helpful to identify spondylolysis. Flexion/extension films are necessary to identify dynamic instability and can assist in identifying appropriate surgical candidates for fusion procedures. Significant degenerative instability usually does not occur before the age of 50, but should be included as a differential diagnosis in patients with clinical symptoms suggestive of advanced facet arthropathy and disc degeneration.[6] *Magnetic resonance imaging (MRI)* of the lumbar spine is used because of its sensitivity to identify abnormalities of the soft tissues and neural structures. It is particularly helpful in identifying various stages of degenerative disc disease as well as annular tears and disc herniation. Other significant sources of back pain such as neoplasms, osteomyelitis, and fractures can also be identified with MRI. *Computerized tomography (CT)* is a valuable diagnostic tool in assessing fractures and other osseous abnormalities of the lumbar spine. CT imaging in combination with myelography (*CT-myelography*) aids with presurgical

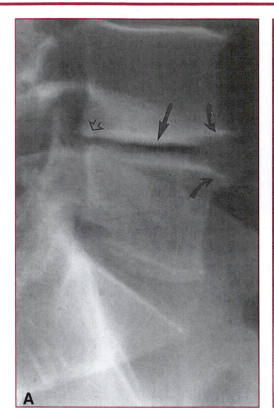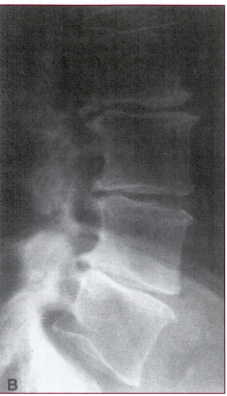

FIGURE 1. Chronic degenerative changes—plain film. On a coned down lateral film (*A*), the L4–L5 motion segment shows a vacuum phenomenon in the disc (*large black arrow*), endplate remodeling with large anterior spurs (*curved arrows*), and grade I retrolisthesis (*open arrow*). A standing lateral film (*B*) shows multilevel degenerative disc disease with large posterior spurs, small anterior osteophytes, endplate remodeling, and moderately severe disc space narrowing at L2–L3, L3–L4, and L4–L5. (From Cole AJ, Herzog RJ: The lumbar spine: imaging options. In Cole AJ, Herring SA (eds): The Low Back Pain Handbook. Philadelphia, Hanley & Belfus, 1997, p 176, with permission.)

planning by allowing identification of osseous structures causing neural compression, especially in spinal stenosis. *Discography* is currently the only technique to correlate structural abnormalities of the intravertebral disc seen on advanced imaging studies with a patient's pain response. Reproduction of painful symptoms with intradiscal injection of dye aids in the localization of specific disc levels as pain generators and can be useful in separating painful disc degeneration from painless degeneration. *Electrodiagnostic studies* may become necessary in cases of peripheral neurological deficits not clarified by physical exam or imaging. They allow for identification of compression neuropathy, radiculopathy, or systemic motor and sensory diseases.

Differential Diagnosis (Table 2)

Radiculopathy

Spinal stenosis

Fractures (e.g., osteoporotic compression fractures)

Spondylolysis, spondylolisthesis

Tumors

Osteomyelitis of the spine, discitis

TABLE 2. Pseudospine Pain—Diagnostic Keys

	Condition	Diagnostic Keys
Vascular	Abdominal aortic aneurysm	Older than 50 yr Abdominal and back pain Pulsatile abdominal mass
Gynecologic	Endometriosis	Woman of reproductive age Cyclic pelvic and back pain
	Pelvic inflammatory disease	Young, sexually active woman Systemically ill (fever chills) Discharge, dysuria
	Ectopic pregnancy	Missed period Abdmonial and/or pelvic pain Positive pregnancy test
Genitourinary	Prostatitis	Men older than 30 yr Dysuria Low back and perineal pain
	Neprolithiasis	Flank and groin pain Hematuria
Gastrointestinal	Pancreatitis	Abdominal pain radiating to back Systemic signs (fever, nausea, vomiting) Elevated serum amylase
	Penetrating or perforated duodenal ulcer	Abdominal pain radiation to back
Rheumatologic	Fibromyalgia	Young to middle age woman Widespread pain Multiple tender points Disrupted sleep, fatigue Normal radiographs and lab values
	Polymyalgia rheumatica (PMR)	Older than 50–60 yr Hip or shoulder girdle pain and stiffness Elevated ESR Dramatic response to low-dose prednisone
	Seronegative spondyloarthropathies (ankylosing spondylitis, Reiter's, psoriatic, enteropathic)	Younger male (AS, Reiter's) Lower lumbosacral pain Morning stiffness ("gel") Improvement with activity Radiographic sacroiliitis
	Diffuse idiopathic skeletal hyperostosis (DISH, Forestier's disease)	Older than 50–60 yr Thoracolumbar stiffness or pain Flowing anterior vertebral calcification
	Piriformis syndrome	Buttock and leg pain Pain on resisted hip external rotation and abduction Transgluteal or transrectal tenderness
	Scheuermann's kyphosis	Age 12–15 yr Thoracic or thoracolumbar pain Increased fixed thoracic kyphosis 3 or more wedged vertebrae with endplate irregularities
	Trochanteric bursitis, gluteal fasciitis	Pain or tenderness over greater trochanter
	Adult scoliosis	Back pain Uneven shoulders, scapular prominence Paravertebral hump with forward flexion
Metabolic	Osteoporosis	Woman older than 60 yr Severe acute thoracic pain (fracture) Severe weight-bearing pelvic pain (fracture) Aching, dull thoracic pain; relieved in supine position (mechanical) Loss of height, increased thoracic kyphosis

(Table continued on next page.)

TABLE 2. Pseudospine Pain—Diagnostic Keys *(Continued)*

	Condition	Diagnostic Keys
Metabolic *(cont.)*	Osteomalacia	Diffuse skeletal pain or tenderness Increased alkaline phosphatase
	Paget's disease	Bone pain: low back, pelvic, tibia Increased alkaline phosphatase Characteristic radiographic appearance
	Diabetic polyradiculopathy	Older than 50 yr Diffuse leg pain, worse at night Proximal muscle weakness
Malignancy		Older than 50 yr Back pain unrelieved by positional change—night pain Previous history of malignancy Elevated ESR

Adapted from Mazanec D: Pseudospine pain: Conditions that mimic spine pain. In Cole AJ, Herring SA (eds): The Low Back Pain Handbook. Philadelphia, Hanley & Belfus, 1997, p 98.

Treatment

Initial

Probably the most important treatment of any low back pain condition is patient education and reassurance. Most of the acute low back symptoms are myofascial in origin and typically resolve within 4 to 6 weeks. The benign nature of degenerative conditions of the spine should be emphasized as well as the fact that acute exacerbations tend to improve over time regardless of therapy. Therapy is directed toward management of the condition rather than "curing" the disease. Initial therapy for lumbar degenerative disease should consist of anti-inflammatory medications; muscle relaxants (Table 3); occasionally, opiate medications for severe symptom exacerbation; and a functionally oriented physical therapy program. Most patients do well with these measures and do not require any invasive procedures. Other useful initial treatments may include trigger point injections as well as heat and cold modalities. Low dose tricyclic antidepressants can help with improvement of sleep. Patients who appear depressed should be identified and treated appropriately.

TABLE 3. Commonly Used Drugs for Muscle Relaxation

Generic Name	Brand Name	Common Doses
Cyclobenzaprine	Flexeril	10 mg qhs to tid
Carisoprodol	Soma	350 mg qhs to tid
Baclofen	Lioresal	10–20 mg q6°
Methocarbamol	Robaxin	500–750 mg tid
Chlorzoxazone	Parafon Forte	250–500 mg tid
Orphenadrine	Norflex	100 mg bid

Adapted from Schofferman J: Medications for low back pain. In Cole AJ, Herring SA (eds): The Low Back Pain Handbook. Philadelphia, Hanley & Belfus, 1997, p 117.

Rehabilitation

Rehabilitation of lumbar degenerative disc disease should include a detailed assessment of functional limitations, and functional goals for every patient. A full assessment of occupational and leisure activity demands and goals should also be implemented. For example, patients with advanced degenerative disc disease may benefit from early vocational rehabilitation and counseling with the goal of avoiding future occupational disability and surgical procedures.

Occasionally, lumbar braces (orthotics/corsets) are prescribed, but these are generally not thought to be very beneficial in the treatment of degenerative low back pain unless there is a significant spondylolisthesis or some other specific indication.

Therapy goals focus on normalization of impairments in flexibility, strength, and endurance and should emphasize healthy lifestyle modifications. A basic lumbar stabilization program with a focus on posture, footwear modifications (if necessary), workplace modifications (if appropriate), and general conditioning works for most patients. Modalities such as ultrasound and electrical stimulation can be used for acute low back pain; however, the focus of supervised therapy should be on an active program rather than the passive treatment that modalities provide.

In patients whose condition does not improve with the outlined initial therapeutic measures, a more intensive, functional restoration approach may be helpful. This commonly includes comprehensive physical rehabilitation with psychologic support. These programs can be called many things (e.g., comprehensive spine program, chronic pain program, work conditioning program). Although most of these programs are traditionally considered later in the course of degenerative diseases, early referral may be helpful in decreasing related disability.[13] Another common functional rehabilitation technique is the dynamic lumbar stabilization approach.[14] This muscular stabilization program uses static and dynamic postural exercises to improve the patient's overall function. Education about proper body mechanics during activities of daily living, improved extremity strength and endurance, and muscle stabilization through gym training and healthy lifestyle activities. The hallmark of this program is that postural control is attained through pelvic tilting to control the degree of lumbar lordosis in a pain-free range. The program is designed to advance the patient toward increasingly demanding exercises and to incorporate these exercises into activities of daily living. The program progresses through the building of static strength into dynamic stabilization for patients with more physically demanding athletic activities and occupational demands. This program is supported by a home exercise program and typically requires 3 months to accomplish.

Procedures

Spinal injection procedures have become an increasingly important part of the overall treatment program for lumbar degenerative disease. These procedures allow for diagnostic, therapeutic, and even prognostic benefits. It is now commonly agreed that injections should ideally be performed with x-ray guidance and contrast enhancement.[15] The most commonly used procedures are *epidural steroid injections*, which have shown benefit primarily for temporary relief of radicular symptoms.[16] Newer injection techniques, such as the transforaminal approach, ensure that the medication, usually a corticosteroid, is delivered into the anterior epidural space.[17] This type of technique may also be beneficial in cases of discogenic pain, in which inflammatory transmitters may leak into the epidural space. Facet joint injections are commonly performed via intra-articular or medial branch injections. *Facet injections* allow for temporary pain relief and establishment of facet mediated pain but commonly lack long-term benefits.[18] *Facet rhizotomies* may provide longer symptomatic relief for patients with clearly identified facet pain.[19] Occasionally, *intradiscal steroid injections* are applied, but their use is debated since intradiscal steroid may cause progression of disc degeneration and calcification of the intervertebral disc.[20] *Semi-invasive intradiscal therapies* (e.g., chemonucleolysis, laser) have been used since the 1970s with various clinical successes. Newer treatment techniques involve controlled thermal application to the posterior annulus through an intradiscal catheter—*intradiscal electrothermal therapy (IDET)* to modify collagen in the posterior annulus in an attempt to seal annular fissures as well as to ablate nociceptive fibers. Short-term data are promising, but long-term data are currently lacking.[21]

Surgery

The surgical indications for degenerative disc disease of the lumbar spine are highly debated and evolving. Surgery is considered when intensive non-surgical therapy as previously outlined, including injection procedures and semi-invasive procedures, have failed and the patient continues to have functionally limiting pain. Confounding psychologic factors and mental disorders should be excluded prior to any surgical procedure.[22] Current data are incomplete to judge the scientific validity of spinal fusion for low back pain syndromes.[23] However, if the intervertebral disc is clearly identified as the source of low back pain, interbody fusion with excision of the diseased disc appears to have favorable results.[24] In general, surgical options include posterior fusion procedures with or without pedicle screw instrumentation, anterior interbody fusion with or without pedicle screws, or a combination of these procedures. In case of additional neural compression, additional decompression procedures may be required.

Potential Disease Complications

In general, degenerative lumbar disease is a benign condition. However, increasing functional limitations can occur, especially if advanced segmental degeneration leads to neural compression and symptoms of spinal stenosis, neural claudication, and segmental instability develop. Persistent neurologic deficits from these conditions are rare and can be avoided if the conditions are diagnosed early and appropriate treatment is begun. A small number of patients may develop chronic pain syndromes. Low back pain is the most common cause of the chronic pain syndrome. Not surprisingly, the incidence of mental disorders, such as depression and somatiform disorders, is high, and these disorders commonly respond better to a behavioral psychology approach than to disease oriented medical treatment approaches. Early detection of patients with mental disorders will help to avoid unnecessary medical treatment and allow for appropriate psychologic and psychiatric interventions.

Potential Treatment Complications

As with any medications, clinicians should be fully aware of their risks and unwanted side effects. Analgesics, NSAIDs, and COX-2 inhibitors have well-known side effects that most commonly affect the gastric, hepatic, and renal systems. Muscle relaxants can cause sedation. Low dose tricyclic antidepressants can cause sedation and urinary retention in men with benign prostatic hypertrophy. Some patients require chronic opioid therapy, and issues of constipation and dependence arise. Risks associated with spinal injection include cortisone flare; hyperglycemia; dural puncture, and rarely, hematoma, infection, and neurologic damage. All potential complications should be thoroughly discussed with the patient prior to their application. Potential surgical complications will vary with the procedure.

References
1. Schwarzer AC, Aprill CN, Bogduk N: The sacroiliac joint in chronic low back pain. Spine 1995;20(1):31–37.
2. Freemont AJ, Peacock TE, Goupille P, et al: Nerve ingrowth into diseased intervertebral disc in chronic back pain. Lancet 1997;350(9072):178–181.
3. Schwarzer AC, Aprill CN, Derby R, et al: The prevalence and clinical features of internal disc disruption in patients withy chronic low back pain. Spine 1995;20(17):1878–1883.
4. Kirkaldy-Willis WH: Managing Low Back Pain. New York, Churchill Livingstone, 1999.
5. Schmorl G, Junghanns H: The Human Spine: Health and Disease, 2nd ed. New York, Grune and Stratton, 1971.
6. Fraser RD, Bleasel JF, Moskowitz RW: Spinal Degeneration: Pathogenesis and Medical Management. In Frymoyer JW (ed): The Adult Spine: Principles and Practice, 2nd ed. Philadelphia, Lippincott-Raven, 1997, pp 735–759.
7. Helms CA: Fundamentals of Skeletal Radiology, 2nd ed. ed. Philadelphia, W.B. Saunders, 1995.
8. Rainville J, Ahern DK, Phalen L, et al: The association of pain with physical activities in chronic low back pain. Spine 1992;17(9):1060–1064.
9. Boden SD, Davis DO, Dina TS, et al: Abnormal magnetic-resonance scans of the lumbar spine in asymptomatic subjects: A prospective investigation. J Bone Joint Surg 1990;72A:403–408.
10. Saal JS: The role of inflammation in lumbar pain [see comments]. Spine 1995;20(16):1821–1827.
11. Rainville J, Sobel JB, Hartigan C: Comparison of total lumbosacral flexion and true lumbar flexion measured by a dual inclinometer technique. Spine 1994;19(23):2698–2701.
12. Waddell G, McCulloch JA, Kummel E, Venner RM: 1979 Volvo award in clinical science. Nonorganic physical signs in low-back pain. Spine 1980;5(2):117–125.
13. Mayer TG, Gatchel RJ, Mayer H, et al: A prospective two-year study of functional restoration in industrial low back injury. An objective assessment procedure [published erratum appears in JAMA 1988;259(2):220]. JAMA 1987;258(13):1763–1767.
14. Saal JA: Dynamic muscular stabilization in the nonoperative treatment of lumbar pain syndromes. Orthop Rev 1990;19(18):691–700.

15. O'Neill C, Derby R, Kenderes L: Precision injection techniques for diagnosis and treatment of lumbar disc disease [review]. Sem Spine Surg 1999;11(2):104–118.
16. Carette S, Leclaire R, Marcoux S, et al: Epidural corticosteroid injections for sciatica due to herniated nucleus pulposus. N Engl J Med 1997;336(23):1634–1640.
17. Lutz GE, Vad VB, Wisneski RJ: Fluoroscopic transforaminal lumbar epidural steroids: an outcome study. Arch Phys Med Rehabil 1998;79(11):1362–1366.
18. Carette S, Marcoux S, Truchon R, et al: A controlled trial of corticosteroid injections into the facet joints for chronic low back pain. N Engl J Med 1998;325(14):1002–1007.
19. Dreyfuss P, Halbrook B, Pauza K, et al: Efficacy and validity of radiofrequency neurotomy for chronic lumbar zygapophysial joint pain. Spine 2000;25(10):1270–1277.
20. Duquesnoy B, Debiais F, Heuline A, et al: [Unsatisfactory results of intradiscal injection of triamcinolone hexacetonide in the treatment of sciatica caused by intervertebral disk herniation (see comments)]. Presse Med 1992;21(38):1801–1804.
21. Saal JA, Saal JS: Intradiscal electrothermal treatment for chronic discogenic low back pain: A prospective outcome study with minimum 1-year follow-Up [in process citation]. Spine 2000;25(20):2622–2627.
22. Carragee EJ, Tanner CM, Khurana S, et al: The rates of false-positive lumbar discography in select patients without low back symptoms. Spine 2000;25(11):1373–1380.
23. Bigos SJ: A literature-based review as a guide for generating recommendations to patients acutely limited by low back symptoms. In Garfin SR, Vaccaro AR (eds): NASS. Orthopaedic knowledge update: Spine, 1st ed. Rosemont, IL, American Academy of Orthopaedic Surgeons, 1997.

45 Lumbar Facet Arthropathy

Ted A. Lennard, MD

Definition

Lumbar facet arthropathy refers to any acquired, traumatic, or degenerative process that distorts the normal anatomy or function of a facet joint. Often these changes disrupt the normal biomechanics of the joint, resulting in hyaline cartilage damage and periarticular hypertrophy. When painful, these joints may limit daily living activities, recreational sports, and work. Lumbar facet joints may be a primary source of pain but are often seen secondary to a diseased or injured lumbar disc.

Symptoms

Patients typically complain of generalized or lateralized spinal pain, sometimes well localized. Pain may be provoked with spinal extension and rotation, either from a standing or prone position. Relief with partial lumbar flexion is common. In the lumbar spine, these joints may refer pain into the buttock or posterior thigh, but rarely below the knee.[1–3]

Physical Examination

A detailed examination of the lumbar spine and a lower extremity neurologic examination are considered standard for those suspected of having a facet arthropathy. Although no portion of the examination has been shown to definitively correlate with the diagnosis of a facet joint disorder, the physical examination can be helpful in elevating the clinician's level of suspicion for this diagnosis.[4,5] The exam starts with simple observation of the patient's gait, movement patterns, posture, and range of motion. Generalized and segmental spinal palpation followed by a detailed neurologic exam for sensation, reflexes, tone, and strength are performed. In the absence of co-existing pathology, such as lumbar radiculopathy, strength, sensation, and deep tendon reflexes should be normal.

Provocative maneuvers and nerve tension tests, including straight leg testing testing, should accompany the evaluation to rule out any superimposed nerve root injury that might accompany a facet disorder. The clinician should note the patient's response when the lower extremity is raised with the hip flexed and the knee extended. This "tension" placed on inflamed or injured lower lumbosacral nerve roots will provoke pain, paresthesias, or numbness down the extremity. Typically, in isolated cases of lumbar facet disorders, this maneuver does not provoke radiating symptoms into the lower extremity, but it may cause lower back pain.

Additional exam techniques may be necessary (e.g., vascular, peripheral joint), depending on the patient's presentation.

Functional Limitations

Patients with lumbar facet joint arthropathy may experience difficulty with prolonged standing, walking, twisting, stairclimbing, and prone lying. Extreme flexion may also be problematic. Since facet problems are common with underlying disc disease, patients often have difficulty with lumbar flexion activities, such as bending, stooping, and lifting.

Diagnostic Studies

Fluoroscopic-guided, contrast-enhanced, anesthetic intra-articular or medial branch blocks are considered the "gold standard" for the diagnosis of a painful lumbar facet joint (Fig. 1).[6,7] Clinical history, examination, x-ray changes, CT, MRI, or bone scan have not been shown to correlate with facet joint pain.[4,5]

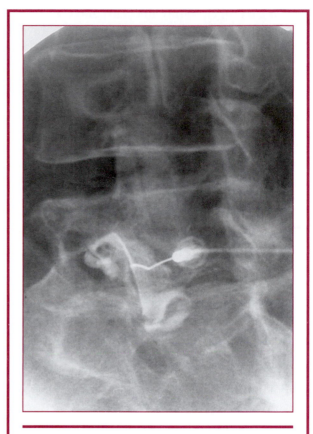

FIGURE 1. Oblique radiograph of an L5–S1 z-joint arthrogram. Superior and inferior capsular recesses are demonstrated. (From Lennard TA: Pain Procedures in Clinical Practice. Philadelphia, Hanley & Belfus, 2000, with permission.)

Differential Diagnosis

Radiculopathy   Spondylolysis/spondylolisthesis
Internal disc disruption   Lumbar stenosis
Myofascial pain syndrome   Spondylosis
Nerve root compression   Sacroiliac joint dysfunction

Treatment

Initial

Initial treatment emphasizes local pain control with ice, oral analgesics and NSAIDs, topical creams, local peri-articular corticosteroid injections, and avoidance of exacerbating activities. Spinal manipulations and acupuncture may also reduce local pain. Temporary use of corsets and limited activity can be used.

Rehabilitation

Physical therapy may include modalities to control pain (e.g., ultrasound), traction, instruction in body mechanics, flexibility training (including hamstring stretching), spinal strengthening, articular mobilization techniques, generalized conditioning, and restoration of normal movement patterns. Critical assessment of the biomechanics of specific activities that may be job related (e.g., working on an assembly line, carpentry work) or sports related (e.g., running, cycling) is important. This assessment can result in prevention of recurrent episodes of pain since changes in a technique or activity may reduce the underlying forces at the joint level.

Procedures

Intra-articular, fluoroscopic-guided, contrast-enhanced facet injections are considered essential in the proper diagnosis and treatment of a painful facet joint.[6,7] Patients can be evaluated before and after injection to determine what portion of their pain can be attributed to the joints injected. After confirmation with contrast, 1 to 2 cc of an anesthetic-corticosteroid mix are injected directly into the joint. An alternative approach is to perform anesthetic medial branch blocks with small volumes (0.1 to 0.3 cc) of anesthetic. If the facet joint is found to be the putative source of pain a medial branch neurotomy may be desirable.[8-10]

Surgery

Surgery is rare in primary and isolated facet arthropathies. Surgical spinal fusion may be performed for discogenic pain, which may affect secondary cases of facet arthropathies.

Potential Disease Complications

Since a common cause of facet arthropathy is degenerative in nature, this disorder is often progressive, resulting in chronic, intractable spinal pain.[11,12] It often co-exists with spinal disc abnormalities, further leading to chronic pain. This subsequently results in diminished spinal motion and weakness.

Potential Treatment Complications

Treatment-related complications may be caused from medications: NSAIDs may cause GI and renal problems, and analgesics may result in liver dysfunction and constipation. Local peri-articular injections and acupuncture may cause local transient needle pain. Often local manual treatments or injections will cause transient exacerbation of symptoms. Intra-articular facet injections will cause transient local spinal pain and swelling and possibly bruising. More serious injection-related complications include an allergic reaction to the medications, injury to a blood vessel or nerve, trauma to the spinal cord, and infection. When more serious injection complications occur, they can usually be attributed to poor procedure technique.[6]

References
1. Dreyer SJ, Dreyfuss P, Low back pain and the zygapophyseal joints. Arch Phys Med Rehabil 1996;77:290–300.
2. Dreyer S, Dreyfuss P, Cole A: Posterior elements and low back pain. Phys Med Rehabil State Art Rev 1999;13:443–471.
3. Fukui S, Ohseto K, Shiotani M, et al: Distribution of referred pain from the lumbar zygapophyseal joints and dorsal rami. Clin J Pain 1997;13:303–307.
4. Dolan AL, Ryan PJ, Arden NK, et al: The value of SPECT scans in identifying back pain likely to benefit from facet joint injection. Br J Rheum 1996;35:1269–1273.
5. Schwarzer AC, Scott AM, Wang S, et al: The role of bone scintigraphy in chronic low back pain: Comparison of SPECT and planar images and zygapophyseal joint injection. Aust NZJ Med 1992;22:185.
6. Bogduk N: International Spinal Injection Society Guidelines for the performance of spinal injection procedures. Part I. Zygapophysial joint blocks. Clinical J Pain 1997;13:285–302.
7. Dreyfuss P, Kaplan M, Dreyer SJ: Zygapophyseal joint injection techniques in the spinal axis. In Lennard TA (ed): Pain Procedures in Clinical Practice. Philadelphia, Hanley & Belfus, 2000.
8. Dreyfuss P, Halbrook B, Pauza K, et al: Lumbar radiofrequency neurotomy for chronic zygapophyseal joint pain: A pilot study using dual medial branch blocks. Int Spinal Injection Soc Sci Newsl 1999;3(2):13–31.
9. Dreyfuss P, Halbrook B, Pauza K, et al: Efficacy and validity of radiofrequency neurotomy for chronic lumbar zygapophyseal joint pain. Spine 2000;25(10):1270–1277.
10. Kleef M, Barendse G, Kessels A, et al: Randomised trial of radiofrequency lumbar facet denervation for chronic low back pain. Spine 1999;24:1937–1942.
11. Cavanaugh JM, Ozaktay AC, Yamashita T, et al: Mechanisms of low back pain: A neurophysiological and neuroanatomic study. Clin Orthop 1997;335:166–180.
12. Lewinnek GE, Warfield CA: Facet joint degeneration as a cause of low back pain. Clin Orthop 1986;213:216–222.

46 Lumbar Radiculopathy

Maury Ellenberg, MD
Joseph C. Honet, MD

Synonyms

Lumbar radiculitis

Sciatica

Pinched nerve

Herniated nucleus pulposus with nerve root irritation

ICD-9 Codes

722.52
Degeneration of lumbar or lumbosacral intervertebral disc

724.2
Low back pain

Definition

Lumbar radiculopathy refers to a pathologic process involving the lumbar nerve root(s). Lumbar radiculitis refers to an inflammation of the nerve root. These terms should not be confused with disc herniation, which is a displacement of the lumbar disc from its anatomic location between the vertebrate (often into the spinal canal) (Fig. 1). Although lumbar radiculopathy is often caused by a herniated lumbar disc, this is not invariably the case. Many pathologic processes, such as bony encroachment, tumors, and metabolic disorders (e.g., diabetes), can also result in lumbar radiculopathy. More importantly, disc herniation is often an incidental finding on cross-sectional imaging of asymptomatic individuals.[1,2]

Symptoms

The most common symptom in lumbar radiculopathy is pain. The pain may vary in severity and location. The pain may be very severe and is often increased or precipitated by standing, sitting, coughing, and sneezing. The location of the pain depends on the nerve root involved, and there is a great deal of overlap among the dermatomes. Most commonly, S1 radiculopathy produces posterior thigh and calf pain; L5, buttocks and anterolateral leg pain; L4, anterior thigh, anterior or medial knee, and medial leg pain. Usually the patient cannot pinpoint the precise onset of pain. It may start in the back, but by the time the patient is evaluated, pain may only be present in the buttocks or limb.

Parasthesias are also common and occur in the dermatomal distribution of the involved nerve root (rarely is complete sensory loss present). Occasionally the patient may present with weakness of a part of the limb. On rare occasion, there is bladder and bowel involvement, especially urinary retention.

A history that includes trauma and cancer, infection, HIV, or diabetes, etc. would be indicative for earlier diagnostic testing.

Physical Examination

The most important elements in the evaluation of lumbar radiculopathy are the history and physical examination.[3]

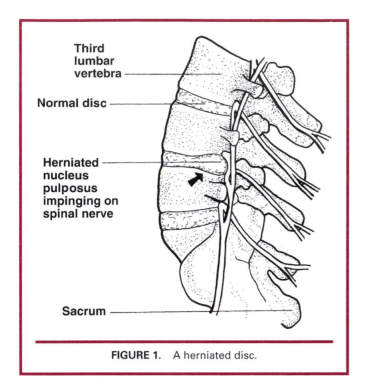

FIGURE 1. A herniated disc.

A thorough musculoskeletal and peripheral neurologic examination should be performed. Examine the back for asymmetry or a shift over one side of the pelvis or the other. Evaluate back motion and see whether radicular symptoms (pain radiating to an extremity) in the distribution of the patient's complaints are produced.

Manual muscle testing (MMT) is a vital part of the examination for radiculopathy. The major muscle weakness in relation to the nerve root involved is: L3—hip flexors; L4—knee extensors and hip adductors; L5—hip abductors, knee flexors, ankle dorsiflexors, and foot everters and inverters; and S1—ankle plantar flexors (Table 1). Try to detect weakness in the distribution of two peripheral nerves arising from the same nerve root.

The straight leg raising (SLR) test can be performed with the patient sitting or supine. The leg is raised straight up, and the test is positive if the patient complains of pain in the extremity (not the back) typically in a specific nerve root distribution. Compare side to side to be sure not to confuse the pain produced with hamstring stretch. There are a number of variations on this test.

Rectal examination and perianal and inguinal sensory testing should be done if there is history of bowel or bladder incontinence or retention or recent onset of erectile dysfunction.

Waddell's signs are a group of indicators that a non-organic process is interfering with the accuracy of the physical examination (see page 233). These signs are often present in patients with compensation, or litigation, or psychoemotional issues.[4] They should be a routine part of the examination in patients with these issues.

TABLE 1. Diagnosing Lumbar Radiculopathy

Nerve Root	Pain Radiation	Gait Deviation	Motor Weakness	Sensory Loss	Reflex Loss
L3	Groin and inner thigh	Sometimes antalgic	Hip flexion	Anteromedial thigh	Patellar (variable)
L4	Anterior thigh or knee, or upper medial leg	Sometimes antalgic Difficulty arising onto a stool or chair with one leg	Knee extension, hip flexion, and adduction	Lateral and/or anterior thigh, medial leg and knee	Patellar
L5	Buttocks, anterior or lateral leg, dorsal foot	Difficulty heel walking; if more severe, then foot slap or steppage gait Trendelenburg gait	Ankle dorsiflexion, foot eversion and inversion, toe extension, hip abduction	Posterolateral thigh, antero-lateral leg and and mid-dorsal foot	Medial hamstring (variable)
S1	Posterior thigh, calf, plantar foot	Difficulty toe walking or cannot arise on toes 20 times	Foot plantar flexion	Posterior thigh, and calf, lateral and plantar foot	Achilles

Functional Limitations

The functional limitations depend on the severity of the problem. Any limitations usually occur because of pain. Standing and walking may be limited, and sitting tolerance is often decreased. Patients with an L4 radiculopathy are at risk of falling down stairs if the involved leg is their "trailing" (power) leg on the stairs. Patients with a severe S1 radiculopathy will be unable to run because of calf weakness, even when the pain resolves. Patients with L5 radiculopathy may catch their foot on curbs, or if severe, on the ground. They may require a brace (ankle dorsiflexion assist).

Diagnostic Studies

Diagnostic testing takes two forms: one to corroborate the diagnoses and the second to determine the etiology. For simple cases, diagnostic testing is usually not needed and the clinical picture can guide the treatment.

Electromyography

Electromyography (EMG) and nerve conduction studies (NCS), when performed by an individual well versed in the diagnoses of neuromuscular disorders, can be valuable in the diagnosis of lumbar radiculopathy. They can also help with differential diagnoses and in patients whose physical examination is not reliable. EMG has the advantage over imaging techniques of high specificity and will rarely be abnormal in asymptomatic individuals.[5] These studies, however, do not give direct information regarding the *cause* of the radiculopathy.

Imaging

Imaging techniques, when related to lumbar radiculopathy, usually refer to lumbosacral spine radiography, CT scan, and MRI (Fig. 2).

Plain x-ray can be useful to exclude traumatic bony injury or metastatic disease. It allows visualization of the disc space but not the contents of the spinal canal or the nerve roots. CT and MRI allow visualization of the disc, spinal canal, and nerve roots. There is a high incidence of abnormal findings in asymptomatic people, with rates of disc herniation ranging from 21% in the 20 to 39 age group to 37.5% in the 60 to 80 age group.[2] To be meaningful, CT and MRI must clearly correlate with the clinical picture and should generally only be performed if tumor is suspected or surgery is contemplated. They also may be useful in locating pathology for selective epidural steroid injection.

Differential Diagnosis

Trochanteric bursitis	Avascular necrosis of the hip
Anserine bursitis	Hip osteoarthritis
Hamstring strain	Shin splints
Lumbosacral plexopathy	Lateral femoral cutaneous neuropathy (meralgia paresthetica)
Diabetic amyotrophy	Spinal stenosis
Peripheral neuropathy	Cauda equina syndrome
Sciatic	Demyelinating disorder
Tibial	
Peroneal	Lumbar facet syndrome
Femoral	Piriformis syndrome

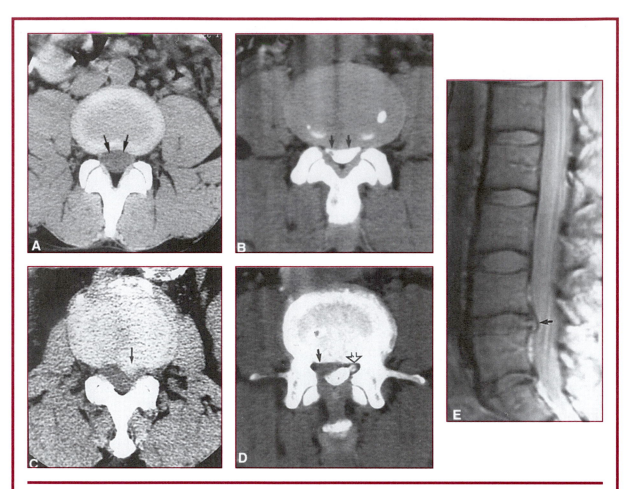

FIGURE 2. *A*, Normal disc. Note the concave posterior margin of the disc (*arrows*). *B*, Bulging disc. Image from a CT-myelogram showing the broad-based margin of the bulging disc (*arrows*) pushing on the anterior thecal sac. *C*, Left posterior disc herniation (*arrow*). *D*, Right posterior disc herniation. The abnormal soft tissue from the herniated disc is seen in the right lateral recess on this CT-myelogram (arrow). Note the normally opacified nerve root sheath on the contralateral side (*open arrow*). *E*, Herniated discs L4–L5 and L5–S1; the L4–L5 herniation is the larger of the two. There is posterior displacement of the low signal posterior longitudinal ligament (*arrow*). (From Barckhausen RR, Math KR: Lumbar Spine Diseases. In Katz DS, Math KR, Groskin SA (eds): Radiology Secrets. Philadelphia, Hanley & Belfus, 1998, pp 322–335, with permission.)

Treatment

Initial

The treatment goal is to reduce inflammation and thereby relieve the pain and resolve the radiculopathy regardless of the underlying anatomic abnormalities. Bed rest, which had been the mainstay of non-operative treatment, is now recommended only for symptom control. In recent studies, bed rest has not been shown to have an effect on the final outcome of the disorder.[6] As long as patients avoid activities such as bending or lifting, which tend to increase intradiscal pressures, they can carry on most everyday activities.

Use nonsteroidal anti-inflammatory drugs (NSAIDs), including COX-2 inhibitors, to help reduce inflammation and provide pain relief. The use of oral steroids is more controversial and has not passed the scrutiny of well controlled studies.

Use opioids as needed for pain relief. There is little concern for addiction in the acute case, and sufficient medication should be provided. The needs range from none to high doses, such as the equivalent of 60 to 100 mg of morphine (MS Contin) a day. Start with hydrocodone or codeine and titrate up as needed. For more severe pain, use a long-acting opioid, such as oxycodone (Oxycontin) or MS Contin, and for breakthrough pain, use a shorter-acting opioid, such as hydrocodone or oxycodone.

Rehabilitation

With a very acute painful radiculopathy, it is generally best to wait for some of the acute stage to subside before ordering physical therapy. In a more longstanding problem, therapy may be the best first approach.

Physical methods are a useful adjunct to the medication treatment. Modalities such as ultrasound and electrical stimulation may be helpful for pain control. Various methods have been tried, which include flexion or extension exercises (often called a lumbosacral stabilization program). Whatever method is used, if radicular pain is produced, the exercises should be stopped. After the radiculopathy resolves, the patient should be placed on a proper exercise regimen to improve flexibility and strength.

Procedures

Epidural steroid injection can be very effective in lumbar radiculopathy with or without disc herniation, especially in patients with acute radiculopathy. A much lower response rate has been found in patients with longstanding problems or those with secondary reinforcers, such as litigation or worker's claims. Although it is unclear whether long-term outcomes are altered, epidural steroids are beneficial during the first 3 months and can allow more rapid pain relief and return to function.[7] These studies ideally should be performed under flouroscopic guidance. If there is no effect with the first injection, selective nerve root injection can be attempted.[8] It is advisable to perform one injection and re-evaluate the patient to determine whether further injections are required. A maximum of three injections should be performed for one episode of radiculopathy, but it is reasonable to repeat this procedure for recurrent episodes of radiculopathy after 3 to 6 months.

Non-operative treatment allows resolution of the radiculopathy in up to 90% of cases.[9] More interestingly, recent studies have demonstrated that when radiculopathy is the result of disc herniation, the actual herniation will resolve in the majority of cases, and even when the herniation remains, the symptoms often will still abate.[10–12]

Surgery

Surgery is appropriate under the following two conditions:

First, when it is done on an emergency basis because a patient presents with a central disc herniation with bowel and bladder incontinence or retention and bilateral lower extremity weakness. In this very rare condition, a neurosurgeon or orthopedic spine surgeon must be consulted immediately and the patient operated on preferably within 6 hours.

Second, surgery is an option if a patient continues to have pain that limits function after an adequate trial of non-operative treatment.

Patient selection is extremely important to achieve a good surgical outcome. The best outcomes occur in patients with single-level root involvement; pain experienced more in the limb than the back; and an anatomic abnormality on imaging that corresponds to the patient's symptoms, physical examination, and EMG findings.[13]

The type of surgery depends on the etiology of the radiculopathy. For cases of disc herniation, simple laminectomy and discectomy suffice. Fusion should be avoided in these instances. With spinal stenosis, a more extensive laminectomy with foraminotomy may be needed. Fusion should be reserved for the relatively infrequent case of well demonstrated spinal instability together with radiculopathy or if the surgical procedure will result in spinal instability.

Potential Disease Complications

Complications relate to involvement of the nerve roots in the cauda equina. The most serious is the "paraplegic disc." In this case, the herniated disc can cause paralysis, but this is very rare. More common, but still unusual, is a disc that causes weakness and involvement of bowel and bladder function. Residual weakness may occur either spontaneously or postsurgery. Patients may progress to a chronic low back pain syndrome.

Potential Treatment Complications

NSAIDs can cause gastrointestinal bleeding, mouth ulcers, and renal and hepatic complications. Newer COX-2 inhibitors avoid the gastrointestinal bleeding.

Epidural steroid injections can (rarely) result in epidural abscess and epidural hematoma. Patients should not take aspirin for 1 week before the injection. Most centers recommend that NSAIDs not be taken for 3 to 5 days prior to the procedure, although there is no literature documenting an increased incidence of complications when patients are taking NSAIDs. The injection can produce local pain, and if performed without fluoroscopy, it can result in spinal headache from piercing the dura and resultant spinal fluid leak.

Surgical complications include infection, nerve root injury, paralysis, local back pain, and the usual postoperative complications (e.g., thrombophlebitis, bladder infection).

References

1. Jensen MC, Brant-Zawadzki, MN, Obuchowski N., et al: Magnetic resonance imaging of the lumbar spine in people without back pain. N Engl J Med 1994;331:69–73.
2. Boden SD, Davis DO, et al: Abnormal magnetic-resonance scans of the lumbar spine in asymptomatic aubjects. JBJS 1990;72-A:403–408.
3. Deyo RA, Rainville J, Kent DL: What can the history and physical examination tell us about low back pain? JAMA 1992;268:760–765.
4. Waddell G, McCulloch JA, et al: Nonorganic physical signs in low-back pain. Spine 1980;5(2):117–125.
5. Robinson, LR: Electromyography, magnetic resonance imaging, and radiculopathy: It's time to focus on specificity. Muscle Nerve 1999;22:149–150.
6. Vroomen P, de Krom M, Wilmink JT, et al: Lack of effectiveness of bed rest for sciatica. N Engl J Med 1999;340:418–423.
7. Carette S, Leclaire R, Marcoux S, et al: Epidural corticosteroid injections for sciatica due to herniated nucleus pulposes. N Engl J Med 1997;336(23):1634–1637.
8. Lutz GE, Vad VB, Wisneski RJ: Flouroscopic transforaminal lumbar epidural steroids: An outcome study. Arch Phys Med Rehabil 1998;79(11):1362–1366.
9. Saal JA, Saal JS: Nonoperative treatment of herniated lumbar intervertebral disc with radiculopathy: an outcome study. Spine 1997;14:431–437.
10. Ellenberg M, Reina N, Ross M, et al: Regression of herniated nucleus pulposus: Two patients with lumbar radiculopathy. Arch Phys Med Rehabil 1989;70:842–844.
11. Ellenberg M, Ross M, Honet JC, et al: Prospective evaluation of the course of disc herniations in patients with proven radiculopathy. Arch Phys Med Rehabil 1993;74:3–8.
12. Saal JA, Saal J.S., Herzog J: The natural history of intervertebral disc extrusions treated nonoperatively. Spine 1990;7:683–686.
13. Finneson BE, Cooper VR: A lumbar disc surgery predictive scorecard. A retrospective evaluation. Spine, 1979:4(2):141–144.

47 Lumbar Sprain/Strain

Darren Rosenberg, DO

Synonyms

Lumbar sprain

Myofascial low back pain

Pulled back

Low back sprain/strain

ICD-9 Codes

724.2
Low back pain

847.2
Sprains and strains of
other and unspecified
parts of back, lumbar

Definition

Lumbar sprain/strain refers to the acute or subacute onset of pain in the region of the lumbar spine due to soft tissue injury of an otherwise normal back. Lumbar sprain/strain is most commonly found in 20- to 40-year-olds and is often related to flexion, side bending, and/or rotation under load or an uncontrolled lift.

Symptoms

Patients typically report pain in their lower back, which may increase with flexion or extension of the lumbar spine. Pain may radiate into the buttocks and is generally relieved with sitting, but symptoms are exacerbated with activities such as prolonged standing or bending (Fig 1). A history of trauma, cancer, recent infection, or bowel or bladder problems often warrants further investigation (Table 1).[1]

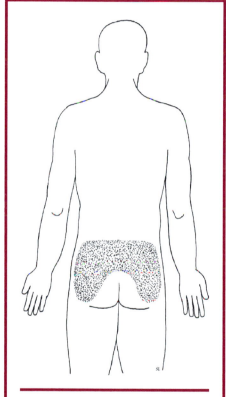

FIGURE 1. This is a typical distribution of pain in a patient with a lumbar sprain/strain injury.

Physical Examination

The essential element in the physical examination is lumbar muscle spasm with a negative neurologic exam. Patients exhibit pain with active movement such as lumbar flexion and rotation and have findings of limited range of motion. Sensation, strength, and reflexes should be normal, but patients might appear weak secondary to pain. Findings of saddle anesthesia, major motor weakness, fever, or severe neurologic deficit in the lower extremity warrant further investigation (see Table 1).[1]

TABLE 1. Red Flags for Potentially Serious Conditions

Possible fracture
Findings from medical history:
Major trauma, such as vehicle accident or fall from height
Minor trauma or even strenuous lifing (in older or potentially osteoporotic patients)

Possible tumor or infection
Findings from medical history:
Age over 50 years or under 20 years
History of cancer
Constitutional symptoms, such as recent fever or chills or unexplained weight loss
Risk factors for spinal infection, recent bacterial infection (e.g., urinary tract infection), intravenous drug use, or immune suppression (from corticosteroid use, transplant, or HIV infection)
Pain that is worse when in supine position, severe nighttime pain

Possible cauda equina syndrome
Findings from medical history:
Saddle anesthesia
Recent onset of bladder dysfunction, such as urinary retention, increased frequency, or overflow incontinence
Severe or progressive neurologic deficit in the lower extremity
Findings from physical examination:
Unexpected laxity of anal sphincter
Perianal/perineal sensory loss
Major motor weakness: quadriceps (knee extension weakness), ankle plantar flexors, evertors, and dorsiflexors (foot drop)

HIV -= human immunodeficiency virus.
From American Family Physician: Acute low back problems in adults: Assessment and treatment. Am Family Physician 1995; 470; with permission.)

Functional Limitations

Functional limitations include difficulty with bending, lifting, and prolonged standing or sitting. These limitations can affect both active and sedentary workers. Commuting in a car may cause increased symptoms. Activities of daily living such as lower extremity bathing and dressing may also exacerbate symptoms.

Diagnostic Studies

No tests are typically necessary during the first 4 weeks of symptoms if the injury is non-traumatic.[2] Pain unresponsive to conservative management generally warrants further investigation with plain films, MRI, bone scan, etc. X-rays are indicated early in the course if there is a history of trauma or to rule out osteoporosis or malignancy.

Differential Diagnosis

Herniated nucleus pulposus (herniated disc)

Spinal stenosis

Spondylosis

Spondylolysis/spondylolisthesis

Lumbar facet syndrome

Sacroiliac joint dysfunction

Osteoarthritis

Discitis

Vertebral fracture

Tumor

Scoliosis

Extraspinal causes (ulcer disease, pancreatititis, nephrolithiasis, ovarian cyst)[3]

Treatment

Initial

Initial treatment involves rest from aggravating activities, medication for pain control, and modalities to decrease pain and inflammation. The use of cold packs to decrease edema during the first 48 hours after sprain/strain and the application of moist heat or cold thereafter to reduce pain and muscle spasm can be helpful. Bed rest for up to 48 hours may be beneficial but prolonged bed rest is discouraged.[4] Relative rest by avoiding activities that exacerbate pain is preferable to complete bed rest. Temporary use of a lumbosacral support when out of bed may reduce pain and muscle spasm and increase activity tolerance.[5] A short course of NSAIDs, acetaminophen, or muscle relaxants may be beneficial. Narcotics are generally not necessary but may be used in the very acute stage. Prolonged use of narcotics should be avoided because they carry the serious risk of addiction.

Rehabilitation

Rehabilitation may include physical therapy consisting of therapeutic lumbar stretching/strengthening and a stabilization program. Light massage (myofascial techniques) can be used to reduce muscle spasm in paraspinal musculature. Body mechanics and posture training are also important parts of the rehabilitation program for lumbar sprain/strain.[6,7] Modalities for pain control should be used sparingly in conjunction with an active stretching and strengthening program. Modalities that include use of superficial and deep heat/cold may help to increase range of motion and decrease pain. Manual medicine (manipulation) may also be used in acute lower back pain to help decrease muscle spasm, increase range of motion, and decrease pain.[8,9]

Work hardening and work conditioning programs can be a useful adjunct to the rehabilitative process in injured workers whose jobs are physically demanding or in workers who are unwilling/unable to return to their former level of activity after an injury.

Procedures

Trigger point injections (TPIs) may help restore range of motion, strength, and balance to the dysfunctional segment.[10,11]

Surgery

Surgery is not indicated in lumbar sprain/strain injuries.

Potential Disease Complications

The primary disease complication is a progression to chronic low back pain syndrome. This is generally avoided by early and appropriate treatment intervention.

Potential Treatment Complications

NSAIDs may cause gastrointestinal side effects. Muscle relaxants can cause somnolence/confusion. Narcotics are potentially addictive. TPIs may cause an allergic reaction to the medications used, bleeding, infection and postinjection soreness. Manipulation is occasionally followed by temporary posttreatment pain or, rarely, by herniation of an intervertebral disc.

References
1. American Family Physician: Acute low back problems in adults: Assessment and treatment. Am Fam Physician 1995;51(2):469–484.
2. Agency of Health Care Policy and Research, Public Health Service: Clinical practice guidelines for acute low back problems in adults, 95-06042. Washington, DC, US Department of Health and Human Services, 1994.
3. Snider RK: Essentials of Musculoskeletal Care. Rosemont, IL, Amereican Academy of Orthopedic Surgeons, 1997.
4. Deyo RA, Diehl AK, Rosenthal M: How many days of bed rest for acute low back pain: A randomized clinical trial. N Engl J Med 1986;315:1064.
5. Nachemson AL: The lumbar spine: An orthopaedic challenge. Spine 1976;1:59.
6. Guccione AA: Physical therapy for musculoskeletal syndromes. Rheum Diseases Clin North Am 1996;22(3):551–562.
7. Turner JA: Educational and behavioral interventions for back pain in primary care. Spine 1996;21:2851–2859.
8. Anderson A, Lucente T, Davis AM, et al: A comparison of osteopathic spinal manipulation with standard care for patients with low back pain. New Engl J Med 1999;341:19.
9. MacDonald RS, Bell CM: An open controlled assessment of osteopathic manipulation in non- specified low-back pain. Spine 1990;15:364–370.
10. Rosen NB: The myofascial pain syndromes. Phys Med Rehabil Clin North Am 1993;4:41–63.
11. Travell JG, Simons DJ: Myofascial Pain and Dysfunction: The Trigger Point Manual, vols 1 and 2. Baltimore, Williams & Wilkins, 1983, 1991.

Diagnostic Studies

Spondylolysis usually can be detected as a defect in the pars interarticularis (a break in the "Scottie dog's neck") on a 45-degree oblique x-ray of the lumbar spine (Fig. 2). Lateral x-rays are used to document the degree of spondylolisthesis.[7]

In children and adolescents, a single photon emission computer tomography (SPECT) is useful to show a pars defect that is not apparent on x-ray and is useful to determine whether a spondylolytic lesion is acute enough to merit immobilization.[8]

CT scan bone windows are considered the most accurate means for demonstrating spondylolysis. Sagittal MRI series are useful for identifying spondylolisthesis. MRI is very useful for evaluating nerve root compression within the neuroforamen or central spinal stenosis in cases of spondylolisthesis and sciatica.[9]

EMG is only infrequently indicated, being limited to cases were symptoms, neurologic findings, and diagnostic studies are inconsistent.

Differential Diagnosis

Degenerative low back pain

Lumbar disc herniation

Spinal stenosis

Vertebral compression fracture

Pathologic fracture from a tumor

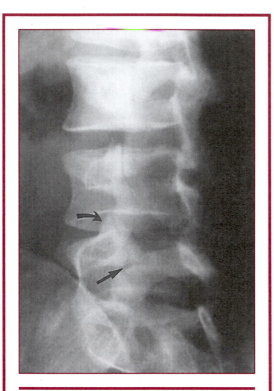

FIGURE 2. Scotty dog spondylolysis. This right posterior oblique radiograph of the lumbar spine demonstrates the linear lucent "collar" at the neck of the scotty dog (straight arrow). The ear of the dog (curved arrow) is the superior articular facet, the foot is the inferior facet, and the head is the right vertebral pedicle. (From Katz DS, Math KR, Groskin SA: Radiology Secrets. Philadelphia, Hanley & Belfus, 1998, with permission.)

Treatment

Initial

In children symptomatic with acute spondylolysis, spinal immobilization with an antilordotic brace for 6 months (23 hours/day) and activity modification are recommended since these have been shown to lead to improvement in symptoms and healing of the spondylolysis in most patients[10]; however, adults rarely need such prolonged bracing.

In adults with degenerative spondylolisthesis, back pain complaints are usually treated similar to those of other back pain disorders—education, analgesics, anti-inflammatory medication, and exercise.

Rehabilitation

Exercise is the major focus of physical therapy for these disorders. Stretches to reduce impairments of trunk mobility, hip flexors, hamstrings, quadriceps, and calves are recommended. Improving back and abdominal strength can help decrease the discomfort associated with the lumbar spine instability.[4,11] Modalities (e.g., ultrasound, electrical stimulation) have not been shown to improve symptoms and are generally of limited value.

Procedures

Epidural spinal injections are occasionally beneficial for symptoms of sciatica or pseudoclaudication associated with degenerative spondylolisthesis. Selective nerve root blocks may help to reduce symptoms from foraminal stenosis. Facet blocks above and below the level of spondylolysis or at the level of degenerative spondylolisthesis may reduce back pain complaints.

Surgery

Lumbar spine fusion is indicated when there is persistence of major back pain symptoms for more than 1 year despite aggressive conservative treatment when the spondylolysis and/or spondylolisthesis is unquestionably the cause of those symptoms. Lumbar spinal fusion may be indicated for persistent sciatica that results from foraminal or central spinal stenosis, especially if neurologic deficits are present.[3]

Potential Disease Complications

The vast majority of cases of spondylolisthesis and spondylolysis are asymptomatic and remain that way.[12] With age, intervertebral disc and facet degeneration are accelerated in the presence of spondylolysis.[13] Because of this, spondylolisthesis can progress and result in nerve root compression or spinal stenosis.

Potential Treatment Complications

Complications from NSAIDs are well known (gastric, renal, and hepatic). Exercise can irritate painful spinal tissue. Spinal injections may result in a temporary increase in pain, spinal headaches, or damage to nerve roots. Surgical decompression and fusion can lead to nerve damage, infection, failed fusion, and persistent back pain.

References
1. Wiltse LL, Newman PH, Macnab I: Classification of spondylolysis and spondylolisthesis. Clin Orthop 1976;117:23–29.
2. Moller H, Sundin A, Hedlund R: Symptoms, signs, and functional disability in adult spondylolisthesis. Spine 2000;25(6):683–689.
3. Amundson G, Edwards CC, Garfin SR: Spondylolisthesis. In Rothman RH, Simeone FA (eds): The Spine. Philadelphia, WB Saunders, 1999, pp 835–885.
4. Sinaki M, Mokri B: Low back pain and disorders of the lumbar spine. In Braddom RL (ed): Physical Medicine and Rehabilitation. Philadelphia, WB Saunders, 1996, pp 813–850.
5. Frennered K: Isthmus spondylolisthesis among patients receiving disability pension under the diagnosis of chronic low back pain syndromes. Spine 1994;19(24):2766–2769.
6. Moller H, Sundin A, Hedlund R: Symptoms, signs, and functional disability in adult spondylolisthesis. Spine 2000;25(6):683–690.
7. Harvey CJ, Richenberg JL, Saifuddin A, Wolman RL: The radiological investigation of lumbar spondylolysis. Clin Radiol 1998;53(10):723–728.
8. Bellah RD, Summerville DA, Treves ST, Micheli LJ: Low-back pain in adolescent athletes: Detection of stress injury to the pars interarticularis. Radiology 1991;180(2):509–512.
9. Jinkins JR, Matthes JC, Sener RN: Spondylolysis, spondylolisthesis, and associated nerve root entrapment in the lumbosacral spine: MR evaluation. Am J Roentgenol 1992;159(4):799–803.
10. Steiner ME, Micheli LJ: Treatment of symptomatic spondylolisthesis and spondylolysis with a modified Boston brace. Spine 1985;10:937–943.
11. O'Sullivan PB, Phyty GD, Twomey LT: Evaluation of specific stabilizing exercise in the treatment of chronic low back pain with radiologic diagnosis of spondylolysis or spondylolisthesis. Spine 1997;22(24):2959–2967.
12. Torgerson WR, Dotter WE: Comparative roentgenograpic study of the asymptomatic and symptomatic lumbar spine. J Bone Joint Surg Am 1976;58(6):850–853.
13. Floman Y: Progression of lumbosacral spondylolisthesis in adults. Spine 2000;25(3):342–347.

49 Lumbar Stenosis

Walter J. Gaudino, MD, MS

Synonyms

Pseudoclaudication

Neurogenic claudication

Spinal claudication

Low back pain

ICD-9 Code

724.02
Spinal stenosis, lumbar
region

Definition

Spinal stenosis is a condition in which the spinal cord, cauda equina, and nerve root structures are compressed due to constriction of the spinal canal, nerve root canal, or the intervertebral foramina. This compression may be due to enlargement of the soft tissues in and around the canal, hypertrophy of the facet joints, intervertebral disc herniation, or ligamentum flavum laxity (Figs. 1 to 4).[1,2]

Lumbar spinal stenosis is a painful and potentially disabling condition. It is most common in older adults, although congenital deformities of the spinal canal may lead to the development of symptoms at an early age. There are two classification systems.[3] One system categorizes lumbar stenosis by the *anatomic site of involvement*. This system classifies the stenosis as either central or lateral. Central stenosis involves narrowing of the spinal canal around the nerve roots of the cauda equina. This is due to an alteration in the normal force distribution system of the lumbar spine. Lateral stenosis may occur from similar mechanisms or from posterolateral disc herniation. Regardless, lateral stenosis connotes an entrapment of the spinal nerve within the nerve root canal or the intervertebral foramina.

The second system delineates lumbar stenosis based on *whether the stenosis is primary or secondary*. Primary stenosis is due to congenital narrowing of the spinal canal. Primary stenosis is uncommon, only occurring in 9% of cases. In secondary lumbar stenosis, the spinal canal is congenitally normal but becomes narrowed due to an acquired condition. The most common causes of secondary lumbar stenosis are degenerative changes within the vertebrae, facets and discs, spondylolisthesis, and postsurgical scarring. Rare causes of acquired stenosis are compression fractures, tumors, Tarlov's cysts, infection, and Paget's disease.

Symptoms

Most patients with lumbar stenosis are older than 50 and have a history of prolonged, recurrent back pain. Leg pain is reported in 90% of the cases and may be either unilateral or bilateral. Katz et al. reported that leg pain in patients with lumbar stenosis is distal to the buttocks in 88% of the cases but only distal to the knees 56% of the time.[4] Many patients are pain free when they are seated. Ambulatory balance is impaired in 70% of patients with lumbar stenosis. *Neurogenic claudication*, the hallmark of

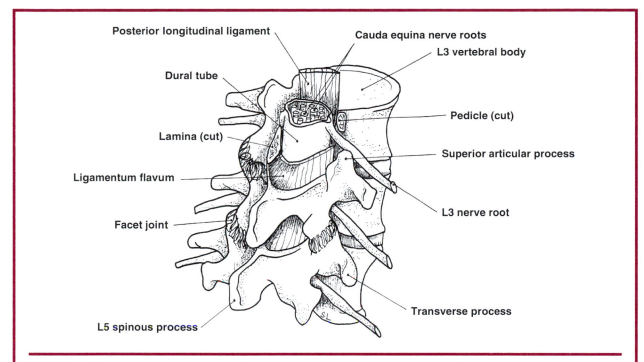

FIGURE 1. Normal anatomic structures of the lumbar spine at the third through the fifth lumbar levels. Note the close association between the nerve roots and the dural tube, the ligamentum flavum, the facet joints, the pedicles and the lamina. The ligamentum flavum (interlaminar ligament) attaches laterally to the facet capsules.

lumbar stenosis, is poorly localized pain, parasthesias, cramping, and weakness of one or both of the lower extremities. It is brought on by walking and is relieved by sitting or flexion of the lumbar spine.

Typically, thigh or leg pain precedes the onset of numbness and leg weakness. Patients may report that they can bicycle extended distances despite their limited walking tolerance. Prone lying may bring on the symptoms. In cases of severe lumbar stenosis, the patient may report urinary incontinence as a result of impingement of sacral nerve roots.[5]

Physical Examination

The physical examination of patients with lumbar stenosis may reveal signs of occult spinal dysraphisms or occult spina bifida. These signs include patches of hair, nevi, hemangiomas, or dimples on the lower back in the midline. These conditions are rare in the adult population. The spine should be observed for signs of scoliosis.

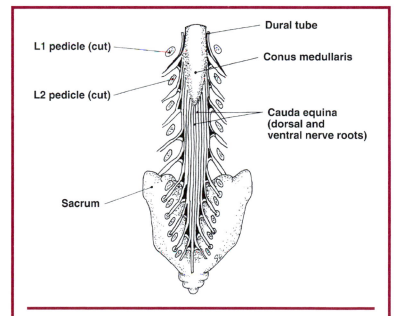

FIGURE 2. Posterior view of the lumbar region of the spinal canal, demonstrating the conus medullaris at the L1 to L2 level and the cauda equina nerve roots inferiorly.

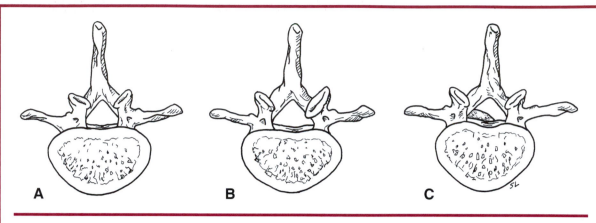

FIGURE 3. Lateral spinal canal stenosis. *A,* normal axial lumbar spine. *B,* osteophyte hypertrophy of the medial edge of the superior facet causing nerve root impingement most commonly in the lateral recess, less frequently in the mid zone (intraforaminal area). *C,* intraforaminal and/or extraforaminal nerve root compression due to osteophytic formation of the vertebral body or from a lateral disc herniation.

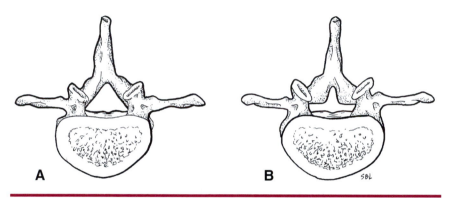

FIGURE 4. Spinal canal stenosis. *A,* normal axial lumbar spine. *B,* the "flattened" or trefoil" canal seen in congenital stenosis.

The patient may assume a Simian stance, with hips and knees slightly flexed when standing erect or with ambulation.[6] Spinal range of motion is usually within normal limits.

Most patients with lumbar stenosis will have a normal neurologic exam at rest. In pure lumbar stenosis, examination of femoral, popliteal, and pedal pulses will be normal. There will be no evidence of limb coolness with elevation, and the patient will have normal capillary refill time of the toes. Skin trophic changes are absent. The neurologic exam at rest is usually quiescent. Neurologic signs can be unmasked by ambulation with the spine in an extended position until the patient complains of claudication symptoms. At that time the neurologic exam may reveal depressed deep tendon reflexes, sensory deficits, weakness or a positive straight leg raise test (Lasegue's sign). The patient may have a positive "stoop test." To perform the "stoop test," the patient walks with an exaggerated lumbar lordosis until claudication symptoms appear or are worsened. At the point of increased symptomatology, the patient is allowed to lean forward. Reduction of symptoms is a positive response and is suggestive of neurogenic claudication.[7] Examining the hips to rule out hip pathology is also important.

Functional Limitations

The patient with lumbar stenosis may develop a progressive reduction of ambulation tolerance. Urinary incontinence may develop and poses a significant detriment to the patient's well being and activities of daily living. The patient may develop atrophy and weakness of the musculature of the legs, thereby limiting mobility.

Diagnostic Studies

The diagnosis of lumbar stenosis depends mostly on history and physical examination. MRI is the best test for radiographic confirmation of the diagnosis. Plain films of the lumbar spine are not sufficiently sensitive but may disclose spondylolisthesis. Spondylolisthesis is a common finding in males with lumbar stenosis. The myelogram is rarely used today due to potential side effects and a poor ability to diagnose lateral stenosis. The CT scan is able to demonstrate the lumbar subarachnoid space, facets, and osteophytes well.

The trefoil canal shape is highly suggestive of lumbar stenosis. The normal A-P diameter of the lumbar canal varies from 15 to 23 mm.[8] An A-P diameter of 10 mm or less is diagnostic of lumbar stenosis, whereas a diameter of 10–12 mm A-P is considered relative stenosis.[3] The MRI has been shown to be the best tool for diagnosing lumbar stenosis because it gives a visualization of both the bony and soft tissue structures of the spinal canal. The MRI also assists in the exclusion of more serious conditions, such as tumors of the conus medullaris and cauda equina. The MRI can also diagnose infectious and inflammatory etiologies of lumbar stenosis.

Ankle/brachial indexes and arterial Doppler studies should be obtained if no abnormalities in the pulses are discovered or if vascular disease is suspected.[6,8] Electrodiagnostic studies are non-specific for the diagnosis of lumbar stenosis; however, they are valuable because they assist in ruling out peripheral neuropathy and entrapment neuropathies. Needle electromyographic testing of the lower extremity may reveal findings of acute and chronic denervation in 50% to 76% of patients.[9,10] There may be some utility for dermatomal somatosensory evoked potentials in the diagnosis of lumbar stenosis.[9,11]

Differential Diagnosis

Peripheral vascular disease

Sciatic claudication[6]

Venous claudication after thrombosis

Myxedema claudication

Peripheral neuropathy

Osteoarthritis of the hips and knees

Conus medullaris and cauda equina neoplasms

Neurofibromas, ependymomas, hemangioblastomas, dermoids, epidermoids, lipomas

Metastatic spread of tumor

Spondylolisthesis

Epidural abscess

Inflammatory arachnoiditis

Lumbar facet syndrome

Pathologic vertebral fracture with bony stenosis (osteoporosis)

Stroke

Treatment

Initial

Conservative treatment is a viable option for many patients with lumbar stenosis.[3,12] The natural history of lumbar stenosis, in most cases, does not necessarily lead to deterioration. Conservative management of lumbar stenosis includes nonsteroidal anti-inflammatory drugs; however, the COX-2 inhibitors may be better tolerated in the geriatric population. Gabapentin has been helpful in decreasing the paresthesias experienced with lumbar stenosis. Gabapentin therapy should be initiated at a low dose of 100 mg tid and titrated up slowly to decrease side effects.

Rehabilitation

Therapeutic exercises are beneficial and should include a lumbar flexion program, modified abdominal strengthening, trunk and lower extremity flexibility, bicycling, and uphill treadmill walking. A treadmill is invaluable when measuring a patient's response to treatment. Assessment on a treadmill will establish an objective record of neurogenic claudication by providing a record of walking speed, tolerance, and distance at which symptoms appear. Response to treatment can be done at weekly follow-up treadmill testing. Physical modalities, such as heat, cyrotherapy, electric modalities, and pelvic traction, are helpful adjuncts to increase tissue flexibility and decrease muscle spasm. Traction should not be used in cases of spondylolisthesis because it may increase the spinal listhesis.

Procedures

The use of epidural steroid injections in the management of lumbar stenosis is controversial. Some studies have shown relief of symptoms for a short period of time.[13] However, sustained pain relief at 6 months was only 0% to 1.5% because the medications did not relieve the underlying stenosis. Epidural steroid injection probably has the best utility in cases in which lumbar stenosis is associated with superimposed acute nerve root irritation. It is also helpful in the management of those patients who are not surgical candidates due to multiple medical risk factors.

Surgery

Surgical management of lumbar stenosis is generally accepted to be an elective course of action. It is more effective in relieving lower extremity symptoms; however, the presence of low back pain alone is rarely an indication for surgery. Lumbar stenosis is treated with a variety of surgical techniques such as decompressive laminectomy with or without instrumented or non-instrumented fusion of the spine.[3] Another type of decompressive procedure is multilevel laminectomy. In this procedure, fenestrations are made in the superior aspect of the inferior lamina and the inferior aspect of the superior lamina at involved levels. This approach is said to allow greater stability to the spine postoperatively.[8] Surgery, in most cases, is usually successful in relieving the leg pain associated with lumbar stenosis.[3,14]

Potential Disease Complications

Lumbar stenosis frequently does not tend to pursue a progressively deteriorating course. Studies have followed the cases of patients with non-treated lumbar stenosis over a period of 2 to 4 years. These reports show little in the way of progressive functional decline in at least 54% of the patients studied. Patients with neurogenic claudication tend to reach a disability plateau and then do not deteriorate further. Nonetheless the natural course of lumbar stenosis may be complicated by a progressive decline in ambulation tolerance, incontinence of bowel and bladder, weakness of the lower extremities, and worsened low back and leg pain.[3,8]

Potential Treatment Complications

Complications of treatment with nonsteroidal anti-inflammatory drugs are well known and include GI bleed, renal insufficiency, and fluid retention. The most common complications of gabapentin include dizziness, ataxia, and somnolence.[15]

Side effects of epidural steroid injections are not common when performed by experienced practitioners. Possible side effects include epidural hematoma, hypercorticism, temporary paralysis, and chemical meningitis. A dural puncture is the most common technical error in epidural steroidal injections. On average, there is a 5% incidence of this mishap.[13] The risk of headache with lumbar epidural steroid injections has been estimated to be 1%.[13]

Complications of surgery include the imposed risks of general anesthesia, wound infection, hematoma formation, dural tears with subsequent cerebrospinal fluid leaks and the risk of meningitis, nerve root damage, and the potential for producing postoperative spinal instability. The overall surgical mortality associated with decompressive laminectomy is 1%; however, it increases to 2.3% for patients older than 80 years of age.[8,16]

References

1. Arnoldi CC, Brodsky AE, Cauchoix J, et al: Lumbar spinal stenosis and nerve root entrapment syndromes. Definition and classification. Clin Orth Rel Res 1976;115: 4–5.
2. Kirkaldy-Willis WH, Paine KWE, Cauchoix J, McIvor G: Lumbar spinal stenosis. Clin Orthop 1974;99:30–50.
3. Fritz JM, Delillo A, Welch WC, Erhard RE: Lumbar spinal stenosis: A review of current concepts in evaluation, management, and outcome measurements. Arch Phys Med Rehabil 1998;79:700–708.
4. Katz JN, Dalgas M, Stucki G, Lipson SG: Degenerative lumbar spinal stenosis. Diagnostic value of the history and physical examination. Arthritis Rheum 1995;38:1236–1241.
5. Johnson B, Stromquist B: Symptoms and signs in degeneration of the lumbar spine: A prospective consecutive study of 300 operated patients. J Bone Joint Surg Br 1993;75:381–385.
6. Porter RW: Spinal stenosis and neurogenic claudication. Spine 1996;21:2046–2052.
7. Dyck P: The Stoop-test in lumbar entrapment radiculopathy. Spine 1979;4:89–92.
8. Alvarez JA, Hardy RH: Lumbar spine stenosis: A common cause of back and leg pain. Am Fam Physician 1998;57:1825–1834.
9. Wilbourn AJ, Aminoff MJ: The electrodiagnostic examination in patients with radiculopathies. Muscle Nerve 1998;21:1612–1631.
10. Seppalainen AM, Alaranta H, Soini J: Electromyography in the diagnosis of lumbar spinal stenosis. Electromyog Clin Neurophysiol 1891;21:55–66.
11. Kraft G: A physiologic approach to the evaluation of lumbosacral stenosis. Phys Med Rehab Clin North Am 1998;9(2): 381–389.
12. Simotas AC, Dorey FJ, Hansraj KK, Cammisa F Jr: Nonoperative treatment for lumbar spinal stenosis. Clinical and outcome results and a 3-year survivorship analysis. Spine 2000;25:197–203.
13. Rydevik BL, Cohen DB, Kostuik JP: Spinal epidural steroids for patients with lumbar stenosis. Spine 1997;22: 2313–2317.
14. Atlas SJ, Keller RB, Robson D, et al: Surgical and nonsurgical management of lumbar spinal stenosis. Spine 2000;25:556–562.
15. Walsh P: Physicians Desk Reference, 55th ed. Montvale, NJ, Medical Economics Company, 2001, pp 2458–2461.
16. Ciol MA, Deyo RA, Howell E, Kreif S: An assessment of surgery for spinal stenosis: Time trends, geographic variations, complications and re-operations. J Geriatrics Society 1996;44:285–291.

50 Sacroiliac Joint Dysfunction

Scott F. Nadler, DO

Synonyms

Sacroiliac sprain

Sacroiliac instability

ICD-9 Codes

846
Sprains and strains of
sacroiliac region

846.0
Lumbosacral (joint)
(ligament)

846.1
Sacroiliac ligament

846.2
Sacrospinatus
(ligament)

846.3
Sacrotuberous
(ligament)

846.8
Other specified sites of
sacroiliac region

846.9
Unspecified site of
sacroiliac region

Definition

The sacroiliac (SI) joints are weight-bearing joints between the articular surfaces of the sacrum and ilium. They are part synovial joint and part syndesmosis, with the synovial portion being the anterior and inferior one-third of the joint. There is hyaline cartilage on the sacral side and fibrocartilage on the ilial side.[1,2] The articular capsule of the sacroiliac joint is attached close to the articulating surfaces of the sacrum and ilium. Also, there is partial interlocking of the bones due to irregular elevations and depressions on the surfaces of the sacrum and ilium. The joints begin to develop uneven opposing surfaces after puberty.[3,4]

There are no muscles that directly control movement of the sacroiliac joints, but many indirectly affect movement. Sacroiliac joint movement is mainly passive in response to the action of surrounding muscles.[1,2] The psoas and piriformis muscles pass anterior to the sacroiliac joints, and imbalance of these muscles in particular may affect SI joint function. Imbalance in the length and strength of the piriformis strongly influences movement of the sacrum.[1] The thoracolumbar fascia extends from the thoracic region to the sacrum and assists in stabilizing the joint in transferring forces from the thoracic cage to the pelvis and lower extremities.[5]

Sacroiliac joint dysfunction occurs when there is an alteration of the structural or positional relationship of the sacrum on a normally positioned ilium.[6] The sacroiliac joint plays a small but significant role in the cause of low back and buttock pain, although the true incidence is unknown. Its extensive innervation from the lumbosacral region accounts for the difficulty in differentiating sacroiliac joint dysfunction from that of surrounding structures. Various medical conditions such as rheumatologic disorders, infection, and neoplasms may also affect the joint. Sacroiliac dysfunction may be symptomatic or asymptomatic and may be acute or chronic. The prevalence of sacroiliac joint dysfunction in the general population has been reported to be from 15% to 30%.[1,7]

Symptoms

The most common presenting symptom in patients with sacroiliac dysfunction is pain or tenderness over the sacroiliac joint posteriorly.[8,9] Radiation may occur into the buttock, groin, posterior proximal thigh, and occasionally, lower leg.[2,8] Pain is often worse with long periods of sitting or standing, turning in bed, or stepping up on the affected leg. This makes it difficult to differentiate from other causes of low back pain, such as a lumbar herniated disc or facet syndrome. Pain may be noted in the buttock, thigh, calf, and foot in patients with sacroiliac dysfunction.[10] Following sacroiliac joint injection, studies have shown pain referral patterns that extended to the medial buttock, lateral buttock to the greater trochanter, and superior lateral thigh. The area of maximal pain was from the medial buttock extending approximately 10 cm caudally and 3 cm laterally from the posterior superior iliac spine (PSIS). From these studies it is suggested that standardized pain diagram be utilized in screening for sacroiliac dysfunction.[11,12]

Physical Examination

Sensory, motor, and reflex examination of the lower extremities should be performed as part of any assessment of the low back, hip, and pelvis, since sacroiliac dysfunction alone should not produce sensory, motor, or reflex deficits.[2] The sacroiliac joint is not directly palpable because it is covered by the posterior aspect of the innominate bone.[14] Examination should include evaluation of true and apparent leg-length discrepancies, symmetry of the iliac crests, PSISs, anterior superior iliac spines (ASIS), gluteal folds, pubic tubercles, ischial tuberosities, and medial malleoli. Palpation of the sacral base is performed by locating the sacral sulcus as the thumb is moved medial to the PSIS and used to press anteriorly. The sacral sulcus and inferior lateral angles should be examined with the patient prone for depth and position. Soft tissue palpation is used to evaluate the skin and subcutaneous tissue, muscles, and ligaments for tissue texture changes.

Along with the aforementioned examination, various provocative maneuvers for SI dysfunction exist. There are two main types of tests: tests for pain and tests for motion or mobility. The more commonly used tests for sacroiliac dysfunction are described in the following section.

Motion Tests

Standing flexion test: The patient stands with the feet 6 inches apart. The clinician stands behind the patient and places the thumbs on the inferior aspects of the PSISs. The patient is instructed to bend forward without bending the knees while the clinician maintains contact with the PSISs. Normally, the PSISs should move equally. If one PSIS moves superiorly and anteriorly to the other, this is the side of restriction and hypomobility and indicates ipsilateral SI joint dysfunction. False positive standing flexion tests can occur from ipsilateral tight quadratus lumborum, contralateral tight hamstrings, sacroiliac joint arthritis, or with hip restriction.[13,14]

Seated flexion test: This is a test of sacroiliac mobility that is used to differentiate sacroiliac from iliosacral dysfunction when compared with the standing flexion test. The patient is seated with the feet firmly supported while the clinician stands or sits behind the patient with the eyes at the level of the iliac crests. The patient bends forward as the clinician maintains contact with the PSISs. If one PSIS moves superiorly and anteriorly to the other, this is the side that is restricted and hypomobile. While the patient is seated, the innominates are fixed in place, thus isolating out sacroiliac motion. A false positive test may occur from tight ipsilateral quadratus lumborum.[2]

Gillet's test (also called the stork or marching test): The patient stands with the feet 6 inches apart while the clinician stands or sits behind the patient. The clinician places one thumb on the PSIS of the side to be tested and the other thumb on the sacral base over S2. The patient flexes the hip and knee to 90 degrees on the side being tested while the clinician notes any movement of the PSIS. Normally the PSIS should move posteriorly and inferiorly as the ilium rotates posteriorly on the sacrum. The joint is considered hypomobile if the PSIS moves superiorly.

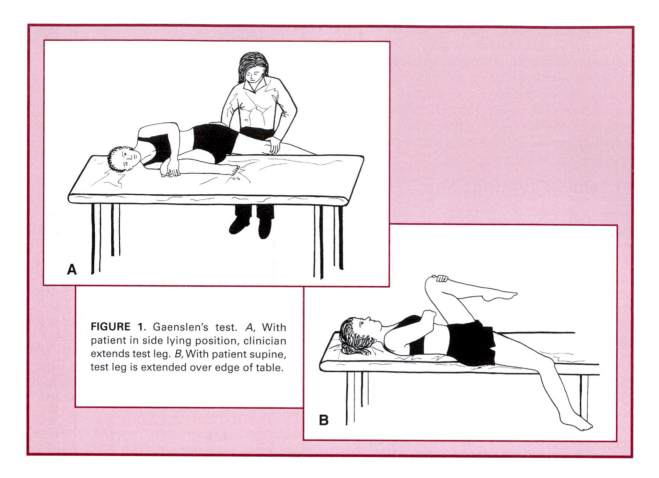

FIGURE 1. Gaenslen's test. *A*, With patient in side lying position, clinician extends test leg. *B*, With patient supine, test leg is extended over edge of table.

Pain Tests

Gaenslen's test: The patient lies supine and moves to the edge of the examination table with the buttock on the side to be tested over the edge (Fig. 1). The patient's leg is dropped off the table so that the thigh and hip are hyperextended, while the opposite knee is maximally flexed. This results in anterior rotation of the innominate and sacroiliac joint on the test side. Pain or discomfort indicates sacroiliac joint pathology, but may also be caused by an L2–L4 nerve root lesion.[8,15]

Patrick's test (also called Fabere's sign): With the patient supine, the hip and knee on one side are flexed, abducted, and externally rotated, and the foot is placed on the opposite knee. The knee is then pushed downward to move the ilium forward, and pressure is applied over the opposite ASIS. Pain or discomfort at the contralateral SI joint reflects sacroiliac pathology; ipsilateral pain indicates hip joint pathology.[8,16]

Distraction test (also called Gapping test): With the patient supine, pressure is applied over both ASISs posterolaterally. This stretches the anterior sacroiliac ligaments, reproducing the patient's pain.[17,18] The test has also been described by compressing medially.[14]

Compression test: The patient lies in the lateral recumbent position with the clinician behind the patient (Fig. 2). Pressure is applied to the uppermost iliac crest, which is directed toward the opposite iliac crest, compressing the pelvis. This stretches the posterior sacroiliac ligaments or compresses the anterior aspect of the joint, reproducing pain.[2]

Functional Limitations

Functional limitations include difficulty with position changes, especially arising from a seated position or bending forward at the waist. Additionally, prolonged ambulation, ambulating on uneven surfaces, or climbing stairs may be painful activities secondary to pain and accompanying muscular imbalances about the pelvis.

Diagnostic Studies

Plain radiographs will help in identifying sacroiliac joint pain resulting from trauma, infection, neoplasm, inflammation, or degenerative arthritis. However, sacroiliac dysfunctions typically reveal no abnormalities on plain radiographs. Bone scan may demonstrate increased uptake in sacroiliac dysfunction.[8] Computed

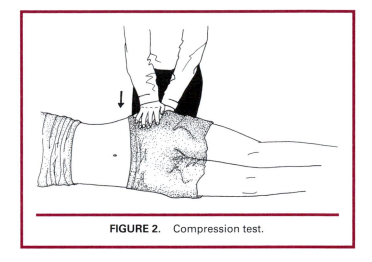

FIGURE 2.   Compression test.

tomography (CT) scan can be used to further identify bony abnormalities, and magnetic resonance imaging (MRI) can be used to identify soft tissue abnormalities if they are suspected.

The radiographic projection of the sacroiliac joint is determined by the shape of the articular surfaces and the inclination of the pelvis, which in turn is determined by the lumbosacral angle and the degree of lumbar lordosis.[19] Projections of the joint should include anteroposterior and oblique views. Other views can include craniocaudal axial projection, inlet views, outlet views, and lithotomy views. The outlet and lithotomy views may provide the best representation of both sacroiliac joints.[19]

Differential Diagnosis

Discogenic low back pain

Lumbosacral radiculopathy

Lumbar facet syndrome

Ankylosing spondylitis and other rheumatologic conditions

Piriformis syndrome

Sacral stress/insufficiency fractures

Spondylosis

Treatment

Initial

Initial treatment of sacroiliac dysfunctions should include limiting or avoiding activities that exacerbate SI joint pain. Pharmacologic intervention with acetaminophen or nonsteroidal anti-inflammatory drugs (NSAIDs), including cyclooxygenase-2 (COX-2) inhibitors, may be used initially to treat acute exacerbations but should not be relied on for long treatment periods. Occasionally, opiate analgesics may be helpful in cases of refractory pain to prevent further compensatory changes with general mobility but are generally discouraged due to their well-known addictive potential. Ice may initially be helpful, but local heat may also provide great comfort. Manipulative treatment may be quite helpful initially to restore functional symmetry during the gait cycle. Controversy exists as to whether manipulation actually changes the position of the SI joint or only work to correct surrounding soft tissue injury.

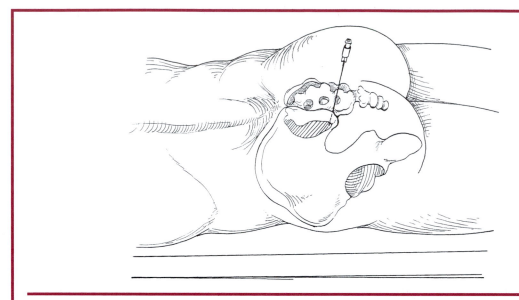

FIGURE 3. Sacroiliac joint injection. The patient is in a prone position, and the needle has been guided into the inferior aspect of the joint employing a direct posterior approach. (From LennardTA (ed): Pain Procedures in Clinical Practice, 2nd ed. Philadelphia, Hanley & Belfus, 2000, p 267.)

Rehabilitation

Physical therapy can be helpful and should include pelvic stabilization exercises, back and lower extremity strengthening, pelvic mobilization, and postural correction exercises. Sacroiliac belts can also be used and provide relief in many patients. Sacroiliac belts usually should be worn in young, hypermobile individuals but not in the elderly, who tend to be hypomobile. Correcting leg-length discrepancy and functional asymmetry in the height of the sacral base with heel lifts and/or orthotics have also shown benefit in improving alignment and decreasing pain.[5] It is recommended that conservative therapy be attempted for a minimum of 6 weeks to 3 months before considering SI joint injection and a minimum of 6 months before consideration of any surgical treatment.

Procedures

Fluoroscopically controlled sacroiliac joint injections with anesthetic or steroid are considered by some to be the "gold standard" in both diagnosing and treating sacroiliac joint dysfunction (Fig. 3).[20] Following the criteria for lumbar epidurals, one may monitor the response to the first injection and perform additional injections only if clinically warranted. In response to compensatory muscle spasm associated with SI joint dysfunction, local trigger point injections (TPIs) may be useful in decreasing pain and restricted motion. Trigger point injections should be used judiciously and in conjunction with a supervised exercise program.

Neuroaugmentation with an electrical stimulator implanted at the third sacral nerve root in a limited number of subjects with sacroiliac joint pain has been successfully used to manage refractory pain.[21]

Surgery

Surgery is very rarely performed for sacroiliac motion dysfunction.

Potential Disease Complications

In the case of refractory pain the subject should be evaluated for underlying sacral insufficiency fracture, and in the young male patient ankylosing spondylitis should be ruled out.

Potential Treatment Complications

Gastrointestinal, hepatic, and renal complications from prolonged use of medications such as acetaminophen or NSAIDs, including COX-2 inhibitors, are well known to occur. Sacral insufficiency fractures may be displaced with manipulation, and aggressive manipulative therapy for rheumatic disease may increase inflammation. Complications from steroid injections include skin depigmentation, fatty atrophy, and/or infection. Additionally, repetitive use of steroids about the SI joint may cause cartilage breakdown within this mobile joint, further restricting motion.

References

1. Greenman PE: Principles of Manual Medicine, 2nd ed. Baltimore, Williams & Wilkins, Baltimore, MD, 1996, pp 305–367, 530–532.
2. Solonen KA: The sacroiliac joint in the light of anatomical, roentgenological and clinical studies. Acta Orthopaedica Scandinavica 1957;(Suppl XXVII):9–127.
3. Beal MC: The sacroiliac problem: Review of anatomy, mechanics, and diagnosis. J Am Osteopathic Assoc 1982;81(10):73–85.
4. Mierau DR, Cassidy JD, Hamin T, Miln RA: Sacroiliac joint dysfunction and low back pain in school aged children. J Manipulative Physiol Therapeutics 1984;7(2):81–84.
5. Harrison DE, Harrison DD, Troyanovich DJ: The sacroiliac joint: A review of anatomy and biomechanics with clinical implications. J Manipulative Physiol Therapeutics 1997:20(9);607–617.
6. Dreyfuss P, Dreyer S, Griffin J, et al: Positive sacroiliac screening tests in asymptomatic adults. Spine 1994;19(10):1138–1143.
7. Ebraheim NA, Xu R, Nadaud M, et al: Sacroiliac joint injection: A cadaveric study. Am J Orthop 1997;26:338–341.
8. Daum WJ: The sacroiliac joint: An underappreciated pain generator. Am J Orthop 1995;24:475-478.
9. Fortin JD, Falco FJE: The Fortin finger test: An indicator of sacroiliac pain. Am J Orthop 1997;26:477–480.
10. Schwarzer AC, Aprill CN, Bogduk N: The sacroiliac joint in chronic low back pain. Spine. 1995;20(1):31–37.
11. Fortin JD, Dwyer AP, West S, Pier J: Sacroiliac joint: Pain referral maps upon applying a new injection/arthrography technique. Part I: Asymptomatic volunteers. Spine 1994;19(13):1475–1482.
12. Fortin JD, Aprill CN, Ponthieux B, Pier J: Sacroiliac joint: Pain referral maps upon applying a new injection/arthrography technique. Part II: Clinical evaluation. Spine 1994;19(13):1483–1489.
13. DiGiovanna EL, Schiowitz S: An Osteopathic Approach to Diagnosis and Treatment. Philadelphia, J.B. Lippincott, 1991, pp 189–212, 221–227.
14. Gross J, Fetto J, Rosen E: Musculoskeletal Examination. Cambridge, MA, Blackwell Science, , 1996, pp 80, 93–94, 96–97, 118–119, 293–294.
15. Magee DJ: Orthopedic Physical Assessment. 3rd ed. Philadelphia, W.B. Saunders, 1997, pp 434–459.
16. Kenna C, Murtagh J: Patrick or Fabere test to test hip and sacroiliac joint disorders. Australian Fam Phys 1989;18(4):375.
17. Laslett M, Williams M: The reliability of selected pain provocation tests for sacroiliac joint pathology. Spine 1994;19(11):1243–1249.
18. Lindsay DM, Meeuwisse WH, Vyse A, et al: Lumbosacral dysfunctions in elite cross country skiers. JOSPT 1993;18(5);580–585.
19. Ebraheim NA, Mekhail AO, Wiley WF, et al: Radiology of the sacroiliac joint. Spine 1997;22(8):869–876.
20. Maigne JY, Aivaliklis A, Pfefer F: Results of sacroiliac joint double block and value of sacroiliac pain provocation tests in 54 patients with low back pain. Spine 1996;21(16):1889–1892.
21. Calvillo O, Esses SI, Ponder C, et al: Neuroaugmentation in the management of sacroiliac joint pain: Report of two cases. Spine 1998;23(9):1069–1072.

51 Hip Arthritis

Jeffrey L. Woodward, MD, MS

Synonyms

Coxarthritis

Coxarthrosis

Hip degenerative joint disease

ICD-9 Codes

715.25
Osteoarthritis, localized secondary (pelvic region and thigh)

715.5
Osteoarthritis, localized, primary (pelvic region and thigh)

716.15
Traumatic arthropathy (pelvic region and thigh)

Definition

Hip osteoarthritis does not represent a single disease entity but consists of a mostly non-inflammatory disorder characterized by deterioration of the articular cartilage. Associated changes include asymmetric joint space narrowing, subchondral bone sclerosis or eburnation under the region of cartilage loss, superficial subchondral bone cyst formation, marginal bone growth (osteophytosis), and associated periarticular bone vascular hypertension.[1] The exact etiology of the degenerative cartilage fibrillation and degradation has not been clearly identified. Osteoarthritis is classified as either primary (idiopathic) or secondary, although this determination can be difficult.

Primary hip osteoarthritis involves degenerative joint changes occurring with no apparent preceding trauma, disease process, or mechanical joint deformity. Prior investigations have indicated that significant generalized primary osteoarthritis often is associated with a positive family history for osteoarthritis, which probably constitutes a polygenic disorder. Recent studies have identified some specific gene loci apparently linked to the development of female hip osteoarthritis, supporting a genetic predisposition for this condition.[2] Primary hip osteoarthritis is more prevalent in women and typically develops in the 50- to 70-year-old age group. There is inconsistent correlation between physical or occupational activity and the development of primary hip osteoarthritis, unlike that of other joints, including hands and knees.[3,4] Interestingly, there is a clear negative association between hip osteoarthritis and femoral neck osteoporosis with females having higher femoral bone mineral density values developing increased incidence of hip osteoarthritis. In one recent study of primary hip osteoarthritis, the average age of onset of symptoms was 61 years, with no significant difference detected in the average body mass indices of these patients as compared with the general population.[5]

Secondary hip osteoarthritis includes hip osteoarthritic changes following localized trauma, such as acetabular or femoral head fracture, or prior hip region abnormality, such as congenital hip dislocation, slipped capital femoral epiphysis, hip avascular necrosis, Paget's disease, or Legg-Calvé-Perthes disease. Prior studies have shown that the risk of developing secondary osteoarthritis in the hip joint is significantly higher if the individual has clinical evidence of primary osteoarthritis with involvement of other joints.[6] The most significant biomechanical joint characteristic associated with the development of secondary osteoarthritis is hip joint space incongruency, which is more clearly related to trauma involving impact or axial loading of the hip joint rather than shear loading.[1] In adults, traumatic hip injury with significant joint disruption has been clearly associated with the onset of hip osteoarthritis. Patients with incomplete hip dislocation or subluxation have a 16% chance of developing hip osteoarthritis, and those who sustain significant acetabular fracture have an 88% chance of subsequent hip osteoarthritis.[7] Hip osteoarthritis presenting in the 20 to 50 year-old age group most likely represents secondary osteoarthritis and any underlying joint mechanical abnormalities contributing to the progressing osteoarthritis should be identified as soon as possible.

Most reviews include a subtype of primary osteoarthritis known as erosive inflammatory, or "destructive," osteoarthritis.[1] These terms designate a relatively aggressive form of osteoarthritis associated with rapid loss of joint cartilage and evidence of at least mild inflammatory changes, including joint synovitis, which can progress quickly to severe joint abnormalities within 1 or 2 years. However, erosive osteoarthritis usually attacks the wrist and finger joints, with hip joint involvement less common.

Symptoms

The most common presenting complaint of hip osteoarthritis is pain. Usually the discomfort is of mild to moderate severity with gradual onset and progression. The initial pain from hip osteoarthritis is most typically only in the hip joint region, usually the anterior hip and the inguinal-groin or lateral hip area. Hip joint stiffness may also be reported, with the most significant symptoms occurring after brief periods of rest and inactivity. Joint aching may be reported in association with significant weather pattern changes. Referred pain can occur as a presenting or progressive symptom, including discomfort in the medial thigh area and knee region pain. Discomfort is often aggravated with repetitive hip movements and strenuous prolonged physical activity involving standing, walking, climbing, and squatting movements. Hip osteoarthritic pain is often relieved significantly with prolonged rest. Hip joint subjective weakness may be a symptom and is usually associated with more chronic and advanced hip osteoarthritis.

Physical Examination

Passive range-of-motion measurements should be performed routinely, and joint motion is often reduced with significant hip osteoarthritic involvement. In some patients, audible or palpable joint crepitus may be noted with passive or active motion. Significant hip joint pain is frequently noted at end range of motion, particularly the internal and external rotation planes. Objective weakness is most commonly noted in active abduction and extension planes. Examination of all other joints, particularly wrist and fingers, should be conducted for evaluation of generalized osteoarthritis. Gait evaluation will often identify an antalgic pattern with decreased stance phase on the affected side and may reveal functional evidence of hip joint contractures. The neurologic examination is generally normal with the exception that strength may be diminished due to pain and/or disuse.

Functional Limitations

Most functional limitations are directly related to a gradual decrease in standing and walking tolerance due to pain. A history of progressive activity restriction in climbing and squatting activities also may be identified primarily due to limitation from pain, but may be secondary to physical joint motion restriction. Gradual development of hip joint and pelvic girdle muscle weakness may also restrict daily activity, particularly rising from a seated position from a chair or commode or getting in and out of the bathtub.

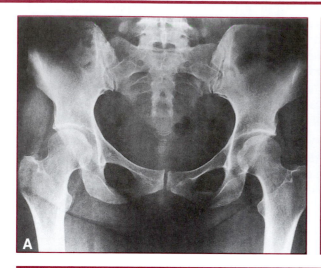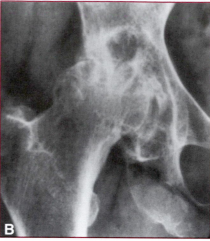

FIGURE 1. *A,* Normal hip joints on plain x-ray AP view. *B,* Osteoarthritic hip joint revealing superior and lateral joint space narrowing, subchondral sclerosis, superior acetabular bone cyst, medial femoral neck, and lesser trochanteric sclerosis with buttressing.

Diagnostic Studies

There is no clinical test that is diagnostic specifically for hip osteoarthritis. Hip osteoarthritis is most commonly diagnosed using routine x-ray studies. Initial x-ray evaluation is usually done with an anterior-posterior (AP) pelvic plain x-ray view. For the best visualization of hip joint space and congruency, the AP view should be performed with about 15 degrees internal rotation of each hip to compensate for the normal anteversion of the femoral neck. Hip joint x-ray findings indicative of osteoarthritis include joint space narrowing with associated femoral head migration, subchondral sclerosis, marginal osteophytes, and subchondral bone cysts (Fig. 1).[8] Identification of underlying structural bone abnormalities contributing to osteoarthritis may also be diagnosed at this time and may include acetabular dysplasia or femoral head/neck deformities. The most common pattern of hip joint osteoarthritic changes includes superior joint cartilage loss and subsequent superior femoral head migration (Fig. 2). Medial femoral head migration may also be seen but is less common with osteoarthritis, whereas severe diffuse joint narrowing along the entire femoral head, known as axial joint space narrowing, may indicate a diagnosis other than osteoarthritis, such as an inflammatory arthritis.[9] The rate of progression of hip osteoarthritis may also be estimated by performing and comparing repeat x-rays at 12-month intervals.

Bone scans are typically *not* helpful for the diagnosis of hip osteoarthritis. However, it may show mild increased activity in the delayed bone phase in the hip joint several years before arthritic changes become evident on plain x-ray (secondary to vascular changes and osteoplastic activity during the early stages of cartilage degeneration with osteoarthritis). Any joint demonstrating significant abnormal uptake on bone scan may develop more rapid and destructive osteoarthritic changes.[10] Hip joint MRI is also not typically required for the diagnosis of hip osteoarthritis, but MRI is indicated for the evaluation of possible avascular necrosis and can be helpful in the noninvasive evaluation of the hip joint cartilage.

At this time, there is no non-radiologic diagnostic test for osteoarthritis. Numerous studies have attempted to identify serum markers for osteoarthritis and have found some assays that may be helpful in future diagnosis.[11] Sedimentation rate values are usually normal, but may be slightly elevated in more aggressive generalized osteoarthritis cases. Synovial joint fluid analysis will demonstrate minimal abnormalities, such as slightly increased cell count, and can be used to rule out other joint diagnoses.

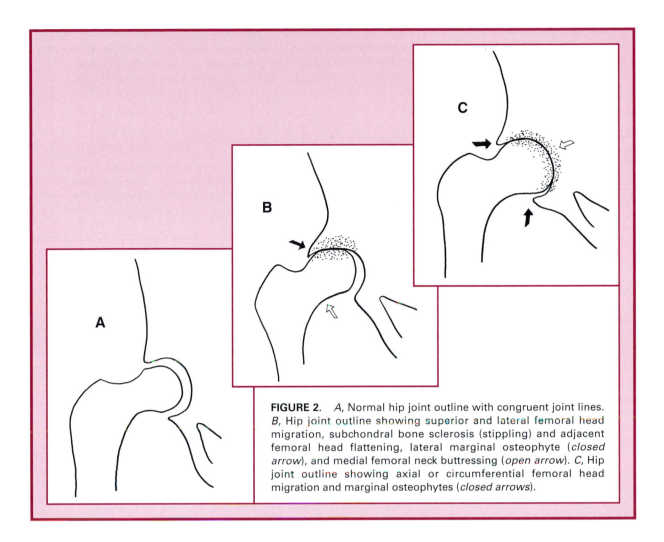

FIGURE 2. *A*, Normal hip joint outline with congruent joint lines. *B*, Hip joint outline showing superior and lateral femoral head migration, subchondral bone sclerosis (stippling) and adjacent femoral head flattening, lateral marginal osteophyte (*closed arrow*), and medial femoral neck buttressing (*open arrow*). *C*, Hip joint outline showing axial or circumferential femoral head migration and marginal osteophytes (*closed arrows*).

Testing such as serum rheumatologic screening to evaluate other possible causes of hip joint arthritic change may be necessary to complete a thorough evaluation and diagnosis following radiologic identification of a hip joint abnormality.

Differential Diagnosis

Inflammatory arthritis:
   rheumatoid arthritis,
   ankylosing spondylitis,
   Reiter's disease
Avascular necrosis of
   the hip

Infectious arthritis
Occult fracture
Paget's disease
Regional bursitis: greater
   trochanteric, iliopectineal,
   ischiogluteal

Congenital hip dysplasia
Primary calcium pyrophosphate
   arthropathy
Pigmented villonodular synovitis
Synovial chondromatosis
Referred pain

Treatment

Initial

Initial medical treatment of hip osteoarthritis usually involves trials of analgesic medications as necessary for pain management. Acetaminophen is often recommended as the initial medication, followed by trials of nonsteroidal anti-inflammatory drugs (NSAIDs), as needed. NSAIDs have not shown significant clinical differences in the treatment of hip osteoarthritis.[12] Moderate potency narcotic analgesics may be appropriate for short-term pain relief only associated with acute flares of osteoarthritic hip pain. Glycosaminoglycan supplements have been studied for years, with most textbook references on the topic indicating that no convincing evidence supports that these compounds modify or arrest the progression of osteoarthritis.[13] However, a very recent meta-analysis report indicates that glucosamine and chondroitin preparations can at least demonstrate moderate to large effects on osteoarthritis symptoms in a significant number of cases.[14]

Rapid symptomatic relief of unilateral hip pain from osteoarthritis may be achieved with prescription of an assistive device, such as a cane or walker. Use of a single-point cane in the hand contralateral to the affected hip joint can reduce reaction forces in the hip by as much as 50%, which may improve both pain and walking tolerance. Hip joint protective behaviors, including activity modification with decreased standing and squatting activities, may also significantly improve symptoms. Weight reduction treatments may gradually reduce hip joint pain.

Rehabilitation

Initial rehabilitation should first promote return of normal hip range of motion with a gradual stretching program. Most importantly, at least 30 degrees of passive hip flexion should be maintained bilaterally to allow for a normal gait pattern. Hip extension contractures can be limited by having the patient lie prone 30 minutes twice daily. Recently, Simpkin reported that patients with hip osteoarthritis showed significant decreases in pain and increases in walking tolerance with aggressive use of continuous passive motion treatment to the hip.[15] Few well-controlled studies have been done to assess the effectiveness of exercise therapy in patients with hip osteoarthritis, although a review of randomized clinical trials did demonstrate a moderate benefit of exercise therapy for osteoarthritis pain management.[16] Early hip joint strengthening can be started with static exercises, which are easily incorporated into a home program. More aggressive dynamic and isokinetic hip exercise can be started when reasonable pain control and hip joint range of motion has been obtained and usually includes lower extremity–closed kinetic chain weight-bearing activities. Intermittent weight-bearing exercise and activity done carefully can be tolerated even by most advanced hip osteoarthritis patients and are important for helping to maintain joint cartilage integrity. For a patient with either severe or recently aggravated hip osteoarthritis pain, the patient may start exercises with reduced hip axial loading force, such as a using a stationary bike or stair-climber along with an aquatic exercise program when available. Patients may tolerate the initial exercise program more comfortably by performing several brief exercise periods throughout the day instead of one prolonged session.

Procedures

Intra-articular hip joint anesthetic and steroid injections may be performed for the treatment of significant unremitting hip joint osteoarthritic pain after appropriate diagnostic workup. Fluoroscopic guidance is recommended for accurate needle placement for either anterior or lateral intra-articular steroid infiltration.[17] Intra-articular hip injection with only anesthetic solution under fluoroscopic guidance can be used as a strictly diagnostic procedure. Improved symptomatic relief from an intra-articular steroid injection may be obtained by providing a brief 1- to 2-week period of non–weight-bearing on the treated side immediately after steroid injection.

Surgery

For the elderly patient presenting with advanced hip osteoarthritis without surgical contraindications, total hip arthroplasty (THA) is the most accepted and efficacious treatment available today (see Chapter 56). This may also be advocated in younger patients who are severely disabled by pain. Clinical factors most closely associated with patients requiring THA are patients who are older than 70 years; female; and have significant superolateral migration of femoral head, hip joint space width measuring less than 2 mm, or an average visual analogue pain scale rating at or greater than the 5/10 level.[18] Due to the failure of THA components over time, younger patients diagnosed with significant hip osteoarthritis may benefit from various surgical acetabular and femoral osteotomies to provide better anatomic positioning of the femoral head and redistribute joint weight bearing, which can postpone the need for THA; however, these procedures are often not curative. In extreme cases of severe osteoarthritis in young individuals, hip arthrodesis traditionally has been considered a treatment option.

Potential Treatment Complications

Since many hip osteoarthritis patients often undergo prolonged courses with acetaminophen and/or NSAIDs, all associated gastric, hepatic, and renal side effect risks known for these specific medications should be monitored. Intra-articular corticosteroid use is associated with possible deleterious effects, including cartilage damage, and these injections into the hip joint should be performed cautiously. An approximate guideline of not more than three joint steroid injections in a 1-year period is often recommended, but cumulative side effects must also be monitored. THA procedures are known to pose a significant risk for the development of proximal and distal deep vein thrombosis, which may be encountered in the postsurgical rehabilitation setting.

Potential Disease Complications

The most significant medical complication directly related to hip osteoarthritis is progressive irreversible joint deterioration. As noted previously, associated joint contracture and weakness may also develop. Significant chronic physical limitations from hip osteoarthritis pain may negatively impact cardiovascular status and bone density in elderly patients. However, hip arthroplasty can often markedly improve a patient's functional status and limit such complications.

References
1. Hough AJ: Pathology of osteoarthritis. In McCarty DJ, Koopman WJ (eds): Arthritis and Allied Conditions. Philadelphia, Lea & Febiger, 1993, pp 1699–1721.
2. Mustafa Z, Chapman K, Irven C, et al: Linkage analyses of candidate genes as susceptibility loci for osteoarthritis-Suggestive linkage of COL9A1 to female hip osteoarthritis. Rheum (Ox) 2000;39:299–306.
3. Cvijetic S, Deknic-Ocegovic D, Campbell L, et al: Occupational physical demands and hip osteoarthritis. Arch Hig Rada Toksikol 1999;50:371–379.
4. Kulkal UN, Katrio J, Sarno S: Osteoarthritis of weightbearing joints of lower limbs in former elite male athletes. Br Med J 1994;308:231.
5. Chitnavis J, Sinsheimer JS, Suchard MA, et al: End-stage coxarthrosis and gonarthrosis: aetiology, clinical patterns and radiological features of idiopathic osteoarthritis. Rheum (Ox) 2000;39:612–619.
6. Doherty M, Watt I, Diepte P: Influence of primary generalized osteoarthritis on the development of secondary osteoarthritis. Lancet 1983;2:8.
7. Rodrigues-Merchan EC: Coxarthrosis after traumatic hip dislocation in the adult. Clin Orthop 2000; 377:92–98.
8. Greenspan A. Orthopedic Radiology, 2nd ed. Philadelphia, Lippincott-Raven, 1996.
9. Resnick D: Patterns of migration of the femoral head in osteoarthritis of the hip. Am J Roent Rad Ther Nucl Med 1975;124:62–74.
10. Hutton CW, Higgs ER, Jackson PC, et al: 99m Tc HMDP bone scanning in generalized nodal osteoarthritis. II. The four hour bone scan image predicts radiographic change. Ann Rheum Dis 1986;45:622–626.
11. Otterness IG, Swindell AC, Zimmerer RO, et al: Cartilage damage after intra-articular exposure to collagenase 3. 2000;8:180–185.
12. Towheed T, Shea B, Wells G, et al: Analgesia and non-aspirin, nonsteroidal anti-inflammatory drugs for osteoarthritis of the hip. Cochrane Database Syst Rev 2000;2:CD000517.
13. Solomon L. Clinical features of osteoarthritis. In Kelley W, Harris E, Ruddy S, Sledge C (eds): Textbook of Rheumatology. Philadelphia, W.B. Saunders, 1997, pp 1383–1393.
14. McAlindon TE, LaValley MP, Gulin JP, et al: Glucosamine and chondroitin for treatment of osteoarthritis. JAMA 2000;283:1469–1475.
15. Simpkin PA, de Lateur BJ, Alquist AD, et al: Continuous passive motion for osteoarthritis of the hip: a pilot study. J Rheum 1999;26:1987–1991.
16. Van Barr ME, Assendelft WJ, Dekker J, et al: Effectiveness of exercise therapy in patients with osteoarthritis of the hip or knee: a systematic review of randomized clinical trials. Arth Rheum 1999;42:1361–1369.
17. Woodward JL, Lennard, TL: Anatomic principles for peripheral joint injection. In Shankar K (ed): Physiatric Anatomic Principles, STAR, vol 10. Philadelphia, Hanley & Belfus, 1996, pp 473–488.
18. Dougados M, Gueguen A, Nguyen M, et al: Requirement of THA: An outcome measure of hip osteoarthritis? J Rheum 1999;26:855–861.

52 Femoral Neuropathy

Earl J. Craig, MD

Synonym

Diabetic amyotrophy

ICD-9 Codes

355.2
Other lesion of femoral nerve

355.8
Mononeuritis of lower limb, unspecified

355.9
Mononeuritis of unspecified site

782.0
Disturbance of skin sensation

Definition

Femoral neuropathy is the focal injury of the femoral nerve causing various combinations of pain, weakness, and sensory loss in the anterior thigh. Diabetic amyotrophy is the most common cause of focal femoral neuropathy, with hemorrhage most often due to anticoagulation therapy also quite common. Table 1 lists other possible etiologies for femoral neuropathy.

The femoral nerve arises from the anterior rami of the lumbar nerve roots 2, 3, and 4. After forming, the nerve passes on the anterolateral border of the psoas muscle, between the psoas and iliacus muscles, down the posterior abdominal wall and through the posterior pelvis until it emerges under the inguinal ligament lateral to the femoral artery (Fig. 1).[1–3] The course continues down the anterior thigh, innervating the anterior thigh muscles. The sensory-only saphenous nerve branches off the femoral nerve distal to the inguinal ligament and courses through the thigh until the Hunter's subsartorial canal where the nerve dives deep. The femoral nerve innervates the psoas and iliacus muscles in the pelvis and the sartorius, pectineus, rectus femoris, vastus medialis, vastus lateralis, and vastus intermedius muscles in the anterior thigh. The femoral nerve provides sensory innervation to the anterior thigh. The saphenous nerve provides sensory innervation to the anterior patella, anteromedial leg, and medial foot (Fig. 2).

TABLE 1. Possible Causes of Focal Femoral Neuropathy[1,2]

Open injuries
Retraction during abdominal/pelvic surgery[4,5]
Hip surgery—heat used by methylmethacrylate—especially when associated with leg lengthening[7,8]
Penetration trauma (e.g., gunshot and knife wounds, glass shards)

Closed Injuries
Retroperitoneal bleeding after femoral vein or artery puncture[6]
Cardiac angiography
Central line placement
Retroperitoneal fibrosis
Injury during femoral nerve block
Diabetic amyotrophy
Infection
Cancer[9]
Pregnancy
Radiation
Acute stretch injury due to a fall or other trauma
Hemorrhage after a fall or other trauma
Spontaneous hemorrhage—generally due to anticoagulant therapy
Idiopathic
Hypertrophic Mononeuropathy[10]

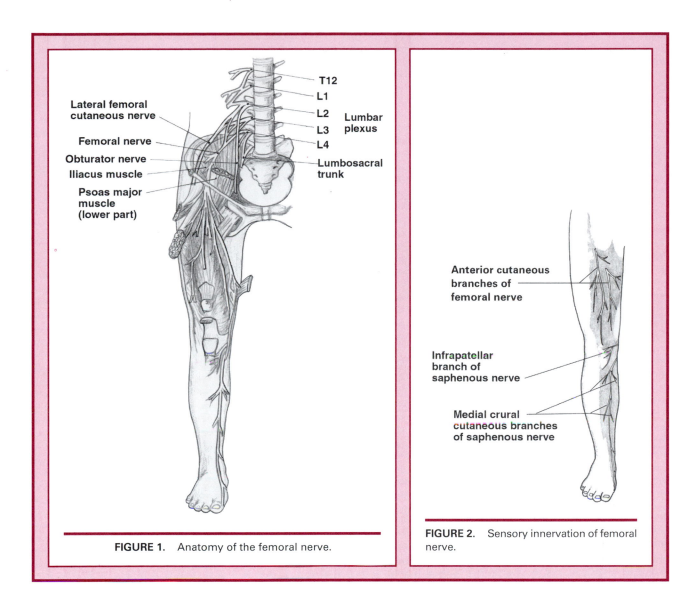

FIGURE 1. Anatomy of the femoral nerve.

Labels in Figure 1:
- Lateral femoral cutaneous nerve
- Femoral nerve
- Obturator nerve
- Iliacus muscle
- Psoas major muscle (lower part)
- T12
- L1
- L2
- L3
- L4
- Lumbar plexus
- Lumbosacral trunk

FIGURE 2. Sensory innervation of femoral nerve.

Labels in Figure 2:
- Anterior cutaneous branches of femoral nerve
- Infrapatellar branch of saphenous nerve
- Medial crural cutaneous branches of saphenous nerve

Symptoms

The symptoms will depend on how acute the injury is and what caused the injury. Often a patient will first complain of a dull, aching pain in the inguinal region, which may intensify within hours. Shortly thereafter, the patient may note difficulty with ambulation secondary to leg weakness. The patient may or may not complain of weakness in the hip or thigh but will often notice difficulty with functional activities, such as getting out of a chair or traversing stairs or inclines.

Numbness over the anterior thigh and medial leg is common. The numbness may extend into the anteromedial leg and the medial aspect of the foot.

Physical Examination

The examination should include a complete neuromuscular evaluation of the low back, hips, and both lower extremities. This should include inspection for asymmetry or atrophy, manual muscle testing, muscle stretch reflexes, and sensory testing for light touch and pinprick.

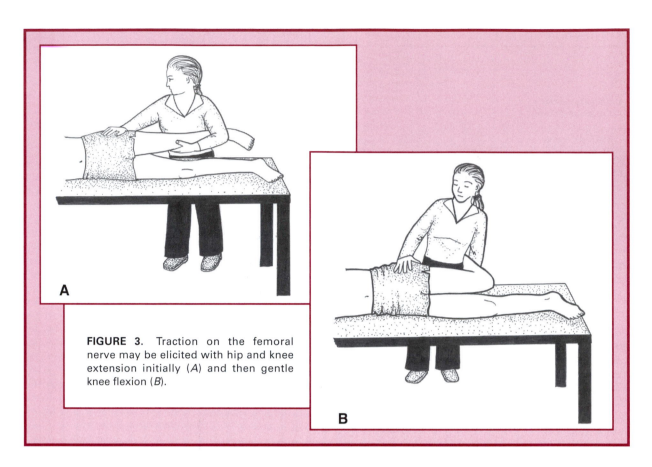

FIGURE 3. Traction on the femoral nerve may be elicited with hip and knee extension initially (*A*) and then gentle knee flexion (*B*).

In the case of femoral neuropathy, the clinician may see atrophy/asymmetry of the quadriceps muscles, and weakness of hip flexion and/or knee extension. Strength testing may be limited due to pain. Quadriceps strength should be compared with adductor strength, which typically is normal. Palpation over the inguinal ligament may reveal a fullness and/or exacerbate the patient's pain symptoms. Often there is a decreased or loss of quadriceps reflex and decreased sensation to the anterior thigh and anterior and medial leg. Palpation may be tender in the thigh and groin. Pain may be exacerbated with hip extension (Fig. 3).[1,2]

Functional Limitations

Functional limitations due to femoral neuropathy are generally a result of weakness and vary depending on the severity of the injury and the functional reserve of the patient. Individuals may have difficulty getting up from a seated position and walking without falling. Inclines and stairs often magnify the limitations. Recreational and work-related activities are often affected, such as running, climbing, jumping, etc.

Diagnostic Studies

Electrodiagnostic studies (nerve conduction studies and electromyography [EMG]) are the "gold standard" to confirm the presence of a femoral nerve injury. These should be performed no earlier than 3 to 4 weeks after the injury. Obviously, in suspected cases of hemorrhage, etc., imaging studies should be done immediately. Imaging studies may include MRI or CT scan of the pelvis in order to look for a hemorrhage or a mass causing impingement.[3,11–13]

In terms of electrodiagnostic studies, nerve conduction studies of the femoral motor component are routinely used. Routine nerve conduction studies are not available for the sensory component of the femoral nerve. Saphenous nerve sensory evaluation is available in routine study but is technically difficult and unreliable.[2] The needle EMG should evaluate muscles innervated by the femoral, obturator, tibial, and peroneal nerves. The needle evaluation therefore should include evaluation of the iliopsoas, at least two of the four quadriceps femoris muscles, one or two adductor muscles, gluteus minimus, three muscles between the knee and the ankle, and paraspinal muscles. The electromyography should be used to rule out other causes of neuropathic thigh pain, including upper and midlumbar radiculopathy, polyradiculopathy, or plexopathy. Serial EMG studies may help with evaluation of the recovery process.

Somatosensory evoked potentials may also be useful.

Differential Diagnosis

Lumbar radiculopathy	Avascular necrosis of the femoral head
Lumbar polyradiculopathy	Polymyalgia rheumatica
Lumbar plexopathy	

Treatment

Initial

Treatment of femoral neuropathy is focused on three separate areas: relief of symptoms, facilitation of nerve healing, and restoration of function. In acute cases in which hemorrhage or trauma is the etiology, surgical intervention may be the initial treatment. Likewise, this is the case when the etiology of the injury is due to a mass lesion, such as a tumor.

Acute, subacute, and chronic relief of the pain and numbness is attempted with modalities and medications. Ice may be helpful acutely, and heat may be helpful in the subacute stage. If an inflammatory component is suspected, NSAIDs/COX-2 inhibitors may help both pain and inflammation. Alternately, oral corticosteroids may be utilized. Narcotics are used when acetaminophen and NSAIDs do not control the pain. Use of anti-seizure medications such as carbamazepine and gabapentin are also of benefit for the neuropathic pain in some individuals.

Transcutaneous electrical stimulation (TENS) may also help with pain control.

Facilitation of healing varies depending on the cause of the injury to the nerve. In the case of diabetes, improved blood glucose control may help recovery. Injury due to impingement may be improved by removal of the mass. Often, little can be done to facilitate healing. Nerves that have sustained a less severe injury (neuropraxia injury) often heal over hours to weeks once the irritant is removed. Nerves that have sustained a more serious injury (neurotemesis or axonotmesis) typically have a much longer healing course due to the time required for wallerian degeneration and regeneration. It is important to educate the patient about the potential for a prolonged (sometimes more than 1 year) course of healing. Also, it is important to counsel patients that healing may not be complete and that there may be permanent loss of strength and sensation as well as continued pain symptoms.

Rehabilitation

Once the damage has been stopped or reversed, the focus turns to improving hip flexion and knee extension strength by maximizing the function of the available neuromuscular components. This is accomplished with the use of physical therapy instruction and a home exercise program. Improving strength in all lower extremity muscle groups is important. Aggressive strengthening should be limited in a nerve that is acutely injured because it may promote further injury and delay healing.

Working on proper gait mechanics is also essential. The physical therapist can help the patient with gait training and gait aides to prevent falls and improve energy utilization.

Range of motion in all lower extremity joints should be addressed.

Neuromuscular electrical stimulation may be of benefit in improving strength in some individuals.

Procedures

Procedures are not indicated for this disease process.

Surgery

In the case of femoral nerve injury due to impingement, mass lesion or hemorrhage surgery may be required to remove the pressure. In the case of a penetrating injury to the femoral nerve, surgery to align the two ends of the nerve and remove scar tissue may be required.

Potential Disease Complications

Potential complications include continued pain, numbness, and weakness despite treatment. In addition, the weakness in the hip and knee increases the risk for falls.

Potential Treatment Complications

Analgesics, NSAIDs, and COX-2 inhibitors have well-known side effects that most commonly affect the gastric, hepatic, and renal systems. Narcotics have the potential for addiction and sedation. Carbamazepine can cause sedation and aplastic anemia. The patient taking carbamazepine should be evaluated with serial complete blood counts and checking of carbamazepine level. Gabapentin can cause sedation. The potential risks of surgical intervention include bleeding, infection, and adverse reaction to the anesthetic agent.

References

1. Kimura J: Electrodiagnosis in Diseases of Nerve and Muscle: Principles and Practice, 2nd ed. Philadelphia, F.A. Davis, 1989.
2. Dumitru D: Electrodiagnostic Medicine. Philadelphia, Hanley & Belfus, 1995.
3. Moore KL: Clinically Oriented Anatomy, 2nd ed, Baltimore, Williams & Wilkins, 1985.
4. Donovan PJ, Zerhouni EA, Siegelman SS: CT of psoas compartment of the retroperitoneum. Semin Roentgenol 1981;16:241–250.
5. Simeone JF, Robinson F, Rothman SLG, et al: Computerized tomographic demonstration of retroperitoneal hematoma causing femoral neuropathy. J Neurosurg 1977;47:946–948.
6. Tysvaer AT: Computerized tomography and surgical treatment of femoral compression neuropathy. J Neurosurg 1982;57:137–139.
7. Dillavou ED, Anderson LR, Bernert RA, et al: Lower extremity iatrogenic nerve injury due to compression during intraabdominal surgery. Am J Surg 1997;173(6):504–508.
8. Kvist-Poulson H, Borel J: Iatrogenic femoral neuropathy subsequent to abdominal hysterectomy: incidence and prevention. Obstet Gynecol 1982;60:516–520.
9. Ho KM, Lim HH: Femoral nerve palsy: An unusual complication after femoral vein puncture in a patient with severe coagulopathy. Anesth Analg 1999;89(3):672.
10. Eggli S, Hankemayer S, Muller ME: Nerve palsy after leg lengthening in total replacement arthroplasty for developmental dysplasia of the hip. J Bone Joint Surg Br 1999;81-B(5):843–845.
11. Oldenburg M, Muller RT: The frequency, prognosis and significance of nerve injuries in total hip arthroplasty. Int Orthop 1997;21:1–3.
12. Gieger D, Mpinga E, Steves MA, et al: Femoral neuropathy: unusual presentation for recurrent large-bowel cancer. Dis Colon Rectum 1998;41(7):910–913.
13. Takao M, Fukuuchi Y, Koto A, et al: Localized hypertrophic mononeuropathy involving the femoral nerve. Neurology 1999;52(2):389–392.

53 Lateral Femoral Cutaneous Neuropathy

Earl J. Craig, MD

Synonyms

Meralgia paresthetica

Barnhardt-Roth syndrome

ICD-9 Codes

355.1
Meralgia paresthetica

355.8
Mononeuritis of lower limb, unspecified

355.9
Mononeuritis of unspecified site

782.0
Disturbance of skin sensation

Definition

Lateral femoral cutaneous neuropathy, commonly called meralgia paresthetica, is the focal injury of the lateral femoral cutaneous nerve causing pain and sensory loss in the lateral thigh of the affected individual.

The lateral femoral cutaneous nerve is a pure sensory nerve that receives fibers from L2–L3 (Fig. 1; see also Figure 1 in Chapter 52, Femoral Neuropathy). After forming, the nerve passes through the psoas major muscle and around the pelvic brim to the lateral edge of the inguinal ligament where it passes out of the pelvis in a tunnel created by the inguinal ligament and the anterior superior iliac spine (ASIS).[1–3] A number of anatomic variations have described the exit of the lateral femoral cutaneous nerve from the pelvis.[4] Approximately 25% of the population has an anomalous course of the lateral femoral cutaneous nerve out of the pelvis.[5] Approximately 12 cm below the ASIS, the nerve splits into anterior and posterior branches. The nerve provides cutaneous sensory innervation to the lateral thigh. The size of the area innervated varies among individuals.

The nerve may be injured as a result of a number of etiologies, as outlined in Table 1. Lateral femoral cutaneous neuropathy is more commonly seen in overweight individuals because of compression of the nerve (due to abdominal girth) when the thigh is flexed in a seated position.

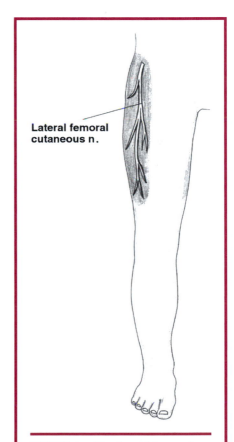

Lateral femoral
cutaneous n.

FIGURE 1. The lateral femoral cutaneous nerve is purely sensory and innervates the anterolateral thigh.

TABLE 1. Causes of Lateral Femoral Cuteneous Neuropathy

Operative and postoperative complications and scarring	Infection
	Pregnancy
	Penetrating injury
	Iliac bone graft
Retroperitoneal tumor	Pressure injury
	Tight clothing
Retroperitoneal fibrosis	Seat belt
	Obesity
Spinal tumor	Idiopathic

Symptoms

Patients typically complain of lateral thigh pain and numbness. The numbness may be described as tingling or a decrease in sensation. The pain is often burning in quality but may be sharp, dull, or aching. The patient may also complain of an itching sensation. In some instances, there will be a precipitating event such as a long car ride in which the patient was seated for a prolonged period, putting stress on the nerve. The patient should not complain of weakness in the lower extremities. The diagnosis requires a high index of suspicion by the evaluating clinician.

Physical Examination

Since the lateral femoral cutaneous nerve is purely sensory, the only finding typical of this condition is decreased sensation, which should be limited to an area of variable diameter in the lateral thigh. In adult males, the clinician may also see an area on the lateral thigh in which the hair has rubbed off. Palpation over the ASIS may exacerbate symptoms.

The physical examination is also used to exclude other possible causes of pain and weakness of the hip, thigh, and knee. The examination should include a complete neuromuscular evaluation of the low back, hips, and the entire lower extremities. This should include inspection for asymmetry or atrophy, manual muscle testing, muscle stretch reflexes, and sensory testing for light touch and pinprick. In the case of lateral femoral cutaneous neuropathy, the clinician should not see muscle atrophy/asymmetry or weakness of lower extremities. Reflexes should remain intact.

Functional Limitations

Typically, there are no functional limitations because this injury is more an annoyance than truly disabling. No true weakness is seen, although prolonged standing and extension at the hip may exacerbate the pain and thus limit the patient in performing tasks, such as standing and walking. The nerve may be further compressed and the symptoms exacerbated when the patient is seated, so long car or plane rides may be difficult. Similarly, individuals who are sedentary at work may experience painful symptoms that limit their ability to function.

Diagnostic Studies

History and physical examination are the most important diagnostic tools, and all other testing should be used as an extension of these. Electromyography is the primary diagnostic tool and should include lateral femoral cutaneous sensory nerve conduction studies and needle EMG of the lower extremity.[2,3] Although routine lateral femoral cutaneous nerve conduction studies have standard normal values with which an individual's study can be compared, it is generally recommended to do comparison studies on the unaffected side, as the studies are technically difficult.[3,6–8] The needle EMG is done to rule out other pathology and should be normal. Serial EMG studies may help with evaluation of the recovery process.

Somatosensory evoked potentials may also be used, but a recent study reports that sensory conduction studies are a more reliable method of evaluation of the lateral femoral cutaneous nerve.[9] Once the diagnosis is made, MRI or CT scan of the pelvis may be required to look for a mass causing impingement.

Differential Diagnosis

Lumbar radiculopathy

Lumbar polyradiculopathy

Lumbar plexopathy

Femoral neuropathy

Treatment

Initial

Treatment of lateral femoral cutaneous neuropathy is focused on symptom relief and facilitation of nerve healing.

Both early and late symptomatic relief of the pain and numbness is attempted with modalities and medications. Both heat and ice can be used. If an inflammatory component is suspected, NSAIDs/COX-2 inhibitors or corticosteroids may be used. Narcotics are used when acetaminophen and anti-inflammatory medications do not control the pain. Use of anti-seizure medications, such as carbamazepine and gabapentin, are also of benefit in some individuals.

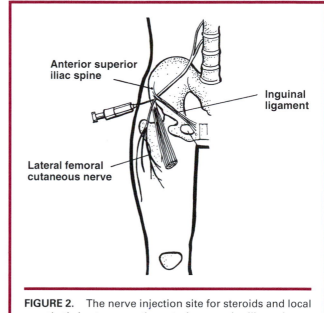

FIGURE 2. The nerve injection site for steroids and local anesthetic is at or near the anterior superior iliac spine.

Facilitation of healing varies depending on the cause of the injury to the nerve. For most individuals this entails removing the cause of the pressure over the anterior iliac region. The pressure may be caused by tight clothing, belts, seat belts, or excess weight. Elimination of the pressure may include weight loss or clothing adjustment. Nerves that have sustained a less serious (neuropraxic) injury often heal over hours to weeks once the irritant is removed. Nerves that have sustained a more severe injury (neurotemesis or axonotemesis) typically have a much longer healing course due to the time required for wallerian degeneration and regeneration. The use of anti-inflammatory medications may also be of benefit in the healing process.

Rehabilitation

Physical therapy may facilitate healing the injured nerve. Gentle stretching of the anterior thigh and groin is indicated. Hot packs and/or ultrasound is often helpful in facilitating the stretching process. Ice may be helpful when the patient continues to have swelling and inflammation around the pelvic brim. In some individuals a general conditioning program to help with weight loss may also be useful. A dietician can assist the patient with weight loss. A skilled therapist may be able to use soft tissue mobilization to help free an impinged and inflamed nerve. Augmented soft tissue mobilization is one of several techniques that may be useful. Electrical stimulation and transcutaneous nerve stimulation (TENS) may be helpful in reducing the perception of pain by the patient during therapy treatments. TENS can be used on a daily basis for pain control.

Procedures

When conservative treatment fails, injection of the nerve at or near the ASIS with steroids and local anesthetic may be helpful (Fig. 2). If the steroid injection is helpful but short lasting, the nerve can be injected with phenol or other neurotoxic agents as a last resort.

Under sterile conditions, the pelvis is palpated and the ASIS and inguinal ligament are identified. A 25-gauge, 2-inch needle is placed perpendicular to the skin approximately 1 inch medial to the ASIS and inferior to the inguinal ligament. The needle is advanced into the soft tissue approximately 1 inch (this may vary depending on the patient's size and amount of excess subcutaneous tissue). At times, paresthesias may be elicited, thereby verifying needle placement; however, it is important to not inject directly into the nerve. Once the area to be injected is located, inject a 5- to 10-cc solution of local anesthetic and steroid (e.g., 2 cc of methylprednisolone, 40 mg/cc, mixed with 5 cc of 1% lidocaine).

Post-injection care may include icing the injected area for 10 to 15 minutes and counseling the patient to avoid pressure on the nerve.

Surgery

In the case of lateral femoral cutaneous nerve injury due to impingement, surgery may be required to remove the pressure. Surgical removal of neuroma or neurectomy proximal to the neuroma may also be helpful if a neuroma is found. Less than half of patients treated with surgery have significant benefit.[3]

Potential Disease Complications

Potential complications include continued pain and numbness despite treatment.

Potential Treatment Complications

Complications of treatment are well recognized. Each medication has potential adverse side effects. NSAIDs have the potential of gastric bleeding, decreased renal blood flow, and decreased platelet function. COX-2 inhibitors may have fewer gastric side effects. Narcotics have the potential for addiction and sedation. Carbamazepine can cause sedation and aplastic anemia. The patient taking carbamazepine should be evaluated with serial complete blood counts. Gabapentin can cause sedation. The injection of the nerve also has potential risks, which include bleeding, infection, and worsening of the pain. The potential risks of surgical intervention include bleeding, infection, and adverse reaction to the anesthetic agent.

References
1. Moore KL: Clinically Oriented Anatomy, 2nd ed. Baltimore, Williams & Wilkins, 1985.
2. Kimura J: Electrodiagnosis in Diseases of Nerve and Muscle: Principles and Practice, 2nd ed. Philadelphia, F.A. Davis, 1989.
3. Dumitru D: Electrodiagnostic Medicine. Philadelphia, Hanley & Belfus, 1995.
4. Williams PH, Trzil KP: Management of meralgia paresthetica. J Neurosurg 1991;74:76–80.
5. de Ridder VA, de Lange S, Popta JV: Anatomic variations of the lateral femoral cutaneous nerve and the consequences for surgery. J Orthop Trauma 1999;13(3):207–211.
6. Bulter ET, Johnson EW, Kaye ZA: Normal conduction velocity in the lateral femoral cutaneous nerve. Arch Phys Med Rehabil 1974;55:31–32.
7. Lagueny A, Deliac MM, Deliac P, et al: Diagnostic and prognostic value of electrophysiologic tests in meralgia paresthetica. Muscle Nerve 1991;14:51–56.
8. Sarala PK, Nishihara T, Oh SJ: Meralgia paresthetica: Electrophysiologic study. Arch Phys Med Rehabil 1979;60–30–31.
9. Seror P: Lateral femoral cutaneous nerve conduction V somatosensory evoked potentials for electrodiagnosis of meralgia paresthetica. Am J Phys Med Rehabil 1999;78(4):313–316.

54 Piriformis Syndrome

Thomas H. Hudgins, MD
Joseph T. Alleva, MD

Synonyms

Hip pocket neuropathy

Wallet neuritis

Sciatica

ICD-9 Code

355.0
Lesion of sciatic nerve

Definition

Piriformis syndrome describes a clinical situation whereby the piriformis muscle is compressing the sciatic nerve, resulting in a sciatic neuropathy. Although the anatomic relationship of these two structures is well documented, this remains a controversial diagnosis. There is no consensus among clinicians on the validity of this and therefore no documentation of the incidence.[1]

The piriformis muscle and sciatic nerve both exit the pelvis through the greater sciatic notch. Numerous anatomic variations of this relationship have been well documented (Fig. 1). Cadaver studies have described the sciatic nerve passing below the piriformis muscle, through the muscle belly, a divided nerve above and through the muscle, and a divided nerve through and below the muscle.[2,3] More recently, a case report of piriformis syndrome described a fifth variation, with an undivided nerve passing above an undivided piriformis muscle.[4] Yeoman was the first to describe the relationship of these two structures in 1928,[5] and Robinson first coined the term piriformis syndrome in 1947.[6]

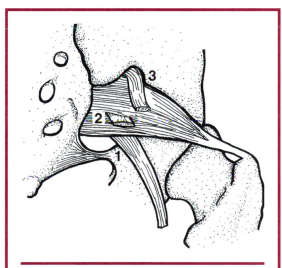

FIGURE 1. Three variations in the course of the sciatic nerve as related to the piriformis muscle.

Symptoms

The patient with piriformis syndrome will complain of buttock pain with or without radiation into the leg. This may be seen in chronic and acute situations. Often, a history of minor trauma may be described, such as falling onto the buttock. Sitting on hard surfaces will exacerbate the

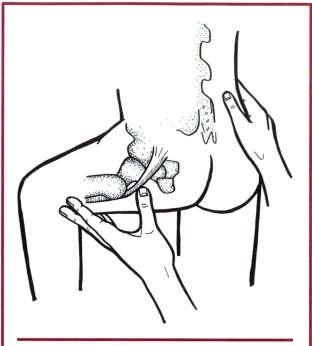

FIGURE 2. The sciatic nerve may be barely palpable at the midpoint between the ischial tuberosity and the greater trochanter. The hip must be flexed to palpate the nerve.

symptoms of pain and occasional numbness and paresthesias without weakness. Activities that produce a motion of hip adduction and internal rotation, such as cross-country skiing and the overhead serve in tennis, may also exacerbate the symptoms.[7,8] Due to the relationship of the piriformis muscle with the lateral pelvis wall, patients may also experience pain with bowel movements and women may complain of dyspareunia.[9]

Physical Examination

The exam will reveal a non-focal neurologic examination with normal sensation, symmetric strength and reflexes. Tenderness to palpation is experienced from the sacrum to the greater trochanter, representing the area of the piriformis muscle. The sciatic nerve is most superficial with the knee flexed (Fig. 2).[10] A palpable taut band is tender with both rectal and pelvic examination because the piriformis muscle sits in the deep pelvic floor.[8] Passive hip abduction and internal rotation may compress the sciatic nerve, reproducing pain (a positive Freiberg's sign). Contraction of the piriformis with resistance to active hip external rotation and abduction may also reproduce pain or asymmetric weakness (a positive Pace's sign).[11] A positive straight leg test may also be appreciated.[12]

Functional Limitations

The patient with piriformis syndrome will experience pain with prolonged sitting and with activities that produce hip internal rotation and adduction. This may include cross-country skiing and one-legged motions such as the overhead serve in tennis or the kicking motion in soccer. Women may have pain with sexual intercourse.

Diagnostic Studies

Piriformis syndrome is a clinical diagnosis. MRI and CT scan are primarily reserved to rule out other disorders associated with sciatic neuropathy, such as a herniated nucleus pulposus. A few case reports have demonstrated hypertrophy of the piriformis muscle on both CT scan and MRI.[13] Electrodiagnostic testing may reveal a prolonged H reflex in symptomatic cases[14] and is helpful in differentiating piriformis syndrome from a lumbosacral radiculopathy.

Differential Diagnosis

Superior and inferior gluteal artery aneurysm
Benign pelvic tumor
Lumbar facet syndrome

L5/S1 radiculopathy
Endometriosis

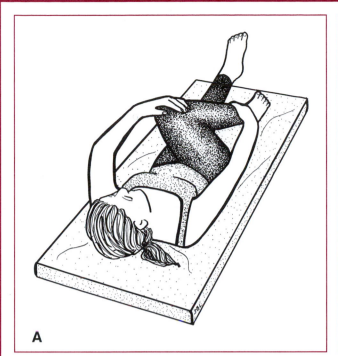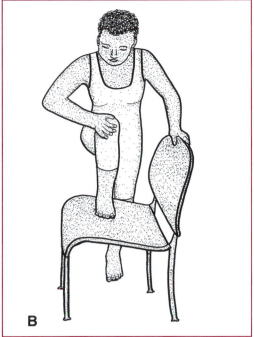

FIGURES 3. Stretching exercises—prolonged stretching of right piriformis muscle by flexion, adduction, and internal rotation of right hip in supine (*A*) and standing (*B*) positions. Patients are instructed to begin holding the stretch for 5 seconds and gradually increase to a 30-second stretch.

Treatment

Initial

NSAIDs/COX-2 inhibitors decrease pain and inflammation. Analgesic medications may also be used for pain. Muscle relaxants and local heat can help to decrease spasm.[8] Low-dose tricyclic antidepressant medications (e.g., 10 to 25mg qhs of nortriptyline) may be used to help with pain and sleep at night. If neuropathic symptoms are prominent, a trial of anti-convulsant medications can be considered (e.g., gabapentin). Avoidance of exacerbating activities and use of soft cushions for prolonged sitting are also advocated initially. TENS units are sometimes helpful for pain as well.

Rehabilitation

Physical therapy can be initiated to decrease pain with modalities (e.g., ultrasound, phonophoresis) and improve flexibility and strength. The use of deep heat therapy such as ultrasound is followed by a gentle stretch of the piriformis muscle. Gentle massage may decrease muscle spasm, but caution should be used not to exacerbate symptoms.

Exercises should focus on improving back and hip flexibility and strength. The piriformis is stretched with hip internal rotation in greater than 90-degree hip flexion (Fig. 3), and with external rotation in less than 90 degrees of hip flexion.[15] Strengthening the hip abductors, in particular the gluteus medius, should be emphasized.

Correction of biomechanical imbalances that may predispose the individual to piriformis syndrome should also be initiated; these include leg-length inequality, increased foot pronation, and hamstring tightness.[7,8]

Procedures

Recalcitrant cases may require a peri-sciatic injection of corticosteroid.[12] Trigger point injections (TPIs) may be used for local muscle spasm.

Surgery

Rarely, surgical release of the piriformis muscle is performed to relieve the compression.[10] Piriformis syndrome carries a favorable prognosis, as the vast majority of patients will respond to a non-operative approach.[7]

Potential Disease Complications

This is a clinical diagnosis that is often overlooked. The primary complication is chronic sciatica.

Potential Treatment Complications

Bleeding and gastrointestinal and renal side effects of NSAIDs are well documented. COX-2 inhibitors may have fewer gastric side effects. Complications of local corticosteroid injections include infection, hematoma/bleeding, and soft tissue atrophy at the site. Care must be taken with surgical techniques to avoid inadvertent injury to the nerves in the buttock. The functional loss resulting from sectioning the piriformis muscle is inconsequential as the other hip abductors may compensate for this movement.[10,16]

References
1. Silver JK, Leadbetter WB: Piriformis syndrome: Assessment of current practice and literature review. Orthopedics 1998;21:1133–1135.
2. Pecina M. Contribution to the etiological explanation of the piriformis syndrome. Acta Anatomica 1979;105:181–187.
3. Beaton LE, Anson BJ. Sciatic nerve and the piriformis muscle: their interrelation as a possible cause of coccydynia. J Bone Joint Surg 1938;20:686–688.
4. Ozaki S, Hamabe T, Muro T: Piriformis syndrome resulting from an anomalous relationship between the sciatic nerve and piriformis muscle. Orthopedics 1999;22:771–772.
5. Yeoman W: The relation of arthritis of the sacroiliac joint to sciatica. Lancet 1978;2:1119–1122.
6. Robinson D: Piriformis syndrome in relation to sciatic pain. Am J Surg 1947;73:355–358.
7. Douglas S. Sciatic pain and piriformis syndrome. Nurse Pract 1997;22:166–180.
8 Parziale JR, Hudgins TH, Fishman LM: The piriformis syndrome. Am J Orthop 1996;12:819–823.
9 Barton PM. Piriformis syndrome: A rational approach to management. Pain 1991;47:345-352.
10. McCrory P, Bell S: Nerve entrapment syndromes as a cause of pain in the hip, groin and buttock. Sports Med 1999;27:261–274.
11. Yuen EC, So YT. Sciatic neuropathy. Neurol Clin 1999;17:617–631.
12. Hanania M, Kitain E: Perisciatic injection of steroid for the treatment of sciatica due to piriformis syndrome. Reg Anesth Pain Med 1998;23:223–228.
13. Jankiewicz JJ, Hennrikus WL, Hookum JA: The appearance of the piriformis muscle syndrome in computed tomography and magnetic resonance imaging. A case report and review of the literature. Clin Orthop 1991;262:205–209.
14. Fishman LM: Electrophysiologic evidence of piriformis syndrome. Arch Phys Med and Rehabil 1992;73:359–364.
15. Greenman PE (ed): Principles of Manual Medicine, 2nd ed. pp 474–475.
16. Vandertop WP, Bosma NJ: The piriformis syndrome. J Bone Joint Surg 1991;73:1095–1096.

55 Quadriceps Contusion

J. Michael Wieting, DO
Ryan C. O'Connor, DO

Synonyms

Traumatic quadriceps strain

ICD-9 Codes

924.00
Contusion of lower limb (thigh)

924.9
Contusion of lower limb (unspecified site)

Definition

An injury resulting from direct trauma to the anterior thigh by a blunt force, such as a football helmet, shoulder pad, elbow, or knee. It is commonly encountered in contact sports, such as football, rugby, and wrestling. Direct trauma to the anterior thigh results in acute damage to muscle tissue, causing hemorrhage and subsequent inflammation. Quadriceps contusions are often graded on a 3–point scale, with a grade 1 injury being mild and a grade 3 injury being severe. At 24 hours after injury, a grade 1 has over 90 degrees preserved knee range of motion, grade 2 has 45–90 degrees range of motion, and grade 3 has less than 45 degrees.[4]

Symptoms

Pain, swelling, and decreased range of motion of the knee, particularly knee flexion, are often seen. Loss of knee range of motion can be the result of muscle and articular edema as well as physiologic inhibition of the quadriceps muscle group and "splinting." Following injury, the quadriceps muscle group will often become stiff and the athlete may have difficulty bearing weight on the affected extremity, resulting in an antalgic (painful) gait. A grade 1 injury describes a mild injury with minimal pain and edema, whereas a grade 3 injury results in significant pain and edema along with hematoma formation and a substantial loss of knee range of motion.

Physical Examination

Visual inspection of quadriceps contusion will show a variable amount of swelling and discoloration present over the anterior thigh due to hematoma formation and intramuscular bleeding. If the contusion is in the distal third of the quadriceps, discoloration and swelling will often track into the knee region due to gravity. Pain of varying intensity will be present upon palpation of the quadriceps muscle group. A firm palpable mass may be noted in the anterior thigh (usually due to hematoma formation); if the hematoma formation is large, an effusion may also be present. The patient will exhibit decreased knee flexion, especially past 90 degrees; knee extension will be less painful than flexion.[6] Check for the presence of distal pulses and capillary refill, and assess range of motion of adjacent joints to be sure that the injury is localized to the anterior thigh. Bony incongruity and tenderness may indicate fracture of the femur, patella, or tibial plateau. Muscle stretch reflexes of the patellar tendon may be inhibited, and serial measurements of thigh circumferences should be made over a 24- to 72-hour period to assess for possible compartment syndrome. Sensory testing should include the saphenous nerve distribution of the distal leg.

Functional Limitations

Initially, gait will be antalgic and weight bearing difficult on the involved extremity. Over a period of days to weeks, running and "kicking" activities will be limited secondary to knee stiffness and pain associated with terminal knee flexion and extension.

Diagnostic Studies

Plain x-rays should initially be obtained in moderate to severe quadriceps contusions to rule out a co-existing fracture. Nuclear bone scan may be ordered in days to weeks following injury to assess for the development of myositis ossificans traumatica, heterotopic bone formation that may develop in up to 20% of injuries. Bone scans are more sensitive for detecting heterotopic bone formation than plain films and can be useful in monitoring its resolution. If compartment syndrome is suspected (see Chapter 64), intracompartmental pressures must be measured.

Differential Diagnosis

Quadriceps tear/strain

Compartment syndrome

Fracture of femur/patella/tibial plateau

Treatment

Initial

Immediately, the patient should cease activity. The knee should be gently elevated and flexed, and ice should be applied to the anterior thigh (for 20 minutes at a time intermittently). An ACE or similar bandage should be placed around the injured leg and thigh and gentle compression applied to decrease hemorrhage formation. Needle aspiration of a formed hematoma may be indicated to relieve pressure and pain.[1] A thigh pad should be worn when ice is not being applied. If the injury is mild, icing should be repeated for 2 to 3 days, and the patient should ambulate with crutches, either non–weight-bearing or partial weight-bearing. If the injury is severe, bed rest may be needed. Massage should be avoided 1 to 2 weeks after injury to lessen the chance of additional hemorrhage. Whirlpool, heat, and ultrasound modalities should be initially avoided for the same reason. If edema persists or becomes severe, surgical referral should be considered to evaluate the possibility of compartment syndrome or ongoing hemorrhage. Nonsteroidal anti-inflammatory drugs (NSAIDs), including cyclooxygenase-2 (COX-2) inhibitors, should be avoided the first 24 hours of injury, because of the hematoma formation. Analgesics may be used for pain without risk of exacerbating hematoma formation.

Rehabilitation

After 48 hours post-injury and for the next 2 to 5 days, range of motion should be tested with the patient in the prone position, and knee flexion exercises should be performed in the "pain-free range" with associated hip flexion. This can be followed with active assisted range of motion exercises. It is important to avoid forced stretching because this may aggravate the injury and slow healing. Static quadriceps exercises can be instituted. Proprioceptive neuromuscular facilitation (PNF) exercises using reciprocal inhibition of the quadriceps and hamstrings can be done as well.[2] Partial weight bearing should be maintained to 90 degrees of knee flexion. Pulsed ultrasound or high velocity galvanic stimulation can be added to the treatment regimen, using continuous 80 to 120 pulses per second at the patient's level of sensory perception for 20- to 25-minute periods. Interferential electrical stimulation can also be used for further edema control.

The next step in treatment should involve active knee range of motion, progressive resistive exercises, and cycling. Pain-free knee range of motion within 10 degrees of the unaffected extremity should be the goal before considering return to activity. Jumping, sprinting and cutting activities should be incorporated into the rehabilitation program at which point functional testing to assess safe return to activity can be done. A thigh wrap, padding, or protective sleeve can be worn following return to play in the case of athletes. Time for return to activity is variable and depends on severity of injury, with full recovery expected in severe contusions by 5 to 8 weeks.[5]

Procedures

Occasionally, needle aspiration of a formed hematoma is performed to alleviate pressure and pain.[1]

Surgery

Surgery is rarely indicated with these injuries, except when associated with a concomitant compartment syndrome.

Potential Disease Complications

If the quadriceps region becomes extremely warm with marked increased edema and the patient complains of paresthesias with an abnormal neurovascular examination and significant quadriceps weakness, consideration must be given to the development of a potential compartment syndrome.

Myositis ossificans traumatica (MOT) usually stabilizes and resorbs spontaneously by 6 months postinjury with conservative care.[7] Plain films may show ectopic bone formation 2 to 4 weeks postinjury, with the most common location being in the midshaft of the femur. Serial bone scans can be performed to monitor resolution of ectopic bone in a symptomatic athlete. Surgical removal of ectopic bone formation is rarely indicated and should not be performed for at least 12 months following injury to allow for adequate maturation; this is to prevent enlargement of ectopic bone and recurrence.

Potential Treatment Complications

Analgesics, NSAIDs, and COX-2 inhibitors have well-known side effects that most commonly affect the gastric, hepatic, and renal systems. Vigorous soft tissue massage and passive stretch should be avoided in the acute period postinjury to prevent further bleeding and hematoma formation (this occurs frequently in a field setting following hamstring injury).

References
1. Delee JC, Drez D: Quadriceps contusion. In Orthopedic Sports Medicine. Philadelphia, W.B. Saunders, 1994.
2. Geraci MC: Rehabilitation of the hip, pelvis, and thigh. In Functional Rehabilitation of Sports and Musculoskeletal Injuries. Gaithersburg, MD, Aspen. 1998.
3. O'Donoghue DH: Treatment of Injuries to Athletes. Philadelphia, W.B. Saunders, 1989.
4. Reid DC. Sports Injury Assessment and Rehabilitation. New York, Churchill Livingstone, 1992.
5. Rothwell, AG: Quadriceps hematoma: A prospective clinical study. Clin Orthop 1982;171:97–103.
6. Ryan JB, Wheeler JH: Quadriceps Contusion. Am J Sports Med 1991;19:299–304.
7. Young JL, Lankowski ER: Thigh injuries in athletes. Mayo Clin Proc 1993;19:299–304.

56 Total Hip Replacement

Robert S. Skerker, MD
Gregory J. Mulford, MD

Synonyms

Total hip replacement
Bipolar hemiarthroplasty
Unipolar hemiarthroplasty
Revision arthroplasty
Austin-Moore endoprosthesis

ICD-9 Codes

715.95
Osteoarthritis hip

733.42
Aseptic necrosis of bone, head and neck of femur

820.09
Fracture of neck of femur, other (head of femur, subcapital)

820.8
Fracture of neck of femur, unspecified part of neck femur, closed

835.00
Dislocation of hip

996.59
Loosening of total hip replacement

V43.64
Total hip replacement

Definition

Arthroplasty involves the reconstruction of a diseased, damaged, or ankylosed joint by natural modification or artificial materials. The most common etiologies of adult hip disease that may require arthroplasy include osteoarthritis, rheumatoid arthritis, avascular necrosis, post-traumatic degenerative joint disease, congenital hip disease, and infectious diseases within the joint or adjacent bone.

The modern era of hip joint replacement began in the late 1960s when Sir John Charnley combined a stainless steel femoral component with a polyethylene socket fixed to the adjacent bone with polymethylmethacrylate (PMMA). Since that time, arthroplasty of the hip joint has become an accepted and standard treatment for common adult hip joint pathology. Modern arthroplasty surgery has resulted in the restoration of pain free motion and improved quality of life for millions of people. Joint arthroplasty has become the most common elective surgical procedure performed in the United States. It is estimated that approximately 150,000 primary total hip arthroplasties (THAs) are performed annually. If one includes partial hip replacements and revision arthroplasty along with unclassified hip arthroplasties, then the figure increases to 289,000 hip surgeries per year in the United States. In recent times, there has been a slow but general increase in yearly hip arthroplasty procedures of about 10,000 per year.

The primary indications for THA include progressive pain and dysfunction and/or a decline in mobility, self-care, and daily living activities despite conservative treatment. Relative contraindications include active or recent joint infection, neurotrophic joints, inability of the patient to cooperate in the immediate postoperative period or with the rehabilitation program following joint implantation, serious co-morbid medical conditions that result in a higher surgical risk or compromised postoperative medical status, rapidly progressive or terminal cancer with shortened survival and/or severe debility, and severe nutritional depletion that jeopardizes postoperative wound healing.

A survey of orthopedic surgeons' opinions regarding indications for THA found ". . . no clear consensus among surgeons." Most surgeons believed THA is necessary if the following symptoms are present: severe pain on a daily basis, rest pain several days per week, and destruction of most of the joint space on a radiograph. Younger age, co-morbidity, technical difficulties, and lack of motivation were factors in the decision against surgery, whereas the desire to return to work and an independent lifestyle swayed the decision for surgery.[1]

Symptoms

The primary symptom of hip pathology is groin pain and, occasionally, pain that radiates to the knee (see Chapter 51). Lateral proximal thigh pain in the region of the greater trochanter is usually not an indicator of hip joint pathology. Pain in this location typically reflects local muscle or bursal inflammation or pathology referred from the pelvis or lumbosacral spine.

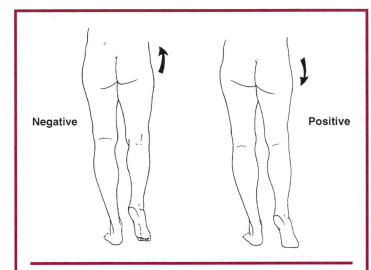

FIGURE 1. Trendelenburg's sign. (From Goldstein B, Chavez F: Applied anatomy of the lower extremities. Phys Med Rehabil State Art Review 10:601–630, 1996, with permission.)

The primary sign of hip pathology is a gait disturbance such as a limp. Patients may complain of difficulty with walking due to pain, limping, or both. Numbness and paresthesias should be absent but if present, suggest an alternative diagnosis (e.g., lumbar radiculopathy).

Physical Examination

Candidates for THA will likely have antalgic (painful) gait patterns that represent a combination of pain that inhibits motion, structural loss of joint motion, and weakness (see also Chapter 51). Hip pain or weakness of the hip abductors results in contralateral pelvic tilt or drop (Trendelenburg sign) with ipsilateral weight bearing (Fig. 1). Passive hip range of motion usually demonstrates significant loss of rotation and moderate loss of abduction and flexion of the involved hip. End ranges of motion are often painful. The manual muscle examination demonstrates mild to moderate weakness of hip flexion, abduction, and extension. The patient may have difficulty with arising from a low seat, crossing the affected leg, and reaching his or her affected foot. A hip flexion contracture may be observed by performing the Thomas test, and accentuated lumbar lordosis may be seen in those with a hip flexion contracture. Neurologic examination is typically normal, except for hip girdle weakness due to guarding or disuse.

Patients who have undergone a THA should be examined for possible complications including deep vein thrombosis (leg swelling and calf tenderness [see Chapter 104]) or infection (fever, wound that appears infected). A hip dislocation should be suspected if the limb is shortened or externally rotated or if gentle hip motion cannot be tolerated because of excessive pain.

Functional Limitations

Functional limitations from severe hip pathology include difficulty with walking and all mobility, even rising from a seated position, due to pain and weakness. This may affect a patient's ability to dress, bathe, perform household chores, participate in recreational activities, and work outside the home.

After returning to the community postoperatively, most patients should be able to ambulate community distances, initially with a walker or a cane, and then advance to ambulating without an assistive device or return to their presurgical baseline within 4 to 12 weeks. The rate of advancement in gait training is usually limited by the weight-bearing status established at the time of surgery. Most people are able to return to activities such as dancing, low impact sports, and presurgical exercise regimens within 12 weeks.[2] Elderly, less active patients should also be able to return to their baseline level of function and in many instances progress to higher levels of activity that had been limited by pain prior to surgery.[3,4] Activities such as cycling, golfing, and bowling after THA should be encouraged, whereas running, jogging, water-skiing, cross-country skiing, football, baseball, handball, hockey, karate, soccer, and racquetball sports (activities that result in high stress or torque through the femur) should be minimized or avoided.[5]

Diagnostic Studies

Plain radiographs remain the primary imaging tool for evaluating the person with hip disease and typically show significant loss of joint cartilage as demonstrated by joint space narrowing, joint incongruity, osteophyte formation, subchondral cysts, and sclerosis. In patients suspected of having a dislocation following THA, radiographs should be obtained urgently since a true dislocation must be relocated expediently (Fig. 2). Plain x-rays are also obtained in patients suspected of having prosthetic loosening (Fig. 3).

Occasionally, a bone scan may be needed to rule out an occult femoral neck fracture, infection, or other bone disorder. Magnetic resonance imaging is often useful when assessing for avascular necrosis (AVN) as the etiology of hip pain.[5] Limb swelling in individuals who have undergone THA should trigger deep vein thrombosis (DVT) surveillance screening with venous imaging ultrasound and Doppler wave signal analysis (commonly referred to as Duplex scanning). Minor calf clots are followed by a repeat study within 7 days to assess for propagation.

Laboratory studies should be performed to monitor for anemia. Wound cultures are performed in patients suspected of having a postoperative infection.

Differential Diagnosis

Prosthetic loosening   Periprosthetic fracture

Infection   Component failure

Treatment

Initial

On the day of surgery, the patient often receives perioperative prophylactic antibiotics; autologous blood transfusions for blood loss–induced anemia; and pain control with narcotics delivered orally, intravenously, or via a patient controlled analgesia (PCA) pump. Within 24 hours postoperatively, a regimen is often initiated to prevent deep venous thrombosis (usually warfarin or a low molecular weight heparin product, such as enoxaparin), and antithrombic calf pumps. If the patient's condition is stable, the patient is ready for discharge from the acute care hospital by the third or fourth postoperative day.[6] By that time, surgical drains have been removed, all perioperative antibiotics have ceased, transfusion therapy has concluded, and the

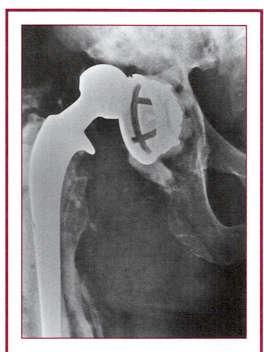

FIGURE 2.   Total hip replacement—dislocation. The femur has dislocated superiorly and laterally relative to the acetabulum. This dislocation is due to abnormal (vertical) position of the acetabular cup which occurred as a result of loosening (see widened cement–bone interface). (From Katz S, et al: Radiology Secrets. Philadelphia, Hanley & Belfus, 1998, p 317, with permission.)

PCA pump has been discontinued in favor of oral analgesic medications. Outpatient, inpatient, or home rehabilitation typically ensues. Adequate pain management must be continuously re-evaluated as the patient progresses through postoperative rehabilitation and recovery. Long-acting oral narcotics (such as oxycodone) combined with rescue doses of immediate release narcotics taken 30 to 60 minutes before a therapy session work well initially. Thereafter, non-narcotic analgesics and NSAIDs/COX-2 inhibitors can be used for pain control if necessary.

Anemia is an important issue to address in the intial treatment period because patients with adequate hemoglobin levels generally progress in rehabilitation more readily than those with low hemoglobin levels. Adequate nutrition; iron supplements; vitamins; and, if needed, erythropoietin can be utilized. Blood transfusions may be necessary if the hemoglobin level continues to drift downward and there is concern of hemodynamic instability or if the patient becomes symptomatic with light-headedness.

It is also important to monitor for deep vein thrombosis. A DVT can occur at the time of surgery or anytime within the first 6 weeks after surgery. The incidence of DVT after total hip implantation without prophylactic anticoagulation is 40% to 70%; the incidence of proximal clot (defined as any thrombosis in the popliteal vein or more proximal) is between 10% to 20%; and the incidence of fatal pulmonary embolism (PE) is between 0.5% and 5%.[7–10] Prophylaxis with warfarin (keeping the INR between 2 and 3) is ideal. However, many orthopedic surgeons are concerned about bleeding complications and prefer an INR of 1.8 to 2. Another accepted prophylactic agent is enoxaparin at a dose of 30 mg subcutaneously every 12 hours.[11,12] Propagating calf clots may be treated with full anticoagulation for 6 weeks to 3 months. Major proximal DVTs are definitively treated with full anticoagulation for 3 to 6 months.

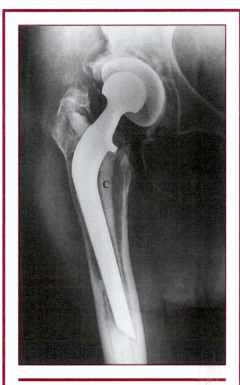

FIGURE 3. Total hip replacement—loose femoral component. There is a wide area of lucency between the opaque cement (*C*) and the adjacent bone at the medial aspect of the proximal femur, in addition to the area of lucency at the metal–bone interface surrounding the acetabular prosthesis. These were new findings, indicative of loosening of both components. (From Katz S, et al: Radiology Secrets. Philadelphia, Hanley & Belfus, 1998, p 317, with permission.)

In the absence of DVT, edema is common after hip arthroplasty due to a combination of disruption of local lymphatic drainage around the hip, dissection of blood and fluids through tissue planes, and loss of the local muscle pump due to pain inhibition. Elevation and compression are the mainstays of treatment. More severe swelling may require transient diuretic therapy and more aggressive compression wraps.

Wound care of the incision line is accomplished with dry sterile dressing changes once or twice per day. Once wound drainage ceases, a dressing is no longer essential. Painting the incision with povidone-iodine (Betadine) provides a drying effect and reduces cutaneous bacterial flora; a non-stick petroleum gauze is then applied, followed by a dry gauze dressing. Tape burns around the surgical incision are a common problem and are treated with a hydrogel pad, such as DuoDerm, for approximately 1 week. Serous drainage without signs of erythema or induration is usually common for 3 to 4 days postoperatively, but persistent drainage necessitates oral prophylactic antibiotics to prevent secondary infection. Surgical clips are routinely removed after 12 to 14 days, at which point the wound is reinforced with steristrips. If the incision develops erythema around the staples, then they are removed sooner. More serious wound problems may require additional management, including cultures, antibiotics, and more invasive intervention if necessary.

Rehabilitation

Hip precautions should be followed and are taught to patients to minimize the possibility of hip dislocation. Patients with weak periarticular tissues, revision surgeries, or previous dislocations are at the highest risk for a dislocation, which is greatest during the first postoperative week. Most surgeons use a posterolateral approach to the hip joint and dislocate the joint by hyperflexion, adduction, and internal rotation. After hip replacement, that combination of movements may increase the risk of redislocation. Therefore, an abduction pillow or wedge is placed between the legs to maintain safe alignment. Patients are taught not to flex at the hip to reach forward. Adaptive equipment such as sock aides, reachers, and dressing sticks are used to perform lower body self-care. Similarly, high toilet seats and tub benches for bathing serve to prevent hip flexion beyond 90 degrees.

Many patients perceive a limb-length discrepancy after THA, and it is important to initially rule out hip dislocation. If a hip dislocation does occur, it often results in a significant functional setback because the patient is often more cautious and fearful of activity. If an abduction hip brace is ordered to prevent recurrent dislocation, this must be worn at all times and results in severe restrictions of motion, bathroom tasks, and mobility. There is little information in the literature to guide the duration of time for maintenance of hip precautions. It is probably wise to enforce strict precautions for at least 6 weeks.

If there is a true leg-length discrepancy—(three fourths of an inch or more)—severe cases are treated with temporary lifts, but in most situations the underlying problem can be identified and ameliorated with ongoing therapy.[13] Some cases are a consequence of an apparent inequality due to pelvic obliquity from muscle imbalances or hip contractures (such as adductor tightness).

A typical total hip replacement clinical pathway/protocol for inpatient rehabilitation is a 9- to 10-day program.[14] Most patients successfully complete this pathway, provided there are no major medical complications (Table 1).[15–18]

Therapeutic exercises to improve hip and knee mobility and strength begin on the first day of the rehabilitation program and continue daily thereafter. By the third postoperative day, the patient should be able to tolerate 2 to 3 hours of therapy a day unless severe anemia or other medical problems result in further functional limitations. Active assisted range-of-motion and strengthening exercises are progressed as tolerated. Strengthening of hip abductors is important, but caution should be taken to avoid overly aggressive abductor strengthening if a trochanteric osteotomy was performed. Ankle pumps, heel slides, quad sets, gluteal squeezes, and straight-leg raises are initiated.

Early protected ambulation is promoted as tolerated by the patient. Weight-bearing aides (e.g., crutches, arm rests) should be used during sit-to-stand maneuvers and stairclimbing in the early postoperative period to minimize these potentially negative forces. Mobility training progresses daily and is advanced as tolerated based on individual response and weight-bearing restrictions.

Out-of-plane loads created during straight-leg raising and stairclimbing generate rotational torque on the femoral stem and may promote femoral loosening.

TABLE 1. Goals of Rehabilitation After Total Hip Arthroplasty

Achieve successful postoperative pain management

Maintain medical stability

Achieve successful surgical incision healing

Guard against dislocation of the implant

Prevent bed rest hazards (e.g., thrombo-phlebitis, pulmonary embolism, decubiti, pneumonia)

Obtain pain free range of motion (ROM) within precaution limits

Strengthen hip and knee musculature

Gain functional strength

Learn transfers and ambulation with assistive devices

Achieve successful progression to prior living situation

Adapted from Rehabilitation after total jointy arthroplasty. In Brotzman SB (ed): Clinical Orthopaedic Rehabilitation. St Louis, Mosby, 1996, pp 284–311.

Procedures

Procedures are not typically performed after THA.

Surgery

There are three common types of hip arthroplasty components: (1) unipolar endoprosthesis, (2) bipolar endoprosthesis, and (3) true total hip (separate femoral and acetabular) components. The unipolar implant (Moore endoprosthesis or Austin Moore endoprosthesis) is a single, machined metal alloy component comprising a femoral stem, neck, and head. The implant head articulates with native acetabular cartilage. This type of prosthesis is commonly used in the minimally mobile elderly patient who sustains an intracapsular (subcapital) displaced femoral neck fracture. The "bipolar" endoprosthesis includes a polished metal alloy acetabular component that is anatomically matched to the patient's acetabulum to provide surface bearing. Within this large spherical head sits a polyethylene liner into which the femoral component is snap fit. This creates an outer bearing interface between the implant and the native acetabulum and an inner bearing interface between the polyethylene liner and the femoral component. This design principle theoretically reduces motion at the native acetabulum (cartilage-metal interface) by increasing motion within the moveable prosthetic parts, thereby reducing stress, wear, or erosion of the acetabular cartilage. It can be used instead of the simpler unipolar (Moore) prosthesis for the same indications. It may also be used for revision arthroplasty. The total hip arthroplasty components include a femoral stem (in various sizes and shapes), a femoral neck (in various angles and lengths), and an acetabular cup with a polyethylene liner of various sizes and inclinations. This allows resurfacing of both sides of the hip joint and allows the highest degree of customization for each individual. It is the most complex device of the three to insert properly but is used most commonly.

Surgical technique is beyond the scope of this text. However, the rehabilitation will be affected by the two common fixation techniques: (1) cemented and (2) cementless or Press-Fit. In general, the cemented technique is used only on the femoral component. After a cement restrictor plug is placed in the distal femoral canal, polymethylmethacrylate (PMMA) cement is freshly made and inserted into the femoral canal utilizing pressurization cementing technique. Insertion of the femoral stem creates an intimate fit of the prosthesis to the intramedullary canal with a small circumferential cement mantle. Cement polymerization rigidly fixates the femoral component. A Press-Fit femoral component usually employs porous surface coating to allow bony in-growth and stability. The Press-Fit technique is most commonly used in the younger, more active patient population. Commonly, the patient with a cemented prosthesis is allowed to weight bear as tolerated immediately, whereas the individual with a non-cemented Press-Fit prosthesis often must wait for 6 to 8 weeks before fully weight bearing to allow for stability by bony in-growth.

In most instances, the acetabular cup is Press-Fit. Porous coating components have resulted in excellent clinical results, whereas non-porous coated acetabular implants have proven unsatisfactory. One or two screws may be placed for added stability. If a trochanteric osteotomy is performed during the surgery, hip abduction resistance exercises are usually restricted.

Potential Disease Complications

Pain and functional limitations including gait deviations and demonstrable hip girdle weakness may persist past the immediate postoperative period (12 weeks). A body of literature suggests that many individuals can benefit from longer term rehabilitation programs that address those impairments.[19,20] The short-term prognosis for modern cemented or uncemented THA is excellent.[21, 22] The long-term prognosis remains good to excellent in most cases.[23,24] A general rule of thumb suggests that a total hip implant should last 10 to 15 years. Lower levels of daily activity often result in an extended life expectancy of the prosthetic components, whereas increased activity may lead to earlier wear and loosening.

Common physical impairments after THA include decreased muscle strength, limited hip range of motion, limited flexibility, and abnormalities of gait. Hip joint weakness has been shown to persist at 2 years following surgery, indicating a need for prolonged exercise. Current data suggest that THA patients continue to experience physical and functional limitations that persist at least 1 year postoperatively. Therefore, it is reasonable to have patients continue with therapeutic exercises to address these limitations well beyond the early recovery period (first 12 weeks).

Potential Treatment Complications

Ultrasound should be avoided over metallic implants and over methyl methacrylate. Overly aggressive anti-coagulation for DVT/PE prophylaxis can have the significant side effect of hemorrhage. Analgesics, NSAIDs, and COX-2 inhibitors have well-known side effects that most commonly affect the gastric, hepatic, and renal systems. Treatment complications from surgical intervention are well known and include iatrogenic infection and injury to a nerve or blood vessel. Significant leg-length discrepancy resulting in an awkward gait is also possible. When this exists, it is important to rule out hip dislocation. Medication side effects include the potential for dependency with narcotics.

References

1. Mancuso CA, Ranawat CS, Esdaile JM, et al: Indications for total hip and total knee arthroplasties. Results of orthopedics surveys. J Arthroplasty 1996;11(1): 34–46.
2. Mont MA, et al: Tennis after total hip arthroplasty. Am J Sports Med 1999;27(1):60–64.
3. Brander VA, et al: Outcome of hip and knee arthroplasty in persons aged 80 years and older. Clin Orthop Rel Res 1997;345:67–78.
4. Gogia PP, et al: Total hip replacement in patients with osteoarthritis of the hip: Improvement in pain and functional status. Orthopedics 1994;17(2):145–150.
5. McGrory BJ, Stuart MJ, Sim FH: Participation in sports after hip and knee arthroplasty: Review of literature and survey of surgeon preferences. Mayo Clin Proc 1995:70:342–348.
6. Munnin MC, Ruby TE, Glynn NW, et al: Early inpatient rehabilitation after elective hip and knee arthroplasty. JAMA 1998;279:847–852.
7. Turpie AGG, Levine MN, Hirsh J, et al: A randomized controlled trial of a low-molecular-weight heparin (enoxaparin) to prevent deep-venous thrombosis in patients undergoing elective hip surgery. N Engl J Med 1986;315(15):925–929.
8. Lieberman JR, Geerts WH: Prevention of venous thromboembolism after total hip and knee arthroplasty. J Bone Joint Surg 1994;76-A:1239–1250.
9. Merli GJ: Deep vein thrombosis and pulmonary embolism prophylaxis in orthopedic surgery. Med Clin North Am 1993;77:397–411.
10. Geerts WH, Heit JA, et al: Prevention of venous thromboembolism. Chest 2001;119(Suppl):132S–175S.
11. Levine MN, Hirsch J, Gent M, et al: Prevention of deep vein thrombosis after elective hip surgery. Ann Intern Med 1991;114:545–551.
12. Spiro TE, Johnson GJ, Christie MJ, et al: Efficacy and safety of enoxaparin to prevent deep venous thrombosis after hip replacement surgery. Ann Intern Med 1994;121:81–87.
13. Edeen J., Sharkey PF, Alexander, AH: Clinical significance of leg-length inequality after total hip arthroplasty. Ame J Orthop 1995;April:347–351.
14. Wang A, et al: Patient variability and the design of clinical pathways after primary total hip replacement surgery. J Qual Clin Pract 1997;17(3):123–129.
15. Aspen Reference Group: Clinical Pathways for Medical Rehabilitation. Gaithersburg, MD, Aspen, 1998.
16. Rehabilitation after total joint arthroplasty. In Brotzman SB (ed): Clinical Orthopaedic Rehabilitation. St Louis, Mosby, 1996.
17. Dowsey MM, et al: Clinical pathways in hip and knee arthroplasty: a prospective randomized controlled study. Med J Aust 1999;170(2):59–62.
18. Mandzuk LL: A total hip arthroplasty critical path: A step in the right direction. Orthoscope 1998;4(3):6–13.
19. Braeker AM, Luchhaas-Gerlach JA, Gollish JD, et al: Determinants of 6–12 month postoperative functional status and pain after elective total hip replacement. International J Qual Informative Health Care 1997;9(6):413–418.
20. Shih C, Du Y, Lin Y, Wu C: Muscular recovery around the hip joint after total hip arthroplasty. Clin Orthop Rel Res 1994;302:115–120.
21. Towheed TE, Hochberg MC: Health related quality of life after total hip replacement. Semin Arthritis Rheum 1996;26(1):483–491.
22. Aarons H et al: Short-term recovery from hip and knee arthroplasty. J Bone Joint Surg 1996;78-B(4):555–558.
23. Rissanen P, et al: Quality of life and functional ability in hip and knee replacements: A prospective study. Quali Life Res 1996;5(1):56–64.
24. Lieberman JR, Dorey F, Shekelle P, et al: Differences between patients' and physicians' evaluations of outcome after total hip arthroplasty. J Bone Joint Surg 1996;78-A(6):835–838.

57 Trochanteric Bursitis

Florian S. Keplinger, MD
Navneet Gupta, MD

Synonyms

Greater trochanteric bursitis

Greater trochanter pain syndrome

Hip bursitis

ICD-9 Codes

726.5
Enthesopathy of hip region (bursitis of hip, trochanteric tendinitis)

Definition

Trochanteric bursitis is a common cause of pain in the hip and lateral aspect of the thigh. It usually occurs in middle-aged to elderly people, with a peak incidence between the fourth and sixth decades of life. Women are 2 to 4 times more commonly affected than men.[1,2]

Three bursae are anatomically associated with the greater trochanter—two major and one minor. The larger major bursa is the subgluteus maximus bursa, which lies lateral to the greater trochanter and underneath the fibers of the gluteus maximus. The other major bursa is the subgluteus medius bursa, which can be found between the gluteus medius tendon and the antero-superior part of the lateral surface of the greater trochanter. The minor bursa is the gluteus minimus bursa, which lies between the gluteus minimus tendon and medial part of the anterior surface of the greater trochanter.[1]

Inflammation or irritation of any or all of these bursae can result in symptoms of trochanteric bursitis.

Symptoms[1–3]

The patient's chief complaint is aching over the trochanteric and lateral thigh areas. It can be sharp and intense, if acute. It is often described as diffuse, especially if chronic. Occasionally, the pain has a radicular quality, with the sensation radiating down the lateral aspect of the thigh and even below the knee, simulating radicular symptoms. Typically the pain is worse at night when sleeping on the affected side and with the first few steps when arising from a chair. Symptoms are also exacerbated with prolonged walking, squatting, or stair-climbing.

The onset can be acute, but is usually gradual, with worsening over time.

Physical Examination

The essential finding is localized tenderness with palpation over the greater trochanter area, greatest at the junction between the upper thigh and the greater trochanter. There may be associated findings of tender points throughout lateral thigh.

Pain can also be elicited by having the patient perform abduction and external rotation of the affected hip against resistance. The neurologic exam should be normal.

Functional Limitations

The patient commonly has difficulty walking. Walking distance and exercise tolerance are decreased. In addition, patients may have limitations in stairclimbing, and sleep may be interrupted when patients shift to the affected side.

Diagnostic Studies

The diagnosis is generally based on the clinical examination; however, imaging studies may be used to rule out other diagnoses. Although imaging studies are rarely necessary to confirm the diagnosis of trochanteric bursitis, plain x-rays may show irregularities of the greater trochanter, or peritrochanteric calcifications.[1,2] Bone scan may show increased uptake in the region of the greater trochanter; this is usually linear and can be seen in the early blood-pooling phase and in the delayed images.[4,5] Magnetic resonance imaging may show high-intensity signal in the region of the greater trochanter.[1]

Laboratory studies may show elevated acute phase reactants (erythrocyte sedimentation rate, C-reactive protein), but again are not generally necessary.

Differential Diagnosis

Osteoarthritis or inflammatory arthritis of the lumbar spine, hip, or knee*

Leg-length discrepancy*

Scoliosis*

Iliotibial band tightness or syndrome*

Tendinitis of the hip external rotators*

Avascular necrosis of the hip

Lumbar radiculopathy, especially of L1–L2–L3 roots

Meralgia paresthetica

Tumor (primary or metastatic)

---

* This condition may actually contribute to trochanteric bursitis by adding stress to the area affected.

Treatment

Initial

Bed rest is rarely necessary; however, patients should try to avoid activities that exacerbate their symptoms. Overweight to obese patients should be advised on gradual weight loss.

Nonsteroidal anti-inflammatory drugs (NSAIDs), including cyclooxygenase-2 (COX-2) inhibitors, are commonly prescribed, for both analgesic and anti-inflammatory effects.

Local application of ice helps to decrease pain and inflammation (20 minutes 2 to 3 times daily is a reasonable regimen). The patient can be taught to use superficial heat for chronic bursitis. This can be done with moistened warm compresses or with a microwaveable/electric heating pad. Precautions should be observed and given to the patient to prevent complications.

Rehabilitation

Physical therapy may be ordered for strengthening of hip muscles, especially the gluteus medius. Additionally, stretching of any tight hip muscles and/or a tight iliotibial band will greatly assist with improving mobility and pain. Correction of leg-length discrepancy, if significant (i.e., greater than 2 cm) may help; a heel lift may be enough, but in cases of larger discrepancies, the entire shoe may need to be lifted and a rocker bottom sole added. Correction of a leg-length discrepancy should be done in stages, and a lift generally does not exceed 50% of the actual discrepancy (e.g., for a 1-inch leg-length discrepancy, start with a ⅛-inch heel lift and work up to a ½-inch lift).

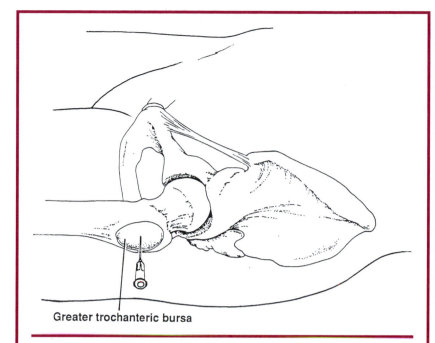

Greater trochanteric bursa

FIGURE 1. Have the patient lie supine or in the lateral recumbent position. Then under sterile conditions, inject a 2 to 4 cc mixture of corticosteroid and local anesthetic (e.g., 1 cc of 1% lidocaine and 2 cc (12 mg) of betamethasone. This can be done using a 22-gauge, 3½-inch needle to ensure that the bursal area is reached. Local anesthetics are sometimes injected just prior to the steroid injection to diminish pain and avoid postinjection steroid flare.[1,2,5,10] Local icing is helpful postinjection. (Adapted from Vander Slam TJ: Atlas of Bedside Procedures. Boston, Little Brown, 1988, with permission.)

Local application of ice helps to decrease pain symptoms and inflammation, especially during the acute stage. Superficial heat in the form of hot packs or compresses are indicated more during the subacute to chronic stages. Deep heat, in the form of ultrasound or diathermy, has not been proven beneficial, and it can possibly worsen the bursitis.

Procedures

Injections are often helpful in decreasing inflammation and symptoms of pain (Fig. 1). Typically no more than three injections are given over a 6- to 12-month period. Persistent hip pain despite injection therapy should alert the clinician to the possibility of an alternative diagnosis.

The patient is generally advised to avoid activity using the area injected for approximately 2 weeks to promote retention of the corticosteroid in the bursa and to avoid systemic absorption.[10]

Surgery

Surgery is rarely necessary and is reserved for patients with chronic trochanteric bursitis that has not responded to the aforementioned management and has led to significant functional limitations for the patient. The operation consists of iliotibial band release, excision of the bursal sac, and removal of calcified tissue.[1,9]

Potential Disease Complications

Potential disease complications include chronic pain, myofascial pain syndrome, deconditioning (local and/or generalized), and falls with possible serious injury.

Potential Treatment Complications

Complications of medications include drug hypersensitivity and gastric, renal, and hepatic side effects from NSAIDs; these side effects are less less with COX-2 inhibitors.[2,9] Hyperglycemia, electrolyte imbalance, and gastric irritation or ulceration may be prevented by intralesional steroids administration, but can still occur from systemic absorption.[2]

Local heat application can result in burns, sedation, and hyperpigmentation,[9] and local ice application can produce hypersensitivity, vasoconstriction in patients with Raynaud's and peripheral vascular disease.[9] Complications resulting from injections include drug hypersensitivity, sterile abscess, infection, nerve injury, tendon rupture, and lipoatrophy from intralesional steroids.[7]

References

1. Shbeeb MI, Matteson EL: Trochanteric Bursitis (Greater trochanteric pain syndrome). Mayo Clin Proc 1996;71(6):86–89.
2. Biundo JJ: Regional Rheumatic pain syndromes. In Schumacher HR (ed): Primer on the Rheumatic Diseases, 10th ed. Atlanta, Arthritis Foundation, 1993, pp 277–287.
3. Reveille JD: Soft tissue rheumatism: Diagnosis and treatment. Am J Med 1997;102(1A):23S–29S.
4. Allwright SJ, Cooper RA, Nash P: Trochanteric bursitis: Bone scan appearance. Clin Nuc Med 1998;13(8):561–564.
5. Schapira D, Nahir M, Scharf Y: Trochanteric bursitis: A common clinical problem. Arch Phys Med Rehabil 1986;67(11):815–817.
6. Little H: Trochanteric bursitis: A common cause of pelvic girdle pain. CMAJ 1979;120(4):456–458.
7. Basford JR: Physical agents. In Delisa JA, Gans BM (eds): Rehabilitation Medicine: Principles and Practice, Philadelphia, Lippincott-Raven, 1993, pp 973–995.
8. Neustadt DH: Intra-articular corticosteroids and other agents: Aspiration techniques. In Katz W (ed): The Diagnosis and Management of Rheumatic Disease, 2nd ed. Philadelphia, J.B. Lippincott, 1988, pp 812–825.
9. Slawski DP, Howard RF: Surgical management of refractory trochanteric bursitis. Am J Sports Med 1997;25(1):86–89.
10. Kaplan H: Therapeutic injection of joints and soft tissues. In Schumacher HR (ed): Primer on the Rheumatic Diseases, 10th ed. Atlanta, Arthritis Foundation, 1993, pp277–287.

58 Anterior Cruciate Ligament Sprain

William Micheo, MD
Eduardo Amy, MD

Synonyms

Anterior cruciate ligament (ACL) sprain

ACL deficient knee

Torn cruciate

Rotary instability of the knee

Anterolateral instability of the knee

ICD-9 Codes

717.83
Old disruption of anterior cruciate ligament

844.2
Sprains and strains of knee and leg (cruciate ligament of knee)

Definition

The anterior cruciate ligament (ACL) is an intra-articular structure essential for the normal function of the knee. Unfortunately, it is commonly injured during sport activities that involve complex movements, such as cutting and pivoting. The injury usually results from a sudden deceleration during a high-velocity movement in which a forceful contraction of the quadriceps muscle is required. Injury to the ligament is also described as a result of a valgus stress, hyperextension, and external rotation, as seen when landing from a jump. In addition, injury may occur with severe internal rotation of the knee or hyperextension with internal rotation. Traumatic injury to the ligament may occur with valgus stress to the knee in association with injury to the medial collateral ligament and the medial meniscus.[1] It has been reported that 70% of the acute ACL injuries are sports related.[2] Recent trends in sports participation has increased the incidence of this injury in the female and the immature athlete.[3,4]

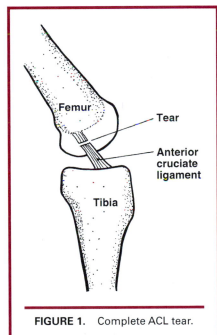

FIGURE 1. Complete ACL tear.

The ACL may be partially or completely torn (Fig. 1). The ACL may be injured alone or in association with other structures—most commonly with a tear of the medial collateral ligament or meniscus.

The ACL is a collagenous structure approximately 38 mm in length and 10 mm in width. The ligament arises from a wide base in the tibia anterolateral to the anterior tibial spine. It then traverses the knee in a posterolateral direction, attaching in a broad fanlike fashion at the posterolateral corner of the intercondylar notch of the femur.

Biomechanical studies using cadaver specimens and more recently robotic units have evaluated the forces that affect the ACL.[5] These forces are the highest in the last 30 degrees of extension; hyperextension; and under other load conditions, including anterior tibial translation, internal rotation, and varus. The ACL is a static stabilizer of the knee with a primary function of resisting hyperextension and anterior tibial translation in flexion and providing rotatory control. It is also a secondary restraint to valgus and varus forces in all degrees of flexion.

Symptoms

Individuals usually present with pain, immediate swelling, and limited range of motion. They may give a history of hearing a "pop." In an acute injury, the individual will have severe pain and difficulty with walking. In a chronic injury, a patient may have a history of recurrent episodes of knee instability associated with swelling and limited motion. Patients may describe the "giving way" phenomenon. They may also give a history of a remote injury to the knee that was not rehabilitated.

Physical Examination

The physical examination has been found to be very sensitive and specific in the diagnosis of anterior cruciate ligament tears.[6] The clinician should observe the knee for asymmetry, palpate for areas of tenderness, measure active and passive range of motion, and document muscle atrophy. Special tests to rule out other pathology such as patellar subluxation, sprains of the collateral ligaments, or meniscal injury should be performed. Testing for the integrity of the ACL in the patient with an acute injury should include Lachman's test in which an anterior force is applied to the tibia with the knee in 30 degrees of flexion, with the clinician trying to reproduce anterior migration of the tibia on the femur (Fig. 2). Another important test in the acute setting is the lateral pivot shift maneuver in which the clinician attempts to reproduce anterolateral rotatory instability by internally rotating the leg and applying a valgus stress to the knee as it is flexed (Fig. 3). In the patient with chronic ACL insufficiency, the anterior drawer test in which an anterior force is applied to the tibia with the knee flexed to 90 degrees may also be used (Fig. 4).

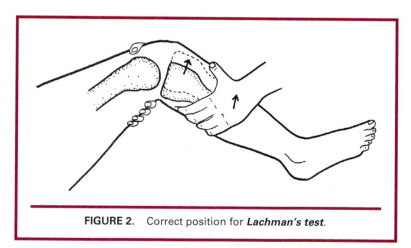

FIGURE 2.   Correct position for *Lachman's test*.

In general, the neurologic exam including strength, sensation, and reflexes should be normal; however, there may be some associated weakness (particularly of knee extension by the quadriceps muscle) due to pain or disuse.

Functional Limitations

Limitations include reduced knee motion, muscle weakness, and pain that interferes with activities involving pivoting and jumping. Recurrent episodes of instability are associated with participation in strenuous sports, such as basketball, soccer, tennis, and volleyball.[7,8] Repeated episodes of knee giving way may result in increased ligamentous laxity, leading to limitations with activities of daily living, such as going down stairs or changing directions while walking.

Diagnostic Studies

Diagnostic studies should include plain x-rays to rule out intra-articular fractures, loose bodies, and arthritic changes. These views should include an AP, lateral, and Merchant. Magnetic resonance imaging (MRI) may be indicated to evaluate associated pathology such as bone bruises, meniscal tears, or other ligamentous injuries. In the pediatric and adolescent age athlete, MRI may also give information about physeal injuries that may go otherwise unnoticed.

Commonly, in an acute injury with a large effusion, arthrocentesis is performed to relieve pressure and pain (Fig. 5). It assists with the diagnosis, as an ACL injury will generally return blood or serosanguinous fluid. If a fat globule is present at the surface of the aspirate, the clinician should be suspicious for a fracture. More than 24 to 48 hours after injury, the blood may be clotted and difficult to aspirate.

Differential Diagnosis

Collateral ligament sprain

Patellar tendon rupture

Fracture (e.g., intra-articular, tibial plateau)

Patellar dislocation

Meniscal tear

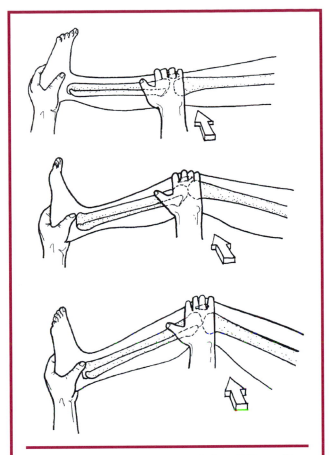

FIGURE 3. Position for the *lateral pivot shift test*. Note that the patient's knee is fully extended. Internally rotate the leg and apply a valgus stress. As the clinician begins to flex the knee, the lateral tibial plateau subluxes. As tension in the iliotibial band is lessened at 45 degrees of flexion, a pivot shift is felt as the tibia reduces. This test is used to identify a rupture of the anterior cruciate ligament.

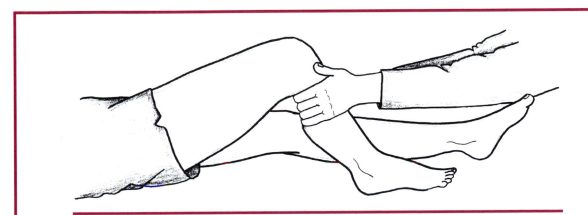

FIGURE 4. Position for *anterior drawer test*. The hip is flexed 45 degrees. The knee is flexed 90 degrees. The tibia is in neutral rotation. Anterior pull can be applied to the proximal tibia with both hands.

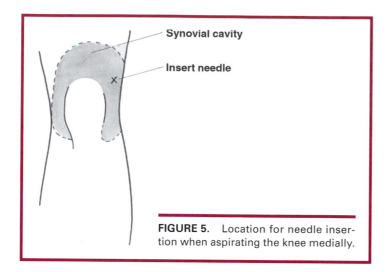

FIGURE 5. Location for needle insertion when aspirating the knee medially.

Treatment

Initial

Immediately after injury, the management of an ACL tear includes relative rest, ice, compression, and analgesic or anti-inflammatory medication. Many patients will benefit from a knee immobilizer and crutches. If the knee is very swollen and painful, arthrocentesis is performed, ideally within the first 24 to 48 hours.

It is very important to establish an accurate diagnosis and the presence of associated injuries, as these might necessitate prompt surgery. These include chondral or osteochondral fractures, meniscal tears, or other injured capsular structures. Generally, in the absence of these other injuries, the acute management can be conservative with early protective rehabilitation.

Treatment of ACL injuries depend on a number of factors including the patient's age; level of activity; presence of associated injuries; and importance of returning to athletic activities that involve acceleration, deceleration, and cutting moves. Surgery is the only definitive treatment for complete ACL injuries, but is generally not necessary for older individuals who do not complain of knee instability with recreational activities or work.

In younger patients, the decision to have surgery is made by the patient and clinician together after a thorough discussion of treatment options and anticipated future activity level. Surgical referral is not necessary in the immediate postinjury period, but should be facilitated as soon as it is clear that an individual desires surgery as a definite treatment measure. When associated injures are present, especially if these cause mechanical symptoms, or in the case of the elite competitive athlete, surgical treatment should be considered as soon as the initial inflammatory phase has passed.[9]

Rehabilitation

The rehabilitation of an ACL tear begins as soon as the injury occurs. Rehabilitation management should focus on reducing pain, restoring full motion, correcting muscle strength deficits, achieving muscle balance, and returning the patient to full activity free of symptoms.[10] The rehabilitation program consists of acute, recovery, and functional phases.

Non-Operated ACL Injury

The patient with the non-operated ACL deficient knee may present with an acute or a recurrent injury. The complaint could vary from a swollen, painful knee to a recurrently unstable joint with associated muscle weakness and atrophy.

In the acutely injured knee, protection of secondary structures is of paramount importance, and progression of rehabilitation will depend on the extent of damage to other knee structures. Early use of closed kinetic chain exercises in which the distal segment of the extremity is fixed and the proximal segments are free to move has allowed progression of strengthening with reduced shear forces to the knee. These exercises allow quadriceps strengthening with hamstring muscle co-contraction without increasing the strain in the ACL and minimizing patellofemoral joint reaction forces (Table 1).[10,11]

The individual with a recurrently unstable knee will benefit from a trial of rehabilitation. Correction of muscle weakness and proprioceptive deficits and functional retraining in combination with activity modification could reduce episodes of instability.

TABLE 1. Non-Operated Anterior Cruciate Ligament Tear Rehabilitation

Acute Phase	Recovery Phase	Functional Phase
Therapeutic Intervention	*Therapeutic Intervention*	*Therapeutic Intervention*
1. Modalities: cryotherapy, electrical stimulation	1. Modalities: superficial heat, pulsed ultrasound, electrical stimulation	1. General flexibility, strengthening training
2. Active assisted flexion and extension	2. Range of motion, flexibility exercises	2. Power and endurance of lower extremities: diagonal and multiplanar motions, plyometrics
3. Isometric quadriceps and hamstring exercise	3. Dynamic lower extremity strengthening	3. Neuromusuclar control, proprioceptive training
4. General conditioning	4. Closed kinetic chain exercises, multiplanar lower extremity joint exercises	4. Return to sports-specific participation with functional bracing
5. Ambulation with crutches	5. General conditioning	
	6. Gradual return to sports-specific training with functional bracing	
Criteria for Advancement	*Criteria for Advancement*	*Criteria for Advancement*
1. Pain reduction	1. Full nonpainful motion	1. No clinical symptoms
2. Recovery of pain-free motion	2. Symmetric quadriceps and hamstring strength	2. Normal running and jumping mechanics
3. Adequate knee muscle control	3. Correction of inflexibility	3. Normal kinematic chain integration
4. Tolerance for strengthening exercises	4. Symptom-free progression in a sports-specific program	4. Completed sports specific program

Acute phase: This phase should focus on treating tissue injury and clinical signs and symptoms. The goal in this stage should be to allow tissue healing while reducing pain and inflammation. Re-establishment of non-painful range of motion, prevention of muscle atrophy, and maintenance of general fitness should be addressed. This phase could last from 1 to 2 weeks.

Recovery phase: This phase should focus on obtaining normal passive and active knee motion, improving knee muscle control, achieving normal hamstrings and quadriceps muscle balance, and working on proprioception. Biomechanical and functional deficits including inflexibilities and inability to run or jump should be addressed. This phase could last from 2 to 8 weeks after the injury occurs.

Functional phase: This phase should focus on increasing power and endurance of the lower extremities while improving neuromuscular control. Rehabilitation at this stage should work on the entire kinematic chain, addressing specific functional deficits. This program should be continuous with the ultimate goal of prevention of recurrent injury. The functional phase could last from 8 weeks to 4 to 6 months after the injury occurs.

If the patient completes a rehabilitation program and is willing to modify the activity level, including limiting sports activity involving cutting and pivoting maneuvers, the functional prognosis for daily living activities is good.[13] In this patient group, functional braces may be used for sports participation that involves changes of direction. These braces may reduce symptoms of instability in individuals who use them and appear to reduce some strain in the ACL in low-demand activities.

Operated ACL Injury

After reconstructive surgery, rehabilitation should begin on the first day postoperation. Early use of cryotherapy, compression, and elevation has been shown to reduce swelling postoperatively. It is very important to achieve full extension and to initiate early active flexion in the first few days postsurgery. Weight bearing with crutches is usually started immediately after the operation.[12]

Rapid progression of the rehabilitation program has reduced complications commonly associated with ACL knee surgery, including stiffness, muscle atrophy, muscle weakness, and patellofemoral pain. In the early rehabilitation period, special precautions need to be taken to avoid excessive strain of the reconstructed ligament with terminal (0 to 30 degrees) extension, resisted quadriceps

TABLE 2. Operated Anterior Cruciate Ligament Tear Rehabilitation

Acute Phase	Recovery Phase	Functional Phase
Therapeutic Intervention	*Therapeutic Intervention*	*Therapeutic Intervention*
1. Modalities: cryotherapy, electrical stimulation	1. Modalities: superficial heat, pulsed ultrasound, electrical stimulation	1. General flexibility training, strengthening exercise program
2. Active assisted flexion, passive	2. Active flexion extension exercises	2. Power and endurance in lower extremities: diagonal and multi-planar motions with tubings, light weight, medicine balls, plyometrics
3. Isometric quadriceps (45 to 90 degrees), dynamic hamstring exercises, straight leg raise (SLR) exercises	3. Dynamic quadriceps (30 to 90 degrees), hamstring strengthening	
	4. Closed kinetic chain exercises, multiplanar lower extremity joint exercises	3. Neuromuscular control, proprioceptive training
4. General conditioning upper extremity ergometer	5. General conditioning: bicycling, swimming	4. Return to sports-specific participation
5. Ambulation with crutches	6. Gradual return to sports-specific training with optional functional brace use	5. Optional functional brace use
Criteria for Advancement	*Criteria for Advancement*	*Criteria for Advancement*
1. Pain reduction	1. Full flexion, knee hyperextension	1. No clinical symptoms
2. Recovery of 90 degrees of flexion, full extension	2. Symmetric quadriceps and hamstring strength	2. Normal running and jumping mechanics
3. Adequate knee muscle control	3. Symptom-free progression in a sports-specific program	3. Normal kinematic chain integration
4. Tolerance for strengthening exercises		4. Completed sports-specific program

exercises. Early use of closed kinetic chain exercises such as mini-squats, steps, and leg press has allowed quadriceps strengthening with reduced shear forces to the graft (Table 2).[10,11,12] Aquatic exercises, which allow progressive weight bearing while benefiting from the effects of buoyancy, can be started as soon as the sutures are removed.

Individuals will vary in the rate in which they achieve full motion, normal strength, normal proprioception, and adequate sports-specific skills. Achievement of these goals should be accomplished prior to allowing the individual to return to sports activity. With accelerated rehabilitation programs, patients usually return to activity in 6 months following surgery.

Procedures

As noted earlier, knee joint aspiration may be attempted to assist with both diagnosis and pain relief. This is generally done in the first 24 to 48 hours of injury.

Under sterile conditions, using a 25-gauge, 1-inch sterile disposable needle, infiltrate the skin with a local anesthetic (e.g., 1% lidocaine) approximately 2 cm proximal and lateral (or medial) to the patella (see Fig. 5). Follow this injection with a second injection using an 18-gauge, 1½-inch needle into the joint capsule. Aspirate any fluid, and note the color and consistency. Without withdrawing the needle, take off the syringe and empty. Repeat this until all of the fluid is aspirated. Use one hand to compress the suprapatellar area to be sure all of the fluid is out. Then (optional) inject 1 to 2 cc of a local steroid preparation (e.g., 40 to 80 mg of methylprednisolone).

Postinjection care includes icing the knee for 15 minutes following the injection and then for 20 minutes 2 to 3 times daily for several days. A compressive dressing or neoprene sleeve is advised to limit future effusions.

Surgery

Surgery is indicated for patients with recurrent episodes of instability in activities of daily living and in active recreational athletes who are symptomatic and do not wish to modify their activities. Surgery is definitely indicated in the high-demand competitive athlete.

The surgical procedure of choice is the endoscopic tendon autograft using the central third of the patellar tendon, which provides the most rigid fixation and permits an aggressive rehabilitation program. Improvement in graft fixation technique has permitted the use of hamstring tendons as a good alternative particularly in patients with history of patellar problems.[8,14] Less commonly used alternatives include the use of cadaver allograft from the patellar or the Achilles tendon and the use of the contralateral patellar tendon. In selected patients with recurrent instability and evidence of osteoarthritis, a surgical reconstruction can still be considered.[15]

Potential Disease Complications

An untreated ACL injury can lead to changes in the knee joint, which may be associated with significant alterations in the patient's lifestyle. Patients who continue participation in strenuous sports have recurrent episodes secondary to anterior laxity and rotatory instability. These may lead to damage of associated structures, such as the meniscus and other secondary restraints. A significant number of patients develop joint space narrowing with evidence of osteoarthritis.[5,15]

Potential Treatment Complications

Medication complications include gastric and renal toxicity with NSAIDs. COX-2 inhibitors may have fewer gastric side effects. Injections carry the risk of infection. Early surgical complications include infection (in approximately 1% to 2% of cases), venous thrombosis, and complications from anesthesia. Fibrous ankylosis and significant loss of motion can be seen in the early rehabilitation stages secondary to poor progression of therapy or patient compliance.[16]

Poor graft placement and fixation can lead to loss of motion and subsequent graft failure with recurrent instability. In patients in whom chondral lesions or meniscal tears are identified at the time of surgery, long-term sequela include the development of arthritis, even after the reconstruction.[15,17]

References

1. Caborn DNM, Johnson BM: The natural history of the anterior cruciate ligament deficient knee: A review. Clin Sports Med 1993;12:625–636.
2. Micheo W, Frontera WR, Amy E, Jordan G: Rehabilitation of the patient with an anterior cruciate ligament injury: A brief review. Bol Assoc Med PR 1995;87:29–36.
3. Arendt E, Dick R: Knee injury patterns among men and women in collegiate basketball and soccer: NCAA data and review of literature. Am J Sports Med 1995;23:694–701.
4. Fehnel DJ, Johnson R: Anterior cruciate injuries in the skeletally immature athlete: A review of treatment outcomes. Sports Med 2000;29:51–63.
5. Woo SLY, Debski RF, Withrow JD, Jannausek MA: Biomechanics of knee ligaments. Am J Sports Med 1999;27:533–543.
6. O'Shea KJ, Murphy KP, Heekin D, Hernzwurm PJ: The diagnostic accuracy of history, physical examination, and radiographs in the evaluation of traumatic knee disorders. Am J Sports Med 1996;24:164–167.
7. Boden BP, Griffin LY, Garrett WE: Etiology and prevention of noncontact ACL injury. Phys Sports Med 2000;28:53–62.
8. Fu F, Bennett CH, Ma B, et al: Current trends in anterior cruciate ligaments reconstruction: Part 2. Operative procedures and clinical correlations. Am J Sports Med 2000;28:124–130.
9. Shelbourne KD, Foulk DA: Timing of surgery in acute anterior cruciate ligament tears on the return of quadriceps muscle strength after reconstruction using an autogenous patellar tendon graft. Am J Sports Med 1995;23:686–689.
10. Gotlin RS, Huie R: Anterior cruciate ligament injuries: Operative and rehabilitative options. PMR Clin North Am 2000;11:895–924.
11. Escamilla RF, Fleisig GS, Zheng N, et al: Biomechanics of the knee during closed kinetic chain and open kinetic chain exercises. Med Sci Sports Exer 1998;30:556–569..
12. Arnold T, Shelbourne KD: A perioperative rehabilitation program for anterior cruciate ligament surgery. Phys Sports Med 2000;28:31–49.
13. Messner K, Maletius W: Eighteen to twenty-five year follow-up after acute partial anterior cruciate ligament rupture. Am J Sports Med 1999;27: 455–459.
14. Brand J, Weiler A, Caborn DNM, et al: Graft fixation in cruciate ligament reconstruction. Am J Sports Med 2000;28:761–774.
15. Clatworthy M, Amendola A: The anterior cruciate ligament and arthritis. Clin Sports Med 1999;18:173–198.
16. Nyland J: Rehabilitation complications following knee surgery. Clin Sports Med 1999;18:905–929.
17. Brown CH, Carson EW: Revision anterior cruciate ligament surgery. Clin Sports Med 1999;18: 109–171.

59 Baker's Cyst

Meryl Stein, MD
Darren Rosenberg, DO

Synonyms

Popliteal cyst

ICD-9 Code

727.51
Synovial cyst of popliteal space (Baker's cyst)

Definition

A Baker's cyst is the most common cyst in the posterior knee, affecting approximately 19% of adults and 6% of children.[1] It results when chronic irritation increases production of synovial fluid, causing one of the six popliteal bursa to distend and then form a palpable mass (usually distention of the gastrocnemius-semimembranosus bursa). Most commonly, the source of this chronic irritation is an inflammatory or degenerative joint disease. Osteoarthritis and rheumatoid arthritis are common culprits. Chodromalacia patellae, chronic ligamentous or meniscal tear, chronic low grade infection, pigmented villonodular synovitis or persistent capsulitis are also common causes.[2] Direct trauma is the most common cause of these cysts in children.[1]

Symptoms

Baker's cyst presents as a fluctuant mass in the popliteal fossa, which is typically not tender (Fig. 1). In fact, often patients with these cysts are asymptomatic. Symptoms are most readily elicited when knee flexion compresses the fluid-filled cyst. Baker's cysts are far more common in older people than in younger people because they result from a chronic injury that produces an effusion. However, Baker's cysts do occur in children due to isolated bursal sac formations.[3] The mass is often accompanied by leg swelling and/or diffuse calf tenderness. Numbness and tingling may be present if there is compression of nerves or blood vessels.

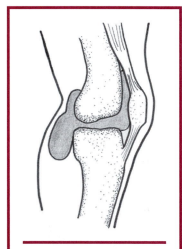

FIGURE 1. Schematic diagram of Baker's cyst.

Physical Examination

Baker's cysts are often visible, or at least palpable, along the medial aspect of the popliteal fossa. The best way to identify a cyst is to lie the patient prone with the knee extended and then have the patient flex the knee. The cyst will be firm with knee extension and soft with knee flexion, a phenomenon known as Foucher's sign.[3] The cyst can extend into the thigh or leg, or it can have multiple satellites along the calf and even into the foot. These satellite cysts may or may not be connected to the primary cyst through channels.[4] When a joint effusion accompanies the cyst, it is often worthwhile to search for the source of chronic irritation. Examine the knee's range of motion, test patellar and tibiofemoral ligamentous laxity, and evaluate for potential patellofemoral pain and meniscal tears.[2] Testing the erythrocyte sedimentation rate (ESR) may also be helpful if an inflammatory process is suspected.

Functional Limitations

The degree of impairment produced by the cyst depends on its size and amount of tenderness. Baker's cysts are usually painless and limit movement minimally, if at all, unless there is an underlying meniscal injury.

Diagnostic Studies

Imaging can help by defining underlying pathology causing continued pain despite medical treatment. Plain films of the knee can be used to diagnose underlying degenerative joint disease but are rarely necessary to diagnose a Baker's cyst.

Ultrasound distinguishes solid from cystic masses and is therefore especially helpful in detecting Baker's cysts when the extensive joint deformities, such as those present with rheumatoid arthritis, obscure the cyst.[4] Magnetic resonance imaging (MRI) delineates the anatomy of the entire joint and is a very sensitive test to identify a Baker's cyst as well as its likely cause. MRIs also help in ruling out suspected solid tumors and defining pathology for possible surgical excision. On these scans, Baker's cysts appear as well circumscribed masses with low signal intensity on T1-weighted images and high signal intensity on T2-weighted images.

Differential Diagnosis

Venous complexes	Neoplasms (sarcoma)
Inflammatory arthritis (rheumatoid)	Thrombophlebitis
Arterial aneurysms	Pseudothrombophlebitis
Fat pads	Compartment syndrome

Treatment

Initial

Intervention is needed only when the Baker's cyst is symptomatic. The simplest treatment is to aspirate the fluid because aspiration collapses the cyst, and the symptoms consequently disappear. However, treating the cyst alone may not be adequate, treating the underlying joint pathology may be necessary. Ice and anti-inflammatory agents (NSAIDs and COX-2 inhibitors), for example, can be used to reduce the inflammatory effusions produced by degenerative joint disease. Quadriceps strengthening exercises can be used for patellofemoral syndrome. In some cases, venous sclerosants are used to prevent recurrence.[3] The cysts tend to involute spontaneously in children.

Rehabilitation

Treatment should be directed towards the cause of the Baker's cyst. The cyst itself will not respond to rehabilitation techniques.

Procedures

Needle aspiration of the cyst is the most effective therapy and, providing the predisposing cause of the cyst resolves, generally results in a cure. The possibility of a vascular malformation must be eliminated either by auscultating the mass with a stethoscope to listen for bruits or by palpating it to feel for a pulse prior to cyst aspiration.[4]

Surgery

Surgical excision is attempted only after all other methods have failed and the cyst is sufficiently large and symptomatic.[5] Occasionally, surgery is necessary to correct the underlying pathology (e.g., arthroscopic surgery for meniscal tears or total knee replacement for intractable degenerative joint disease).

Potential Disease Complications

The most common complications of Baker's cysts are dissection into the calf or rupture. When the cyst ruptures, it produces a "pseudothrombophlebitis syndrome," meaning that it results in intense calf pain and swelling without an associated deep venous thrombosis. Less commonly, a Baker's cyst produces a compartment syndrome; a peripheral neuropathy; or calf, foot and ankle ecchymoses.[3] More rarely, if the cyst is infected, it can result in septic arthritis of the knee.[6]

Potential Treatment Complications

Analgesics, NSAIDs, and COX-2 inhibitors have well-known side effects that most commonly affect the gastric, hepatic, and renal systems. Aspiration can result in recurrence, infection, and bleeding.

References
1. De Maeseneer M, Debaere C, Desprechins B, Osteaux M: Popliteal Cysts in children: prevalence, appearance and associated findings at MR imaging. Pediatr Radiol 1999;29:605–609.
2. Tinker RV: Orthopaedics in Primary Care. Baltimore, Williams & Wilkins, 1979, p 221.
3. Langsfeld M, Matteson B, Johnson W, et al: Baker's cysts mimicking the symptoms of deep vein thrombosis: Diagnosis with venous duplex scanning. J Vasc Surg 1997;25(4):658–662.
4. Katz WA (ed): Diagnosis and Management of Rheumatic Diseases, 2nd ed. Philadelphia: JB Lippincott, 1988, p 193.
5. Birnbaum JS: The Musculoskeletal Manual. New York, Academic Press, 1982, p 104.
6. Drees C, Lewis T, Mossad S: "Baker's cyst infection: Case report and review. Clin Infect Dis 1999;29:276–278.

60 Collateral Ligament Sprain

Paul Lento, MD
Venu Akuthota, MD

Synonyms

Knee ligamentous injuries

Medial or lateral collateral knee injury

Knee valgus or varus instability/insufficiency

ICD-9 Codes

717.81
Old disruption of lateral collateral ligament

717.82
Old disruption of medial collateral ligament

844.0
Sprains and strains of knee and leg (lateral collateral ligament)

844.1
Sprains and strains of knee and leg (medial collateral ligament)

Definition

The medial and lateral collateral ligaments are very important structures that predominantly prevent valgus and varus forces, respectively, through the knee (Fig. 1). As with other ligamentous injuries, knee collateral ligament sprains can be defined using three grades of injury. With a first-degree sprain, there is localized tenderness without frank instability. Anatomically, only a minimal number of fibers are torn. On physical examination, the joint space opens less than 5 mm (i.e., 1+ laxity). With a moderate, or second-degree sprain, there is more generalized tenderness without frank instability. Grade 2 sprains can cover the gamut from a few fibers torn to nearly all fibers torn. The joint may gap 5 to 10 mm (i.e., 2+ laxity) when force is applied. Finally, a severe or grade 3 sprain, by definition, is a complete disruption of all ligamentous fibers with the joint space gapping greater than 10 mm (i.e., 3+ laxity) upon stressing the ligament.[1]

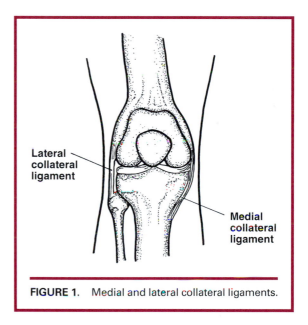

FIGURE 1. Medial and lateral collateral ligaments.

Medial Complex Injury and Resultant Instability

The medial collateral ligament (MCL) is the most commonly injured ligament of the knee.[2] Usually this ligament is injured when valgus forces are applied to the knee. Contact injuries often produce grade 3 MCL deficits, whereas noncontact MCL injuries typically result in lower-grade injuries. Although MCL injury can occur in isolation, valgus forces typically instigate injury to other medial structures.[3] Findings of a rotational component to medial joint instability should prompt a search for cruciate ligament injury or meniscal or posterior oblique ligament involvement.[4,5]

Lateral Complex Injury and Resultant Instability

The lateral collateral ligament (LCL) is much less commonly injured than the MCL. True isolated injury to the LCL is very rare. True straight lateral instability requires a large vector force. Thus, a complete knee dislocation with possible damage to neurovascular structures should be suspected if straight lateral instability is present.[6] Posterolateral rotatory instability appears to be a more common cause of lateral instability than straight lateral instability. Most authors feel that posterolateral rotatory instability requires disruption of the arcuate complex, posterior cruciate ligament, and the LCL. The mechanism of posterolateral rotatory instability usually occurs when the knee is forced into hyperextension and external rotation.[6,7]

Symptoms

Medial or lateral knee pain is the most common symptom related to knee collateral ligament injury. Interestingly, grade 1 and 2 injuries cause more pain than grade 3 injuries.[2,3] Pain is often accompanied by a sensation of knee locking.[5] This may be due to hamstring spasm or concomitant meniscal injury. Though more common with anterior cruciate ligament injuries, patients may also report an audible pop.[2] A give-way sensation or a feeling of instability is often reported with high-grade injuries. Moreover, patients with high-grade injuries may also have neurovascular damage.[8] Therefore, these individuals may complain of a loss of sensation or strength below the knee.[6]

Physical Examination

Physical examination begins with the uninjured knee to obtain a baseline. Palpatory examination can be as important as instability testing. Palpation can reveal tenderness along the length of the collateral ligament, localized swelling, or a tissue defect.[5] With pure joint line tenderness, an underlying meniscal injury should be suspected. A true knee joint effusion may also be present with collateral ligament injuries; however, it is more prevalent with meniscal or cruciate injury.[9]

Instability of the medial joint ligaments is determined by the *abduction stress test* (Fig. 2), performed by examining the knee at 0 and 30 degrees of joint flexion. If negative, a firm endpoint

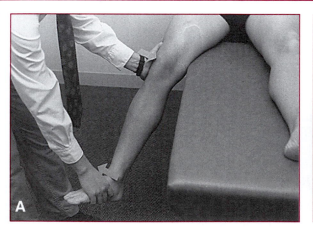
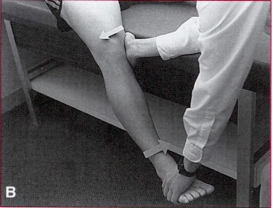

FIGURE 2. *A*, Abduction stress test of right knee at 30 degrees tests for medial collateral ligament injury. *B*, Adduction stress test of the knee at 30 degrees tests for lateral collateral ligament injury. (From Mellion MB, et al: The Team Physician's Handbook, 2nd ed. Philadelphia, Hanley & Belfus, 1997, pp 558–559, with permission.)

will be reached. If the test is grossly positive, the femur and tibia will gap with valgus stress and "clunk" back when the stress is removed.[10] Although controversial, increased medial joint laxity of the fully extended knee with a valgus force implies not only damage to the superficial and deep fibers of the MCL but also indicates rupture of the posterior cruciate ligament or posterior oblique ligament.[11,12] If laxity occurs at 30 degrees but not at 0 degrees, then one may confidently conclude that MCL injury is present with sparing of the posterior capsule and posterior cruciate ligament.[3,10] Although classically used for chronic anterior cruciate ligament tears, the anterior drawer test can be a useful adjunctive test for detecting MCL or posterior oblique ligament injury.[3]

Instability of the lateral knee joint ligaments is determined by the *adduction stress test* (which is also performed both at 0 and 30 degrees of knee flexion and compared with the opposite "normal" knee). Gapping of the lateral joint line at 30 degrees of knee flexion indicates damage to the LCL and arcuate ligament complex.[9,12] However, joint opening with the knee in full extension indicates damage not only to the LCL but also the middle third of the capsular ligament, cruciates, iliotibial band, and/or arcuate ligament complex.[7,13] When LCL injury is associated with rotational instability, the *reverse pivot shift* may be helpful.[14] This maneuver is performed by applying a varus force to an initially flexed knee. A positive

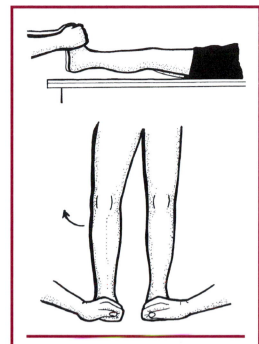

FIGURE 3. *External rotation recurvatum test.* Both knees are passively held in extension by holding the forefoot. If the tibia on the affected side externally rotates more than the normal side, the test is considered positive and indicates damage to posterolateral knee structures.

test reveals a "clunk" as the knee is passively extended from a flexed position. The "clunk" is a result of a subluxed knee in flexion, relocating with extension[8,12] Rotational instability may also be detected using the *external rotation recurvatum test* (Fig. 3).

Functional Limitations

The functional limitations for patients with both medial and lateral collateral ligament injuries occur as a result of instability. In general, sagittal plane movements are better tolerated than frontal or transverse plane motions. Most patients with grade 3 tears of the MCL are able to walk comfortably without an assistive device. Few, however, are able to traverse steps or do a full knee squat.[3] Patients may also report difficulty with transfers and "cutting" sports activities. Some individuals with posterolateral ligament injuries may have pain with prolonged standing or knee hyperextension. Eventually this posterolateral laxity may result in significant genu recurvatum as well as tibia vara, producing pain with even basic activities, such as walking or standing.[7]

Diagnostic Studies

Plain radiographs are usually normal in acute sprains of the collateral ligaments. X-rays may be particularly useful for detecting avulsion and tibial plateau fractures.[4] For example, an avulsion fracture of the proximal fibula can be detected after a varus-type injury—the so-called Segond fracture.[10] The current "gold standard" diagnostic test is MRI. MRIs can be useful to detect concomitant injury as well as the severity of collateral ligament damage.[15] Bone bruises not evident on plain films, may be detected utilizing MRI. This can be an important finding particularly in a patient who is experiencing persistent pain.

Differential Diagnosis

Medial knee pain:
- Medial meniscus injury
- ACL injury
- Medial compartment osteoarthritis
- Pes anserine bursitis
- Medial tibial plateau fracture
- Vastus medialis obliquus injury
- Medial plica band syndrome

Medial or lateral knee pain:
- Patella subluxation or dislocation
- Bone bruise
- Osteochondral injury
- Referred or radicular pain

Lateral knee pain:
- Lateral meniscus tear
- ITB syndrome
- Lateral compartment osteoarthritis
- Popliteus or biceps tendinitis
- Lateral gastrocnemius strain

Treatment

Initial

After determining whether concomitant injury is present, all grades of collateral ligament injuries are treated initially in the same manner. The basic principles of PRICE (pressure/protection, rest, ice, and elevation) apply. Patients with grade 2 and 3 injuries may need crutches and/or a hinged knee brace locked between 20 to 60 degrees to provide additional support for an unstable knee. Allowable brace range of motion (ROM) should be increased as tolerated to prevent arthrofibrosis.[4,9,16] Nonsteroidal anti-inflammatory medications may be prescribed to provide pain relief and reduce local inflammation associated with acute injury.

Rehabilitation

The goals of rehabilitation for the knee with a collateral ligament injury are to restore range of motion, increase stability, and return to pain-free activity. Within the first 24 to 48 hours after injury, static quadricep contractions and electrical stimulation can be instituted to reduce local tissue swelling and retard muscular atrophy.[10,16] ROM and gentle stretching activities are introduced after the first day.[4] Early weight bearing should also be encouraged. Aerobic conditioning can be maintained by utilizing upper body ergometry, stationary bicycle, or swimming with gentle flutter kicks. Maintenance phase rehabilitation should emphasize exercises in multiple planes. Rehabilitation should eventually progress to functional or sport-specific activity. A combination of closed and open kinetic chain exercises is utilized. Typically, individuals with mild collateral ligament injuries return to activity after 3 to 4 weeks, whereas patients with severe injuries typically return to activity after 8 to 12 weeks.[18] Prophylactic hinged knee brace use has been advocated, although its effectiveness remains controversial.[19–21]

Procedures

Procedures are not typically indicated in collateral ligament injuries.

Surgery

The treatment for grade 1 and 2 injuries of the medial and lateral collateral ligaments is nonsurgical. Grade 3 injuries, especially when associated with concomitant injuries, may be treated surgically. However, most clinics treat isolated grade 3 MCL injuries nonsurgically due to the high healing rates.[10,16,22,23]

Repair of an MCL tear without repair of an associated anterior cruciate ligament injury may lead to a high failure rate.[5] In contrast, grade 3 LCL injuries or posterolateral complex tears with or without associated cruciate ligament injuries have been shown to heal poorly with nonsurgical measures.[4,24,25] In this case, surgical intervention within 2 weeks, addressing deficits of the arcuate ligament complex, lateral meniscus, and cruciates, provides optimal outcomes.[4]

Potential Disease Complications

The most significant disease complication is chronic knee instability. This most commonly occurs with undetected injury to the posterolateral joint complex. Another cited complication is an increased risk of osteoarthritis. Osteoarthritis occurs more commonly with combined MCL and anterior cruciate ligament ruptures rather than with pure MCL injury.[26] Pellegrini-Steida disease may also be a rare complication. This condition consists of focal calcium deposition in the area of the injured ligament, typically on the femoral side of the MCL. Massage or manipulation may worsen this condition. Instead, calcium reabsorption may be stimulated by dry needling .[4,9]

Potential Treatment Complications

Analgesics, NSAIDs, and COX-2 inhibitors have well-known side effects that most commonly affect the gastric, hepatic, and renal systems. If the injured knee is immobilized for too long or if ROM does not proceed in an appropriate fashion, stiffness may result with possible loss of full extension. Similarly, if a surgeon reattaches the deep or superficial components of the MCL to the femoral condyle as opposed to the epicondyle, ankylosis of the joint may result, restricting flexion as well as extension.[5]

References

1. Committee on the Medical Aspects, American Medical Association: Standard nomenclature of athletic injuries. American Medical Association, 1968, pp 99–101.
2. Linton RC, Indelicato PA: Medial ligament injuries. In Delee JC, Drez D (eds): Orthopedic Sports Medicine Principles and Practice, vol. 2. Philadelphia: W.B. Saunders, 1994, pp 1261–1274.
3. Hughston JC, Andrews JR, Cross MJ, et al: Classification of knee ligament instabilities Part I. The medial compartment and cruciate ligaments. J Bone Joint Surg 1976;58A(2):159–172.
4. LaPrade R:. Medial ligament complex and the posterolateral aspect of the knee. In Arendt EA (ed): Orthopedic Knowledge Update. Rosemont, American Academy of Orthopedic Surgeons, 1999, pp 327–347.
5. Bocell JR: Medial collateral ligament injuries. In Baker CL (ed): The Hughston Clinic Sports Medicine Book. Media, PA, Williams & Wilkins, 1995, pp 516–525.
6. Jakob RP, Warner JP: Lateral and posterolateral rotatory instability of the knee. In Delee JC, Drez D (eds): Orthopedic Sports Medicine Principles and Practice, vol. 2. Philadelphia, W.B. Saunders, 1994, pp 1275–1312.
7. Hughston JC, Andrews JR, Cross MJ, et al: Classification of knee ligament instabilities. Part II. The lateral compartment. J Bone Joint Surg 1976;58A(2):173–183.
8. DeLee JC, Riley MB, Rockwood CA: Acute posterolateral rotatory instability of the knee. Am J Sports Med 1983;11:199–207.
9. Simon RR, Koenigsknecht SJ: The knee. In Simon RR, Koenigsknecht SJ (eds): Emergency Orthopedics, The Extremities. East Norwalk, Appleton and Lange, 1995, pp 437–462.
10. Reider B: Medial collateral ligament injuries in athletes. Sports Med 1996;21(2):147–156.
11. Swenson TM, Harner CD: Knee ligament and meniscal injuries: Current concepts. Orthop Clin North Am 1995;26(3):529–546.
12. Magee DJ: Knee. In Magee DJ (ed): Orthopedic Physical Examination, 2nd ed. Philadelphia, W.B. Saunders, 1992, pp 372–447.
13. Grood ES, Noyes FR, Butler DL, et al: Ligamentous and capsular restraints preventing straight medial and lateral laxity in intact human cadaver knees. J Bone Joint Surg 1981;63A(8):1257–1269.
14. LaPrade RF, Glenn TC: Injuries to the posterolateral aspect of the knee. Am J Sports Med 1997;25(4):433–438.
15. Stoller DW, Cannon, WD, Anderson LJ: The knee. In Stoller DW (ed): Magnetic Resonance Imaging in Orthopaedics and Sports Medicine, 2nd ed. Philadelphia, Lippincott, 1997, pp 203–442.
16. Richards DB, Kibler BW: Rehabilitation of knee injuries. In Kibler BW, Herring SA, Press JM (eds): Functional Rehabilitation of Sports and Musculoskeletal Injuries. Gaithersburg, Aspen, 1998, pp 244–253.
17. Shelbourne KD, Klootwyk TE, DeCarlo MS: Ligamentous injuries. In Griffin LY (ed): Rehabilitation of the Injured Knee, 2nd ed. St. Louis, Mosby, 1995, pp 149–164.
18. Brukner P, Kahn K: Acute knee injuries. In Brukner P, Kahn K (eds): Clinical Sports Medicine. New York, McGraw-Hill, 1997, pp 337–371.
19. Rovere GD, Haupt HA, Yates CS: Prophylactic knee bracing in college football. Am J Sports Med 1986;14:262–266.
20. Teitz CC, Hermanson BK, Kronmal RA, et al: Evaluation of the use of braces to prevent injury to the knee in collegiate football players, J Bone Joint Surg Am 1988;70A:422–427.
21. Hewson GF, Mendini RA, Wang JB: Prophylactic knee bracing in college football. Am J Sports Med 1986;14:262–266.
22. Indelicato PA: Non-operative treatment of complete tears of the medial collateral ligament ruptures. J Bone Joint Surg 1983;65A(3):323–329.
23. Reider B, Sathy MR, Talkington J, et al: Treatment of isolated medial collateral ligament injuries with early functional rehabilitation. A five-year follow-up study. Am J Sports Med 1994;22(4):470–477.
24. Kannus P: Nonoperative treatment of grade II and III sprains of the lateral ligament compartment of the knee. Am J Sports Med 1989;17(1):83–88.
25. LaPrade RF, Hamilton CD, Engebretson L: Treatment of acute and chronic combined anterior cruciate ligament and posterolateral knee ligament injuries. Sports Med Arth Rev 1997;5:91–99.
26. Lundberg M, Messner K: Ten-year prognosis of isolated and combined medial collateral ligament ruptures. Am J Sports Med;25(1):2–6.

61 Compartment Syndrome

Karen P. Barr, MD

Definition

Compartment syndrome is defined as an acute or chronic condition in which there is increased tissue pressure within an enclosed fascial space.

Acute Compartment Syndrome

Acute compartment syndrome, by definition, is a rapid rise in pressure caused by swelling of injured tissue. If the pressure is high enough and maintained long enough, decreased blood flow causes necrosis of the muscles and nerves in the involved compartment. If fasciotomy is not performed, patients may suffer contractures, foot drop, myoglobinuria, and kidney failure or gangrene, necessitating amputation.[3] Acute compartment syndrome is most commonly caused by a tibial fracture[4,5] and can occur in as many as 17% of these fractures.[5] It can also be caused by other forms of trauma, such as crush injuries, muscle ruptures, a direct blow to a muscle, or circumferential burns.[5]

Other causes of acute compartment syndrome are hemorrhage into a compartment, as can occur in anticoagulated patients; ischemia and then hyperperfusion caused by prolonged surgery in the lithotomy position (especially when Trendelenburg is added); and direct pressure, such as from a cast or antishock garment.[6]

Chronic Compartment Syndrome

In chronic compartment syndrome, the fascia in the lower leg does not accommodate to the increase in blood flow and fluid shifts that may occur with heavy exercise.[4] An increase in compartmental pressure can interfere with blood flow, leading to ischemia and pain.[7]

Symptoms

The area where symptoms occur depends on which compartment is involved.

Acute Compartment Syndrome

Patients may present with pain out of proportion to the injury and swelling or tenseness in the area. Other symptoms include severe pain with passive movement of the muscles within the compartment, loss of voluntary movement of the muscles involved, and sensory changes and paresthesias of the nerve involved.[4,5]

Chronic Compartment Syndrome

In chronic compartment syndrome, symptoms start gradually, usually with an increase in training or training on hard surfaces. The pain is described as aching, burning, or cramping and occurs with repetitive movements, most commonly running, but also with activities such as dancing, cycling, and hiking. The pain usually occurs around the same time each time the patient participates in the activity (e.g., after 15 minutes of running) and increases or stays constant if the activity continues. The pain disappears or dramatically lessens after a few minutes of rest.

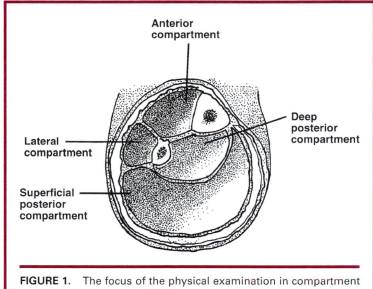

FIGURE 1. The focus of the physical examination in compartment syndrome is the anterior, lateral, superficial posterior and deep posterior compartments.

As symptoms progress, a dull aching pain may persist. Pain may be localized to a particular compartment, although often multiple compartments can be involved. Numbness and tingling may occur in the nerves that travel within the involved compartment. Chronic compartment syndrome can be seen with other overuse syndromes (e.g., concurrent with tibial stress fractures).

Physical Examination

The exam should be focused on the following four compartments of the leg (Fig. 1).

1. *Anterior compartment*—contains the tibialis anterior, which dorsiflex the ankle; long toe extensors, which dorsiflex the toes, the anterior tibial artery; and the deep peroneal nerve, which supplies sensation to the first web space.

2. *Lateral compartment*—contains the peroneus longus and brevis, which evert the foot, and the superficial peroneal nerve, which supplies sensation to the dorsum of the foot.

3. *Superficial posterior compartment*—contains the gastrocnemius and soleus muscles, which plantarflex the foot, and part of the sural nerve, which supplies sensation to the lateral foot and distal calf.[2,3,10]

4. *Deep posterior compartment*—contains the tibialis posterior, which plantarflexes and inverts the foot; long toe flexors, which plantarflex the toes; the peroneal artery; and the tibial nerve, which supplies sensation to the plantar surface of the foot. This compartment may contain several subcompartments.[11]

Acute Compartment Syndrome

In acute compartment syndrome, patients present with a swollen, tense leg. They have weakness or paralysis of the muscles involved in the affected compartment and numbness in the area supplied by the nerve involved in the affected compartment. Pulses and capillary refills are generally normal, as these are involved only with extremely high pressures.[4,5,8,9]

Chronic Compartment Syndrome

In chronic compartment syndrome, patients may have pain with palpation of the muscles involved or may be asymptomatic at rest. The compartment may feel firm. In approximately 40% of cases, muscle herniation in the compartment can be palpated, especially in the anterior and lateral compartments where the superficial peoneal nerve pierces the fascia.[12] In severe cases, numbness may occur in the area supplied by the nerve involved, but usually this is normal at rest.[4] The following types of weakness may be present: *dorsiflexion* weakness if the *anterior compartment* is involved, *foot eversion* weakness if the *lateral compartment* is involved, and *plantarflexion* weakness if one of the *posterior compartments* is involved.

Pain is reproduced by repetitive activity, such as toe raises, or running in place. Compartment syndrome occurs more commonly in patients who pronate during running, so pronation is a common finding on physical exam.[3,4,13]

Functional Limitations

Acute Compartment Syndrome

Functionally, the sequelae of new compartment syndrome may be foot drop, severe muscle weakness, and contractures—all of which can lead to abnormal gait and difficulties with activities of daily living.

Chronic Compartment Syndrome

With chronic compartment syndrome, functional limitations usually occur around the same point each time during exercise, at that individual's ischemic threshold. For example, runners may start to develop symptoms each time they reach the half-mile mark or cyclists may develop symptoms each time they climb a large hill.

Diagnostic Studies

The "gold standard" for diagnosis is compartmental tissue pressure measurements. Several different devices are available for this. The most common are the slit and wick catheters (Fig. 2).[4]

The following is one set of values[4,9] commonly used to diagnose *anterior compartment syndrome*:
- Pre-exercise pressure > 15 mm Hg
- 1 minute postexercise > 30 mm Hg
- 5 minutes postexercise > 20 mm Hg

Values for *posterior compartments* are more controversial. Normal resting pressures are less than 10 mm Hg, and values should return to resting levels after 1 to 2 minutes of exercise.[9]

It is important that the patient's symptoms correlate with the compartment in which there is elevated pressure. Pressure should increase in the symptomatic compartment with exercise and remain elevated for an abnormal period of time.[7,10]

Drawbacks to measuring pressures include the following:
- They are invasive and can be complicated by bleeding or infection.
- Because of the anatomy, it is more difficult to test the deep posterior compartment.
- Pressures are dependent on the position of the leg and the technique used, so strict standards should be followed.
- It is time consuming because each compartment must be tested separately, and all compartments should be tested because often multiple areas are involved.
- It is often difficult for patients to exercise with the catheter in place.[13,14]

Because of those drawbacks, alternative tests to confirm the diagnosis have been sought. The most promising is 201-thallium testing. The patient exercises to the point of symptoms, the thallium is injected, and exercise is continued for another minute. This is promising because it actually shows ischemia (as compared to pressure only), much as it has been used to show myocardial perfusion for many years. In small studies, this testing has been found to be both sensitive and specific and may be a good way to assess the patient because it is less invasive, readily available, and can be ordered without referring the patient to a specialist who does pressure measurements place.[3,13,14]

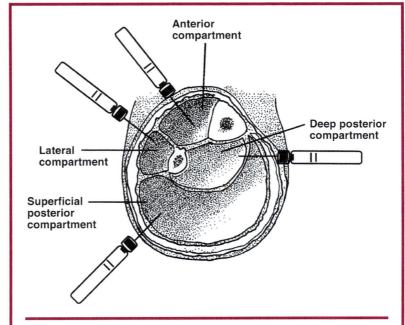

FIGURE 2. Compartmental tissue pressure measurements are the "gold standard" for diagnosis of compartment syndrome. The most common devices are the slit and wick catheters.

Acute Compartment Syndrome

For acute compartment syndrome, tissue pressures between 30 and 45 mm Hg are normally used as the cutoff to perform fasciotomy, although the exact number is controversial.[4] Normal pressure is less than 10 mm Hg.

Chronic Compartment Syndrome

For chronic compartment syndrome, pressures should be performed at rest, during, and after exercise. Interestingly, there does not seem to be a particular threshold compartmental pressure in which symptoms occur, and patients with higher pressures do not necessarily have worse symptoms than patients with lower-but-still abnormal pressures.[7]

MRI is currently not helpful for making this diagnosis, but further research is needed in this area, as proton density changes with ischemia, so specific protocols may be developed in the future. Ultrasound only shows the size of the muscles, so is not helpful.[2,3] Plain x-rays, bone scans and CT scans are useful only for ruling out other conditions.

Differential Diagnosis

Acute Compartment Syndrome
    Arterial occlusion
    Neuropraxia of the common, deep, or
      superficial peroneal or tibial nerve
    Deep venous thrombosis
    Cellulitis

Chronic Compartment Syndrome
    Stress fractures
    Shin splints

Treatment

Initial

Acute Compartment Syndrome

Initial treatment for acute compartment syndrome is surgery.

Chronic Compartment Syndrome

For chronic compartment syndrome, the initial treatment consists of rest, ice, and NSAIDs. Control of pronation with orthotics is important. The patient should be counseled to avoid running on hard surfaces and to wear running shoes with the appropriate amount of cushion and a flared heel.[4] Massage has been shown in small studies to be promising, but more research needs to be done in this area to see whether long-term significant changes can be made with either manual therapy or massage.[15]

Rehabilitation

Acute Compartment Syndrome

The rehabilitation of acute compartment syndrome is limited to the postfasciotomy stage. Rehabilitation depends on the extent of the injury. Proper skin care for either the open area left to close by secondary intent or skin grafts that have been applied is imperative. Often an ankle/foot orthosis to correct foot drop is needed. Physical therapy is needed for gentle range of motion to prevent contractures. Other measures include strengthening in muscles that may only be partially affected and gait training, possibly with an assistive device. If the patient has deficits in activities of daily living, such as dressing or transfers, occupational therapy may be helpful in addressing these areas.

Chronic Compartment Syndrome

The rehabilitation of chronic compartment syndrome has not been fully explored.

Because it is an overuse injury that is aggravated by pronation, rehabilitation focuses around establishing normal muscle lengths throughout the kinetic chain, especially lengthening the gastrocnemius and posterior tibialis, and strengthening the anterior tibialis.[15]

If fasciotomy is done for chronic compartment syndrome, postsurgical rehabilitation should follow. Weight bearing as tolerated and gentle range of motion are begun 1 to 2 days postoperatively. Strengthening and gradual return to activity begin at 1 to 2 weeks. Full return to activity, such as running, usually takes 8 to 12 weeks.[16]

Procedures

Procedures are not typically done in compartment syndrome except as stated earlier to measure compartmental pressures as a diagnostic procedure.

Surgery

Acute Compartment Syndrome

Fasciotomy should be performed for acute compartment syndrome as soon as possible. Large longitudinal incisions are made in the affected compartment. These incisions are left open to be closed gradually or split-thickness skin grafts are applied. Results of the surgery are variable and depend on the length of time of ischemia and other injuries involved.[17]

If treatment is delayed for more than 12 hours, it is assumed that permanent damage has occurred to the muscles and nerves in the involved compartment. Sometimes, patients are managed with supportive care: pain management, following renal status and monitoring fluids. This is because increased morbidity, especially infection and loss of limb, and increased mortality have been shown with delayed fasciotomy. Late reconstruction procedures can be done, if necessary, to correct muscle contractures or perform tendon transfers for foot drop.[17]

Chronic Compartment Syndrome

Fasciotomy is also the mainstay of surgical treatment for chronic compartment syndrome, and some authors state that there is a 100% failure rate with conservative treatment. This may be because the patient population that specialists see for this problem has already failed conservative management by the time the diagnosis is made. The average time from the onset of symptoms to the time that the diagnosis is made is 22 months.[4]

For chronic compartment syndrome, different techniques for fasciotomy have been described. Most consist of making a small incision in the skin and then releasing the fascia as far proximally and distally as possible while avoiding nerves and vessels.

Results of surgery are usually good, with average success rates of 80% to 90%.[16]

Potential Disease Complications

Acute Compartment Syndrome

In acute compartment syndrome, ischemia of less than 4 hours usually does not cause permanent damage. If ischemia lasts greater than 12 hours, severe damage is expected, including muscle necrosis, muscle contractures, loss of nerve function, infection, gangrene, myoglobinuria, and renal failure.[3–5] Recurrence has also been known to occur.[17] Calcific myonecrosis can also be a late side effect.[18]

Chronic Compartment Syndrome

Chronic compartment syndrome may cause some damage to the muscle and nerves, but this has not been definitively proven.

Potential Treatment Complications

Analgesics, NSAIDs, and COX-2 inhibitors have well-known side effects that most commonly affect the gastric, hepatic, and renal systems. Complication rates are about 11% to 13% from surgery and include bleeding, infection, nerve damage, or recurrence of pain. Recurrence of pain is usually secondary to an incorrect diagnosis, inadequate fasciotomy, or scarring.[12] In the case of the latter two, repeat decompression using fasciectomy is usually curative.[4]

References
1. Mabee RJ, Bostwick TL, et al: Pathophysiology and mechanisms of compartment syndrome. Orthop Rev 1993; 22:175–181.
2. Blackman P, et al: A review of chronic exertional compartment syndrome in the lower leg. Med Sci Sports Exerc 2000;32:S4–S10.
3. Swain R, Ross D, et al: Lower extremity compartment syndrome: When to suspect acute or chronic pressure buildup. Postgrad Med J 1999;105:159–168.
4. DeLee JC, Drez D, et al: Orthopaedic Sports Medicine: Principles and Practice, vol. 2. Philadelphia, W.B. Saunders, pp 1612–1619.
5. Gulli B, Templeman D, et al: Compartment Syndrome of the Lower Extremity. Orthopedic Clinic of America, 1994, pp 677–684.
6. Horgan AF, Geddes S, Jinlay IG, et al: Lloyd-Davies Position with Trendelenburg—A Disaster Waiting to Happen. United Kingdom, Deptartment of Coloproctology and Anestheisas, 1998, pp 916–920.
7. Mannarino F, Sexson S, et al: The Significance of Intracompartmental Pressures in the Diagnosis of Chronic Exertional Compartment Syndrome, vol. 12. Orthopedic Section, Wright State University, and Ports Medicine Center, 1989.
8. Mars M, Hadley GP, et al: Failure of pulse oximetry in the assessment of raised limb intracompartmental pressure. Kunjury 1994;25:379–381.

9. Mubarak SJ, Horgans AR, Owen CA, et al: The wick catheter technique for measurement of intramuscular pressure. A new research clinical tool. J Bone Joint Surg 1977;58A:1016–1102.

10. Styf JR, Korner LM, et al: Diagnosis of chronic anterior compartment syndrome in thelower leg. Acta Orthop Scand 1998;58:139–144 .

11. Cheney RA, Melaragno PG, Prayson MJ, et al: Anatomic investigation of the deep posterior compartment of the leg,foot and ankle. Foot Ankle Int 1998;2:98–101.

12. Detmar DE, Sharpe K, Sufit RL, et al: Chronic compartment syndrome: Diagnosis, management and outcomes. Am J Sports Med 1985;13:162–167.

13. Hayes A, Bower G, Pitstock K, et al: Chronic (exertional) compartment syndrome of the legs diagnosed with thallous chloride scintigraphy. J Nuclear Med 1995;36:1618–1624.

14. Takebayashi S, Takazawa H, Sasaki R, et al: Chronic exertional compartment syndrome in lower legs: Localization and follow-up with thallium-201 SPECT imaging. J Nuclear Med 1997;38:972–976.

15. Blackman PG, Simmons LR, Crossley KM, et al: Treatment of chronic exertional anterior compartment syndrome with massage: A pilot study. Clin J Sport Med 1998;8(1):14–17.

16. Schepsis AA, Sanjitpal SG, Foster, TA, et al: Fasciotomy for exertional anterior compartment syndrome: Is lateral compartment release necessary? Am J Sports Med 1999;27:430–435.

17. Finkelstein J, Hunter G, Hu R, et al: Lower limb compartment syndrome: Course after eelayed fasciotomy. J Trauma: Injury, Infection and Critical Care 1996;40:342–344.

17. Kotak PB, Bendall SP, et al: Recurrent acute compartment syndrome. Injury, Int J Care Injured 2000;31:66–67.

18. Synder BJ, Oliva A, Bencke H, et al: Calcific myonecrosis following compartment syndrome: Report of two cases, review of the literature, and recommendations for treatment. J Trauma: Injury, Infection, and Critical Care 1995;39:792–795.

62 Hamstring Strain

Anne Zeni, DO, PT
Erasmus G. Morfe, DO

Synonyms

Pulled hamstring

Torn hamstring

Hammy

Delayed onset muscle soreness (DOMS) of the posterior thigh

Stretch-induced injury to the hamstring

ICD-9 Code

843.9
Sprains and strains of hip and thigh, unspecified site

Definition

The hamstrings refer to the semimembraneous and semitendinosous muscles medially, and the long and short heads of the biceps femoris muscle laterally. Hamstring muscle strains are among the most common injuries in athletes and often occur due to an imbalance between the quadriceps and hamstring muscles (Fig. 1). These injuries are generally non-contact injuries that occur due to violent eccentric contraction of the muscle.

Hamstring strains constitute a range of injuries, from delayed onset muscle soreness to partial tears to complete rupture of the muscle.[1] Since the hamstrings cross two joints (hip and knee), they are at increased risk for an acute muscle strain injury. This typically occurs at the myotendinous junction during eccentric actions when the muscle lengthens while developing tension.[2] Injuries are most likely to occur at high running speeds. The higher the running speed, the less time in stance phase.[3] This shorter interval subjects the hamstrings to higher angular velocities and greater forces at heel strike.[4] Sprinters, wide receivers, and gymnasts running for a vault are particularly vulnerable to this type of injury. Complete avulsion of the proximal hamstring origin from the ischial tuberosity has been described

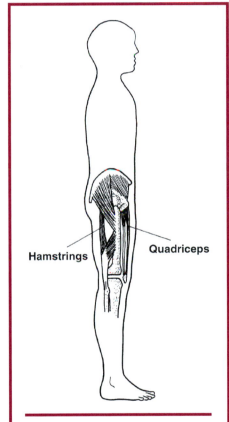

FIGURE 1. Tight hamstring muscles may lead to an imbalance between the quadriceps and hamstring muscles, placing an athlete at increased risk for injury.

in water skiers.[5] In these cases the patients sustained a forced hip flexion while the knee remained in complete extension type injury.

A common clinical presentation for a hamstring strain injury involves a single muscle, most commonly the long head of the biceps femoris.[1] More severe injuries may include more than one of the hamstring muscles, with complete ruptures occurring typically near the common origin at the ischial tuberosity. Hamstring strains are graded as follows:

1. *First degree:* Minimal muscle damage (less than 5% of muscle fiber disruption). There is associated pain, but no loss of strength.

2. *Second degree:* Incomplete muscle tear. Again, pain is present, but there is also loss of knee flexion strength.

3. *Third degree:* Complete muscle rupture, including avulsion injury of the ischial tuberosity. This injury presents with severe pain and marked loss of knee flexion strength.

Symptoms

At the time of injury, patients typically report a sudden, sharp pain in the back of the thigh. Some describe a "popping or tearing" sensation associated with severe pain. This is followed by tightness, weakness, and impaired range of motion. The patient may or may not be able to weight bear on the affected limb. Swelling and ecchymosis are variable and may be delayed for several days.

If the patient complains of symptoms of numbness, tingling, and distal weakness, further investigation into a sciatic nerve injury (rarely associated with complete tears) or lumbar disc herniation with a resultant S1 radiculopathy is warranted.

Physical Examination

The physical examination should begin with assessing gait abnormalities—including a shortened walking and running stride associated with a limp. Swelling and ecchymosis may not be detectable for several days after the initial injury, and the amount of bleeding depends on the severity of the strain. Unlike direct muscle contusions in which the ecchymosis remains confined to the muscle proper, the bleeding in a hamstring strain can escape through the ruptured fascia with resultant ecchymosis into interfascial and interstitial spaces.[6] This explains the common finding of ecchymosis, which may spread distal to the site of injury into the calf and ankle.

The posterior thigh should be inspected for atrophy, asymmetry, swelling, or ecchymosis. The entire length of the hamstrings should be palpated, including the proximal origin near the ischial tuberosity and distal insertions at the posterior knee. The presence of a palpable defect in the posterior thigh indicates a more severe injury with possible complete rupture of the muscle.

Active and passive range of motion of the hamstrings should be tested and compared with the contralateral side, with the hip at neutral in the supine position and flexed to 90 degrees in the sitting position. Deficits in knee and hip range of motion are common, and the point at which pain limits range of motion should be noted (Fig. 2). Concentric and eccentric muscle strength testing of the hamstrings should also be performed with the patient both sitting and prone. Weakness of knee flexion and hip extension is common. Asymmetry of the hamstrings can sometimes be accentuated with active resisted static muscle contraction. A soft tissue defect with distal bulging of the retracted muscle belly indicates a partial or complete rupture.

The neurologic exam should be normal except for strength testing of the hamstring group and in rare cases when there is an associated sciatic nerve injury. In these cases, there may be weakness, particularly notable in plantarflexion and loss of the affected Achilles reflex.

Functional Limitations

Depending on the severity of the injury, some patients may have no residual deficits. However, others may experience difficulty with walking or running, time lost from occupation, and delayed return to sports. Some patients may take up to 1 year to resume pre-injury activities, and in some cases of complete ruptures, never return to their previous level of function.[7]

Diagnostic Studies

The common hamstring strain usually requires no additional testing because the diagnosis is made by history and clinical exam. However, more severe cases may warrant diagnostic imaging. If the injury localizes near the origin of the hamstrings, plain x-rays may help identify irregularities of the ischial tuberosity; further findings on x-ray include bony avulsions and ectopic calcification.[1] MRI or CT may help determine the degree of injury by identifying a complete versus partial tear.

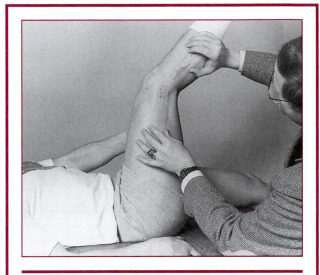

FIGURE 2. Measuring hamstring tightness. With the patient supine and hip flexed 90 degrees, the knee should extend fully if the hamstrings are flexible. If the knee will not extend completely, the residual knee flexion angle is measured and recorded as hamstring tightness. (From Mellion MB: Office Sports Medicine, 2nd ed. Philadelphia, Hanley & Belfus, 1996, p 275, with permission.)

Differential Diagnosis

S1 radiculopathy
Piriformis syndrome
Referred pain from sacroiliac
   joint or lumbar spine

Bony avulsion/apophysitis of the ischial tuberosity
Ischial bursitis (weaver's bottom)
Stress fracture in the pelvis, femoral neck, or femoral shaft
Adductor magnus strain

Treatment

Initial

Initial management of a hamstring strain consists of the PRICE principle (*p*rotection, *r*est, *i*ce, *c*ompression, and *e*levation). Relative rest and protection may involve weight bearing as tolerated or with higher-grade injuries (grades 2 and 3) cane or crutch walking. Ice massage as often as 20 minutes every 2 hours for the first 48 hours is indicated to limit the amount of pain and swelling. For high-grade injuries, taping or ACE-wrapping the thigh combined with elevation may help control edema and pain. NSAIDs/COX-2 inhibitors are commonly used to limit the inflammatory reaction and for pain control in the first few days. Soft tissue mobilization to the site of pain should be avoided for at least 5 days, since this may exacerbate the inflammatory response.

Rehabilitation

The elements of a hamstring rehabilitation program involve stretching, strengthening, and sports-specific activities. In the acute phase, pain-free range of motion should be achieved as soon as possible. To achieve a full stretch of the hamstring muscle, the hip must be flexed to 90 degrees

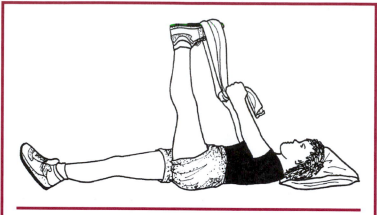

FIGURE 3. Stretching the hamstring fully requires the hip be at 90 degrees and the ankle dorsiflexed. However, forceful stretching should be avoided.

and the knee fully extended. This stretch is best achieved in the supine position; a towel can be used to facilitate hamstring lengthening (Fig. 3). It is also critical to improve flexibility throughout the spine and lower extremities.

Strengthening can begin when the patient is pain free. It is best to start with static contractions and progress to concentric, eccentric, and sports-specific activities as tolerated. Return to sport is allowed when motion is restored and pain free, strength is at least 90% of the uninjured side, and the hamstring/quadriceps strength ratio is symmetric.[3] Aerobic conditioning should be maintained throughout the rehabilitation process. Bicycling *without* toe clips (toe clips increase use of hamstrings), swimming, and upper body ergometry are recommended.

It is critical to educate patients about how to prevent recurrent hamstring injuries. This includes a good warmup period with stretching prior to engaging in sports. Full return to play must occur gradually because the risk of recurrent injury is high. Additionally, training errors, such as an abrupt switch to a hard surface or increase in training intensity, should be avoided.

Procedures

Procedures are not typically done in hamstring strain injuries.

Surgery

Routine hamstring strains do not require surgery and respond well to a conservative rehabilitation program. However, for complete hamstring avulsions from the ischial tuberosity, surgical repair may be appropriate. Treatment for hamstring strains associated with scarring around the sciatic nerves has been successful with surgical neurolysis.[8]

Potential Disease Complications

Complete hamstring tears may be associated with scar formation around the sciatic nerve in the proximal posterior thigh. Patients typically present with a dynamic foot drop and paresthesias in the lower extremity. Recurrent injury is not uncommon.

Potential Treatment Complications

NSAIDs are known to have gastrointestinal, renal, and liver side effects. COX-2 inhibitors may have fewer gastric side effects. Ultrasound therapy should be avoided in the acute treatment of high-degree strains, especially if hematoma formation is suspected because it may extend the hematoma.[9]

References

1. Kujala UM, Orava S, Järvinen M: Hamstring injuries: Current trends in treatment and prevention. Sports Med 1997;23(6):397–404.
2. Garrett WE: Muscle strain injuries. Am J Sports Med 1996;24(6):S2–S8.
3. Young JL, Laskowski ER, Rock M: Thigh injuries in athletes. Mayo Clin Proc 1993;68:1099–1106.
4. Agre JC: Hamstring injuries: proposed aetiological factors, prevention, and treatment. Sports Med 1985;2:21–33.
5. Blasier RB, Morawa LG: Complete rupture of the hamstring origin from a water skiing injury. Am J Sports Med 1990;18:435–437.
6. Best TM: Soft-tissue injuries and muscle tears. Clin Sports Med 1997;16(3):419–434.
7. Salley PI, Friedman RL, Coogan PG, et al: Hamstring muscle injuries among water skiers: Functional outcome and prevention. Am J Sports Med 1996;24(2):130–136.
8. Street CC, Burks RT: Chronic complete hamstring avulsion causing foot drop. Am J Sports Med 2000;28:1–3.
9. Cross MG, Vandersluis R, Wood D, Banff M: Surgical repair of chronic complete hamstring tendon rupture in the adult patient. Am J Sports Med 1998;26(6):785–788.

63 Iliotibial Band Syndrome

Venu Akuthota, MD
Sonja K. Stilp, MD
Paul Lento, MD

Synonyms

Iliotibial band friction syndrome

Iliotibial tract friction syndrome

Snapping hip

ICD-9 Code

719.65
Snapping hip

728.89
Iliotibial band syndrome

Definition

The iliotibial band (ITB) is a dense fascia on the lateral aspect of the knee and hip.[1] Traditionally, the gluteus maximus and tensor fascia lata were thought to be the proximal origin of the ITB. Further anatomic dissections have demonstrated that the gluteus medius also has direct and indirect contributions to the ITB (Fig. 1).[2] In the distal thigh, the ITB passes over the lateral femoral epicondyle and attaches to the Gerdy's tubercle of the anterolateral proximal tibia. The ITB also has aponeurotic connections to the patella and the vastus lateralis.[3] An anatomic pouch can be found underlying the posterior ITB at the level of the lateral femoral epicondyle. Controversy exists whether this pouch is a bursa, a synovial extension of the knee joint, or degenerative tissue.[4,5]

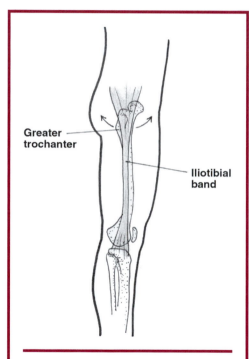

FIGURE 1. Anatomy of the iliotibial band, which can cause "snapping" as it slips anteriorly and posteriorly over the prominent greater trochanter.

Iliotibial band syndrome (ITBS) is an overuse injury that causes lateral knee and hip pain, typically a result of the ITB impinging over the lateral femoral epicondyle. The ITB passes over the lateral femoral epicondyle with knee flexion and extension. Maximum friction occurs when the posterior fibers of the ITB pass over the lateral femoral epicondyle at 20 to 30 degrees of knee flexion—the putative "impingement zone."

Friction has been implicated as the most important factor in ITBS.[6,7] As previously mentioned, friction is greatest in the impingement zone between 20 and 30 degrees of knee flexion. Repeated knee flexion and extension, particularly with increased running mileage per week, has been shown to predispose an individual to lateral knee pain.[8] Increased ground reaction force, as with running in old shoes, may also increase frictional forces.[6] Although not extensively studied, poor neuromuscular control appears to be an important *modifiable* risk factor for ITBS. Specifically, neuromuscular control is needed to attenuate the valgus/internal rotation vectors at the knee after heel strike. If appropriate control is not available, the ITB may have an abrupt increase in tension at its insertion site. Strengthening the gluteus medius and tensor fascia lata, decelerators of the valgus/internal rotation vectors at the knee, has been shown to ameliorate ITBS.[9] Lack of dynamic flexibility, particularly of the ITB, has been implicated with ITB injury susceptibility. Yet, no research study has revealed a correlation between ITB tightness and ITB injury. Theoretically, however, tightness of the ITB or its constituent muscles increases impingement of the ITB on the lateral femoral epicondyle.[6] Further risk factors, which may be attenuated with proper shoe wear or foot orthoses, include excessive foot/ankle pronation or supination.[8,10,11] Intrinsic or non-modifiable factors, such as bony malignment or a wide distal ITB, may also contribute to the development of ITBS. Finally, repeated direct trauma to the lateral knee, particularly with soccer goalies, appears to be injurious to the ITB impingement area.[12]

Symptoms

Symptoms of ITBS can emanate at three typical sites—at the proximal lateral hip, over the lateral femoral epicondyle, or at Gerdy's tubercle. Most commonly, individuals present with sharp or burning lateral knee pain that is aggravated during repetitive activity. This pain may radiate up into the lateral thigh or down to Gerdy's tubercle.[13] Runners often describe a specific, reproducible time when their symptoms commence.[14] Pain usually subsides after a run; however, in severe cases, persistent pain may cause restriction in distance.[15] Runners also note more pain with downhill running because of the increased time spent in the impingement zone.[6] Paradoxically, runners state that faster running and sprinting often does not produce pain. Fast running allows the athlete to spend more time in knee angles greater than 30 degrees.[6] Cyclists present with rhythmic, stabbing pain with pedaling. Specifically, they complain of pain at the end of their downstroke or the beginning of their upstroke. Bikers with improper saddle height and cleat position may experience greater symptoms.[16]

ITBS symptoms may also occur as a lateral snapping hip. An external or lateral snapping hip occurs as the iliotibial band rapidly passes anteriorly over the greater trochanter as the femur passes from extension to flexion.[17] Athletes, particularly dancers, sometimes experience an audible painful snap when landing in poor turnout (decreased external rotation at the hip) and with excessive anterior pelvic tilt.[18,19]

Physical Examination

Physical examination should begin with a screening examination of the joints above and below the site of injury. Hip girdle examination includes an assessment for joint range of motion, asymmetries,[20] muscle strength (particularly hip abductors),[9] and lumbopelvic somatic dysfunctions.[21] The modified Thomas and Ober tests are used to assess flexibility of the ITB and related musculature at the hip and knee (Figs. 2 and 3).[22,23]

The knee examination includes palpation, patellar accessory motion,[24] and the Noble compression test (Fig. 4).[7] Knee tenderness is noted either at the lateral femoral epicondyle (above the lateral joint line) or at Gerdy's tubercle. Palpatory examination should also include a thorough assessment for myofascial restrictions and trigger points along the lateral thigh musculature.[14] On rare occasion, ITB swelling and crepitus accompany tenderness. Pain can also be frequently elicited by the Noble compression test.[7] Other conditions are effectively ruled out by performing appropriate ligamentous or provocative maneuvers.

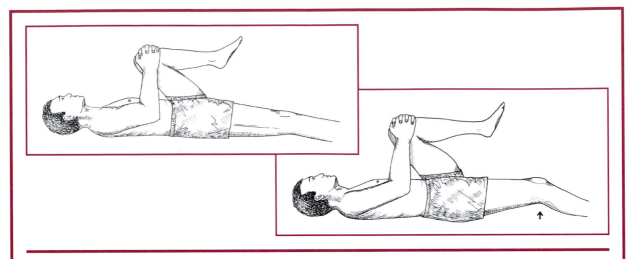

FIGURE 2. Thomas test. This test is used to assess a hip flexion contracture. The patient lies supine while the clinician flexes one of the patient's hips, bringing the knee to the chest to flatten the lumbar spine. The patient holds the flexed knee and hip against the chest. If there is a flexion contracture of the hip, the patient's other leg will rise off the table.

The foot and ankle examination is particularly useful in the determination of gastrocsoleus inflexibility, subtalar motion restrictions and specific foot type (e.g., hindfoot varus). Finally, a biomechanical assessment of sports-specific activity can be done. Walkers and runners are observed for abnormalities such as excessive foot/ankle pronation, inability to attenuate shock at the knee, Trendelenburg frontal plane gait at the pelvis, and forward trunk lean. Bicyclers are observed for proper foot placement on the pedal, saddle height, and knee angles with pedaling revolution.[16] Dancers can be observed performing *rond de jambe* or *grand plie* for proper turnout and pelvic stabilization.[18]

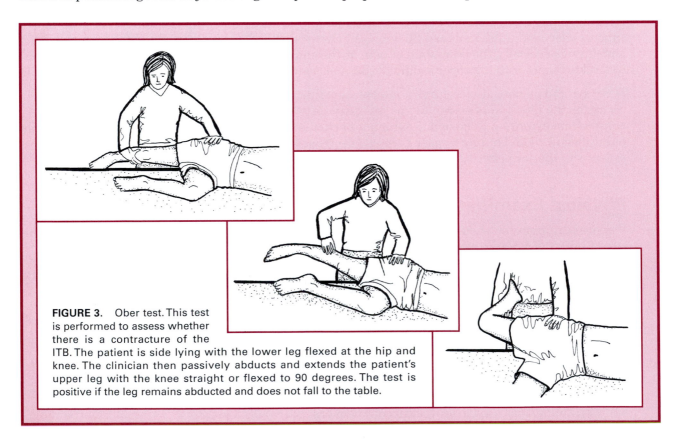

FIGURE 3. Ober test. This test is performed to assess whether there is a contracture of the ITB. The patient is side lying with the lower leg flexed at the hip and knee. The clinician then passively abducts and extends the patient's upper leg with the knee straight or flexed to 90 degrees. The test is positive if the leg remains abducted and does not fall to the table.

Neurologic examination including strength, sensation, and reflexes is typically normal. Strength may be affected by disuse or guarding due to pain—particularly in the hip abductors and external rotators.

Functional Limitations

ITBS pain usually restricts athletes from their sports activity but does not typically cause limitations of daily activities. Yet, a vicious cycle is set forth in which biomechanical deficits (e.g., gluteal weakness and ITB tightness) cause ITB tissue injury with resultant functional adaptions to avoid the pain of the tissue injury (e.g., externally rotating the hip).[20]

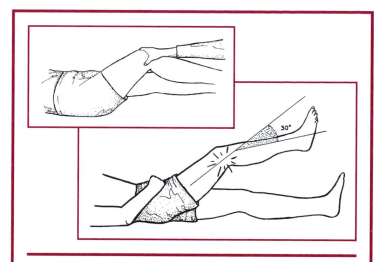

FIGURE 4. Noble compression test. This test is used to determine whether there is ITB friction at the knee. The patient lies supine and the knee is flexed to 90 degrees (the hip flexes as well). The clinician then applies pressure with the thumb at the lateral femoral epicondyle while the patient slowly extends the knee. The test is positive if the patient complains of severe pain over the lateral femoral epicondyle at 30 degrees.

Diagnostic Studies

Imaging has a limited role in ITBS. X-rays are rarely helpful. Diagnostic ultrasound has been used in some centers to confirm injuries.[25] When definitive diagnosis is needed or other diagnoses need to be excluded, MRI has emerged as a potentially useful test.[26] MRI may show a thickened ITB and/or high intensity on axial T2-weighted images.[26,27]

Differential Diagnosis

Hip joint pathology
Meralgia paresthetica
Trochanteric bursitis
Internal snapping hip
Referred/radicular pain from
   lumbar spine
Primary myofascial pain

Popliteus tendinitis
Lateral collateral ligament injury
Lateral hamstring strain
Lateral meniscus tear
Patellofemoral pain
Common peroneal nerve injury
Fabella syndrome
Lateral plica
Stress fracture
Primary myofascial pain

Treatment

Initial

Acute phase treatment is akin to that of other musculoskeletal injuries. Relative rest is more appropriately defined as activity modification. In most instances, this does not mean a complete cessation of activity. The clinician needs to emphasize the positive aspects of relative rest and provide alternative training regimens. ITB can be relatively off-loaded if an individual can keep his or her activity below the threshold of pain. Frequently, this can be achieved by simply decreasing intensity or training duration. Medications such as NSAIDs/COX-2 inhibitors may help to reduce pain and inflammation in the first few weeks of injury. If swelling is present, some authors advocate a local corticosteroid injection in the initial stages.[14] As well, modalities such as ice massage can be helpful in the early period.

It is critical early on to address the biomechanical cause of ITB injury.

Rehabilitation

Ultrasound, phonophoresis, and electric stimulation may also be used to reduce early inflammation and pain.

The subacute phase of rehabilitation addresses the biomechanical deficits found on physical examination. Typically, flexibility deficits are seen in the ITB, iliopsoas, quadriceps, and gastrocsoleus.[14] Proper stretching addresses all three planes and incorporates proximal and distal musculotendinous fibers. Some muscle groups do not respond to stretch unless myofascial and joint restrictions are concomitantly addressed by experienced therapists or by self-administered techniques.[14] Proper facilitation of hip girdle musculature can be achieved be addressing antagonistic tight structures, such as tight hip flexors or anterior hip capsule.[28] Subtalar mobilizations are often needed to prevent excessive valgus/internal rotation forces from transferring to the knee and ITB.[29] In conjunction with a flexibility and joint mobilization program, strengthening of weak or inhibited muscles can be started. Strengthening regimens ultimately need to move away from the plinth to more functional activities such as single squats and lunges with an emphasis on proper pelvic/core stabilization.

Finally, the maintenance phase focuses on returning patients to their respective activity with confidence in their functional ability. In this phase, athletes are ideally observed or videotaped in their sporting environment. Frequently, runners have form deviations that lead to a sine qua non of uncontrolled valgus/internal rotation of the knee. These abnormalities include excessive pronation, inability to shock attenuate at the knee, and Trendelenburg frontal plane gait at the pelvis. Changing to shock-absorbing or motion-control shoes respectively can accommodate supination and overpronation.[30] Foot orthoses have also been advocated for runners with lower limb injuries. Their benefit is as yet empirical. Cyclists can often correct their ITB problems with equipment and bicycle adjustments.[13] Dancers, performing *rond de jambe* or *grand plie*, can be cued on maintaining turnout and neutral pelvic position.[28] After sports-specific adjustments have been made, athletes need to be reintroduced to activity gradually and individually.

Procedures

Corticosteroid injections may be performed at different locations along the ITB. Directing the injection into the anatomic pouch at the lateral femoral epicondyle is a relatively simple procedure and is advocated for patients with persistent pain and swelling.[14] A mixture of anesthetic (e.g., 1 cc of 1% lidocaine) and long-acting steroid (e.g., 1 cc of betamethasone) is instilled to the affected site. Steroid injections should be repeated only if adequate relief is obtained after the initial injection. Patients can return to play as their pain allows.

Surgery

Surgical treatment for ITBS is rarely needed. Surgery involves either excising the posterior half of the ITB where it passes over the lateral femoral epicondyle or removing the underlying putative bursa.[31] These procedures appear to have mixed results and should be contemplated only for patients who have exhausted all other options, including a comprehensive rehabilitation program as previously outlined.

Potential Disease Complications

If ITBS is not properly addressed, biomechanical adaptions can occur.[20] Chronic pain leading to progressive disability is a potential complication.

Potential Treatment Complications

Rehabilitation complications are rare. NSAID use for a short course does not lead to many long-term sequela. However, patients may commonly complain of gastrointestinal distress. COX-2 inhibitors may cause fewer gastric side effects. Corticosteroid injections have a plethora of potential complications including infection, depigmentation of skin, and flare of symptoms at the site of injection. Surgical procedures for ITBS carry inherent risks. Postoperative infection and other standard risks should be explained to patients prior to surgical interventions. Overall, interventional procedures toward the ITB carry few risks or complications.

References

1. Porterfield J, DeRosa C: Mechanical Low Back Pain: Perspectives in Functional Anatomy, 2nd ed. Philadelphia, W.B. Saunders, 1998.
2. Gottschalk F, Kourosh S, Leveau B: The functional anatomy of tensor fasciae latae and gluteus medius and minimus. J Anat 1989;166:179–189.
3. Terry GC, Hughston JC, Norwood LA: The anatomy of the iliopatellar band and iliotibial tract. Am J Sports Med 1986;14(1):39–45.
4. Nemeth WC, Sanders BL: The lateral synovial recess of the knee: anatomy and role in chronic Iliotibial band friction syndrome. Arthroscopy 1996;12(5): 574–580.
6. Orchard, JW, et al: Biomechanics of iliotibial band friction syndrome in runners. Am J Sports Med 1996;24(3):375–379.
7. Noble CA: The treatment of iliotibial band friction syndrome. Br J Sports Med 1979;13(2):51–54.
8. Messier SP, et al: Etiology of iliotibial band friction syndrome in distance runners. Med Sci Sports Exerc 1995;27(7): 951–960.
9. Fredericson M, et al: Hip abductor weakness in distance runners with iliotibial band syndrome. Clin J Sport Med 2000;10(3):169–175.
10. James SL: Running injuries to the knee. J Am Acad Orthop Surg 1995;3(6):309–318.
11. Schwellnus MP: Lower limb biomechanics in runners with iliotibial band friction syndrome, abstracted. Med Sci Sports Exerc 1993;25(5):S68.
12. Xethalis J, Lorei M: Soccer injuries In Nicholas J, Hershman E (eds): The Lower Extremity and Spine in Sports Medicine. Mosby, St Louis, 1995, pp 1509–1557.
13. Holmes J, Pruitt A, Whalen N: Cycling injuries. In Nicholas J, Hershman E (eds): The Lower Extremity and Spine in Sports Medicine. 1995, Mosby, St Louis, 1995, pp 1559–1579.
14. Fredericson M, Guillet M, DeBenedictis L: Quick solutions for iliotibial band syndrome. Physician and Sportsmedicine 2000;28(2):53–68.
15. Lindenberg G, Pinshaw R, Noakes T: Iliotibial band friction syndrome in runners. The Physician and Sportsmedicine 1984;12(5):118–130.
16. Holmes JC, Pruitt AL, Whalen NJ: Lower extremity overuse in bicycling. Clin Sports Med 1994;13(1):187–205.
17. Allen WC, Cope R: Coxa saltans: The snapping hip revisited. J Am Acad Orthop Surg 1995;3(5):303–308.
18. Khan K, et al: Overuse injuries in classical ballet. Sports Med 1995;19(5):341–357.
19. Sammarco GJ: Dance injuries. In Nicholas J, Hershman E (eds): The Lower Extremity and Spine in Sports Medicine. Mosby, St Louis, 1995, pp 1385–1410.
20. Press J, Herring S, Kibler W: Rehabilitation of the combatant with musculoskeletal disorders. In Dillingham T, Belandres P (eds): Rehabilitation of the Injured Combatant. Washington, DC, 1999, Office of the Surgeon General, 1999, pp 353–415.
21. Greenman P: Principles of Manual Medicine, 2nd ed. Baltimore, Williams & Wilkins, 1996.
22. Geraci M, Alleva J: Physical examination of the spine and its functional kinetic chain. In Cole A, Harring S (eds): The Low Back Pain Handbook. Philadelphia, Hanley & Belfus, 1996.
23. Kendall F, McCreary E, Provance P: Muscles Testing and Function, 4th ed. Baltimore, Williams & Wilkins, 1993.
24. Puniello MS: Iliotibial band tightness and medial patellar glide in patients with patellofemoral dysfunction. J Orthop Sports Phys Ther 1993;17(3):144–148.
25. Martens M, Libbrecht P, Burssens A: Surgical treatment of the iliotibial band friction syndrome. Am J Sports Med 1989;17(5): 651–654.
26. Bergman AG, Fredericson M: MR imaging of stress reactions, muscle injuries, and other overuse injuries in runners. Magn Reson Imaging Clin North Am 1999;7(1):151–174, ix.
27. Ekman EF, et al: Magnetic resonance imaging of iliotibial band syndrome. Am J Sports Med 1994;22(6):851–854.
28. Geraci M: Rehabilitation of the hip, pelvis, and thigh. In Kibler W, Herring S, Press J (eds): Functional Rehabilitation of Sports and Musculoskeletal Injuries. Gaithersburg, MD, Aspen, 1998.
29. Gray G: Chain reaction festival. Adrian, MI, Wynn Marketing, 1999.
30. Barber FA, Sutker AN: Iliotibial band syndrome. Sports Med 1992;14(2):144–148.
31. Drogset JO, IRossvoll I, Grontvedt T: Surgical treatment of iliotibial band friction syndrome. A retrospective study of 45 patients. Scand J Med Sci Sports 1999;9(5):296–298.

64 Knee Arthritis

Ashok N. Nimgade, MD, MPH
Edward M. Phillips, MD

Synonyms

Degenerative joint
disease (DJD) of the knee
joint

Degenerative arthritis

Joint destruction of the
knee

Osteoarthrosis

ICD-9 Codes

715.16
Osteoarthrosis, localized,
primary, lower leg

715.26
Osteoarthrosis, localized,
secondary, lower leg

716.16
Traumatic arthropathy,
lower leg

Definition

More than 20 million Americans[1] have *osteoarthritis* (OA), the leading
cause of disability in the United States. For these individuals, the knee is
the body part most commonly involved by OA. Knee OA results from
mechanical and idiopathic factors that alter the balance between
degradation and synthesis of articular cartilage and subchondral bone. The
disease characteristically involves axial and peripheral joints.

OA can involve any of the three major knee compartments: medial,
patellofemoral, or lateral. The medial compartment is most often involved
and quite often leads to medial joint space collapse and thus to a genu
varum (bowleg) deformity. Lateral compartment involvement may lead to a
genu valgum (knock-knee) deformity. Arthritis in one compartment might,
through altered biomechanical stress patterns, eventually lead to
involvement of another compartment.

The prevalence of OA increases with age, usually affecting people older than
55 years. OA can derive from a long-term response to cumulative trauma
to the knee over a period of years or decades. Obesity and a positive family
history are often associated with OA. While the role of physical activity and
sports in OA has been long debated, it appears that low-to-moderate levels
of sporting activity are not associated with increased risk for OA, but high
levels[2] of sports, such as running more than 20 miles per week, may be
associated with OA. The type of sporting activity may also make a difference;
one retrospective study,[3] for example, found increased OA in men with a
high level of exposure to contact sports, such as soccer and hockey. This
association was attributed to acute, direct joint impact from contact with
other participants, playing surfaces, and equipment. There was no
association with recreational jogging, which actually seemed protective.

Osteoarthritis can open a Pandora's box of pain generators for the patient.
Associated changes leading to pain include pseudogout,
microfractures/subchondral fractures, chondromalacia patellae, bursitis
(pes anserine or prepatellar), and periosteal elevation by spurring.

Symptoms

Knee OA is characterized by joint pain; tenderness; decreased range of
motion; crepitus; occasional effusion; and often, inflammation of varying

degrees. Initial OA symptoms are generally minimal, given the gradual and insidious onset of the condition. Pain typically occurs in the affected region, particularly during weight bearing, and decreases with rest. But with progression of the disease, pain can even persist at rest. Patients often report higher pain levels in the morning, but usually for less than 30 minutes. Barometric changes such as those associated with damp, rainy weather will often increase pain intensity.

Pain may also radiate to adjacent sites as OA indirectly alters the biomechanics of other anatomic structures. These include: ligaments (e.g., laxity of overstretched collateral ligaments), muscles (e.g., from spasm or from compensatory overuse), nerves, and even veins.

Patients often experience limitation of movement because of joint stiffness or swelling. Many patients report a "locking" or a "catching" sensation, which is likely due to a variety of causes, including debris from degenerated cartilage or meniscus in the joint, increased adhesiveness of the relatively rough articular surfaces, or even tissue inflammation. Joint stiffness may occur after periods of inactivity, such as after awakening in the morning. Stiffness can discourage mobility, thus starting a vicious cycle that culminates in deconditioning; decreased function; and, paradoxically, even increased pain.

Physical Examination

The entire quadrant from the hip to the ankle should be examined. It is important to identify findings such as quadriceps weakness or atrophy and knee flexion contractures. Gait should be observed for presence of a limp, functional limb-length discrepancy, or buckling. Genu varum or valgum is often better appreciated when the patient is standing.

The affected knee should be compared with the contralateral uninvolved knee. Knee exam may reveal decreased knee extension or flexion secondary to effusion or osteophytes (both of which may be palpable). Osteophytes along the femoral condyles may be palpated, especially along the medial distal femur. Palpation may reveal patellar or parapatellar tenderness. Crepitation, resulting from juxtaposition of roughened cartilage surfaces, may be appreciated along the joint line when the knee is flexed or extended. A mild effusion and tenderness may be appreciated along the medial joint line or at the pes anserine bursa. Ligament testing may reveal laxity of one or both of the collateral ligaments. Lateral subluxation of the patella may be found in patients with genu valgum.

The neurologic examination is typically normal with the exception of decreased strength, particularly in the quadriceps, due to disuse or guarding due to pain.

Functional Limitations

Joint stiffness and pain during weight bearing lead directly to difficulties with prolonged standing, transfers, and walking. Involvement of the patellofemoral compartment may lead to difficulty with climbing stairs, as well as to a buckling sensation. Disability is further compounded by secondary factors such as depression, poor aerobic capacity, and co-existing chronic conditions.[4] Radiographic evidence of knee OA, even without symptoms, increases the risk for dependence with activities of daily living.[5] The risk of dependence with stairclimbing and walking attributed to knee OA is comparable to that with cardiovascular disease and greater than any other medical condition in elders.[6]

Diagnostic Studies

Radiographic evidence of osteoarthritis is not well correlated with symptoms.[7] Note that osteophytes *alone* are associated with aging, rather than with OA. Indications for plain x-ray films include trauma, effusion, symptoms not readily explainable by physical exam findings, severe pain, presurgical planning, and failure of conservative management. Recommended films are

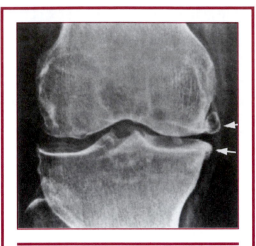

FIGURE 1. Knee radiograph demonstrating osteophytes (*arrows*) and medial joint space narrowing consistent with degenerative arthritis. (From West SG, et al: Rheumatology Secrets. Philadelphia, Hanley & Belfus, 1997, p 58, with permission.)

weight-bearing (standing) AP, lateral, and patellar views. X-ray films taken during weight bearing with the knee in full extension and partial flexion may reveal a constellation of findings associated with OA, including asymmetric narrowing of the joint space (typically medial compartment), osteophytes, sclerosis, and subchondral cysts (Fig. 1). A Merchant's view specifically evaluates the patellofemoral space. Non–weight-bearing lateral views may help in the evaluation of the patellofemoral and tibiofemoral joint spaces. Tunnel views can help visualize loose osteochondral bodies. MRI usually adds little but cost to the entire evaluation.

Lab testing is typically normal, but may be undertaken especially for elder patients for establishing a baseline (e.g., BUN, creatinine, or liver function tests prior to NSAIDs or acetaminophen use) or for excluding other conditions such as rheumatoid arthritis. Synovial fluid analysis should not be undertaken unless suspicion for destructive, crystalline, or septic arthritis exists.

Differential Diagnosis

Osteonecrosis of femur or tibia

Bursitis

Meniscal tear

Primary hip or ankle pathology

Lyme disease

Tendinitis

Midlumbar radiculopathy

Septic arthritis

Tumor

Treatment

Initial

The *PRICE* regimen may help provide initial relief for patients in pain: *p*rotection with limited weight bearing by using a cane or modifying exercise to reduce stress; relative *r*est (or taking adequate rests throughout the day, avoiding prolonged standing, climbing stairs, kneeling, deep knee bending); *i*ce (applied while protecting the skin with a towel for up to 15 minutes at a time several times a day; note, however, that some patients with chronic pain may find better relief with moist heat); *c*ompression (if swelling exists, ACE wrapping or a sleeve may help); and *e*levation (may help diminish swelling, if present).

Acetaminophen may provide pain relief for many patients and is an appropriate initial pharmacologic treatment. NSAIDs can perhaps prevent degenerative changes such as chondromalacia but might worsen the osteoarthritic process.[8] Selective COX-2 inhibitors provide comparable pain relief as NSAIDs[9] with potentially fewer side effects and may therefore be kept in mind for elderly patients or those with GI considerations. Capsaicin ointment may provide relief in some patients. Assistive devices such as a walker or a cane held in the contralateral hand can help maintain function, especially in patients with a history of falls or gait deviations. If pain persists even at rest, then less conservative measures should be considered.

Nutritional intervention may include supplementation with glucosamine sulfate (1500 mg po qd) and chondroitin sulfate (1200 mg po qd) in divided doses. Glucosamine was found to have symptom modifying and potentially disease modifying effects on knee OA.[10] Vitamin C as an antioxidant was associated with reduced progression of radiographic osteoarthritis and pain in one study.[11] Even moderate weight loss can dramatically reduce the risk of knee OA.[12]

Rehabilitation

Randomized studies indicate the benefits of exercise, even if home-based, on pain and function in patients with OA.[13] Attempts to maintain function can be helped through non–weight-bearing strengthening, especially of the quadriceps; for patients with greater pain, this can be done with static exercise or through water aerobics, which allows for motion at the knee with reduced joint loads. Exercise bicycles and walking should be recommended. Deep knee bends in the presence of effusions should be avoided. Particular attention must be paid to strengthening the medial quadriceps in patients with genu valgum who have lateral subluxation of the patella. Exercise load should be increased gradually: by 10% per week with the goal of almost daily exercise of 1 hour or more each day. Maintaining activity is critical to maintaining function. Even those patients scheduled for total knee arthroplasty should pursue static and dynamic strengthening as well as cardiovascular conditioning to ease the postoperative rehabilitation.

Supervised therapy should restore strength, range of motion, and function and also address pain relief. Physical therapists may use additional therapeutic modalities such as electrical stimulation or massage. Therapists may also review postural alignment and joint positioning techniques, especially for when the patient is sleeping. In particular, the use of a pillow under bent knees, much favored by many patients when supine, should be avoided since resulting knee flexion contractures, even if small, can significantly increase stresses on the knee during gait. Stretching of the hamstrings and quadriceps may also prove beneficial. Patients should be counseled against prolonged wearing of high heels, which is associated with medial knee osteoarthritis.[14] Knee deformity can be corrected through addition of shoe wedges (medial for valgum; lateral for varum). Heel lifts or built-up shoes may be required in the presence of leg-length discrepancy to prevent compensatory knee flexion gait on the longer side. In the presence of knee deformity, therapists can also evaluate for the presence of altered biomechanics (e.g., genu varum may lead to femoral internal torsion, resulting in compensatory external rotation of the tibia, which predisposes the patient to increased arthritic changes). Therapists can also visit patient homes and workplaces to suggest adjustments such as raised toilet seats, grab bars, reachers, etc.

Procedures

Intra-articular corticosteroid injections (e.g., 20 to 40 mg methylprednisolone) may prove helpful in reducing local inflammation (Fig. 2). These should be given no more than 2 or 3 times a year to reduce potential damage to cartilage from the steroids. Administration of steroids through *iontophoresis* may be an alternative for patients hesitant to undergo injections. Patients may also be referred for acupuncture. Viscosupplementation with hyaluronic acid available as naturally occurring hyaluronan or synthetic hylan G-F 20 may be helpful. Hyaluronan is administered in a series of five weekly injections, whereas the hylan G-F 20 is given in three weekly injections. One randomized, blinded comparison study[15] indicated better results on all outcome measures for hylan G-F 20. The entire series of injections can be repeated in 6 months, if necessary, for further amelioration of pain. The hyaluronic acid is injected into the knee in the same manner as the intra-articular steroid is administered.

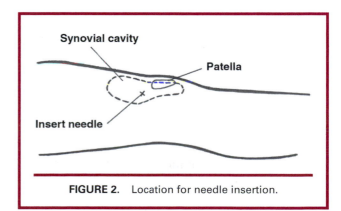

FIGURE 2. Location for needle insertion.

With the patient supine, under sterile conditions using a 25-gauge needle, inject 2 to 3 cc of local anesthetic (e.g., 1% lidocaine) just posterior to the upper lateral pole of the patella. Alternatively, ethyl chloride spray can be used. Then, using a 1½-inch 22- to 25-gauge needle, inject either local steroid (e.g., 20 to 40 mg methylprednisolone) or hyaluronic acid in the same region (these products are available in 2 ml vials or prefilled syringes—one injection per vial).

If a knee effusion exists, it may be necessary to drain the effusion to avoid dilution of the medications. This is ideally done with an 18- to 20-gauge needle. The needle can remain in place, and then switching the syringes to inject the medication prevents additional trauma.

Postinjection care should include local icing for 5 to 10 minutes. Patients are advised to avoid excessive weight bearing for 24 to 48 hours after an injection.

Surgery

Arthroscopic debridement may provide pain relief in patients with internal derangements, such as presence of loose bodies or articular surface irregularities. But with success rates of about 50%—far less than that for replacement surgery—arthroscopy is often viewed as a temporary measure. *Total knee replacements*, with a quarter century track record, have generally provided most patients with good pain relief (see Chapter 74). While joint replacement surgery has been found in numerous studies to provide pain relief, it paradoxically may lead to increase of services as patients become more mobile.[16] *Osteotomy* is a less drastic measure than knee replacement and is often favored by younger active patients with unicompartmental symptoms. In osteotomy, a wedge-shaped piece of bone is removed from either the femur or tibia to bring the knee joint back into a more physiologic alignment; mechanical stress in the diseased compartment is thus reduced and patients can resume an active lifestyle until OA progression may necessitate total knee replacement. Patients with severe chondromalacia may necessitate patellectomy (patella excision). Knee *arthrodesis* today is generally reserved for patients in whom knee replacement surgery fails. Other less commonly utilized surgical options such as synovectomy or small prostheses (to correct deformity) are also possible.

Potential Disease Complications

Progressive knee osteoarthritis may result in reduced mobility and the general systemic complications of immobility and deconditioning. Antalgic gait can result in contralateral hip pathology (e.g., greater trochanteric bursitis). The risk of falls will be increased by decreased mobility at the knee. Complaints of chronic pain may result from the initial knee osteoarthritis if inadequately treated.

Potential Treatment Complications

Complications of anti-inflammatory mediation and steroid injections are well known. Repeated steroid injections can lead to further cartilage destruction as well as sepsis. Infection is a rare but possible result of joint injection or surgery. Cryotherapy or heat therapy can, of course, lead to frostbite or burns. Hyaluronic acid injections may result in localized transient pain or effusion.

Arthroscopy may damage the articular surface membrane, thus initiating damage to uninvolved cartilage. Excessive arthroscopic scraping has sometimes been associated with persistent pain. The possibility of infection and deep venous thrombosis and the small-but-real possibility of intraoperative mortality limit the use of surgery to a last line option. One series of patients *not* taking anticoagulants experienced a 50% rate of proximal deep venous thrombosis (DVT), 14.5% of which was proximal DVT,[17] thus indicating the importance of anticoagulation, which reduces the risk to less than 5%. In any case, mechanical wear and prosthesis loosening, especially for cement prostheses, often lead to the need for revision after a decade or so.

References

1. Centers for Disease Control and Prevention. Targeting arthritis: The nation's leading cause of disability. At-A-Glance, 1999. www.cdc.gov/nccdphp/art-aag.htm.
2. Cheng Y, Macera CA, Davis DR, et al: Physical activity and self-reported, physician-diagnosed osteoarthritis: Is physical activity a risk factor? J Clin Epidemiol 2000;53(3):315–322.
3. Sandmark H, Vingard E: Sports and risk for severe osteoarthritis of the knee. Scand J Med Sci Sports 1999;9:279–284.
4. Felson D, Lawrence R, et al: NIH Conference: Osteoarthritis: new insights. Ann Int Med 2000;133(8):635–646.
5. Guccione A, Felson D, Anderson J: Defining arthritis and measuring functional status in elders: methodological issues in the study of disease and physical disability. Am J Public Health 1990;80:945–949.
6. Guccione A, Felson D, Anderson J, et al: The effects of specific medical conditions on the functional limitation of elders in the Framingham Study. Am J Public Health 1994;84:351–358.
7. Lawrence J, Bremner J, Bier F: Osteo-arthrosis. Prevalence in the population and relationships between symptoms and x-ray changes. Ann Rheum Dis 1966;25:1–24.
8. Newman N, Ling R: Acetabular bone destruction related to non-steroidal anti-inflammatory drugs. Lancet 1985;2:11–14.
9. Cannon GW, Caldwell JR, Holt P, et al: Rofecoxib, a specific inhibitor of cyclooxygenease 2, with clinical efficacy comparable with that of diclofenac sodium. Arthritis Rheum 2000;43(5):978–987.
10. Reginster J, Deroisy R, Rovati L, et al: Long-term effects of glucosamine sulphaste on osteoarthritis progression: A randomised, placebo-controlled clinical trial. Lancet 2001;357:251–256.
11. McALindon TE, Jacques P, Zhang Y, et al: Do antioxidant micronutrients protect against the development and progression of knee osteoarthritis? Arthritis Rheum 1996;39:648–656.
12. Felson D, Zhang Y, Anthony J, et al: Weight loss reduces the risk for symptomatic knee osteoarthritis in women. The Framingham Study. Ann Intern Med 1992;116:535–539.
13. O'Reilly SC, Muir KR, Doherty M: Effectiveness of a home exercise on pain and disability from osteoarthritis of the knee: A randomised controlled trial. Ann Rheum Dis 1999;58(1):15–19.
14. Kerrigan D, Todd M, O'Reilly P: Knee osteoarthritis and high heeled shoes. Lancet 1998;351(9113) 1399–1401.
15. Wobig M, Bach G, Beks P, et al: The role of elastoviscosity in the efficacy of viscosupplementation for osteoarthritis of the knee: a comparison of hylan G-F 20 and a lower-molecular-weight hyaluronan. Clin Ther 1999;21:1549–1562.
16. Orbell S, Espley A, Johnston M, Rowley D: Health benefits of joint replacement surgery for patients with osteoarthritis. J Epidemiol Community Health 1998;52(9):564–570.
17. Fujita S, Hirota S, Oda T, et al: Deep venous thrombosis after total hip or total knee arthroplasty in patients in Japan. Clin Orthop 2000;375:168–174.

65 Knee Bursitis

Florian S. Keplinger, MD
Navneet Gupta, MD

Florian S. Keplinger, MD
Navneet Gupta, MD

Synonyms

Prepatellar bursitis (housemaid's knee)

Infrapatellar bursitis (vicar's knee)

Anserine bursitis

No name, no fame bursitis

Semimembranosus bursitis

ICD-9 Codes

726.60
Enthesopathy of knee, unspecified bursitis of knee

726.61
Pes anserinus tendinitis or bursitis

726.62
Tibial collateral ligament bursitis

726.63
Fibular collateral ligament bursitis

726.65
Prepatellar bursitis

726.69
Other bursitis: infrapatellar; subpatellar

Definition

Knee bursitis can arise from inflammation of any bursa in the region of the knee joint. Eleven (11) bursae are found within this region (Fig. 1).[1]

Three bursae communicate with the knee joint: quadriceps or suprapatellar, popliteus, and medial gastrocnemius. Four more are associated with the patella: superficial and deep prepatellar, and superficial and deep infrapatellar. Two are related to the semimembranosus tendons, and two are related to the collateral ligaments of the knee (one of which is under the pes anserinus, or the conjoined tendons of the sartorius, gracilis, and semitendinous muscles).[1]

In the posterior knee, a bursa is located between the medial head of the gastrocnemius and semimembranosus tendon. Swelling in this area is also called a Baker's cyst and may actually be due to other conditions (see Chapter 59). For this chapter's purpose, discussion is limited to knee bursitis arising from inflammation of the previously mentioned bursae.

The most common knee bursitis conditions are the following:

1. Prepatellar bursitis (housemaid's knee)—caused by direct trauma, such as falling on a bent knee or frequent kneeling.[1]
2. Infrapatellar bursitis (vicar's knee)—usually due to repetitive knee flexion in weight bearing, such as deep knee bends, squatting, or jumping; it can be associated with patellar/quadriceps tendinitis.[2,3]
3. Anserine bursitis—commonly seen in overweight older women who also have osteoarthritis of the knees and in individuals who participate in sports that require running, side-to-side movement, and cutting.[2,4]
4. No name, no fame bursitis—refers to inflammation of a bursa located between the deep and superficial parts of the medial collateral ligament.[2]
5. Semimembranosus bursitis—usually seen in runners and may be associated with hamstring tendinitis.[2]

Symptoms

The patient will usually complain of local pain, tenderness, and/or swelling in the affected site. The pain is worse with flexion and usually occurs at

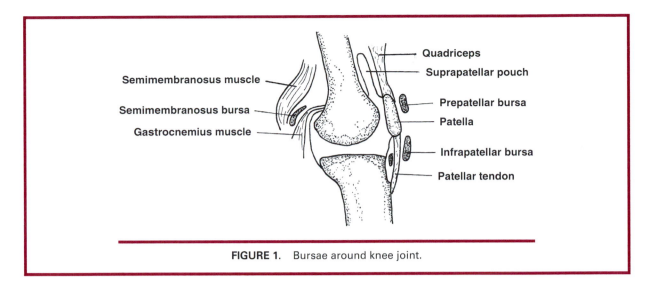

FIGURE 1. Bursae around knee joint.

night or after activity. The pain also may be more prominent and accompanied by stiffness upon waking in the morning. Limping may or may not be present.

Physical Examination

The patient may have an antalgic gait, with a shortened stance phase on the affected side. There is discrete tenderness to palpation associated with fullness at the site of the bursa involved. If the bursa connects with the knee joint, there may be an associated effusion. There is often limited range of motion in the knee. Neurologic exam should be normal.

Functional Limitations

The patient may have difficulty with prolonged walking. Decreased balance is often seen in older patients, sometimes necessitating assistive devices (e.g., walker, crutches, cane, or wheelchair). If there is limitation in knee range of motion, patients may have difficulty bending their knees to drive or sit at their desk at work. They will also have problems stooping, crawling, climbing, etc., which may interfere with vocational and recreational activities. Athletes such as runners may have diminished performance or may be sidelined altogether.

Diagnostic Studies

The diagnosis is based mainly on history and clinical examination. Aspiration is rarely needed but may be necessary if an infection is suspected. Radiologic studies are usually performed to rule out other diagnoses, but may show exostosis in areas related to the bursa. Plain x-rays should be done if a tumor is suspected, particularly in patients with night pain. Arthrography, which is rarely done, may show the connection to the knee joint, if it is involved. Magnetic resonance imaging may be needed to rule out a tumor or malignancy; this will show a fluid collection in the involved bursa.[1,2]

Differential Diagnosis

Infection (e.g., septic knee)

Arthritis (osteoarthritis, rheumatoid arthritis, psoriatic arthritis)

Tumor

Patellar fracture

Meniscal tear

Collateral ligament sprain or tear

Saphenous nerve entrapment

Treatment

Initial

Restriction of activity that provokes or aggravates symptoms is important.[1-5] In athletes, this may mean a substitution of their usual athletic activities while the healing process proceeds. Local application of ice helps with decreasing pain and inflammation. The patient can be taught to use superficial heat for chronic bursitis. This can be done with moistened warm compresses or with a microwaveable/electric heating pad. Precautions should be observed and given to the patient to prevent burns and other complications (see Potential Treatment Complications).

Nonsteroidal anti-inflammatory drugs (NSAIDs) can be prescribed to decrease pain and inflammation. COX-2 inhibitors may also be used, especially in elderly patients since these have fewer gastrointestinal side effects and are easier to administer (i.e., smaller-sized pills, taken once or twice a day). Oral steroids are generally not indicated as initial treatment.

Rehabilitation

Splinting/bracing of the knee can assist in preventing/avoiding movement and further inflammation, as well as providing comfort. However, long-term use of splints is not advised because it promotes muscle weakness.

Formal physical therapy may address stretching of the quadriceps, hamstrings, iliotibial band, and hip adductor muscles if these muscles are tight. Strengthening exercises are often needed in chronic knee bursitis because of disuse weakness and/or atrophy. Correcting gait abnormalities (e.g., leg length discrepancy with a heel lift or pes planus with orthotics) is also important. Therapists should also counsel patients to protect their knees from further trauma (e.g., by avoiding bending or kneeling or by using knee pads).

Modalities such as ultrasound have not been proven to be more effective than a combination of the aforementioned measures. Ultrasound should be avoided when an effusion is present because it can worsen an effusion. The use of phonophoresis and iontophoresis may have merit, but they are still controversial.[6]

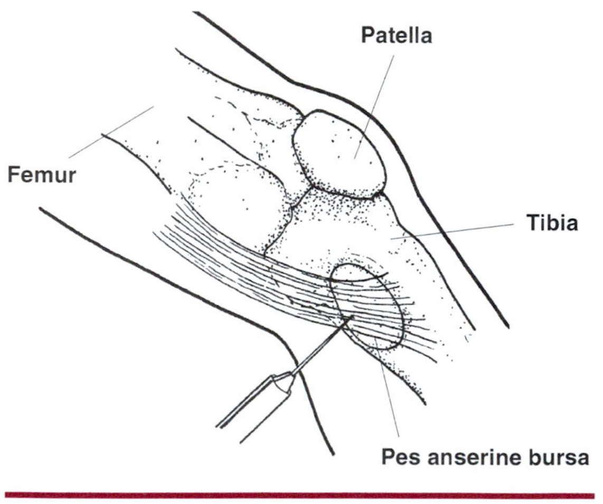

FIGURE 2.   Under sterile conditions, using a 1½-inch 22 gauge needle, inject the bursa at the point of maximal tenderness. A 1- to 3-cc combination of local anesthetic and corticosteroid is used (e.g., 1 cc of 1% lidocaine mixed with 1 cc of 80 mg of methylprednisolone. Local anesthetics may be injected just prior to the steroid to diminish pain and prevent postinjection steroid flare.[1-4,7] Postinjection ice application is helpful in decreasing pain at the site of injection.

Procedures

Intrabursal corticosteroid injection is appropriate if there is no response to conservative management or if the patient demonstrates significant functional limitations (Fig. 2). Typically no more than three injections are done in a 6- to 12-month period. Alternative diagnoses should be considered for patients with refractory symptoms.

The patient is generally advised to avoid activity involving the area injected for approximately 2 weeks to promote retention of the corticosteroid in the bursa and avoid systemic absorption.[7]

Surgery

Surgery is generally not indicated and should be undertaken only in refractory cases. Excision of a bursa can be considered if the disease does not respond to conservative measures, the problem persists for more than 6 weeks despite treatment, and it greatly limits the patient's activities.

Potential Disease Complications

Possible complications include chronic pain, deconditioning, disuse muscle atrophy, and knee flexion contracture.

Potential Treatment Complications

Potential complications from medications include drug hypersensitivity; prolonged bleeding; gastric, renal, and hepatic side effects from NSAIDs (less so with COX-2 inhibitors). Hyperglycemia, electrolyte imbalance, and gastric irritation or ulceration from intrabursal steroid injection are not as common as with orally administered corticosteroids, but can still occur from systemic absorption. Local ice application may produce hypersensitivity and vasoconstriction in patients with Raynaud's and peripheral vascular disease, and local heat application may produce burns, sedation, skin discoloration, and vascular compromise. Injections may result in drug hypersensitivity, sterile abscess, infection, nerve injury, tendon rupture, lipoatrophy from intralesional steroids.[7,8]

References
1. Cailliet R: Knee Pain and Disability, 3rd ed. Philadelphia, F.A. Davis, 1992.
2. Biundo JJ: Regional rheumatic pain syndromes. In Schumacher HR (ed): Primer on the Rheumatic Diseases, 10th ed. Atlanta, Arthritis Foundation, 1993, pp 277–287.
3. Larson RL, Grana WA (eds): The Knee: Form, Function, Pathology, and Treatment. Philadelphia, W.B. Saunders, 1993, pp 329–330.
4. Slaten W: The knee. In Young BO, Young MA, Stiens SA (eds): Physical Medicine and Rehabilitation Secrets. Philadelphia, Hanley & Belfus, 1997, p 295.
5. Kang I, Han SW: Anserine bursitis in patients with osteoarthritis of the knee. Southern Med J 2000;93(2):207–209.
6. Basford JR: Physical agents. In Delisa JA, Gans BM (eds): Rehabilitation Medicine: Principles and Practice, 2nd ed. Philadelphia, Lippincott, 1993, pp 404–424.
7. Neustadt DH: Intra-articular corticosteroids and other agents: Aspiration techniques. In Katz W (ed): The Diagnosis and Management of Rheumatic Disease, 2nd ed. Philadelphia, J.B. Lippincott, 1988, pp 812–825.
8. Handy JR: Anserinebursitis: A brief review. Southern Med J 1997;90(4):376–377.

66 Meniscal Injuries

Paul Lento, MD
Venu Akuthota, MD

Synonyms

Cartilage tears

Locked knee

ICD-9 Codes

717.3
Other and unspecified
derangement of medial
meniscus

717.4
Derangement of lateral
meniscus

717.40
Derangement of lateral
meniscus, unspecified

717.41
Bucket handle tear of
lateral meniscus

717.42
Derangement of anterior
horn of lateral meniscus

717.43
Derangement of
posterior horn of lateral
meniscus

717.49
Other

717.5
Derangement of
meniscus, not elsewhere
classified

717.9
Unspecified internal
derangement of knee

836.0
Acute tear of medial
meniscus of knee

836.1
Acute tear of lateral
meniscus of knee

Definition

The menisci serve important roles in maintaining proper joint health, stability, and function.[1] The anatomy of the medial and lateral menisci helps explain its functional biomechanics. When viewed from above, the medial meniscus appears C shaped, whereas the lateral meniscus appears O shaped.[1] Each meniscus is thick and convex at its periphery (the horns) but becomes thin and concave at its center. This contouring provides a larger area for the rounded femoral condyles and the relatively flat tibia. In addition, menisci do not move in isolation. They are connected to each other anteriorly and also to the anterior cruciate ligament (ACL), patella, femur, and tibia via ligaments (Fig. 1).[2,3]

The medial meniscus is less mobile than the lateral meniscus. This is due to its firm connections to the knee joint capsule and the medial collateral ligament. This decreased mobility, in conjunction with the fact that the medial meniscus is wider posteriorly, is cited as the usual reason for the

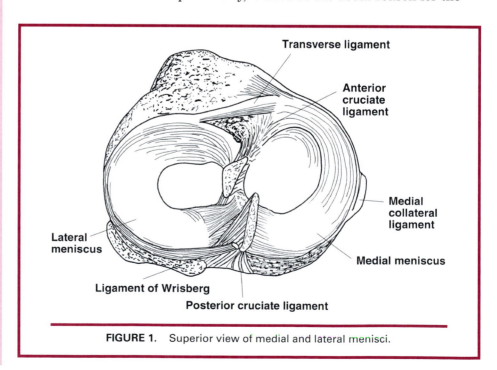

FIGURE 1. Superior view of medial and lateral menisci.

higher incidence of tears seen within the medial rather than the lateral meniscus.[1] The semimembranosus muscle (via attachments from the joint capsule) helps to retract the medial meniscus posteriorly, serving to prevent entrapment and injury to the medial meniscus as the knee is flexed.[3]

The lateral meniscus is not as adherent to the joint capsule. Also, unlike the medial meniscus, the lateral meniscus does not attach to its respective collateral ligament. The lateral meniscus's posterolateral aspect is separated from the capsule by the popliteus tendon. Therefore, the lateral meniscus is more mobile than the medial meniscus.[1,3] The popliteus's tendon attachment to the posterolateral meniscus ensures dynamic retraction of the lateral meniscus when the knee internally rotates to return out of the screw-home mechanism.[2] Therefore, both the medial and the lateral menisci, by having attachments to muscular structures, share a common mechanism that helps prevent injury.

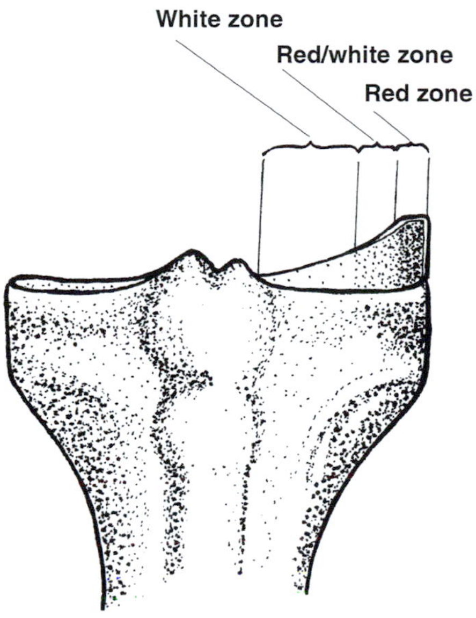

The vascular supply scheme to the meniscus has important healing implications..[1,4] Capillaries penetrate the menisci from the periphery to provide nourishment. After 18 months of age, as increased weight bearing occurs, the blood supply to the central part of the menisci recedes. In fact, research has shown that eventually only the peripheral 10% to 30% of the menisci, or the red zone, receives this capillary network[5] (Fig. 2). Therefore, the central portions, or white zone, of these fibrocartilaginous structures become avascular with age, relying on nutrition received via diffusion from the synovial fluid. Because of this vascular arrangement the peripheral meniscus is more likely to heal than the central and posterolateral aspects.[4]

The primary but not sole function of the menisci is to distribute forces across the knee joint and enhance stability.[1,6–8] Multiple studies have shown that the ability of the joint to transmit loads is significantly reduced if the meniscus is partially or wholly removed.[1,6,7,9] Fairbank, with a seminal article in 1948, suggested that the menisci were vital in protecting the articular surfaces. He reported that individuals who had undergone total meniscectomies demonstrated premature osteoarthritis.[10]

Meniscal tears are classified by their complexity, plane of rupture, direction, location, and overall shape. Tears are commonly defined as vertical, horizontal, or oblique in relation to the tibial surface (Fig. 3).[11] The bucket-handle tear is the most common type of vertical (or longitudinal) tear (Fig. 4).[12] Tears are also described as complete, full-thickness or partial. Complete, full-thickness tears are so named as they extend from the tibial to femoral surfaces. In addition, medial meniscus tears outnumber lateral meniscus tears anywhere from 2:1 to 5:1.[13,14]

White zone
Red/white zone
Red zone

FIGURE 2.   Vascular zones of the meniscus. Tears within the red zone have a higher healing potential.

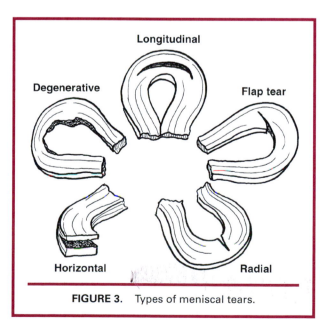

Longitudinal

Degenerative

Flap tear

Horizontal

Radial

FIGURE 3.   Types of meniscal tears.

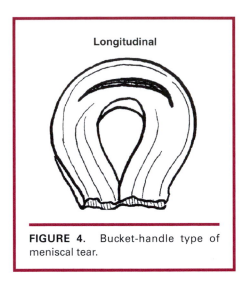

FIGURE 4. Bucket-handle type of meniscal tear.

Meniscal injuries may result from an acute injury or from gradual degeneration with aging.[15] Vertical tears (e.g., bucket-handle tears) tend to occur acutely in individuals 20 to 30 years old and are usually located in the posterior two thirds of the meniscus.[12,16] Sports commonly associated with meniscal injuries include soccer, football, basketball, baseball, wrestling, skiing, rugby, and lacrosse. Injury commonly occurs when an axial load is transmitted through a flexed or extended knee that is simultaneously rotating.[15] Degenerative tears, in contrast, are usually horizontal and are seen in older individuals with concomitant degenerative joint changes.[12,17]

The majority of acute peripheral meniscal injuries are associated with some degree of ACL laxity.[18] In addition, true ACL tears are associated with lesions of the posterior horns of the menisci.[18] Lateral meniscal tears appear to occur with more frequency with acute ACL injuries, whereas medial meniscal tears have a higher incidence with chronic ACL injuries. With chronic ACL injuries, the medial meniscus may be more commonly damaged because its posterior horn serves as an important secondary stabilizer of anteroposterior instability.[19]

Symptoms

The history will help diagnose a meniscal injury 75% of the time.[20,21] Young patients who experience meniscal tears will recall the mechanism of injury 80% to 90% of the time and may report a "pop" or a "snap" at the time of injury. Deep knee bending activities are often painful, and mechanical locking may be present in 30% of patients.[22] Bucket-handle tears should be suspected in cases of mechanical locking with loss of full extension.[15] If locking is reported approximately 1 day after the injury, this may be due to "pseudolocking," which occurs as a result of hamstring contracture.[13] Knee swelling and hemarthrosis may also occur acutely, especially if the vascularized, peripheral portion of the meniscus is involved. In fact, 20% of all cases of acute traumatic knee hemarthrosis are caused by isolated meniscal injury.[23] More typically, however, knee swelling occurs approximately 1 day later as the meniscal tear creates mechanical irritation within the intra-articular space, resulting in a reactive effusion. Typically, this effusion is secondary to a lesion more in the central portion of the meniscus.[15]

In contrast, degenerative meniscal tears are not classically associated with a history of trauma. In fact, the mechanism of injury, which may not be reported by the patient, can occur with simple daily activities, such as rising from a chair and pivoting on a planted foot.[15] Patients with degenerative tears often also report recurrent knee swelling, particularly after activity.

Physical Examination

Physical examination aids in the diagnosis of a meniscal injury accurately in 70% of patients.[24] Gait evaluation may reveal an antalgic gait with decreased stance-phase and knee extension on the symptomatic side.[23] A knee effusion is observed in about half of individuals with a known meniscal tear.[25] Quadriceps atrophy may be noted a few weeks after injury. On palpation, joint line tenderness is commonly present. Tenderness posteromedially or laterally is most suggestive of a meniscal tear.[20] A positive "bounce home" test may be present. This test is positive when pain or a mechanical blocking is appreciated as patient's knee is passively forced into full extension.[13] Classically, McMurray's test is positive 58% of the time in the presence of a tear but is also reported to be positive in 5% of individuals without a tear (Fig. 5).[12] The Apley grind or

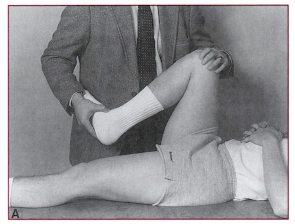
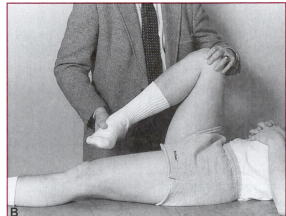
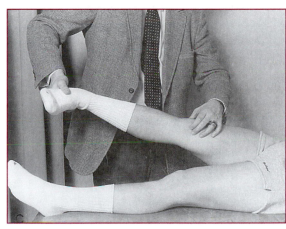

FIGURE 5. McMurray test. *A*, Starting position for testing the medial meniscus. The knee is acutely flexed, with the foot and tibia in external rotation. *B*, Starting position for testing the lateral meniscus. The knee is acutely flexed and the foot and tibia are internally rotated. *C*, Ending position for the lateral meniscus. The knee is brought into extension while rotation is maintained. Ending position for medial meniscus would be the same, but with external rotation. If pain and/or a "clunk" is elicited, the test is considered positive. (From Mellion MB: Office Sports Medicine, 2nd ed. Philadelphia, Hanley & Belfus, 1996, p 258, with permission.)

compression test is an insensitive indicator of meniscal injury. With this test, the prone knee is flexed to 90 degrees and an axial load is applied (Fig. 6). A painful response is considered a confirmatory test with a reported sensitivity of 45%.[23] No singular meniscal provocation test has been shown to be predictive of meniscal injury when compared with findings on arthroscopy. Physical exam findings become even less reliable in patients with concomitant ACL deficiencies.[13]

In some instances, patients will present with a locked knee or "pseudolocked" knee due to meniscal pathology.

Neurologic exam including sensation and deep tendon reflexes should be normal. Strength should also be normal unless there is associated guarding due to pain or disuse weakness, particularly of knee extension (quadriceps muscles).

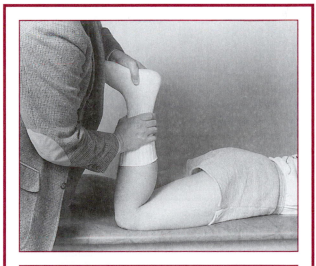

FIGURE 6. Apley compression test. Patient is prone. The examiner applies pressure on the sole of the foot toward the examination table. The tibia is rotated externally and internally. (From Mellion MB: Office Sports Medicine, 2nd ed. Philadelphia, Hanley & Belfus, 1996, p 259, with permission.)

Functional Limitations

Patients with meniscal injuries may have difficulty with deep knee bending activities such as traversing stairs, squatting, or toileting. In addition, jogging, running, and even walking may become problematic, particularly if any rotational component is involved. Laborers who repetitively squat may report mechanical locking with loss of full knee extension upon arising.

Diagnostic Studies

Standing plain radiographs are usually negative in isolated meniscal injuries. Presence of osteoarthritis, as with degenerative meniscal tears, can be detected with weight-bearing AP and lateral knee films. With non-degenerative tears, MRI has largely replaced plain radiographic examination in detecting injury.[20] Sagittal views demonstrate the anterior and posterior horns of the menisci, and coronal images can be vital in diagnosing bucket-handle and parrot-beak tears.[1,13] There are three grades of meniscal injury as graded by location of T2 signal intensity within the black cartilage. By definition, only grade 3 tears qualify as true meniscal tears; however, a few grade 2 lesions seen on MRI will be found to be true tears on arthroscopy (Fig. 7).[26] Using arthroscopy as the "gold standard," the sensitivity of MRI varies from 64% to 95% with an accuracy of 83% to 93%.[15] MRI appears to have a false positive rate of 10%.[1,24] A 5% false negative

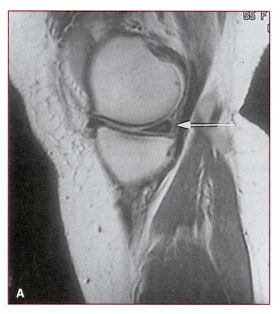
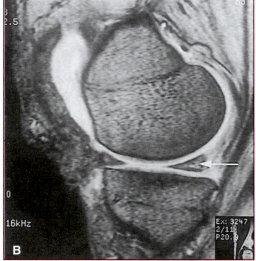
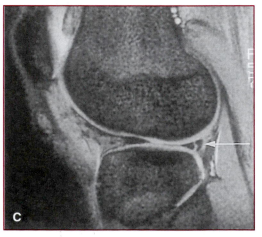

FIGURE 7. MRI grading of meniscal tears. *A*, poorly defined "globular" zone of increased signal intensity (*arrow*) corresponding to grade I change. *B*, linear zone of hyperintensity (*arrow*), not communicating with the articular surface, corresponding to grade II change. *C*, linear band of hyperintensity (*arrow*) communication with both articular surfaces corresponding with grade III change; that is, a complete tear. (From Mellion MB: Office Sports Medicine, 2nd ed. Philadelphia, Hanley & Belfus, 1996, p 263, with permission.)

rate is also reported and may be due to the incidence of missed tears at the meniscosynovial junction.[29]

Interestingly, despite the recent accessibility and advancement in magnetic resonance imaging, clinical examination by experienced clinicians is cheaper and appears to be as accurate as MRI for the diagnosis of meniscal tears.[26] However, MRI may be particularly helpful when history and physical examination are equivocal and the clinician is required to establish an expedient diagnosis.[12,23]

Knee aspiration is also performed acutely for diagnostic purposes. When aspirating the knee, the presence of blood (hemarthrosis) is suggestive of a meniscal injury. Marrow fat is suggestive of an occult fracture.

Differential Diagnosis

Anterior or posterior cruciate ligament tear

Medial collateral ligament tear

Osteoarthritis

Plica syndromes

Popliteal tendinitis

Osteochondritic lesions

Loose bodies

Patellofemoral pain

Fat pad impingement syndrome

Inflammatory arthritis

Fracture (e.g., anterior tibial spine, osteochondral, physeal)

Tumors

Treatment

Initial

The truly locked knee resulting from a meniscal tear should be reduced within 24 hours of injury. Otherwise, acute tears of the meniscus may initially be treated with rest, ice, and compression, with weight bearing as tolerated. Patients may need to use crutches acutely. A knee splint may be applied for patient comfort, particularly in the case of unstable knees with underlying ligamentous injury.[22]

Analgesics can be used for pain and NSAIDs/COX-2 inhibitors can be used for pain and inflammation.

Arthrocentesis can be performed (ideally in the first 24 to 48 hours) for both diagnostic and treatment purposes when there is a significant effusion.

Rehabilitation

Non-surgical options for meniscal injuries exist. In fact, some meniscal lesions have gradual resolution of symptoms over a 6-week period and may have normal function by 3 months.[11] In general, only meniscal injuries that are persistently symptomatic should be referred for surgical intervention.

Both non-surgical and partial meniscectomy patients undergo similar rehabilitation protocols. Crutches may be utilized to off-load the affected limb. Usually these can be discontinued when patients are ambulating without a limp.[28] The goal during the first week is to decrease pain and swelling while increasing range of motion and muscle conditioning. Instituting static strengthening exercises in conjunction with electrical stimulation can retard quadriceps atrophy. Aerobic conditioning can begin as long as the patient can tolerate bicycle training or aqua jogging. As time progresses, a combination of open and closed kinetic chain exercises in all three planes (sagittal, coronal, and transverse) can be performed in conjunction with stretching of the lower limb. Gradually, over the ensuing weeks, more functional activities are introduced. More challenging proprioceptive and balancing activities also can be started as deemed appropriate. Finally, plyometric training is begun, and the individual is gradually introduced back into sport-specific activities.

Multiple rehabilitation protocols for the surgically repaired meniscus have been described. Rehabilitation programs ideally need to be individualized to the specific type of repair performed. In addition, there has been considerable controversy among clinicians regarding the patient's weight-bearing and immobilization status soon after repair surgery.[29-32] In general, however, initial exercises are non-aggressive, avoiding dynamic shear forces that may occur from joint active range of motion. Therefore, exercises are initially static, targeting hip abductors, adductors, and extensors. Static quadriceps exercises are performed with care to prevent terminal knee extension. While superior and medial patella mobilization is begun, stretching of the lower limb musculature in multiple planes is emphasized. After 2 to 3 weeks, goals are to increase range of motion and advance weight-bearing status while introducing a resistance program. With the absence of effusion and significant pain, improved knee range of motion from 5 to 110° should be achieved. More aggressive active range of motion may be started, particularly if the repair was to the outer peripheral or vascular zone of the meniscus, since the success rate for healing in these areas is higher.[29] Gradually, more functional activities utilizing resistive bands may be introduced. With time and treatment success, resistance can be increased and proprioceptive neuromuscular facilitation activities can be implemented, ensuring that the individual is rehabilitated in the coronal, transverse, and sagittal planes.[33]

By 6 to 8 weeks, low impact functional activities that entail components of the patient's sport or activity are introduced. Brace protection, if used, now may be discontinued, particularly when the patient demonstrates success with proprioceptive testing. Running, cutting, and rotational activities are avoided. Athletes may be able to return their individual activities at about 16 weeks for those with repairs in the vascular zone and 24 weeks for those with repairs in the non-vascular zone.

Procedures

Patients presenting after an acute injury with an effusion may benefit from joint aspiration not only to help relieve discomfort and stiffness but also to aid in discerning whether a hemarthrosis or marrow fat (to rule out an occult fracture) is present.

Surgery

Specific types of tears may not require surgical repair, which include longitudinal partial thickness tears, stable full thickness peripheral tears (less than 5 mm long), or short radial tears (less than 5 mm).[28] These are usually stable and may not require either suture fixation or immobilization. However, arthroscopy may still be necessary to determine stability and to stimulate healing via perimeniscal abrasion.[11] Some larger longitudinal, radial, and degenerative meniscal tears are less likely to heal without surgical intervention. Although first line treatment for these lesions is aggressive rehabilitation, recalcitrant cases may necessitate a partial meniscectomy that preserves as much of the meniscus as possible.[31] In addition, the inner aspect of the cartilage, which may be ragged, may be rasped or shaved, providing a smooth surface that eliminates mechanical symptoms.

Occasionally, other tears of the menisci, because of their size and location, are best treated by primary approximation utilizing primary repair.[30] Typically, longitudinal tears longer than 5 mm in the periphery of the meniscus are best suited for this since they have a high rate of successful healing.[28] In older individuals, the mere presence of a horizontal or degenerative cleavage tear is insufficient to justify removal since these meniscal portions may still participate in significant load transmission but not necessarily cause symptoms.[11] Treatment of these degenerative tears is usually non-surgical; however, unstable portions may be removed during arthroscopy.

Potential Disease Complications

Once a meniscal tear occurs, the joint inherently becomes less stable. This instability may promote further extension of the initial tear, turning a non-surgical lesion into one in which arthroscopic repair may be necessary. Chronically, the resultant increased abnormal motion that occurs secondary to the meniscal injury may also lead to damage of the articular surface and predispose the patient to premature osteoarthritis.[20]

Potential Treatment Complications

Analgesics, NSAIDs, and COX-2 inhibitors have well-known side effects that most commonly affect the gastric, hepatic, and renal systems. If the clinician is unfamiliar with appropriate rehabilitation strategies, an overaggressive regimen may lead to extension of the tear or failure of the meniscus to heal. A rehabilitative program that is too conservative, in contrast, may lead to a significant loss of strength with muscular atrophy and decreased range of motion. If the surgical approach resulted in a significant amount of cartilage removal, the knee may be predisposed to developing osteoarthritis as originally described by Fairbank.[10] Saphenous nerve injuries as well as infection are also common complications following meniscal repair surgery and arthroscopy.[20]

References

1. Renstrom P: Anatomy and biomechanics of the menisci. Clin Sports Med 1990;9(3):523–538.
2. Norkin C, Levangie P: The knee complex. In Norkin C, Levangie P (eds): Joint Structure and Function, 2nd ed. Philadelphia, F.A. Davis, 1992, pp 337–378.
3. Maitra, RS, et al: Meniscal reconstruction. Part I: Indications, techniques, and graft considerations. Am J Orthop 1999;28(4):213–218.
4. Gray JC: Neural and vascular anatomy of the menisci of the human knee. J Orthop Sports Phys Ther 1999;29(1):23–30.
5. Arnoczky SP, Warren RF: The microvasculature of the meniscus and its reponse to injury. Am J Sports Med 1983;11:131–141.
6. Walker PS, Erkman MJ: The role of the menisci in force transmission across the knee. Clin Orthop 1975;109:184.
7. Seedholm BB: Transmission on the load in the knee joint with special reference to the role of the menisci: I. Anatomy, analysis and apparatus. Eng Med 1979;8:207–219.
8. Ahmed AM, Burke DL: In vitro measurement of static pressure distribution in synovial joints: I. Tibial surface of the knee. J Biomech Eng 1983;105:216–225.
9. Krause WE, Pope MD, Johnson RJ, et al: Mechanical changes in the knee after menisectomy. J Bone Joint Surg 1976;58A:599.
10. Fairbank TJ, et al: Knee joint changes after meniscectomy. J Bone Joint Surg 1948;30(4):664–670.
11. Newman AP, Daniels AU, Burke RT: Principles and decision making in meniscal surgery. Arthroscopy 1993;9(1):33–51.
12. Oberlander MA, Pryde JA: Meniscal injuries. In Baker CL (ed): The Hughston Clinic Sports Medicine Book. Media, Williams & Wilkins, 1995, pp 465–472.
13. Hardin GT, et al: Meniscal tears: Diagnosis, evaluation, and treatment. Orthop Rev 1992;21(11): 1311–1317.
14. Metcalf RW: The torn medial meniscus. In Parisien JS (ed): Arthroscopic Surgery. New York, McGraw-Hill, 1988, pp 93–110.
15. Tuerlings L. Meniscal injuries. In Arendt EA (ed): Orthopaedic Knowledge Update Sports Medicine 2. Rosemont, Ill, AAOS, 1999, pp 349–354.
16. Baker BE, Peckham AC, Pupparo F. Review of meniscal injury and associated sports. Am J Sports Med 1983; 11: 8-13.
17. Rodkey WG: Basic biology of the meniscus and response to injury. AAOS Instructional Course Lectures 2000;49:189–193.
18. Poehling GG, Ruch DS, Chabon SJ: The landscape of meniscal injuries. Clin Sports Med 1990;9:539.
19. Bellabarba C, et al: Patterns of meniscal injury in the anterior cruciate-deficient knee: A review of the literature. Am J Orthop 1997;6(1):18–23.
20. Fu,FH, Baratz M: Meniscal injuries. In Delee JC, Drez D (eds): Orthopedic Sports Medicine Principles and Practice, vol 2. Philadelphia, W.B. Saunders, 1994, pp 1146–1162.
21. Casscells SW: The place of arthroscopy in the diagnosis and treatment of internal derangement of the knee: an analysis of 1000 cases. Clin Orthop 1980;151:135–142.
22. Simon RR, Koenigsknecht SJ: The knee. In Simon RR, Koenigsknecht SJ (eds): Emergency Orthopedics The Extremities. Norwalk, CT, Appleton & Lange, pp 437–462.
23. Muellner T, Nikolic A, Vecsei V: Recommendations for the diagnosis of traumatic meniscal injuries in Athletes. Sports Med 1999;27(5):337–345.
24. Rose NE, Gold SM: A comparison of accuracy between clinical examination and magnetic resonance imaging in the diagnosis of meniscal and anterior cruciate ligament tears. Arthroscopy 1996;12(4):398–405.
25. Anderson AF, Lipscomb AB: Clinical diagnosis of meniscal tears. Description of a new manipulative test. Am J Sports Med 1986;14:291–293.

26. Baratz ME, Rehak DC, Fu FH, et al: Peripheral tears of the meniscus. The effect of open versus arthroscopic repair on intra-articular contact stresses in the human knee. Am J Sports Med 1988;16:1.
27. DeHaven, KE, et al: Meniscus repair: Basic science, indications for repair, and open repair. AAOS Instructional Course Lectures 1994;43:65–76.
28. DeHaven KE, Bronstein RD: Injuries to the menisci of the knee. In Nicholas JA, Hershman EB (eds): The Lower Extremity and Spine in Sports Medicine, 2nd ed. Saint Louis, Mosby, 1995, pp 813–823.
29. Auberger SS, Mangine RE: Innovative approaches to surgery and rehabilitation. In Mangine RE (ed): Physical Therapy of the Knee, 2nd ed. New York, Churchill Livingstone, 1995, pp 233–249.
30. Brukner P, Kahn K: Acute knee injuries. In Brukner P, Kahn K (eds). Clinical Sports Medicine. Roseville, Australia, McGraw-Hill, pp 343–353.
30. Rispoli DM, et al: Options in meniscal repair. Clin Sports Med 1999;18(1):77–90.
31. Shelbourne KD, Patel DV, Adsit WS, et al: Rehabilitation after meniscal repair. Clin Sports Med 1996;15(3):595–612.
32. Swenson TM, Harner CD. Knee ligament and mensical injuries. Orthop Clin North Ame 1995;26(3):535–546.
33. Gray GW: Lunge tests. In Gray GW (ed). Lower Extremity Functional Profile. Adrian, MI, Wynn Marketing, 1995, pp 100–108.

67 | Patellar Tendinitis (Jumper's Knee)

Tommy Hudgins, MD
Alexandra R. Bunyak, MD

Definition

"Jumper's knee," first described by Blazina in 1973,[2] is primarily a chronic overuse injury of the patellar tendon resulting from excessive stress on the knee extensor mechanism. Athletes involved in sports requiring repetitive jumping, running, and kicking (e.g., volleyball, basketball, tennis, track) are at greatest risk. In volleyball players, the incidence ranges from 22% to 39%.[3] Acceleration, deceleration, takeoff, and landing generate eccentric forces that can be three times greater than conventional concentric and static forces. These eccentric forces may exceed the inherent strength of the patellar tendon, resulting in microtears anywhere along the bone-tendon interface.[1,3,4] With continued stress, a cycle of microtearing, degeneration, and regeneration weakens the tendon and may lead to tendon rupture.

Similar to other overuse injuries, the predisposing factors in jumper's knee include extrinsic causes such as errors in training and intrinsic causes such as biomechanical flaws. Training errors include improper warmup or cool-down, rapid increase in frequency or intensity of activity, and training on hard surfaces.[1,4] Biomechanical flaws such as muscle strength/flexibility imbalances—in jumper's knee, tight hamstrings and increased femoral anteversion[1]—and jumping mechanics[3,5] also have been implicated. Finally, an increased incidence of Osgood-Schlatter defect and idiopathic anterior knee pain during adolescence have been identified in patients with jumper's knee.[1]

Because histologic studies of the patellar tendon reveal collagen degeneration with little or no evidence of acute inflammation, many authors argue that "patellar tendinosis" is a more accurate description than "patellar tendinitis."[6–8] This distinction has important implications for rehabilitation. In treatment of patellar tendinosis and other chronic overuse tendinopathies, the treatment team should emphasize restoration of function rather than control of inflammation.

Symptoms

Patients typically report a dull, aching anterior knee pain, initially noted after a strenuous workout or competition, that is insidious in onset and well localized.[7] The bone-tendon junction at the inferior pole of the patella is

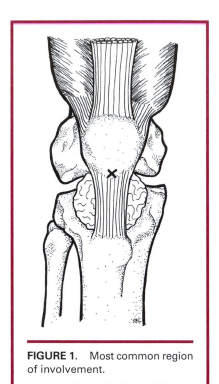

FIGURE 1. Most common region of involvement.

most commonly affected (65% of cases) (Fig. 1), followed by the superior pole of the patella (25%), and the tibial tubercle (10%).[6] Other symptoms may include stiffness or pain after prolonged sitting or climbing stairs,[1] a feeling of swelling or fullness over the patella, and knee extensor weakness.[2] Mechanical symptoms of instability, such as locking, catching, or give-away, weakness, are uncommon. The following four phases have been described in the progression of jumper's knee[2]:

Phase 1: Pain is present after activity only and is not associated with functional impairment.

Phase 2: Pain is present during and after activity but does not limit performance and resolves with rest.

Phase 3: Pain is present continually and is associated with progressively impaired performance.

Phase 4: Complete tendon rupture.

As the disease progresses, the pain becomes sharper, more severe, and constant (present not only with athletic endeavor but also with walking and other everyday activities). If not treated, the disorder may result in tendon rupture, a sudden painful event associated with immediate inability to extend the knee.[7]

Physical Examination

The hallmark of jumper's knee is tenderness at the site of involvement, usually the inferior pole of the patella.[7] This sign is best elicited on palpation of the knee in full extension,[7] and the pain typically increases when the knee is extended against resistance.[1] Occasionally, there may be swelling of the tendon or the fat pad, although a frank effusion is not typically present.[1] Mild patellofemoral crepitus and pain with compression of the patellofemoral joint have been noted.[1] In advanced disease, patients may have quadriceps atrophy without detectable weakness on manual muscle testing and hamstring tightness.[1,7] The clinician should also expect a normal, non-focal neurologic examination.

Functional Limitations

Most patients experience little functional limitation in the early stages of jumper's knee. As the disease progresses, however, increasing disability from persistent pain and inhibition of knee extension impairs performance. Eventually walking and the ability to perform basic activities of daily living, such as ascending or descending stairs, may be compromised. In the event of patellar tendon rupture, complete functional impairment with inability to extend the affected knee, limiting weight bearing and ambulation, necessitates surgical repair.

Diagnostic Studies

Radiographic changes are rarely present during the first 6 months of jumper's knee, limiting the usefulness of radiographs during initial evaluation.[4] When performed, the examination generally includes anteroposterior, lateral, intercondylar, and skyline tracking patellar views.[1] Documented findings include radiolucency at the site of involvement, elongation of the involved pole, and occasionally, a fracture at the junction of the elongation with the main portion of the patella. Occasionally, calcification of the involved tendon and irregularity or even avulsion of the involved pole may be seen.[2]

Ultrasound has the advantage of allowing early diagnosis and dynamic imaging of the tendon, while remaining inexpensive, noninvasive, reproducible, and sensitive to changes as small as 0.1 mm.[4] Many authors feel ultrasonography to be the preferred method for evaluating jumper's knee. It has been used to confirm the diagnosis, guide steroid injections, and examine tendons after surgery.[4] Ultrasound should be considered in cases that do not respond to a trial of conservative treatment after 4 to 6 weeks and in which the diagnosis is questioned. Findings on ultrasound include thickening of the tendon.[4,9] A hypoechoic focal lesion at the area of greatest thickening correlates well with the lesion on MRI, CT, and histologic findings.[1,10] However, critics of ultrasound have noted abnormalities in asymptomatic athletes. This phenomenon may be explained by a preclinical or postclinical stage of the disease.[4] Plain MRI, MRI with intravenous gadolinium, and MRI with arthrography gadolinium have been used to corroborate the clinical diagnosis of jumper's knee. Increased thickening of the patella tendon on MRI is present in all patients resistant to conservative therapy..[12] MRI is also advantageous in excluding other intrinsic joint pathology. MRI arthrography is particularly useful in examining the chondral surfaces of the patella and femur when osteochondritis dessicans or other pathology in these areas is suspected.

Differential Diagnosis

Patellofemoral maltracking

Retinacular pain

Fat pad lesion

Infrapatellar bursitis

Partial ACL tear

Meniscal injuries

Chondromalacia patella

Plica syndrome

Entrapment of the saphenous nerve

Traction apophysitis at the tibia tubercle (Osgood-Schlatter lesion)

Sinding-Larsen syndrome

Treatment

Initial

Since the syndrome is progressive and associated with difficult and slow rehabilitation, the importance of early diagnosis and treatment cannot be overemphasized.[13] Initial interventions include controlling inflammation and pain with NSAIDs/COX-2 inhibitors, ice, and relative rest from aggravating activities. Analgesics can be used for pain as well.

Rehabilitation

The first goal of rehabilitation is to decrease pain. Judicious use of passive modalities such as ultrasound and iontophoresis is utilized to control pain. When pain has improved, a comprehensive rehabilitation program can address the biomechanical flaws found on the musculoskeletal examination. These include the functional deficits (inflexibilities in joints, tendons, etc. that lead to altered biomechanics) and subclinical adaptations (muscular substitution patterns that compensate for the functional deficits).[15] This approach may be utilized when addressing all overuse syndromes. Hamstring and quadriceps range of motion and strength need to be addressed.[15] As the rehabilitation program advances and pain abates, eccentric strengthening exercises should be emphasized. This type of strengthening exercise is optimal for rehabilitating tendinopathies because it places maximal tensile load on the muscle and tendon

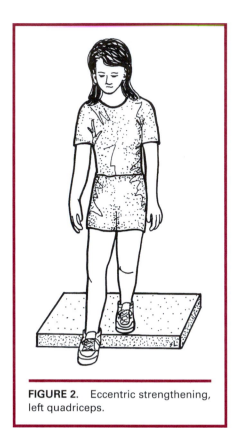

FIGURE 2. Eccentric strengthening, left quadriceps.

unit (Fig. 2).[13,14] This final phase of rehabilitation should also encompass sports-specific drills/training. Return to play should occur gradually, with careful monitoring of the patient's symptoms. Absence of pain is normally used as the guide to progress athletes in physical therapy and with return to play. Knee supports and straps, such as the Chopat strap, have been used to alleviate pain and change the force dynamics through the patella tendon with variable results.[4,17]

Procedures

Some authors recommend a peritendinous injection of steroid if non-invasive conservative therapy fails.[1,4] Decreased pain with injection of the fat pad rather than the tendon itself has been documented.[1] As histologic studies have shown a minimal inflammatory component in surgical specimens, the mechanism of action of these approaches is unknown.[4] It is important to note that studies have associated tendon ruptures with steroid injection.[4,16]

Surgery

Surgery is rarely necessary for the management of jumper's knee. However, in advanced-stage jumper's knee, if a well-documented conservative therapy trial fails or if the tendon ruptures, surgery may be indicated. It is incumbent upon the clinician to ensure that a comprehensive rehabilitation program has been followed thoroughly, as previously outlined, before one declares a patient a "conservative management failure." Several surgical approaches have been utilized with mixed success; resection of the tendon pathology and resuturing of the tendon are most often cited, with authors reporting good or excellent results 77% to 93% of the time.[18,19]

Potential Disease Complications

Stress reaction of the patella, stress fracture, and patellar tendon rupture are some of the advanced complications. Others include formation of accessory ossicles, avulsion apophysis, and bony growth acceleration or arrest in adolescents.[20] Chronic intractable pain may occur, leading to impaired athletic performance and functional limitations.

Potential Treatment Complications

Gastrointestinal, bleeding, and renal side effects of NSAIDs are well documented. COX-2 inhibitors may cause fewer gastric side effects. Complications of corticosteroid injections include bleeding, infection, and soft tissue atrophy at the site of injection. Tendon weakening with possible increased incidence of tendon rupture has also been cited. Surgery can lead to inadvertent tibial or peroneal nerve injury.

References

1. Duri ZAA, Aichroth PM, et al: Patellar tendonitis and anterior knee pain. Am J Knee Surg 1999;12:99–108.
2. Blazina ME, Kerlan RK, et al: Jumper's knee. Orthop Clin North Am 1973;4:665–678.
3. Ferretti A, Puddy G, et al: The natural history of jumper's knee. International Orthopaedics 1985;8:239–242.
4. Fredberg U, Bolvig L: Jumper's knee. Scand J Med Sci Sports 1999;9:66–73.
5. Colosimo AJ, Bassett FH: Jumper's knee diagnosis and treatment. Orthopaedic Review 1990;19:139–149.
6. Popp JE, Yu JS, et al: Recalcitrant patellar tendinitis. Am J Sports Med 1997;25:218–222.
7. Lian O, Engebretsen L, et al: Characteristics of the leg extensors in male volleyball players with jumper's knee. Am J Sports Med 1996;24:380–385.
8. Richards DP, Ajemian SV, et al: Knee joint dynamics predict patellar tendinitis in elite volleyball players. Am J Sports Med 1996;24:676–683.
9. Visentini PJ, Khan KM, et al: The VISA score: An index of severity of symptoms in patients with jumper's knee (patellar tendinosis). J Sci Med Sport 1998;1:22–28.
10. Khan MK, Cook JL, et al: Patellar tendon ultrasonography and jumper's knee in female basketball players: A longitudinal study. Clin J Sport Med 1997;7:199–206.
11. Davies SG, Baudouin CJ, et al: Ultrasound, computed tomography, and magnetic resonance imaging in patellar tendinitis. Clin Radiol 1991;43:52–56.
12. Khan KM, Bonar F, et al. Patellar tendinosis (jumper's knee): findings at histopathologic examination, US, and MRI imaging. Radiology 1996;200:821–827.
13. Jensen K, Di Fabio R: Evaluation of eccentric exercise in treatment of patellar tendinitis. Phys Ther 1989;69:211–216.
14. Stanish, WD, Rubinovich RM, et al: Eccentric exercise in chronic tendinitis. Clin Orthopaedics Rel Res 1985;4:65–68.
15. Gotlin RS: Effective rehabilitation for anterior knee pain. J Musculoskeletal Med 2000;17:421–432.
16. Ismail AM, Balakrishnan R, et al: Rupture of patellar ligament after steroid infiltration. J Bone Joint Surg 1969;51:503–505.
17. Palumbo PM: Dynamic patellar brace: A new orthosis in the management of patellofemoral disorders. Am J Sports Med 1981;9:45–49.
18. Verheyden F, Geens G, et al: Jumper's knee: Results of surgical treatment. Acta Orthopaedica Belgica 1997;63:102–105.
19. Pierets K, Verdonk R, et al: Jumper's knee: Postoperative assessment. Surg Sports Traumatol, Arthrosc 1999;7:239–242.
20. Cood JL, Khan KM, et al: A cross sectional study of 100 athletes with jumper's knee managed conservatively and surgically. Br J Sports Med 1997;31:332–336.

68 Patellofemoral Syndrome

Thomas H. Hudgins, MD
Joseph T. Alleva, MD

Synonyms

Anterior knee pain
Chondromalacia patella
Patellofemoral arthralgia
Patellar pain
Maltracking
Patellagia

ICD-9 Codes

717.7
Chondromalacia of patella

719.46
Pain in joint, knee

Definition

Patellofemoral syndrome is the most common ailment involving the knee in both the athletic and nonathletic population.[3–5] Twenty-five percent of patients complaining of knee pain in sports medicine clinics are diagnosed with this syndrome, and it affects women twice as often as men.[3] Yet, despite the common occurrence of this disorder, there is no clear consensus on its definition, etiology, and pathophysiology.[6] The most common theory is that the syndrome is an overuse injury from repetitive overload at the patellofemoral joint (Fig. 1). This increased stress results in physical and biomechanical changes of the patellofemoral joint.[6] The literature has focused on identifying risk factors that lead to altered biomechanics, producing maltracking of the patella in the femoral trochlear groove and thus stress at the patellofemoral joint. Possible pain generators in this scenario include the subchondral bone, retinacula, and capsule and the synovial membrane.[7] Historically, the histologic diagnosis of chondromalacia had been associated with patellofemoral syndrome (PFS). However, chondromalacia is poorly associated with the incidence of PFS.[5]

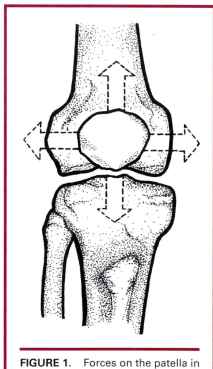

FIGURE 1. Forces on the patella in patellofemoral syndrome.

Symptoms

The patient with PFS will complain of a diffuse, vague ache of insidious onset.[3] The anterior knee is the most common location for pain, but some patients describe posterior knee discomfort in the popliteal fossa area.[4]

The discomfort is aggravated by prolonged sitting with the knees flexed (positive "theater" sign) as well as by ascending and descending stairs and squatting because these positions place the greatest force on the patellofemoral joint.[8] The patient may also complain of swelling and may experience symptoms of instability, such as pseudolocking, in which the knee momentarily locks in an extended position.[9,10] Symptoms of true locking and instability, such as with ligamentous and meniscal injuries, are usually absent.

Physical Examination

The examination should focus on identifying risk factors that contribute to malalignment and ruling out other pathology associated with anterior knee pain. The neurologic exam should be normal. There is often tenderness to palpation at the medial and lateral borders of the patella.[3] A minimal effusion may also be present. Manual testing for intra-articular pathology, such as Lachman's and McMurray's tests, will be negative.

The presence of femoral anteversion; tibia internal rotation; excessive pronation at the foot; an increased Q angle; and inflexibility of the hip flexors, quadriceps, iliotibial band, and gastrocsoleus should be determined.[11] The patella position (baja/alta, squinting/grasshopper) should also be assessed with the patient sitting and standing. Each of these factors has either a direct or indirect influence on the tracking of the patella with the femur (see Fig. 1).

The Q angle is the intersection of a line from the anterior sacroiliac spine (ASIS) to the patella, with a line from the tibia tubercle to the patella (Fig. 2). This angle is typically less than 15 degrees in males and less that 20 degrees in females. An increased angle is associated with increased femoral anteversion and thus patellofemoral joint torsion.[9] However, a consensus on the importance of an increased Q angle is lacking.[6] Tight hip flexors, quadriceps, hamstrings, and gastrocsoleus muscles will increase knee flexion and thus patellofemoral joint reaction force. A tight iliotibial band will increase the lateral pull of the patella through the lateral retinacula fibers.[12,13] It is imperative to assess each of these components in the lower extremity kinetic chain to prescribe a tailored physical therapy program for each individual.

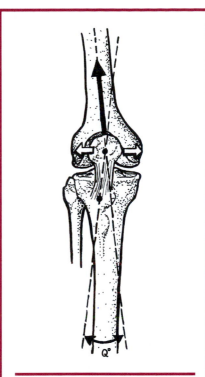

FIGURE 2. Measurement of Q angle. A line is drawn from the anterior iliac spine to the center of the patella. A second line is drawn from the center of the patella to the tibial tubercle. An angle between these two lines is called the Q angle.

Functional Limitations

The patient with PFS will avoid activities that provoke the discomfort initially, such as stairclimbing. Prolonged sitting in a car or at work may be difficult. In chronic, progressive cases, ambulation may be enough to incite the pain, making all mobility difficult.

Diagnostic Studies

PFS is a clinical diagnosis. Plain films may be used to evaluate Q angle and patella alta/baja. Advanced imaging such as MRI is reserved for recalcitrant cases that do not respond to conservative care to rule out intra-articular pathology.

Differential Diagnosis

Patella fracture

Patella dislocation

Quadriceps rupture

Patellar tendinitis

Peripatellar bursitis

Osgood Schlatter disease

Meniscal lesions

Ligamentous lesions

Plica syndromes

Osteochondritis dessicans

Treatment

Initial

Similar to other overuse injuries, the initial treatment focuses on decreasing pain. Icing is beneficial, particularly after activities. NSAIDs/COX-2 inhibitors may be used to decrease inflammation and pain. Analgesics may be utilized in a judicious manner. Relative rest from activities that cause pain combined with non–weight-bearing aerobic activity (e.g., swimming) may also be necessary initially. A knee sleeve with an opening for the patella is helpful to increase proprioceptive feedback.

Rehabilitation

With no consensus on the etiology and pathophysiology of PFS, numerous treatment protocols and therapies have been utilized in the literature.[17] Despite the lack of consensus, most patients respond to a directed rehabilitation approach with therapeutic exercise.[12,13] Initially, the physical therapist can teach the patient McConnell's taping method to reduce pain and increase tolerance of a therapeutic exercise program.[13–16]

Biomechanical imbalances identified during the physical examination should be addressed with strength, flexibility, and proprioception training. Strength training can be achieved with both open kinetic chain and closed kinetic chain exercises. Open kinetic chain exercises occur when the distal link, the foot, is allowed to move freely in space (e.g., such as when running or doing a leg extension exercise with weights). During closed kinetic chain exercises, the foot maintains contact with the ground or pedal, resulting in a multiarticular closed kinetic exercise (e.g., as in cycling or performing a leg press or wall sit).[13] Closed kinetic chain exercises are less stressful than open chain exercises at the patellofemoral joint in the functional range of 0 to 45 degrees knee flexion.[18] Thus, a rehabilitation program generally focuses first on closed chain exercises.

These exercises can be performed in multiple planes in a "functional" rehabilitation program. This may entail having the patient perform a lunge in the coronal, saggital, and transverse planes, simulating positions applied during activities (Fig. 3). These exercises can also stress patients' balance by having patients perform lunges with the eyes closed. Through this functional, or skill, training, the clinician is preparing the patient for all functional tasks by achieving efficient nerve-muscle interactions.[8]

Many studies have focused on selectively strengthening the vastus medialis oblique (VMO) as a dynamic medial stabilizer on the patella. Selective VMO strengthening may be achieved with combined hip adduction because the fibers of the VMO originate on the adductor magnus tendon and to a lesser extent, the adductor longus. However, attempts at proving isolated recruitment of the VMO in relation to the vastus lateralis have failed.[3] Nevertheless, quadriceps strengthening, in general, should be incorporated in the rehabilitation program through closed chain and "functional" exercises, as mentioned previously.

Procedures

Injections are not indicated because this is primarily a maltracking phenomena without a clear consensus on the pain generator.

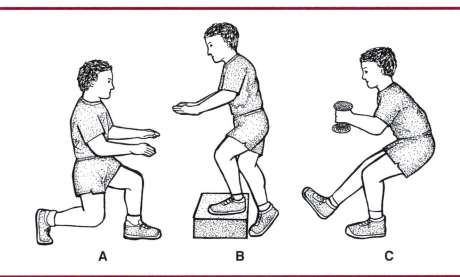

FIGURE 3. Skill training can help resolve anterior knee pain by improving strength and neuromuscular coordination. The lunge (*A*), step-down (*B*), and knee bend (*C*) are examples of force-absorbing skill-training exercises that are particularly valuable for improving strength, which, in turn, promotes stability. For the most benefit during the knee bend, the patient's knee should be aligned with the shoelaces.

Surgery

Surgery is rarely indicated, and a directed rehabilitation program is often successful.[4] However, several techniques have been illustrated in the literature. These include lateral retinacular release to decrease the lateral force, proximal and distal realignment procedures, and elevation of the tibia tubercle.[1]

Potential Disease Complications

Recalcitrant, chronic cases of anterior knee pain may show progressive degenerative changes at the patellofemoral joint, such as severe (grade IV) chondromalacia patella. Chronic intractable pain may also occur.

Potential Treatment Complications

Renal and gastric side effects are well known with NSAIDs. COX-2 inhibitors may cause fewer gastric side effects. Overcompensating the malalignment may occur with the surgical techniques, such as the lateral retinacular release. The surgeon may lyse too many fibers, leading to increased medial tracking. Many of the realignment procedures should also be reserved for the skeletally mature patient.[1]

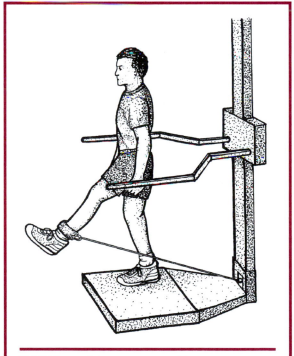

FIGURE 4. The standing cable column is an example of a skill-training exercise. The patient uses strength to exercise against resistance offered by a cable and simultaneously refines balancing skills.

References

1. Thomee R, Augustsson J, Karlsson J: Patellofemoral pain syndrome: A review of current issues. Sports Med 1999;28:245–262.
2. Beckman M, Craig R, Lehman RC: Rehabilitation of patellofemoral dysfunction in the athlete. Clin Sports Med 1989;8:841–860.
3. Powers CM: Rehabilitation of patellofemoral disorders: A critical review. J Orthop Sports Phys Ther 1998;5:345–354.
4. Goldberg B: Patellofemoral malalignment. Pediatr Ann 1997;26:32–35.
5. Sanchis-Alfonso V: Pathogenesis of anterior knee pain syndrome and functional patellofemoral instability in the active young. Am J Knee Surg 1999;12:29–40.
6. Baker MM, Juhn MS: Patellofemoral pain syndrome in the female athlete. Clin Sports Med 2000;19:314–329.
7. Papagelopoulos PJ, Sim FH: Patellofemoral pain syndrome: Diagnosis and management. Orthopedics 1997;20:148–157.
8. Gotlin RS: Affective knee rehabilitation for anterior knee pain. J Muscle Med 2000;July:421–432.
9. Hilyard A: Recent developments in the management of patellofemoral pain. Physiotherapy 1990;76:559–565.
10. Kannus P, Niitymaki S: Which factors predict outcome in the non-operative treatment of patellofemoral pain syndrome? A prospective follow up study. Med Sci Sports Exerc 1993;289–296.
11. Insall J: Chondromalacia patella. J Bone Joint Surg 1976;58:1–8.
12. Juhn MS: Patellofemoral pain syndrome: A review and guidelines for treatment. Am Fam Physician 1999;60:2012–2018.
13. Press JM, Young JA: Rehabilitation of patellofemoral pain syndrome. In Kebler WB, Herring SA, Press JM (eds): Functional Rehabilitation of Sports and Musculoskeletal Injuries. Gaithersburg, MD, Aspen, 1998, pp 254–264.
14. McConnell J: The management of chondromalacia patellae: A long term solution. Aust J Phys 1986;32:215–233.
15. Kowall MG, Kolk G, Nuber GW: Patellar taping in the treatment of patellofemoral pain. Am J Sports Med 1996;24:61–65.
16. Larsen B: Patellar taping: A radiographic examination of the medial glide technique. Am J Sports Med 1995;23:465–471.
17. Arroll B: Patellofemoral pain syndrome. Am J Sports Med 1997;25:207–212.
18. Steinkamp LA: Biomechanical considerations in patellofemoral joint rehabilitation. Am J Sports Med 1993;21:438–442.

69 Peroneal Neuropathy

Alice V. Fann, MD

Synonyms

Peroneal palsy

Compression neuropathy of the peroneal nerve

Peroneal mononeuropathy

ICD-9 Codes

355.3
Common peroneal neuropathy

355.8
Mononeuritis of lower limb, unspecified

Definition

Peroneal neuropathy is a focal disorder that affects the peroneal nerve. The usual causes include compromise of nerve function by compression, entrapment, ischemia, or direct trauma. Entrapment or compression of the peroneal nerve occurs most commonly at the fibular head, where the nerve is superficial and covered only by skin and subcutaneous tissue (Fig. 1). Stretch injury to the peroneal nerve commonly occurs at the point of its tethering as it passes through the peroneus longus muscle.

Symptoms begin generally after a recent weight loss, plaster casting of the leg, ice application around the knee, or use of a knee brace or tight bandage at the knee. Symptoms may emerge as the patient is ambulated after an operation or after having been immobilized, paralyzed, or comatose during a prolonged hospitalization. Occupational squatting (e.g., as seen in roofers, carpetlayers, and farmers), squatting during child birth, and prolonged crossed-legged positions (e.g., as seen in religious and ceremonial practices, habit) carry a risk of injury to the peroneal nerve. Trauma to the nerve may result from dislocation, knee surgery (including arthroscopy), lacerations, blunt injury to the knee, fibular fracture, and severe ankle inversion injury (stretch injury).

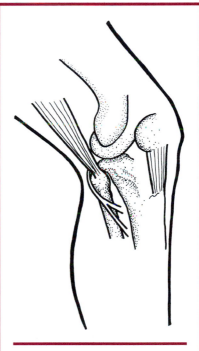

FIGURE 1. The peroneal nerve is superficial and subject to compression as it passes over the fibular head.

Symptoms

The patient with peroneal neuropathy typically presents with an acute foot drop, although in some cases the foot drop may develop slowly over a period of several days or weeks.[1] The foot drop may be complete or partial.

The salient complaints caused by the condition are those of frequent tripping, falls, or near-falls. The patient may report parasthesias in the lower lateral leg and dorsum of the foot, with or without accompanying numbness. Pain in peroneal neuropathy is rare, but when present, it is usually reported as occurring in or around the knee.

Physical Examination

Manifestations of the neuropathy will vary depending on the chronicity of the condition. In long-term cases there may be atrophy in the anterior and lateral compartments of the leg. The popliteal fossa and fibular head should be inspected and palpated for a Baker's cyst, nerve tumor, ganglion, and lipoma—each of which can compress the nerve. Tinel's sign with percussion at the fibular head may elicit pain or radiation in the distribution of the nerve.

The evaluation for a peroneal neuropathy should include a neurologic examination. The superficial peroneal nerve is relatively spared in most cases because of its topography, which protects it.[4,5] As a result, foot strength tests will demonstrate more weakness in dorsiflexion and great toe extension than in foot eversion. Foot inversion will be weak unless it is tested with the foot in plantarflexion, in which case it will have normal strength. Toe flexion; plantarflexion; knee flexion and extension; and hip flexion, extension, abduction, and adduction will be normal in uncomplicated cases of peroneal neuropathy.

Sensory testing will be abnormal in the distribution of the peroneal nerve. Sensation will be diminished more in the distribution of the *deep peroneal nerve* (first web space) but relatively spared over the distribution of the *superficial peroneal nerve* and *common peroneal nerve* distribution because of protective topography (Figs. 2 and 3). The overall sensory distribution for the L5 dermatome will be normal except where it overlaps with the peroneal distribution.

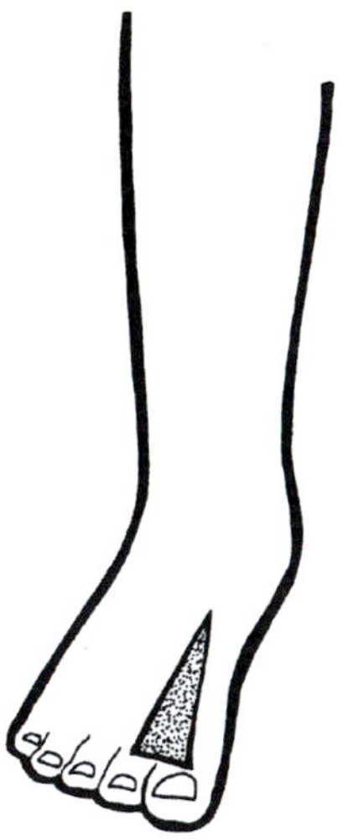

Testing of the lower extremity deep tendon reflexes should be normal.

On ambulation, the patient should demonstrate a foot slap or steppage gait and a hip hike. With a steppage gait, the patient will have increased flexion of the hip and knee and hiking of the pelvis for clearance of the toe and foot during the swing phase of the gait cycle. Due to weakness of the tibialis anterior muscle, the foot will slap down at heel contact.

Functional Limitations

Gait abnormalities, the major impairment from peroneal neuropathy, may lead to difficulty with activities of daily living, and vocational and recreational activities. Tasks that may be affected are those that require balance (since the anterior tibialis helps stabilize the ankle), such as lower extremity dressing, stepping in/out of the bathtub, and

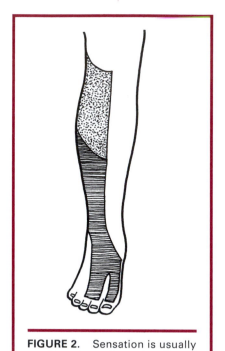

FIGURE 2. Sensation is usually unaffected or only mildly affected in the distribution of the *superficial peroneal nerve.*

FIGURE 3. Loss of sensation is most pronounced in the first web space, which is supplied by the *deep peroneal nerve.*

driving (especially if the right peroneal nerve is affected). The patient will also have difficulty climbing stairs and running, and may report injuries due to falls.

Diagnostic Studies

For suspected peroneal nerve injuries, electrodiagnostic studies are the "gold standard" for diagnosis and will help with the differentiation between other causes of a foot drop.[1,4]

Imaging studies are not usually indicated for the diagnosis of a peroneal neuropathy. An MRI of the knee, fibular head, and peroneal nerve region should be considered when a thorough history and physical examination have been unable to elucidate an etiology for the peroneal neuropathy.[6]

Differential Diagnosis

Sciatic mononeuropathy	Motor neuron disease
Lumbosacral plexopathy	Cerebral lesion
L5 radiculopathy	Triorthocresylphosphate toxicity

Treatment

Initial

The nerve needs to be protected from further injury and compression. The patient should be educated to avoid compressive postures such as leg crossing and to avoid external compression through the use of protective pads around knees, especially while sleeping. The patient should also be instructed on heel cord stretches to prevent contractures in the affected leg. Since pain is rarely an issue, medications are not typically prescribed. However, if pain is a problem, the usual medications may be utilized (e.g., NSAIDs/COX-2 inhibitors, analgesics, etc.).

Rehabilitation

Depending on the severity of the deficit and gait dysfunction, the patient may require a brace such as an ankle foot orthosis (AFO) and/or other assistive devices such as a cane to normalize gait and decrease falls or risk of falls. The typical AFO prescribed for a foot drop includes a dorsiflexion assist device such as a posterior leaf spring for a plastic AFO or spring in the posterior channel of a double upright AFO. A peroneal neuropathy secondary to a conduction block will be expected to heal spontaneously in 2 to 3 months, whereas a neuropathy due to an axonopathy at the fibular head may require 4 to 6 months to heal. Healing may be incomplete. Additional physical therapy, including intensive gait training, may be indicated for the patient for whom the neuropathy has become chronic and who has persistent gait abnormalities even with an AFO.

Procedures

Procedures are not indicated for peroneal neuropathy.

Surgery

Surgical intervention is appropriate if the nerve is lacerated; if compression is due to nerve tumor, ganglion, cyst, or lipoma; or if true entrapment of the nerve is suspected.

Potential Disease Complications

Potential disease complications include injury secondary to falls, back pain due to gait abnormalities, and plantarflexion contracture. Additionally, weakness and loss of sensation may be permanent.

Potential Treatment Complications

Analgesics, NSAIDs, and COX-2 inhibitors have well-known side effects that most commonly affect the gastric, hepatic, and renal systems. Skin breakdown brought on by malfitting orthotic devices is possible.

References
1. Katirji B: Peroneal neuropathy. Neurol Clin 1999;17:567–591.
2. Campbell WW: Diagnosis and management of common compression and entrapment neuropathies. Neurol Clinic 1997;15:549–567.
3. Esselman PC, Tomski MA, Robinson LR, et al: Selective deep peroneal nerve injury associated with arthroscopic knee surgery. Muscle Nerve 1993;16:1188–1192.
4. Wilbourn AJ. AAEM Case Report #12: Common peroneal mononeuropathy at the fibular head. Muscle Nerve 1986;9:825–836.
5. Levin KH, Stevens JC, Daube JR: Superficial peroneal nerve conduction studies for electrodiagnostic diagnosis. Muscle Nerve 1986;9:322–326.
6. Weig SG, Waite RJ, McAvoy K: MRI in unexplained mononeuropathy. Pediatr Neurol 2000;22:314–317.

70 Posterior Cruciate Ligament Sprain

Peter Bienkowski, MD
Lyle J. Micheli, MD

Synonyms

Posterior cruciate ligament tear

ICD-9 Codes

717.84
Old disruption of posterior cruciate ligament

844.2
Acute posterior cruciate ligament tear

Definition

Posterior cruciate ligament (PCL) tears represent 5% to 20% of all knee ligament injuries.[1] The PCL arises from the posterior aspect of the tibial plateau, crosses ("cruciate") behind the anterior cruciate ligament (ACL), and inserts into the lateral portion of the medial femoral condyle (Fig. 1). The main function of the PCL is to resist posterior displacement of the tibia on the femur. It also acts as a secondary restraint to external tibial rotation. Together with the ACL, it functions in the "screw home" mechanism of the knee by which the tibia glides to its exact position at terminal knee extension. Generally, PCL tears occur in a flexed knee when the tibia is displaced

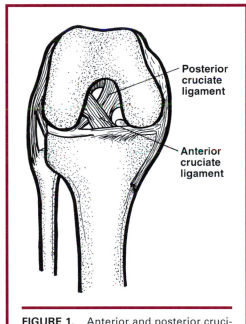

FIGURE 1. Anterior and posterior cruciate ligament structures.

posteriorly. This can occur in a motor vehicle accident–dashboard injury or during a fall on a flexed knee with the foot in plantarflexion. The PCL may also rupture due to hyperextension and rotation on a planted foot or due to forced hyperflexion. PCL injuries may occur in isolation, but generally they occur with other injuries (e.g., ACL tear, collateral ligament tear, and meniscal injuries).

The long-term sequelae of posterior instability of the knee may include the development of degenerative arthritis.[2]

Symptoms

It is important to obtain information about the nature of the injury. Typically, patients report that they have fallen on a flexed knee or have

TABLE 1. Classification of Posterior Cruciate Ligament Injuries

Grade	Definition	Laxity (mm)
I	PCL partially torn	< 5
II	PCL partially torn	5–9
III	PCL completely torn	> 10
IV a	PCL and LCL, posterolateral injury	> 12
IV b	PCL and MCL, posteromedial injury	> 12
IV c	PCL and ACL injury	> 15

NOTE: Grades I–III are isolated injuries; grade IV is a combined injury.
Adapted from Janousek AT, Jones DG, Clatworthy M, et al: Posterior cruciate ligament injuries of the knee joint. Sports Medicine 1999;28(6): 429–441.

sustained a blow to the anterior knee when it was flexed (e.g., on the dashboard of a car). Some patients may recall feeling or hearing a "pop" at the time of injury.

Patients may report pain along the medial and patellofemoral regions of the knee, instability, and an inability to weight bear and walk. Swelling can range from insignificant to very swollen.

Physical Examination

In an acute injury there may be contusions of the anterior tibia, and popliteal ecchymosis may be present. Swelling and effusions will vary and may not be present at all. See Table 1 for the general classifications of PCL injuries.

It is essential during the examination of the knee to thoroughly evaluate all knee ligaments in order to identify combined ligamentous injury. The goal of PCL evaluation is to exploit posterior subluxation of the tibia, which occurs with PCL insufficiency.

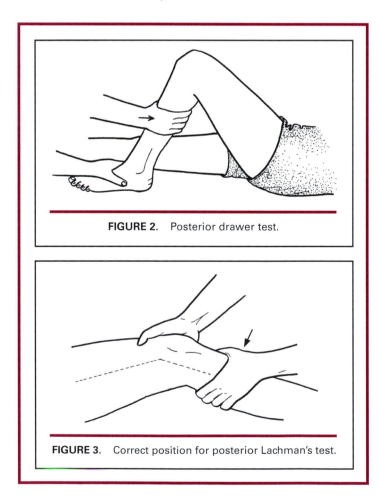

FIGURE 2. Posterior drawer test.

FIGURE 3. Correct position for posterior Lachman's test.

The "gold standard" of PCL examination is the posterior drawer test (Fig. 2). During this test, the knee is flexed at 90 degrees with the hip held at 45 degrees flexion. It is essential to appreciate a normal 1 cm step-off of the medial tibial plateau anterior to the medial femoral condyle. The absence of the step-off should alert the clinician to a possibility of PCL injury. Posterior pressure is applied to the tibia while the amount of displacement of the medial tibial step-offs and the quality of the endpoint in comparison with the contralateral knee are noted. Posterolateral instability may be evaluated using the *posterior drawer test* with the foot externally rotated 15 degrees. Similarly, posteromedial instability is assessed with the posterior drawer test with the foot internally rotated 15 degrees.

The *posterior Lachman test* involves positioning the knee at 30 degrees flexion with posterior pressure applied to the proximal tibia (Fig. 3). The extent of displacement and the quality of the endpoint are evaluated and compared with the contralateral knee.

The *posterior sag test* is performed with the patient supine with the hips and knees at 90 degrees flexion (Fig. 4). The clinician grasps both heels and inspects for posterior tibial translation consistent with an insufficient PCL.

The *reverse pivot shift* includes a valgus loaded, externally rotated knee moved from 90 degrees flexion to full extension (Fig. 5). A positive test is indicated by a pivot shift felt at 20 to 30 degrees when the posteriorly subluxated tibia is reduced.

The *dynamic posterior shift test* is implemented by extending the knee from 90 degrees flexion to full extension with 90 degrees hip flexion. A positive result is indicated if the tibia reduces with a "clunk" near full extension.

The *quadriceps active test* is achieved with the knee flexed at 60 degrees while the foot is secured by the clinician. The patient attempts to extend the knee isometrically. PCL insufficiency is demonstrated by anterior tibial translation from a subluxated position.

The neurologic examination should be normal with the possible exception of apparent weakness with strength testing due to pain.

Functional Limitations

Functional limitations of PCL tears may include difficulty with walking and a decrease in the level of functioning because of pain, as well as apprehension of instability. Athletes may be unable to complete cutting movements.

Diagnostic Studies

Diagnostic testing is useful as an adjunct to the clinical examination. The KT-1000 arthrometer is highly specific in the detection of high-grade PCL tears.[3] Stress radiographs may be obtained to document the extent of posterior

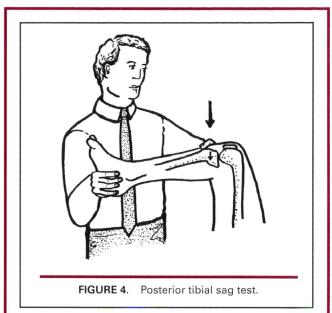

FIGURE 4.   Posterior tibial sag test.

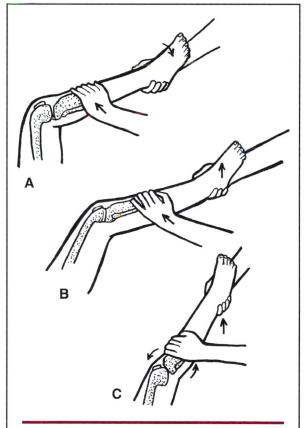

FIGURE 5.   Reverse pivot shift test. *A*, The knee is flexed to 90°. A valgus, external rotation force is applied to the knee. *B*, The knee is extended while the valgus, external rotation is maintained. *C*, Near full extension, the lateral tibia shifts forward, reducing the knee and confirming PCL deficiency.

instability. After an acute injury, plain x-rays must be performed to rule out fractures, including PCL avulsions (the tunnel view is best to visualize this). MRI assessment is highly specific and sensitive in assessment of PCL injuries.[4] Finally, diagnostic arthroscopy allows direct visualization of the PCL.

Differential Diagnosis

Anterior cruciate ligament tear

Collateral ligament tear

Meniscal tear

Osteochondral fracture

Patellar tendon rupture

Patellofemoral dislocation

Tibial plateau fracture

Treatment

Initial

Initial treatment consists of protection, rest, ice, compression, and elevation (PRICE); crutches; and short-term NSAIDs/COX-2 inhibitors. Analgesics may be used to control pain if this is an issue. Currently, non-operative treatment is advocated for those with isolated PCL injuries with mild (grade I or II) laxity.[3] Some recommend conservative treatment for all acute isolated PCL injury as well as chronic, isolated, asymptomatic PCL injury when newly diagnosed with no history of prior rehabilitation.[5]

Surgical intervention is advocated for patients with bony avulsion fractures, combined ligament injuries, and chronic symptomatic PCL laxity.[6]

Rehabilitation

Non-operative rehabilitation consists of early motion and aggressive quadriceps rehabilitation while preventing posterior tibial sag. The use of a PCL functional brace has not been proven to be effective, although some may find it useful.[6] Management includes immobilization in extension with a Velcro knee immobilizer and avoidance of hamstring exercise. After acute symptoms have subsided, or immediately if dealing with a chronic tear, daily stationary bicycle exercises can be initiated. After 3 months, closed-chain exercises are started, with the exception of isolated hamstring strengthening, which is done later in the course.[7]

Postoperative PCL rehabilitation includes initial bracing in full extension to prevent posterior tibial translation. Continuous passive motion, straight leg raising, and quadriceps static exercises are initiated soon after surgery. The day following surgery, partial weight bearing with crutches is initiated as tolerated. In the early phase of rehabilitation, gravity assisted flexion exercises to 90 degrees and closed-chain exercises emphasizing quadriceps strengthening are pursued. The progression to greater than 90 degrees of flexion is delayed until after 6 weeks following surgery. At 9 to 12 months following surgical intervention, the patient with full range of motion, equal strength compared with the contralateral leg, and a stable knee is allowed to return to full activity.

Procedures

Arthrocentesis is performed for painful effusions (hemarthrosis). As mentioned earlier, KT-1000 arthrometer testing is done for diagnostic purposes and to document the degree of instability.[3]

Surgery

Various surgical techniques have been developed for the repair of the PCL. Controversy exists regarding the most effective procedure.[7] The aim of surgery is to replace the PCL with a graft inserted into a tunnel drilled through the tibia and femur. Allograft or autograft tissue are most commonly used. Donor sites include the patellar tendon; hamstring tendons; and rarely, the quadriceps tendon. Achilles tendon allograft is also useful. PCL reconstruction is performed arthroscopically, arthroscopically-assisted, or open.[5]

Potential Disease Complications

Potential disease complications include pain, limitation of function and activity, and onset of degenerative arthritis. Patients with isolated PCL tears tend to fare better than patients with combined ligamentous injuries.[8] Recent studies suggest that non-operatively treated PCL injuries allow many athletes to return to their sport independent of level of laxity.[8] However, late degenerative arthritis has been reported as a consequence of PCL instability.[9]

Potential Treatment Complications

Treatment complications include the well-known side effects of NSAIDs that may be mitigated with the newer COX-2 inhibitors. Prolonged bracing can lead to significant muscular weakness and atrophy. The risks of surgery, although uncommon, are also well known. These include the risks of anesthesia. In addition, bleeding is controlled with the use of a tourniquet and surgical hemostasis. Infection is limited with diligent sterile technique as well as antibiotics. Damage to nerve and vascular structures, the popliteal vessels in particular, is a slight risk. Postoperative laxity of the PCL graft may occur. The theoretic risk of disease transmission with the use of allograft tissues is extremely low.

References
1. Hannus P, Bergfeld J, Jarvinen M, et al: Injuries to the posterior cruciate ligament of the knee. Sports Medicine 1991;12(2):110–131.
2. Janousek AT, Jones DG, Clatworthy M, et al: Posterior cruciate ligament injuries of the knee joint. Sports Medicine 1999;28(6):429–441.
3. Rubinstein RA Jr, Shelbourne KD, McCarroll JR, et al: The accuracy of the clinical examination in the setting of posterior cruciate ligament injuries. Am Orthop Soc Sports Med 1994;22(4):550–557.
4. Gross ML, Grover JS, Bassett LW, et al: Magnetic resonance imaging of the posterior cruciate ligament: Clinical use to improve diagnostic accuracy. Am J Sports Med 1992;20:732–737.
5. Margheritini F, Mariani PF, Mariani PP: Current concepts in diagnosis and treatment of posterior cruciate ligament injury. Acta Orthopaedica Belgica 2000;66(3):217–228.
6. St. Pierre P, Miller MD: Posterior cruciate ligament injuries. Clin Sports Med 1999;18(1):199–221.
7. Barber FA, Fanelli GC, Matthews LS, et al: The treatment of complete posterior cruciate ligament tears. Arthroscopy 2000;16(7):725–731.
8. Shelbourne KD, Davis TJ, Patel DV: The natural history of acute, isolated, nonoperatively treated posterior cruciate ligament injuries. Am J Sports Med 1999;27(3):276–283.
9. Boynton MD, Tietjens BR: Long-term follow-up of untreated isolated posterior cruciate deficient knees. Am J Sports Med 1996;24:306–310.

71 Quadriceps Tendinitis

Peter Bienkowski, MD
Lyle J. Micheli, MD

Synonyms

None

ICD-9 Codes

726.60
Enthesopathy of knee, unspecified

844.8
Sprains and strains of knee and leg, other specified sites

959.7
Injury, other and unspecified, knee, leg, ankle, and foot

Definition

The quadriceps tendon is located at the insertion of the quadriceps muscle into the patella and functions as part of the knee extensor mechanism. Quadriceps tendinitis is an overuse syndrome characterized by repetitive overloading of the quadriceps tendon. The common mechanism of injury is microtrauma, in which the basal ability of the tissue to repair itself is outpaced by the repetition of insult.[1] Quadriceps tendinitis often occurs in athletes participating in running and jumping sports, as well as in persons who perform frequent kneeling, squatting, and stairclimbing.[2]

Symptoms

Patients usually report an insidious onset of knee pain and may note painful clicking. A burning sensation at the bone-tendon junction may be experienced.[3] The pain is aggravated by activity that challenges the extensor mechanism, including bending, stairclimbing, running, and jumping. Severe weakness, an inability to extend the knee or the report of acute trauma with a "pop" should alert the clinician to the possibility of a quadriceps tendon partial or complete rupture.

Physical Examination

On examination of the knee, point tenderness is localized along the superior pole of the patella and along the quadriceps tendon. Quadriceps tendon pain may be elucidated with extreme knee flexion and by resisted knee extension. The clinician should also be on the lookout for a palpable defect, suggesting partial rupture of the quadriceps tendon. Neurologic exam should be normal with the possible exception of strength testing, which may be limited by pain or partial tendon rupture.

Functional Limitations

Quadriceps tendinitis may interfere with activities of daily living. Pain is usually felt with stairclimbing, kneeling, and rising from a chair. Athletes may be unable to participate in running and jumping activities.

Diagnostic Studies

Quadriceps tendinitis is a clinical diagnosis, and diagnostic investigations are not generally necessary. If a partial tear of the quadriceps tendon is suspected but not apparent clinically, MRI may be of assistance in confirming the diagnosis.

Differential Diagnosis

Patellar tendinitis

Patellofemoral syndrome

Prepatellar bursitis

Quadriceps tendon rupture

Quadriceps strain

Quadriceps contusion

Quadriceps tear

Patellar fracture

Apophysitis

Anterior fat pad syndrome

Chondromalacia patella

Osteochondritis dissecans

Plica

Treatment

Initial

Initial treatment includes rest from aggravating activities. Activity modification should include protection from eccentric or high-load knee extension (e.g., going up and down stairs, bending, jumping). Proper warmup and stretching should be conducted prior to activity. Also, the application of ice to the injured area for 20 minutes, 2 to 3 times daily and before and after athletics can be useful. NSAIDs/COX-2 inhibitors may be used for pain and inflammation. In some instances, knee immobilizers are used but may promote weakness and disuse atrophy.

Rehabilitation

The main treatment modality includes muscle strengthening and stretching. All muscle-strengthening exercises are conducted in the pain-free range. Static exercises may be utilized to minimize compressive forces across the patellofemoral joint.[2] Therapeutic modalities including ultrasonography, phonophoresis, or iontophoresis may be employed.[2] The use of icing immediately after activity or work has been advocated.[4] A general conditioning program is recommended.

Procedures

Local steroid injections are not typically done because of the risk of tendon rupture, but may be necessary in some cases.

Surgery

Quadriceps tendinitis is mostly managed non-operatively. Surgical intervention may be necessary in rare cases. If partial tendon rupture is suspected, surgical consultation is advised.

Potential Disease Complications

Functional deterioration with the development of chronic symptoms may occur. A high level of functioning in patients with quadriceps tendinitis is usually regained and maintained.[2] In rare cases of progressive microtrauma to the injured area, rupture of tendon may result.

Potential Treatment Complications

The complications related to NSAID use include the development of gastritis, as well as renal and hepatic involvement. COX-2 inhibitors may reduce the risk of gastric complications. Steroid injection may predispose the tendon to rupture. Repeated injections of corticosteroids may increase the risk for mucoid degeneration, fibrinoid necrosis, mineralization, fibroblastic degeneration, and capillary proliferation within the tendon.[5]

References

1. Micheli LJ, Fehlandt AF JR: Overuse injuries to tendons and apophyses in children and adolescents. Clin Sports Med 1992;11(4):713–726.
2. Westrich GH, Haas SB, Bono JV: Occupational knee injuries. Orthop Clin North Am 1996;27(4):805–814.
3. Yost JG Jr, Ellfeldt HJ: Basketball injuries. The Lower Extremity and Spine in Sports Medicine. 1986;43:1440–1466.
4. Antich TJ, Randall CC, Westbrook RA, et al: Treatment of knee extensor mechanism disorders: Comparison of four treatment modalities. J Orthop Sports Phys Ther 1986;8:225–259.
5. Key J, Johnson D, Jarvis G, Ponsonby D: Knee and Thigh Injuries. Sports Medicine of the Lower Extremity. 1989;17:297–310.

72 Shin Splints

Michael J. Woods, DO

Synonyms

Medial tibial stress syndrome

Periostitis

Medial tibial periostalgia

ICD-9 Codes

730.3
Periostitis without mention of osteomyelitis

844.9
Sprains and strains of knee and leg, unspecified site

Definition

Shin splints is defined as pain and discomfort in the anterior portion of the foreleg from repetitive activity on hard surfaces, or due to forcible, excessive use of the foot flexors. The diagnosis should be limited to musculoskeletal inflammations, excluding stress fractures and ischemic disorders.[1]

Shin splints most commonly occur in athletes who have sudden increases or changes in their training activity. This disorder occurs in dancers, gymnasts, runners, and in athletes who participate in court or field sports. The etiology of shin splints is not clearly defined, but it likely is multifactorial and involves biomechanical abnormalities of the foot/ankle, poor footwear and shock absorption, hard playing surfaces, and training errors.

Symptoms

It is important for the clinician to differentiate shin splints, which is a fairly benign condition, from acute compartment syndrome which is an emergency and stress fractures, which is a more serious condition (see Chapters 61 and 73). Patients presenting with shin splints are usually athletes or dancers and complain of a localized area of posteromedial tibial pain that is dull and aching in quality. This is usually near the junction of the mid to distal one third of the tibia (Fig. 1). Symptoms are commonly bilateral, occur with exercise, and are relieved with rest.[2] Initially the pain may ease with continued running and recur after prolonged activity. Those with more severe symptoms may have persistent pain with normal walking or at rest.

Contributing factors include weakness of anterior and posterior compartment musculature, training errors such as running in poor footwear or on hard surfaces, inadequate warmup, and increasing training intensity too quickly. Lower extremity biomechanical malalignments may play a role, including hyperpronation, pes cavus, tarsal coalition, leg-length discrepancy, tibial torsion, excessive femoral anteversion, and increased Q-angle.[3,4]

In school-age athletes and adults who participate in seasonal sports, shin splints can occur when they resume their sport or start a new sport (e.g., high school or college athletes who go from playing basketball to cross country or track).

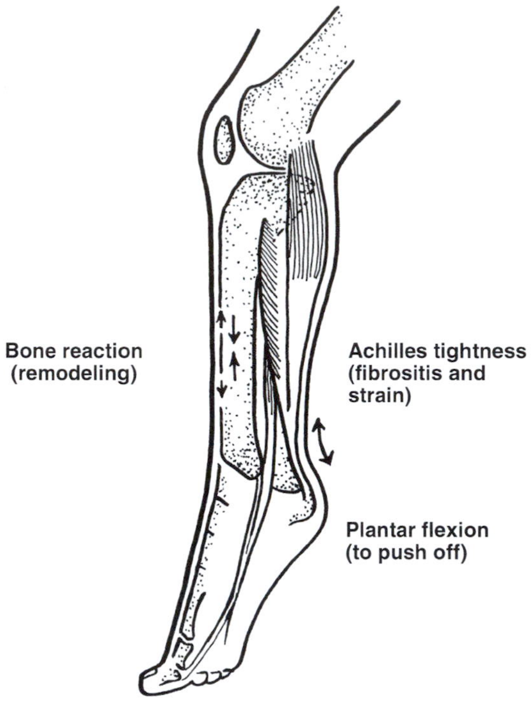

FIGURE 1. Repetitive microtrauma and overuse in running leads to soft tissue and even bony breakdown, a process commonly called "shin splints." Muscle overpull can lead to periostitis, strain, or trabecular breakdown. The area approximately 13 cm proximal to the tip of the medial malleolus along the posterior tibial cortex appears to be maximally at risk.

Labels in figure:
- Bone reaction (remodeling)
- Achilles tightness (fibrositis and strain)
- Plantar flexion (to push off)

Physical Examination

Physical examination typically reveals generalized tenderness along the medial tibia. Mild swelling may also be present. Resisted plantarflexion, toe flexion, or toe raises may aggravate symptoms. Striking a tuning fork and placing it on the tibia may reproduce the pain associated with stress fractures (see Chapter 73). Patients with stress fractures will usually have point tenderness over the bone, whereas those with shin splints will have more widespread tenderness to palpation. Patients must also be examined for signs of co-existing lower extremity problems that may be contributing to their symptoms including forefoot pronation (flat feet) and excessive heel valgus. Inflexibility may also contribute to shin splints, and the clinician should note tight Achilles tendon, hamstrings, etc. The neurologic exam, including strength, sensation, and deep tendon reflexes, should be normal.

Functional Limitations

In early stages of shin splints, activity limitations occur most often while running or participating in ballistic activities or dancing. When more severe, symptoms may occur with walking or at rest, thus causing further functional limitations. Athletes may be unable to participate in their sport.

Diagnostic Studies

Plain x-rays are typically negative early in the disease process. Later, there may be evidence of periosteal thickening. Radionucleotide bone scanning helps to differentiate shin splints from stress fracture. Diffuse radioisotopic uptake along the medial or posteromedial tibia on the delayed phase is the pattern usually seen with shin splints. A focal defined area of uptake in all phases is more consistent with a stress fracture.[5] MRI can also help diagnose a stress fracture, but is not usually necessary. Exertional compartment syndrome is uncommon, but if clinical suspicion is high, compartment pressure measurements must be done to rule it out.

Differential Diagnosis

Stress fracture

Chronic exertional compartment syndrome

Tendinitis

Muscle strain

Vascular and muscular abnormalities

Primary muscle disease

Peroneal nerve entrapment

Fascial defect

Muscle herniation

Lumbar radiculopathy

Treatment

Initial

Relative rest—that is participation in only those activities that can be done without pain—is the key to initial management. If reducing running intensity or mileage allows the athlete to remain pain-free, continuing the activity may be acceptable. Generally, however, even in mild cases, the athlete should avoid repetitive lower extremity stress for at least 1 to 2 weeks. In more serious cases, athletes may need to stop running entirely for a longer period of time. If walking is painful, crutches are indicated. An air stirrup brace may also decrease pain associated with weight bearing.[4]

Stretching and ice or ice massage to the involved areas can be helpful. NSAIDs/COX-2 inhibitors can reduce inflammation and help manage pain. Analgesics can be taken for pain as well.

In addressing malalignments of the lower extremities, orthoses, such as longitudinal arch supports with or without a medial heel wedge, may be indicated in select patients.

Rehabilitation

In individuals who continue to have pain despite initial conservative treatment, physical therapy may be indicated to decrease pain and further educate the patient about the disorder. Modalities such as electrical stimulation and ultrasound may be used. Advising the patient to ice after exercise is helpful.

Once the symptoms have diminished, the rehabilitation program focuses on improving strength, flexibility, and endurance and preventing recurrence of the injury.[6]

The primary muscles involved in shin splints are the flexor digitorum longus and the soleus. Others have implicated the tibialis posterior, but its attachment is more posterior than the area of typical shin splint symptoms, and it actually attaches more to the interosseous membrane, rather than the medial tibia.[7] The deep crural fascia also attaches to the posteromedial tibia. Rehabilitation for shin splints involves improving the flexibility, strength, and endurance of the involved muscles.

Anterior compartment stretching exercises, Achilles tendon stretching, and overall lower extremity flexibility exercises are important. Eccentric strengthening of antagonistic muscle groups is also useful. Pain can be a guide in the advancement of the rehabilitation program.

Athletes should have full range of motion that is symmetric to the uninvolved side and have near full strength before returning to their prior activity or to competition. Plyometrics should be avoided until a high level of strength, endurance, and flexibility have been attained.

Cardiovascular fitness should be maintained through lower impact activities, such as biking, swimming or water running.

Return to previous activity level should be a gradual process and should be individualized, based on the athlete's response to increasing intensity of training. Proper footwear is essential. Running shoes lose greater than 60% of their shock absorption after 250 miles of use.[3] Orthotics are often necessary in those individuals with foot abnormalities, such as pes planus.

Procedures

There is really no proven benefit noted in the literature to support any type of procedure, such as local cortisone injection, in the treatment of shin splints.

Surgery

Surgery is rarely indicated, but would involve a posteromedial fasciotomy with release of the fascial bridge of the medial soleus and the fascia of the deep posterior compartment, with periosteal cauterization.[5] Surgery is very effective in relieving pain, but it frequently leaves the patient with persistent strength deficits.

Potential Disease Complications

If shin splints are not treated and biomechanical malalignments are not addressed, stress fractures and potentially true fractures may occur. This would result in further morbidity and more time lost from the desired physical activity.

Potential Treatment Complications

Complications involving the gastrointestinal system, liver, and kidneys may result from treatment with NSAIDs. COX-2 inhibitors may have fewer gastric side effects. Fasciotomy may result in residual weakness. Overly aggressive rehabilitation may progress the injury.

References
1. Subcommittee on Classification of Injuries in Sports and Committee on the Medical Aspects of Sports: Standard nomenclature of athletic injuries. Chicago, American Medical Association, 1966.
2. Andrish JA: The leg. In DeLee JC, Drez D (eds): Orthopedic Sports Medicine: Principles and Practice. Philadelphia, W.B. Saunders, 1994, pp 1603–1607.
3. Touliopolous S, Hershman EB: Lower leg pain: Diagnosis and treatment of compartment syndromes and other pain syndromes of the leg. Sports Med 1999;27(3):193–204.
4. Reid DC: Sports Injury Assessment and Rehabilitation. New York, Churchill Livingstone, 1992, pp 269–300.
5. Barry NN, McGuire JL: Acute Injuries and specific problems in adult athletes. Rheum Dis Clin North Am 1996;22(3):531–549.
6. Windsor RE, Chambers K: Overuse injuries of the leg. In Kibler WB, Herring SA, Press JM (eds): Functional Rehabilitation of Sports and Musculoskeletal Injuries. Gaithersburg, MD, Aspen, 1998, pp 265–267.
7. Beck BR, Osternig LR: Medial tibial stress syndrome: The location of muscles in the leg in relation to symptoms. J Bone Joint Surg Am 1994;76-A(7):1057–1061.

73 Stress Fractures

Sheila Dugan, MD

Definition

Stress fractures are complete or partial bone fractures caused by the accumulation of microtrauma.[1] Normal bone accommodates to stress via ongoing remodeling; if this remodeling system does not keep pace with the force applied, stress reaction (micro fractures) and, finally, stress fracture can result. Both extrinsic and intrinsic factors have been implicated in this imbalance between bone resorption and bone deposition.[2] Malalignment and poor flexibility of the lower extremities (intrinsic factors) and inadequate footwear, changes in training surface, and increases in training intensity and duration without an adequate ramp-up period (extrinsic factors) can lead to stress fractures.[3]

Stress fractures in athletes are most common in the lower extremities.[4] The most common sites include the tibia, metatarsals, and fibula and most commonly affect runners and dancers. The fracture site is the area of greatest stress, such as the origin of lower leg muscles along the medial tibia.[5] A narrower mediolateral tibial width was a risk factor for femoral, tibial and foot stress fractures in a study of military recruits.[6]

Stress fractures may be related to abnormalities of the bone, such as in female athletes with low bone density due to exercise-induced menstrual abnormalities.[7–10] Premature osteoporosis leads to an increased risk for stress fractures. One study looked at premenopausal female runners and collegiate athletes and concluded that those with absent or irregular menses were at increased risk of musculoskeletal injuries while engaged in active training.[10] Muscular deficits in the gastrocnemius-soleus complex in jumping athletes have also been implicated in causing tibial stress fractures. Bone injury may be a secondary event following a primary failure of muscle function.[11]

Symptoms

Patients may report a recent increase in training or activity level preceding the onset of symptoms. Due to pain in the affected region of the bone, patients may seek medical attention during the micro fracture or stress reaction phase of injury. Should they forego resting the area (avoiding the pain-provoking activity), their injury can progress to stress fracture. The pain will gradually increase with activity and may occur with less intense exercise, such as walking, or even at rest. In general, however, the pain will improve with rest. The pain can lead to a decline in

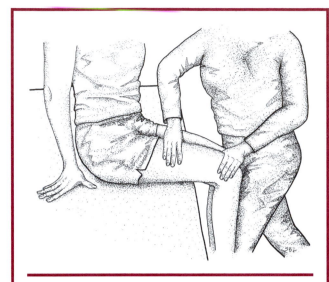

FIGURE 1. Physical examination technique to evaluate for femoral stress fracture. The examiner applies a downward pressure on the distal femur, using the examination table as a fulcrum, to increase the force across the fracture site. A positive test reproduces the individual's pain.

performance. The individual may also note swelling in the affected region of the bone. Symptoms of paresthesias and numbness should alert the clinician that an alternative diagnosis should be considered.

Physical Examination

On physical examination, the clinician will find an area of exquisite, well-localized tenderness, warmth, and edema over the affected region of the bone. Ecchymosis may be present with foot involvement. Percussion of the nearby region can cause pain. Placing a vibrating tuning fork over the fracture site intensifies the pain.[12] In the tibia, stress fractures primarily occur along the medial border; the frequency, in order, is upper, lower, and midshaft. In the fibula, they usually occur one hand-breadth proximal to the lateral malleolus.[2] Tarsal or metatarsal stress fractures present with localized foot tenderness. Weight-bearing activity, such as a one legged-hop test, can provoke the pain by increasing the ground reaction forces. For a presumed femoral stress fracture, the clinician can provoke pain by applying a downward force on the distal femur while the affected individual is seated with the distal femur extending beyond the edge of the seat (Fig. 1).

The physical examination must include an examination of the lumbar spine and lower limbs to evaluate for any biomechanical abnormalities. For instance, an individual with rigid supinated feet or weak foot intrinsic muscles may transmit more ground reaction forces to the tibia. On physical exam, one can identify problems that must be addressed in treatment planning.

Strength should be normal but occasionally is limited by pain. Sensation and deep tendon reflexes should also be normal.

Functional Limitations

Recreational and athletic activities requiring weight bearing through the affected lower limb may be limited by pain. For instance, running results in the transmission of increased ground reaction forces through the leg. These forces can increase if one runs on a concrete surface versus an all-weather track. In acute cases, ambulation can be painful.

Diagnostic Studies

Plain films may take as long as 6 weeks to demonstrate fracture. Technetium-99m diphosphonate bone scanning will yield the earliest confirmatory data for stress fractures, demonstrating a "hot spot" in 1 to 4 days.[12] The fracture site may not return to normal on a bone scan for 5 months or longer. CT is necessary for differentiating stress fractures of the sacrum and pelvis. MRI provides soft tissue definition, which can be helpful in the setting of stress reaction or tendinitis; although it can confirm the diagnosis in the acute phase, it is generally not indicated initially. One should consider bone density testing in women with a history of amenorrhea.[13]

Differential Diagnosis

Medial tibial stress syndrome

Osteoid osteoma

Compartment syndromes

Deep vein thrombosis

Knee pathology (e.g., pes anserine bursitis)

Bone neoplasm

Osteomyelitis

Treatment

Initial

Pain and edema should be managed initially with PRICE (protection, rest, ice, compression, and elevation) and oral nonsteroidal anti-inflammatory drugs (NSAIDs). There is ongoing controversy regarding the negative impact of NSAIDs on healing.[14] Activities that provoke pain are eliminated. Fractures with the propensity to progress to non-union may require immediate immobilization, such as midshaft tibial stress fractures. Femoral neck fractures on the tension (superior) aspect can become displaced and require strict non–weight-bearing status with axillary crutches initially.[15] Metatarsal stress fractures can be treated with a stiff shoe and a straight cane or a rigid orthosis. Navicular fractures may require immobilization in a short leg cast.[14]

In the setting of female athletes with exercised-induced amenorrhea, nutritional counseling and correction of any energy debt must be included in the stress fracture treatment program. If the menstrual cycle does not return with these interventions, there is controversy regarding the use of an oral contraceptive pill to restore menses. Fewer athletes with fractures were using oral contraceptive pills than athletes without fractures in one study.[16] In addition, women without stress fractures had a higher intake of calcium than those with stress fractures. Nine elite runners with stress fractures were compared with matched controls without stress fractures, and significant differences in the number of menses per year (less in fracture group) and the age of onset of menses (delayed in fracture group) were identified.[17]

Rehabilitation

Physical therapy modalities, such as heat and interferential electrical stimulation, are used to increase local blood flow and promote healing; however, there is a lack of controlled studies to prove their efficacy. Deep soft tissue massage, including transverse friction massage, may be indicated and complement stretching for the muscles that originate along the medial tibia. Ongoing cardiovascular and strengthening activities should continue if they produce no pain; aqua jogging, stationary bicycling, or use of the elliptical machine can be substituted for running. An athlete can return to running once pain free with ambulation and cross training activities; however, training schedules should be modified and pain should be used as the guide to progressing the program.[18] Sports-specific training must be addressed prior to return to play.

Careful attention to the training surface and equipment is mandatory. In the setting of significant forefoot or rearfoot biomechanical abnormalities, custom foot orthotics may be indicated. Taping may be utilized temporarily to provide stability of the ankle and foot. Specific lower extremity strengthening is progressed from static exercises to concentric to eccentric training, based on symptoms. Plyometric (weight-bearing eccentric) training should precede return to play. Shock absorbing insoles and running on softer surfaces, such as grass, decrease the ground reaction forces transmitted to the bones of the lower extremity. In a prospective study of athletes without control subjects, immobilization with a pneumatic leg brace was utilized to allow for participation in a modified training schedule earlier. The authors concluded that the brace promoted healing and limited the forces across the fracture site.[19]

Procedures

There is no specific non-surgical procedure for this injury.

Surgery

Conservative management successfully treats lower extremity stress fractures with a few exceptions. Femoral neck stress fractures on the tensile (superior) aspect may require pinning if they do not heal after a course of non–weight bearing. Midshaft tibial fractures are at risk of non-union and must be immobilized and followed closely; an open bone grafting procedure may be indicated in the setting of non-union.

Potential Disease Complications

Recurrent stress fractures can occur if biomechanical and training principles are not addressed during treatment. In female athletes with menstrual abnormalities and premature osteoporosis, failure to treat these conditions might also lead to recurrent stress fractures.

Potential Treatment Complications

Immobilization can lead to loss of joint range of motion and muscle strength. Complications of surgery include non-union and other typical infrequent complications such as infection, bleeding, etc. NSAID treatment risks include gastrointestinal, hepatic, and renal side effects. Treatment of amenorrhea with oral contraceptive pills involves increased risk for blood clots and their sequelae. Treatment of premature osteoporosis with bisphosphonates includes risk for esophageal erosion or ulceration.

References

1. McBryde AM: Stress fractures in runners. Clin Sports Med 1985;4:737–752.
2. Reid DC: Exercise induced leg pain. In Reid DC (ed): Sports Injury Assessment and Rehabilitation. New York, Churchill Livingstone, 1992.
3. Sullivan D. Stress fractures in 51 runners. Clin Orthop 1984;187:188.
4. Bennell KL, Brukner PD: Epidemiology and site specificity of stress fractures. Clin Sports Med 1997;16:179–196.
5. Markey KL: Stress fractures. Clin Sports Med 1987;6(2):405–425.
6. Giladi M, Milgrom C, Simkin A, et al: Stress fractures: Identifiable risk factors. Am J Sports Med 1991;19:647–652.
7. Myburgh DH, Bachrach LK, et al: Low bone mineral density at axial and appendicular sites in amenorrheic athletes. Med Sci Sports Exerc 1993;25:1197–1202.
8. Barrow G, Saha S: Menstrual irregularity and stress fracture in collegiate female distance runners. Am J Sports Med 1988;16:209–216.
9. Marcus R, Cann C, et al: Menstrual function and bone mass in elite women distance runners: Endocrine and metabolic factors. Ann Intern Med 1985;102:158–163.
10. Lloyd T, Triantafyllou SJ, et al: Women athletes with menstrual irregularity have increased musculoskeletal injuries. Med Sci Sports Exerc 1986;18:374–379.
11. Keats TE: Radiology of Musculoskeletal Stress Injury. Chicago, Year Book Medical Publishers, 1990.
12. Young JL, Press JM: Rehabilitation of running injuries. In Buschbacher R, Braddom R (eds): Sports Medicine and Rehabilitation: A Sports Specific Approach. Philadelphia, Hanley & Belfus, 1994.
13. Nattiv A, Armsey TD: Stress injury to bone in the female athlete. Clin Sports Med 1997;16(2):197–219.
14. Snider RK (ed): Essentials of Musculoskeletal Care. Rosemont, IL, American Academy of Orthopedic Surgery, 1997, pp 485–486.
15. Windsor RE, Chambers K: Overuse injuries of the leg. In Kibler WB, Herring SA, Press JM (eds): Functional Rehabilitation of Sports and Musculoskeletal Injuries. Gaithersburg, Aspen, 1998, pp 186–187.
16. Myburgh KH, Hutchins J, et al: Low bone density is an etiologic factor for stress fracture in athletes. Ann Intern Med 1990;113:754–759.
17. Carbon R, Sambrook PN, et al: Bone density of elite female athletes with stress fractures. Med J Austral 1990;153:373–376.
18. Brody DM: Techniques in the evaluation and treatment of the injured runner. Orthop Clin North Am 1982;13:541.
19. Whitelaw GP, Wetzler MJ, Levy AS, et al: A pneumatic leg brace for the treatment of tibial stress fractures. Clin Orthop 1991;207:301–305.

74 | Total Knee Replacement

Robert J. Kaplan, MD

Synonyms

Total knee arthroplasty

Total knee implant

Unicompartmental knee arthroplasty

Revision knee arthroplasty

ICD-9 Codes

715.16
Osteoarthrosis, localized, primary, lower leg

715.26
Osteoarthrosis, localized, secondary, lower leg

V52.1
Fitting and adjustment of prosthetic device and implant, artificial leg (complete) (partial)

Definition

Arthroplasty involves the reconstruction by natural modification or artificial replacement of a diseased, damaged, or ankylosed joint.

There are three basic types of total knee arthroplasty: *totally constrained, semi-constrained,* and *totally unconstrained*. The amount of constraint built into an artificial joint reflects the amount of stability the hardware provides. As such, a totally constrained joint has the femoral portion physically attached to the tibial component and requires no ligamentous or soft tissue support. The semi-constrained total knee arthroplasty has two separate components that glide on each other, but the physical characteristics of the tibial component prevent excessive femoral glide. The totally unconstrained device relies completely on the body's ligaments and soft tissues to maintain the stability of the joint.

The semi-constrained and totally unconstrained knee implants are most often utilized. In general, the totally unconstrained implants afford the most normal range of motion and gait.

In unicompartmental knee arthroplasty, only the joint surfaces on one side of the knee (usually the medial compartment) are replaced. Unicompartmental knee arthroplasty provides better relief than does a tibial osteotomy and greater range of motion than does a total knee arthroplasty, as well as improved ambulation velocity.

The principal diagnoses most commonly associated with total knee replacement procedures are osteoarthrosis and allied disorders (90.9%), followed by rheumatoid arthritis and other inflammatory polyarthropathies (3.4%).[8] The knee is the joint most often replaced in arthroplasty procedures. The most common age group for total knee replacements is 65 to 84. Women in this age range are more likely to undergo total knee arthroplasty than their male counterparts.

Symptoms

Refractory knee pain is the most common symptom among patients who undergo total knee arthroplasty. Stiffness, deformity, and instability are symptoms also commonly seen in advanced osteoarthrosis or inflammatory polyarthropathy. In the postoperative period, acute surgical pain manifests and is most intense during the first 2 weeks. Disruption and inflammation of the periarticular soft tissues present as a soft tissue stiffness pattern that differs from the preoperative rigid stiffness of advanced arthrosis. Joint proprioception impairment may give rise to a sense of mild knee instability in the postoperative period. Uncommonly, debris may generate a sense of cracking, popping, or locking. (See also Chapter 64.)

Physical Examination

The findings of advanced arthrosis on examination are joint hypertrophy, joint line tenderness, and reduced passive and active range of motion associated with crepitus. Valgus deformity is common in osteoarthrosis. Varus deformity is more common in rheumatoid arthritis. Ligamentous laxity is more commonly encountered in rheumatoid arthritis as compared with osteoarthritis. Additional findings include joint effusion and concomitant suprapatellar or pes anserine bursitis. In the postoperative period, staples or sutures appose the incision margins. A serosanguineous discharge may be present during the first week postoperatively. There is marked effusion of the knee joint. Increased warmth and erythema are prominent features along with hyperpathia/allodynia. Muscle inhibition of the quadriceps and hamstrings interferes with manual muscle testing. Range of motion is most often guarded secondary to pain. (See also Chapter 64.)

Functional Limitations

Advanced osteoarthrosis of the knee compromises functional activities as the patient's knee pain becomes recalcitrant and unresponsive to conservative therapeutic interventions. In the immediate postoperative period the inhibited quadriceps and hamstrings may not adequately stabilize the knee and the patient may require a knee immobilizer for transfers and walking.

The patient will require a two-handed assistive device (e.g., walker or axillary crutches) for gait training initially. Adaptive equipment for bathing and dressing (e.g., tub or shower seat, grab bars, dressing sticks, sock aid) is generally necessary. The patient may not have sufficient range of motion during the first week postoperatively to negotiate stairs. The motor reactions normalize by the third week; therefore, patients may return to driving activities if they can perform car transfers independently and can tolerate sitting for prolonged periods.

After reintegration into the community, patients require up to 1 year to achieve 80% of normal muscle strength; walking speeds remain 10% to 20% less than age-matched controls, and stairclimbing is 40% to 50% slower than age-matched controls (even at 1 year). Most patients who participated in sports prior to surgery are able to return to low impact sport activities and exercise regimens. Patients are able to return to sedentary, light, and medium work categories. Patients who are on sick leave for more than 6 months preoperatively are less likely to return to work.

Diagnostic Studies

Diagnostic studies are necessary to address potential complications of total knee arthroplasty.

Preoperative diagnostic testing appropriate for the evaluation of the patient with endstage arthropathy of the knee includes standing AP and lateral x-rays to assess joint space compromise and valgus or varus deformity. If infection is suspected, arthrocentesis should be performed with synovial fluid analysis for gram stain and culture sensitivity studies.

Postoperative diagnostic testing initially includes non–weight-bearing x-rays PA and lateral. During follow-up at 8–12 weeks, standing x-rays should be obtained to assess component and alignment integrity.

Diagnostic testing for suspected prosthetic loosening includes plain x-rays of the knee (Fig. 1). If infection is suspected, joint fluid can be analyzed.

Differential Diagnosis

Prosthetic loosening   Periprosthetic fracture

Infection   Component failure

Treatment

Initial

Medical therapeutic interventions address the following:

1. Warfarin, low molecular weight heparin, and pneumatic compression boots are the most common and efficacious agents for DVT prophylaxis in the postoperative period after TKA.

2. Postoperative pain management—During the first 48 to 72 hours, patients often receive controlled analgesia therapy administered via the intravenous or epidural route. Subsequently, patients are then given oral opioids. Controlled release and short acting opioids may be utilized. Depending on clinician and patient preference, fixed and/or rescue dose opioid medications are selected. The opioids can be titrated to achieve balance of analgesia vs emerging side effects.

3. Incision site care—Dry, sterile gauze dressings are applied as long as drainage is present. Staples and sutures can safely be removed 10 to 14 days after surgery.

4. Postoperative swelling—Properly fitting, thigh-high elastic compression stockings, the use of a continuous passive motion machine, and possibly the use of local cryotherapy are used to manage swelling.

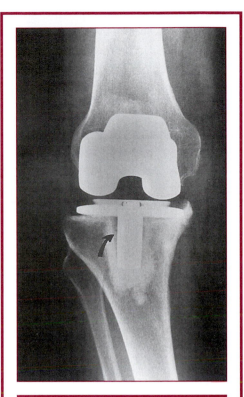

FIGURE 1. Total knee replacement—subsidence. The medial aspect of the tibial plateau component has sunk into the tibia, with a rim of bone at its medial aspect. This finding, combined with the radiolucency at the lateral metal–cement interface (*curved arrow*), indicates loosening of the prosthesis.

5. Postoperative anemia—The overall blood lost following unilateral total knee arthroplasty has been estimated at 2.2 units. Blood loss is greater for uncemented than cemented prosthesis. Patients are often advised prior to surgery to donate 1 to 3 units of packed red blood cells for autotransfusion. Additionally, the use of postoperative blood collection and reinfusion via the surgical drain have been shown to be effective in reducing the need for bank blood and have a low morbidity rate when used with current techniques. If the patient is receiving anticoagulation therapy, serial stool guaiac tests should be performed. If the anemia is macrocytic, vitamin B_{12} and folic acid levels should be obtained. If the anemia is microcytic, a serum iron level, total iron-binding capacity, and/or a ferritin level should be obtained along with a reticulocyte count.

Rehabilitation

Rehabilitation programs that use clinical pathways enhance the efficiency of postoperative rehabilitation for the patient with TKA.

The rehabilitation program can be conceptualized as occurring in stages, or phases. The first stage commences in the immediate postoperative period. The final stage concludes when the patient returns to the community and pursues optimal independent functional living.

See Table 1 for an example of a clinical pathway that addresses the schedule of progression during the first phase. Note that there are numerous protocols for the use of continuous passive motion

TABLE 1. Clinical Pathway for First Phase Rehabilitation

Postoperative Day	Exercise	Mobility	Ambulation	Activities of Daily Living
0	Deep breathing Incentive spirometer Quadriceps and gluteal sets Straight leg raise Hip abduction Ankle pumps	Sits to chair transfer Education on continuous passive motion machine		
1	Deep breathing Lower extremity static resistance exercises Ankle pumps and circles Continuous passive motion	Bed mobility Bed to chair transfers with knee immobilizer		Assess adaptive equipment: reachers, long-handled sponges, and shoehorns
2	Continue previously described exercises Short arc quads Straight leg raise with knee immobilizer Upper extremity strengthening	Continue bed mobility and transfers Begin toilet transfers	Assisted ambulation in Rome partial weight bearing or weight bearing as tolerated with knee immobilizer	Raised toilet seat Grooming and dressing well while seated
3	Continue previously described exercises Sitting full bark motion: flexion and extension Passive flexion and extension	Decreased assistance in basic transfers	Independent ambulation with walker or crutches in Rome partial weight bearing for weight bearing is tolerated with knee immobilizer	Independent toileting and grooming Education on joint protection and energy conservation techniques
4	Continue previously described exercises with increased intensity Initiate active assistance range-of-motion exercises and quadriceps and hamstrings self-stretch	Independent in basic transfers	Gait training to improve pattern and endurance Discontinue knee immobilizer (if quadriceps strength is greater than 3/5)	Continue previously described ADLs
5–6	Continue previously described exercises Transition from passive to active assistive range-of-motion exercises		Independent ambulation on nursing unit Begin stairs with railing cane	Independent dressing out

machines during the first phase of TKA rehabilitation. Flexion can be increased approximately 7 degrees each day according to patient tolerance, unless otherwise indicated. The continuous passive motion apparatus is helpful in controlling swelling and reduces the frequency of later knee manipulation with anesthetic use.

Ideally, a range of motion of 5 to 75 degrees should be achieved after 1 week.

During the second stage of TKA rehabilitation (weeks 2 to 6), the patient progresses to low resistance dynamic exercise therapy for the involved lower extremity. This can be carried out using a stationary bicycle. Some patients may prefer aquatic based exercise regimens during this period. The patient should be independent in ambulating with a two-handed or single-handed device if they are full weight bearing on level surfaces up to 500 feet. They should be supervised when negotiating stairs. Electrical stimulation of the quadriceps can be considered for patients who have inhibited recruitment. Soft tissue mobilization can be introduced to facilitate patellar glide. Most patients have a strength ratio favoring the hamstrings. During this period, the patient should be independent in all basic activities of daily living.

During the third stage of TKA rehabilitation (weeks 6 to 12), the available range of motion should reach 0 to 115 degrees. Patients are able to advance their dynamic resistance exercise regimens and more freely pursue both open and closed kinetic chain and dynamic balance exercises. Patients advance to a single-handed device or no device for ambulation and at different speeds and on different terrain. They should be independent in negotiating stairs. Patients advance to independence in instrumental activities of daily living.

In the final stage (weeks 12 to 24), patients may return to their preoperative exercise regimens and recreation activities and kneeling. Contact sports are advised against, and caution should be considered with high impact aerobic activities.

Procedures

Manipulation

Some patients with unsatisfactory gains in knee range of motion may be candidates for manipulation. The role of manipulation for the patient with a TKA contracture remains controversial. Outcome studies are divided about whether functional outcomes and quality of life are enhanced as a result of manipulation. When an orthopedic surgeon performs the procedure, it is carried in an operating room with the use of general or epidural anesthesia. The goal is to overcome articular lesions with minimal force after quadriceps resistance is eliminated. Manipulation is most commonly performed during the second or third postoperative week if the range of motion of the involved knee is less than 75 degrees.

Arthrocentesis

Aspiration of the knee for aerobic and anaerobic cultures and sensitivities is the most reliable method of diagnosing infection. Strict sterile technique must be used throughout the aspiration procedure.

Surgery

Presently, the most common materials used in replacement joints are cobalt chromium or titanium on ultra high molecular weight polyethylene. In total knee arthroplasties, cobalt chromium is always used on femoral weight-bearing surfaces due to its superior strength. Total knee arthroplasties can be stabilized with or without cement. In some cases, hybrid total knee arthroplasties are utilized.

There are three major surgical approaches for the standard total knee arthroplasty: the medial parapatellar retinacular approach, the midvastus approach, and the subvastus or southern approach. The medial parapatellar retinacular approach compromises the quadriceps tendon in its medial one third, and this gives rise to more postoperative patellofemoral complications. The midvastus approach does not compromise the extensor mechanism of the knee joint. The subvastus approach also preserves the integrity of the extensor mechanism but does not expose the knee as well as the other two approaches do. The type of arthrotomy used will influence postoperative management. After a standard anteromedial arthrotomy between the vastus medialis and rectus tendons with eversion of the patella, active and passive range of motion may begin immediately. Protected ambulation with crutches or a walker is recommended for 4 to 6 weeks to allow healing of the arthrotomy repair and for quadriceps strength to recover. Although recovery following the subvastus approach may be more rapid than after the standard anteromedial approach, protected weight bearing with ambulatory aids for 3 to 6 weeks is still recommended to allow soft tissue healing. In the patient with limited preoperative range of motion, either tibial tubercle osteotomy or a V-Y quadricepsplasty needs to be performed.

Following tibial tubercle osteotomy, early range of motion and full weight bearing within 1 week of surgery is recommended.

Weight-bearing status depends on the details of the surgical reconstruction and whether the components were inserted with or without cement. For the otherwise uncomplicated primary cemented total knee arthroplasty, the patient can tolerate weight bearing within the confines of safety. Protected weight bearing can be performed only after the patient demonstrates adequate control of the limb to prevent falling. The time to weight bearing after total arthroplasty varies, depending on the use of cement or cementless fixation and whether large structural bone grafting was required. No differences in the incidence of radiolucent lines have been observed between cemented total knees with immediate weight bearing or protected weight bearing for 12 weeks. Although weight bearing after cementless fixation might increase micromotion, many surgeons allow early weight bearing.

The tibial and femoral components presently in use have a life expectancy of 10 to 20 years. This lifespan depends on the surgical technique, the components used, the bone stock, and the level of physical activity after TKA. Revision TKA is a surgical procedure that the patient with TKA may encounter several years after the original surgery.

Potential Disease Complications

Potential disease complications of conditions involving the knee such as osteoarthritis, rheumatoid arthritis, or osteonecrosis of the femoral epicondyle or tibial condyle include intractable pain, swelling, stiffness, contracture, and valgus or varus deformity.

Potential Treatment Complications

Potential treatment complications include (1) local complications, (2) patellar complications, (3) inadequate motion, (4) instability, (5) infection, and (6) loosening:

1. Local complications include DVT and peroneal nerve palsy. The incidence of deep venous thrombosis following total knee arthroplasty is 40% to 80%. Distal DVT has a rate of occurrence of 50% to 70%, whereas proximal DVT has a rate of occurrence of 10% to 15%. Pulmonary embolism following total knee arthroplasty has an estimated rate of occurrence of 1.8% to 7%.[3] In the patient who does not receive anticoagulation therapy, the thrombus develops within the first 24 hours and peak development is at 5 to 7 days of surgery. The growth ceases by day 10, and resolution of the thrombus (intrinsic thrombolysis) commences by day 14. Venogram, Doppler ultrasound imaging, or impedance plethysmography are utilized to diagnose the presence of DVT. Doppler ultrasound studies are most commonly used in clinical practice. Currently, anticoagulation with warfarin, low molecular weight heparin, and continuous IV heparin are recommended for active DVT treatment. Please see Chapter 104 for further details.

   The incidence of postthrombotic syndrome is low in the TKA patient population. Peroneal nerve injury occurs in less than 1% of patients in most series.[11] Most patients experience partial resolution of their nerve palsy within the first few months postoperatively. Few patients require use of a plastic or double metal upright ankle-foot orthosis.

2. Patellar complications include subluxation and dislocation. These are often due to excessive tracking of the patella, which is difficult to correct with conservative treatment after the initial surgery. These complications are often recognized during the initial operative procedure. When they are not recognized early, revision surgery is often needed. Patella fractures can be traumatically induced or stress induced. These fractures are generally treated conservatively unless closed reduction is problematic.

3. Inadequate motion may result in a flexion contracture of the knee. Aggressive pain management, early continuous passive motion, and mobilization of the patient can reduce the likelihood of contracture. A dynamic locking knee brace may help reduce small flexion

contractures (less than 20 degrees). The need for manipulation depends on the available ROM of the knee. The required range of motion for the knee during functional activities is shown in Table 2.

Manipulation can be considered if the knee range of motion is less than 85 degrees.

4. Instability is usually due to surgical error and requires surgical revision rather than bracing.

5. The overall infection rate for initial TKAs is 1%.[7] This is higher in patients with advanced rheumatoid arthritis, revision TKA, and constrained prostheses. Deep infection can occur anytime from days to months after surgery. Musculoskeletal infection usually presents as increase in pain with or without weight bearing, increase in swelling, and fever. Diagnosis is confirmed by joint fluid analysis, as described earlier. The patient requires a 6-week course of antibiotic treatment between the period of component removal and reimplantation. The most successful technique for treating the infected total knee replacement is a two-stage reimplantation of the TKA components. The success rate with this technique is 80% to 97%.[4] Infection must never be overlooked as a cause of implant loosening. Infection can occur early or late and can present with or without signs of systemic toxicity. The symptoms are commonly the same as those seen with aseptic loosening. A progressive radiolucency between prosthesis and its adjacent almost always is considered an infection until proven otherwise. Negative aspirate from the knee, normal sedimentation rates and C-reactive protein, and negative gallium or indium scans cannot rule out infection or prosthetic device. The patient should be advised that even in the presence of normal tests, infection may be discovered intraoperatively and necessitate the removal of the prosthetic device.

6. The most common reason for total arthroplasty failure has been loosening of the implant (Fig. 2). Factors associated with loosening include infection, implant constraint, failure to achieve neutral mechanical alignment, instability, and cement technique. The prodromal features of impending loosening and failure of the components are an increase in pain and swelling with or without angular deformity of the knee. The radiographic features include a widening radiolucent zone between the implant and the adjacent bone and subsidence of the implant. Loosening may occur at the component cement interface or bone cement interface. Implant loosening can be attributed to mechanical and biologic factors. The mechanical factors include limb alignment, ligamentous balance, and the preservation of a contracted posterior cruciate ligament. Implant loosening can occur early or late. Early implant loosening usually occurs within the first 2 years and represents a mechanical failure of the interlock of the implant and host to bone. This early implant loosening is more appropriately called *fixation failure* and is

TABLE 2. Range of Motion Needed	
Activity of Daily Living	**Extension-Flexion**
Walking in stance phase	15–40 degrees
Walking in swing phase	15–70 degrees
Stairclimbing step over step	0–83 degrees
Standing up from a chair	0–93 degrees
Standing up from a toilet	0–105 degrees
Stooping to lift an object	0–117 degrees
Tying a shoelace	0–106 degrees

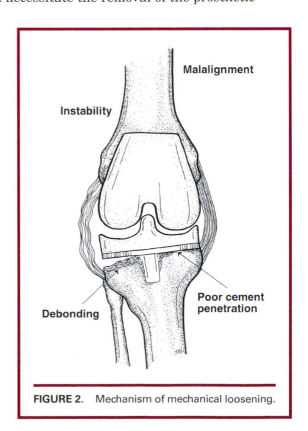

FIGURE 2. Mechanism of mechanical loosening.

often secondary to errors in judgment at the time of surgery or to problems with the technical aspects of the surgical procedure. Extremity malalignment, soft tissue imbalance, and poor cement technique individually or in combination contribute to loosening. Biologic factors are largely responsible for the phenomenon of late loosening. Late loosening of total knee implants is often secondary to the host biologic response to the implant's debris that weakens the mechanical bond of implant to bone established during surgery. Mechanical factors may contribute to late loosening, but they do not alone explain the loss of fixation device that has been stable for many years. The volume of particles generated from the articulation is influenced by patient weight and activity level, duration of implantation, polyethylene thickness, and contact stresses. Wear may be accelerated by malalignment, instability, and ligament imbalance, resulting in increased volume of particulate released into the joint.

References

1. McInnes I, Daltroy LH: A controlled evaluation of CPM in patients undergoing TKA. JAMA 1992;268(11):1423–1426.
2. Martin SD, Thornhill TS: Current concepts of total knee arthroplasty. J Orthop Sports Phys Ther 1998;28(4):252–261.
3. Stulberg BN, Williams GW: DVT following TKR: An analysis of 638 arthroplasties. J Bone Joint Surg 1984;66A:194–199.
4. Hecht PJ, Booth RE: Effects of thermal therapy on rehabilitation after TKA: A prospective randomized study. Clin Orthop Related Res 1983;178:199–201.
5. Goldstein T: Geriatric Orthopedics, 2nd ed. Gaithersburg, MD, Aspen, 1999.
6. Schai PA: Kneeling ability after total knee arthroplasty. Clin Orthop Related Res 1999;367:195–200.
7. Wilde A: Management of infected knee and hip prosthesis. Curr Opin Rheumatol 1993;6(3):317–321.
8. Praemer MA, Rice D: Musculoskeletal conditions in the United States. AAOS, 1999.
9. Bradbury N, Spoo G, Cross MJ: Participation in sports after total knee replacement. Am J Sports Med 1998;26(4): 530–535.
10. Jorn LP: Patient satisfaction, function and return to work after knee arthroplasty. Acta Orthop Scand 1999;70(4): 343–347.
11. Asp JP: Peroneal nerve palsy after total knee arthroplasty. Clin Orthop Related Res 1990;261:233–237.
12. Walsh M: Physical impairments and functional limitations: A comparison of individuals 1 year after total knee arthroplasty with control subjects. Phys Ther 1998;78(3):248–258.
13. Semkiw LB: Post operative blood salvage using the cell saver after total joint arthroplasty. J Bone Joint Surg 1989;6(71A):823–327.
14. Walker RH, Angulo DL: Post operative use of CPM, TENS and cryotherapy following TKA. J Arthroplasty 1991;6(2): 151–156.
15. Lonner JH, Scott RD: Prodromes of failure in total knee arthroplasty. J Arthroplasty 1999;331:140–145.
16. Sharma L: Prognostic factors for functional outcome of total knee replacement: A prospective study. J Gerontol A Biol Sci Med Sci 1996;51(4):152–157.

75 Achilles Tendinitis

Robert P. Nirschl, MD, MS

Definition

A more accurate name for Achilles tendinitis is Achilles tendinosis or peritendinitis. This is a painful, swollen, and tender area of the Achilles tendon and peritenon secondary to repetitive overuse. The histopathology of this overuse is angio-fibroblastic hyperplasia (tendinosis) of the body of the tendon (a degenerative process) and an inflammatory response in the peritenon.[1,2] The maladies often occur simultaneously but may occur individually.

Symptoms

Pain and tenderness in the Achilles tendon are predominant symptoms, usually in association with running sports and fitness activities.[3] In some patients the pain actually improves with exercise. Typically the pain occurs with a change in the athletic training schedule. The most common location for tendinosis symptoms is at the apex of the Achilles tendon curvature. A history of an acute traumatic event in which the patient reports a "pop" should make the clinician suspicious for an Achilles tendon partial or complete rupture.

Physical Examination

The essential element in the physical examination is the localization of swelling and tenderness in the critical zone of the Achilles tendon (at the apex of the Achilles curve approximately 2½ inches proximal to the os calcis insertion). Exquisite tenderness to palpation is classic. Palpable heat is usually not evident unless peritendinitis is a major component. The Achilles is usually tight with ankle dorsiflexion rarely extending beyond 90 degrees. Associated findings may include abnormal foot posture (pes planus or cavus), tight hamstrings, and muscle weakness of the entire hip and leg. Neurologic evaluation, including strength, sensation and deep tendon reflexes, is normal.

The examination should also include observation for a palpable defect and the Thompson test (squeezing the calf, which should result in plantarflexion in an attached tendon) to rule out rupture of the Achilles tendon (Fig. 1).

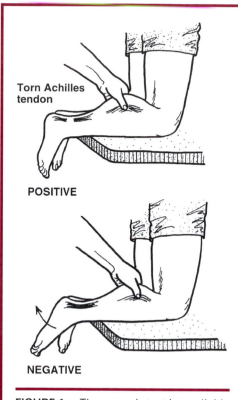

FIGURE 1. Thompson's test is a reliable clinical test to identify the presence of a complete tear in the Achilles tendon. When the Achilles tendon is torn, a positive test is elicited by squeezing the calf and seeing no plantarflexion of the foot. A negative test occurs when the calf is squeezed and plantar flexion occurs in the foot.

Functional Limitations

Impact weight-bearing activities such as jogging, fast walking and running, are usually limited. Non-impact fitness activities, such as cycling and using an elliptical trainer, may also result in symptoms. Patients may complain of pain with daily ambulatory activities, such as walking at work or climbing stairs.

Diagnostic Studies

Unless a special form of calcified Achilles tendinosis occurs at the os calcis insertion, regular x-rays are usually normal. Ultrasonography or MRI exam is capable of defining the extent of both tendinosis and peritendinitis. These studies are generally only recommended to help define the prognosis or in patients who are unresponsive to rehabilitation and surgery is being considered.

Differential Diagnosis

Haglund's deformity   Achilles tendon rupture

Retrocalcaneal bursitis   Tibial stress fracture

Adventitial bursitis   Medial gastrocnemius tear

Treatment

Initial

The initial treatment goal is to decrease pain and reduce inflammation. Therefore, rest from aggravating activities is critical. Icing (20 minutes, 2 to 3 times daily) and NSAIDs/COX-2 inhibitors can be used for pain and inflammation. Oral analgesics can be used for pain alone. Counterforce bracing is often helpful. A simple heel lift (⅛ to ½ inch) can decrease some of the stress on the tendon. Warmup before any weight-bearing activity and cooling with ice afterward are recommended.

Rehabilitation

The rehabilitative process focuses on curative efforts (e.g., biologic improvement of the damaged tendon and peritenon) rather than the comfort efforts of the initial treatment phase. These biologic goals include neovascularization; fibroblastic infiltration; collagen production; and the restoration of strength, endurance, and flexibility.

Rehabilitation is best initiated in a structured physical therapy program followed by home therapeutic exercise. Modalities including electrical stimulation and/or ultrasound often comfort and may enhance the biologic goals. Therapeutic exercise needs to be directed to the entire leg, including the hip, because strength, endurance, and flexibility deficits are common in a global fashion. Isokinetic strength and endurance testing usually aid in monitoring the rehabilitation progress.

Control of abusive force loads can be accomplished by counterforce bracing the Achilles and/or orthotics to minimize abnormal foot posture. Gradual, controlled return to running might be initiated by running in water programs. General fitness may be maintained by utilizing upper body land programs, such as arm ergometry; resistance training; and water programs dedicated to the entire body. Return to sport or running is transitional, including plyometric and eccentric exercises. Full return generally requires normal strength, endurance, and flexibility.

Procedures

Control of pain by cortisone injections is not recommended because cellular death and tendon weakness with potential progression to tendon rupture are significant concerns.

Surgery

Rehabilitation failure may invite surgical intervention for ultimate problem resolution versus acceptance of the malady and alteration of activity level. The concepts of surgery include removal of symptomatic peritendinitis tissue and resection of the abnormal tendinosis tissue in the body of the Achilles tendon with subsequent repair of the remaining adjacent normal tendon. Surgery is highly successful if all pathologic tissue is removed and appropriate postoperative rehabilitation is implemented.

In cases of suspected tendon rupture, a surgical consultation is also warranted.

Potential Disease Complications

Chronic signs and symptoms can result in weakening and subsequent complete rupture of the Achilles tendon. Chronic intractable pain may also develop.

Potential Treatment Complications

Side effects of NSAIDs are well known and include gastric, renal, and hepatic complications. COX-2 inhibitors may cause fewer gastric side effects. Bracing for prolonged periods of time may lead to disuse weakness and atrophy. Significant alterations in gait by using too high of a heel lift can cause knee, hip, and low back pain. Overly aggressive physical therapy may cause tendon weakness and potential rupture. Surgical complications are well known.

References
1. Kraushaar B, Nirschl R: Current concepts review. Tendinosis of the elbow (tennis elbow). Clinical features and findings of histological, immunohistochemical, and electron microscopy studies. J Bone Joint Surg 1999;81-A(2):259–278.
2. Puddu G, Ippolito E, Postacchini F: A Classification of Achilles tendon disease. Am J Sports Med 1976;4:145–150.
3. Nirschl R: Surgical Considerations of Ankle Injuries. In O'Connor F, Wilder R (eds): The Complete Book of Running Medicine. New York, McGraw-Hill, 2001.

76 Ankle Arthritis

David Wexler, MD
Todd A. Kile, MD

Synonym

Degenerative joint disease (DJD) of the ankle joint

ICD-9 Codes

715.17
Osteoarthrosis, localized, primary, ankle and foot

715.27
Osteoarthrosis, localized, secondary, ankle and foot

716.17
Traumatic arthropathy, ankle and foot

Definition

Ankle arthritis can result from a wide range of causes; however, the most common cause is *post-traumatic degenerative joint disease (DJD)*. An acute injury or trauma sustained a number of years prior to presentation or less severe, repetitive, minor injuries sustained over a longer period of time can lead to a slow-but-progressive destruction of the articular cartilage, resulting in DJD.[2] Other common types of arthritis include rheumatoid arthritis (RA) and septic arthritis. Osteoarthritis (OA) is usually less inflammatory than RA but can also involve many joints simultaneously.

Symptoms

As with most types of arthritis, the presenting symptoms are pain (which may be variable at different times of the day and exacerbated by weight bearing), swelling, stiffness, and deformity.[2] In the inflammatory types of arthritis, the joints can become warm and red. Pieces of the cartilage can break off, forming a loose body, and the joint can "lock" or "catch," sticking in one position and causing acute, excruciating pain until the loose body moves from between the two irregular joint surfaces. A further symptom is that of "giving way" or instability of the joint, which may be a result of surrounding muscle weakness or ligamentous laxity. With progression of the arthritis, night pain can become a major complaint.

Physical Examination

As with any arthritic joint, there are likely to be signs of deformity on inspection; swelling, tenderness, and possibly increased temperature on palpation; and reduced range of motion in plantar and dorsiflexion. The tenderness is usually maximal along the anterior talocrural joint line. With inflammatory arthropathy, a boggy swelling can be palpated anteriorly due to synovitis. The patient may also exhibit an antalgic (painful) gait or a limp.

Functional Limitations

Pain with walking distances and difficulty negotiating stairs or inclines are particular functional disabilities. Even prolonged standing can become intolerable with advanced joint deterioration. Night pain can lead to difficulties with sleep.

Diagnostic Studies

Plain AP and lateral standing radiographs provide sufficient information in the latter stages of the disease (Figs. 1 and 2). An MRI may show damage to articular cartilage and a joint effusion earlier in the course. When assessing the x-rays, attention should also be paid to the other joints in the hindfoot since these will affect management options; generalized bone density and alignment should also be noted.

In some cases, patients present with varying degrees of degeneration of other, adjacent joints. By performing differential blocks with local anaesthetic and under radiographic control, the clinician may determine which of these is symptomatic.

Differential Diagnosis

Edema (e.g., edema secondary to congestive cardiac failure)

Subtalar joint pathology

Posterior tibial tenosynovitis

Treatment

Initial

Nonsteroidal anti-inflammatory drugs (NSAIDs), including COX-2 inhibitors, or simple analgesics are used to alleviate the pain. Pre-fabricated orthoses ranging from flexible neoprene braces to canvas lace-up or wrap-around ankle supports, to more rigid braces or ankle walking boots, can be prescribed to enhance stability and reduce movement in the ankle joint, thus reducing pain levels.

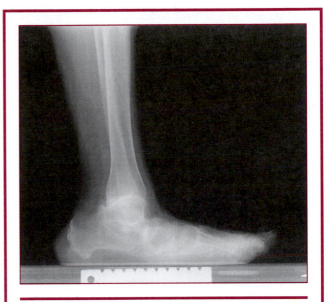

FIGURE 1. Lateral standing radiograph of the ankle in a patient with rheumatoid arthritis. This demonstrates loss of joint space and bony destruction of the ankle joint.

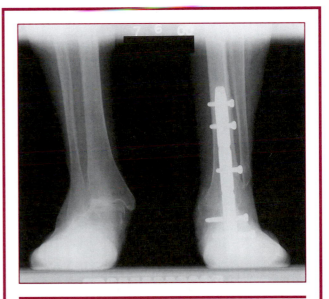

FIGURE 2. AP standing radiograph of bilateral ankles in a patient with rheumatoid arthritis. This demonstrates the degenerative, destroyed joint on the left and one method of fusion with an intramedullary nail on the right.

Rehabilitation

A custom-molded rigid ankle-foot orthosis (AFO) fabricated by a skilled orthotist can provide dramatic pain relief for the vast majority of patients with ankle arthritis. A physical therapist can instruct a patient in the proper technique for using a walking stick or cane in the opposite hand. This is a simple but effective aid in reducing the forces across the ankle joint when the patient is up and about.

Mobilization, stretching techniques, and range-of-movement exercises may help alleviate pain and stiffness. Non–weight-bearing exercises are important, and, if accessible, hydrotherapy has been shown to be an extremely useful and productive adjunct. Distraction and gliding mobilization techniques improve range of movement. Strengthening of surrounding muscle groups and proprioceptive rehabilitation will enhance stability.

Procedures

Other than the blocks that are done to determine the location of the pathology in confusing cases, injections are not typically done for ankle arthritis. The use of corticosteroid injection is generally of only limited duration, and steroids are chondrotoxic (cause cartilage damage). However, they can provide excellent temporary pain relief in patients with joints at end-stage disease.

Surgery

Surgery is indicated in patients who fail to respond to non-operative management and especially in those with unremitting pain . In the earlier stages of arthritis, an arthroscopic washout and cartilage debridement of the ankle joint may provide significant improvement in pain levels. As the disease progresses, more extensive surgery is required. Many different variations and techniques for fusion have been described, ranging from minimally invasive arthroscopic arthrodesis to open fusion with metal work.[1–3,5,7,8] Total ankle joint replacement (arthroplasty) is gaining popularity once again as newer and more reliable prostheses are available.[6] In the past, however, they were prone to early failure and unpredictable results.[9] Patient selection is of paramount importance as those with high demands must be realistic in their expectations.

Potential Disease Complications

Progressive immobility, permanent loss of motion of the ankle joint, bony collapse leading to leg-length discrepancy, and chronic intractable pain can result from ankle arthritis.

Potential Treatment Complications

Analgesics, NSAIDs, and COX-2 inhibitors have well-known side effects that most commonly affect the gastric, hepatic, and renal systems. Arthroscopy can be complicated by nerve damage or, rarely, septic arthritis. Occasionally with arthrodesis, fusion can fail to occur.[11] An alteration in gait is common.[10] Arthroplasty complications include infection, thromboembolism, and implant failure.

References

1. Thordarson DB: Ankle and hindfoot arthritis: Fusion techniques. In Craig EV (ed): Clinical Orthopaedics, 1st ed. Philadelphia, Lippincott, Williams & Wilkins, 1999, pp 883–890.
2. Richardson EG: Arthrodesis of ankle, knee and hip. In Canale ST (ed): Campbell's Operative Orthopaedics, 9th ed. St Louis, Mosby, 1998, pp 165–182.
3. Mann RA, VanMannen JW, et al: Ankle fusion. Clin Orthop 1991;268:49–55.
4. Hertling D, Kessler RM: The leg, ankle and foot. In Hertling D, Kessler RM (eds): Management of Common Musculoskeletal Disorders, 3rd ed. Lippincott, Williams & Wilkins, 1996, pp 435–438.
5. Morgan CD, Henke JA, et al: Long-term results of tibiotalar arthrodesis. J Bone Joint Surg 1985;67A:546–550.
6. Balton-Maggs BG, Sudlaw RA, et al: Total ankle arthroplasty: A long term review of the London Hospital experience. J Bone Joint Surg 1985;67-B:785–790.
7. Kile TA, Ankle arthrodesis. In Morrey B, et al (eds): Reconstructive Surgery of the Joints, 2nd ed. New York, Churchill Livingstone, 1996, pp 1771–1787.
8. Kile TA, Donnelly RE, et al: Tibiotalocalcaneal arthrodesis with an intramedullary device. Foot Ankle 1994;15:669–673.
9. McGuire MR, Kyle RF, et al: Comparative analysis of ankle arthroplasty versus ankle arthrodesis. Clin Orthop 1988; 226:174–181.
10. Mazur JM, Schwartz E, et al: Ankle arthrodesis: long-term follow-up with gait analysis. J Bone Joint Surg 1979;61-A:964–975.
11. Smith RW: Ankle arthrodesis. In Thompson RC, Johnson KA (eds): Master Techniques in Orthopaedic Surgery—The Foot and Ankle, 1st ed. Philadelphia, Raven Press, 1994, pp 467–482.

77 Ankle and Foot Bursitis

Rene Cailliet, MD

Synonyms

Fluid-filled sac of fibrous tissue

Glandular sac (a pouch at a joint to lessen friction)

ICD-9 Code

726.71
Achilles bursitis or tendinitis

Definition

A bursa is a lubricating sac of synovial fluid that minimizes friction between moving parts of an extremity. These moving parts may be bone against bone with intervening cartilage or tendons moving between adjacent bones at an articulation.

In bursitis, the bursa, not normally palpable when not inflamed, becomes swollen, tender, and painful. Pain is aggravated by movement of that specific joint and/or tendon.

The stages of bursitis are acute, recurrent, and chronic. A bursa facilitates gliding of adjacent anatomic tissues because the two surfaces of the bursa, enclosing synovial fluid, glide upon the two adjacent bursal surfaces that are each connected to the moving tissues. This action minimizes friction. During the acute phase of bursitis, however, inflammation thickens the synovial fluid and results in painful movement, both active and passive. Movement is therefore limited.

Acute and chronic tendinitis need to be differentiated from bursitis, although these conditions commonly co-exist, as tendinitis precedes and accompanies bursitis. A tendon is readily palpable, and the space behind it usually contains the bursa.

Symptoms

Patients typically complain of pain and tenderness at a specific anatomic area of the foot or ankle. Patients may also complain about swelling and inflammation.

Physical Examination

Locating the bursa is imperative; otherwise, a diagnosis of tendinitis may be made since the area of concern is mostly adjacent to tendons. There are numerous sites that must be considered when inflammation, tenderness, pain, and limitation are experienced (Fig. 1). Every tendon in the foot and ankle has a bursa between it and the underlying bone. Of the various bursa, several are more prominent. These include the bunion bursa, which overlies the hallux valgus, and the pre-Achilles and post- Achilles tendons (Fig. 2).

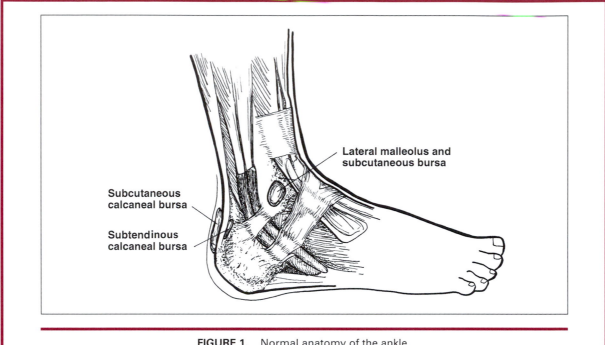

FIGURE 1. Normal anatomy of the ankle.

In addition to swelling, residual inflammatory changes may persist with less pain and tenderness but residual limited movement remains as the layers of the bursa remain thickened. In the chronic phase, the two adjacent layers of the bursa may adhere and prevent any movement. This is considered adhesive bursitis.

Functional Limitations

Adhesions of the surfaces of a bursa limit the degree of movement of the joint to which it is attached. The patient may be limited in ambulation, climbing stairs, and sports activities.

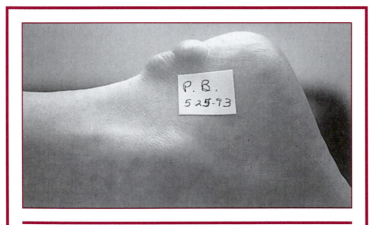

FIGURE 2.. Pump bump. (From Mellion MB: Office Sports Medicine, 2nd ed. Philadelphia, Hanley & Belfus, 1996, p 327, with permission.)

Diagnostic Studies

Bursitis is typically a clinical diagnosis. Normal radiologic studies fail to discern the presence of an inflamed bursa, but MRI and CT scanning studies identify the presence and the degree of inflammation.

Differential Diagnosis

Plantar fasciitis	Fracture
Tendinitis	Arthritis
Acute synovitis	

Treatment

Initial

Initially the application of ice (cryotherapy) relieves the pain and aching and decreases the inflammation and minimizes the chance of adhesive bursitis. Avoiding painful activities is important. Splinting with an ankle brace for several days is generally beneficial but prolonged immobilization is contraindicated because it fosters adhesions. NSAIDs including COX-2 inhibitors can be used for pain and inflammation. Analgesics are used to treat pain only.

Rehabilitation

Evaluating footwear is necessary. Sometimes custom orthotics to correct foot deformities are useful.

In the chronic phase, when there is firm adhesion, manipulation may relieve the limitation and allow normal joint motion. Passive and active exercises by a physical therapist are effective and are often done in conjunction with heat, ice, and ultrasound.

Procedures

Local injection with an anesthetic/corticosteroid mixture is advocated. Upon entering the bursa, aspiration of fluid for diagnostic evaluation of the fluid is indicated because the presence of infection denies the use of the injected material.

Surgery

Surgical release is warranted when adhesive bursitis presents severe debilitating joint motion. During surgery the adhered bursa is removed and the contiguous tissues are released.

In the management of bunion bursitis, when the hallux valgus persists and cannot be managed by orthotic changes in the shoe, surgery may be indicated to correct the hallux valgus.

Potential Disease Complications

The primary disease complication is chronic bursitis with intractable pain that may limit footwear and all mobility.

Potential Treatment Complications

Analgesics, NSAIDs, and COX-2 inhibitors have well-known side effects that most commonly affect the gastric, hepatic, and renal systems. Injection complications include infection and an allergic reaction to the medication used. Surgical complications are well known and will vary with the specific procedure used.

References
1. Cailliet R: Foot and Ankle Pain, 3rd ed. Philadelphia, F.A. Davis, 1997.
2. Milgram JE: Office measures for relief of the painful foot. J Bone Joint Surg 1994;46A:1095.
3. Root ML, Orien WP, Weed JM: Normal and Abnormal Functions of the Foot. Clinical Biomechanics, vol II. Los Angeles, Clinical Biomechanics Corporation, 1977.
4. O'Young B, Young MA, Steins SA: PM&R Secrets. Philadelphia, Hanley & Belfus, 1997.

78 Ankle Sprain

Wayne Stokes, MD

Synonym

Inversion sprain

ICD-9 Code

845.00
Sprains and strains of
the ankle and foot

Definition

Ankle sprains are a common cause of morbidity in the general population, and the ankle is the most commonly injured joint complex among athletes.[1,2] It is estimated that more than 23,000 ankle sprains require medical care in the United States per day.[3] Of these, 85% are lateral ankle sprains (anterior talofibular [ATFL] and calcaneofibular [CFL] ligaments)

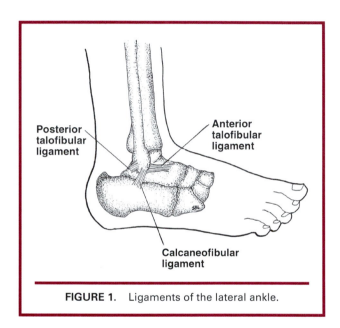

FIGURE 1. Ligaments of the lateral ankle.

(Fig. 1). Another 5% to 10% are syndesmotic injuries, which involve a partial tear of the distal anterior tibiofibular ligament. This is also called a *high* ankle sprain and may have a prolonged recovery. The medial deltoid ligament is strong, sprains less frequently, and is involved in approximately 5% of ankle sprains. Of the ankle sprains, 20% to 40% can progress to chronic problems.[4] The ankle sprain that does not heal may be caused by injuries to other structures that may later cause symptoms.[5]

Ligamentous injuries are categorized into three gradations. Grade I is a partial tear without laxity and only mild swelling. Grade II is a partial tear with mild laxity and moderate pain, tenderness, and instability. Grade III is a complete rupture resulting in considerable swelling, increased pain, significant laxity, and often an unstable joint (Fig. 2).

Symptoms

Pain over the injured ligaments and associated swelling and tenderness are noted. There can be difficulty walking secondary to pain. The patient may have heard a "pop" at the time of injury. Decreased function and range of motion along with instability are seen more often in grade II and grade III injuries. There may be sensory symptoms in the superficial or deep peroneal nerve territory. The patient may report previous ankle sprains.

Physical Examination

Examine for swelling and ecchymosis laterally (most common) as well as around the entire ankle joint. Palpate the ATFL and CFL ligaments, syndesmotic area, and medial deltoid ligament. Bony avulsion/fracture should be sought by palpation of the medial and lateral malleoli, base of the fifth metatarsal, cuboid, lateral process of the talus (snow boarders' fracture), and epiphyseal areas. An anterior force is applied to the calcaneous while stabilizing the tibia. Increased translation compared with the other side implies ATFL injury. The talar tilt test (Fig. 3) done with the ankle in neutral assesses the CFL and is compared with the other side. The squeeze test (Fig. 4) can help diagnose the syndesmotic injury. Squeezing the fibula and tibia at midcalf can cause pain in the syndesmotic area. Dorsiflexion of the ankle with external rotation of the tibia may cause pain in

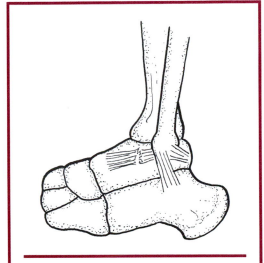

FIGURE 2. Grade III ankle sprain with a complete tear of the anterior talofibular ligament.

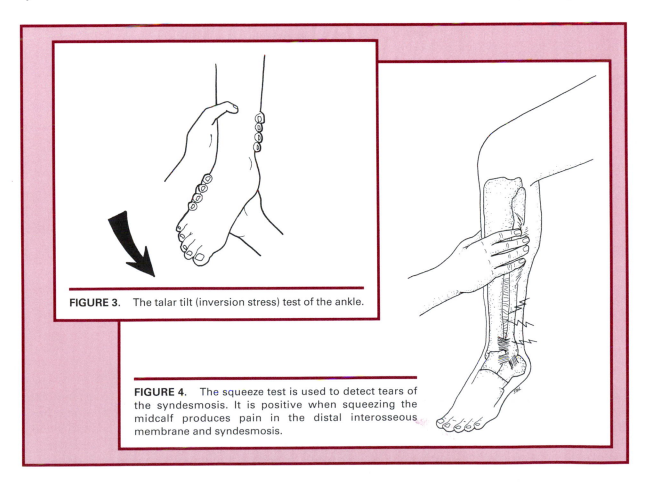

FIGURE 3. The talar tilt (inversion stress) test of the ankle.

FIGURE 4. The squeeze test is used to detect tears of the syndesmosis. It is positive when squeezing the midcalf produces pain in the distal interosseous membrane and syndesmosis.

the syndesmotic area. This coupled with tenderness in the distal tibiofibular joint implies a high ankle sprain and usually a significantly longer recovery. Ankle inversion injuries are associated with peroneal nerve injury and may result in sensory changes on the dorsum of the foot (superficial peroneal nerve) or the first web space (deep peroneal nerve). Deep peroneal nerve injury could result in decreased strength in dorsiflexion and eversion, yet is not common. The peroneal tendon may be tender along its course behind and below the medial malleolus and have associated swelling and fullness (tenosynovitis) and tenderness to palpation that may be increased with resisted eversion.

Functional Limitations

The patient may have difficulty walking, secondary to pain and swelling. The athlete will have difficulty with return to play until swelling and pain have diminished and rehabilitation is nearly completed. Abnormal proprioception, balance, or peroneal weakness in ankle sprains may predispose the patient to re-injury. Chronic ankle sprains can result in mechanical instability with objective instability/laxity noted upon exam. Functional instability (or a sense of giving way with activity) may be present as well, without the extent of instability noted on exam (as in mechanical instability).

Diagnostic Studies

Standard AP and lateral x-rays should be considered in grade II and grade III injuries and in cases in which there is tenderness over the lateral malleolus, ankle joint, syndesmosis, or other bony structure to rule out fracture. At 4 to 6 weeks, a slowly healing lateral ankle injury without significant pain resolution or improvement should be x-rayed again to rule out other pathology. Mortise views allow for a clearer view of the talar dome and osteochondral lesions by eliminating the overlap of the fibula on the lateral talus. A MRI scan can help identify the soft tissue pathology as well as evaluate osteochondral joint surface when the ankle does not heal despite good rehabilitation. Stress x-rays are optional and have questionable reliability because of the great spectrum of normal.

Differential Diagnosis

High ankle sprain, syndesmotic sprain

Osteochondral fracture of the talar dome

Neuropraxia of the superficial or deep peroneal nerve

Fracture of the lateral process of the talus (snow boarders' fracture)

Avulsion/fracture of the tip of the fibula, base of the fifth metatarsal

Peroneal tendon damage

Subtalar joint instability[6]

Posterior impingement/fracture of the os trigonum

Treatment

Initial

Protection, rest, ice, compression, and elevation (PRICE) are the mainstay of initial treatment and are initiated immediately. Crutches should be utilized if weight bearing causes pain; they can be discontinued as walking pain declines (usually 2 to 3 days). Patients should be cautioned to avoid hanging the ankle in a plantar flexed position because it may stretch the injured ATFL. Plastic removable walking castboots/air splints are occasionally used in higher grade injuries. Local ice applications for 20 to 30 minutes 3 to 4 times daily combined with compression immediately after injury is very effective in decreasing swelling, pain, and dysfunction. Nonsteroidal anti-inflammatory drugs (NSAIDs) are employed to decrease pain and inflammation.

Rehabilitation

Rehabilitation is aimed at minimizing swelling, decreasing pain, and preventing chronic ankle problems. Various modalities, such as ultrasound and electrical stimulation, are utilized as needed during the rehabilitative phase to decrease pain and swelling. Achilles stretching is begun to avoid disuse shortening. Active range of motion is initially performed without resistance. Dorsiflexion and peroneal strengthening can be started with static exercises and progress to concentric and eccentric exercises with tubing. These muscles are responsible for activity resisting an inversion/plantar flexion injury.[7] Double leg toe raises progress to single leg and can be done in water if not tolerated on land. Endurance and lower extremity strengthening are incorporated and are increased as functional exercises are begun. Proprioception training can begin in a seated position and then increased to standing balance exercises. Poor proprioception is a major cause of repeat sprain and functional instability.[8] In athletes, when forward running is pain free, agility drills that mimic their sport or activity are added. Skipping rope may be beneficial in the later stages. In general, functional skills that gradually stress the patient will be added as strength and range of motion are obtained and balance is improved.

The use of orthotic bracing may decrease re-injury rate in the previously injured ankle.[9] Bracing and proprioception training, along with peroneal muscle strengthening are strongly recommended to decrease re-injury. These may play a beneficial role in preventing first-time injuries as well.

Procedures

Procedures are generally not done in ankle sprains.

Surgery

Surgery is rare for ankle sprains. Most grade III ankle sprains with complete tears of the ATFL and instability are *not* treated surgically. If necessary, surgical repair may be completed after the sports season and is usually successful. Reconstruction of the lateral ankle ligaments involves anatomic reconstruction of the ligament (modified Bronstrom) and tendon weaving through the fibula (Watson-Jones, Chrisman-Snook).[10] The direct repair of the ligament, even years after the injury, can be highly successful.

Occasionally the patient with an ankle sprain that does not heal with proper time and rehabilitation may undergo arthroscopic evaluation for other sources of pathology.

Potential Disease Complications

Recurrent sprains may lead to both mechanical (gross laxity) and functional instability (giving way). The patient may present with hidden secondary sources of pain and these must be sought (see Differential Diagnosis). Chronic intractable pain is another potential complication.

Potential Treatment Complications

Lack of recognition of the prevalence of chronic problems with ankle sprains may lead to undertreatment and subsequent chronic pain or instability. NSAIDs, including COX-2 inhibitors, may cause gastric, hepatic, or renal complications. Return to work, sport, or activity prior to adequate healing and rehabilitation may result in chronic pain and giving way (functional instability) and gross laxity (mechanical instability).

References

1. Braun B: Effects of ankle sprain in a general clinic population six to 18 months after medical evaluation. Arch Fam Med 1999;8:143–148.
2. Berndt AL, Harty M: Transchondral fracture of the talus. J Bone Joint Surg 1959;41-A:988–1029.
3. Garrick JG, Regina RK: The epidemiology of foot and ankle injuries in sports. Clin Sports Med 1988;17:29–36.
4. Safran MR, et al: Lateral ankle sprains: A comprehensive review. Part I: Etiology, pathoanatomy, histopathogenesis, and diagnosis. Med Sci Sports Exerc 1999;31(Suppl 7):S492–S437.
5. Renstrom PAFH: Persistently painful sprained ankle. J Am Acad Orthop Surg 1994;2:270–280.
6. Hertel J, Denegar C, Monroe M, Stokes W: Talocrural and subtalar joint instability after lateral ankle sprain. Med Sci Sports Exerc 1999;31(11):1501–1507.
7. Brotzman SB, Brasel J: Foot and ankle rehabilitation. In Brotzman SB (ed): Clinical Orthopaedic Rehabilitation. St Louis, Mosby, 1996; p 253.
8. Hurwitz S, Ernst G, Yi S: The foot and ankle. In Canavan P (ed): Rehabilitation and Sports Medicine. Stamford, CT, Appleton & Lange, 1998, p 346.
9. Shapiro M, Kabo JM, Mitchell PW, et al: Ankle sprain prophylaxis: An analysis of the stabilizing effects of braces and tape. Am J Sports Med 1994;22:78–82.
10. Liu SH, Baker CL: Comparison of lateral ankle ligamentous reconstruction procedures. Am J Sports Med 1992;20:594–600.

79 Bunion/Bunionette

David Wexler, MD
Todd A. Kile, MD

Synonyms

Hallux valgus

Lateral deviation of the great toe

ICD-9 Codes

727.1
Bunion

735.0
Hallux valgus (acquired)

Definition

A bunion is a common deformity of the forefoot, often causing pain (Figs. 1 and 2). The etiology is multifactorial and can be either intrinsic or extrinsic.[1] The intrinsic causes are essentially genetic and are related to hypermobility of the first ray (hallux or great toe metatarsal) at its articulation with the medial cuneiform. A further contributory factor is metatarsus primus varus, or medial deviation of the first metatarsal.[8] The principal extrinsic cause is inappropriate, non-conforming footwear with abnormal forces creating deformity.[6] This is particularly notable in women who wear high heeled shoes with narrow toe boxes.

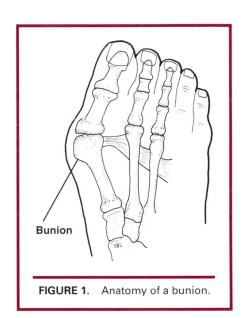

FIGURE 1. Anatomy of a bunion.

The proximal phalanx deviates laterally on the head of the first metatarsal, exacerbated by the pull of the adductor hallucis muscle. The lateral capsule becomes contracted and the medial structures attenuated. The metatarsal head deviates medially but the underlying sesamoids remain in their relationship to the second metatarsal, thus creating dissociation in the metatarsal-sesamoid complex, a prominent medial eminence, lateral deviation, and pronation of the great toe. Depending on the amount of axial rotation of the first metatarsal and forefoot pronation, the first metatarsophalangeal (MTP) joint and great toe become dysfunctional, leading to weight bearing on the more lateral metatarsal heads and "transfer metatarsalgia," causing pain under the plantar aspect of the forefoot.[2]

Symptoms

Presenting symptoms can vary. The patient may only complain of a painless prominence on the inner aspect of the foot. However, more commonly, there will be pain, which is worse when shoes are worn and

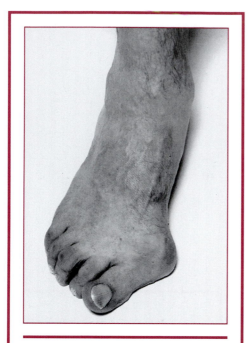

FIGURE 2. Clinical photograph demonstrating a bunion or hallux valgus deformity. Note also the pronation of the digit.

relieved by walking barefoot. The bunion may become red and inflamed. The patient will have difficulty in finding comfortable shoes. As the hallux deviates into the increased valgus, it tends to impinge onto the medial aspect of the pulp of the second toe, causing pressure and soreness.[3]

Physical Examination

There is generally an obvious medial enlargement overlying the metatarsal head, with occasional signs of inflammation. The great toe will be laterally deviated and, with progression of deformity, it will be pronated (axially rotated). There may be splaying of the forefoot and callosities visible under the metatarsal heads of the lesser toes. Passive hyperextension of the hallux MTP joint will reveal any limitation of range of motion (normally approximately 70 degrees). This may indicate concomitant degenerative joint disease of the MTP joint (see Chapter 84). Mobility of the hallux at the first metatarsal-medial cuneiform joint is assessed in relation to the second ray. Hammer toes are commonly noted as a consequence to the crowding in the shoe by the great toe.

Functional Limitations

Limitations are principally walking long distances and wearing shoes with a narrow toe box or high heels for prolonged periods.

Diagnostic Studies

Weight-bearing plain radiographs will provide most of the necessary information. The AP view (Fig. 3) demonstrates the angle (Fig. 4) between the first and second metatarsals (intermetatarsal angle [IMA]) and the angle between the first metatarsal and the hallux itself (hallux valgus angle [HVA]). The congruency of the first MTP joint can also be assessed and any evidence of arthritis. These all have a bearing on any proposed surgery.[4,5]

Differential Diagnosis

Gout

Hallux rigidus

Rheumatoid arthritis

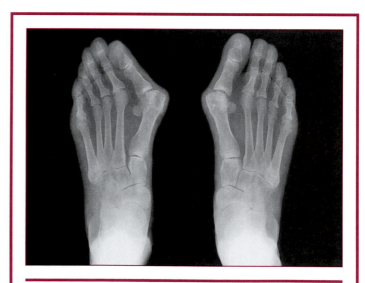

FIGURE 3. Standing AP radiograph of both feet in a patient with bilateral hallux valgus. This is more pronounced on the left. Note also the lateral deviation of the sesamoid bones.

Treatment

Initial

Nonsteroidal anti-inflammatory medications (NSAIDs) and analgesics may be used to alleviate pain. However, key preventative measures include education about footwear, namely shoes with low heels, well cushioned soles, extra depth, and broad toe boxes. Many orthoses are available of varying efficacy. These include sponge wedges to be placed in the first web space; more formal braces, which attempt to pull the hallux into a more neutral position; and custom molded orthotic appliances to resist foot pronation and encourage larger shoes.

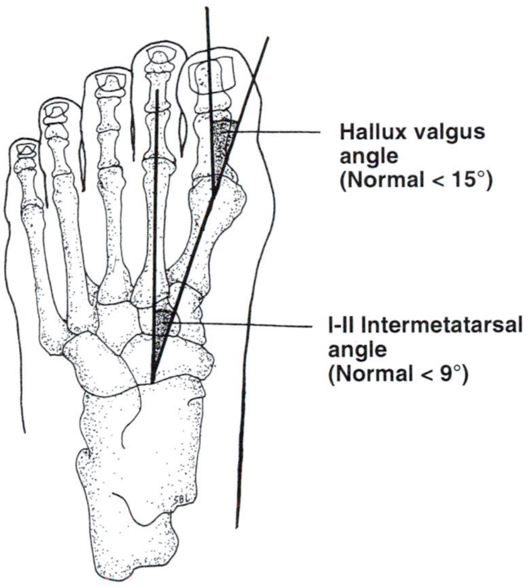

Rehabilitation

Once the structural deformity has progressed, physical therapy has a limited role. This would include mobilization of the first MTP joint and strengthening of the intrinsic muscles of the foot, which may improve symptoms. Distraction techniques may also be useful.

FIGURE 4. Measure the above angles from the patient's standing AP radiograph.

Labels in figure:
Hallux valgus angle (Normal < 15°)
I-II Intermetatarsal angle (Normal < 9°)

Procedures

Local anaesthetic and steroid injection into the first MTP joint may provide short-term pain relief, but is certainly not curative and generally not recommended.

Surgery

Over the years a vast array of different surgical procedures have been described.[8,9] Furthermore, no single procedure has provided sufficient evidence of being superior to any other. *The complication and recurrence rates can be relatively high and patient satisfaction difficult to achieve.* Thus, it is very important to counsel patients preoperatively, explaining these facts and especially that there can be no guarantees that they will be able to return to wearing high heel fashionable footwear.[10] The principal goal of surgery is to relieve pain and provide a foot capable of wearing a shoe.

The type of surgery itself, whether it be a distal soft tissue procedure (DSTP)[11] combined with a proximal metatarsal osteotomy or a distal metatarsal osteotomy alone, is dependent on the presenting anatomic deformity and its complexity.

Potential Disease Complications

Disease complications include ulceration of the medial eminence, metatarsalgia, callosities, hammer toe deformity, and stress fractures of the lesser toes.

Potential Treatment Complications

Analgesics, NSAIDs, and COX-2 inhibitors have well-known side effects that most commonly affect the gastric, hepatic, and renal systems. Treatment can result in recurrent hallux valgus deformity, hallux varus from surgical overcorrection,[12] and hallux extensus (cock-up toe). Procedures in which the first metatarsal is excessively shortened may result in transfer metatarsalgia. Osteonecrosis of the first metatarsal head can occur if the blood supply is disrupted significantly.

References

1. Pedowitz W: Hallux valgus. In Craig EV (ed): Clinical Orthopaedics, 1st ed. Philadelphia, Lippincott, Williams & Wilkins, 1999, pp 904–912.
2. Richardson EG, Donley BG: Disorders of hallux. In Canale ST (ed): Campbell's Operative Orthopaedics, 9th ed, vol 2. St Louis, Mosby, 1998, pp 1621–1711.
3. Hertling D, Kessler RM: The leg, ankle and foot. In Hertling D, Kessler RM (eds): Management of Common Musculoskeletal Disorders, 3rd ed. Philadelphia, Lippincott, Williams & Wilkins, 1996, pp 435–438.
4. Mann RA: Decision making in bunion surgery. Instr Course Lect 1990;39:3–13.
5. Bordelon RL: Evaluation and operative procedures for hallux valgus deformity. Orthopaedics 1987;10:38–44.
6. Seale KS: Women and their shoes: Unrealistic expectations? Instr Course Lect 1995;44:379–384.
7. Antrobus J: The primary deformity in hallux valgus and metatarsus primus varus. Clin Orthop 1984;184:251–255
8. Austin D, Leventen E: A new osteotomy for hallux valgus: a horizontally directed V displacement osteotomy of the metatarsal head for hallux valgus and primus varus. Clin Orthop 1981;157:25–30.
9. Donnelly RE, Saltzman CL, et al: Modified osteotomy for hallux valgus. Foot Ankle 1994;15:642–645.
10. Hattrup SJ, Johnson KA: Chevron osteotomy: Analysis of factors in patients' dissatisfaction. Foot Ankle 1985;5:327–332.
11. Mann RA, Rudicel S, et al: Repair of hallux valgus with a distal soft-tissue procedure and proximal metatarsal osteotomy. J Bone Joint Surg 1992;74-A:124–129.
12. Tourné Y, Saragaglia D, et al: Iatrogenic hallux varus surgical procedure: A study of 14 cases. Foot Ankle 1995;16:457–463.
13. Johnson KA: Chevron osteotomy. In Thompson RC, Johnson KA (eds): Master Techniques in Orthopaedic Surgery—The Foot and Ankle, 1st ed. Philadelphia, Raven Press, 1994, pp 31–48.

80 Chronic Ankle Instability

Michael D. Osborne, MD

Synonym

Weak ankle

ICD-9 Codes

715.17
Osteoarthritis, localized, primary, foot and ankle

718.87
Ankle/foot instability

719.47
Pain in joint; foot and ankle

726.79
Peroneal tendinitis

Definition

Chronic ankle instability is a disease state that is characterized by a constellation of symptoms (typically including pain, weakness, and a feeling that the ankle episodically gives way) that persist following an acute lateral ankle sprain. It has been reported to occur in up to 40% of individuals with a history of ankle sprain and as late as 6.5 years following initial injury.[1] Anatomic lateral ankle ligament laxity (mechanical instability), peroneal muscle weakness, and ankle proprioceptive deficits are three primary factors classically thought to cause and perpetuate symptoms. These causative factors may co-exist with other pathologic processes of the ankle that may serve to amplify and perpetuate symptoms of functional instability. Establishing additional diagnoses (see Differential Diagnosis later in the chapter) does not preclude a diagnosis of chronic ankle instability.

Symptoms

Usual symptoms are ankle pain, swelling, weakness, and a feeling that the ankle is episodically unstable. The term "functional instability" describes the subjective sensation of "give way" that often persists following ankle sprains.[2] Functional instability may occur in the absence of true mechanical ligament laxity and vice versa. Symptoms can continue for months or years following the original injury, range from mild to severe, and often manifest as recurrent acute lateral ankle sprains.

Physical Examination

Objective findings are quite variable and can often be minimal. Potential exam findings in patients with chronic ankle instability may include reduced passive or active ankle range of motion, lateral ankle swelling, ecchymosis, lateral ankle tenderness (typically over the lateral ligament complex or peroneal tendons), weakness of the peroneal muscles, proprioceptive deficits (manifested by decreased ability to perform a single leg stance), and mechanical laxity (demonstrated by increased motion on anterior drawer or talar tilt test compared with the contralateral ankle). Examination of the affected ankle should always be compared with the contralateral unaffected ankle.

A limp may also be observed. Neurologic examination including sensation and deep tendon reflexes is commonly normal. Manual muscle testing

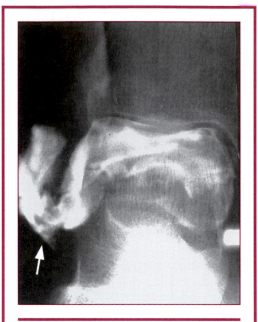

FIGURE 1. Ankle arthrogram. AP view after ankle injection demonstrates extravasation laterally (*arrow*) resulting from anterior talo-fibular ligament tear. There is no filling of the peroneal tendon sheath. (From Berquist TH: Radiology of the Foot and Ankle. © Mayo Foundation, 2000.)

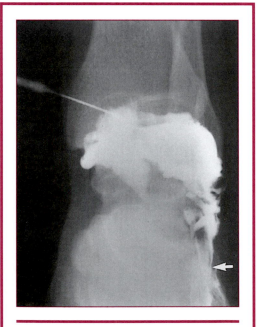

FIGURE 2. Ankle arthrogram. AP view taken during ankle injection demonstrates filling of the peroneal tendon sheaths (*arrow*) result-ing from calcaneofibular ligament disruption. (From Berquist TH: Radiology of the Foot and Ankle. © Mayo Foundation, 2000.)

should also be normal, with the exception of muscles surrounding the ankle that may exhibit weakness due to disuse or due to pain.

Functional Limitations

Affected persons may have difficulty participating in sports, particularly high demand sports that require quick starts and stops, cutting, and jumping (such as soccer, football, and basketball), as well as sports that involve a lot of lateral movement (such as tennis). When symptoms are severe, limitations can include difficulty with climbing steps, ambulation, and activities that require prolonged standing.

Diagnostic Studies

Diagnosis is made by confirming a history of prior sprain with subsequent development of typical symptoms of functional instability, in conjunction with consistent examination findings. Adjunctive diagnostic testing can be helpful in establishing the diagnosis, particularly by identifying pathology and conditions that may produce similar symptomatology. Testing that may be useful when the diagnosis of chronic ankle instability is being considered includes routine x-rays, stress x-rays, computed tomography, bone scans, magnetic resonance imaging, ankle arthrography (Figs. 1 and 2) and magnetic resonance arthrography.

Routine x-rays are useful to rule out old or chronic fractures (most commonly of the fibula, tibia, talus, and fifth metatarsal), to assess the integrity of the ankle mortise, and to assess for ankle arthritis. A routine x-ray series should include AP, lateral, and mortise views. Widening of the ankle mortise may indicate a syndesmotic disruption or significant deltoid ligament tear. X-rays should be obtained in all cases with a history of significant trauma at initial injury.

Stress x-rays may be helpful in determining the presence of chronic mechanical instability. Though the routine use of stress radiographs remains controversial, a finding of greater than 5 mm of anterior displacement of the talus during anterior drawer testing is typically considered to be abnormal.[3] Inversion stress x-rays are considered abnormal with a finding of greater than 5 degrees of side-to-side difference in tibiotalar tilt.[3] However, a recent review found the published data regarding stress radiographs too variable to determine accepted normal values for acute and chronic sprains.[4] The sensitivity of stress radiographs in diagnosing chronic lateral ligament tears (surgically confirmed) is low, though specificity is high.[4]

Computed tomography can be useful for identifying subtle talus fractures and other bony pathology, such as tumors. Bones scans are particularly helpful in identifying stress fractures and can be a useful screening tool to evaluate for ongoing ankle pathology, such as significant arthritis, infection, tumors, and reflex sympathetic dystrophy. MRI and MR arthrography generally give the most information regarding soft tissue injury, though they also can be helpful in identifying fractures (such as osteochondral fractures), tumors, and chronic infections. MRI and MR arthrography both have high specificity for identifying chronic ligament tears, though MR arthrography has higher sensitivity.[5] The appropriate timing of advanced imaging is variable, though is typically governed by the clinical suspicion of further injury or pathology not evident on routine x-rays or persistent symptoms despite appropriate treatment. Figures 1 and 2 demonstrate anterior talofibular and calcaneofibular ligament tears as observed with ankle arthrography.

Differential Diagnosis

Peroneal tendinopathy: subluxation, tear, chronic tendinitis

Ankle impingement syndrome

Sinus tarsi syndrome

Subtalar instability

Sprain: midfoot, subtalar

Fracture: distal tibia/fibula, talar, osteochondral, stress fracture, fifth metatarsal, physeal

Arthropathy: degenerative, inflammatory, crystalline, infectious

Treatment

Initial

The initial treatment regimen depends, in part, on symptom acuity and whether a recent sprain has occurred. Initial treatment considerations include ice massage, compression, elevation, taping/bracing, NSAIDs/COX-2 inhibitors, and/or analgesics. The goal with bracing at this juncture is to prevent recurrent sprains and further tissue trauma. Many patients can successfully wean from their brace following rehabilitation. However, high demand athletes may choose to brace/tape during athletic participation, indefinitely.

A thin lateral heel wedge will put the ankle in slight valgus alignment and potentially diminish symptoms of instability and the tendency for spontaneous ankle inversion with activity. High top sneakers may help reduce symptoms as well.

Rehabilitation

Rehabilitation first starts by normalizing ankle range of motion, with primary emphasis on restoring ankle dorsiflexion and eversion. This typically includes heel cord stretching with the knee straight (to stretch the gastrocnemius) and flexed 30 degrees (to stretch the soleus), as well as eversion (posterior tibialis) stretching. Care must be taken to avoid recurrent inversion stress to the ankle, which can perpetuate lateral capsuloligamentous laxity.

As symptoms allow, the patient begins an ankle group strengthening program with an emphasis on ankle evertor strengthening. Resistance exercises can begin when there is no pain through the available range of motion, with full weight bearing.[6] The rehabilitation program may start with low level strengthening, such as submaximal static exercises, and progress in a pain free fashion to dynamic and isokinetic strengthening. Typically a combination of open and closed kinetic chain strengthening is employed in the rehabilitation process. Open chain exercises include the use of ankle weights and resistance tubing. Closed chain exercises are more functionally based, in which the foot is planted on the ground and the patient engages in an activity that requires the activation of antagonistic muscles that stabilize the ankle. Since eccentric muscle contractions place the greatest force on the muscle, this mode of strengthening should be reserved for the final stages of the rehabilitation program.

Balance challenge/proprioceptive exercises are a very important part of chronic ankle instability rehabilitation and have been found to decrease symptoms of functional instability as well as reduce the rate of re-injury.[7,8] Ankle disks/wobble boards are devices that facilitate proprioceptive training. These exercises can be started without specialized equipment by having the patient perform a single leg stance on the affected ankle and then increasing the skill level by having the patient close his or her eyes or stand on a pillow.

Functional exercises and sport specific drills can begin when the patient has full range of motion, no pain, and at least 85% peroneal strength compared with the contralateral ankle.[9] These exercises add progressively difficult challenges and facilitate the attainment of dynamic strength and balance. Examples of these exercises include jogging, running, double leg jumping, single leg hopping, skipping rope, figure eight drills, lateral cutting drills, and plyometrics. Patients should start at a low level of intensity and progress with increased intensity and difficulty only if they remain pain free while performing the exercise and have no pain or swelling following the training session.

Adjunctive modalities may be helpful throughout the rehabilitation process. These may include regular ice application (ice massage, ice pack, ankle Cryo/Cuff) following therapy sessions or heat application (superficial heat or ultrasound) to facilitate range of motion of a stiff joint. Electrical stimulation may be helpful for pain and edema control.

Procedures

No procedures are typically indicated for chronic ankle instability.

Surgery

Surgery should be considered for patients who sustain recurrent lateral ankle sprains or exhibit significant symptoms of functional instability despite appropriate rehabilitation interventions. The goal with surgery is to restore mechanical stability to the ankle and thereby significantly reduce or eliminate chronic symptoms of instability. Late ankle reconstruction for chronic lateral instability is successful in approximately 85% of patients, regardless of the type of surgical procedure performed.[10] Primary anatomic repair of the anterior talofibular and calcaneal fibular ligaments is often preferred.[10] However, in cases in which there is excessive joint laxity, peroneal weakness, hindfoot varus, or significant tibiotalar osteoarthritis, reconstructions such as the Chrisman-Snook or Watson-Jones procedures may be perferred.[10,11]

Potential Disease Complications

Potential long-term sequelae of chronic ankle instability include the development of ankle impingement syndrome; chronic peroneal tendinopathy or subluxation; tibiotalar osteochondral injury; degenerative arthritis; superficial peroneal neuropathy; or chronic pain syndromes, such as complex regional pain syndrome type I (reflex sympathetic dystrophy; see Chapter 132).

Potential Treatment Complications

Potential treatment complications include frostbite from overly aggressive use of ice; exacerbation of edema from inappropriate ankle taping/wrapping/bracing; and pain exacerbation or re-injury during physical therapy. Analgesics, NSAIDs, and COX-2 inhibitors have well-known side effects that most commonly affect the gastric, hepatic, and renal systems. Surgical complications include failed repair, wound or bone infection, loss of ankle range of motion from an aggressive reconstruction, and persistent ankle pain despite appropriate rehabilitation or surgical repair/reconstruction.

References

1. Verhagen R, de Keizer G, van Dijk CN: Long term follow-up of inversion trauma of the ankle. Arch Orthop Trauma Surg 1995;114:92–96.
2. Freeman M: Instability of the foot after injuries to the lateral ligaments of the foot. J Bone Joint Surg Br 1965;47-B:669–677.
3. Miller MD, Cooper DE, Warner JP: Review of Sports Medicine and Arthroscopy. Philadelphia, W.B. Saunders, 1995.
4. Frost SC, Amendola A: Is stress radiography necessary in the diagnosis of acute or chronic ankle instability? Clin J Sports Med 1999;9(1):40–45.
5. Chandnani VP, Harper MT, Ficke JR, et al: Chronic ankle instability: evaluation with MR arthrography, MR imaging, and stress radiography. Radiology 1994;192:189–194.
6. Demaio M, Paine R, Drez D: Chronic lateral ankle instability-inversion sprains: Part I. Orthopedics 1992;15(1):87–96.
7. Gauffin H, Tropp H, Odenrick P: Effect of ankle disk training on postural control in patients with functional instability of the ankle joint. Int J Sports Med 1988;9:141–148.
8. Tropp H, Askling C, Gillquist J: Prevention of ankle sprains. Am J Sports Med 1985;13:259–262.
9. Demaio M, Paine R, Drez D: Chronic lateral ankle instability-inversion sprains: Part II. Orthopedics 1992;15(1):87–96.
10. Colville MR: Surgical treatment of the unstable ankle. JAAOS 1998;6(6):368–377.
11. Peters JW, Trevio SG, Renstrom PA: Chronic lateral ankle instability. Foot Ankle 1991;12(3):182–191.

81 | Claw Toe

Elise H. Lee, MD
Sheila Dugan, MD

Synonyms

None

ICD-9 Codes

735.5
Claw toe (acquired)

735.8
Other acquired
deformities of toe

Definition

Claw toe refers to hyperextension of the metatarsophalangeal (MTP) joint with abnormal flexion posture of the proximal interphalangeal (PIP) joint (Fig. 1). The deformity typically affects all of the toes and can be either fixed or flexible. Pathogenesis involves an imbalance between the extrinsic and intrinsic foot muscles. Such an imbalance leads to simultaneous contraction of the extensor digitorum longus upon its insertion at the MTP joint and the flexor digitorum longus at the interphalangeal joints. Hence, an additional flexion deformity at the distal interphalangeal (DIP) joint commonly accompanies the claw deformity.

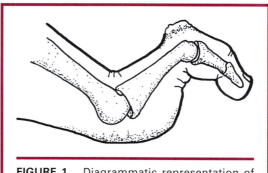

FIGURE 1. Diagrammatic representation of claw toe.

Etiology is commonly unknown. However, an association with neuromuscular diseases is noted, in particular, Charcot-Marie-Tooth (hereditary sensorimotor neuropathy I), stroke, and polio. Other precipitating conditions include rheumatoid arthritis, diabetes, and deep posterior compartment syndrome. Mechanical factors such as pes cavus can also cause claw toes. Correction of the foot deformity often leads to resolution of the claw deformity as well. Age is another contributing factor as decreased muscle tone results in an increased reliance on toe gripping for balance in the elderly.[1,2]

Symptoms

The chief complaint is usually pain as a result of corn formation over the dorsal aspect of the PIP joint from shoe compression. End corns may develop just distal to the nail if a flexion deformity is also present at the DIP joint. In more severe cases, the extension posture of the claw toes increases pressure over the metatarsal heads. Metatarsalgia with subsequent callus formation underneath the metatarsal heads occur secondary to their plantar displacement.[3] Cosmetic complaints are also common.

Physical Examination

On inspection, determine the degree of MTP hyperextension and PIP flexion. Also note accompanying foot deformities such as pes cavus, plantar ulcerations, and hyperkeratosis. A focused exam directed at the factors that bear upon the diagnosis of claw toe is key.

Next, determine whether the clawing is fixed or flexible. This can be done by assessing toe flexibility with the ankle in dorsiflexion and plantarflexion. Correction of the deformity upon plantarflexion signifies a flexible deformity.[1]

Claw pattern should also be examined during gait. An exacerbation of clawing during swing signifies weak ankle dorsiflexors and overcompensation of toe extensors. Worsening of clawing during stance indicates a weakened gastrocnemius and soleus complex with overcompensation of the long toe flexors.

Functional Limitations

Functional limitations primarily result from pain incurred by corn and callus formation. Walking and other weight-bearing activities can be painful. The ability to tolerate shoe gear with a narrow toe box is also impaired.

Diagnostic Studies

Claw toe is a clinical diagnosis; therefore, history and physical exam are sufficient. Should radiographs be taken, weight-bearing views should be obtained. An apparent joint space narrowing corresponds to subluxation of the proximal phalanx on the metatarsal head at the MTP joint.[1,3]

Differential Diagnosis

Hammer toes

Mallet toes

Interdigital neuroma

Non-specific synovitis of the metatarsophalangeal joint

Triggering of the toes (lower limb analog of trigger finger)[4]

Treatment

Initial

The first treatment step involves fitting for shoes with an adequate toe box to accommodate the increased toe dorsiflexion. A soft insole can also be used. In particular, a soft metatarsal pad placed just proximal to the metatarsal head region is useful for pressure relief.[5] Nonsteroidal anti-inflammatory drugs (NSAIDs) and analgesic medications can reduce pain. Ulcer and callus management may be required, and patients should be educated in monitoring their skin for breakdown, especially in the setting of peripheral neuropathy.

Rehabilitation

The clinician should prescribe shoes with deep, wide toe boxes. Alternatively, extra depth can be achieved in a standard shoe by trimming the existing shoe insert just distal to the metatarsal heads.[6] An external metatarsal bar and rocker bottom shoe are additional comfort-enhancing options.

Stretching, friction massage, manipulation, and taping of the MTP joints in neutral may be useful in correcting a flexible foot deformity.

Strengthening of the intrinsic foot muscles should also be part of the rehabilitation regimen. Exercises may include towel rolling or picking up marbles or rolls of tape with the toes.[5]

Procedures

Non-surgical procedures are not typically done in treating claw toe.

Surgery

Operative treatment should only be pursued if the patient remains symptomatic after all the aforementioned conservative approaches have failed. Cosmesis alone is not a good indication for surgery. The approach taken for surgical correction varies depending on whether the deformity is fixed or flexible.

In a flexible claw toe, in which contractures do not exist, soft tissue procedures are the procedures of choice. The Girdlestone flexor tendon transfer, involving transposition of the flexor digitorum longus to the dorsal extensor hood of the proximal phalanx, provides increased plantarflexion pull at the MTP joint. Extensor tenotomy may be added as an adjunct.

In the more severe fixed deformity, bone and joint procedures are used. Resection arthrodesis of the distal third of the proximal phalanx is indicated in joint subluxation. Extensor digitorum longus (then brevis) tenotomy, dorsal MTP capsulotomy, and collateral ligament sectioning release the fixed contractures. Some or all of the procedures discussed may be necessary to achieve full correction.[2,7] It should be noted, moreover, that proper correction places the PIP joint in slight plantarflexion to avoid rigidity.

Postoperatively, full weight-bearing status in a postoperative shoe or appropriate pedal splinting device is generally allowed. Bandaging is continued for its compression and splinting effects until healing.[1]

Potential Discease Complications

The complications of claw toe include metatarsalgia, plantar and point-of-contact ulcerations in the insensate foot, arthralgia and joint stiffness if subluxation has occurred, and toenail deformities. Bursitis/synovitis, gait abnormalities with proximal structural symptoms, and degenerative joint disease are additional complications.

Potential Treatment Complictions

Analgesics, NSAIDs, and COX-2 inhibitors have well-known side effects that most commonly affect the gastric, hepatic, and renal systems. Potential treatment complications are primarily postsurgical and include toe ischemia; digital nerve palsy; non-union; malalignment; reduced toe range of motion; rigid, excessively straight toe; persistent edema; flail foe; and osseous regrowth.

References
1. Wheeless CR. Wheeless' Textbook of Orthopaedics. www.medmedia.com, 1996.
2. Canale ST (ed): Campbell's Operative Orthopedics, 9th ed, vol 2. Mosby, 1998.
3. American College of Foot and Ankle Surgeons: Preferred Practice Guidelines. Hammer toe syndrome. J Foot Ankle Surg 1999;38(2):166–178.
4. Martin MG, Masear VR: Triggering of the lesser toes at a previously undescribed distal pulley system. Foot Ankle Int 1998;19(2):113–117.
5. Hunt GC, McPoil TG (eds): Physical Therapy of the Foot and Ankle, 2nd ed. New York, Churchill Livingstone, 1995.
6. Kaye RA: The extra-depth toe box: A rational approach. Foot Ankle Int 1994;15(3):146–150.
7. Myerson MS, Shereff MJ: The pathological anatomy of claw and hammer toes. J Bone Joint Surg Am 1989;71(1):45–49.

82 Corns

Robert J. Scardina, DPM
Sammy M. Lee, DPM

Synonyms

Clavus

Heloma

Helomata

Callosity

Callositas

ICD-9 Code

700
Corns and calluses

Definition

A corn is a circumscribed, focal thickening of epidermis composed of impacted, dead keratinocytes,[1] usually located over dorsally prominent digital interphalangeal joints (hammer toes). Corns form in response to excessive and repetitive pressure and/or friction from shoe gear. These lesions are usually hard and ovoid or circular with a polished or translucent center, like a kernel of a corn (from which they take their name), and they may become painfully inflamed or ulcerated.[2]

There are two types of corns. Heloma durum (hard corn) is the most common (Fig. 1). These develop dorsally over digital interphalangeal joints and distally on toes and are caused primarily by toe deformity and may be accentuated by improper or ill-fitting shoes. The second type (Fig. 2) is known as heloma molle (soft corn), occurring primarily interdigitally and most commonly in the web space between toes four and five. These are usually the result of tight-fitting shoes and/or adjacent bone (phalangeal) abnormalities, including exostoses.[3]

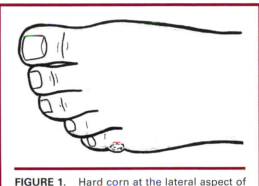

FIGURE 1. Hard corn at the lateral aspect of the PIP joint of the small toe.

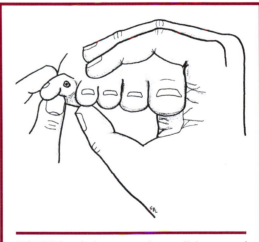

FIGURE 2. Soft corn on the medial aspect of the small toe.

Symptoms

Symptoms range from sharp, shooting pain to dull, aching soreness, aggravated by wearing closed shoe gear. If secondary ulceration develops, infection may ensue with subsequent local and systemic manifestations.

Physical Examination

On inspection, these cutaneous lesions are typically hard (or in the case of heloma molle, soft or macerated) with thickened skin and a yellowish or translucent nidus or center. In contrast to warts (verrucae), which are typically painful with lateral compression, corns are more painful to direct pressure.

Typically, corns are associated with digital deformities, including hammer toe, claw toe, or mallet toe, or combined interphalangeal joint deformities.[4] Hammer toe or claw toe deformities may contribute to "retrograde" lesser metatarsalgia. Associated forefoot deformities include bunion with hallux abductus.

Functional Limitations

Corns can result in difficulty with walking (primarily with closed shoe gear), pain associated with running or athletic activities, and residual non–weight-bearing or nocturnal pain.

Diagnostic Studies

The diagnosis of a corn (or clavus) is done primarily on a clinical basis. However, plain radiographic analysis may be helpful in identifying underlying primary structural digital deformity or associated contributing forefoot deformities (i.e., hallux abductus/bunion).

Differential Diagnosis

Verruca (wart)
Subcutaneous bursa
Benign or malignant cutaneous neoplasm
Superficial foreign body

Tinea pedis (fourth web space lesions)
Keratoderma
Porokeratoma

Treatment

Initial

Conservative measures for symptomatic relief include efforts to reduce or eliminate direct friction or pressure at the involved site by the use of various padding or shielding methods (e.g., moleskin pads, aperture pads, silicone sleeves); orthodigital (toe-straightening) devices for reducible deformity only; and proper shoe gear, allowing adequate toe box room.[5] The patient should be counseled to avoid narrow shoes and high heels.

Use of over-the-counter keratolytic agents (including salicylic acid) is a common self-care measure; however, this should be discouraged due to lack of tissue specificity and potential for ulceration and/or infection.

Possible skin breakdown and ulceration with infection, especially in the diabetic neuropathic or dysvascular patient, may occur, often requiring local wound care and/or systemic antibiotics.

NSAIDs/COX-2 inhibitors and analgesics may be used acutely for pain.

Rehabilitation

There are no true rehabilitative modalities for corns. However, should these cutaneous lesions respond to initial conservative measures, one may consider custom shoe gear (e.g., extra depth, moulded), orthodigital devices, and custom orthotics to improve foot biomechanics and decrease pressure on the painful area.

Procedures

Trimming or paring of a corn should be done under aseptic technique, to a proper level, and with appropriate instrumentation (Fig. 3). This type of palliative treatment is traditionally provided for patients who are not surgical candidates, either by individual choice or medical

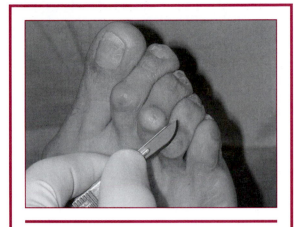

FIGURE 3. Trimming of hard corn on hammer toe.

contraindication. The interval for this type of ongoing care generally ranges from every 4 to 12 weeks, depending on the nature and extent of the lesion(s), as well as the patient's activity level.

Other invasive, non-surgical procedures include subcutaneous injection of a local anesthetic/soluble corticosteroid preparation for *acute* conditions with bursitis.[6] These injections should not be performed more than a few times, as they may lead to dermal atrophy.

Surgery

Surgical correction involves addressing the underlying structural deformity, including hammer toes, claw toes, or mallet toes.[7,8]

Potential Disease Complications

Potential disease complications include refractory or intractable pain, secondary functional limitation, superficial or deep skin ulceration, infection, and shoe gear restrictions.

Potential Treatment Complications

Analgesics, NSAIDs, and COX-2 inhibitors have well-known side effects that most commonly affect the gastric, hepatic, and renal systems. Treatment complications from conservative care include skin ulceration or infection due to overly aggressive debridement or use of keratolytic agents. Postsurgical complications include infection, wound problems, nerve injury/numbness, chronic digital edema, and recurrent deformity.

References
1. Harkless LB: Podiatric dermatology. Clin Podiatr Med Surg 1996;13:73–84.
2. Neale D: Common Foot Disorders: Diagnosis and Management. New York, Churchill Livingstone, 1981.
3. Birrer RB, et al: Common Foot Problems in Primary Care. Philadelphia, Hanley & Belfus, 1998.
4. Oliver TP, Armstrong DG, et al: Digital surgery. Clin Podiatr Med Surg 1996;13:263–268.
5. Gould JS: The Foot Book. Baltimore, Williams & Wilkins, 1988.
6. Yale JR: Yale's Podiatric Medicine. Baltimore, Williams & Wilkins, 1987.
7. Bordelon RL: Surgical and Conservative Foot Care. Thorofare, NJ, Slack, 1988.
8. Day RD, Reyzelman AM, Harkless LB: Digital surgery. Clin Podiatr Med Surg 1996;13:201–206.

83 Foot and Ankle Ganglia

Jeffrey T. Brodie, MD

Synonyms

Cyst of joint capsule
Cyst of tendon
Cyst of tendon sheath
Myxomatous cyst
Mucoid cyst

ICD-9 Code

727.43
Ganglion and cyst of synovium, tendon, and bursa, unspecified

Definition

Ganglia are benign cystic fibrous lesions that are contained by thin walls of connective tissue, are often multilocular, and contain relatively colorless fluid that is thickened and gelatinous.[1] Many authors believe that ganglion cysts are due to myxoid degeneration of surrounding connective tissue.[2,3] They are most commonly found in the hand; however, the foot and ankle are also common sites for these benign lesions to occur, especially on the dorsolateral surface.[3] They are most commonly seen in the soft tissues of young and middle age adults and have a preponderance for females. Ganglia rarely connect with a joint and can occasionally be seen within tendons and bone.[4]

Symptoms

Whereas the majority of patients present with a painful mass in the soft tissues of the foot or ankle, a small percentage of patients are asymptomatic and are more concerned about the possibility of malignancy or simply cosmesis. The symptoms are often brought about only by certain types of shoe gear that may cause direct compression of the mass or indirectly through traction of the adjacent skin. If the mass is compressing a sensory nerve, it can lead to burning, radiating neuritic pain.[5] If this occurs in the posteromedial aspect of the ankle, it can cause symptoms consistent with tarsal tunnel syndrome due to compression of the posterior tibial nerve.[6]

Physical Examination

Evaluation of a soft tissue mass on the foot and ankle should include a complete history, careful physical examination, and radiographic studies. These lesions are generally less than 2 centimeters in diameter. They can be soft, firm, or hard depending on their size and location. Although they may be found on the plantar aspect of the foot, they are most commonly seen on the dorsal aspect.[4,7] If they are compressing a nerve, Tinel's sign may be present or there may be a region of dysesthesia or anesthesia.[8] Transillumination may be possible if the ganglion is close to the skin surface. These lesions are not associated with a particular foot type; however, foot abnormalities should be noted (e.g., pes planus or flat feet).

Functional Limitations

Because these lesions are rarely symptomatic outside of shoe gear, the only significant limitations are due to inability to tolerate certain types of shoes. This could limit walking; running; or sports that involve kicking, such as soccer.

Diagnostic Studies

Plain radiographs are typically normal, but AP and lateral planes should be obtained in most cases to rule out bony exostoses or soft tissue calcification. In most cases, the diagnosis is confirmed with aspiration of the lesion, which will reveal the classic clear, gelatinous fluid and provide definitive diagnosis. However,

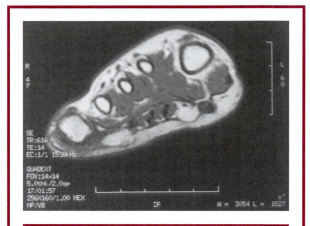

FIGURE 1. MRI of a ganglion cyst below the skin, inferior and lateral to the fibular sesamoid.

if the lesion is too small or if the fluid too thick to aspirate, MRI can help provide useful and often diagnostic information regarding these masses. Ganglia visualized on MRI will demonstrate low to intermediate signal intensity on T1-weighted images and high signal intensity on T2-weighted images (Fig. 1). They are commonly septated or lobulated in appearance.[8,9]

Differential Diagnosis

Giant cell tumor of tendon sheath	Hypertrophic synovial cysts	Lipoma
Pigmented villonodular synovitis	Soft tissue calcifications	Malignant sarcoma
Benign synoviomas	Bony exostoses	

Treatment

Initial

Shoe gear modification can alleviate the pressure exerted on many of these lesions. Many times, alteration of lacing patterns in athletic shoes can eliminate these symptoms. Oral medications have not been demonstrated to be of benefit in the treatment of ganglion cysts; however, if pain is acute, then traditional analgesics or NSAIDs/COX-2 inhibitors can be used.

Rehabilitation

No formal rehabilitative techniques have been demonstrated as effective treatment options for ganglia. However, for the rare mass on the plantar aspect of the foot, biomechanical unloading can be accomplished with the use of custom orthoses.

Procedures

Simple aspiration of ganglion cysts has resulted in recurrence rates as high as 60% to 100%.[4,5,7,10] The addition of steroid injection after aspiration can reduce the rate of recurrence to 33% to 50%.[5,11]

After preparation of the skin, ethyl chloride spray can be used as a local anesthetic. Then, under sterile conditions, a large bore needle (e.g., 18 gauge) should be used with a 5 or 10 cc syringe to apply sufficient suction and allow the thick material to pass into the syringe. Without removing the needle, usually less than 0.5 cc to 1.0 cc of a local corticosteroid (e.g., triamcinolone) is injected into the evacuated cyst. Compression and ice can be applied after this procedure. This process can be

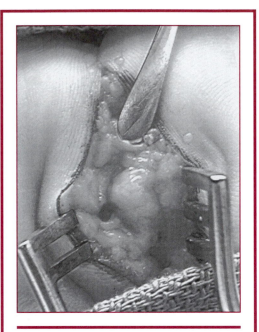

FIGURE 2. Surgical exposure of the lesion seen in Fig. 1. Note the round mass in the center of surgical field seen just below the surgical instrument. This cyst was compressing the plantar digital nerve in this web space.

repeated a second time after at least 4 to 6 weeks, if necessary. If no fluid can be aspirated, a solid tumor should be considered and further workup including CT scan, MRI, or possibly biopsy may be considered.[2]

Postinjection care includes local icing for 5 to 10 minutes and avoidance, if possible, of direct pressure on the injected site for 24 to 48 hours.

Surgery

If conservative treatment of ganglia has failed, surgical excision can be curative (Fig. 2). Because there is a high rate of failure of conservative treatment, approximately one third to one half of symptomatic ganglia go on to require surgery. Unfortunately, recurrence rates can still run as high as 10% to 27% after excision; therefore, it is imperative that careful, meticulous dissection of the entire mass be performed to minimize this risk.[1,7,10]

Potential Disease Complications

The main disease complication is chronic pain. This may lead to an inability to wear certain types of shoes.

Potential Treatment Complications

Analgesics, NSAIDs, and COX-2 inhibitors have well-known side effects that most commonly affect the gastric, hepatic, and renal systems. As previously noted, recurrence of the cyst is the most common complication from surgical excision. Painful scars and keloids can occur as with any surgical procedure. If the cyst is located in the vicinity of a motor or sensory nerve, injury to the nerve is possible. In addition, incisions near the anterior aspect of the ankle can lead to joint stiffness from scar contracture.[1,4,7] Care should be taken with cortisone injections to reduce the risk of fat necrosis in the subcutaneous tissues. Small amounts of cortisone should be used (less than 1 cc), and attempt to keep the needle within the potential space of the evacuated cyst.

References
1. Rozbruch SR, Chang V, et al: Ganglion cysts of the lower extremity: An analysis of 54 cases and review of the literature. Orthopedics 1998;21:141–148.
2. Walling AK, Gasser SI: Soft-tissue and bone tumors about the foot and ankle. Clin Sports Med 1994;13:909–938.
3. Carnesale PG. Soft tissue tumors and nonneoplastic conditions simulating bone tumors. In Crenchaw AH (ed): Campbell's Operative Orthopaedics, 8th ed. St. Louis, Mosby, 1992, pp 299–300.
4. Kliman ME, Freiberg A: Ganglia of the foot and ankle. Foot Ankle 1982;3:45–46.
5. Slavitt JA, Beheshti F, et al: Ganglions of the foot: A six-year retrospective study and a review of the literature. J Am Podiatr Med Assoc 1980;70:459–465.
6. Takakura Y, Kitada C, et al: Tarsal tunnel syndrome: causes and results of operative treatment. J Bone Joint Surg 1991;73-B:125–128.
7. Pontious J, Good J, Maxian SH: Ganglions of the foot and ankle: A retrospective analysis of 63 procedures. J Am Podiatr Med Assoc 1999;89:163–168.
8. Steiner E, Steinbach LS, et al: Ganglia and cysts around joints. Radiol Clin North Am 1996;34:395–425.
9. Wetzel LH, Levine E: Soft-tissue tumors of the foot: Value of MR imaging for specific diagnosis. Am J Radiol 1990;155:1025–1030.
10. Johnston JO: Tumors and metabolic diseases of the foot. In Mann RA, Coughlin MJ (eds): Surgery of the Foot and Ankle, 6th ed. St. Louis, Mosby, 1993, p 997.
11. Derbyshire RC: Observations on the treatment of ganglia: With a report on hydrocortisone. Am J Surg 1966;112:635–636.

84 Hallux Rigidus

David Wexler, MD
Todd A. Kile, MD

Synonyms

Osteoarthritis or degenerative joint disease of the first metatarsophalangeal joint

Osteoarthritis of the great toe[1]

ICD-9 Code

735.2
Hallux rigidus

Definition

Degenerative joint disease or loss of articular cartilage from the first metatarsophalangeal (MTP) joint leads to a painful restriction of its range of motion. The normal range is from 30 to 45 degrees of plantarflexion to almost 90 degrees of dorsiflexion (hyperextension). Generally, 45 to 60 degrees of dorsiflexion are required for normal activities of daily living. The limited range of motion is exacerbated by overgrowth of bone (osteophytes or "bone spurs") on the dorsal aspects of the bases of the proximal phalanx and the head of the metatarsal, which impinge on one another as the great toe dorsiflexes.[2]

In general, the cause is unknown, although it is associated with generalized osteoarthritis of other joints and repeated microtrauma (e.g., in soccer players). Sustaining repetitive turf toe-type injuries may lead to this form of early joint degeneration.[10]

Symptoms

Patients typically report pain on walking, especially going up stairs. It is associated with stiffness, swelling, and sometimes inflammation. There can be occasional locking due to a cartilaginous loose body. Patients may notice that they are walking on the outside of the foot to avoid pushing off with the great toe during the terminal stance and toe-off phases of the gait cycle. As the degeneration increases, the pain may intensify and result in a limp.

Physical Examination

On inspection, there will usually be swelling around the MTP joint with tenderness of the joint line. Pain is reproduced with forcible dorsiflexion of the great toe, which is also restricted in range. There may be an antalgic (painful) gait, and single stance toe raise may be difficult. Neurologic exam including strength, sensation, and reflexes is typically normal.

Functional Limitations

Functional limitations include walking long distances, running any distance, and ascending stairs. Wearing flexible shoes may prove too uncomfortable.

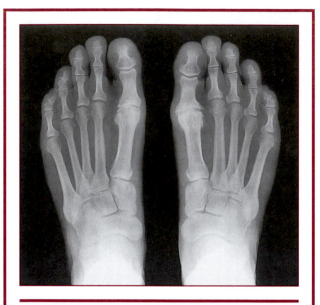

FIGURE 1. Standing AP radiograph of both feet. This demonstrates bilateral hallux rigidus or degenerative joint disease of the hallux MTP joints. The signs are narrowing of the joint space, osteophyte formation, and sclerosis. This is more pronounced on the right.

Diagnostic Studies

Plain AP and lateral standing radiographs will usually suffice in confirming the diagnosis (Fig. 1). The signs are consistent with degenerative joint disease, namely loss of joint space and congruency, large dorsal osteophytes (bone spurs), sclerosis (increased density of bone), and subchondral cysts. There may be evidence of a loose body.

Differential Diagnosis

Gout

Hallux valgus

Turf toe

Treatment

Initial

Nonsteroidal anti-inflammatory drugs (NSAIDs) may provide symptomatic relief. Footwear modifications or use of orthotics to limit stresses at the MTP joint are good initial treatment measures. These include avoiding high-heeled shoes and shoes with very flexible soles.[3]

Rehabilitation

More advanced shoe modifications can be made by a certified pedorthist. These include a steel shank or possibly a rocker bottom that may be applied to the soles of many different types of shoes, particularly athletic shoes.

If there is evidence of other foot deformities such as pes planus (flat foot), orthotic inserts may provide correction and help with gait biomechanics.

Physical therapy is not generally indicated, but may include basic mobilization and distraction techniques, as well as strengthening exercises of the flexor and extensor hallucis muscles to enhance joint stability. Modalities such as contrast baths and ice may help with pain control.

Procedures

Intra-articular injection of local anaesthetic with steroid may provide short-term relief.

Surgery

The principal indications for surgery are continuing pain and failed non-operative management. Depending on the severity of the degeneration, there are two broad approaches to surgery. The first is joint preserving, by excising the impinging dorsal osteophytes, thereby debulking the joint and improving dorsiflexion.[7,8,12] The second approach is joint sacrificing and ranges from resection arthroplasty (resulting in a floppy or flail shortened toe) to arthrodesis (resulting in a stiff, rigidly fixed toe).[5,6,13] A number of manufacturers have tried to produce artificial great toe joints, made of silastic,[4] metal, and polyethylene or ceramic,[9,11] but the long-term results of these have not lived up to expectations. Arthroscopic surgery has also been attempted.

Potential Disease Complications

Hallux rigidus may produce intractable pain and reduced mobility.

Potential Treatment Complications

Analgesics, NSAIDs, and COX-2 inhibitors have well-known side effects that most commonly affect the gastric, hepatic, and renal systems. Steroid injection can rarely introduce infection.

Complications of surgery can range from failure of improvement with insufficient osteophyte resection, to toe shortening and transfer metatarsalgia (pain under the metatarsal heads of the lesser toes) and implant failure, silicone wear, foreign body reaction, and osteolysis following arthroplasty. Surgical complications of fusion include mal-union and non-union.

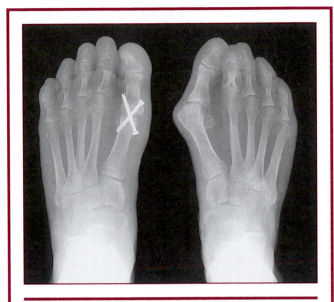

FIGURE 2. Standing AP radiograph of both feet. This demonstrates, on the left foot, one of the techniques for fusing the MTP joint, with crossed cannulated screws. The right foot shows a hallux valgus deformity.

References

1. O'Malley MJ: Hallux rigidus. In Craig EV (ed): Clinical Orthopaedics, 1st ed. Media, PA, Williams & Wilkins, 1999, pp 913–919.
2. Richardson EG, Donley BG: Disorders of hallux. In Canale ST (ed): Campbell's Operative Orthopaedics, vol 2, 9th ed, St Louis, Mosby, 1998, pp 1621–1711.
3. Hertling D, Kessler RM: The leg, ankle and foot. In Hertling D, Kessler RM (eds): Management of Common Musculoskeletal Disorders, 3rd ed. Philadelphia, Lippincott, Williams & Wilkins, 1996, pp 435–438.
4. Cracchiolo A, Swanson A, et al: The arthritic great toe metatarsophalangeal joint: A review of flexible silicone implant arthroplasty from two medical centres. Clin Orthop 1981;157:64–69.
5. Coughlin MJ: Arthrodesis of the first metatarsophalangeal joint. Orthop Rev 1990;19:177–186.
6. Curtis MJ, Myerson M, et al: Arthrodesis of the first metatarsophalangeal joint: A biomechanical study of internal fixation techniques. Foot Ankle 1993;14:395–399.
7. Geldwert JJ, Rock GD, et al: Cheilectomy: Still a useful technique for grade I and grade II hallux limitus/rigidus. J Foot Surg 1992;31:154–159.
8. Hattrup SJ, Johnson KA: Subjective results of hallux rigidus following treatment with cheilectomy. Clin Orthop 1988;226:182–189.
9. Wenger RJ, Whalley RC: Total replacement of the first MTP joint. J Bone Joint Surg 1978;60-B:88–92.
10. Mann RA: Disorders of the first metatarsophalangeal joint. J Am Acad Orthop Surg 1995;3:34–40.
11. Townley CO, Taranow WS: A metallic hemiarthroplasty resurfacing prosthesis for the hallux metatarsophalangeal joint. Foot Ankle Int 1994;15:575–580.
12. Pfeffer GB: Cheilectomy. In Thompson RC, Johnson KA (eds): Master Techniques in Orthopaedic Surgery—The Foot and Ankle, 1st ed. Philadelphia, Raven Press, 1994, pp 119–133.
13. Alexander IA: Hallux metatarsophalangeal arthrodesis. In Thompson RC, Johnson KA (eds): Master Techniques in Orthopaedic Surgery—The Foot and Ankle, 1st ed. Philadelphia, Raven Press, 1994, pp 49–64.

85 Hammer Toe

Robert J. Krug, MD
Elise H. Lee, MD
Sheila Dugan, MD
Katherine Mashey, DPM

Synonyms

Flexion contracture of the proximal interphalangeal joint

Lesser toe deformity

Hammer toe syndrome

ICD-9 Codes

735.4
Hammer toe (acquired)

735.8
Other acquired deformities of toe

Definition

Hammer toe refers to an abnormal flexion posture at the proximal interphalangeal (PIP) joint of one of the lesser four toes. A hammer toe involves hyperextension of the metatarsophalangeal (MTP) joint, flexion of the PIP joint, and extension of the distal interphalangeal (DIP) joint (Fig. 1). In severe cases, the MTP joint becomes hyperextended, mirroring the situation seen in claw toe deformity. In contrast to clawing, which tends to involve all toes, hammer toe deformity usually affects only one or two toes.[1] Hammer toes are classified as either flexible or rigid. The most commonly affected toe is the second, although multiple digits can be involved.[2]

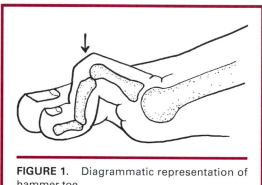

FIGURE 1. Diagrammatic representation of hammer toe.

Hammer toe is the most common of the lesser toe deformities and occurs primarily in the sagittal plane. It is arguably the most common toe disorder that presents to the foot and ankle surgeon's office. Women are more commonly affected, and the incidence of hammer toe increases with age.[3,4]

The most common etiology for hammer toe deformity is flexor stabilization in a pronated foot. The pronated foot requires more effort from the intrinsic muscles of the toes to stabilize the foot during toe-off.[5] Hammer-toe deformities progress from flexible to rigid over time. Contributing factors include long term wear of poorly fitting shoes, especially those with tight, narrow toe boxes. Crowding and overlapping from hallux valgus are other causes. A long second ray with subsequent buckling of the toe may also lead to the deformity. Other predisposing factors are diabetes, connective tissue disease, and trauma.[4] Importantly, no foot intrinsic imbalance or neuromuscular disease association, such as seen in claw toes, is found.[1] Contracture of the flexor digitorum longus, however, may be present in some cases.

Symptoms

Patients commonly complain of pain or tenderness in the area of the PIP joint, especially when wearing shoes or during weight-bearing activities. Patients also commonly present with cosmetic complaints. Pain may be the result of corn formation over the dorsal aspect of the PIP joint from shoe compression. In cases in which hyperextension of the MTP joint has occurred, there is also increased pressure over the metatarsal heads. Metatarsalgia with subsequent callus formation underneath the metatarsal heads may occur secondary to their plantar displacement.[1]

Physical Examination

The diagnosis is confirmed by the presence of MTP joint hyperextension, PIP joint flexion, and DIP joint extension in the affected toe. Palpation of the PIP joint usually causes tenderness, with the plantar aspect more commonly affected.

On inspection, determine the degree of PIP flexion. Also note accompanying foot deformities such as ulcerations and callus formation over the PIP joint and tip of the toe. Hammer toe deformities become more prominent in stance, when intrinsic muscles are silent.[1] This observation provides corroborating evidence for the absence of intrinsic imbalance in the majority of cases.

Next, determine whether the hammer toe deformity is fixed or flexible. Flexor digitorum longus contracture is assessed with the ankle in dorsiflexion and plantarflexion. Correction of the deformity upon plantarflexion signifies a flexible hammer toe. Dorsiflexion, in turn, accentuates the deformity.[6]

Perform a joint range-of-motion examination of the affected toe to determine flexibility and presence or absence of crepitus. The *Kelikian push-up test* is used to assess the degree of flexibility. Press upward on the plantar aspect of the metatarsal head; in flexible deformities, the MTP joint will align and the proximal phalanx will assume a more normal position.

Also assess for signs of swelling, temperature change, or erythema that might indicate the presence of an infectious or rheumatic process responsible for the deformity.

Inspection of the patient's footwear is necessary to determine the ability of the toe box to accommodate the forefoot. The presence of clavi or corns over the PIP joint, which may ulcerate, is often indicative of poorly fitting footwear.

Standard neurologic and vascular examinations will reveal no abnormal findings in uncomplicated hammer toe deformities. If there is a superficial peroneal nerve injury causing a dropfoot deformity, hammer toes will result due to extensor substitution. Likewise, a weakness of the gastrocnemius can lead to flexor substitution, causing a hammer toe.

If the patient has peripheral vascular disease or atherosclerosis, ulceration over a PIP joint may lead to toe loss unless the toe is revascularized.

Functional Limitations

Functional limitations mostly result from pain incurred by corn and callus formation. Walking and other weight-bearing activities can be painful. The ability to tolerate footwear with a narrow toe box is also impaired.

Diagnostic Studies

The diagnosis is primarily a clinical one. However, radiographs can be useful in assessing a rigid hammer toe, with weight-bearing views preferred. An apparent joint space narrowing corresponds to subluxation of the proximal phalanx on the metatarsal head at the MTP joint.[4,6]

Differential Diagnosis

Claw toes

Mallet toes

Interdigital neuroma

Non-specific synovitis of the metatarsophalangeal joint

Triggering of the lesser toes (lower limb analog of trigger finger)[7]

Rheumatoid or psoriatic arthritis

Plantar plate rupture

Treatment

Initial

Patient education is critical. The first step involves fitting for shoes with an adequate toe box to accommodate the dorsiflexed position of the proximal phalanx. High heels should be avoided as much as possible. A soft insole can also be used—particularly a soft metatarsal pad placed just proximal to the metatarsal head region, which is useful for pressure relief.[7] NSAIDs/COX-2 inhibitors can help with pain and inflammation, if present. Analgesic medications may be taken for pain relief. Ulcer and callus management may be necessary, and patients should be educated regarding monitoring their skin for breakdown, especially in the setting of peripheral neuropathy.

Local icing may also help with acute pain (20 minutes, 2 to 3 times a day). However, ice should be avoided in patients with significant peripheral vascular disease due to its vasoconstrictive properties and in individuals with impaired sensation due to the risk of frostbite.

Initial treatment is palliative rather than corrective and predominantly consists of attempts to accommodate the toe deformity by changing the patient's footwear. This may include stretching the shoes or switching to shoes with a deeper toe box or to extra-depth shoes. Padding, such as toe crest pads or custom or premade hammer toe regulators, may relieve pressure over the involved joints. Patients with clavi on the PIP joint may benefit from digital caps or silicone cushions.

Rehabilitation

Formal physical therapy is usually not required, although some patients might benefit from a supervised paraffin treatment, which should be followed by stretching exercises. Paraffin baths are contraindicated if ulcers or sensory deficits are present.

Stretching exercises can relieve the "tight" sensation in patients with a flexible or semiflexible deformity. Exercises such as picking up a towel with the toes are recommended for both stretching and strengthening of the intrinsic foot muscles.

Functional orthotics will provide flexor stabilization and, in some instances, symptomatic relief to overpronators with a flexible hammer toe deformity. Orthotics have not, however, been found to alter the progression of the deformity.

The clinician may prescribe shoes with deep, wide toe boxes. Alternatively, extra depth can be achieved in a standard shoe by trimming the existing shoe insert just distal to the metatarsal heads.[9] Lamb's wool or felt around the toes provides extra padding. An external metatarsal bar and rocker bottom shoes are additional comfort enhancing options.

Daily stretching, manipulation, and taping of the PIP joints in neutral may be useful in correcting a flexible foot deformity. Specific strapping devices and hammer toe straightening orthoses are available.

Procedures

Steroid injections may be indicated for patients with painful PIP joint capsulitis or arthritic flare secondary to a hammer toe deformity. Combine steroid injections with padding or splinting for optimal relief. Using a 27-gauge needle and corticosteroid with local anesthetic mixture, introduce the solution into the joint capsule through the dorsomedial or dorsolateral aspect of the joint. Performing a surgical prep prior to injecting the joint is recommended. The patient should be advised about the possibility of a steroid flare.

Surgery

Operative treatment should be pursued only if conservative treatment fails. Cosmesis alone is not a good indication for surgery. Associated deformities must also be corrected for optimal surgical outcome (e.g., hallux valgus).[6]

For a mild deformity in which contractures do not exist, soft tissue procedures are preferred. Flexor digitorum longus tenotomy in isolation is one such option.[10] The Girdlestone flexor tendon transfer, involving transposition of the flexor digitorum longus to the dorsal extensor hood of the proximal phalanx, provides increased plantarflexion pull at the joint.[11]

For the more severe deformity, bone and joint procedures are used. Resection arthroplasty of the distal third of the proximal phalanx with intramedullary Kirschner wire fixation is necessary for a dislocated metatarsal head. Extensor digitorum longus (then brevis) tenotomy, dorsal matatarsophalangeal capsulotomy, and collateral ligament sectioning are performed. Flexor digitorum longus split, transfer, or release can also be considered. Some or all of the previously described procedures are performed until correction is obtained.[1,2] It should be noted that proper correction should result in slight plantarflexion of the PIP joint. Full weight-bearing status in a postoperative shoe or an appropriate pedal splint device is generally permissible immediately following the surgery.[4]

If the toe fails the Kelikian test, remodeling of the soft and bony tissue has taken place, and a stabilizing arthrodesis will probably be indicated.

Arthroplasty of the PIP joint is the usual surgical treatment for digits with flexible or semiflexible deformities.[10] Shortening the toe lessens the extensor and flexor tension. The soft tissue and head of the proximal phalanx are resected, enough tissue and bone are removed to relieve tension, and the length of the neighboring toes is approximated. Because the toe retains flexibility, this may provide better functional and cosmetic results for some patients. Recognize that if the cause of the deformity is still present or continues after the surgical correction, the deformity will likely recur. Postsurgical treatment should include use of a Darco device or splinting to prevent complications.

For patients in need of additional joint stability or in instances of a rigid deformity, an arthrodesis procedure may be a better choice.[10] In severe deformities, an arthrodesis is sometimes combined with a flexor tendon release. The arthrodesis may be either an end-to-end type or the joint may be remodeled into a peg-in-hole arthrodesis. The peg-in-hole technique has the advantage of shortening the toe to reduce tension on the joint. Postsurgical treatment for arthrodesis should also include use of a Darco device or splinting to prevent complications.

Potential Disease Complications

Potential disease complications include chronic intractable pain that limits all mobility. Other complications may include metatarsalgia, plantar and point of contact ulcerations in the insensate foot, arthralgia and joint stiffness if subluxation has occurred, toenail deformities, and bursitis/synovitis.[4] Gait abnormalities may contribute to more proximal pain symptoms (e.g., low back and hip pain).

Potential complications for non-surgical treatment also include deviation of the toes, especially overlapping second toes. This can be prevented by splinting or using a Darco device. Diabetic neuropathy and advanced peripheral vascular disease are relative contraindications for splinting.[10]

Common potential complications include PIP joint ulceration due to excessive pressure, fixed foot deformity, and postural changes resulting from pain induced gait deviations.

Potential Treatment Complications

Local icing can cause vasoconstriction and frostbite. Analgesics, NSAIDs, and COX-2 inhibitors have well-known side effects that most commonly affect the gastric, hepatic, and renal systems. Postsurgical complications include toe ischemia, digital nerve palsy, non-union, malalignment, reduced toe range of motion, rigid and excessively straight toe, persistent edema, flail toe, and osseous regrowth. Potential complications of surgical correction include flail or "floppy" toes, which can be repaired by collateral ligament repair. Infection, and in severe cases osteomyelitis can occur either prior to or as a complication of surgery. If intravenous antibiotic treatment is unsuccessful, partial or total toe amputation may be required.

References
1. Canale ST (ed): Campbell's Operative Orthopedics, 9th ed, vol 2. St Louis, Mosby, 1998.
2. Myerson MS, Sherefff MJ: The pathological anatomy of claw and hammer toes. J Bone Joint Surg Am 1989;71(1): 45–49.
3. Preferred Practice Guidelines, Hammertoe Syndrome. J Foot Ankle Surg 1999;38:1067–2516.
4. Hammer toe syndrome. J Foot Ankle Surg 1999;38(2):166–178.
5. Mann R, Inman VT: Phasic activity of the intrinsic muscles of the foot. J Bone Joint Surg 1964;46A:469.
6. Wheeless CR: Wheeless' Textbook of Orthopaedics. www.medmedia.com, 1996.
7. Martin MG, Masear VR: Triggering of the lesser toes at a previously undescribed distal pulley system. Foot Ankle Int 1998;19(2):113–117.
8. Hunt GC, McPoil TG (eds): Physical Therapy of the Foot and Ankle, 2nd ed. New York, Churchill Livingstone, 1995.
9. Kaye RA: The extra-depth toe box: A rational approach. Foot Ankle Int 1994;15(3):146–150.
10. McGlamry ED, Banks AS, Downey, MS (eds): Comprehensive Textbook of Foot Surgery, Baltimore, Williams & Wilkins, 1992, p 341.
11. Padanilam TG: The flexible hammertoe; flexor-to-extensor transfer. Foot and Ankle Clin 1998;3(2):259.

86 | Mallet Toe

Julie K. Silver, MD
Robert J. Krug, MD
Katherine Mashey, DPM

Synonyms

Lesser toe deformity

Mallet toe syndrome

ICD-9 Code

735.8
Other acquired
deformities of toe

Definition

Mallet toe refers to an abnormal flexion deformity at the distal interphalangeal (DIP) joint (Fig. 1). Typically there is normal alignment of the metatarsophalangeal (MTP) and proximal interphalangeal (PIP) joints. The most commonly affected toe is the second, although multiple digits can be involved. The third and fourth toes are also

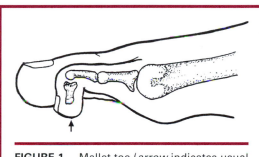

FIGURE 1. Mallet toe (*arrow* indicates usual area of callus formation).

commonly involved. The deformity may be fixed or flexible, and the condition may occur in both feet. High heeled or narrow toe box shoes aggravate the deformity.[1] There is some observational evidence to suggest that a toe longer than adjacent toes is at increased risk for developing lesser toe deformities.[2]

Symptoms

Patients typically complain of pain or tenderness in the area of the DIP joint. This is often most prominent when wearing shoes, particularly shoes with high heels or a narrow toe box. The symptoms are also worse during weight bearing, and activities such as running may promote symptoms. Patients also complain of cosmetic issues, which can include a toenail deformity. Pain may be the result of corn formation over the dorsal aspect of the PIP or DIP joint from shoe compression.

Physical Examination

On inspection, determine the degree of DIP flexion. Also note accompanying foot deformities, such as ulcerations and callus formation. Note whether the deformity changes with standing and whether it is fixed or flexible.

Perform a joint range-of-motion examination of the affected toe to determine flexibility and presence or absence of crepitus. Also assess for signs of swelling, temperature change, or erythema that might indicate the presence of an infectious or rheumatic process responsible for the deformity.

Inspection of the patient's footwear is necessary to determine the ability of the toe box to accommodate the forefoot. The presence of clavi or corns, which may ulcerate, is often indicative of poorly fitting footwear.

Standard neurologic and vascular examinations will reveal no abnormal findings in uncomplicated mallet toe deformities. If the patient has peripheral vascular disease or atherosclerosis, ulceration over a joint may lead to toe loss unless the toe is revascularized.

Functional Limitations

Functional limitations mostly result from pain, particularly with weight-bearing activities. Thus, walking may be limited and high impact activities such as running may be altogether too painful. Women may complain that they are unable to dress appropriately for work because high heels are uncomfortable.

Diagnostic Studies

The diagnosis is primarily a clinical one. However, radiographs can be useful in assessing a rigid mallet toe, with weight-bearing views preferred.

Differential Diagnosis

Claw toe

Hammer toe

Interdigital neuroma

Non-specific synovitis of the metatarsophalangeal joint

Triggering of the lesser toes (lower limb analog of trigger finger)[3]

Rheumatoid or psoriatic arthritis

Plantar plate rupture

Treatment

Initial

Patient education is critical. The first step involves fitting for shoes with an adequate toe box to accommodate the deformity. High heels should be avoided as much as possible. A soft insole can also be used—particularly a soft metatarsal pad or bar placed just proximal to the metatarsal head region is useful for pressure relief.[4] NSAIDs/COX-2 inhibitors can help with pain and inflammation if present. Analgesic medications may be taken for pain relief. Ulcer and callus management may be required, and patients should be educated regarding monitoring their skin for breakdown, especially in the setting of peripheral neuropathy.

Local icing may also help with acute pain (20 minutes, 2 to 3 times a day). However, ice should be avoided in patients with significant peripheral vascular disease due to its vasoconstrictive properties and in individuals with impaired sensation due to the risk of frostbite.

Initial treatment is palliative rather than corrective. This predominantly consists of attempts to accommodate the toe deformity by changing the patient's footwear. This may include stretching the shoes or switching to shoes with a deeper toe box or extra-depth shoes. Padding such as toe crest pads or custom or pre-made mallet toe regulators may relieve pressure over the involved joints. Patients with clavi may benefit from digital caps or silicone cushions. Ulcer and callus management may be required, and patients should be educated in monitoring their skin for breakdown, especially in the setting of peripheral neuropathy.

Rehabilitation

Formal physical therapy is usually not required, although some patients might benefit from a supervised paraffin treatment. Paraffin baths are contraindicated if ulcers or sensory deficits are present and should be followed by stretching exercises.

Stretching exercises can relieve the "tight" sensation in patients with a flexible or semi-flexible deformity. Exercises such as picking up a towel with the toes are recommended for both stretching and strengthening of the intrinsic foot muscles.

Functional orthotics will provide flexor stabilization and, in some instances, symptomatic relief to overpronators with a flexible mallet toe deformity. Orthotics have not, however, been found to alter the progression of the deformity.

The clinician may prescribe shoes with deep, wide toe boxes. Alternatively, extra depth can be achieved in a standard shoe by trimming the existing shoe insert just distal to the metatarsal heads.[5] Lamb's wool or felt around the toes provide extra padding. An external metatarsal bar or rocker bottom shoe are additional comfort-enhancing options.

Daily stretching, manipulation, and taping of the proximal interphalangeal joints in neutral may be useful in correcting a flexible foot deformity. Specific strapping devices and mallet toe straightening orthoses are available.

Procedures

Steroid injections may be indicated for patients with painful PIP joint capsulitis or arthritic flare secondary to a mallet toe deformity. Combine steroid injections with padding or splinting for optimal relief. Using a 27-gauge needle and corticosteroid with local anesthetic mixture, introduce the steroid into the joint capsule through the dorsomedial or dorsolateral aspect of the joint. Performing a surgical prep prior to injecting the joint is recommended. The patient should be advised about the possibility of a steroid flare.

Surgery

Operative treatment should only be pursued if conservative treatment fails. Cosmesis alone is not a good indication for surgery. Associated deformities must also be fixed for optimal surgical outcome (e.g., hallux valgus). In some instances, surgical management will need to address a combined mallet toe-hammer toe deformity.

For a mild deformity, in which contractures do not exist, soft tissue procedures are the procedures of choice. For the more severe deformity, bone and joint procedures are used. Full weight-bearing status in a postoperative shoe or an appropriate pedal splint device are generally permissible immediately following the outpatient surgery.

Due to the progressive nature of this deformity, most patients eventually are treated with surgical options. Surgical treatment depends on the etiology, extent, and severity of the deformity.

In younger patients, a flexor tenotomy alone is often sufficient to treat the mallet toe deformity. For patients in need of additional joint stability or in instances of a rigid deformity, an arthrodesis procedure may be a better choice. In severe deformities, an arthrodesis is sometimes combined with a flexor tendon release. Retrospective studies have shown that an excisional arthroplasty of the DIP joint that achieves DIP fusion, with a simultaneous flexor tenotomy, optimizes the chance for a good outcome.[6] Postoperative AP and lateral weight-bearing radiographs can illustrate whether an actual fusion of the DIP joint has been achieved. In the setting of a stiff joint without actual fusion, the outcome is still usually satisfactory. The arthrodesis may be either an end-to-end type or the joint may be remodeled into a peg-in-hole arthrodesis. The peg-in-hole technique has advantages in which shortening the toe can reduce tension on the joint. Postsurgical treatment for arthrodesis should also include use of a Darco device or splinting to prevent complications.

Potential Disease Complications

Potential disease complications include chronic intractable pain that limits all mobility. Other complications may include metatarsalgia, plantar and point of contact ulcerations in the insensate foot, arthralgia and joint stiffness if subluxation has occurred, toenail deformities, and bursitis/synovitis. Gait abnormalities may contribute to more proximal pain symptoms (e.g., low back and hip pain).

Potential complications for non-surgical treatment also include deviation of the toes, especially overlapping second toes. This can be prevented by splinting or using a Darco device. Diabetic neuropathy and advanced peripheral vascular disease are relative contraindications for splinting.

Common potential complications include PIP joint ulceration due to excessive pressure, fixed foot deformity, and postural changes resulting from pain-induced gait deviations.

Potential Treatment Complications

Local icing can cause vasoconstriction and frostbite. Analgesics, NSAIDs, and COX-2 inhibitors have well-known side effects that most commonly affect the gastric, hepatic, and renal systems. Postsurgical complications include toe ischemia, digital nerve palsy, non-union, malalignment, reduced range of motion, rigid and excessively straight toe, persistent edema, flail toe, and osseous regrowth. Potential complications of surgical correction include flail or "floppy" toes, which can be repaired by collateral ligament repair, and hyperextension of the DIP joint. Infection, and in severe cases osteomyelitis, can occur either prior to or as a complication of surgery. If intravenous antibiotic treatment is unsuccessful, partial or total toe amputation may be required.

References
1. Birrer RB, DellaCorte MP, Grisafi PJ (eds): Common Foot Problems in Primary Care. Philadelphia, Hanley & Belfus, 1992.
2. Coughlin M, Mann R: Lesser toe deformities. In: Surgery of the Foot, 6th ed. St. Louis, Mosby, 1993, pp. 341–412.
3. Martin MG, Masear VR: Triggering of the lesser toes at a previously undescribed distal pulley system. Foot Ankle Int 1998;19(2):113–117.
4. Hunt GC, McPoil TG (eds): Physical Therapy of the Foot and Ankle, 2nd ed. New York, Churchill Livingstone, 1995.
5. Kaye RA: The extra-depth toe box: A rational approach. Foot Ankle Int 1994;15(3):146–150.
6. Coughlin MJ: Operative repair of the mallet toe deformity. Foot Int 1995;16(3):109–116.

87 Metatarsalgia

Alice V. Fann, MD

Synonyms

Pain in the metatarsal heads

Forefoot pain

ICD-9 Code

726.70
Enthesopathy of ankle and tarsus, unspecified; metatarsalgia

Definition

Metatarsalgia refers to pain in the plantar aspect of the foot in the region of the metatarsal heads. It may be a primary or secondary condition and cause acute or chronic pain. Intrinsic or extrinsic biomechanical conditions that increase stress on the metatarsal heads may result in metatarsalgia.[1] Primary metatarsalgia is usually due to biomechanical reasons, such as excessive foot pronation ("flat foot"), wearing high-heeled or pointed shoes, wearing shoes with poor padding, obesity, or pes planus (splayed foot with loss of metatarsal arch).[2] Primary metatarsalgia can also be congenital or may be due to recent surgery for other foot conditions. Secondary metatarsalgia may be due to conditions such as gout, rheumatoid arthritis, sesamoiditis, trauma, or stress fractures.

Symptoms

Metatarsalgia is pain in the forefoot that occurs with weight bearing. Patients typically report severe pain in the metatarsophalangeal region of the foot during prolonged weight-bearing activities and ambulation; however, in severe metatarsalgia pain can be present with initial weight-bearing. Pain is often described "like walking with a pebble in the shoe." The patient usually cannot describe a precipitating cause, but rather recounts the pain as gradual in onset.

Physical Examination

The clinician should evaluate the foot in both weight-bearing (functional position) and non–weight-bearing positions. In a non–weight-bearing position, the clinician should inspect for swelling, masses, and calluses (see Fig. 1). Calluses are in response to abnormal weight bearing and are good indicants of stress and pressure. The clinician should observe the toes. A relative long second metatarsal with a short first metatarsal (Morton's foot) may result in increased loading of the second metatarsal head. Hammer or claw toes may be indicative of a collapsed transverse arch. With the patient standing, the foot should be examined for collapse of the arches, especially the transverse (or metatarsal) one. The hindfoot should be examined for varus and valgus deformities that will affect placement of the forefoot. Evaluation should include the lower limb for rotational deformities that may affect placement of the forefoot.

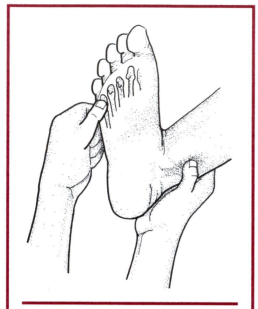

FIGURE 1. The metatarsal heads should be palpated with the thumb on the plantar surface and the forefinger on the dorsal surface. Palpate each head individually.

The foot should be palpated for calluses (that may not be obvious to inspection), swelling, and masses (Fig. 1). Pain with palpation between metatarsal head and metatarsal neck may be indicative of an intermetarsal bursitis. Pain with the metatarsal compression test may indicate irritation of a Morton's neuroma. Pain with palpation under the first metatarsal head may be due to sesamoiditis. Laxity in the first metatarsal-cuneiform joints, resulting in a hypermobile first ray, will increase weight bearing under the second and third metatarsals and predispose the patient to metatarsalgia. A tight Achilles tendon will increase forefoot load in the late stance phase and increase the biomechanical stress on the forefoot.

Diffuse pain and swelling along with stiffness of the metatarsophalangeal (MTP) joints may be due to an inflammatory arthropathy such as rheumatoid arthritis and gout. Because of destruction of the joint capsule and stretching of the plantar intertarsal ligaments, rheumatoid arthritis–induced synovitis of MTP joints is associated with volar subluxation of metatarsal heads. In this condition, the shortening of the long toe extensors and the excess tension of the long toe flexors may lead to hammer toes.[3]

In metatarsalgia, the neurologic portion of the overall evaluation should be normal (e.g., normal strength, sensation, and deep tendon reflexes). If there are parasthesias within the adjacent border of the affected toes (in the digital nerve distribution), the clinician should be suspicious of Morton's neuroma.

The patient with metatarsalgia requires evaluation for any postural abnormalities or asymmetries that may be extrinsic biomechanical causes of the condition. These abnormalities and/or asymmetries include pelvic obliquity/leg-length discrepancy; scoliosis; rotation of hip, femur, and knee; and valgus and varus deformities of the knee and ankle. These may lead to displacement of the forefoot and contribute to metatarsalgia.[3,4]

During ambulation, the patient with extrinsic biomechanical causes of metatarsalgia may have increased abduction of forefoot at toe-off:

> The foot is in its maximum position of flexibility at foot flat and then becomes rigid at heel rise as the subtalar joint inverts and the transverse tarsal joint becomes locked. It is during this period of forefoot rigidity in late stance phase that the forefoot experiences most of its stresses. During heel rise and toe off, the hallux and lesser toes reach their maximum dorsiflexion. Toe dorsiflexion places traction on the plantar fascia and helps to elevate the medial longitudinal arch through the windlass mechanism of the plantar fascia.[1]

At foot flat and heel rise, there is rapid acceleration of pressure initially located in the central heel then across the midfoot to the forefoot where the pressure center is under the second metatarsal head. The center of pressure shifts to the hallux at toe-off.[1]

Functional Limitations

Metatarsalgia may severely restrict ambulation. This may affect patients' ability to perform activities of daily living and vocational activities. This condition may also affect their ability to exercise and/or compete in athletic events.

Diagnostic Studies

Metatarsalgia remains a diagnosis made by clinical evaluation. If, however, the history and physical examination raise the suspicion of a fracture, radiographs may be indicated. If stress fracture is suspected, a technetium bone scan may prove useful. Electromyography and nerve conduction studies may provide diagnostic clarity if tarsal tunnel syndrome or a S1 radiculopathy is in the differential diagnosis.

Differential Diagnosis

Intermetatarsal ligament strain

Intermetarsal bursitis

Morton's neuroma

Stress fracture

Metatarsal head avascular necrosis (Freiberg's infarction)

Sesamoiditis

Tarsal tunnel syndrome

S1 radiculopathy

Treatment

Initial

Initial treatment of metatarsalgia includes analgesics, nonsteroidal anti-inflammatory drugs (NSAIDs), orthotics for correction of pronated feet (if present), and posting of the metatarsal arch with a metatarsal pad (e.g., proximal to metatarsal heads).[5,6] It is also important to include modification of activities (avoidance of running and jumping activities) and change of footwear (e.g., avoiding high-heeled shoes and promoting shoes with proper cushioning and extra depth). Rocker bottom soles should be considered if hallux rigidus is present.

Rehabilitation

The goals of rehabilitation should be the correction of postural dysfunction that may be contributing to the metatarsalgia. Postural problems that can affect the forefoot include pelvic obliquity/leg-length discrepancy, which can be corrected with heel lifts. Correction of pronated feet by gradually augmenting arches of orthotics may help to reduce functional rotational deformities of the hip and knee, as well as correct the position of the foot.

Realignment by strengthening alone is of limited value and needs to be done in conjunction with biomechanical correction, appropriate stretching, orthotics, and surgery to improve alignment. Strengthening exercises for the intrinsic muscles of the foot include using the toes to pick up small objects and transfer them to a container and rolling a tennis ball under the feet.[3] Instruct the patient to perform the exercises to fatigue. Strengthening exercises need to be progressed to closed-chain activities since most of the symptoms of metatarsalgia and most of the functional demands of the foot are during weight-bearing activities.[3] The patient should be instructed in stretching exercises to include the Achilles tendon, digits, and other lower extremity muscles, as needed, to improve posture.

Modalities such as ultrasound may have some limited value.

Procedures

Procedures are generally not indicated in metatarsalgia.

Surgery

Surgery may be indicated when conservative management fails to relieve the pain with ambulation. Several procedures can be performed for resection of the involved metatarsal heads and proximal phalanges, which are beyond the scope of this chapter.[3]

Potential Disease Complications

Disease-related complications might include deconditioning due to the patient's difficulty with ambulation and chronic intractable pain. Patients who are diabetic or who have metatarsalgia due to faulty foot mechanics are at higher risk for skin ulceration.[7]

Potential Treatment Complications

Analgesics, NSAIDs, and COX-2 inhibitors have well-known side effects that most commonly affect the gastric, hepatic, and renal systems. Orthotics are generally well tolerated but may cause skin breakdown.

References

1. Hockenbury RT: Forefoot problems in athletes. Med Sci Sports Exerc 1999;31S:S448–S458.
2. Pyasta RT, Panush RS: Common painful foot syndromes. Bulletin Rheum Dis 1999;48:1–4.
3. Kisner C, Colby LA: The ankle and foot. In Kisner C, Colby LA (eds): Therapeutic Exercise: Foundations and Techniques, 2nd ed. Philadelphia, F.A. Davis, 1990, pp 385–408.
4. Donatelli RA: Abnormal biomechanics. In Donatelli RA (ed): The Biomechanics of the Foot and Ankle, 2nd ed. Philadelphia, F.A. Davis, 1996.
5. Kelly A, Winson I: Use of ready-made insoles in the treatment of lesser metatarsalgia: Prospective randomized controlled trial. Foot Ankle 1998;19:217–220.
6. Hodge MC, Bach TM, Carter GM: Orthotic management of plantar pressure and pain in rheumatoid arthritis. Clin Biomech 1999;14:567–575.
7. Mueller MJ, Minor SD, Diamond JE, Blair VP: Relationship of foot deformity to ulcer location in patients with diabetes mellitus. Phys Ther 1990;70:356–362.

88 Morton's Neuroma

Robert J. Scardina, DPM
Sammy M. Lee, DPM

Synonyms

Metatarsal neuralgia

Perineural fibroma

Plantar neuralgia

Morton's neuralgia

Intermetatarsal neuroma

Pseudoneuroma

Metatarsal neuroma

Interdigital neuroma

Morton's toe syndrome

ICD-9 Code

355.6
Mononeuritis of lower limb; lesion of plantar nerve

Definition

Morton's neuroma is not a true neoplasm but rather an enlargement of the third intermetatarsal nerve with associated perineural fibrosis[1] that is caused by an accumulation of collagenous material within the sheath of Schwann, usually as a result of repetitive trauma (Fig. 1). The exact etiology has never been clearly identified or proven conclusively, but the following have been postulated: flat (pes planus) foot; anterior splay foot; high arch (pes cavus) foot; ill-fitting (tight or high heel) shoe gear; abnormal proximity of neighboring metatarsal heads[2]; and associated forefoot deformities, including hallux abductus/bunion, and hammer toes.

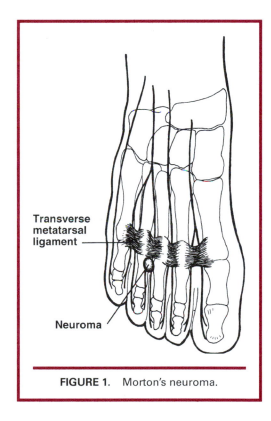

FIGURE 1. Morton's neuroma.

Intermetatarsal nerves are purely sensory at the level of the metatarsophalangeal joints, as they course through a fibro-osseous canal comprised of neighboring metatarsal heads and the overlying deep transverse intermetatarsal ligament.[3]

Anatomic (cadaver) studies have identified the third intermetatarsal nerve as most commonly receiving proximal innervation from a branch of the medial plantar and lateral plantar nerves, both from the common posterior tibial nerve. Therefore, anatomically, the third intermetatarsal nerve is normally enlarged when it receives proximal trunks from not one but two nerves branches. This may or may not be a causative factor.

Although the classic "Morton's neuroma" occurs in the third intermetatarsal space, a similar nerve pathology occurs in the second intermetatarsal space, but less commonly. This is treated in a similar fashion.

Symptoms

Morton's neuroma may present in a variety of ways, including a localized sharp or lancinating pain, paresthesias, numbness, or toe cramping. Radiation of symptoms is typically distal involving the opposing sides of the third and fourth toes, but toe pain exclusively in the fourth toe is not uncommon.

The pain may be described as burning, tingling, or the sensation of a "hot poker" between the involved metatarsal heads and/or toes. Unilateral presentation is most common, whereas bilateral occurrence is extremely rare. Symptoms occur predominantly during weight-bearing activities, but residual non–weight-bearing or nocturnal pain is possible. Often, patients complain of experiencing symptoms while driving an automobile with the foot held in a slightly dorsiflexed position. A characteristic and suggestively pathognomonic sign is the overwhelming desire to remove one's shoe and massage or manipulate the forefoot, creating transient relief of symptoms.[4]

Physical Examination

On inspection, the foot may appear normal but may demonstrate a slight or subtle divergence of the third and fourth toes, enhanced by weight bearing. Palpable pain about the site is predominantly plantar. The lateral forefoot squeeze test may mimic a tight shoe, reproducing symptoms. In longstanding cases, hypesthesia may be noted in the third web space and distal toes.

The most diagnostic clinical test is the Mulder's sign (or click),[5] performed with alternate lateral compression of the forefoot combined with dorsal-to-plantar compression of the involved intermetatarsal space with the forefinger and thumb (Fig. 2).[4] This maneuver may reproduce symptoms, radiating distally into the toes with a palpable and audible click. Localized areas of hypesthesia or anesthesia may be identified in the interdigital web space, opposing sides of the involved toes, or plantar region just distal to the metatarsal heads.

Generally, there are no signs of proximal nerve involvement, vasomotor instability, or arterial insufficiency. Predisposing foot types such as pes planus or pes cavus may be evident on clinical examination. Range of motion of the neighboring metatarsophalangeal joints are usually pain free without crepitus. Unilateral antalgic (pain-avoiding) gait may be evident.

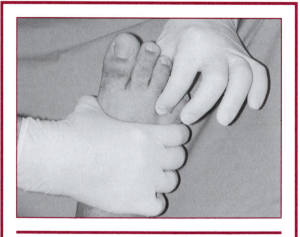

FIGURE 2. Technique to elicit Mulder's sign/click.

Functional Limitations

Functional limitations include difficulty with walking or running any significant distance and difficulty with other physical activities resulting in forefoot loading as well as the inability to wear dress shoes (particularly women's high heeled shoes).

Diagnostic Studies

The diagnosis of Morton's neuroma is generally made from history and clinical examination. However, several diagnostic studies may be helpful when considering surgical intervention.

Ultrasonography is a relatively simple, inexpensive, and helpful diagnostic tool.[6,7] In the evaluation of a primary neuroma, a positive finding is a 5 mm or greater hypoechoic mass, visualized in the coronal (frontal) plane projection, between and beneath the neighboring metatarsal heads. Magnetic resonance imaging (MRI), although generally not recommended in the initial evaluation, may also be utilized, particularly in the presence of equivocal or negative ultrasonographic findings and when surgical incision is being consided.[8] Both ultrasonography and MRI are used in the diagnosis of recurrent or "stump" neuroma, postsurgical excision.[9–11]

The neuroma itself is not visible by plain radiographic imaging. Plain radiographs are performed to rule out metatarsal stress fracture, metatarsophalangeal joint disease (degenerative or inflammatory), or contributing anomalous morphology of neighboring metatarsal heads. At the metatarsophalangeal level, "positional" phalangeal changes may be seen that are consistent with overall foot configuration in pes planus or pes cavus.

Sensory nerve conduction studies can be utilized, but due to the difficulty in isolating individual nerve trunks, results are not consistently accurate or helpful. Lastly, local anesthetic injections can be useful in supporting the diagnosis.

Differential Diagnosis

Metatarsal stress fracture

Metatarsal head avascular necrosis (Freiberg's infarction)

Osseous neoplasm

Soft tissue neoplasm

Localized mechanical synovitis

Systemic synovitis (e.g., rheumatoid arthritis)

Arthritic changes (e.g., degenerative, posttraumatic)

Submetatarsal head bursitis/capsulitis

Localized ischemia

Tarsal tunnel syndrome

Proximal nerve root syndrome (e.g., radiculopathy)

Peripheral neuritis

Peripheral neuropathy (e.g., diabetic, alcoholic)

Treatment

Initial

Conservative treatment modalities include shoe gear modifications (e.g., wider toe box), adhesive tape strapping and/or padding of the foot, and use of orthoses. NSAIDs/COX-2 inhibitors and/or oral analgesics may provide some relief of acute symptoms but are not recommended for long-term treatment.

Rehabilitation

Physiotherapy modalities, including both iontophoresis and phonophoresis, may help manage acute pain. If symptoms respond to initial conservative "mechanical" measures, more individualized therapies such as custom foot orthoses and custom shoe gear (wider toe box) may provide additional symptomatic relief and usually require referral to podiatrists or pedorthists for fabrication.

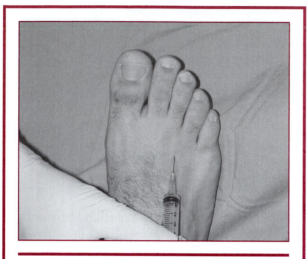

FIGURE 3. Technique of injection of a Morton's neuroma.

Procedures

Injections with sclerosing agents, such as alcohol,[12] phenol or vitamin B_{12}, may be utilized if conservative non-invasive treatments fail. Local anesthetic/corticosteroid injections,[13] however, are more commonly used and may provide transient (but rarely long-term) relief of symptoms (Fig. 3). These injections are limited to no more than three within a 3- to 6-month period, due to the potential for plantar fat pad atrophy.

Surgery

Conservative measures do not always result in symptomatic improvement.[14] The neuroma as well as the distal digital branches and proximal nerve trunk may be too large for their confined space. In these cases, surgical excision may be necessary.[15] Surgical excision success rate is approximately 85%, and surgical revision consistently carries a poor prognosis.[16]

Less traditional surgical techniques include neurolysis, dorsal nerve transposition, transection of the deep transverse intermetatarsal ligament, laser treatment, and distal lesser metatarsal osteotomies.[17–19]

Potential Disease Complications

Potential disease complications include persistent refractory or intractable pain, reduced mobility, functional limitation, and shoe gear restrictions.

Potential Treatment Complications

Few complications may arise from conservative measures, such as padding, strapping, orthoses, and shoe modifications. Occasionally, ipsilateral or contralateral knee, ankle, hip, or even low back pain may be encountered, but these respond rapidly to discontinuing treatment. Likewise, there are no significant treatment complications from physiotherapy measures when used and applied properly. Long-term use of NSAIDs may lead to gastrointestinal irritation, but newer NSAIDs (e.g., COX-2 inhibitors) have demonstrated a lower incidence.

Injection therapy with corticosteroid/local anesthetic agents may result in plantar fat pad atrophy and secondary metatarsalgia. Injection therapy with sclerosing agents may result in perineural irritation, inflammation, and pain.

Postsurgical complications include hematoma, vascular compromise, infection, dorsal cutaneous nerve injury, incomplete resection, recurrence,[20,21] "stump" neuroma, plantar fat pad atrophy, painful hypertrophic scar formation, and reflex sympathetic dystrophy.[20,21]

References

1. Addante JB, Peicott PS, et al: Interdigital neuromas: Results of surgical excision of 152 neuromas. J Am Podiatr Med Assoc 1986;76:493–495.
2. Levitsky KA, Alman BA, et al: Digital nerves of the foot: Anatomic variations and implications regarding the pathogenesis of interdigital neuroma. Foot Ankle 1993;14:208–214.
3. McMinn RM, et al: Foot and Ankle Anatomy. London, Mosby-Wolfe, 1996.
4. Wu KK: Morton's interdigital neuroma. A clinical review of its etiology, treatment, and results. J. Foot Ankle Surg 1996;35:112–119; discussion 187–188.
5. Mulder JD: The causative mechanism in Morton's metatarsalgia. J Bone Joint Surg 1951;33B:94–95.
6. Pollak RA, Bellacosa RA, et al: Sonographic analysis of Morton's neuroma. J Foot Surg 1992;31:534–537.
7. Read JW, Noakes JB, et al: Morton's metatarsalgia: Sonographic findings and correlated histopathology. Foot Ankle Int 1999;20:153.
8. Biasca N, Zanetti M, Zollinger H: Outcomes after partial neurectomy of Morton's neuroma related to preoperative case histories, clinical findings, and findings on magnetic resonance imaging scans. Foot Ankle Int 1999;20:568.
9. Levine SE, Myerson MS, et al: Ultrasonographic diagnosis of recurrence after excision of an interdigital neuroma. Foot Ankle Int 1998;19:79–84.
10. Resch S, Stentstrom A, Jonnsson K: The diagnostic efficacy of magnetic resonance imaging and ultrasonography in Morton's neuroma: A radiological-surgical correlation. Foot Ankle Int 1994;15:88–92.
11. Terk MR, Kwong PK, et al: Morton neuroma: Evaluation with MR imaging performed with contrast enhancement and fat suppression Radiology 1993;189:239–241.
12. Dockery GL: The treatment of intermetatarsal neuromas with 4% alcohol sclerosing injections. J Foot Ankle Surg 1999;38:403–408.
13. Greenfield J, Read J, Lifeld FW: Morton's interdigital neuroma: Indication for treatment by local injections versus surgery. Clin Orthop 1984;185:142–144.
14. Bennett GL, Graham CE, Mauldin DM: Morton's interdigital neuroma: A comprehensive treatment protocol. Foot Ankle Int 1995;16:760–763.
15. Miller SJ: Intermetatarsal neuromas and associated nerve problems. In Butterworth R, Dockery GL (eds): Color Atlas and Text of Forefoot Surgery. London, Mosby-Wolfe, 1996, pp 159–182.
16. Mann Roger A (ed): Surgery of the Foot. St Louis, Mosby, 1986.
17. Delon AL: Treatment of Morton's neuroma as a nerve compression. The role for neurolysis. J Am Podiatr Med Assoc 1992;82(8):389–402.
18. Dibold PF, et al: Current topics in International foot and anklesurgery—True epineural neurolysis in Morton's neuroma: A 5-year follow up. Orthopedics 1996;19:397–400.
19. Gauthier G: Thomas Morton's disease: A nerve entrapment syndrome. A new surgical technique. Clin Othop 1979;142:90–92.
20. Amis JA, Siverhus SW, Liwnicz BH: An Anatomic basis for recurrence after Morton's neuroma excision. Foot Ankle 1992;13:153–156.
21. Banks AS, Vito GR, Giorgi TL: Recurrent intermetatarsal neuroma. A follow-up study. Northlake Regional Medical Center. Tucker, GA 30084, USA. J Am Podiatr Med Assoc 1996;86:299–306.

89 Plantar Fasciitis

Paul F. Pasquina, MD

Synonyms

Plantar tendinitis
Plantar tendinosis
Plantar fasciosis

ICD-9 Code

728.71
Plantar fascial
fibromatosis; plantar
fasciitis (traumatic)

Definition

The plantar fascia is a multi-layered fibrous aponeurosis that originates from the medial calcaneal tuberosity and extends distally, both wider and thinner, splitting into five bands (Fig. 1). Each band then divides into a superficial and deep layer to insert onto the transverse tarsal ligament, flexor sheath, volar plate, and periosteum of the base of the proximal phalanges.[1]

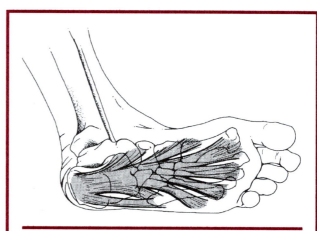

FIGURE 1. Plantar fascia. (From Mellion MB, et al: The Team Physician's Handbook, 2nd ed. Philadelphia, Hanley & Belfus, 1997, p 610, with permission.)

Plantar fasciitis is an overuse injury resulting from repetitive microtears of the plantar fascia at its origin on the calcaneus. It is classically described as a local inflammatory reaction, although recent research has demonstrated the relative absence of inflammatory cells in the injured tissue, suggesting more of a degenerative process and therefore advocating the use of the terms "tendinosis" or "fasciosis."[2]

Plantar fasciitis is one of the most common injuries of runners. The condition typically is precipitated by a change in the athlete's training program. Such changes may include an increase in intensity, frequency, decreased recovery time, or change in terrain or running surface. In the non-athlete, an increase in the amount of walking, standing, or stairclimbing may also precipitate symptoms.

Biomechanical factors such as pes planus (flat feet), pes cavus with rigid high arches, excessive pronation, or poor footwear (usually a loose heel counter and inadequate arch support) all may contribute to the development of this condition.

Symptoms

Patients typically complain of sharp, knifelike pain in the plantar aspect of the heel at the base of the fascial insertion to the calcaneus (see Fig. 1). Pain is generally worse with standing or during the initial steps upon awakening or after prolonged sitting. Pain also typically worsens at the beginning of a workout, but decreases during exercise. The athlete may describe being able to "run through" the pain. Complaints of numbness, paresthesias, and/or weakness are atypical for plantar fasciitis, and therefore if present, the clinician should be suspicious of an underlying nerve injury.

Physical Examination

Palpation reveals tenderness at the origin of the fascia of the medial calcaneal tubercle, but the majority of the fascia may be tender. Range of motion often reveals limited great toe dorsiflexion from a tight plantar fascia as well as decreased ankle dorsiflexion from a tight Achilles tendon. Dorsiflexion should be tested with the knee straight (gastrocnemius on stretch) and with the knee bent (gastrocnemius relaxed, soleus on stretch) in order to better differentiate tightness of the gastrocnemius versus soleus muscles. The neurologic exam should reveal normal strength, sensation, and deep tendon reflexes, unless a concomitant neuropathy is present.

Functional Limitations

Depending on the severity of disease, patients may only complain of symptoms when they try to increase their running intensity or distance. More severe cases may significantly limit a patient's ability to ambulate during daily activities or climbing stairs. Professions requiring extensive walking or standing, such as those of postal workers, nurses, or waitresses may require job modification as well as more aggressive splinting or even casting during the initial phase of treatment.

Diagnostic Studies

X-rays of the foot may be helpful in ruling out other potential causes of heel or foot pain. However, it is a common misconception that the pain of plantar fasciitis is the direct result of the often (50%) associated anterior calcaneal spur ("heel spur"). In fact, a study of 461 asymptomatic patients showed x-ray evidence of heel spurs in 27% of those studied.[3]

Electrodiagnostic testing (EMG and nerve conduction studies) may be useful when considering the possibility of a nerve entrapment.

Ultrasound and MRI studies may be helpful prior to considering surgical intervention since these studies may demonstrate signal changes or swelling within the fascia.

Differential Diagnosis

Inflammatory
    Juvenile rheumatoid arthritis
    Rheumatoid arthritis
    Ankylosing spondylitis
    Reiter's syndrome
    Gout
Metabolic
    Migratory osteoporosis
    Osteomalacia

Traumatic
    Calcaneal fracture
    Calcaneal malunions
    Traumatic arthritis
    Fat pad injury

Degenerative
  Osteoarthritis
  Atrophy of the heel fat pad
Nerve Entrapment
  Tarsal tunnel syndrome
  Entrapment of the medial calcaneal
    branch of the posterior tibial nerve
  Entrapment of the nerve to abductor
    digiti quinti

Overuse syndromes
  Stenosing tenosynovitis of flexor digitorum longus
    and flexor hallucis longus
  Calcaneal apophysitis (Sever's disease)
  Subcalcaneal bursitis
  Periostitis
  Calcaneal stress fracture
  Achilles tendinitis and peritendinitis
  Haglund's deformity

Treatment

Initial

As with most overuse injuries, initial treatment should follow the *PRICE* principles. This is an acronym that refers to *P:* protect, *R:* rest, *I:* ice, *C:* compression, *E:* elevation. Protection and rest usually involve "relative rest," which has the patient avoid aggravating activities while maintaining cardiovascular and muscular fitness by participating in low-impact activities such as swimming, bicycling, and weight lifting. Ice massage to the plantar fascia can easily be performed by the patient at home. Have the patient put a Styrofoam or paper cup full of water into the freezer. Once the water becomes ice, the patient may massage the block of ice along the origin of the plantar fascia for approximately 10 to 15 minutes. Icing is most helpful after activities or at the end of the day. Compression by way of taping the sole of the foot or applying an ACE wrap around the foot may offer comfort to the patient as may soft gel heel cups, which may be placed in the patient's shoes. Keeping the foot elevated while sitting or lying may also be helpful at reducing any local inflammation and swelling. Frequently used medications include nonsteroidal anti-inflammatory drugs (NSAIDs) and analgesics.

Rehabilitation

The key elements of rehabilitation include stretching and strength training of the plantar fascia, gastroc-soleus complex, quadriceps, hamstrings, and hip flexors and extensors.

Increased flexibility is achieved through performing frequent stretching during the day. Each stretch should be held for 30 seconds. It is beneficial to tell patients that muscles need to be reminded to stay elongated, therefore it is better to stretch for 30 seconds 10 times per day than to dedicate 1 hour once a day to perform stretches. This is also very helpful at achieving patient compliance.

Strengthening of the foot intrinsic muscles may be achieved by placing a towel on the floor and having the patient crunch up the towel into a ball and then spread it back out by flexing and extending the toes.

Alternate aerobic exercises or "cross-training" should be prescribed in order to minimize the effects of deconditioning. This can generally be achieved with running or swimming in the pool, as well as bicycling.

Modalities often prescribed include local ultrasound, iontophoresis, and phonophoresis. Although there is little evidence in the literature to suggest these modalities hasten the resolution of the underlying problem, they may be helpful in controlling the patient's pain symptoms, thus allowing better participation in a rehabilitation exercise program.

In an athlete, as symptoms resolve and the patient has achieved good flexibility and strength, a gradual return to running is attempted. An appropriate return to a running program should be established by the clinician together with the patient. This can generally be achieved by having the patient start at half of the time/distance and intensity he/she was running before the injury, divided into equal walk/jog intervals. An example would be if a patient was running up to 30 minutes before the injury, an appropriate return to running schedule might include the following: alternate 4 minutes of walking with 1 minute of jogging for a total of 15 minutes. The patient should then add another 5 minute walk/jog interval every week as tolerated until he/she has reached 30 minutes of 4 minutes walk–1 minute jog intervals. Next, have the patient decrease the walk time intervals to 3 minutes each and increase the jog time intervals to 2 minutes. Each week the patient should diminish walk-time intervals by 1 minute and add 1 minute to the jog interval. Walk/jog sessions should be performed 3 times per week, allowing 24 hours of rest between workouts. If at any time the symptoms begin to reappear, have the patient return to the walk/jog intensity of the previous week for another week until advancing again. It is generally accepted to first build endurance before intensity and to start on level surfaces before introducing hills. Patients must be cautioned to not overdo it and to stay within a structured rehabilitation program since reinjury is common.

Management of excessive foot pronation is essential to correcting a common contributing biomechanical factor.[5] This may be achieved simply by stretching the Achilles tendon; however, a change in footwear often is indicated. In both athletes and non-athletes, running shoes are excellent footwear. Numerous running shoes are on the market and a good running shoe store with a knowledgeable staff may be very helpful in finding the appropriate shoe for a particular type of foot. Essential components include a good heel counter and reasonable midfoot flexibility. Patients who demonstrate excessive hindfoot and forefoot varus deformities typically benefit from custom-made orthotics that incorporate medial side wedging. Patients should be cautioned about wearing high-heeled shoes, especially those with hard soles since this type of shoe increases the forces across the plantar fascia as well as promotes Achilles tendon shortening.

Posterior night splinting may prove effective in resistant cases. Off-the-shelf devices are available or fabrication of a posterior splint is simple utilizing fiberglass casting tape. The patient's foot should be splinted in maximum dorsiflexion to allow maximum lengthening of the plantar fascia and to prevent the stiffening and contraction that normally occurs during sleep. The splint should be applied every evening and worn throughout the night for two to three weeks.[6] If the patient finds that wearing the splints is uncomfortable at first, a gradual break in the wearing of the splints may be necessary, with the goal of wearing the splints throughout the night in 1 to 2 weeks.

Procedures

Corticosteroid injections can often be avoided if an effective treatment plan is adhered to. In refractory cases, however, a local steroid injection may be helpful to allow the patient to be more compliant with the established rehabilitation program (Fig. 2). Injections should be recommended with caution because they may promote fat pad atrophy with loss of cushioning of the heel.

Potential Disease Complications

Athletes who continue their activity untreated and "run through" their pain typically have progressive symptoms, which begin to interfere with their activities of daily living and may lead to irreversible fascial degeneration and damage.

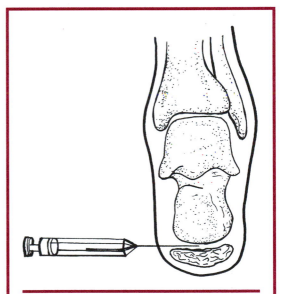

FIGURE 2. Proper medial approach for injection of plantar fascia. Under sterile conditions, a mixture of a local anesthetic (e.g., 2 cc of 1% lidocaine) and a corticosteroid (e.g., 2 cc of 10 mg/cc triamcinolone) may be injected into the heel with a 25-gauge, 1–1½-inch needle. A medial approach is used since the patient generally better tolerates it. The needle is aimed toward the medial tubercle of the calcaneus or most tender point, ensuring that the injection is above the fat pad in order to avoid potential fat pad atrophy.

Potential Treatment Complications

Because of the risk of gastrointestinal bleeding, long-term use of NSAIDs should be avoided and should be used with caution in elderly patients or those with a prior history of gastrointestinal or bleeding disorders. The use of NSAIDs is counterindicated in patients with a known hypersensitivity to them.

Although corticosteroid injections may be helpful in selected patients to help them participate in a more effective rehabilitation program, this procedure should be performed with reservation because it may lead to heel fat pad atrophy or even plantar fascia rupture.[7] Therefore the application of a walking splint or cast for several days following an injection may be helpful.

References

1. Karr SD: Subcalcaneal heel pain. Orthop Clin North Am 1994;25(1):161–174.
2. Nirschl RP: Plantar fasciitis—A new perspective. Am Med Joggers Assoc Q 1996; Summer:9–11.
3. Rubin G, Witten M: Plantar calcaneal spurs. Am J Orthop 1963;5:38.
4. Kwong PK, Kay D, Voner RT, White MW: Plantar fasciitis—Mechanics and pathomechanics of treatment. Clin Sports Med 1988;7(1):119–126.
5. Kibler BW, Goldberg C, Chandler TJ: Functional biomechanical deficits in running athletes with plantar fasciitis. Am J Sports Med 1991;19(1):66–71.
6. Ryan J: Use of posterior night splints in the treatment of plantar fasciitis. Am Fam Phys 1995;52 (3):891–898.
7. Sellman JR: Plantar fascia rupture associated with corticosteroid injection. Foot Ankle Int 1994;15(7):376–381.

90 Posterior Tibial Dysfunction

David Wexler, MD
Todd A. Kile, MD

Synonyms

Chronic tenosynovitis

Tibialis posterior tendon insufficiency

Asymmetrical pes planus

Adult acquired flat foot deformity[1]

ICD-9 Code

726.72
Tibialis tendinitis
(posterior)

Definition

Posterior tibial dysfunction is a condition characterized by the loss of function of the posterior tibialis tendon. Posterior tibial dysfunction can be a disabling affliction of the lower extremity caused by trauma, degeneration, or secondary to inflammatory arthritis.[2] These pathologies lead to loss or reduction of effective excursion of the tendon of tibialis posterior behind the medial malleolus, resulting in the characteristic loss of the medial arch or "asymmetrical adult flat foot" deformity. Spontaneous rupture can occur in patients receiving long-term steroid therapy or as a result of trauma.

Symptoms

Patients primarily complain of pain on the inner or medial aspect of the ankle and the hindfoot. As the insufficiency progresses, pronation increases, leading to pain over the dorsolateral aspect of the midfoot.[3,4] Rarely, there is a history of a rapid collapse following an acute injury.[5,6] More commonly, there is a gradual loss of the arch associated with a gradual increase in pain.

Physical Examination

The physical examination reveals swelling confined to the area around the medial malleolus (Fig. 1). Generally there is tenderness along the course of the tendon, and there may be exquisite tenderness just distal to the medial malleolus where the tendon most commonly tears.[7,8]

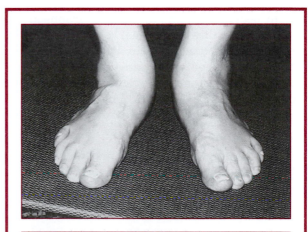

FIGURE 1. Clinical photograph of a patient with bilateral tibialis posterior tendon dysfunction—anterior view. Note the flattened arches and "rolled in" ankles.

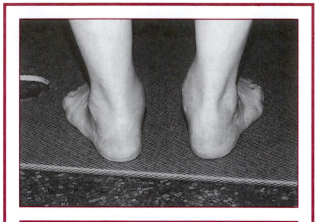

FIGURE 2. Clinical photograph of the same patient in Fig. 1—posterior view. Note the swelling, or "fullness," in the gutter medial to the Achilles tendon bilaterally and the valgus posture of the calcaneum. Note also the "too-many-toes" sign due to relative abduction of the forefoot, making it possible to see more than the normal one to two toes when observing from behind.

Assessing the lower extremity in the weight-bearing position best demonstrates the essential elements of the deformity. These are a valgus hindfoot (calcaneovalgus) and midfoot abduction and forefoot pronation, all of which occur at the midtarsal joint. The severity of these findings depends on the chronicity of the insufficiency and the magnitude of the tendon dysfunction. The medial longitudinal arch of the foot may be entirely lost. These are believed to be a result of tightening of the tendo-Achilles with an eventual "too many toes sign" (i.e., when the feet are viewed from behind, there appear to be more toes on the affected side than on the unaffected side (Fig. 2).

The tendon of tibialis anterior may become more visible than on the normal side as the patient, subconsciously, tries to regain the arch. Patients may have difficulty walking on their tip toes or have difficulty performing a one-sided toe-stand while holding onto the clinician's hands. The heel fails to invert into a varus position. Asking the patient to invert the plantar-flexed foot against resistance can be overcome by the clinician's hand. Assessing the patient on the couch reveals altered posture of the foot, due to the unopposed action of peroneus brevis. A callosity can be seen in the region of the medial, plantar aspect of the midfoot.

Functional Limitations

Patients may experience fatigue after only limited activity and, as the foot "rolls out," difficulty finding well-fitting footwear. Pain may limit walking and sports-related activities.[9]

Diagnostic Studies

Weight-bearing foot and ankle radiographs are usually quite helpful, depending on the severity of the clinical findings. In the earlier stages of tenosynovitis, the roentgenograms are usually normal, even if there is some mild clinical flattening of the medial longitudinal arch. As the problem progresses, radiographic changes occur, including—on the anteroposterior view—uncovering of the head of the talus (as the navicular moves laterally) and increase of the angle between the bodies of the talus and the calcaneum. On the lateral view, plantar flexion of the talus, collapse of the navicular-cuneiform joint, and overlapping of the four medial metatarsals are noted.

Ultrasonography has been used in the past to visualise the tendon of tibialis posterior both statically and dynamically and to demonstrate excursion. Currently, though, the "gold standard" is MRI, which provides a reasonably accurate view of the degree of inflammation and synovial fluid present within the tendon sheath, as well as whether a tear of the tendon is present.

Differential Diagnosis

Tarsal coalition—spastic flat foot

Degenerative arthritic deformity

Idiopathic flexible pes planus

Neuropathic arthropathy (e.g., secondary to diabetes mellitus)

Midtarsal collapse

Congenital pes planus

Lisfranc's dislocation

Treatment

Initial

The first line of management, in the early stages of tibialis posterior insufficiency, is with orthoses. Custom orthotic appliances to insert into the shoes, UCBL inserts, rigid ankle-foot orthoses (AFOs), and even double upright braces may be necessary. Occasionally, a short leg cast is applied for 4 to 6 weeks for rest. Unfortunately, there is no proof that any orthotic device can halt progression of the disorder.

Anti-inflammatory medication may help alleviate some of the pain from the tenosynovitis.

In obese individuals, weight loss can be critical.

Rehabilitation

Once the acute inflammation has settled, an exercise program may be started to strengthen the tibialis posterior. This can include active-resisted exercise routines with elastic materials (such as Clini-band or Thera-band) and an exercise akin to trying to "pick up carpet with the sole of the foot" or "grasping a towel." Further methods include muscle stretching and strengthening techniques, particularly aimed at the Achilles tendon and heel cord. Proprioceptive drills on the wobble board and gait re-education are also important.

Postoperatively, therapy can be ordered for range-of-motion exercises after tenosynovectomy and most certainly following tendon transfer surgery to strengthen the muscle-tendon complex. Following any fusion, the patient will have had a lengthy period of cast immobilization, and therefore, gait re-education can be beneficial.

Procedures

Injection of local anesthetic and steroid into the tendon sheath is a contentious subject and is not recommended due to the possibility of tendon rupture.

Surgery

Different surgical procedures are recommended, depending on the stage of the disease. Continuing pain and failure of non-operative management of tenosynovitis are the main indications for tenosynovectomy to remove all the inflamed synovium. This is followed by a period of cast immobilization.

Repair of incomplete tears of the tendon may also be indicated and can be augmented by tendon transfers. Complete tendon disruption, in the absence of bony collapse, can be treated with split tendon transfers; combining a flexor digitorum longus transfer with a calcaneal medial slide osteotomy. Subtalar or triple arthrodesis may be indicated for patients with progressively worsening deformity and lateral hindfoot pain.[10,11]

Potential Disease Complications

Posterior tibial dysfunction can result in progressive pain and deformity, restriction of mobility, valgus deformity of the knee, and medial longitudinal arch ulceration.

Potential Treatment Complications

Analgesics, NSAIDs, and COX-2 inhibitors have well-known side effects that most commonly affect the gastric, hepatic, and renal systems. Steroid injection can cause tendon rupture. Complications of surgery include wound infection (in an area that can be notoriously slow to heal) and non-union or failure of fusion in attempted arthrodesis.

References
1. Deland JT: Posterior tibial tendon dysfunction. In Craig EV (ed): Clinical Orthopaedics, 1st ed. Philadelphia, Lippincott Williams & Wilkins, 1999, pp 883–890.
2. Richardson EG: Disorders of tendons and fascia. In Canale ST (ed): Campbell's Operative Orthopaedics, vol 2, 9th ed. St Louis, Mosby, 1998, pp 1889–1923.
3. Hertling D, Kessler RM: The leg, ankle and foot. In Hertling D, Kessler RM (eds): Management of Common Musculoskeletal Eisorders, 3rd ed. Philadelphia, Lippincott, Williams & Wilkins, 1996, pp 435–438.
4. Mann RA: Biomechanics of the foot and ankle. In Mann RA, Coughlin RJ (eds): Surgery of the Foot and Ankle, 6th ed. St Louis Mosby, 1993, pp 3–44.
5. Myerson MS: Adult acquired flatfoot deformity. J Bone Joint Surg 1996;78-A:780–792.
6. Mann RA, Thompson FM: Rupture of the posterior tibial tendon causing flat foot. Surgical treatment. J Bone Joint Surg 1985;67-A:556–561.
7. Johnson KA, Strom DE: Tibialis posterior tendon dysfunction. Clin Orthop 1989;239:196–206.
8. Johnson KA: Tibialis posterior tendon rupture. Clin Orthop 1983;177:140–147.
9. Pedowitz WJ, Kovatis P: Flatfoot in the adult. J Am Acad Orthop Surg 1995;3:293–302.
10. Myerson MS, Corrigan J: Treatment of posterior tibial tendon dysfunction with flexor digitorum longus tendon transfer and calcaneal osteotomy. Orthopaedics 1996;19:383–388.
11. Johnson KA: Tibialis posterior tendon release-substitution. In Thompson RC, Johnson KA (eds): Master Techniques in Orthopaedic Surgery—The Foot and Ankle, 1st ed. Philadelphia, Raven Press, 1994, pp 271–283.

91 Tibial Neuropathy (Tarsal Tunnel Syndrome)

David R. Del Toro, MD

Synonyms

Tibial neuropathy at the ankle

Compression or entrapment neuropathy of the tibial nerve

Posterior tarsal tunnel syndrome

Posterior tibial nerve entrapment

ICD-9 Code

355.5
Tarsal tunnel syndrome

Definition

Tarsal tunnel syndrome (TTS) may be described as a constellation of signs and symptoms caused by entrapment or compression of the tibial nerve or any of its branches in the region beneath the flexor retinaculum (Fig. 1). The tibial nerve branches that may be involved deep to the tarsal tunnel include the medial or lateral plantar nerve, the first branch of the lateral plantar nerve (also called Baxter's nerve or inferior calcaneal nerve), or the medial calcaneal nerve. Anatomically, the tarsal tunnel is a fibro-osseous structure that begins just posterior to the medial malleolus, with the roof being the flexor retinaculum (also called the laciniate ligament) and the floor being formed by the tendons of the posterior tibialis, flexor digitorum longus, and the flexor hallucis longus muscles. The tibial nerve usually divides into three branches at the level of the ankle: the medial and lateral plantar nerves and the medial calcaneal nerve. The first branch of the lateral plantar nerve usually branches from the lateral plantar nerve or the tibial nerve just distal to the origin of the medial calcaneal nerve at the level of the tarsal tunnel; it traverses laterally across the anterior aspect of the heel and terminates with motor branches to the abductor digiti quinti pedis muscle.[1] It is likely that true TTS occurs very infrequently when compared with other focal entrapment neuropathies, such as carpal tunnel syndrome, ulnar neuropathy at the elbow, or peroneal neuropathy.

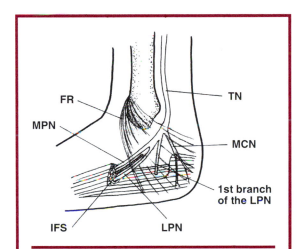

FIGURE 1. The medial aspect of a right foot. Note that the MCN branches pierce the FR as they course toward the medioplantar aspect of the heel. TN = tibial nerve; MCN = medial calcaneal nerve; QP = quadratus plantar muscle; LPN = lateral plantar nerve; MPN = medial plantar nerve; IFS = interfascicular septum; AH = abductor hallucis muscle; FR = flexor retinaculum.

There are generally considered to be five basic categories that may account for the etiology of tarsal tunnel syndrome: (1) trauma and post-traumatic changes, (2) space occupying lesions causing compression, (3) systemic diseases, (4) biomechanical causes related to joint structure/deformity, and (5) idiopathic causes. In addition, the underlying pathophysiology of tarsal tunnel syndrome remains elusive since a portion of the literature supports the process of demyelination, whereas other case reports implicate axonal degeneration as the primary process.[2,3] It is believed that the tibial nerve may be entrapped proximally within the tarsal tunnel, or distally one of the branches (e.g., the medial plantar nerve or lateral plantar nerve) may be entrapped individually in its own calcaneal chamber.[4] Also, entrapment of the first branch of the lateral plantar nerve has been described as a cause for heel pain.[5,6] Therefore, in a case of suspected tarsal tunnel syndrome, the tibial nerve and its major terminal branches should be thoroughly evaluated.

Symptoms

The patient usually presents with pain and/or paresthesias along with numbness over the sole of the foot. The pain is usually described as burning or a dull ache, but may also be expressed as throbbing, cramping, or even tightness and may radiate proximally up the medial calf. Symptoms are often exacerbated by prolonged standing or walking and may be worse at night, but may not be well localized. However, if limited to a particular region of the foot, the distribution of symptoms might correspond to a specific tibial nerve branch that is involved. Weakness in the foot is uncommon and may only present itself if the resulting foot deformity is so severe that it causes an unstable gait pattern. Patients with true TTS generally present with unilateral symptoms.

Physical Examination

A patient with TTS often has a Tinel's sign over the tibial nerve or one of its branches in the tarsal tunnel (Fig. 2). Occasionally, percussion over the tibial nerve at the ankle will elicit pain extending proximally along the course of the tibial nerve, this sign is called the Valleix phenomenon. There may also be palpable tenderness over the tibial nerve in the tarsal tunnel. Two other provocative maneuvers that may reproduce symptoms in the foot/ankle include extension of the great toe and sustained passive eversion of the ankle.[4] Sensory exam might reveal decreased light touch and/or pinprick over the plantar aspect of the foot in the distribution of one or all of the tibial nerve branches (Fig. 3). Motor examination of the intrinsic foot muscles is challenging since it is often very difficult for patients to selectively activate these muscles. However, one may be able to appreciate muscle atrophy about the foot that is asymmetric when compared with the other side.[4] Muscle stretch reflexes in the lower extremity (including patellar, medial hamstring, and Achilles) should be normal and symmetric when compared with the unaffected side. Peripheral pulses (posterior tibial and dorsalis pedis) are usually palpable and full. Also, if the biomechanical configuration of the foot is altered severely enough, then gait deviations could be observed.

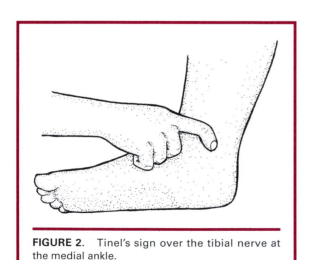

FIGURE 2. Tinel's sign over the tibial nerve at the medial ankle.

Functional Limitations

Impaired balance or a perception of instability due to diminished sensation on the sole of the foot may be the only functional impairment that is noted by the patient. As a consequence, limited walking tolerance/distance or falls may be noted.

Diagnostic Studies

Electrodiagnostic testing should be performed on all patients with suspected TTS since this is the only objective study that evaluates the physiologic function of the tibial nerve. Both needle electromyography and nerve conduction studies (i.e., motor, sensory, and/or mixed nerve study) should be done since abnormal findings may be present in one or both of these parts of the electrodiagnostic evaluation. In addition, it is imperative that the tibial nerve be meticulously evaluated from an electrophysiologic standpoint, since the tibial nerve or only one of its branches may be involved in a case of suspected tarsal tunnel syndrome. A magnetic resonance (MR) imaging study may be useful in detecting a space occupying lesion or mass that is impinging on or compressing the tibial nerve within the tarsal tunnel. The MR imaging can provide a "road map" for surgical exploration of the tarsal tunnel and then direct the procedure toward suitable anatomic decompression of the nerve.[7] Plain x-rays and a bone scan may be needed to rule out a possible fracture.

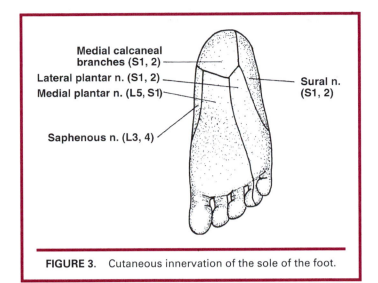

FIGURE 3. Cutaneous innervation of the sole of the foot.

Differential Diagnosis

Plantar fasciitis

Peripheral neuropathy

Sciatic neuropathy

Lumbosacral plexopathy

Posterior tibial dysfunction

Lumbosacral radiculopathy

Treatment

Initial

Conservative measures are often effective in the majority of TTS cases, and therefore most patients should be given an adequate trial, which is generally at least 3 to 6 months. Initial management should include NSAIDs/COX-2 inhibitors and possibly a neuropathic pain medication (such as gabapentin). If there is a biomechanical foot condition, which can be corrected or supported, then the patient could benefit from a medial arch support (for a pronated foot) or a foot orthosis (for hindfoot valgus).[5] Also, a short leg walking cast or boot in some patients can be used to provide symptomatic relief.[8]

Rehabilitation

Physical therapy can be useful in certain cases, most typically with modalities such as iontophoresis to reduce symptoms of inflammation, deep massage to mobilize scar tissue, desensitization, and stretching exercises. Strengthening exercises may also be prescribed, as well as gait training, if necessary. The patient may require extra depth shoes to accommodate a medial arch support or a custom made foot orthosis. An orthotist or pedorthist may provide custom orthotics or footwear, if necessary.

Procedures

For diagnostic and therapeutic purposes, a local anesthetic/steroid injection into the tarsal tunnel can give relatively immediate relief of local swelling and inflammation around the tibial nerve.

Surgery

Surgical management consists of releasing the flexor retinaculum and possibly exploring for a mass or space occupying lesion and neurolysis of the tibial nerve, depending on the surgeon.[4] In addition, some surgeons advocate release of the superficial and deep fascia of the abductor hallucis to more completely decompress the tibial nerve and its branches. The success rate (good to excellent outcome) for tarsal tunnel release is variable and reported to be 44% to 78%, depending on the study.[7] Endoscopic release of the tarsal tunnel may be a potential surgical option in some cases.[7]

Potential Disease Complications

There are several potential disease complications that may result as a consequence of TTS. Skin breakdown, including ulcerations, due to impaired sensation can occur over the plantar aspect of the foot. An altered gait pattern may develop with possibly a "feeling of unsteadiness" due to impaired sensation, particularly with respect to proprioception and light touch/pressure in the foot, or due to the biomechanical configuration of the foot being distorted. Also, low back pain may arise subsequently as a result of a gait deviation.

Potential Treatment Complications

NSAIDs may cause, most commonly, gastric or renal complications. COX-2 inhibitors may have fewer gastric side effects. Skin breakdown can develop over the foot/ankle from a poorly fitting orthotic device. Tendon rupture may occur after steroid injection into the incorrect location (e.g., flexor tendon sheath). In addition, the symptoms of pain, numbness, or paresthesias in the foot can be exacerbated after a local anesthetic/steroid injection or after surgical decompression of the tarsal tunnel.

References
1. Sarrafian SK: Anatomy of the Foot and Ankle. Philadelphia, J.B. Lippincott, 1983.
2. Kraft GH: Tarsal tunnel entrapment. In Course E: Entrapment Neuropathies. Boston, AAEE Ninth Annual Continuing Education Course, 1986, pp 13–18.
3. Spindler HA, Reischer MA, Felsenthal G: Electrodiagnostic assessment in suspected tarsal tunnel syndrome. Phys Med Rehabil Clin North Am 1994;5:595–612.
8. Mann RA: Diseases of the nerves. In Coughlin MJ, Mann RA (eds): Surgery of the Foot and Ankle. St Louis, Mosby, 1999, pp 502–524.
4. Park TA, Del Toro DR: Electrodiagnostic evaluation of the voot. Phys Med Rehabil ClinNorth Am 1998;9:871–896.
5. Przylucki H, Jones CL: Entrapment neuropathy of muscle branch of lateral plantar nerve. J Am Podiatr Med Assoc 1981;71:119–124.
6. Schon LC, Baxter DE: Heel pain syndrome and entrapment neuropathies about the foot and ankle. In Gould JS (ed): Operative Foot Surgery. Philadelphia, W.B. Saunders, 1994, pp 192–208.
7. Haddad SL: Compressive neuropathies of the foot and ankle. In Myerson MS (ed): Foot and Ankle Disorders. Philadelphia, W.B. Saunders, 2000, pp 808–833.

SECTION 2

Rehabilitation

92 | Acquired Immunodeficiency Syndrome

Farrukh Hamid, MD

Synonyms

HIV disease

AIDS

ICD-9 Code

042
Human immunodeficiency
virus (HIV) disease

Definition

Acquired immunodeficiency syndrome (AIDS) is the final stage of a viral infection that affects the immune system, primarily the T4 lymphocytes. As defined by the Centers for Disease Control and Prevention (CDC), only human immunodeficiency virus (HIV)–infected persons who have an AIDS-indicator condition or a CD4 count of less than 200/mm^3 (normal range is typically 500 to 1500) actually have AIDS. The clinical illness results from an infection by a human retrovirus, causing a profound cellular immune system dysfunction with direct and indirect damage to multiple body systems from either HIV itself or opportunistic infections or malignancies. There are no risk groups for AIDS, only risk behaviors. Unprotected sex, intravenous drug use, and mother-to-fetus exposure are the main modes of transmission. Although the life expectancy for patients with AIDS is increasing, new problems such as drug resistance, drug side effects, and new long-term impairments continue to challenge health care providers. Sexually active men and women are the target population for this disease with a high incidence in gay men and minority women, mostly from the lower socioeconomic class. Infants born to HIV-positive mothers are also at high risk for transmission.

The spectrum of potential complications from AIDS is vast. Table 1 gives a brief overview.

Symptoms

The spectrum of clinical manifestation is widespread and ranges from flulike symptoms of initial HIV infection to severe wasting, multiple opportunistic infections, and multisystem involvement of terminal AIDS. Thus, the history of the presenting complaint is critical in a patient with previously established HIV infection.

Symptoms depend not only on the system involved but also the primary etiology and the stage of the disease. The majority of AIDS patients present with *Pneumocystis carinii* pneumonia as the initial feature. Kaposi's sarcoma (a lymphoendothelial malignancy) is commonly seen in AIDS patients. Other common associated conditions include peripheral neuropathies, arthropathies, cardiomyopathies, gastrointestinal disorders, chronic pain and fatigue, and cognitive dysfunction. Table 2 provides a list of some common problems but certainly is not meant to be all-inclusive.

TABLE 1. AIDS-Related Complications

Neurologic
Toxoplasmosis
Progressive multifocal leukodystrophy
Cytomegalovirus (CMV) encephalitis or
   polyradiculopathy
Mononeuritis multiplex
Diffuse symmetrical neuropathy
HIV myelopathy
Cryptococcal meningitis
CNS lymphoma
Medication induced neuropathies
Autonomic neuropathy

Pulmonary
Pneumocystis pneumonia
Bacterial pneumonia (e.g., *Streptococcus*,
   Haemophilus influenzae)
Viral pneumonia (e.g., CMV, herpes simplex)
Fungal infections (e.g., *Cryptococcus
   neoformans, Histoplasma capsulatum*)
Tuberculosis pneumonia
Malignancies (e.g., non-Hodgkin's
   lymphoma, Kaposi's sarcoma)
Pleural effusion

Cardiac
Cardiomyopathy
Pericardial disease
Valve dysfunction

Musculoskeletal and Rheumatologic
Rheumatoid arthritis
Systemic lupus erythematosus
Polyarthritis
HIV or drug-induced myopathy
Tendinitis or bursitis
Plantar fasciitis
Fibromyalgia
Vasculitides
Osteonecrosis

Physical Examination

Universal precautions should be observed during the entire examination. General mood and constitution should be assessed. A thorough examination of the skin and joints with the clinician assessing for rashes, lesions, contractures, swelling, and effusions is important. A complete neurologic exam should precede a focal exam of the involved region due to the simultaneous involvement of multiple areas of the nervous system (i.e., the layering and parallel tracking of multiple systems).[1] The distribution of neurologic deficits helps the clinician determine the impairment. The clinical distribution of sensory loss helps in the identification of the type of peripheral neuropathy. Similarly, the pattern of motor weakness indicates whether a nerve, plexus, or root or the central nervous system is involved.

Musculoskeletal system examination may reveal symmetric or asymmetric joint swelling, tenderness, warmth, erythema, and decreased range of motion of the joint. Pain to palpation in periarticular structures and muscle weakness and wasting may also be present. Examination should not be limited by the description of the patient since overlapping neurologic and musculoskeletal impairments are common. For example, in clinically described peripheral neuropathy, plantar fasciitis should be excluded as the cause of foot pain since it is commonly present concomitantly. It is important to remember that in this often young and highly functional population, early deficits are easily missed, especially when checking for weakness.

Thorough chest auscultation and percussion should be performed to rule out pulmonary pathology. Standard cardiac exam and abdominal palpation and percussion are indicated to assess for organomegaly or other masses. Pulmonary, gastrointestinal, and other exams should be performed with an emphasis, again, on the patient's presenting symptoms. Since depression is common, mood and affect should be assessed.

Functional Limitations

As expected, functional limitations depend on the severity of the illness. Many factors can cause functional limitations, including pain, fatigue, and neurologic or orthopedic impairments.[2] Cognitive deficits may further limit function.

Early on, there may be no limitations. Later, functional limitations are disease-based.[3] If the musculoskeletal system is involved, limited range of motion may impair reach, grip, overhead activities, and gait. Muscle weakness affects motor function, lifting, pulling, pushing, carrying, and gripping activities. Sensory deficits limit fine motor function and proprioception.

Typical functional limitations include difficulty with dressing, bathing, doing household chores, work, and recreational activities. Limitations of driving and returning to work may be similar to those of young stroke patients.

Patients may not function at optimal levels due to embarrassment and/or fear both at work and at home. The vast majority of HIV-infected individuals continue to work during the initial years of infection. However, as their disease progresses, time lost from work due to illness, chronic pain and fatigue, and cognitive dysfunction all contribute to out-of-work disability issues. Depression is commonly encountered in AIDS patients and may contribute to decreased function in all aspects of life. At home, sexual dysfunction and the inability to maintain intimate and/or supportive relationships may contribute to functional losses.

TABLE 2. Common Symptoms in AIDS

Organ/System	Common Problems
Constitutional	Fatigue, malaise, asthenia, wasting, anorexia
Musculoskeletal	Arthralgia, myalgia, connective tissue inflammations, muscle weakness, tendinitis, contractures, edema, chronic pain, joint swelling/effusion
Neurologic	Ataxia, aphasia, dysarthria, cranial nerve deficits, swallowing disorders, paralysis, movement disorders, peripheral neuropathy, polyradiculopathy, myelopathy, hemiplegia
Psychiatric	Anxiety, depression, irritability, dementia, cognitive dysfunction
Cardiac and pulmonary	Dyspnea, angina, hypertriglyceridemia

Diagnostic Studies

HIV antibody test or HIV virus test are both commercially available to diagnose HIV infection. CD4 count and viral load are the current parameters used to grade severity and to monitor treatment response or drug resistance. A normal CD4 count (500 to 1500) and an undetectable viral load are good prognostic indicators and a goal for successful antiretroviral therapy.

In general, diagnostic studies are based on presenting signs and symptoms, and all potential etiologies for the symptoms should be systematically ruled out using the appropriate diagnostic tools. For example in a patient with an antalgic gait, an MRI may confirm the presence of avascular necrosis of the hip(s) (Fig. 1). MRI of the head is indicated for focal neurologic deficits.

Sensory loss or suspected neuropathies can be evaluated with EMG/nerve conduction studies.

Nerve and muscle biopsy are the next step for undiagnosed neuromuscular illnesses and bone scan for undiagnosed skeletal problems.

Hemoglobin, oxygen saturation, testosterone, and thyroxine levels are required for proper evaluation of fatigue. Similarly, chest x-ray and oxygen saturation and arterial blood gas measurements are indicated when the patient has respiratory complaints. Uric acid level, rheumatoid factor, antinuclear antibody, joint aspirate, and joint x-ray studies are useful in the diagnosis of arthritis. Muscle pain can be evaluated with creatine kinase, erythrocyte sedimentation rate, aldolase, and thyroid function tests.

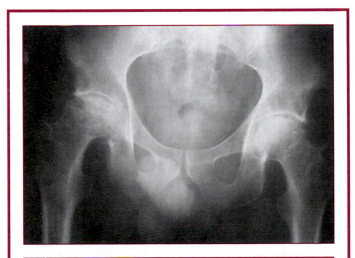

FIGURE 1. Advanced bilateral avascular necrosis (AVN) in a 32-year-old male with HIV disease with no other known risk factor for AVN.

TABLE 3. Antiviral Medications Used to Treat HIV	
Non-nucleoside reverse transcriptase inhibitors	Nevirapine, efavirenz, delavirdine
Nucleoside analogs	3TC (lamivudine), d4T (stavudine), ddC (zalcitabine), ddI (didanosine), zidovudine (AZT)
Protease inhibitors	Indinavir, saquinavir, nelfinavir, ritonavir, amprenavir

Differential Diagnosis

None

Treatment

Initial

Treatment for AIDS is rapidly improving with the addition of new agents in the armamentarium against the disease.[6] The standard is combination therapy.

The agents used to treat HIV are classified into three major groups, but new combinations of these agents are being developed to make the treatment easier, more effective, and better tolerated. The three groups of antiretrovirals are listed in Table 3.

Treatment of a specific constellation of symptoms depends on the etiology and severity. It ranges from the use of antibiotics to treat the infection to the use of adjuvant pharmacologic agents to treat symptoms as well as rehabilitative approaches to prevent and treat impairments. For example, testosterone and epoetin alfa are used to treat fatigue related to low testosterone level or anemia, respectively. Oxandrolone[8] and growth hormone are used for the treatment of AIDS wasting.

A detailed discussion of treatment for all complications is beyond the scope of this chapter. Pain management options include oral medications and NSAIDs for inflammatory etiologies; tramadol can be used for pain that does not respond to NSAIDs. Narcotics are used for refractory cases only. Use of narcotics should not be stringent for any patient population with severe pain. However, too liberal use of narcotics in the HIV population is also not advocated. The assumption that life expectancy among HIV patients is very limited as a rule is not true anymore, and therefore care should be exercised regarding the dosage of narcotics prescribed to patients who have non-specific musculoskeletal pain complaints.

For neuropathic pain, however, tricyclics, gabapentin or carbamazepine should be the first choice. In the management of diffuse symmetric neuropathy, low dose amitriptyline (10 to 50 mg qhs), trazodone (15 to 50 mg qhs), or nortriptyline (10 to 50 mg qhs), or using gabapentin (100 to 600 mg tid) alone or in combination with the previously mentioned agents provides good results.[7]

Non-pharmacologic alternatives for pain control include transcutaneous electrical nerve stimulation (TENS) or galvanic stimulation for neuropathic pain. Using hot/cold packs may alleviate musculoskeletal pain as well. Psychotherapy may be used for patients with chronic pain or with obvious findings of anxiety or depression related to pain.

Fatigue should be appropriately worked-up, and treatable causes such as anemia, thyroid dysfunction, and sleep disorders should be assessed. Depression may also contribute to symptoms of fatigue. Education on pacing and sleep hygiene (e.g., avoiding caffeine and alcohol, maintaining a regular bedtime) is important.

Rehabilitation

Rehabilitation for HIV disease involves addressing the specific problems that an individual faces. There are no specific guidelines because of the wide spectrum of syndromes found in HIV and AIDS. Patients may benefit from skilled physical therapy, occupational therapy, and/or speech therapy, depending on the spectrum of their illness. Physical and occupational therapists can be instrumental in helping patients manage pain through the use of modalities such as ultrasound, cold therapy, or myofascial release techniques. Therapists can also suggest appropriate adaptive equipment and mobility aides when necessary. Orthotics (braces) may improve ambulation.

Supervised exercise programs can focus on strength training, stretching, gait, cardiovascular conditioning, and posture training. Some patients will benefit from learning energy conservation and task simplification techniques. Therapists can also provide information about joint and nerve protection. In some instances, having a therapist visit a patient's home or workplace to make recommendations may be useful.

Speech therapists can address swallowing and speech issues, as well as safety and cognitive retraining. Speech therapists can also provide treatment regarding communication and memory aides.

Social workers, psychologists, vocational rehabilitation specialists, and other health care providers all may have a role in the care of HIV-infected patients, depending on their specific needs and the stage of their illness.

Procedures

Many procedures can be utilized in AIDS patients, depending on the specific problem. Clinicians should use the same criteria for procedures that they use for other illnesses (i.e., weighing the risk/benefit ratio for the patient). Universal Precautions should be adhered to in all instances in which procedures are performed. Examples of potentially helpful procedures include injections for tendinitis, bursitis, or trigger points that generally respond well to injected corticosteroid and/or anesthetic medications. Similarly, spasticity in a focal area can be appropriately treated with phenol blocks or botulinum toxin injections (see chapter on spasticity). End stage patients may necessitate procedures such as the insertion of feeding tubes.

Surgery

Surgery may be recommended for a variety of reasons in AIDS patients. For example, contractures can be treated surgically to improve hygiene, function, or mobility. Similarly, joint replacement in severe avascular necrosis produces dramatic improvement in function and pain relief. Surgical interventions, again, should be approached with the usual risk/benefit considerations that are assessed in any patient population.

Potential Disease Complications

Untreated, AIDS affects many organ systems and ultimately results in death. Permanent damage to a part of the neuraxis, as in progressive multifocal dystrophy, causes severe debilitating paralysis and motor function loss. Severe cardiopulmonary disease, or cardiomyopathy,[11] is often the cause of death in a young HIV patient. In the musculoskeletal system, irreversible skeletal damage may present as avascular necrosis, whereas unusual widespread malignancies such as Kaposi's sarcoma or lymphomas may cause severe disfiguring or neurologic deficits. Severe wasting is not an uncommon complication and results in the typical look of a terminally ill AIDS patient.

Potential Treatment Complications

The addition of new agents in the fight against AIDS also brings new side effects. For example, ddI, ddC, and d4T are all known to cause neuropathy, as are some of the agents used to treat opportunistic infections. Plenty of liquids may still not prevent the ability of indinavir (Crixivan) to cause nephrolithiasis.

Protease inhibitors are an excellent group of agents to suppress HIV but collectively produce hypertriglyceridemia and increase the risk of cardiac disease. Due to the co-existence of multiple illnesses along with the symptomatic treatment and anti-HIV medications, drug interactions and polypharmacy are common problems.

References

1. Berger JR, Levy RM: AIDS and the Nervous System, 2nd ed. Philadelphia, Lippincott-Raven, 1977.
2. Soucy MD: Fatigue and depression: Assessment in human immunodeficiency virus disease. Nurse Pract Forum 1997;8:121–125.
3. O'Dell MW (ed): HIV-related disability: Assessment and management. Phys Med Rehabil 1993;7:(Special Issue).
4. O'Dell MW, Hubert H, Lubeck DP, et al: Pre-AIDS disability: Data from the AIDS Time Health-Oriented Study. Arch Phys Med Rehabil 1998;79:1200–1205.
5. O'Dell MW, Riggs RV: Correlates of HIV-related fatigue: A pilot study. Disabil Rehabil 1996;18:249–254.
6. Deeks SG, Smith M, Holodnly M, et al: HIV protease inhibitors: A review for clinicians. JAMA 1997;277:145–153.
7. Levinson SF, Fine SM: Rehabilitation of individuals with human immunodeficiency virus. In DeLisa JA, Gans BM (eds): Rehabilitation Medicine: Principles and Practice. Philadelphia, Lippincott-Raven, 1998, pp 1319–1335.
8. Berger JR, Pall L, Hall CD, et al: Oxandrolone in AIDS wasting myopathy. AIDS 1996;10:1657–1662.
9. Darko DF, Milter MM, Miller JC: Growth hormone, fatigue, poor sleep, and disability in HIV infection. Neuroendocrinology 1998;67:317–324.
10. O'Dell MW: Rehabilitation in HIV infection: New applications for old knowledge. Phys Med Rehabil 1993;Supplement:S1–S8.
11. Yunis NA, Stone VE: Cardiac manifestations of HIV/AIDS: A review of disease spectrum and clinical management. J AIDS Hum Retrovirol 1998;18:145–154.
12. Safai B, Diaz B, Schwartz J: Malignant neoplasms associated with human immunodeficiency syndrome infection. CA Cancer J Clin 1992;42:74–95.

93 Amputation: Upper Limb

Timothy R. Dillingham, MD

Definition

Upper limb amputations are devastating occurrences for individuals and result in profound functional and vocational consequences. The primary reason for upper limb loss is trauma, with cancer being the next most common cause.[1] Upper limb amputations occur in 3.9 individuals per 100,000, with finger amputations being the most common (3.2 per 100,000) followed by hand amputations (0.5 per 100,000).[2] These rates of amputation are far lower than the incidence rates for lower limb dysvascular amputations, which occur in 47 per 100,000 individuals.[3] Fortunately the rates for traumatic amputation declined during the last decade.[2]

Machinery and power tools are the most common reasons for traumatic amputation. Men are at far greater risk for traumatic amputation than women and demonstrate about 6.6 times the female rate for minor amputations of the finger and hand.[2]

The level of amputation is the single most important determinant of postamputation function. The primary surgical principle is to save as much limb as possible while ensuring removal of devitalized tissues and residual limb wound healing. Saving the most distal joint possible dramatically improves the amputee's function. The elbow joint for instance, when preserved, allows the arm to function in carrying and supporting activities. For the mangled hand, saving any fingers or remnants provides reconstructive hand surgeons the possibility of creating a hand with two-finger opposition and grip.

Symptoms

Patients may present with phantom pain (i.e., pain perceived in the missing part of the limb), phantom sensation (i.e., non-painful perceptions of the missing part of the limb), discomfort with prosthetic fit, and skin breakdown on the residual limb.

Physical Examination

Upper limb amputees require a thorough musculoskeletal examination that includes motor strength testing, sensory testing, and examination of the contralateral limb. Persons with traumatic amputations of the upper limb can have brachial plexus injuries that weaken the residual upper limb muscles. Insensate skin can predispose a patient to breakdown at the site of contact with a prosthesis. Joint range of motion should be assessed. In particular, the scapulothoracic motion is important since protraction of the scapulae provides the force for a dual-control cable system for body-powered prostheses. Reduced elbow or shoulder range of motion from heterotopic ossification, joint capsule contracture, or muscle contracture can severely impede rehabilitation.

Functional Limitations

An upper limb amputee's functional status depends on the level of amputation. Persons with finger loss (not including the thumb) are quite functional without a prosthesis. Persons with thumb amputations lose the ability to grip large objects as well as fine motor skills that require opposition with another finger. Reconstructive surgery with pollicization using another remaining finger dramatically improves hand function.[4]

Below elbow and above elbow amputees lose hand function and have limitations in basic and higher level activities of daily living, such as dressing. They frequently sustain new vocational limitations that can preclude return to their previous work activities. Most persons can adapt to almost all basic daily activities using the intact contralateral hand and upper limb. Prosthetic devices may or may not improve function. Some amputees find upper limb prosthetic devices cumbersome, discarding their use altogether. Other amputees require a specialized prosthesis to continue their work-related activities.

Diagnostic Studies

No special diagnostic testing is generally required beyond a careful physical examination. If there is weakness of the limb, then electrodiagnostic testing (EMG and nerve conduction studies) may clarify whether a plexopathy is also present. X-rays may be necessary to evaluate for osteomyelitis, heterotopic ossification, or a bone spur in the distal limb causing poor prosthetic fit.

Differential Diagnosis

None

Treatment

Initial

Management of persons with upper limb amputations involves a continuum of care.[1,4] This begins with provision of pre-operative information when the amputation is elective, as in the case of cancer. The overriding concern when planning the amputation is to save all possible length, particularly the elbow joint. This preserves elbow flexion and prevents the need for a dual-control cable system. The early input of a physiatrist, nurse, and therapist with expertise in this area is highly advantageous. Early involvement of the rehabilitation team can provide helpful information about prosthetic options; the rehabilitation continuum; and what can be expected after amputation, such as phantom sensations.

Residual limb pain and *phantom pain* are two conditions that can affect patients with upper limb amputations.[5] Phantom sensations are common, yet fortunately, disabling phantom pain occurs in only about 5% of amputees.[1,5] Despite the many interventions used for phantom pain, there are no uniformly effective treatments. Medication and physical modalities must be tried in a rational fashion to determine the most effective intervention. Physical modalities include a transcutaneous electrical stimulation (TENS) unit and physical manipulation and massage of the residual limb.[5]

Fitting a comfortable prosthesis can often help reduce these painful sensations. Antidepressant and anti-epileptic (gabapentin) medications are frequently used with variable results.[1,5] Beta blockers (propranolol and atenolol) have been found to be somewhat effective in treating phantom pain.[5] If patients require cardiac or hypertension medications, the choice of a beta blocker may serve two purposes for amputees with phantom pain. Opiates may be effective for these problems when other methods fail to relieve phantom pain. If it is anticipated that the person with phantom pain will need analgesia for a long period, then long-acting opiates should be used because they have less habituation and addiction potential. Most amputees with phantom pain have intermittent severe pain that can be treated with as-needed small doses of a short-acting opiate. For the few patients with severe, unremitting phantom and residual limb pain, referral to a pain center is suggested.

Rehabilitation

Persons sustaining upper limb amputations present complex rehabilitative needs that are ideally managed in a rehabilitation center with therapists, prosthetists, and physicians possessing specialized knowledge and experience. Proper rehabilitation and a comfortable and functional prosthesis will facilitate functional restoration. Vocational counseling and vocational retraining are vital aspects of any program, as this condition often afflicts young, vocationally productive persons, primarily men.

A continuum of care is vital to successful rehabilitation and patients must be transitioned effectively from the inpatient postsurgical unit, sometimes to an inpatient rehabilitation unit, and always to a long-term outpatient rehabilitation and prosthetic program.

After amputation the primary goal is wound healing, edema control, and prevention of contractures and deconditioning. Persons sustaining upper limb amputations due to trauma or cancer generally have normal underlying blood supply and can readily heal most surgical sites. Edema is prevented by using a shrinker sock, ACE wrapping with a figure-eight technique that provides pressure distally without choking the limb, or by means of a rigid dressing system. In sophisticated centers, immediate postoperative prosthesis (IPOP) fitting in the operating room is implemented. The IPOP is placed over the limb after the skin is padded with soft dressings. The IPOP accommodates surgical drains, yet prevents the formation of edema. Prosthetic components can be attached to the IPOP, and early training can be implemented.

Prevention of contractures in the residual limb and prevention of generalized deconditioning are important goals of early rehabilitation. Any other injuries, as are common in persons sustaining severe trauma, should be identified and rehabilitation efforts directed at their remediation. For body-powered prostheses, scapulothoracic motion provides power through a cable system to operate the prosthesis. Likewise, elbow or shoulder contractures or capsulitis will severely impede maximal prosthetic use, and these problems should be aggressively addressed. Early training in activity of daily living skills should be pursued as well. Therapies should be directed toward ameliorating weakness through exercises or contractures through active assistive range-of-motion exercises and prolonged stretching.

A detailed discussion of prosthetic devices is beyond the scope of this chapter, and consultation with a skilled prosthetist and physiatrist is desirable. In general, there are two types: body-powered and myoelectric devices.[1,4] Body-powered devices are usually less cosmetic, yet are less expensive and much more durable. Myoelectric prostheses are controlled by electrical signals generated in muscles from the remaining residual limb or shoulder girdle. These devices are expensive and require special prosthetic skills to fabricate and maintain, but are generally more cosmetic in appearance. Skin breakdown can occur over bony prominences, where there are skin grafts or where skin is adherent to underlying bone. Alteration of the prosthetic socket and suspension systems or temporarily discontinuing prosthetic use until the skin has healed may be necessary.

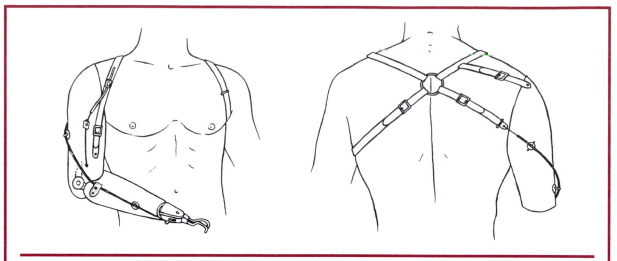

FIGURE 1. Above-elbow prosthesis. (From Jebson PJL, Kasdan ML: Hand Secrets. Philadelphia, Hanley & Belfus, 1998, p 188.)

Procedures

Appropriate management of phantom limb pain should include early intervention and the prevention of prolonged periods of pain. However, if desensitization techniques and traditional pharmacologic agents don't work, then nerve blocks, steroid injections, or neuroma resections can be entertained. The success of these interventions is limited. Surgery is rarely done and generally is not successful for phantom limb pain.

Surgery

Revision surgeries are sometimes necessary to remove bone spurs that interfere with prosthetic fitting. The initial surgery should spare all length possible, particularly the elbow joint. A well-healed surgical site with good distal soft tissue coverage of the bony end is an optimal result and facilitates prosthetic use.

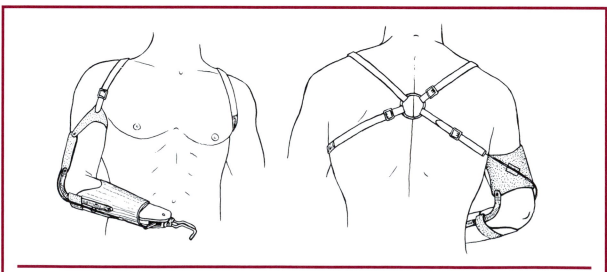

FIGURE 2. Below-elbow prosthesis. (From Jebson PJL, Kasdan ML: Hand Secrets. Philadelphia, Hanley & Belfus, 1998, p 187.)

Potential Disease Complications

Upper limb amputations may result in pain in the residual limb, joint contractures in the remaining part of the limb, and severe phantom and residual limb pain.

Potential Treatment Complications

Possible complications include postoperative infections, postoperative failure of the surgical wounds to heal, side effects from drugs used to manage phantom pain, skin breakdown from a poorly fitting prosthesis, and depression brought on by the difficulties of adjusting to limb loss.

References

1. Leonard J, Meier R: Upper and lower extremity prosthetics. In Delisa J, Gans BM (eds): Rehabilitation Medicine: Principles and Practice. Philadelphia, Lippincott-Raven, 1998, pp 669–696.
2. Dillingham TR, Pezzin LE, MacKenzie EJ: Incidence, acute care length of stay, and discharge to rehabilitation of traumatic amputee patients: an epidemiologic study. Arch Phys Med Rehabil 1998;79(3):279–287.
3. Dillingham TR, Pezzin LE, MacKenzie EJ: Racial differences in the incidence of limb loss secondary to peripheral vascular disease: A population-based study (unpublished observations).
4. Dillingham TR: Rehabilitation of the upper limb amputee. In Dillingham TR, Belandres P (eds): Rehabilitation of the Injured Combatant. Washington, DC, Office of the Surgeon General, 1998, pp 33–77.
5. Vaida G, Friedmann LW: Postamputation phantoms: A review. Phys Med Rehabil Clin North Am 1991;2(2):325–353.

94 Amputation: Lower Limb

Michelle Gittler, MD

Definition

Approximately 70% of lower extremity amputations in adults are the result of complications of diabetes and peripheral vascular disease. Most of these amputations occur in people age 60 years and older. Trauma is the next most common cause of lower extremity amputation (22%) followed by tumors (5%). However, in children ages 10 to 20 years, tumor is the most common cause of both upper and lower extremity amputations. Male amputees outnumber female amputees in disease 2.1:1 and trauma 7.2:1.[1] While the exact number of lower extremity amputations performed in the United States is not known, it is estimated that approximately 24,000 are at the below knee level and 30,000 are above the knee.

Symptoms

Obviously, the postoperative or post-traumatic sequela of an amputation is that the patient is missing all or part of a limb. Additionally there may be associated symptoms such as phantom limb sensation and/or pain, stump pain, and pain from skin breakdown.

Phantom limb sensation is a phenomenon that includes the perception that the extremity is still present and occasionally distorted in position. Phantom limb pain is differentiated as a painful perception within the absent body part. Phantom limb sensation typically fades away within the first year after amputation, usually in a "telescoping" phenomenon. This includes the perception that the distal aspect of the limb that is the foot is moving closer and closer to the site of amputation.

The incidence of phantom limb pain is variable and has been reported from 0% to virtually 100%. Patients may describe the foot or the absent limb as cramping, or they may describe a stabbing feeling. Stump and residual limb pain is perceived in the residual limb in the region of the amputation. The incidence of stump pain has been reported between 10% to 25% but may be diffuse or focal and is commonly associated with neuroma, which is palpable around the amputation site.

Physical Examination

Wound healing, range of motion, muscle strength, incisional integrity, and visualization of the contralateral foot are mandatory components of the examination. The unaffected foot is assessed for areas of (potential) breakdown, including toes, plantar surface of the foot, and web spaces. Referral for podiatry care and appropriate shoes (e.g., extra depth toe box, rocker bottom) may prevent major limb amputation.

Skin breakdown is typically a result of pressure or shear forces applied in a residual limb and/or at the amputation (i.e., incisional) site. Skin breakdown can range from abrasions from tape or the unraveling or unwrapping of an ACE wrap to true partial- or full-thickness pressure sores from an improperly positioned limb. Pressure sore phenomenon typically occurs at bony prominences. The fibular head, hamstring tendons, patellar tendon, medial-lateral femoral condyle, and anterior distal tibia should routinely be examined for skin breakdown.

Joint contractures are a loss of range of motion at a joint. They may be conceptualized as functional or mechanical. Functional contractures are the result of (inappropriate) positioning. A below knee amputee may develop knee flexion contractures merely by sitting with the knee flexed. Similarly, a hip flexion contracture may occur simply from sitting. A mechanical contracture may occur as the result of unopposed muscle action. In the above knee amputee, the insertion of the hip adductors are sacrificed, leaving the unopposed (and firmly attached) hip abductors. This results in an abduction contracture.

In the above knee (AK) amputee, the range-of-motion evaluation should include hip flexion/extension adduction/abduction. An AK prosthesis can functionally accommodate up to a 20-degree flexion contracture; a contracture greater than this makes prosthetic fitting and successful ambulation less likely. Strength should also be assessed, and grades of ≥ 4/5 in hip flexion/extension and abduction will help to facilitate ambulation.

For the below knee (BK) and Syme's amputee, knee flexion and extension are evaluated, as are medial and lateral knee stability. Knee extension muscle strength should be ≥ 4/5 for successful ambulation with a prosthesis.

Stump or residual limb pain is assessed first by inspection. Areas of obvious necrosis indicating poor blood flow may require surgical debridement. Non-healing incisions are manifestations of ischemia, underlying hematoma, or frank abscess. The surrounding area should be palpated and assessed for induction and discharge; an attempt should be made to "milk" drainage or fluctuance. Sutures (if present) may need to be removed to facilitate evacuation of the abscess or hematoma. In some instances, the incision may need to be reopened for drainage and healing to take place.

Stump pain without signs or symptoms of infection should be evaluated for neuroma (careful palpation, etc.). Stump pain with or without skin breakdown may be also be due to poor prosthetic fit, so the fit of the prosthesis ought to be evaluated. Non-blanchable erythema is a pressure sore until proven otherwise, and the prothesis should not be worn until appropriate adjustments are made. Bruising at the distal aspect of the stump in the prosthetic wearer may be indicative of a poor prosthetic fit (i.e., loss of total contact or a choke phenomenon); this can progress to venous hyperplasia, which predisposes the individual to fissuring and infection.

Functional Limitations

Functional limitations are largely dependent on the premorbid status of the individual.

An otherwise healthy person who has sustained a traumatic limb amputation or an individual who had been ambulating with crutches or another assistive device prior to having an amputation (often because of a non–weight-bearing status on the affected limb) will probably be discharged from the acute care setting to home with outpatient services, at an "ambulatory" level with the appropriate assistive device.

An older individual or person with multiple co-morbidities may be at the wheelchair level secondary to deconditioning and/or inadequate cardiopulmonary reserve to ambulate with an assistive device. This person may have had an acute or subacute rehabilitation hospital stay after the acute care hospitalization.

Functional limitations due to pain are associated with an inability to participate in ongoing activities of daily living. In general, symptoms of phantom sensation tend not to be an issue, whereas phantom pain can be severely limiting, preventing a person from participating in pre-prosthetic and prosthetic rehabilitation. Functional limitations related to stump or residual limb pain include inability to tolerate stump shrinkage via appropriate modalities as well as an ability to tolerate gait training with a prosthesis. To accommodate stump pain, the patient may develop gait deviations to decrease pressure under the aspect of the residual limb and may find functional ambulation significantly curtailed.

Joint contractures may result in an inability to wear a prosthesis which would obviously limit mobility.

Diagnostic Studies

There are no specific indicated tests for the outpatient management of the amputee.

The individual with phantom limb pain may benefit from diagnostic as well as therapeutic sympathetic nerve block. Occasionally, electrodiagnostic tests (EMG and nerve conduction studies) are helpful to differentiate symptoms of radiculopathy or other pathology in the phantom limb.

In the younger amputee, it is occasionally necessary to obtain plain x-rays of the residual limb to assess the bony overgrowth; however, this is typically visually evident upon inspection.

Differential Diagnosis

None

Treatment

Initial

Initial treatment focuses on edema control and shaping of the residual limb as well as wound healing, prevention of contractures, and pain management.

Options for edema control are listed in Table 1.[2,3]

Patients with a BK amputation have the potential for knee flexion and hip flexion contractures as a result of positioning (usually, sitting in wheelchair or in bed). Therefore, avoiding pillows under the knee and promoting lying prone in bed can be helpful.

Persons with an AK amputation may also develop hip flexion contractures as a result of sitting. Additionally, there is the tendency for hip abduction contractures to develop, so positioning the hip in relative adduction, avoiding pillows under the residual limb, and promoting the prone position are essential.

Phantom sensation is not typically painful, although it can be frightening for the patient. The best treatment is to reassure that patient that this is a normal reaction after amputation. Patient education and reassurance as well as ongoing tactile input (i.e., massaging the distal residual limb and utilizing the limb) will enhance the treatment of phantom sensation pain. There are many proposed treatments for phantom pain; however, there is no one definitive treatment that seems to work best. Pharmacologic intervention includes non-narcotic and narcotic analgesics; nonsteroidal anti-inflammatory drugs (NSAIDS); anti-convulsants, particularly carbamazepine and gabapentin; and antidepressants.

TABLE 1. Treatment Options for Edema Control

In a BK amputee, options include:

• **_An above knee cast_**

ADVANTAGES	DISADVANTAGES
Prevents knee flexion contracture	Bulky, awkward, heavy to move
Provides protection	Unable to visualize wound
No patient "skill" or management necessary to remove	Unable to remove
Very low cost	Potential for skin breakdown

• **_A "stump shrinker"_**

ADVANTAGES	DISADVANTAGES
Easy to don/doff	Cost—may need to be replaced after stump has begun to shrink
Enables visualization of wound	
Accustoms individual to using a sock	
Provides shaping of residual limb	

• **_Rigid removable dressing_** (Fig. 1)

ADVANTAGES	DISADVANTAGES
Excellent for preparing residual limb for eventual prosthesis	Therapist, physician, or prosthetist must be skilled in fabrication
Fosters patient independence in assessing need for stump socks	Potential for skin breakdown if applied incorrectly
Good edema management	
Provides some soft tissue protection	
Able to view wound	

• **_Elastic bandage (ACE wrap)_**

ADVANTAGES	DISADVANTAGES
Easily available	Requires excellent dexterity for patient to don/doff
Able to visualize wound	Potential for shear injury as/if wrap unravels
Accommodates all shapes and sizes	Must be reapplied multiple times/day secondary to potential loosening
Good edema control	

In an AK amputee, options include:
    Stump shrinker
    ACE wrap

Same advantages and disadvantages as described for BK amputee

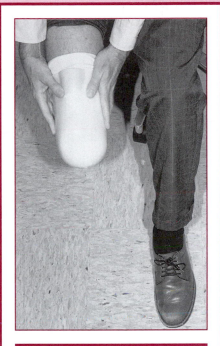

FIGURE 1. Application of the removable rigid dressing. (From Lennard TA: Pain Procedures in Clinical Practice, 2nd ed. Philadelphia, Hanley & Belfus, 2000, p 79.)

Rehabilitation

In physical therapy, pre-prosthetic training focuses on independence in mobility from the ambulatory or wheelchair level, avoidance of hip and knee contractures, and residual limb management. Prosthetic training is initiated once the limb is ready and the prosthesis is fabricated. Description of prostheses is beyond the scope of this chapter.[4] When the prosthesis has been fabricated, an outpatient appointment should be scheduled that is attended by the patient and prosthetist. A basic evaluation of the fit of the prosthesis is conducted, and referral for physical therapy that focuses on prosthetic training is made at that time. Either the prosthetist or the physical therapist should teach the patient how to put on and take off the prosthesis as well as when to add socks for a better fit. The patient should also be encouraged to routinely inspect the skin on the stump (often done best with a long-handled mirror).

Occupational therapy can include pre-prosthetic training that consists of identifying necessary equipment (e.g., toilet safety frame, tub transfer bench) and establishing independence in self-care from the wheelchair or ambulatory level using just the unaffected limb (single limb stance). Occupational therapy can also be ordered when the patient is independent with the prosthesis to establish independence in self-care, particularly with lower extremity dressing and homemaking while wearing the prosthesis.

Procedures

Other treatments for postamputation phantom pain include sympathetic blocks.

Surgery

Surgery is indicated when a residual limb requires wound revision or higher level of amputation. Hamstring releases have a limited or no role since they would inhibit the ability to walk. There does not appear to be any rule for surgical stump revision as a procedure for phantom pain.

There are little data to promote dorsal root entry zone, dorsal rhizotomy, dorsal column tractotomy, thalamotomy, or cortical resection.

Potential Disease Complications

The most common complications include dehiscence/breakdown of the incision or nonhealing wound(s). Wound infection is the most likely etiology for dehiscence or nonhealing. A trial of conservative management including antibiotics (after obtaining culture) and appropriate local wound care is reasonable. Increasing wound necrosis, foul drainage, or fever/chills warrant re-evaluation by the surgeon.

Other potential complications may involve cardiac ischemia, as a heretofore inactive (i.e., energy conservative) individual begins using 100% more energy for gait training.[5] A reasonable guideline for gait training includes assessment of an individual's ability to ambulate with the intact lower extremity with crutches or another assistive device. This consumes approximately 60% more energy than normal walking. A person who is not able to gait train (hop on one foot) using an assistive device is probably not a potential ambulator.

Potential Treatment Complications

Once the prosthesis has been fabricated, skin breakdown is the most common complication. Breakdown commonly occurs at the distal anterior tibia (clapper-in-bell phenomenon—a result of continued forward motion of the residual limb in the socket during swing phase), the hamstring tendons (tight brim), and the patellar tendon.

Patients should be instructed to inspect these areas and immediately report to the prosthetist signs of persistent, non-blanchable erythema. The prosthesis should not be worn until modifications are made.

Medication side effects are well known and depend on the particular medication being used.

References
1. Leonard EI, McAnelly RD, Lomba M, Faulker VW: Lower limb prosthesis in physical medicine and rehabilitation. Ed. Braddom, 200 p. 279
2. Mueller MS: Comparison of rigid removable dressings and elastic bandages in preprosthetic management of patients with below-knee amputations. Phys Ther 1982;62:1438–1441.
3. Wu Y, Krick H: Rigid removable dressings for below knee amputees. Clinical Prosthetics Orthotics 1987;11:33–44.
4. Bowker JH (ed): Atlas of Limb Prosthetics. American Association of Orthopedic Surgery. St. Louis, Mosby, 1981.
5. Esquenazi A: Gait analysis and the metabolic energy expenditure of amputee ambulation. Seattle, AAPMR 1998.
6. Loesner J: Pain after amputation. In Bonica J (ed): The Management of Pain, 2nd ed. Baltimore, Williams & Wilkins, 1990, pp 244–256.
7. New Developments in Prosthetics and Orthotics. Phys Med Rehabil Clin North Am 2000;11:559–568.
8. Prosthetics. Phys Med Rehabil Clin North Am 1991;2:253–436 (complete volume).

95 Ankylosing Spondylitis

Steven E. Braverman, MD

Synonyms

Seronegative
spondyloarthropathy

Seronegative arthritis

Seronegative
spondyloarthritides

ICD-9 Code

720.0
Ankylosing spondylitis

Definition

Ankylosing spondylitis (AS) is one of a group of rheumatic disorders that affect the spinal column, sacroiliac (SI) joints, and the peripheral joints. It involves inflammation of the enthesis (tissues attaching tendons, ligaments, and joint capsules to bone)—called *enthesitis*—and inflammation of the synovium—called *synovitis*.

It is not associated with the presence of rheumatoid factor or antinuclear antibodies. The onset of symptoms is usually in late adolescence or early adulthood and is three times more common in men than women. There is a genetic association with the HLA-B27 histocompatability antigen, but this marker is neither specific to the disease nor necessary to make the diagnosis.

The most common sites of involvement are sacroiliac, apophyseal, and discovertebral joints of the spine; costochondral and manubriosternal joints; paravertebral ligaments; and attachments of the Achilles tendon and plantar fascia. Peripheral joint involvement is less common but occurs in the more severe forms of the disease.[1]

Symptoms

Ankylosing spondylitis should be considered in any young adult patient who complains of insidious onset of worsening, dull, lumbosacral back pain with progressive morning stiffness. Pain in the area of the SI joints is common, as is prolonged stiffness after inactivity. Neurologic symptoms such as parasthesias and motor weakness are absent. Tendon and ligament attachment sites may become painful and swollen. One third of patients may develop hip or shoulder pain. Chest pain with deep breathing and eye pain with blurred vision are late symptoms of more severe disease.

Physical Examination

The most typical findings involve signs of decreased spine mobility as measured by the modified Schober's test, finger to floor distance, occiput to wall distance, and chest expansion. A Gaenslen's test may be positive (Fig. 1).

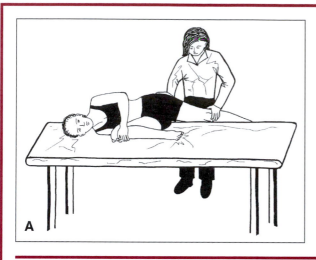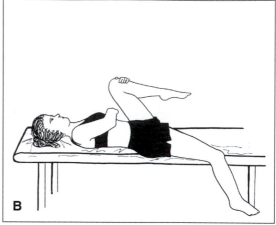

FIGURE 1. Gaenslen's test. *A*, With patient in side lying position, clinician extends test leg. *B*, With patient supine, test leg is extended over edge of table. Pain in the SI joints indicates a positive test.

On palpation, the lower paraspinal muscles and SI joints are tender. Ligamentous and tendinous attachment sites are tender in areas of enthesitis, particularly around the heel and tibial tuberosity.

Peripheral joint swelling and pain with decreased range of motion are found in about one third of patients. A discolored and edematous iris with circumferential corneal congestion occurs in iritis and anterior uveitis.

Functional Limitations

The AS patient's functional limitations are typically related to spine mobility and dysfunction. The three best predictors of decreased function are cervical rotation, modified Schober's test, and pain.[2] The Bath Ankylosing Spondylitis Functional Index[3] is a functional assessment measurement index utilized by clinicians specializing in the care of AS patients.

Early on, decreased spine range of motion is secondary to pain and spasm and improves with treatment. Most dysfunction is mild and self-limiting, with 90% of AS patients remaining employed.

In severe disease, positioning from hip flexion contractures, thoracic kyphosis, and loss of cervical rotation decrease patients' ability to view activities in front of them and side to side. Limitations in chest-wall motion lead to a reliance on diaphragmatic breathing and a secondary drop in aerobic capacity.

Diagnostic Studies

Standard spine and SI joint radiographs show ossification of spinal ligaments and apophyseal joints with eventual ankylosis, leading to the classical bamboo spine appearance. SI joint findings are symmetric with bony erosions, sclerosis, and blurring of the subchondral bone plate eventually progressing to complete ankylosis. Bony erosions at entheses are common. Hip x-rays demonstrate symmetric and concentric joint narrowing with subchondral sclerosis. Ankylosis is found in very severe disease. Computed tomography (CT) scans and magnetic resonance images (MRIs) are more sensitive in early disease.

HLA-B27 is positive in 90% of AS patients. A negative test suggests milder disease with a better prognosis. Rheumatoid factor and ANA are negative. Erythrocyte sedimentation rate and C-reactive protein levels correlate with disease activity.

Differential Diagnosis

Rheumatoid arthritis

Other seronegative spondyloarthropathies (e.g., Reiter's syndrome, psoriatic arthritis, enteropathic spondylitis, Behçet's syndrome)

Treatment

Initial

The primary medical treatment for AS is nonsteroidal anti-inflammatory drugs (NSAIDs). NSAIDs provide symptomatic relief but do not halt progression of the disease. No single NSAID is more effective than any other in AS. The choice of NSAID is based on individual therapeutic response, compliance, and side effects. COX-2 inhibitors are not more effective than other NSAIDs but may have less gastrointestinal toxicity. Intermittent NSAID dosing (taking the medication only during periods of exacerbation) is as effective as continuous dosing and results in fewer side effects.[4] Pulsed methyl prednisolone at 15 mg/kg for 3 days may be effective for NSAID resistant flares.[5] Sulfasalazine is ineffective except in cases with a predominance of peripheral disease, inflammatory bowel disease, or psoriasis.[6]

Iritis is treated with pupillary dilatation and corticosteroid drops. Low-dose amitriptyline (10–50 mg qhs) may help with pain and sleep.

Rehabilitation

Physical therapy and home exercise programs may improve spine mobility and lead to improvements in flexibility.[7,8] The benefit to these programs is lost once the exercise is discontinued. Hip range of motion increases with regular stretching utilizing the contraction/relaxation/stretching technique.[7] Strengthening of back and hip extensors should follow the flexibility exercises. Aerobic activities may maintain chest expansion. However, an exercise stress test should be considered prior to an aerobic program if aortic insufficiency is suspected.

In general, splinting and spinal orthoses are not effective, but foot orthotics may help with calcaneal enthesopathies. A firm mattress may help with sleep. Wide mirrors assist drivers with limited cervical mobility.[8]

Procedures

Periarticular corticosteroid injections and fluoroscopic guided SI joint injections may help during NSAID resistant flares or when NSAIDs are contraindicated.[9] Local injections for enthesopathies may be effective, but injections in and around the Achilles tendon insertion should be avoided.

Surgery

Hip and knee arthroplasties should be considered prior to joint ankylosis. Spinal osteotomy is a risky procedure for patients with severe kyphosis.[10]

Potential Disease Complications

Potential complications include iritis/uveitis, inflammatory bowel disease, aortic insufficiency and aortic root dilatation, osteoporosis (best evaluated with bone densitometry of the femur), spine fracture with spinal cord injury (rare).

Potential Treatment Complications

NSAIDs may produce gastrointestinal and renal toxicity, and corticosteroids increase risk of osteoporosis. Total hip arthroplasty increases the risk of anterior dislocations, and spinal osteotomy carries the risk of paralysis and a mortality rate of up to 4%.[10]

References

1. Klippel JH: Primer on Rheumatic Disease. Arthritis Foundation, 1999, pp 189–193.
2. Dalyan M, Guner A, Tuncer S, et al: Disability in ankylosing spondylitis. Disability Rehabilitation 1999;21(2):74–79.
3. Calin A, Garrett S, Whitelock H, et al: A new approach to defining functional ability in ankylosing spondylitis: The development of the Bath Ankylosing Spondylitis Functional Index. J Rheum 1994;21:2281–2285.
4. Koehler L, Kuipers J, Zeidler H: Managing seronegative spondarthitides. Rheumatology 2000;39: 360–368.
5. Peters ND, Ejstrup L: Intravenous methyl prednisolone pulse therapy in AS. Scand J Rheumatology 1992;21:134–138.
6. Clegg DO, Reda DJ, Abdellatif M: Comparison of sulfasalazine and placebo for the treatment of axial and peripheral articular manifestations of the seronegative arthropathies: A Department of Veterans Affairs Comparative Study. Arthritis Rheum 1999;42:2325–2329.
7. Viitanen JV, Lehtinen K, Suni J, Kautiainen H: Fifteen months' follow-up of intensive inpatient physiotherapy and exercise in ankylosing spondylitis. Clin Rheumatol 1995;14(4):413–419.
8. Gall V: Exercise in the spondyloarthropathies. Arthritis Care Research 1994;7(4):215–220.
9. Luukainen R, Nissila M, Sanila M, et al: Periarticular corticoid treatment of the sacroiliac joint in patients with seronegative spondyloarthropathy. Clin Exp Rheum 1999;17:88–90.
10. Van Royen BJ, de Gast A. Lumbar osteotomy for correction of thoracolumbar deformity in ankylosing spondylitis: a structure review of three methods of treatment. Ann Rheum Dis 1999;58:399–406.

Note: The opinions in this article are those of the author and not necessarily those of the U.S. Army or Department of Defense.

96 Burns

M. Catherine Spires, MD

Definition

Burn injury can result from flame, electrical exposure, chemical injury, or radiation. In the United States, the number of burn injuries has declined significantly. However, approximately 1.25 million persons are treated for burns each year, and 4% of these individuals require hospitalization and specialized burn care.[1] Injuries covering less than 10% of the body surface area typically do not cause death or hemodynamic instability, except in the elderly, the very young, or those with inhalation injury.[2,3]

Burn injury can be classified in a number of ways. The most typical is to grade the injury by the depth of tissue damage. Superficial injuries, or *first degree burns*, disrupt the epidermis without injuring deep layers of skin. Erythema, but no blistering, is present. Once healed, typically in 1 to 3 days, no scarring results.

Superficial partial thickness burns, also sometimes called superficial *second degree burns*, injure the superficial dermis as well as the epidermis. Blistering is present, and the wound usually heals within 14 days. Pigment changes may be observed once healing is complete.

Deep superficial burns result in damage to the dermis but spare skin appendages. These wounds may take up to 21 days to heal, and skin grafting may be performed to speed healing and reduce scarring. These injuries result in severe scarring, skin fragility, sensory loss, and impaired apocrine function.

Third degree burns result in full thickness skin loss. Grafting is required unless the wound is small and amenable to excision and primary closure. In addition to the aforementioned sequelae, areas of grafting are fragile and lack normal moisture and lubrication since normal skin appendages are absent.

Burns affecting bone, tendon, and muscle were previously termed fourth degree burns. Skin grafting and reconstruction are necessary, and often amputation is required if the limb is not viable.[4]

Symptoms

The symptoms of burn injury are a direct result of changes in the skin structure and function. Because full thickness burns and those involving the deep dermis disturb or destroy oil and sweat glands, patients experience problems with dry, friable skin, which is intolerant of mechanical irritation. Pruritus is a common complaint. The skin does not tolerate sun exposure, perfumes, and other chemical irritants. Because the skin's role in thermal regulation is disrupted, many patients are intolerant of heat or cold.

In deep partial and full thickness burns, scar tissue replaces normal skin. Scars appear a few weeks after wound closure. Excessive scar tissue may develop, creating hypertrophic scars, which are characteristically red and raised. These scars may prevent normal joint motion. If loss of motion is due to true joint dysfunction and not from overlying scarring, heterotopic ossification should be considered. This occurs commonly in patients with major burns and can affect any joint. The elbow is the most common site affected.

Lastly, patients can present with symptoms of weakness, numbness, or paresthesias. Mononeuropathies are not unusual in this population. Mononeuropathy may result from poor positioning, ill fitting splints, local scarring, and heterotopic ossification.[4,5]

During the acute period, pain is a major issue, especially with injuries that preserve cutaneous nerve endings. Full thickness burns are not painful during the acute period. As healing occurs, patients may experience pain associated with nerve injury, joint contracture, and scarring. Pruritus can be a major source of discomfort as well.

Generalized deconditioning is often seen after an acute injury. Because the physiologic demands of surviving a major insult such as a burn, patients fatigue easily, even when performing basic mobility, transfer, and gait activities. Poor endurance is particularly evident in the patient with pre-morbid diseases of the cardiopulmonary, musculoskeletal, or neurologic systems.

After a life threatening injury such as a major burn, the clinician must keep in mind post traumatic stress disorder (PTSD). Symptoms of nightmare, flashbacks, exaggerated startle response, and avoiding reminders of the accident that persist greater than 1 month postinjury are indicative of PTSD.[6]

Fatigue may be a result of an underlying anemia from multiple surgical procedures, metabolic causes, or deconditioning from bed rest or inactivity. Fatigue may indicate depression or other mental health problems.

Sleep difficulties may be due to airway changes from an inhalation injury, substance abuse, depression, or a post-traumatic stress disorder.

Physical Examination

On acute examination of the burn survivor, assessing the airway and taking vital signs should be priorities. Examination of the upper airway is best assesssed by nasopharyngoscopy. If the exam is normal during the first 4 hours, it still may need to be repeated 6 hours later, since edema can present over time. The lower airway can be assessed by fiberoptic bronchoscopy. It is also critical to monitor pulses acutely and to assess the extent of the soft tissues injured.

In the post-acute setting, the focus will be on scarring that presents over any area that sustained deep partial thickness or full thickness injury to the skin. Scarring will also be present over areas of skin grafting. Occasionally, skin donor sites will scar but typically mildly. Scarring may occur over areas that will interfere with joint mobility, change body contours, and alter one's appearance.

Once the wounds are closed, the initial scars are flat and reddened. A few weeks later the scar grows above the skin's normal contour, creating an irregular surface. The hypertrophic scar that develops is firm and reddened but blanches with pressure.

As the scar maturation progresses, the patient will complain of dry pruritic skin. Burn trauma can disrupt or destroy oil gland, preventing normal lubrication of the skin. The skin is dry, fragile, and easily traumatized.

Patients who have sustained a severe injury should have a complete neurologic examination to assess for peripheral neuropathy, mononeuropathy, and the extent of sensory loss due to skin grafting and scarring.

Scarring, prolonged immobilization, or underlying process such as heterotopic ossification can precipitate joint contracture. Range of motion, actively and passively, should be assessed and monitored regularly. If range of motion is being lost, the clinician should maintain a low threshold for evaluating the patient for heterotopic ossification.

Functional Limitations

The location of the scarring is critical. If it is present over a joint, the scar can limit joint range of motion, impairing the patient's ability to ambulate, perform activities of daily living, and engage in work or recreational activities.

Depending on the location and extent, scarring can create a cosmetic crisis for the injured individual. The appearance of some patients may be totally altered, interfering with their ability to go out in public or relate to family, peers, or co-workers. Burn scars are more than skin deep and may precipitate many psychosocial problems, including depression, anxiety, and sexual dysfunction.

Because severe burn injury disrupts the sweat glands and impairs normal perspiration, patients have difficulty tolerating heat and cold. This is problematic if the injury is extensive and covers a large body surface area.

Burn specialists may be asked to rate the patient's final level of impairment. These patients are among the most difficult to obtain work disability. Many impairment scales do not acknowledge the individual's intolerance of chemicals, heat and cold sensitivity, sensory impairment, or reduced endurance. Mental health disorders, such as PTSD and adjustment disorders related to returning to the site of injury or similar settings, are also often underrecognized. In the end, it is the clinician's responsibility to determine when the patient is ready for school or work. The decision is complex and requires consideration of not only the physical impairments and the sequelae of such, but also assessment of the patient's pre-morbid health, age, schooling, social situation, and mental health.[4]

Diagnostic Studies

Diagnostic workup is dependent on the patient's complaints, history, and examination. The patient who complains of impaired range of motion may have this difficulty not only because of the restriction of the skin secondary to scarring over a joint, but joint pathology must be considered as well. Burn patients are at risk for heterotopic ossification, which most often occurs in the posterior lateral elbow, the shoulder, and hips. It is often bilateral. Bone scan may demonstrate increased activity 2 to 3 weeks before radiographic changes of abnormal ossification are evident. Serum alkaline phosphatase level is often increased in burn patients as it is in individuals with spinal cord or traumatic brain injuries. Underlying arthritis can also be a problem.

Patients may complain of signs and symptoms consistent with a peripheral mononeuropathy. These may result from poor positioning techniques during acute hospitalization, improper use of splints, or as a result of the original injury. Patients who sustained an electrical injury may develop mononeuropathy as a late effect. These mononeuropathies do not necessarily occur at the site of the electrical injury. When a mononeuropathy is suspected, electrodiagnostic testing is indicated.

Pre-existing peripheral neuropathies can complicate the picture. Patients who have previous condition, such as diabetes mellitus or alcoholism, are at increased risk for peripheral mononeuropathies as well as exacerbation of the pre-existing peripheral neuropathy. It must also be remembered that patients who have been critically ill from burn injury may demonstrate the residua of a critical peripheral neuropathy or myopathy.

Patients reporting symptoms of anxiety should have a workup for metabolic causes and psychologic evaluation.

Patients who have experienced a significant inhalation injury should be questioned regarding their pulmonary endurance. Those with residual effects on history or examination should undergo pulmonary function testing for the presence of pulmonary problems, such as a diffusion abnormality.

Differential Diagnosis

None

Treatment

Initial

Tables 1 and 2 list some of the agents used to initially treat an acute chemical injury. Wounds are typically treated with silver sulfadiazine. Other agents include betadine, silver nitrate, and mafenide. Wound care is generally done 1 to 2 times daily.

Pain control is critical in the initial stages because it causes a rise in heart rate, blood pressure, and metabolic rate. Also, poor pain control will cause the patient to fear movement, thereby increasing the risk of severe contractures. Inadequate pain control will also contribute to anxiety and depression. Narcotics are the first line agents acutely.

Limb edema and scarring are also priorities in the initial stages and are generally managed with elevation; excellent wound care; and later, specialized garments. Range of motion is also important throughout the care of the burn patient. Commercially available mouth appliances for the prevention of microstomia are available.

During the acute period it is important to educate the patient about the injury and to encourage the patient's independence in exercise and mobility. This will facilitate the patient's role in his or her recovery and reestablish a sense of control over his or her life.

Because of the systemic impact of serious burn injuries, nutrition is a major concern. The extensive damage created by a burn challenges the homeostasis and nutritional status of the body. Increased energy expenditure needed for rebuilding lost tissue and warding off infection markedly increases the caloric needs of the seriously burned patient. As a result, patients require supplemental nutrition and often require tube feeding to supplement oral intake. The undernourished patient will require a longer time to heal and will experience higher infection and complication rates.

TABLE 1. Chemical Agents

Agent	Common Use	Characteristics	Agent to Remove or Dilute	Systemic Effects
Oxidizing agents				
Chromic acid	Metal cleansing	Ulcerates, blisters	Water lavage	
Potassium permanganate	Bleach, deodorizer, disinfectant	Thick, brownish purple eschar	Water lavage, eggwhite solution	
Sodium hypochlorite	Bleach, deodorizer, disinfectant	Local irritation, inflammation	Water lavage, milk, eggwhite solution, paste, starch	
Corrosive agents				
Phenol	Deodorant, sanitizer, plastics, dyes, fertilizers, explosives, disinfectants	Soft white eschar, brown stain when eschar removed, mild to no pain	Copious water lavage, polyethylene glycol solution, vegetable oil	Minor exposure: tachycardia, arrhythmias Significant exposure: depression, hypothermia, cardiac depression, respiratory depression
Phosphorus (white)	Explosives, poisons, insecticides, fertilizers	Necrotic with yellowish color, garlic odor, glows in dark, pain	Lavage with 1% copper sulfate, cover with castor oil	Nephrotoxic, hepatic necrosis
Sodium metal, lye, KOH, NaOH, NH$_4$OH, LiOH, Ba$_2$(OH)$_3$, CA(OH)$_3$	Cleaning agent (washing powder, drain cleaner, paint remover), cement	Soft, gelatinous, brown eschar	Sodium metal: oil immersion Lye: water lavage	
Protoplasmic poisons				
Salt formers (acids), Tungstic, picric, sulfasalicylic, tannic, cresylic, acetate, formic, trichloroacetic	Industrial	Thin, hard eschar	Water lavage	Nephrotoxic, hepatic necrosis
Metabolic competitor/inhibitor Oxalic acid	Industrial	Chalky white ulcers	Large volume calcium salts, copious water lavage, intravenous calcium	Hypocalcemia
Hydrofluoric	Industrial	Painful, deep ulcerations	Water lavage, subcutaneous calcium, subcutaneous magnesium sulfate	Hypocalcemia, hypomagnesemia

Patients often have chronic problems with pruritus and dry, friable skin. Treatments initiated during the acute phase may need to be lifelong. Pruritus is controlled by using skin moisturizers. Patients need to use moisturizers that are hypoallergenic and do not contain perfumes. Typically, the patient needs to use topical moisturizers at least twice a day. Often, oral medications are necessary to control these symptoms, such as diphenhydramine or hydroxyzine. In severe cases, patients may require training in relaxation or other techniques to minimize the discomfort associated with pruritus.

Skin fragility is also a factor. Working in sunlight, extreme temperatures, or around chemicals is to be avoided. Extra protection will be needed to prevent skin breakdown and tissue disruption.

Sensory loss or impairment must be also considered. Like other patients with sensory impairment, burn patients must protect their limbs and skin from trauma, stress, shear or thermal injury, and heated or frozen materials.

Patient education should address skin care and protection. Patients should be counseled to avoid ultraviolet light exposure. They are at increase risk for sunburn and the ill effects of ultraviolet light. Sun blocking agents of SPF 35 or higher should be used. Clothing, including hats, that cover injured areas should be recommended.

TABLE 2. Treatment Measures for Specific Chemical Burns

Irrigation with water

Chromic acid	Sulfosalicylic acid	Dichromate salts
Cantharides	Acetic acid	Tungstic acid
Lyes and alkalis	Cresylic acid	Picric acid
Potassium hydroxide	Potassium permanganate	Tannic acid
Sodium hydroxide	Dimethyl sulfoxide (DMSO)	Trichloroacetic acid
Ammonium hydroxide	Sodium hypochlorite	Formic acid
Barium hydroxide	Phenol	Gasoline
Calcium hydroxide	Hydrofluoric acid	

Calcium salts irrigation and/or injection: hydrofluoric acid

Cover burn with oil: sodium metal, lithium metal, mustard gas

Special measures for certain chemicals

Sodium and lithium metals: pieces must be excised

Hydrofluoric acid: calcium gluconate injection

Phenol: Polyethylene glycol wipe

White phosphorus: copper sulfate irrigation

Alkyl mercury agents: debride and remove blister fluid

At times, patients require medications, such as a tricyclic antidepressant for depression. Group therapy with other burn survivors or one-to-one counseling with an experienced mental health professional may be needed.

Return to work or to school is an important step in the recovery of an individual who has sustained a severe burn injury. A number of factors must be considered in the timing of this return. The clinician must consider if any open wounds persist or are likely to recur. Obviously, these individuals cannot return to situations requiring food handling, patient care, child care, or settings requiring the use of chemicals.

Rehabilitation

Physical and occupational therapy is essential during the acute period to prevent the complications of immobilization. Early ambulation is essential to maintain mobility and strength. Maintaining joint range of motion is crucial during the acute period as well as through the entire recovery period. For burns that are deep partial thickness or deeper over a joint, therapy is prescribed to fabricate and fit splints to increase or maintain range of motion. Therapy is also prescribed for early exercise and to address problems with self-care and other daily activities.

Aggressive scar suppression begins once the wounds have healed. Hypertrophic scarring is controlled using burn suppression garments, silicone, and splinting. Scar suppression is achieved using elasticized garments that are custom fitted to provide at least 24 mm Hg of pressure to the site at risk for hypertrophic scarring. Several manufacturers of these garments exist. Scar suppression garments are worn 24 hours a day, except during bathing, for 12 to 24 months. These garments are no longer needed once the scar is supple and no longer red in color.[7] Typically, occupational therapists are skilled in measuring patients for customized garments as well as fabricating custom splints.

For areas that are difficult to apply pressure with a garment, such as the web spaces between the fingers, silicone sheeting can be cut to fit the area and placed under the garment.

Facial scar suppression is challenging. An experienced orthotist or occupational therapist can make a custom fitted clear thermoplastic face mask to cover the injured areas of the face. It is critical that the face mask be custom fabricated and must accurately fit the contours of the face to achieve appropriate compression to decrease scar formation.

Scarring about the mouth can result in loss of the normal mouth opening (microstomia). Commercial splints and custom mouth splints can be fitted to prevent loss of the normal mouth aperture. The patient must wear the device at all times, except during eating and oral hygiene, to prevent contracture of the oral aperture. These devices are necessary until scar maturation is achieved.

Therapy also addresses endurance training, and any ongoing problems with mobility or gait. Emphasis on correct posture and positioning will help to prevent gait deviations. Therapists can play a major role in helping a patient return to work, particularly if adaptive equipment is necessary.

Procedures

For the patient with serious burn injury, major debridement is typically surgically performed. Simple sharp debridement or mechanical debridement can be performed in the clinic with a scalpel or gauze. Hydrotherapy, using agitation, can also be a convenient means of debriding devitalized tissue.[8] Sometimes, enzymatic agents are indicated to remove tissue debris, but this can be uncomfortable for the patient and must be limited to small areas.

Temporary wound dressing may also be applied. Allograft (cadaver skin) is generally considered the best temporary dressing because it provides good vascularization of the wound bed. However, it is costly, and there is a concern over potential for viral infection transmission. These grafts generally last 2 to 3 weeks. Xenograft (pig skin) is less expensive but does not last as long or provide vascularization of the wound bed. There are also a number of synthetic dressings available.

Surgery

Initial surgeries typically involve grafts—often either split thickness or full thickness skin grafts. If non-surgical efforts to maintain or achieve normal range of motion fail, surgery should be considered. Surgery is indicated to release contracted skin and joint. Surgical procedures include simple releases, such as a Z-plasty or sophisticated reconstruction of a facial body contour.[9] For the patient with recurrent ulceration or skin breakdown, additional repeat skin grafting may be needed.[10]

Cosmesis can be a major indication for surgery as well as functional limitations. Plastic surgery to reconstruct an ear, reduce scarring over the face, or allow adolescent female breast development are critical reasons to proceed with surgery. However, this requires a collaborative relationship with the surgeon as well as an extensive discussion with and education of the patient. Often, patients who have sustained a major burn injury are unwilling to pursue further surgery even if the clinician believes significant functional or cosmetic gains are possible.

Potential Disease Complications

Scarring is the most common sequela of burn injury. Depending on the location and the extent of the scarring, other problems can develop. Loss of skin and soft tissue flexibility over a joint impairs range of motion.

Scarring can be disfiguring, negatively affecting the patient's sense of attractiveness and self-esteem. A burn injury can precipitate mental illness or exacerbate any pre-existing psychologic conditions.

Skin that sustains a significant burn injury does not tolerate sun exposure or chemical irritants. Because the skin's role in thermal regulation is disrupted, many patients are intolerant of heat or cold.

Heterotopic ossification can be severe enough to cause complete loss of joint function and cause joint ankylosis. Peripheral nerve entrapments, such as an ulnar mononeuropathy at the elbow, can occur as a result of heterotopic ossification.

Limb loss can occur with burn injury, especially injury secondary to high voltage electrical injury. Like other amputees, these patients require amputee rehabilitation and prosthetic restoration. Many burn patients require prostheses with liners that minimize the skin irritation and complications that are sometimes associated with prosthetic use.

Potential Treatment Complications

Treatment complications often result from a lack of aggressive treatment of burn scarring and the associated complications of loss of joint range of motion. The patient who does not receive aggressive range-of-motion exercise and scar suppression treatment develops limitations that affect independence in daily activities and mobility.

The use of oral medications to control pruritus may cause sedation and the risks associated with decreased alertness and impaired judgment.

Ill fitting splints or inappropriate positioning of a limb can lead to compression of peripheral nerves, causing a mononeuropathy, such as a peroneal mononeuropathy.

Overlooking signs and symptoms of depression, PTSD, and other psychosocial complications can lead to the further disability, additional injury, loss of psychosocial health and independence, suicide, and unintentional death.

References

1. Bringham PA, McLoughlin E: Burn incidence and medical care use in the United States: Estimate, trends, and data sources. J Burn Care Rehabil 1996;17:95–107.
2. Sheridan RL, Hinson MI, Laing MH, et al: Long-term outcomes of children surviving massive burns. JAMA 2000;283:69–73.
3. Saffle JR, Davis B, American Burn Association Registry Participant Group: Recent outcomes in the treatment of burn injury in the United States: A report from the American Burn Association Patient Registry. J Burn Care Rehabil 1995;16:219–232.
4. Spires MC: Rehabilitation of patients with burns. In Braddom R, Dumitru D (eds): Physical Medicine and Rehabilitation. Philadelphia,W.B. Saunders, 2000.
5. Helm PA, Kevorkian GC, Lusbaugh MS, et al: Burn injury: Rehabilitation management. Arch Phys Med Rehabil 1982;63:6–16.
6. Watkins PN, Cook E, May SR, Ehleben CM: Psychological stages in adaptation following burn injury: A method for facilitating psychological recovery of burn victims. J Burn Care Rehabil 1998;9:376–381.
7. Ward RS: Pressure therapy for the control of hypertrophic scar formation after burn injury: A history and review. J Burn Care Rehabil 1991;12:257–262.
8. Richard RL, Staley MJ: Burn Care and Rehabilitation: Principles and Practice. Philadelphia, F.A. Davis, 1994.
9. Achauer BM: Reconstructing the burned face. Clin Plastic Surg 1992;19:623–636.
10. Monafo WW: Initial management of burns. N Engl J Med 1996;335:1581–1586.

97 Cardiac Rehabilitation

Alan M. Davis, MD, PhD

Synonyms

None

ICD-9 Codes

410.00–410.92
Acute myocardial
infarction

411.0–411.89
Other acute and
subacute forms of
ischemic heart disease

412
Old myocardial infarction

413.0–413.9
Angina pectoris

414.0–414.9
Other forms of chronic
ischemic heart disease

429.2
Cardiovascular disease,
unspecified

V45.81
Aortocoronary bypass
status

Definition

Cardiac rehabilitation is the integrated treatment of individuals after cardiac events or procedures with the goals of maximizing physical function, promoting emotional adjustment, modifying cardiac risk factors, and addressing return to previous social roles and responsibilities. Cardiovascular diseases affect more than 5.9 million Americans. Cardiac diseases accounted for 41.2% of all deaths in 1997,[1] the leading cause of mortality in both men and women.

Outpatient cardiac rehabilitation may benefit individuals in the following diagnostic categories:

1. Acute myocardial infarction
2. Coronary artery bypass surgery
3. Coronary angioplasty
4. Cardiac transplant
5. Cardiac reduction surgery
6. Compensated congestive heart failure
7. Cardiac disease in addition to debility due to other medical illness

Symptoms

The individual with a recent cardiac event or procedure frequently complains of decreased endurance for walking or climbing stairs, increased dyspnea during physical activity, and fatigue. If arrhythmia is present, the patient may feel palpitations. Chest pain may accompany physical exertion or emotional stress. Pain due to surgical incisions of the extremities or chest wall may also be present. The person may feel anxious about any type of physical exercise, resumption of sexual activities, and his or her returning to work. Symptoms of heart failure, such as orthopnea and paroxysmal nocturnal dyspnea, may also be present.

Physical Examination

During the examination of the cardiac patient, the clinician should search for signs of complications following the myocardial infarction or cardiac procedure. Findings of congestive heart failure, such as rales, peripheral edema, or elevated jugular venous distention, should be evaluated. Surgical wounds, such as vascular harvest sites, arterial puncture sites, and sternotomy wounds, need evaluation before exercise programs are prescribed. Manual muscle testing of the extremities provides an indication of the degree of skeletal muscle atrophy due to decreased physical activity.

Functional Limitations

Functional limitations due to cardiac disease alone are related to the workload the myocardium can sustain before signs of cardiac dysfunction result. The workload achieved before symptom onset is generally decreased. Overall endurance is decreased. Most patients with uncomplicated cardiac cases are able to ambulate slowly and perform self-care upon discharge from the hospital. This alone does not guarantee quality of life for the treated individual. The degree and severity of cardiac impairment may limit a patient's physical progress and ultimate maximum level of function. Decreased endurance for walking, independent living skills, physically demanding labor, and recreational activities are addressed during cardiac rehabilitation. The patient may return to physically demanding activity such as heavy labor or competitive singles tennis after rehabilitation following coronary angioplasty or stenting without myocardial infarction. However, for the patient who experienced myocardial infarction complicated by congestive heart failure and arrhythmia, walking to a neighbor's home or performing the household chores may be limited by dyspnea. Further compromise of progress is related to the common co-morbidities of intrinsic lung disease, diabetes mellitus, and peripheral vascular disease. Advanced rheumatologic or orthopedic skeletal degeneration may require specific adaptations to allow for conditioning exercise.

Emotional stress and an individual's response to it may also produce functional limitations when considering return to social roles and responsibilities. Dysfunction such as ischemia or arrhythmia may be produced by either physical or emotional demands.[2] This may range from anxiety about physical exertion to major reactive depression. It has been argued that the best predictors of cardiac rehabilitation outcome are psychosocial rather than physiological.[3]

Diagnostic Studies

The clinician should evaluate the patient's lipid profile to guide pharmacologic and dietary management of hyperlipidemia and hypercholesterolemia. Tight diabetic control may decrease the rate of atheroma formation and glycosylated hemoglobin (hemoglobin A_{1C}) is used to ascertain the recent success of blood glucose control.

For the individual with dyspnea on exertion and the co-morbidity of lung disease, pulmonary function testing will clarify the contribution of obstructive or restrictive lung disease at rest. Treatable conditions such as reactive airways and hypoxia during exercise should be addressed before beginning cardiac rehabilitation for maximal benefit.

A sub-maximal exercise test may be administered prior to or immediately after hospital discharge for risk stratification.[4] *This does not guide the therapeutic exercise prescription.* Sub-maximal exercise testing is usually limited to 5 METS for patients older than 40 years or to 7 METS for patients 40 years old or younger. A symptom limited exercise test administered at 2 to 6 weeks after cardiac event or procedure provides the best guide to exercise prescription. The specific timing of exercise testing depends on the amount of myocardium damage, the need for return to work, and the practice pattern of the clinician administering the test. Typical functional exercise testing documents work capacity and cardiopulmonary function. Treadmill testing following a modified Naughton, a Naughton/Balke, or a ramp protocol is especially well suited to guide cardiac rehabilitation exercise training because these protocols use smaller increments of workload that more accurately portray functional capacity. Alternatively, bicycle ergometer protocols may also use smaller gradations of workload. These suggested protocols usually start at a lower level than common diagnostic protocols, such as the Bruce protocol, and increase fewer METS per stage. Bicycle ergometry should be considered for individuals with balance deficits, mild neurologic impairment, or orthopedic limitations.

Echocardiogram, pharmacologic, or nuclear medicine stress exercise testing should be considered for patients with marked lower extremity limitations, severe debility, or electrocardiograms that are difficult to interpret. Combined use of ventilatory gas analysis with electrocardiographic monitoring may be used to differentiate cardiac versus pulmonary exercise-induced dyspnea.

Most patients have had many electrocardiograms (ECGs) during their hospital stay or evaluation. In the outpatient setting, ECGs should be ordered if there is a change in clinical status such as new symptoms (e.g., the resumption of angina). For the most part, patients are also ECG monitored during the initial part of their cardiac rehabilitation.

Treatment

Initial

Cardiac rehabilitation begins with *risk factor reduction*. The initial medical management focuses on optimizing the cardiac medication regimen to control or prevent hypertension, ischemia, arrhythmia, hyperlipidemia, or other complications following the patient's cardiac event. Concurrent with medical management, the clinician prescribing cardiac rehabilitation must promote choices for healthy living. Each cardiac patient has control of smoking, diet, and stress management.

Smoking cessation has the highest rates of success by combining participation in a smoking cessation support group with pharmacologic management of the craving due to nicotine addiction. Bupropion combined with either a nicotine patch or nicotine gum work well. Have the patient begin taking the bupropion hydrochloride (150 mg qd for the first 3 days then 150 mg bid) 1 to 2 weeks before the chosen date to quit smoking, and begin using the nicotine supplement at the time of smoking cessation. This should coincide with the first smoking cessation support group meeting.

Dietary modification has been documented to improve the lipid profile. Ask the patient to keep a food diary for at least 3 days, and refer the patient to a registered dietician for evaluation and education on appropriate dietary choices. The American Heart Association (AHA) diet recommends consuming less than 30% of dietary calories from fat and less than 10% of calories from saturated fat. The dietician may recommend the AHA diet, but other choices could be the Mediterranean diet or the lactoovovegetarian diet. None of these three diets have been shown to be superior, and the choice of which diet to recommend is based primarily on the patient's ability to follow the diet.

The individual with cardiac disease often needs to learn tools to *decrease emotional stress*. A referral for counseling from a mental health professional can provide patients with an assortment of tools to learn relaxation and provides a forum for the discussion of anxiety surrounding cardiac events in their life. Women have a higher rate of anxiety and psychosomatic complaints than do men beginning cardiac rehabilitation.[5] In the busy clinic, the clinician can also teach the individual a simple stress reduction technique. A relaxation response documented by augmented parasympathetic activity has been noted during the simple exercise of paced breathing. Ask the patient to pace his or her breathing, using a clock, for 5 to 10 minutes twice daily. The patient should time inhalation and exhalation equally for 3 seconds each while avoiding air hunger or hyperventilation. Once he or she performs this exercise with facility, additional relaxation can be achieved from further slowing the breathing rate or prolonging the period of exhalation.[6]

Return to sexual activity should be frankly discussed with patients and their sexual partners to decrease their anxiety regarding sexual activity after cardiac event.[7] Sexual activity between couples with a longstanding relationship requires 3 to 5 METS. A simple test is the two-flight stair test. After a few minutes of level walking, the patient rapidly ascends and descends two flights of stairs. If this does not produce cardiac symptoms, then sexual relations can be resumed.[8] Extramarital sex causes higher energy demands.

Return to work and recreational activities should be based on patients' clinical status and their previous work. The exercise test performance predicts the level of vocational work capacity. If the patient's work capacity is only 3 to 4 METS or less, then returning to work may be unrealistic. Even self-care activities are likely to produce symptoms at this low level. With a 5 to 7 MET capacity the person should be able to perform sedentary work and most domestic roles. If the person can exercise beyond 7 METS, most types of work can be performed without restriction, except those involving heavy physical labor. For recreational activity, the MET level required should be evaluated before recommending return to play. The following are some common recreational activities and their MET requirements: tennis, 4 to 7 METS; golf, 2 to 5; skiing, 7 to 18; bowling, 4 to 5; and volleyball, 3 to 4.

Rehabilitation

If the patient is unable to begin a supervised exercise training program upon discharge from the hospital due to potential complications (Table 1), recommend a self-directed walking program. The patient should walk primarily on level surfaces with the goal of 15 to 30 minutes of walking at least 3 to 5 times per week at an intensity that will allow talking. Ask patients to keep a walking journal, and review it with them. If no significant cardiac damage has occurred, such as after angioplasty, then the period of convalescence may be shortened based on the clinician judgment and considerations such as the individual's need to return to previous pursuits.

Physical training begins at the end of the convalescence period ideally, based on functional exercise testing previously described in diagnostic testing discussion. Arguments have been made that exercise testing at this stage does not improve the outcome or safety of a supervised cardiac rehabilitation therapy program.[9] Prescription includes type, target intensity, frequency, and duration of exercise. Aerobic exercises, such as walking or bicycling, are the mainstay of most programs. Passive resistive exercises and weight training develop skeletal muscle mass but remain somewhat controversial for patients with congestive heart failure. Prescribe aerobic exercise *intensity* based on heart rate (HR), workload (METS), or perceived exertion (Table 2). The visual analog Borg scale rates perceived exertion (Fig. 1) that has been shown to correlate linearly with heart rate and oxygen consumption.[10] The *frequency* of exercise sessions is usually 3 to 5 times per week.

Aerobic exercise sessions begin with a *warmup phase* of 2 to 5 minutes at a lower intensity of exercise to limber the joints, open collateral circulation, and decrease peripheral vascular resistance. The *stimulus*, or *conditioning phase* may be continuous or discontinuous with the 3 to 12 month goal of at least 20 to 30 minutes of aerobic exercise. This may be broken down as a discontinuous exercise with rest breaks between periods of conditioning exercise. A *cool down phase* at a lower intensity of exercise will prevent hypotension and, later, joint pain. *Duration* of aerobic exercise sessions will vary depending on the individual's level of fitness. For the poorly debilitated patient, 3 to 5 minutes in the target range will provide benefit initially. The deconditioned individual should be progressed over 4 to 12 weeks to this stimulus duration. ECG monitoring during aerobic exercise is recommended for patients with low ejection fraction, abnormal blood pressure response to exercise, ST segment depression during low level exercise testing, or serious ventricular arrhythmia.[11,12]

Strength training or circuit training with resistance exercises adds skeletal muscle strength and facilitates building local muscular endurance for those with good left ventricular function. This

TABLE 1. Possible Contraindications for Entry into Inpatient or Outpatient Exercise Programs

According to the *American College of Sports Medicine*, contraindications are:
- Unstable angina
- Resting systolic BP > 200 mm Hg
- Resting diastolic BP > 100 mm Hg
- Orthostatic BP drop or drop during exercise training of ≥ 20 mm Hg
- Moderate to severe aortic stenosis
- Acute systemic illness or fever
- Uncontrolled atrial or ventricular dysrhythmias
- Uncontrolled sinus tachycardia (120 bpm)
- Uncontrolled congestive heart failure
- Third-degree A-V block
- Active pericarditis or myocarditis
- Recent embolism
- Thrombophlebitis
- Resting ST displacement (> 3 mm)
- Uncontrolled diabetes
- Orthopedic problems that prohibit exercise

From American College of Sports Medicine: Guidelines for Exercise Testing and Prescription, 4th ed. Malvern, PA, Lea and Febiger, 1991.

TABLE 2. Cardiac Rehabilitation Exercise Prescription

Type: Aerobic   Treadmill   Bicycle   (circle one)

Include: Strength training?   Yes   No   (circle one)

Intensity: Based on heart rate
- Target heart range 70% to 85% of maximum heart rate if patient not taking beta adrenergic blockade
- 85% maximum completed on treadmill if patient taking beta adrenergic blockade
- High resting heart rate, using exercise testing results (Kavonen formula): Target heart rate = Resting HR + [(HR$_{max}$ – HR$_{rest}$) × (60 + MT$_{max}$/100)].

Intensity: Based on workload
- Target 66% MET level completed on treadmill testing
- Target 25 watts or 150 KPM less than completed stage on bicycle ergometer testing

Intensity: Based on perceived exertion
- Borg scale target 11 to 15

Warmup phase
- Treadmill ambulation at ____ speed ____ grade for ____ minutes.
- Bicycle ergometry at ____ KPM/watts for ____ minutes.
- Check blood pressure, pulse rate, and perceived exertion.
- Advance to stimulus phase.

Stimulus phase
- Treadmill ambulation at ____ speed ____ grade ____ minutes with/without rest. Repeat ____ sets.
- Bicycle ergometry at ____ KPM/watts for ____ minutes with/without rest. Repeat ____ sets.
- Check blood pressure, pulse rate, and perceived exertion.
- Advance to cool down phase.

Cool down phase
- Treadmill ambulation at ____ speed ____ grade for ____ minutes.
- Bicycle ergometry at ____ KPM/watts for ____ minutes.
- Check blood pressure, pulse rate.

Frequency: 3 times per week.

Duration: 1 hour per visit for 12 weeks.

6	
7 ____	Very, very light
8	
9 ____	Very light
10	
11 ____	Fairly light
12	
13 ____	Somewhat hard
14	
15 ____	Hard
16	
17 ____	Very hard
18	
19 ____	Very, very hard
20	

This scale is used to indicate the self-assessed level of exertion for the individual performing exercise.

FIGURE 1. Borg's Scale of Perceived Exertion. (Used with permission.)

should especially be considered for the cardiac patient who may be returning to a physically demanding job. Static exercise has generally been avoided for cardiac patients due to an exaggerated hypertensive response. Patients who use free weights should begin with the lowest weight that produces a perceived exertion of 11 to 13 after 10 to 15 repetitions (Fig. 1). One to three sets will build strength. This should involve enough different exercises to include all major muscle groups of the upper and lower extremities.

The clinic-based supervised exercise program typically lasts 1 to 3 months, with the exercise prescription upgraded monthly. Monthly re-evaluation should include consideration of increasing the stimulus phase intensity and/or duration of aerobic exercise. After 2 to 3 months on a conditioning exercise program the individual should have the ability to achieve 7 to 8 METS of sustained exercise. Once the patient has achieved this goal, repeating the exercise test will show the level of improvement and guide the transition to a self-directed maintenance program. The patient may choose his or her own target heart rate or exertion level during exercise.

The benefits of exercise training include increased maximum oxygen uptake (VO$_{2max}$), increased endurance for activities of daily living, increased work capacity, decreased heart rate during exercise, decreased rate pressure product, decreased fatigue, decreased dyspnea, and decreased symptoms of heart failure. Exercise training reduces atherogenic and thrombotic risk factors by managing or preventing excess body weight, increasing high-density lipoprotein (HDL) cholesterol, decreasing plasma triglycerides, decreasing platelet aggregation, and improving glucose levels. Myocardial perfusion may be improved by increased coronary blood flow. The progress of coronary atherosclerosis may be slowed or possibly reversed.[13-15]

Procedures

Medically stabilized cardiac patients need few procedures. Thoracentesis for pulmonary effusion will greatly enhance physical performance. Interventional cardiology procedures may be needed for acutely occluded stents, angioplasty, or grafts. The patient with worsening cardiac symptoms may need to repeat coronary angiography if medication adjustment is unsuccessful.

Surgery

Surgical interventions may be needed for failed coronary bypass vascular grafts.

Potential Disease Complications

The potential complications of cardiac disease include death as the most common cause of mortality in the United States. Decreased exercise tolerance and decreased work capacity are the most common functional impairments. Complications include congestive heart failure; arrhythmia; re-infarction; and possible closure of coronary artery grafts, stents, or angioplasties. Despite referral to cardiac rehabilitation, individuals may still experience loss of social roles, vocational barriers, and difficulty with emotional adjustment despite excellent physical improvement and appropriate psychosocial interventions.

Potential Treatment Complications

There exists a slight risk of precipitating a cardiac event during exercise testing and training. In one study, non-fatal myocardial infarction occurred in approximately 1 per 300,000 person hours of exercise and resulted in 1 death per 800,000 person hours of exercise.[16] Preventing the enrollment of patients into cardiac rehabilitation who are not medically stabilized can minimize the risk. Exercise testing has relative and absolute contraindications that should be followed; these contraindications have been elucidated in great detail elsewhere.[4] Generally, however, do not test patients with unstable angina, malignant cardiac arrhythmia, pericarditis, endocarditis, severe left ventricular dysfunction, severe aortic stenosis, or any other acute non-cardiac disease.

References

1. Cardiovascular disease statistics. American Heart Association Web site, 2000.
2. Davis AM, Natelson BH: Brain-heart interactions. The neurocardiology of arrhythmia and sudden cardiac death. Tex Heart Inst J 1993;20(3):158–169.
3. Thompson DR, Lewin RJ: Coronary disease. Management of the post-myocardial infarction patient: Rehabilitation and cardiac neurosis. Heart 2000;84(1):101–105.
4. ACC/AHA guidelines for exercise testing. Circulation 1997;96:345–354.
5. Brezinka V, Kittel F: Psychosocial factors of coronary heart disease in women: A review. Soc Sci Med 1996;42(10): 1351–1365.
6. Davis AM: Respiratory modulation of heart rate variability and parasympathetic influence on the heart. Doctoral dissertation, UMDNJ-NJ Medical School, Department of Neurosciences.
7. Friedman S: Cardiac disease, anxiety, and sexual functioning. Am J Cardiol 2000;86(2A):46F–50F.
8. Larsen JL, McNaughton MW, KennedyJW, et al: Heart rate and blood pressure response to sexual activity and a stair climbing test. Heart Lung 1980;9:1025–1030.
9. McConnell TR, Klinger TA, Gardner JK, et al: Cardiac rehabilitation without exercise tests for post-myocardial infarction and post bypass surgery patients. J Cardiopulm Rehabil 1998;18(6):458–463.
10. Borg G: Perceived exertion as an indicator of somatic stress. Scand J Rehabil Med 1970;2-3:92–98.
11. Hamm LF, Leon AS: Exercise training for the coronary patient. In Wnger NK, Heller Stein HK (eds): Rehabilitation of the Coronary Patient, 2nd ed. New York, Churchill Livingstone, 1992, pp 267–402.
12. American Association of Cardiovascular and Pulmonary Rehabilitation: Guidelines for Cardiac Rehabilitation Programs. Champaign, IL), Human Kinetics, 1991.
13. Ignaszewski A, Lear SA: Cardiac rehabilitation programs. Can J Cardiol 1999;15(Suppl G):110G–113G.
14. Leon AS: Exercise following myocardial infarction. Current recommendations. Sports Med 2000;29(5):301–311.
15. Ades PA, Coello CE: Effects of exercise and cardiac rehabilitation on cardiovascular outcomes. Med Clin North Am 2000;84(1):251–265, x–xi.
16. Thompson PD, Moore GE: The cardiac risks of vigorous physical activity. In Leon AS (ed): National Institutes of Health. Physical Activity and Cardiovascular Health: A National Consensus. Champaign, IL, Human Kinetics, 1997, pp 137–142.

98 Cancer

Andrea Cheville, MD
Lora Beth Packel, PT

Synonyms

Cancer-related fatigue syndrome

Perineoplastic dysfunction

ICD-9 Codes

357.6
Polyneuropathy due to drugs

780.79
Other malaise and fatigue

781.2
Abnormality of gait

Definition

Cancer rehabilitation eludes a reductive, algorithmic approach given the tremendous heterogeneity in prognosis, natural history, management strategies, and treatment responsiveness that characterize different malignancies. Related impairments vary with location and stage of cancer, as well as the type of antineoplastic therapy. For example, cancers of the head and neck may require radical neck dissection and subsequent irradiation. Common adverse sequelae include shoulder dysfunction and fibrosis of cervical soft tissue. In contrast, surgical resection and radiation of axillary lymph nodes for breast cancer may cause chronic upper extremity swelling. The reader is referred to chapters specific to these conditions and anatomic locations (e.g., scapular winging, lymphedema).

A more uniform approach can be applied to the management of exertional intolerance, which affects up to 80% of cancer patients.[1] Despite the inconsistency of presentation, disease management, and clinical course, the majority of cancer patients will develop deconditioning and fatigue during their illness. A constellation of symptoms, including motor weakness, cognitive dysfunction, imbalance, dyspnea on exertion, and globally reduced functional capacity, may contribute to these phenomena. Deconditioning arises from many potential etiologies: cancer-related cachexia, inactivity, poor nutrition, fatigue, steroid use, or as a direct side effect of the cancer therapy.[2] Advanced age and extensive medical co-morbidity may contribute as well.

Symptoms

A characteristic constellation of symptoms should not be anticipated. Patients' malignancies, treatment regimens, and disease trajectories are extremely variable. Deconditioning may, therefore, present differently contingent on the unique particulars of each case. Any of the following subjective complaints should raise concern over possible cancer related fatigue: weakness (generalized or proximal hip and shoulder), dyspnea on exertion, sedation, hypersomnolence, fatigue, exertional intolerance, and cognitive compromise (e.g., attention/concentration deficits, short term memory dysfunction). Symptoms of depression should also be assessed.

A comprehensive history is essential, with particular attention paid to the precise symptoms underlying the patient's complaint. Since many symptoms associated with deconditioning are subjective, accurate description is essential in the formulation of an appropriate differential diagnosis. The patient's cancer history should be collected in detail, including prior and ongoing radiation therapy and chemotherapy, and any surgical procedures. Knowledge of each patient's primary cancer will shift the focus toward particular etiologies. For example, pancreatic cancer is more likely to produce cachexia, whereas breast or lung cancers are associated with a high incidence of hypercalcemia and neurologic compromise.[3] Attention should be paid to whether radiation fields encompass thyroid, lung, adrenal, or cardiac tissue. Medications and nutritional patterns must be carefully reviewed.

Physical Examination

The physical examination may reveal evidence of congestive heart failure or pulmonary compromise. Stigmata of hypothyroidism should be sought, particularly in head and neck cancer patients. Neurologic examination should be normal beyond chemotherapy related peripheral neuropathy. Weakness in proximal hip and shoulder musculature suggests steroid myopathy. Identification of new neurologic deficits should trigger evaluation for malignant progression or emerging treatment toxicity.[4] Mental status examination may reveal evidence of compromised arousal, attention, memory, and/or concentration. A brief screen for depression or other mood disorders is essential.[5]

Functional evaluation will clarify the extent to which symptoms are interfering with mobility and performance of activities of daily living. Assessment of skin integrity, balance, ambulation, and joint excursion may lead to the identification of factors contributing to functional debility and potential therapeutic targets. Useful objective measures include the 6-minute walk test, "get up and go" test, fatigue scale, and manual muscle testing.

Functional Limitations

Functional limitations will depend on which symptoms are present. Patients may demonstrate difficulty with transfers, bed mobility, or stairclimbing. Ambulating moderate distances may produce severe dyspnea in patients with cancer related cardiac or pulmonary dysfunction. Patients with steroid myopathy or generalized muscle weakness may have difficulty arising from low surfaces, such as a toilet, soft chair, or car seat. They may also demonstrate a decreased ability to independently complete their activities of daily living in a reasonable time frame. Patients may describe generalized heaviness of their limbs and a global decrement in their activity level without precise functional limitations. Finally, a component of postural instability and compromised balance may complicate severe deconditioning.

Patients with cognitive deficits related to radiation therapy or chemotherapy may experience difficulty maintaining their vocational productivity. Financial and domestic management skills may be compromised as well.

Dysfunction in social, vocational, psychologic, and personal domains may be present. Patients should be questioned about compromised social interactions, sleep, and intimacy, as well as vocational and avocational pursuits.

Diagnostic Studies

Diagnostic tests will vary contingent on the patient's presentation. Deconditioning associated with dyspnea should be assessed with pulse oximetry, chest x-ray, and electrocardiogram. Patients may exhibit shortness of breath with minimal activity while maintaining normal oxygen saturation. Pulmonary parenchymal disease or fibrosis may require a CT scan for adequate evaluation. Cancer patients are at an elevated risk for venous thrombosis; therefore a venous duplex study, and possibly a VQ-scan, should be considered for persistent shortness of breath. Patients who have received adriamycin or herceptin should be evaluated with a MUGA scan to rule out possible chemotherapy related cardiac toxicity. Most patients will have undergone screening prior to the administration of chemotherapy. The results of these tests can be compared with those of new evaluations for evidence of deterioration. Pericardial effusions may occur as a consequence of malignant spread, radiation-induced irritation, or as a perineoplastic phenomenon. An echocardiogram should be obtained for patients with a suggestive history and physical.

Serologic evaluation may include TSH (thyroid myopathy in patients who have received radiation to the anterior neck), calcium, electrolytes (Addison's disease may occur with adrenal metastases or radiation), hemoglobin, and hematocrit. Hypercalcemia or persistent mechanical pain should be evaluated with a bone scan. *Clinicians must be cognizant that multiple myeloma and malignancies producing lytic metastases may fail to generate a positive bone scan despite diffuse skeletal involvement.* Serologic levels of centrally acting medications (e.g., tricyclic antidepressants, anticonvulsants) should be checked in patients who describe fatigue with a significant cognitive dimension. Steroids administered in conjunction with chemotherapy may cause myopathy. Electrodiagnostic studies are used to rule in/out myopathy.

For patients with focal neurologic deficits, imaging of those portions of the neural axis implicated on physical examination should be performed. Magnetic resonance images should be obtained with contrast to elucidate enhancing lesions.

Patients complaining of generalized cognitive dysfunction may benefit from neuropsychologic evaluation. Subtle cognitive deficits have been detected following chemotherapy. Multifocal brain metastases may present with a global decrement in mental acuity and capacity to attend. Head CT with contrast may be warranted when there is a high clinical probability of brain metastases (e.g., patients with melanoma, breast or lung cancers).

Differential Diagnosis

Depression	Steroid myopathy	Pleural effusion
Nutritional insufficiency	Medication side effects	Adriamycin or herceptin related cardiotoxicity
Anemia	Chemotherapy- or radiation therapy-induced cognitive dysfunction	
Infection		Disturbed sleep-wake cycles
Metabolic/endocrine abnormality (e.g., hypercalcemia, hypothyroidism)	Cachexia	Neural axis compromise (e.g., brain metastasis, epidural metastasis, brachial plexopathy)
	Pulmonary parenchymal disease/ bleomycin toxicity/radiation fibrosis	

Treatment

Initial

It is important to address any endocrine, hematologic, metabolic, or reversible physical abnormalities prior to initiating an exercise program. Uncontrolled pain mandates the initiation or modification of an analgesic regimen. Opioid-based pharmacotherapy has emerged as the cornerstone of cancer pain management. Secondary infections related to cancer therapy-induced neutropenia must be treated before aerobic conditioning can begin. Leukopenia will resolve more rapidly with granulocyte colony stimulating factor (GCSF). The discovery of progressive disease may warrant initiating or altering an antineoplastic regimen or the administration of radiation therapy. Cardiac toxicity may improve following the initiation of digoxin and/or medication(s) to reduce afterload. Anemia generally responds to therapy with subcutaneous, recombinant erythropoietin. Patients with radiation therapy or chemotherapy-induced pulmonary fibrosis or those who have undergone lobectomy or pneumonectomy may require supplemental oxygen during rehabilitative efforts. Nutritional evaluation may be needed for cachectic or hypoproteinemic patients.

A psychiatric consultation may be indicated if depression is a concern. All nonessential centrally acting drugs should be eliminated. Pain medications should be chosen to minimize neuropsychologic toxicity. Among the opioids, hydromorphone, fentanyl, and oxycodone have fewer active metabolites that morphine sulfate. Therefore, these agents may be associated with a more tolerable side effect profile in the elderly and patients with renal impairment. Pharmacologic approaches for cancer fatigue center predominantly around the administration of psychostimulants.[1] The utility of these agents is supported by studies of methylphenidate and pemoline.[6,7]

Rehabilitation

Most of the research on exercise in the person with cancer has looked at the effect of aerobic exercise on functional capacity and quality of life. Presently, there is no consensus on an ideal type, frequency, intensity, duration, or mode of exercise. The trend of these studies indicates that there is a good cardiopulmonary response to interval training at 50% to 70% of the heart rate reserve or while working at an exertion of 11 to 14 on the 6 to 20 perceived rate of exertion scale.[8,9] The intensity of the exercise program is dependent on baseline fitness levels, intensity of cancer treatment, and stage of cancer treatment. While the patient is undergoing treatment, most studies recommend decreasing the intensity to the lower end of the heart rate range. Once active therapy is over, the program should be progressed toward the higher end of the range. The intensity must also take into account daily lab values and patterns of fatigue associated with treatment. For example, fatigue seems to peak within the middle and end of the radiation cycle, and the program should account for this pattern. Finally, duration and frequency should closely match the American College of Sports Medicine guidelines, which recommends that patients exercise for a total of 20 to 30 minutes, three to five times per week.

Exercise precautions for cancer patients are seldom evidence based. They vary significantly between institutions and clinicians. The following limitations are conservative suggestions and should not be interpreted as absolute exercise contraindications.[10] Aerobic and resistive exercise should be discontinued when platelets fall below 10,000. Light exercise is allowed when hemoglobin is less than 8, with patients closely monitored for symptoms. Contact and high impact sports should be avoided when platelets fall below 50,000 or in those with primary or metastatic bone disease. Exercise should be deferred for febrile patients with temperatures greater that 101.5° F. Therapeutic activities should be restricted to indoor exercise for nadiring patients with an absolute neutrophil count less than 500.

In addition to aerobic conditioning, referral to occupational and physical therapy for training in energy conservation strategies, use of adaptive equipment, and progressive resistive exercise will benefit appropriate patients. Non-fatiguing exercise should be used. Instruction in compensatory strategies for mobility and performance of activities of daily living should be explored to optimize autonomy within the constraints imposed by disease. Adaptive equipment such as canes, crutches, or walkers may be geared toward enhancing mobility. Provision with adaptive devices such as long-handled shoehorns and reachers may facilitate the independent performance of self-care activities. Conservative interventions geared toward optimizing mobility and independent performance of activities of daily living have demonstrated benefit even in end stage cancer patients.[11] For these patients, education and empowerment of caretakers may emerge as the primary therapeutic focus.

Procedures

Patients with pleural or pericardial effusions will benefit from percutaneous drainage of the fluid. Pleurocardiodesis or pericardiodesis may be required to prevent the reaccumulation of effusions with associated exertional intolerance. Percutaneous stinting procedures have become commonplace when tumor compression narrows the lumen of ureters, bile ducts, bronchi, or blood vessels with adverse physiologic sequelae. When cancer pain cannot be adequately managed with systemic therapy or if side effects become untenable, delivery of spinal analgesics may restore normal arousal, energy, and cognition. Radiation therapy may be used palliatively to treat pain or reduce tumor bulk that is compressing neurologic structures.

Surgery

Cancer patients with deconditioning and fatigue may require surgical debulking of tumor or resection of isolated lung, liver, bone, or brain metastases. If focal sensory or motor deficits result from tumor compression of neural pathways, emergent resection may be required.

Potential Disease Complications

Patients commonly deteriorate functionally or develop progressive morbidity as their cancers advance. Consequences of malignant progression may include new or worsening neurologic deficits, dyspnea, cognitive deterioration from intracranial metastases or radiation-induced changes, pathologic fractures, and visceral or somatic pain syndromes.

Potential Treatment Complications

Potential complications of anticancer modalities are extensive. Radiation therapy can cause fibrosis, neurologic compromise, and worsening fatigue. Chemotherapy can similarly exacerbate fatigue. Various chemotherapeutic agents have the capacity to impair cognitive, renal, pulmonary, cardiac, and neurologic function. The myriad pharmacologic agents used to manage cancer associated symptoms and pain can adversely affect gastrointestinal and urinary systems, as well as worsen peripheral edema.

Complications associated with rehabilitative interventions are few when strategies are deployed appropriately. Patients with osseously avid cancers (e.g., lung, prostate, breast, thyroid, multiple myeloma, and renal) are at risk for pathologic fractures, particularly those with lytic metastases. A recent bone scan or skeletal survey should be reviewed before an exercise program is initiated. Overly aggressive aerobic conditioning or strengthening programs may lead to worsening fatigue. Uncustomary exertion may aggravate chemotherapeutically induced electrolyte and fluid imbalances. Cancer patients should generally be considered more prone to common exercise-induced complications. Their therapeutic regimens should be adapted and scrutinized accordingly.

Reference

1. Portenoy RK, Miaskowski C: Assessment and management of cancer-related fatigue. In Berger AM, Portenoy RK, Weissman DE (eds): Supportive Oncology. Philadelphia, Lippincott-Raven, 1998, pp 109–118.
2. Gillis TA: The role of the physiatrist. In Winningham ML, Barton-Burke M (eds): Fatigue in cancer. Baltimore, Jones and Bartlett, 2000, pp 295–301.
3. Posner J: Neurologic Complications of Cancer. Philadelphia, F.A. Davis, 1995, p 284.
4. Posner J: Neurologic Complications of Cancer. Philadelphia, F.A. Davis, 1995, pp 10–22.
5. Payne DK, Massie MJ: Depression and anxiety. In Berger A, Portenoy R, Weissman D (eds): Principles and Practice of Supportive Oncology. New York, Lippincott-Raven, 1998, pp 497_511.
6. Bruera E, Chadwick S, Brenneis C, et al: Methylphenidate associated with narcotics for the treatment of cancer pain. Cancer Treat Rep 1987;71:67–70.
7. Krupp LB, Coyle PK, Doscher C, et al: Fatigue therapy in multiple sclerosis: A double-blind, randomized, parallel trial of amantidine, pemoline and placebo. Neurology 1995;45(11):1956_1961.
8. Dimeo FC, Tilman MH, Bertz H, et al: Aerobic exercise in the rehabilitation of cancer patients after high dose chemotherapy and autologous peripheral stem cell transplantation. Cancer 1997;79:1717–1722.
9. Winningham ML, Nail L, Barton-Burke M, et al: Fatigue and the cancer experience: The state of the knowledge. Oncol Nurs Forum 1994;21:23–36.
10. Gerber L, Hicks J, Klaiman M, et al: Rehabilitation of the cancer patient. In DeVita VT, Hellman S, Rosenberg SA (eds): Cancer: Principles & Practice of oncology, 5th ed. Philadelphia, Lippincott-Raven, 1997, pp 2925–2956.
11. Yoshioka H: Rehabilitation for the terminal cancer patient. Am J Phys Med Rehabil 1994;73:199–206.

99 Cerebral Palsy

Patrick Brennan, MD

Synonyms

Little's disease

ICD-9 Codes

343
Infantile cerebral palsy

343.0
Diplegic

343.1
Hemiplegic
Congenital
hemiplegia

343.2
Quadriplegic

343.3
Monoplegic

343.4
Infantile hemiplegia
Infantile hemiplegia
(postnatal) NOS

343.8
Other specified
infantile cerebral palsy

343.9
Infantile cerebral
palsy, unspecified

V54.8
Orthopedic aftercare:
changes, check or
removal of casts, splint
(external)

Definition

Cerebral palsy is a clinical syndrome resulting from a static lesion of an immature brain that primarily affects motor functioning and posture.[1] A commonly accepted criteria for having an immature brain is younger than 4 years of age, and therefore a child who sustains a static lesion (e.g., traumatic brain injury, meningitis) prior to 4 years of age meets the definition of cerebral palsy. Its range of severity is as wide as the list of etiologies associated with it. Reported incidence varies from 2 to 3 per thousand live births.[2] Impairments ranging from mild gait abnormalities to severe mental retardation and wheelchair dependence are its hallmark; the majority of patients exhibit upper motor neuron findings.

Neurologic classification divides the syndrome into three types: spastic (pyramidal), dyskinetic (extrapyramidal), and mixed. The spastic group can be further specified by body region involved: monoplegia, diplegia, triplegia, quadriplegia, and hemiplegia.

Although the neurologic lesion itself is nonprogressive, deterioration of function commonly occurs with aging as a result of muscle spasticity superimposed upon growth, resulting in worsening contractures and very often chronic joint pain.

There is a paucity of literature on the long-term sequelae of cerebral palsy in adulthood. Basic demographic characteristics of the affected population are lacking.[3] Prevalence in the United States is estimated at 400,000 adults and is expected to increase.[4] Ninety-five percent of children with diplegia and 75% of children with quadriplegia survive until the age of 30 years.[5] Lack of basic functional skills (mobility and feeding) were found to be key predictors of reduced life expectancy, as short as 11 years in the worst functioning groups.[6] A recent study showed higher-than-expected mortality from ischemic heart disease, cancer, and stroke in adults with cerebral palsy.[7] A lack of early detection and periodic health care were implicated. Comprehensive care of an adult with cerebral palsy is complex and requires ongoing evaluation by a mutidisciplinary team of physicians, therapists, psychologists, and social workers.

Symptoms

Symptoms vary widely depending on disease severity and chronicity. A cross-sectional survey of 63 adult women ages 20 to 74 with cerebral palsy living in the community revealed a high incidence of mental retardation (34%), learning disabilities (26%), seizure (40%), pain (84%), hip and back deformities (59%), bowel problems (56%), bladder problems (49%), poor dental health (43%), and gastroesophageal reflux (28%).[8]

Musculoskeletal

Common presenting symptoms include neck pain (abnormal tonicity or movements of the neck, especially in athetotic cerebral palsy, can be associated with early cervical spine degeneration and instability)[9,10]; low back pain (anecdotally reported as a long-term consequence of hamstring tightness); back deformity (scoliosis is especially common in non-ambulatory patients and can progress beyond skeletal maturity[11]); hip pain (hip deformities are common especially in the non-ambulatory, are often present in childhood, and can result in disabling osteoarthritis); knee pain (anecdotally reported as a long-term consequence of a crouched [bent-knee] gait pattern, resulting in disabling osteoarthritis at an early age); and loss of range of motion of lower extremity joints due to musculotendinous unit shortening and/or joint capsule contracture.

Neurologic

Symptoms include spasticity, weakness, and deterioration of upper extremity function. Visual problems exist in 25% to 39% of adult patients, hearing deficits in 18%.[12,13] These symptoms commonly worsen with aging.[14] Cognitive deficits may be absent and can range from mild to profound mental retardation. Communication disorders can be severe in athetotic cerebral palsy; these patients are often labeled mentally retarded, although the majority have normal cognition. Thirty percent of individuals with cerebral palsy have a seizure disorder, which is most common in spastic quadriplegia.

Presenting symptoms of spasticity and underlying weakness (partially attributable to antagonist co-contraction of the muscles)[15] consistent with an upper motor neuron lesion are common. Any worsening of baseline spasticity should prompt an investigation into noxious stimuli, such as impacted bowel or other intra-abdominal processes, urinary tract infection, and musculoskeletal disorders.

Functional deterioration of the upper extremity, especially in athetotic cerebral palsy, warrants consideration of cervical myelopathy or radiculopathy.

The etiology of visual deficits in adults is likely associated with cataracts, optic atrophy, or retinitis known to be present in children.[16]

Cardiopulmonary

Symptoms include shortness of breath, irritability, and pallor that may comprise a subtle picture of cardiac ischemia. Lower extremity swelling, coolness, and discoloration are common in non-ambulatory patients. Chronic gastroesophageal reflux can be associated with symptoms of aspiration pneumonia.

Gastrointestinal/Nutritional

Feeding difficulties are common in severely neurologically impaired individuals, and the time required to feed patients can negatively affect the patient's and the caregivers' quality of life. Nutritional problems include malnutrition associated with dysphagia and obesity due to inactivity and overeating. Constipation, diverticula, and hemorrhoids are common, as are dental problems, due to difficulties with hygiene, spasticity of oral musculature, and abnormal development.[15]

Delayed gastric emptying, gastroesophageal reflux, and constipation are all commonly seen.

Urinary

Although uncommon in children and not well studied in adults, urinary urgency and frequency with small output is seen, as well as a hypotonic enlarged bladder pattern. Urinary tract infection; reflux; and spastic, flaccid, or dyssynergic bladder should be considered.

Psychosocial

Depression is often associated with the social isolation that is a consequence of limited independence.

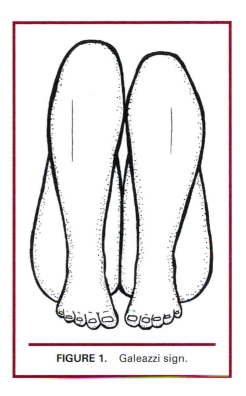

FIGURE 1.   Galeazzi sign.

Physical Examination

The physical examination of an adult with cerebral palsy should focus on range of motion and spasticity to differentiate functional limitations as a result of contracture versus motor control issues. Deep tendon reflexes are increased (Ashworth spasticity scale; see p. 787). Sensation is usually not impaired, and strength testing may reveal weakness that is partly attributable to antagonist muscle co-contraction. Skin should be inspected for decubiti, especially in the non-ambulatory patient.

Hips should be examined for symmetry of abduction and external and internal rotation. Common findings include asymmetry and a positive Galeazzi sign (Fig. 1). One knee is less prominent than the other with the patient supine, hips and knees flexed to 90 degrees, and pelvis neutral, which implies hip subluxation on the less prominent side.

Loss of knee range of motion is common. Inability to fully extend the knee while supine implies posterior joint capsule tightness, especially when the hamstrings are palpably slack. An increased popliteal angle combined with full knee extension when supine indicates hamstring contracture and/or spasticity.

Examination of the foot is complex, and structural abnormalities are common, including pes planus and pronation with weight bearing.

Observational gait analysis that shows a disparity between available (passive) and utilized range of motion indicates spasticity and/or weakness and can guide therapeutic alternatives. Common gait abnormalities include initial contact with the forefoot, an exaggerated knee extension moment, lack of full knee extension at midstance, a narrow base of support with scissoring, and a shortened stride length.

Cognitive testing, when appropriate, is helpful with school- or work-related problems. An evaluation by a neuropsychologist skilled in working with this population is essential.

Five or more positive responses to the SIGECAPS screen (deterioration in sleep, interests; feelings of guilt; decreased energy, concentration, appetite; psychomotor symptoms or suicidal thoughts) are consistent with depression. The presence of anhedonia (lack of pleasure) increases sensitivity further.

Functional Limitations

Functional limitations correlate with the degree of severity of cerebral palsy, and investigation into functional status should focus on mobility, self-care, and activities of daily living.

Forty percent of adults with cerebral palsy are non-ambulatory, 40% require assistance (e.g., walkers, orthotics, caregivers), and 20% ambulate independently; approximately one third of adults with cerebral palsy live at home.[12] Depending on the degree of impairment, patients may or may not be able to work outside the home. Recreational activities and hobbies may be limited by cognitive and physical impairments. Impairments may affect intimacy and also result in social embarrassment.

Diagnostic Studies

Musculoskeletal

Radiographs of the symptomatic joints are indicated to confirm a clinical presentation of osteoarthritis. MRI of the cervical spine is indicated when new neurologic symptoms are present, especially in the athetotic patient. Computerized gait analysis has proven useful in guiding surgical and rehabilitative treatments in pediatric cerebral palsy patients; its use in adults is not widely reported.

Neurologic

Electrodiagnostic testing (e.g., EMG/nerve conductionstudies) is indicated in cases of new focal neurologic deficits. Results of IQ testing that are fine motor dependent should be interpreted with caution since the majority of patients with cerebral palsy have fine motor deficits.

Cardiopulmonary

ECG and stress testing are indicated when cardiac dysfunction is suspected.

Gastrointestinal

Upper GI imaging and contrast studies, pH probe, and gastric emptying studies may be indicated in patients with symptoms of aspiration pneumonia.

Urinary

Urodynamic testing can distinguish between upper motor neuron and lower motor neuron patterns of bladder dysfunction and thus helps to direct treatment.

Differential Diagnosis

Familial spastic paraparesis

Treatment

Initial

Treatment of musculoskeletal conditions, including osteoarthritis, should be based on the specific diagnosis. The goal, however, is to preserve function and minimize pain as much as possible. Traditional methods of treating musculoskeletal conditions such as the use of NSAIDs/COX-2 inhibitors, analgesics, local icing, etc. are all appropriate interventions in the adult patient with cerebral palsy.

The initial treatment of contracture includes relief of underlying spasticity with oral medications or injections (see Chapters 103 and 136) and application of low-load prolonged stretch with serial casting or dynamic splinting. The use of superficial heat or ultrasound can be an important adjunct to a stretching program. Clear, functional goals should be established prior to treatment.

Visual and hearing deficits should be managed by referral to the appropriate specialists.

Educating patients, family members, and caregivers about the rights of the disabled encourages advocacy. Resources including *Exceptional Parent* magazine and United Cerebral Palsy (www.ucpa.org) provide information about employment opportunities, research, and treatment providers specializing in the care of patients with cerebral palsy.

Rehabilitation

Inquiries into the home environment and a home visit by therapists, when appropriate, can help focus interventions that create the least-restrictive and safest environment. Assistive devices provided with input from physical and occupational therapists are essential, and powered mobility should be considered for community access (e.g., walkers and wheelchairs for community mobility and mobility of longer distances are important).

Speech/language pathologists as well as augmentative equipment providers are essential in assisting patients and their caregivers to maximize communication. Vocational rehabilitation services can help patients access appropriate training and job placement.

If there is a decline in a patient's functional abilities, a supervised exercise program of graded closed chain exercises, which has been shown to increase strength in children and to not worsen spasticity, may be considered. Its efficacy in adults, however, has not been studied. Supervised therapy can also be helpful in maintaining joint range of motion and in educating both patients and care providers on how to correctly perform stretching and strengthening exercises at home. Superficial and deep heating modalities during stretch may relax tone and allow a more permanent elongation of the musculotendinous unit.

Bracing may be an option for some patients. Lower extremity orthotics such as an ankle foot orthosis (AFO) may improve ambulation. In patients with scoliosis, bracing has been shown to slow progression but not to prevent progressive deformity; early referral to an orthopedist is generally indicated.

Procedures

Many procedures may be helpful to manage pain and spasticity and to improve contractures. These are described throughout this text and are based on the specific diagnosis or condition. Joint and soft tissue injections (e.g., trigger point injectons) can be helpful in managing pain and improving function. Phenol blocks and botulinum toxin injections may assist in managing spasticity and preventing or improving contractures when combined with low-load prolonged stretch, as provided by serial casting or dynamic splinting.

Surgery

Surgery may be an option for patients with advanced osteoarthritis that limits function and/or causes pain. Arthroplasty in early or midadulthood has been shown to be beneficial.[15] Spinal stenosis due to advanced cervical degenerative disease warrants referral to a neurosurgeon in some cases. Longstanding contracture may not respond to conservative measures, and referral to an orthopedic surgeon for surgical lengthening or release is often necessary.

Potential Disease Complications

The spectrum of potential disease complications is vast for individuals with cerebral palsy. As aging occurs, it is important to try and maintain as much function as possible. Progressive weakness, spasticity, and contractures all lead to increasing disability. Pain can also limit function. Cognitive changes do not typically occur, but if present should be worked-up to rule out co-existing pathology (e.g., dementia, hydrocephalus).

Potential Treatment Complications

Botulinum toxin injections that are repeated more often than every 4 to 6 months may be associated with antibody production, leading to decreased efficacy. Transient weakness of the injected muscles, malaise, and inflammation at the injection site can occur. Phenol injection of a mixed nerve can result in painful dysesthesias. Overly aggressive stretching can lead to pain, inflammation, and joint damage. Surgical complications are generally well known and depend on the type of surgery performed.

References

1. Bax MCO: Terminology and classification of cerebral palsy. Dev Med Child Neurol 1964;6:295.
2. Paneth N, Kiely J: The frequency of cerebral palsy: A review of population studies in industrialized nations since 1950. In Stanley F, Alberman E (eds): The epidemiology of the cerebral palsies. Oxford, England, Blackwell Scientific, 1984, pp 46–56.
3. Overeynder J, Turk M, Dalton AJ, Janicki MP: I'm worried about the future: The aging of adults with cerebral palsy. Albany, NY, New York State Developmental Disabilities Planning Council, 1992.
4. Murphy KP, Molnar GE, Lankasky K: Medical and functional status of adults with cerebral palsy Dev Med Child Neurol 1995;37:1075–1084.
5. Crichton J, MacKinney M, Light CP: The life expectancy of persons with cerebral palsy. Dev Med Child Neurol 1995;37:567–576.
6. Strauss D, Shavelle R: Life expectancy of adults with cerebral palsy. Dev Med Child Neurol. 1998; 40(6): 369–375.
7. Strauss D, Cable W, Shavelle R: Causes of excess mortality in cerebral palsy. Dev Med Child Neurol 1999; 41:580–585.
8. Turk MA, Geremski CA, Rosenbaum PF, Weber RJ: The health status of women with cerebral palsy. Arch Phys Med Rehabil 1997;78(12 Suppl 5): S10–S17.
9. Ko HY, Park-Ko I: Spinal cord injury secondary to cervical disc herniation in ambulatory patients with cerebral palsy. Spinal Cord 1998;36(4):288–292.
10. Nagashima T.: Late deterioration of functional abilities in adult cerebral palsy. Clin Neurol 1993;33(9):939–944.
11. Thometz JG, Simon SR: Progression of scoliosis after skeletal maturity in institutionalized adults who have cerebral palsy. J Bone Joint Surg Am 1988;Oct:1290–1296.
12. Granet KM, Balaghi M, Jaeger J: Adults with cerebral palsy. N J Med 1997;94:51–54.
13. Janicki NP: Aging, cerebral palsy and older persons with mental retardation. Aust N Z J Dev Disabil 1989;15:311–330.
14. Currie DM, Gershkoff AM, Cifu DX: Geriatric Rehabilitation. 3. Mid- and late-life effects of early-life disabilities. Arch Phys Med Rehabil 1993;74:S413–S414.
15. Brown MC, Bontempo A, Turk MA: Secondary consequences of cerebral palsy: Adults with cerebral palsy in New York State. Albany, NY, Developmental Disabilities Planning Council; 1992.
16. Ingram TTS: Pediatric Aspects of Cerebral Palsy. Edinburgh, Scotland, E&S Livingstone 1964.

100 Chronic Fatigue Syndrome

Deborah Reiss Schneider, MD

Synonyms

Chronic fatigue and immune dysfunction syndrome (CFIDS)[1]

ICD-9 Code

780.71
Chronic fatigue syndrome

Definition

A syndrome of chronic fatigue was first described as early as 1750.[2] The definition of chronic fatigue syndrome (CFS) was originally formulated in 1988[3] and then revised in 1994. The 1994 revision occurred because the original criteria did not effectively distinguish CFS from other types of unexplained fatigue. An international panel of experts met to better differentiate it from other causes of fatigue.[4]

The most current criteria defining chronic fatigue syndrome are as follows:

1. Severe chronic fatigue for 6 months or longer with no other known condition as the cause.
2. Four or more of the following that did not pre-date the fatigue: significant impairment in short-term memory or concentration, sore throat, tender lymph nodes, muscle pains, joint pain in multiple joints without inflammatory signs of swelling or redness, new headaches, unrefreshing sleep, postexertional malaise lasting more than 24 hours.[5]

Chronic fatigue syndrome is defined by a grouping of nonspecific symptoms and is a diagnosis of exclusion. A central issue in CFS research is whether the syndrome is a specific disease entity or a nonspecific condition shared by many different entities.

Recent data suggest that women are up to three times more commonly affected than men, and prevalence appears to be greater than 400 per every 100,000 persons in the United States.[1] Evaluation to rule out a treatable cause of fatigue is of paramount importance. Twenty-four percent of adults in the United States have reported having experienced fatigue of 1 month or longer. Studies have revealed that the recovery from CFS was 31.4% during the first 5 years of illness and 48.1% during the first 10 years.[1] Recovery episodes are more likely during the early years, but if this does not occur, many continue to suffer with debilitating fatigue.[6]

A subset of individuals, diagnosed with the following conditions, may have symptoms consistent with chronic fatigue syndrome: vapors, neurasthenia, effort syndrome, hyperventilation syndrome, chronic brucellosis, epidemic neuromyasthenia, myalgic encephalitis, hypoglycemia, multiple chemical sensitivity syndrome, chronic candidiasis, chronic mononucleosis, chronic Epstein-Barr virus, and postviral fatigue syndrome.[7]

Symptoms

History, physical examination, and diagnostic testing are directed toward determining whether symptoms represent a detectable infection; autoimmune disease; endocrine abnormality; absorption or nutrient problem; toxic exposure; sleep disorder; medication side effect, central nervous system (CNS) disease; drug or alcohol abuse; or other chronic illness of the heart, lung, digestive system or other bodily system. Symptoms of chronic fatigue syndrome include severe disabling fatigue of 6 months duration or longer, short-term memory impairment, difficulty with concentrating on tasks, sore throat, new-onset headaches, unrefreshing sleep, postexertional malaise lasting more than 24 hours, joint and muscle aches, tender lymph nodes, abdominal and chest pain, chills, low-grade fevers, vertigo, nausea, emotional lability, photophobia, allergies, hot flashes, and rashes.[1,3–11]

Infection and psychologic or physical stress have been noted to commonly precede fatigue.[11] More than 45% of patients reported sore throat, fever, tender lymph nodes, general weakness, and muscle pain at onset. For those with sudden onset of CFS, common additional symptoms reported include hypersomnia, difficulty with thinking or concentration, and depression.[6]

Physical Examination

Chronic fatigue syndrome is a diagnosis of exclusion.[7,11] Each organ is examined systematically to assess for abnormalities in vital signs, including temperature; rashes; nodal enlargement; pharyngitis; other upper or lower respiratory symptoms or signs; irregularities in the cardiac, digestive, or urologic systems; or abnormalities in the pelvis or extremities. Examination of the CNS is crucial to rule out other causes of fatigue, headaches, or cranial nerve abnormalities, such as Lyme disease or multiple sclerosis.

Functional Limitations

Functional limitations depend on the severity of the fatigue and which of the diagnostic criteria are present. Presentations may differ at onset; progression varies; and individual responses, both physical and psychologic, will result in an entire spectrum of functional limitations expressed.[12]

Fatigue commonly diminishes endurance.[13] Individuals may be able to begin but not complete mental or physical tasks that were previously easily accomplished. Combinations of weakness, achiness, inability to concentrate, memory difficulties, dizziness, depression, or other symptoms may determine whether an individual feels safely independent. Symptoms may be severe enough to make driving or even walking difficult tasks.

Work may require strength or endurance that is no longer present or affect concentration or memory, causing errors and inconsistent performance. Job modifications may allow a patient to continue to function effectively at work. Active employment diminishes the risk of social isolation. Allowing even limited participation can strongly influence an individual's perception of support and help with stress which may accompany a person's change in function. Modifications to accommodate achiness, dizziness, or lack of strength may include working fewer hours each day, altering positions regularly, improving the ergonomics of a work station, or providing aids one may need to help with memory and concentration.

Most individuals are able to perform their activities of daily living and live independently with chronic fatigue syndrome. Some may require assistance if weakness or pain predominate or if memory or concentration abnormalities become severe. If ability to think significantly changes, tests of mental status or neuropsychologic testing may better define mental functioning and help determine whether modifications, such as memory aids, can improve functioning.

Fatigue itself can cause social isolation and depression. The rate of depression among individuals with CFS is increased when compared with other chronic illnesses. Depression can diminish one's will to function. Socialization may require initiation from others because individuals may lose their desire to participate.

Diagnostic Studies

There is no specific test at present that clearly diagnoses chronic fatigue syndrome as a distinct clinical entity. At one time, Epstein-Barr virus (EBV) antibodies were thought to have correlated with disease activity, but this has been proven incorrect.

Since fatigue can be caused by a large spectrum of diseases, routine blood work and evaluation must be complete but directed appropriately toward differentiating chronic fatigue syndrome from other known causes of fatigue. Serum for complete blood count (CBC) with differential, erythrocyte sedimentation rate (ESR), total protein, albumin, globulins, calcium, electrolytes, glucose, phosphorus, blood urea nitrogen (BUN), creatinine, thyroid function tests such as thyroid-stimulating hormone (TSH) for screening, amylase and liver function tests including alanine aminotransferase (ALT), aspartate aminotransferase (AST), gamma-glutamyl transferase (GGT), and alkaline phosphatase have been recommended on initial evaluation, along with urinalysis for multiple substances including blood, sugar, protein, electrolytes, ketones, osmolality, and myoglobin. Further tests may be chosen on an individual basis to confirm or exclude other diagnoses. Testing may be appropriate for entities such as multiple sclerosis, Lyme disease, Epstein Barr virus, autoimmune disease, parasites, fungal infections, human immunodeficiency virus (HIV) related diseases, bacterial infection or mycoplasma, drug use, absorption issues, toxic exposures, or psychiatric illnesses.[4,14,15] Brain abnormalities have been found to be present in many patients who were initially diagnosed with chronic fatigue syndrome.[16]

MRI and spinal taps are useful in determining abnormalities of the CNS exhibiting fatigue, but should be used judiciously. Nutritional deficiencies have been implicated, but deficiencies of various B vitamins, vitamin C, magnesium, sodium, zinc, L-tryptophan, L-carnitine, coenzyme Q10, and essential fatty acids as a cause for chronic fatigue syndrome have yet to be proven. Empiric treatment with a general high-potency vitamin/mineral supplement has been suggested.[17] PET and SPECT examinations are used in research only and have not been proven helpful in the diagnosis of chronic fatigue syndrome.[18] Searches for immunologic markers have been undertaken, but none have been found.[19,20]

Testing involving Profile of Mood Status Questionnaire (POMS), Sickness Impact Profile, Composite International Diagnostic Instrument, General Health Questionnaire and Hospital Anxiety and Depression Scale have been used to assess treatment and rehabilitation results. No one test of cognitive or physical function has been determined ideal for monitoring outcomes.

Differential Diagnosis

Bacterial infection—local or systemic
    Occult abscesses
    Lyme disease
    Syphilis
    Endocarditis
Mycoplasma
Mycobacteria
Viral infection
    Enteroviruses
    Polio
    Aseptic meningitis
    Encephalitis
    HIV and other retroviruses
    Epstein Barr virus

Fungal infection
    Candidiasis
    Coccidioidomycosis
    Histoplasmosis
Parasitic infection
    Amebiasis
    Giardiasis
    Helminths
Endocrine abnormality
    Diabetes
    Thyroid function abnormalities
    Cortisol function abnormalities
Fibromyalgia

(Continued on next page.)

Autoimmune disease
   Rheumatoid arthritis
   Lupus
   Vasculitis
Malignancy
Toxic exposure
   Environmental chemicals—formalde-
      hyde toluene, organophosphates
   Heavy metals
   Pesticides (lindane, dieldrin)
Psychiatric disease
   Anxiety

Psychiatric disease *(cont.)*
   Hypochondriasis
   Depression
   Somatization
Drug or alcohol abuse
Sleep disorders
Medicine side effects
CNS disease
Other chronic disease of the lung, heart, liver
   kideny, blood, or gastrointestinal tract, or
   nutritional deficiencies

Treatment

Initial

No clear treatment has been proven to shorten the course of the syndrome. Symptom moderation has occurred with varying success when moderate exercise, healthy diet, adequate vitamin supplementation, stress reduction, support groups, and counseling have been employed. Symptomatic treatment, with or without counseling for coping with a chronic debilitating disease, has been a common approach to therapy. Cognitive behavioral therapy(CBT), a nonpharmacologic treatment emphasizing self-help by changing thought patterns and behavior, has been extensively studied with mixed results. Some individuals have reported CBT to be helpful.[24,25] Treatment of depression in this syndrome has been noted to respond to the stimulant antidepressants, such as sertraline and appropriate counseling.

Educating the individual as to what is known and not known about CFS, addressing impact on function at work and home, and providing information regarding prognosis are beneficial. Patients are better prepared for coping on a daily basis, have more realistic expectations, and feel the physician is not ignoring their concerns. In addition, when appropriate, the individual should be informed that periodic reassessment, for a possible treatable underlying process, may ensue. This may help relieve anxiety about abandonment.

Symptomatic treatment for headache, pain, and fever is accomplished using nonsteroidal anti-inflammatory drugs (NSAIDs). Treating rhinitis or sinusitis with antihistamines or decongestants and treating depression successfully can improve mood, help with sleep disorders, attenuate fatigue, and diminish frustration.

Avoiding heavy meals, alcohol, caffeine, and total rest can help as well as minimizing intake of substances that alter sleep patterns or alter one's self-image.[2]

Low-dose amitriptyline may be used for achiness—similar to treatments employed for fibromyalgia.[9]

Rehabilitation

Rehabilitation for chronic fatigue syndrome is based on symptomatic treatment. Exhaustive exercise has proven to decrease cognitive functioning and compliance. Therefore, a graduated exercise program to tolerance is recommended.[9,13] If severe fatigue follows, lasting more than 24 hours, then the exercise prescription is adjusted so it is less demanding; there are no specific and firm guidelines due to the wide spectrum found in this syndrome. It is key to continue to maintain fitness and avoid excessive weight gain. Patients may find themselves ingesting more calories and exercising less due to the fatigue, and many must be warned to watch for excessive weight gain. Loss of fitness can accelerate an individual's loss of functioning and should be carefully monitored.

Procedures

Treatment is symptomatic, therefore procedures may be chosen to help with trigger points, dizziness, headache, or other symptoms as they occur. If trigger points are noted, appropriate therapy may be initiated. Both the use of spray and stretch techniques, dry needling, or trigger point injection using a local anesthetic or small amount of steroid have all met with some success.[9]

Surgery

No specific surgery is performed for chronic fatigue syndrome.

Potential Disease Complications

Chronic fatigue syndrome will resolve in up to 48% of individuals. However, a few of these individuals, as well as others, will continue with some mixture of debilitating fatigue and other intermittent symptoms. The primary complication of the disease is continued fatigue and loss of function, which commonly occur despite treatment. Social isolation can result in increasing disability. Maintaining enough function to continue participation in work and social events is extremely important for an individual's quality of life. Total rest should be discouraged because it results in increasing weakness and decreasing function.[7] At the other end of the spectrum, exhaustion and exercising to exhaustion also need to be avoided because they can result in decreasing mental functioning and an aversion to continuing such a regimen.[13]

Potential Treatment Complications

Physicians should be aware that conveying understanding and compassion to patients, despite the lack of a known "cure," can still alter a patient's quality of life. Fear, or the perception of being abandoned, can markedly accentuate frustration and accelerate a decline in function. Medication side effects should be reviewed on an intermittent basis, to be certain that accentuation of the nonspecific symptoms found in chronic fatigue syndrome, are not occurring. Care to avoid too strenuous an exercise program should be included because the fatigue which may ensue can be both physically and mentally debilitating. Despite optimal care, depression, fatigue, and a loss of function may still occur. Physicians and patients should both be aware that symptoms found in CFS may persist for months or years but that remittance or recovery is still possible.

References
1. CFIDS Association of America web site. Available at http://www.cfids.org/ (accessed 9/6/00).
2. Manningham R: The Symptoms, Nature and Causes, and Cure of the Febricula, or Little Fever. London, J. Robinson, 1750.
3. Holmes GP, Kaplan JE, Gantz NM, et al: Chronic fatigue syndrome: A working case definition. Ann Int Med 1988;108:387–389.
4. Fukuda K, Straus SE, Hickie I, et al, including the International CFS Study Group: The chronic fatigue syndrome: A comprehensive approach to its definition and study. Ann Intern Med 1994;121:953–959..
5. Fukuda K: Development of the 1994 chronic fatigue syndrome case definition and clinical evaluation guidelines. In Yehuda S, Mostofsky D (eds): Chronic Fatigue Syndrome. New York, Plenum Press, 1997, pp 29–94.
6. Reyes M, Dobbins JG, Nisenbaum R, et al: Chronic fatigue syndrome progression and self-defined recovery: Evidence from the CDC surveillance system. J Chronic Fatigue Syndrome 1999;5(1):17–27.
7. Fauci AS, et al: Harrison's Principles of Internal Medicine, 14th ed. New York, McGraw-Hill, 1998, pp 2483–2485.
8. Centers for Disease Control and Prevention: Available at http://www.cdc.gov/ncidod/diseases/cfs/publicat.txt (accessed 9/6/00).
9. Braddom RL: Physical Medicine and Rehabilitation. Philadelphia, W. B. Saunders, 1996, pp. 908–912.
10. Griffith's Five Minute Clinical Consult, 8th ed.
11. Levine PH: Chronic fatigue syndrome comes of age. Am J Med 1998;105(3A):2s–4s.
12. Lloyd A: Chronic fatigue and chronic fatigue syndrome: Shifting boundaries and attributions. Am J Med 1998;105(3A):7s–10s.
13. La Manca, et al: Influence of exhaustive treadmill exercise on cognitive functioning in chronic fatigue syndrome. Am J Med 1998;105(3A):59s–65s.
14. Nasralla M, Haier J, Nicolson GL: Multiple mycoplasmal infections detected in blood of patients with chronic fatigue syndrome and/or fibromyalgia syndrome. Eur J Clin Microbiol Infect Dis 1999;18(12):859–865.

15. Bell R, et al: Illness from low levels of environmental chemicals: Relevance to chronic fatigue syndrome and fibromyalgia. Am J Med 1998;105(3A):74s–90s.
16. Lange G, DeLuca J, Maldjian JA, et al: Brain MRI abnormalities exist in a subset of patients with chronic fatigue syndrome; J Neurol Sci 1999;171(1):3–7.
17. Werbach MR: Nutritional strategies for treating chronic fatigue syndrome. Altern Med Rev 2000;5(2):93–108.
18. Tirelli U, et al: Brain positron emission tomography (PET) in chronic fatigue syndrome: Preliminary data. Am J Med 1998;105(3A):54s–58s.
19. Natelson BH, et al: Immunologic parameters in chronic fatigue syndrome, major depression and multiple sclerosis. Am J Med 1998;105(3A):43s–49s.
20. Whiteside TL, et al: Natural killer cells and natural killer cell activity in chronic fatigue syndrome. Am J Med 1998;105(3A):27s–34s.
21. Bruno RL, et al: Parallels between post-polio fatigue and chronic fatigue syndrome: A common pathophysiology? Am J Med 1998;105(3A):66s–73s.
22. Heneine W, Woods TC, Sinha SD, et al: Lack of evidence for infection with known human and animal retroviruses in patients with chronic fatigue syndrome. Clin Infect Dis 1994;18(Suppl 1):121–125.
23. Mawle AC, Reyes M, Schmid DS: Is chronic fatigue syndrome an infectious disease? Infectectious Agents and Disease 1994;2:387–389.
24. Sharpe M, et al: Cognitive Behavioral Therapy for chronic fatigue syndrome: Efficacy and implications. Am J Med 1998;105(3A):104s–109s.
25. Lloyd AR, Hickie I, Brockman A, et al: Immunologic and psychologic therapy for patients with chronic fatigue syndrome: A double-blind, placebo-controlled trial. Am J Med, 1993;94:197–203.

101 Chronic Pain Syndrome

Heechin Chae, MD
Joseph F. Audette, MD

Synonyms

Behavioral
maladaptations to
chronic pain

ICD-9 Codes

None

Definition

Chronic pain syndrome can be defined as longstanding complaints of trauma-induced discomfort and pain that have persisted beyond the expected healing time and have resisted more conservative and traditional health care intervention strategies.[1] It is important to differentiate patients with chronic pain syndrome from those who experience chronic pain due to an unresolved or permanent localized injury.

The Office of Disabilities of the Social Security Administration uses the following criteria to establish the diagnosis of chronic pain syndrome (must meet *all* the criteria): (1) any intractable pain of more than 6 month's duration; (2) marked alteration in behavior with depression or anxiety; (3) marked restriction in daily activities; (4) excessive use of medication and frequent use of medical services; (5) no clear relationship to organic disorder; and (6) history of multiple, nonproductive tests, treatment, and surgeries.

Studies suggest that women are up to four times more affected than men.[2] There is a high incidence of chronic pain syndrome in people with a history of abuse in childhood, borderline personality disorder, narcissistic personality disorder, and lower income.[3,4]

In patients with chronic pain syndrome, there is no clear relationship between pain and tissue damage and the degree of functional loss or impairment.[5,6] Pain behavior, such as limping, grimacing, restricting movement, and avoidance of physical activities, also contributes to impairments and functional limitations independent of the initial physical problem. These behaviors persist when they are rewarded, such as increased attention from friends and family; reinforcement from health care providers; or avoidance of disliked activities such as work.

Patients with chronic pain syndrome have low activity levels compared with their premorbid levels and those of normally functioning controls.[8] Patients are often instructed by their family and health care providers to "stop when it hurts" or to "let pain be your guide" and thus limit their activity levels. These low activity levels, however, are not usually associated with significant physical limitations or with reduction in chronic pain. Frequently, patients have tried to resume normal activity, only to experience increased pain. Fear of pain plays a central role in the lives of patients with chronic pain syndrome. They learn to anticipate the painful consequences of engaging in activities and avoid these activities because they are afraid they will harm themselves by becoming more active. This fear-avoidance behavior results in a downward spiral of further deconditioning and decline in function.[9]

Chronic pain syndrome is a diagnosis of exclusion. Therefore, history, physical examination, and diagnostic testing are directed toward determining whether the symptoms represent a treatable condition.

Symptoms

Patients with chronic pain syndrome experience pain that is often not well localized, lasts longer than anticipated, and is more severe than typically expected. Common pain complaints include headaches, muscle aches, and/or joint aches. Symptoms of weakness, paresthesias, and sensory loss may or may not be present. Cognitive complaints such as short-term memory impairment and difficulty with concentrating on tasks may be reported. Mood disturbances are very common and can include depression, anxiety, and emotional lability. Sleep disturbances are also common and contribute to the vicious cycle of physical and psychologic disability. Other symptoms may include sweating, chills without fever, cold intolerance, shortness of breath, fatigue, and avoidance of physical activity. There may also be a tendency to view the world catastrophically. See Table 1.

Physical Examination

Thorough musculoskeletal and neurologic examinations are desirable but often cannot be completed effectively due to the patient's complaint of severe pain. If this is the case, an abbreviated specific neurologic exam is performed to aid the clinician about the need for further diagnostic tests. Typically during the examination, patients will demonstrate behaviors that imply misery, such as grimacing, sighing, or a dramatic presentation. Almost all patients have tender points where muscles attach to bones, especially the spinal axial muscle groups. These tender points are found to be inconsistent in their locations and tend to be absent when the patient's attention is focused elsewhere on his or her body. The patient with true tenderness on pressure

TABLE 1. Difference in Findings Between Patients with Chronic Pain and Patients with Chronic Pain Syndrome[7]

Assessment Methods	Chronic Pain	Chronic Pain Syndrome
Pain drawing	Localized with appropriate neuro-anatomic features	Magnified, covering diffuse regions of body
Symptoms		
Pain	Localized	Whole leg pain
Numbness	Dermatomal	Whole leg
Weakness	Myotomal	Whole leg giving away
Time pattern	Varies	Never free of pain
Response to treatment	Variable benefit	Intolerance of treatments Frequent ER visits
Signs		
Tenderness	Localized	Superficial, non-anatomical
Axial loading	No lumbar pain	Lumbar pain
Straight-leg raise	Limited on distraction	Improves with distraction
Sensory	Dermatomal	Regional
Motor	Myotomal	Jerky, give away weakness
Tenderness	Appropriate pain	Over-reaction

flinches with a spinal reflex, which is immediate, whereas the patient with chronic pain syndrome has a flinching response on a cortical reflex basis, which is delayed.

To assess for inconsistencies in the neurologic and musculoskeletal examination (see Table 1), the clinician should re-examine the involved area at the end of the examination or during the next visit to note any changes in physical findings.

Functional Limitations

Patients with chronic pain syndrome typically function at a much lower level than would be anticipated for their age and reported injury. They frequently complain of pain with even the most minor activities, so they limit themselves at home and work. Often, they are not gainfully employed and decline to work due to pain. It is no surprise that they often have difficulty with relationships with family members, friends, and colleagues. They may avoid both physical and psychologic intimacy.

Diagnostic Studies

Chronic pain syndrome is a clinical diagnosis. Diagnostic studies reveal either no pathology, or degenerative/congenital conditions that do not fully explain the patient's symptoms.

Psychologic testing such as the Minnesota Multiphasic Personality Inventory (MMPI) can be helpful in assessing for characterologic and axis II diagnoses. Other tests such as MRI, electrodiagnostic studies, and laboratory tests may be indicated if other diagnoses are suspected. Sometimes, a diagnostic study can be a useful tool in helping the patient to shift the focus from the diagnosis to restoring his or her function.

Differential Diagnosis

Malingering

Depression

Cultural differences

Somatoform disorder

Conversion disorder

Treatment

Initial

Initial treatment includes patient education, pharmacologic treatment, and psychotherapy. Patient education includes individual or/and group classes that review the physiology of chronic pain, define acute pain versus chronic pain, and define the patient's role in the treatment plan. Any environmental, physical, and psychologic factor that maintains fear-avoidance behavior should be addressed. Patients can attempt to make sense of their pain through past experiences. Therefore, anticipated consequence of a behavior is as important as the actual consequence of the behavior. Negative thoughts stemming from pain and fear can influence mood, physiology, and behavior (e.g., anxious thoughts producing disturbed sleep, and results in depressed mood).

It is important for patients to maintain some level of function to prevent the worsening cycle of activity avoidance. To address the patient's persistent fear of self-harm with increased activity, the clinician may need to order diagnostic tests that can alleviate this fear. Behavioral treatment by a mental health professional with a pain subspecialty that addresses factors which maintain or exacerbate fear-avoidance behavior is essential.

The goal of the pharmacologic treatment is *not* to eliminate pain (Table 2), rather it is to improve functional tolerance to rehabilitation, restore sleep, and improve mood, if indicated.

TABLE 2. Medications Used for Chronic Pain Syndrome

Non Opioid Analgesics

Generic Name	Brand Name	Common Unit Dose	Dosage Frequency
Acetaminophen	Tylenol	650 mg	tid to qid
Aspirin		325 mg	q 2 h
Celecoxib	Celebrex	200 mg	qd to bid
Diclofenac	Voltaren	75 mg	bid
Diflunisal	Dolobid	500 mg	bid
Etodolac	Lodine	400 mg	bid
Fenoprofen	Nalfon	600 mg	qid
Flurbiprofen	Ansaid	100 mg	tid
Ibuprofen	Motrin	800 mg	qid
Indomethacin	Indocin	25 mg	tid
Ketoprofen	Orudis	75 mg	tid
Ketorolac	Toradol	10 mg	qid
Meclofenamate	Meclomen	100 mg	tid
Nabumetone	Relafen	500 mg	2 qd
Naproxen	Naprosyn	500 mg	bid
Oxaprozin	Daypro	600 mg	2 qd
Piroxicam	Feldene	20 mg	qd
Salsalate	Disalcid	750 mg	qid
Sodium salicylate		650 mg	Q 4 h
Rofecoxib	Vioxx	25 mg	qd
Sulindac	Clinoril	200 mg	bid
Tolmentin	Tolectin	400 mg	tid

Opoid Analgesic

Generic Name	Brand Name	Morphine Equivalent Dose	Starting Dose	Dosage Frequency
Propoxyphene	Darvon Darvocet	NA	Darvocet: N50–100 Darvon: 65 mg	qid
Hydrocodone	Vicodin, Vicodin ES, Vicoprofen	30 mg	1 tablet	q 4 h
Hydromorphone	Dilaudid	7.5/5.6 mg	2 mg	q 3–4 h
Morphine	MSIR MS Contin Kadian Duragesic patch Oramorph	30/45 mg	MSIR: 15 mg MSContin: 15 mg Kadian: 20 mg Duragesic patch: 25 mcg/hr Oramorph: 15 mg	MSIR: q 4 h MS Contin: tid Kadian: qd Duragesic patch: 72 h Oramorph: tid
Oxycodone	Percocet Roxicet Oxycontin	30 mg	Percocet: 5mg Oxycodone: 5mg Oxycontin: 10 mg	Percocet or oxyco: done: q 4 h Oxycontin: bid
Methadone	Dolophine	10/20 mg	2.5–5 mg	q 18–24 h
Levorphanol	Levo-Dromoran	4 mg	2 mg	q 6–8 h

bid, twice a day; qd, each day; qid, 4 times a day; tid, 3 times a day; q 2–4 h, every 2 to 4 hours; 2 qd, 2 once a day; q 4 h, every 4 hours.

(Table contined on next page.)

TABLE 2. Medications Used for Chronic Pain Syndrome (*Continued*)

Adjuvant Medications

Generic Name	Brand Name	Starting Dose	Dosage Frequency
Tricyclic Antidepressants			
Amitriptyline	Elavil	10–25 mg	qhs
Nortriptyline	Pamelor	10–25 mg	qhs
Doxepin	Sinequan	10–25 mg	qhs
Anticonvulsants			
Carbamazepine	Tegretol	100 mg	bid (titrate up by 100 mg q 5 days)
Gabapentin	Neurontin	100 mg	tid (titrate up by 100 mg q 4 days)
Topiramate	Topamax	25 mg	bid (titrate up by 25 mg q 7 days)
Lamotrigine	Lamictal	50 mg	bid (titrate up by 25 mg q 4-7 days)
Other			
Tizanidine (α-2 agonist)	Zanaflex	2 mg	qhs then bid–tid (titrate up by 1–2 mg q 3 days)

Evaluation by an experienced pain mental health professional is important before initiating opioid treatment. As part of the evaluation process, the patient's substance abuse history should be determined. The presence of a past substance abuse problem is not an absolute contraindication for opioid therapy. However, it is recommended that all patients have had reasonable pain management treatment, such as rehabilitation therapies, medical techniques, and cognitive-behavioral techniques. Opioid medication should be started after the patient reads and signs an informed consent form.

Once the decision has been made to use opioid medication, consider using long-acting opioid medication in a fixed-dosing schedule. Frequent follow-up visits to titrate the dosage and assess for functional improvement are recommended. The patient should also continue to follow up with a mental health practitioner.

Medications should be reviewed intermittently since side effects can accentuate symptoms, thus leading to further decline in function. Unscheduled medication use (i.e., on an as-needed basis) can create unwanted dependency on the medications, which can lead to further functional decline.

Rehabilitation

A comprehensive rehabilitation program that focuses on functional restoration by modifying maladaptive behaviors, physical reconditioning, and drug minimization is essential in treating patients with chronic pain syndrome. Clinicians should be aware that treatments focused only on symptomatic relief are bound to fail. Treatments that reinforce passive and compliant behavior should be avoided. Any strenuous exercise program that can significantly worsen the pain, thus accentuate fear-avoidance behavior, should be avoided. Instead, functionally oriented exercise programs are used. A typical program can be anywhere from 4 to 8 weeks long, 3 to 5 days per week, and 3 to 6 hours per day. The program involves a clinician, mental health practitioner, and a physical therapist. Occupational therapists and other rehabilitation clincians are also often involved.

Physical therapy is utilized to increase the patient's activity level. This is accomplished through education in the use of proper body mechanics, postural re-education, endurance training (e.g., walking, swimming), and the incorporation of pain control modalities. Occupational therapy aims at helping patients develop new, non-pharmacologic skills to decrease pain, improve function and endurance in all areas of living, and to prevent injury despite persistent pain.

Mental health professionals play an important role in reducing suffering and in helping the patient cope more effectively with life stressors by teaching the patient about the role of thoughts, feelings, and behaviors in maintaining the pain experience. Cognitive and behavioral strategies such as transformative imagery, biofeedback-assisted relaxation, cognitive restructuring, and stress inoculation are employed as well.

Rehabilitation in an inpatient setting may be indicated when the home environment appears likely to enforce maladaptive behaviors more strongly than the outpatient program can reinforce positive behaviors and/or when there is a significant medication dependency that requires detoxification. Other reasons for inpatient treatment include co-morbid conditions, such as heart or pulmonary disease, that may make participation in an outpatient program difficult.

Procedures

Procedures can be considered if a specific functional outcome is to be achieved, and both the patient and the rehabilitation team are aware that this is the goal of the procedure.

Trigger point injections are sometimes used by injecting a local anesthetic into the myofascial trigger point to reduce pain and improve the range of motion. If patients have specific diagnoses, such as facet syndrome, bursitis, or nerve entrapments, specific therapeutic blocks or injections to treat these disorders can be used to reduce pain and increase participation in the rehabilitation program.

Surgery

Surgery is not indicated.

Potential Disease Complications

Chronic pain syndrome can limit all aspects of a patient's ability to function. Profound depression and suicide are important disease complications.

Potential Treatment Complications

Medication side effects are well documented. Opiates can cause physical and psychologic dependence and should be used only after careful consideration of other pharmacologic agents. Clinicians who are dismissive of a patient's symptoms without providing information on available treatment programs and objectives for this illness may increase the likelihood of continued disability.

References
1. Fordyce WE: Behavioral Methods for Chronic Pain and Illness. St. Louis, Mosby, 1976.
2. Unruh AM: Gender variations in clinical pain experience. Pain 1996;65:123–167.
3. Craig TK, Boardman AP, Mills K: The South London somatisation study. Br J Psychiatry 1993;163:579–588.
4. Craig TK, Drake H: The South London somatisation study II. Br J Psychiatry 1994;165:248–258.
5. Waddell G, Somerville D: Objective clinical dvaluation of physical impairment in chronic low back pain. Spine 1992;17:617.
6. Vasudevan S: Impairment, Disability and Functional Capacity Assessment. Handbook of Pain Assessment. New York, Guilford, 1992.
7. Waddell G, Pilowski I: Clinical assessment and interpretation of abnormal illness behavior in low back pain. Pain 1989;39:41.
8. Vlayen JWS, Kole-Snijders AMJ, et al: Fear of movement/(re)injury in chronic low back pain and its relation to vehavioral performance. Pain 1995;62:363.
9. Fordyce WE, et al: Pain complaint-exercise performance relationships in chronicpain. Pain 1981;10:311.

102 Chronic Renal Failure

Ajay K. Singh, MD

Synonyms

Chronic kidney disease

Chronic kidney failure

Pre-ESRD (end stage renal disease)

ICD-9 Codes

585
Chronic renal failure

586
Renal failure (unspecified)

593.9
Unspecified disorder of kidney and ureter

Definition

Chronic renal failure is a syndrome characterized by a progressive decline in kidney function such that the kidney's ability to adequately excrete waste products and to contribute to the constancy of the body's homeostatic functions is severely impaired. Chronic renal failure at its mildest stage is asymptomatic, whereas at its most severe stage is characterized by uremia. End-stage renal disease is the term used to denote chronic renal failure that necessitates renal replacement therapy (dialysis or transplantation).

The incidence of renal failure in the United States is approximately 268 cases per 1 million population per year.[1] However, incidence of chronic renal failure is greater among African-Americans (829 per million population per year, as compared with 199 per million population per year among Caucasian Americans). The major causes of chronic renal failure in the United States are diabetes mellitus (40%), hypertension (30%), glomerular disease (15%), polycystic kidney disease, and obstructive uropathy (Table 1).[1] Elsewhere in the world, where the incidence of diabetes mellitus has not reached epidemic proportions (e.g., in Europe and parts of the developing world), chronic glomerulonephritis (20%) and chronic reflux nephropathy (25%) are the most common causes of chronic renal failure. The progressive decline in renal function in individuals with chronic renal failure is variable and depends on both the cause of the underlying insult and patient specific factors. Furthermore, evidence also points to the importance of several factors in modulating renal progression. These include proteinuria, the presence of systemic hypertension, age, gender, genetic factors, and smoking.[2]

TABLE 1. Etiologies for Chronic Renal Failure

Prerenal
  Cardiogenic
    Severe cardiac failure
  Vascular
    Renal artery stenosis
Renal
  Immunological
    Glomerulonephritis (primary or secondary)
  Neoplastic
    Multiple myeloma
  Toxic
    Gold, pencillamine, cyclosporine
  Tubulointerstitial
  Infection and/or reflux
  Cystic diseases
    Polycystic kidney disease
Postrenal
  Stones
  Pelvi-uretic obstruction
  Retroperitoneal fibrosis
  Prostatic hypertrophy
  Urethral stricture

In the United States, an arteriovenous (AV) graft is the most common form of vascular access for dialysis—outnumbering AV fistulas in some centers by 3 to 1. In contrast, in Europe, Canada, and even some American centers, AV grafts are in the minority. The reasons behind this variation include a higher rate of patients with diabetes with chronic renal failure in the United States, a higher rate of small vessel disease (because of the higher prevalence of diabetes mellitus coupled with an older population), and a higher level of time and skill to create an AV fistula compared with an AV graft.

At an early stage, insidious effects on target organs may become manifest. For example, patients may have mild to moderate hypertension, mild anemia, left ventricular hypertrophy, and subtle changes in bone structure due to renal osteodystrophy. It is imperative to investigate the abnormal renal function and to refer the patient to a nephrologist. As renal function gradually declines further—with glomerular filtration rates reaching 10 to 30 ml/min, hypertension is usually present and subtle biochemical and hematologic abnormalities may become evident, such as mild hyperkalemia, mild hypobicarbonatemia (from uremic acidosis), and anemia of chronic disease.[3]

As renal dysfunction becomes severe—GFR in the 10 to 15 ml/min range—the syndrome of uremia is invariably present. Uremia reflects the accumulation of metabolic toxins, some characterized and others unknown, that influences the functioning of a variety of organ systems. In this late stage, the need for renal replacement therapy is imminent and dialysis and/or transplantation are required to sustain life. The indications for initiating renal replacement therapy include severe refractory abnormalities in biochemistry (severe hyperkalemia and acidosis), severe pulmonary edema, bleeding, metabolic encephalopathy, and the presence of pericarditis.[4] More subtle but no less important indications include malnutrition and severe disability (marked tiredness and lethargy).

Symptoms

Chronic renal failure may be asymptomatic when renal function is only mildly impaired, whereas when the glomerular filtration rate (GFR) is markedly reduced the patient is usually very symptomatic and may be severely disabled. Early in renal disease, individuals may present simply with elevated serum creatinine and blood urea nitrogen (BUN) levels but no symptoms. These individuals are usually unaware that they have any abnormalities in their renal function and usually fail to register on the "radar screen" of their clinicians. Edema may also be observed for the first time, reflecting the kidney's inability to excrete salt and water. With a further decline in renal function, there is often a concomitant decline in cognitive and physical functioning. This is usually due to anemia, renal osteodystophy, and the onset of the uremic syndrome. In addition, appetite declines and there is often a significant loss of lean body mass.

Physical Examination

The physical examination in patients with chronic renal failure may manifest as one or more of a spectrum of abnormalities that reflect the multisystem nature of the uremic syndrome. Patients may appear generally ill, gaunt, and pale. Mucous membraness may be pale from anemia, and poor platelet function may result in easy bleeding of the gums. The cardiovascular system may exhibit either no abnormality or there may be evidence of hypertension, extracellular fluid overload (elevated jugular venous pressure, pulmonary venous congestion manifested by rales, and the presence of pitting edema), and acute pericarditis. The presence of a pericardial rub on physical examination is usually highly suggestive of uremic pericarditis. The pulmonary system may demonstrate rales from fluid overload on physical examination. Gastrointestinal abnormalities include stomatitis, cheilosis, and halitosis. Patients may also experience epigastric tenderness compatible with gastritis secondary to uremia. Abnormalities in the musculoskeletal system may include generalized weakness on physical examination.

Proximal weakness may be an early sign of renal osteodystrophy. Patients with dialysis associated amyloidosis may experience bone tenderness, carpal tunnel syndrome, and amyloid accumulations or tumors in various parts of the body, such as the skin. Hematologic abnormalities evident on physical examination may include bruising from platelet function abnormalities. Findings of the neurological examination may, quite commonly, be abnormal in patients with uremia. Patients may manifest mild abnormalities, such as intermittent confusion, or more severe manifestations, such as delirium, seizure activity, and psychosis. In exteme cases, the patient may become comatose. Common abnormalities on physical examination include evidence of confusion, a flapping tremor (asterixis), and fasciculations. A peripheral neuropathy is quite rare since most patients have started dialysis treatment before a neuropathy has time to present.

It is unclear why some patients demonstrate the "full-blown" physical abnormalities of the uremic syndrome, whereas others exhibit relatively mild findings on physical examination. The physical examination is important in the diagnosis of uremia. In particular, abnormalities such as the presence of an encephalopathy, acute pericarditis, or pulmonary edema are indications for initiation of renal replacement therapy.

Functional Limitations

Functional limitations in individuals with chronic renal failure depend on the degree of lethargy, fatigue, and neuropsychologic symptoms that are present. Individuals may go from being mobile to non-mobile because of weakness. Elderly individuals with underlying co-morbidities may be the most affected. Endurance and the ability to perform activities of daily living may be reduced, and modifications in lifestyle may become necessary, including changing from a full-time to part-time job, reducing travel, and discontinuing driving.[5–7] In diabetic patients, the onset of symptomatic chronic renal failure in the setting of other underlying complications of diabetes mellitus, including impaired visual acuity and peripheral neuropathy, become challenging functional limitations.

Diagnostic Studies

Diagnostic testing in individuals with chronic renal failure essentially focuses on two areas: monitoring the progression of chronic renal failure and assessing the complications of chronic renal failure. Monitoring renal progression involves regular measurement of the following: serum creatinine, BUN, electrolytes, calcium, phosphorous, albumin, and magnesium. A complete blood count is also necessary.

Creatinine and urea have several major limitations in estimating renal function accurately.[8] Muscle mass is perhaps the single most important factor for the limited accuracy of creatinine as a measure of renal function. This is because creatinine is a by-product of creatine metabolism, which is a product of muscle breakdown. Thus, individuals with large muscular mass generate greater amounts of endogenous creatine and therefore creatinine and have a higher steady state serum creatinine level, even though their renal function as measured by GFR is in the normal range.[9] On the other hand, individuals with smaller muscle mass, such as elderly patients, will have a serum creatinine within the normal range but will have lower than normal renal function as measured by the GFR.[9] Urea levels reflect the metabolic state of the body. In highly anabolic individuals, a "normal" level may even suggest significant abnormality in renal function (e.g., pregnant women will have blood urea levels that are markedly depressed). In contrast, a very high urea level may be observed in highly catabolic patients, such as those who are critically ill or are receiving high doses of corticosteroids. Therefore, interpretation of a very high BUN level should be done in concert with the serum creatinine measurement.

Renal function can be measured more accurately by calculation of the creatinine clearance and urea clearance using 24-hour collection of urine. These methods also have limitations because they are dependent on the compulsiveness of the patient in collection procedures; however, they are very useful in practice—often more so than a serum creatinine measurement. A creatinine clearance measurement is reasonably accurate until renal function is severely impaired. This is because, as alluded to earlier, creatinine is both filtered freely by glomeruli and secreted by the proximal tubule. Thus, as renal function declines, the proportion of creatinine that is secreted over that which is filtered increases. Hence, as renal function declines the creatinine clearance tends to underestimate the impairment of GFR. In contrast, urea clearance is an overestimation of GFR. This is because despite the fact that urea is freely filtered by the glomerulus and not secreted by the proximal tubule, it undergoes a variable degree of reabsorption in the distal nephron—its reabsorption being crucial for the maintenance of an hyperosmolar medullary interstitium. In low flow states, such as dehydration, urea is reabsorbed in the collecting duct of the distal nephron. Consequently, urea clearance values overestimate impairment in GFR.

More accurate measurement of renal function is feasible through the measurement of inulin clearance and iothalamate or ethylenediaminetetraacetic acid (EDTA) clearance. These methods are not widely available, are expensive, and may be inconvenient for the patient to have performed. Most recently the use of cimetidine-blocked creatinine clearance and the use of the MDRD formula have become popular.[10,11]

Approximately every 3 months, measurement of iron stores (serum iron, ferritin, and total iron binding capacity) and parathyroid hormone (PTH) is warranted. In patients with early to moderate renal dysfunction, measurement of proteinuria, using either a spot protein-to-creatinine ratio or a 24-hour collection for protein, is necessary, given the important role that proteinuria plays as a risk factor in renal progression.

Screening for complications of chronic renal failure is very important to reduce morbidity and mortality. In assessing for cardiovascular complications, an annual cardiac echocardiogram is increasingly being recommended to assess for early left ventricular hypertrophy.[12] An electrocardiogram may also be utilized for this purpose, but its sensitivity is limited, particularly for early detection. Measurement of serum total cholesterol, LDL, HDL, triglycerides, and homocysteine levels is recommended since nearly 50% of individuals with end stage renal disease die from cardiovascular causes—commonly coronary artery disease. To screen for malnutrition, regular assessment by a dietitian is also recommended. Individuals with chronic renal failure spontaneously eat less than healthy age-matched controls. Furthermore, the majority of patients who reach end stage renal failure in the United States have hypoalbuminemia, despite good evidence that suggests the importance of albumin as a marker for a poor outcome among patients receiving dialysis. Although anemia is a common complication in individuals with chronic renal failure, as a result of erythropoietin deficiency, it is important to rule out other causes of anemia, particularly if the patient has erythropoietin resistance. Screening for fecal occult blood and measurement of iron stores and serum folate are recommended.

Differential Diagnosis

Acute renal failure

Treatment

Initial

The timely referral of the patient with chronic renal failure to a nephrologist is of great importance.[13] Studies demonstrate that early referral is associated with more optimal management of the complications of chronic renal disease.[14,15] As well, there is time to electively create an arteriovenous fistula rather than resorting to either a temporary catheter or a synthetic graft. In addition, early referral saves money and reduces the days of hospitalization.

The focus of treatment before dialysis becomes necessary is slowing the progression of chronic renal failure and managing complications. The main thrusts of antiprogression therapy are the use of an ACE inhibitor (or, if the patient cannot tolerate an ACE inhibitor, the use of an angiotensin receptor blocker), the optimal management of hypertension targeting a mean arterial blood pressure of 92 mm Hg (120/80 mm Hg), particularly in patients who have chronic renal failure associated with significant (more than 1g/24 hour) proteinuria; strategies to reduce proteinuria; and the judicious use of a low protein, high caloric diet. In addition, the use of a hypolipidemic agent and early treatment of anemia with epoetin are important. The use of a protocol to comprehensively manage the protean manifestations of chronic renal failure is highly recommended. One such protocol focuses on the 10 *A*'s of chronic renal failure: *a*nemia, *a*therosclerosis (cardiovascular disease), *a*nti-angiotensin therapy, *a*lbumin (nutrition), *a*nions and cations (acidosis, hyperkalemia, hypermagnesemia), *a*rterial blood pressure, *a*rterial calcification (calcium x phosphorous product), *a*ccess (vascular access), *a*voidance of nephrotoxic drugs, and *a*llograft (timely referral for a renal transplant evaluation).

Rehabilitation

Rehabilitation ensures that the patient remains intact both physically and psychologically as major changes in health and life status occur. In this regard, rehabilitation strategies have emerged as adjuncts in managing patients with chronic renal failure, especially those nearing the initiation of dialysis.[16–24] These strategies focus on two issues: an assessment of function and then a prescriptive component targeted at muscle strengthening and restoration of function. This is accomplished in some dialysis programs with exercise machines.

Referral to a physical or occupational therapist as an outpatient is an important part of the overall management. Initially a physical medicine consult is sought to assess the degree of physical and functional impairment. Evaluation of the patient in the home setting is particularly valuable and is usually orchestrated by the social worker in concert with the physical therapist, occupational therapist, and a visiting nurse. Adaptations in the home may be necessary, particularly for elderly patients. These could range from obtaining new housing for patients who need ground floor accommodation or more space to facilitate equipment such as a dialysis machine to adaptations in the bathroom (e.g., raised toilet seat, railings to steady the patient, and shower adaptations). Modifications such as a bed with railings, safety adaptations to the kitchen, and a chair-lift may also become necessary.

Education of patients with chronic renal failure is of crucial importance.[22–24] In addition to improving a patient's understanding of the treatment protocol, an informed patient is likely to make better choices about dialytic options and about whether he or she wishes to be considered for kidney transplantation. Many options for education are now available, including the "People Like Us" program by the National Kidney Foundation.[24]

Procedures

Temporary line insertion procedures are a much less desirable method to obtain vascular access for dialysis and should be contemplated only in patients who cannot undergo creation of an AV fistula or placement of an AV graft. Occasionally, because patients present late or in cases in which chronic renal failure ensues after a devastating acute renal insult, insertion of a tunneled internal jugular double-lumen dialysis catheter is necessary. It is important to insert the catheter into the jugular vein and not a subclavian vein because studies demonstrate that the latter has a substantially higher risk of stenosing in the setting of an indwelling line.

Surgery

The most common surgical procedure in patients with chronic renal failure is dialysis access. An early assessment of the patient's vascular access options by a vascular surgeon is very important. Patients are asked to save their non-dominant veins during blood draws to facilitate future creation of vascular access.

Although once the patient reaches end stage renal disease, transplantation is the preferred option, this may not be feasible. Individuals may have co-morbidities that preclude transplantation (e.g., there may be no readily available living related or unrelated donor and the patient may have to wait 3 to 4 years for a cadaveric kidney). Alternatively, the patient may prefer dialysis over transplantation as a lifestyle option. Because the failure and complication rates of an AV fistula are much lower than those of an ateriovenous synthetic graft—approximately 80% of AV grafts have failed 3 years after placement, whereas the reverse is true for AV fistulas—creation of an AV fistula is highly recommended. Surgery is usually performed when the GFR has reached 25 to 30 ml/min and can be done on an outpatient basis. An arteriovenous fistula takes approximately 6 months to mature before it can be used, and therefore surgery should be planned at least 6 to 9 months before the anticipated initiation of dialysis treatment.

If the patient is to start hemodialysis, then the dialysis access is either an arteriovenous fistula or an arteriovenous graft. In a minority of patients in whom dialysis is required emergently or in whom surgical creation or insertion of a dialysis accesss is not feasible, the use of a tunneled double-lumen catheter is the treatment of choice. On the other hand, in patients targeted to start peritoneal dialysis, surgical insertion of a tunneled peritoneal dialysis catheter (Tenckhoff catheter) into the anterior abdominal wall is necessary.

Vascular accesss for hemodialysis requires early planning, rigorous counseling of the patient on the choice available for dialysis access, and a good vascular surgeon. Access via an AV fistula is preferred in all patients receiving hemodialysis because of its advantage of long-term patency (more than 80% are patent at 3 years postcreation) and a low complication rate. An AV fistula is the native anastomosis of an arm vein with an arm artery (e.g., the cephalic vein in the arm with the radial artery). In contast, AV grafts have a low patency rate (nearly 80% fail by 3 years postsurgery) and a higher complication rate. An AV graft is the surgical connection of a native vein and a native artery (e.g., an AV graft connects the cephalic vein with the radial artery).

If the patient is a viable candidate for renal transplantation, this procedure is the treatment of choice from medical, patient quality-of-life, and cost perspectives. Potential contraindications include cardiopulmonary disease that places the patient at risk from the surgery; an underlying malignancy; active infection, including positive HIV status; and active intravenous drug abuse. Age is not considered an absolute contraindication, although very few elderly patients undergo transplantation. The inability to comply with medications and/or psychiatric disability are also relative contraindications. The work-up for a renal transplant recipient consists of a thorough physical examination; screeing for infections, including HIV; and screening for underlying malignancy. In patients with diabetes mellitus, formal cardiac testing, such an exercise tolerance stress test and a cardiac echo, is recommended. Many centers also perform pulmonary function testing.

Potential Disease Complications

Chronic renal failure may be associated with protean disease complications. However, complications in the cardiovascular system, bone and mineral metabolism, and the hematologic system are of the greatest significance.

Life expectancy for a 49-year-old patient with chronic renal failure is approximately 7 years—lower than in colon and prostate cancer and one quarter that of the general population.[25] This staggering reduction in life expectancy is largely attributable to cardiovascular complications.[26,27] Nearly 50% of all deaths in patients with end stage renal failure are due to cardiovascular causes.[27] The risk is 17 times that of the general population. Remarkably, this gap is largest in young patients with end stage renal disease.[27,28] The risk factors for cardiovascular disease in individuals with chronic renal failure include, but are not limited to, the magnitude of the calcium/phosphorous product with its attendant risk of coronary calcification and the presence of dyslipidemia, hypertension, hyperhomocystemia, and left ventricular hypertrophy.[26,27] The clinical manifestations of cardiovascular disease in patients with chronic renal failure include left ventricular hypertrophy; left ventricular dilatation; diastolic dysfunction; macrovascular and microvascular disease; and abnormalities in autonomic function, including increased sympathetic discharge and increased circulating catecholamine levels. Vascular disease may involve calcification of coronary vessels and valve disease. Calcification of the mitral valve annulus and the aortic valve cusps is common among patients with chronic renal failure.

Abnormalities in bone and mineral metabolism are common in individuals with chronic renal failure.[29] Patients may manifest both biochemical and skeletal abnormalities. Hypocalcemia, hyperphosphatemia, hypermagnesemia, and hyperparathyroidism are usually observed in some combination. In addition, bony effects may range from an abnormally high to an abnormally low bone turnover.[30] Renal osteodystrophy is characterized by increased osteoclast and osteoblast activity coupled with peritrabecular fibrosis. Bone pain is the single most common manifestation of renal osteodystrophy; it occurs mostly in the hips, lumbosacral spine, and legs and is usually non-specific in nature. Acute periarthritis from metastatic calcification may also occur. Muscle weakness is also common. Other clinical manifestations of renal osteodystrophy include pruritus, metastatic calcification, and calciphylaxis. All of these clinical manifestations progressively impair the patient's strength and functionality.

Anemia is an early and easily recognized complication of chronic renal failure. Erythropoietin is produced predominantly by renal interstitial cells and to a lesser degree by the liver. Erythropoietin production is markedly decreased in individuals with chronic renal failure and, as a consequence, anemia ensues. Other causes of anemia in chronic renal failure include direct marrow suppression by uremic toxins, shortened red cell survival, increased blood loss, and iron deficiency. The benefits of treating anemia with epoetin have been well established in the literature and include a better sense of well-being, enhanced cognitive function, regression of left ventricular hypertrophy, improved sleep pattern, and reduced hospitalizations. Current recommendations center on a target hemoglobin level of 11 g/dL and a hematocrit level of 33 to 36%.

Potential Treatment Complications

Strategies to slow progression are now the centerpiece to managing chronic renal failure. Nevertheless, treatment complications may occur. Because ACE inhibitor therapy is a central component to anti-progression therapy (i.e., all patients with chronic renal insufficiency and chronic renal failure should be targeted for ACE inhibitor therapy), complications include, most commonly, hyperkalemia, a dry cough, and a feeling of lassitude. In patients who have not reached the stage of advanced chronic renal failure, the use of the resin polystyrene in conjunction with a low potassium diet allows continued use of an ACE inhibitor. Often, the patient's potassium level may stabilize in the high side of the normal range when polystyrene is taken every other day. Patients who experience a dry cough—about 15% of the ACE inhibitor treated population—can instead be sufficiently treated with an angiotensin receptor blocker. It is important to remember that ACE inhibitors may result in hemodynamically associated acute renal failure in patients with bilateral renal artery stenosis.

The use of low protein diets in patients who are borderline malnourished may precipitate even worse malnutrition. Withdrawl of the low protein diet in these circumstances is important. In addition, ensuring that the patient is consuming sufficient calories is also important. Referral to a dietitian is an important adjunct to management that specifically addresses the aforementioned issues.

Complications of AV grafts (and to a lesser extent AV fistulas) include, most commonly, thrombosis and infection. Thrombosis of an AV graft is probably the most common reason for a patient with end stage renal disease to be admitted to the hospital.

Renal transplantation is very successful. One-year renal survival rates are more than 95% for transplants from living related and unrelated donors, whereas the 1-year rate is 90% to 95% for cadaveric renal transplantation. Longer-term survival is in the 80% range at 5 years. The most common complications are early non-function; acute rejection; mechanical issues, such as obstruction of the allograft; and chronic allograft rejection. As well, depending on the underlying renal disease, recurrent disease in the allograft may present as a complication. Immunosuppressive treatment includes a calcineurin inhibitor (cyclosporine or FK 506), mycophenolate mofetil (CellCept), and prednisone. Treatment of rejection involves pulsing with methylprednisone acutely and a "rescue" strategy with either muromonab-CD3 (OKT3) or antithymocyte globulin (ATG).

References

1. USRDS: 1998 Annual Data report. The national Institutes of Health, national Institutes of Diabetes and Digestive and Kidney Diseases, Bethesda, MD. Incidence and prevalence of ESRD. Am J Kidney Dis 1998;32:S38–S49.
2. El Nahas M: Progression of chronic renal failure. In Johnson RJ, Freehally J (eds): Comprehensive Clinical Nephrology. Mosby, London, UK, 2000, pp 67.1–67.10.
3. Winearls CG: In Johnson RJ, Freehally J (eds): Comprehensive Clinical Nephrology. Mosby, London, UK, 2000, pp 68.1–68.14.
4. Hakim RM, Lazarus JM: Initiation of dialysis. J Am Soc Nephrol 1995;6(5):1319–1328.
5. Furr LA: Psycho-social aspects of serious renal disease and dialysis: a review of the literature. Soc Work Health Care 1998;27(3):97–118.
6. Iborra MC, Pico VL, Montiel CA, Clemente R:. Quality of life and exercise in renal disease. EDTNA ERCA J 2000;26(1):38–40.
7. Fitts SS, Guthrie MR, Blagg CR: Exercise coaching and rehabilitation counseling improve quality of life for predialysis and dialysis patients. Nephron 1999;82(2):115–121.
8. Levey AS: Measurement of renal function in chronic renal disease. Kidney Int 1990;38(1):167–184.
9. Perrone RD, Madias NE, Levey AS: Serum creatinine as an index of renal function: New insights into old concepts. Clin Chem 1992;38(10):1933–1953.
10. Walser M: Assessing renal function from creatinine measurements in adults with chronic renal failure. Am J Kidney Dis 1998;32(1):23–31.
11. Levey AS, Bosch JP, Lewis JB, et al: A more accurate method to estimate glomerular filtration rate from serum creatinine: A new prediction equation. Modification of diet in Renal Disease Study Group. Ann Intern Med 1999;130(6):461–470.
12. Murphy SW, Parfrey PS: Screening for cardiovascular disease in dialysis patients. Curr Opin Nephrol Hypertens. 1996;5(6):532–540.
13. Pereira BJ: Optimization of pre-ESRD care: The key to improved dialysis outcomes. Kidney Int 2000;57(1):351–365.
14. Obrador GT, Ruthazer R, Arora P, et al: Prevalence of and factors associated with suboptimal care before initiation of dialysis in the United States. J Am Soc Nephrol. 1999;10(8):1793–1800.
15. Arora P, Obrador GT, Ruthazer R, et al: Prevalence, predictors, and consequences of late nephrology referral at a tertiary care center. J Am Soc Nephrol. 1999;10(6):1281–1286.
16. Tawney KW, Tawney PJ, Hladik G, et al: The life readiness program: a physical rehabilitation program for patients on hemodialysis. Am J Kidney Dis. 2000;36(3):581–591.
17. Thornton TA, Hakim RM: Meaningful rehabilitation of the end-stage renal disease patient [Review]. Semin Nephrol 1997;17(3):246–252.
18. Cowen TD, Huang CT, Lebow J, et al: Functional outcomes after inpatient rehabilitation of patients with end-stage renal disease. Arch Phys Med Rehabil. 1995;76(4):355–359.
19. Oberley ET, Sadler JH, Alt PS: Renal rehabilitation: Obstacles, progress, and prospects for the future. Am J Kidney Dis 2000;35(4 Suppl 1):S141–S147.
20. Kutner NG, Cardenas DD, Bower JD: Rehabilitation, aging and chronic renal disease. Am J Phys Med Rehabil. 1992;71(2):97–101.
21. Callahan MB, LeSage L, Johnstone S: A model for patient participation in quality of life measurement to improve rehabilitation outcomes. Nephrol News Issues 1999;13(1):33–37.
22. Orr ML: Pre-dialysis patient education. J Nephrol Nurs 1985;2(1):22–24.
23. Gorrie S. Patient education: A commitment. ANNA J 1992t;19(5):506, 504.
24. King K: People like us, live: An interactive patient education program. EDTNA ERCA J 1997;23(3):34–35, 50.
25. Port FK: Morbidity and mortality in dialysis patients. Kidney Int 1994;46:1728–1737.
26. Levey AS, Beto JA, Coronado BE, et al: Controlling the epidemic of cardiovascular disease in chronic renal disease: What do we know? What do we need to learn? Where do we go from here? National Kidney Foundation Task Force on Cardiovascular Disease. Am J Kidney Dis 1998;32(5):853–906.
27. Foley RN, Parfrey PS, Sarnak MJ: Clinical epidemiology of cardiovascular disease in chronic renal disease. Am J Kidney Dis 1998;32(5 Suppl 3):S112–S119.
28. Raine AE, Margreiter R, Brunner FP, et al: Report on management of renal failure in Europe, XXII, 1991. Nephrol Dial Transplant 1992;7(Suppl 2):7–35.
29. Llach F, Yudd M: Pathogenic, clinical, and therapeutic aspects of secondary hyperparathyroidism in chronic renal failure. Am J Kidney Dis 1998;32(2 Suppl 2):S3–S12.
30. Sherrard DJ, Hercz G, Pei Y, et al: The spectrum of bone disease in end-stage renal failure—an evolving disorder. Kidney Int 1993;43(2):436–442.

103 Contractures

Fae Garden, MD

Synonyms

Contracture deformity

Soft tissue contracture

Muscle, tendon, capsule, ligament. or skin shortening

ICD-9 Codes

718.4
Contracture of joint

727.81
Contracture of tendon (sheath)

728.85
Spasm of muscle

Definition

Contractures are shortenings of muscle, connective tissue, tendons, ligaments, or skin. A contracture develops when normally elastic connective tissues become replaced with inelastic fibrous tissues.[1] Contractures prevent normal movement of the associated body part. Permanent impairments and deformity can ensue. Contractures may occur due to immobilization or as a result of spasticity and excessive muscle tone or prolonged bed rest (Fig. 1). Contracture may also occur following orthopedic procedures, including anterior cruciate ligament repair and total joint arthroplasty. They occur when normal range of motion is not restored following a traumatic joint injury, such as an elbow injury in throwing athletes. Shoulder contractures can occur in persons with diabetes, connective tissue disorders, vascular disturbances, and rotator cuff injuries. Children with Duchenne muscular dystrophy may develop contractures of the heel cords, hamstrings, iliotibial bands, and elbows by age 5 or 6 years. Neurologic conditions, including stroke, traumatic brain injury, and multiple sclerosis, can be complicated by the development of contractures.[1]

Contractures can begin with unequal loss of strength in opposing muscle groups or by reduced range of motion in joints. Loss of mobility in a joint can be caused from immobilization in a cast or splint, by spasticity, or when a person is just too weak to move. Improper stretching and exercise techniques can favor one muscle group over another, leading to unopposed muscle/tendon shortening.[2]

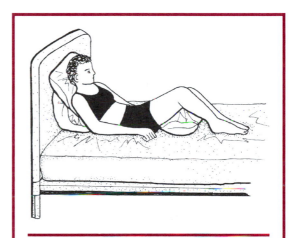

FIGURE 1. Individuals who have experienced prolonged bed rest are susceptible to contractures of multiple areas due to their chronically flexed posture.

Symptoms

The main symptom is loss of range of motion of a joint. When a joint is painful, the body's natural reaction is to "splint" or immobilize the area. A cycle of pain, reduced movement, pain on movement, and further restriction of mobility to avoid pain ensues.

Physical Examination

The physical examination of a patient with contractures should take into account the underlying medical or surgical problem and its resultant anatomic changes.

A thorough neuromuscular examination with documentation of active and passive range of motion is necessary. The most effective tool for joint measuring is a universal goniometer. Spinal range of motion can be assessed with an inclinometer. Standard methods of measuring and recording joint motion as well as a range of normal values have been published.[1] Most reference textbooks utilize a 180 degree system.[3]

The clinician should inspect the patient to observe for abnormalities of limb shape, size, and symmetry. Improper positioning of the joints as well as the presence of marked imbalance of muscle strength should be noted. The presence of abnormally brisk reflexes, sustained clonus, or increased muscle tone occur with spasticity. When increased tone is present, the clinician should apply gentle, prolonged passive stretch (sometimes utilizing therapeutic heating modalities) to determine whether full range of motion can be achieved or whether there is a true contracture.

Swelling of the joints should be noted if present. Skin should also be assessed for any areas of breakdown.

Functional Limitations

Functional limitations depend on the underlying medical condition and the body parts affected. Contractures produce restrictions on mobility and the performance of activities of daily living.

Adhesive capsulitis of the shoulder (frozen shoulder) is one example of a contracture that results in reduced movement and function. In this disorder, shoulder pain and stiffness are followed by decreased range of motion and an inability to raise the affected arm. Functional limitations when performing basic grooming skills and reaching to obtain objects occur, especially if the dominant extremity is affected. Fortunately, most cases of adhesive capsulitis are marked by a recovery stage, in which some, if not all, of the lost movement is regained.[4]

Upper extremity contractures of the elbow, wrist, and fingers impair the performance of all basic activities of daily living as well as advanced skills requiring fine motor coordination.

Hip flexion contractures alter gait pattern and increase the energy expenditure of walking. Hip and knee extension contractures can interfere with wheelchair mobility and car transfers.

Patients with multiple joint contractures are at risk for developing hygiene problems due to inability to obtain proper bed positioning and access for cleaning. Areas of skin breakdown (decubiti) are more likely to occur near the site of joint contracture due to increased pressure on the skin and underlying soft tissue (Table 1).

TABLE 1. Types of Contractures

Joint Contractures
Cartilage damage, joint incongruency
  (e.g., osteoarthritis)
Synovial proliferation, effusion
  (e.g., rheumatoid arthritis)
Capsular fibrosis (e.g., trauma)

Soft Tissue Contractures
Soft tissues surrounding the joint
  (e.g., immobilization)
Skin, subcutaneous tissue (e.g., burns)
Tendon and ligaments (e.g., tendinitis)

Muscle Contractures
Intrinsic (e.g., trauma, inflammation,
  atrophy, ischemia)
Extrinsic (e.g., spasticity, paralysis)

Mixed Contractures

Diagnostic Studies

The diagnosis of contracture is made clinically. Radiographic evaluation with plain x-rays can be done if contributing conditions, such as bone spurs, heterotopic ossifications, or ankylosis, are suspected.

Differential Diagnosis

Spasticity

Heterotopic ossification

Degenerative joint disease

Fracture

Dislocation

Loose body in a joint

Meniscal tears

Psychogenic

Treatment

Initial

The initial "treatment" for contractures is prevention. Contractures are prevented by moving muscles and joints through their full range on a daily basis. Active exercise is preferable, but if passive range of motion exercises are needed, a therapist or family member can do them under a clinician supervised program.

If spasticity is thought to be promoting contractures, then treating the spasticity is advisable (refer to Chapter 136).

Pain control is essential in the prevention and treatment of contractures. NSAIDs/COX-2 inhibitors and oral prednisone are used for treatment of acute painful conditions that, if left untreated, could result in contractures. Non-narcotic analgesics may be used for pain. In selected cases, the use of opioid analgesics is appropriate to promote patient comfort and compliance with rehabilitation measures.

Splints and therapeutic positioning are also important in preventing contractures.[8] These measures help to maintain the correct length of connective tissue. Examples of therapeutic positioning include lying prone occasionally to stretch the hip joint. Standing upright will help to stretch the hip and knee joints. The use of pillows, trochanteric rolls, and footboards for patients experiencing prolonged bed rest should be considered.

Rehabilitation

Once contractures have developed, rehabilitation includes range of motion exercises and sustained stretching. Adequate treatment of pain is essential to ensure patient comfort and compliance with therapeutic exercise. Active range of motion accomplished by the patient is preferable, but in extreme cases of debility or obtundation/sedation, active assisted or passive range of motion may be necessary. Muscles and joints that are resistant to stretch should be further evaluated for the presence of heterotopic ossification.[5]

Along with therapeutic stretching exercises, massage may assist in improving contractures. Splints are also commonly prescribed, as they provide a gentle sustained stretch (e.g., night splints used to stretch the Achilles tendon).

Modalities are an essential part of treating contractures. The therapeutic modality most commonly used to treat contractures in large joints is ultrasound. Heating the joint to a therapeutic temperature range of 40°C to 43°C will compliment the effects of manual stretching. Ultrasound and manual stretching exercises are best done simultaneously. With adequate pain control, patients should be encouraged to perform daily therapeutic exercises. Small joints may be heated by the use of paraffin bath dips or fluidotherapy.[5] Paraffin baths are used particularly in

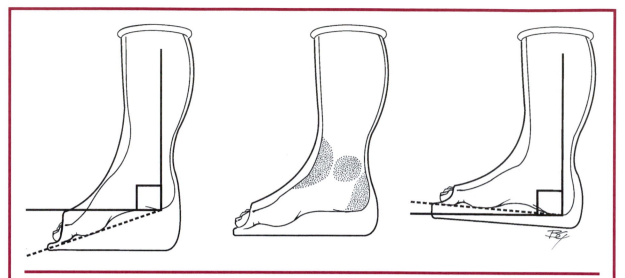

FIGURE 2. Serial short leg casts depicting a reduction of plantar flexion contracture of 20° to a final holding cast at 5° of dorsiflexion. Several intermediate casts between the initial and final holding cast may be required to achieve a gradual lengthening of the contracted gastrocsoleus muscle. (From Lennard TA: Pain Procedures in Clinical Practice, 2nd ed. Philadelphia, Hanley & Belfus, 2000, p 84, with permission.)

the treatment of contractures of the hand (e.g., in patients with scleroderma or with a hand injury).

Procedures

When therapeutic heating and stretching are not effective, procedures to be considered include motor point or nerve blocks. The use of these injection techniques can be diagnostic as well as therapeutic since they can help differentiate a true contracture from spasticity. Following anesthetic block, the affected area can be stretched to its maximal extent and a cast is applied. The cast is removed every 2 or 3 days. Stretching is repeated and the cast is re-applied. This process, known as "serial casting" (Fig. 2) should not be performed on patients with circulatory or sensory compromise.[6]

Surgery

Surgical treatments for contractures include tenotomy, tendon lengthening, and joint capsule release. These procedures are reserved for patients in whom less aggressive methods of treatment have *failed* and when the persistence of contractures is felt to be affecting hygiene, skin care, or mobility.[7]

Potential Disease Complications

Contracture related complications include permanent loss of range of motion and the associated loss of functional mobility. Pressure sores can develop under the bony prominences of contracted joints. Skin breakdown and infection by bacteria fungal agents can occur in the skinfolds if contractures prevent adequate access for cleaning.

Potential Treatment Complications

Medication reactions are generally well known and are specific to the drug used. Analgesics, NSAIDs, and COX-2 inhibitors have well-known side effects that most commonly affect the gastric, hepatic, and renal systems. Opioids may cause dependency. Over-aggressive stretching can inadvertently result in muscle, ligament, or capsular tears. These complications are especially serious when they occur in patients receiving anticoagulation. Splinting and casting can result in ischemia or skin ulceration if patients are not appropriately selected for the procedure and if the procedure is not closely supervised. Complications from motor point and nerve blocks include tendon rupture, nerve injury, infection, and skin atrophy.

References

1. McPeak L: Physiatric history and examination. In Braddom RL (ed): Physical Medicine and Rehabilitation, 2nd ed. Philadelphia, W.B. Saunders, 2000, pp 3–45.
2. Halar EM, Bell KR: Contracture and other deleterious effects of immobility. In DeLisa JA (ed): Rehabilitation Medicine Principles and Practice. Philadelphia, J.B. Lippincott, 1988, pp 448–462.
3. Norkin CC, White DJ: Measurement of Joint Motion: A Guide to Goniometry, 2nd ed. Philadelphia, F.A. Davis, 1995.
4. Sandor R: Adhesive Capsulitis: Optimal Treatment of Frozen Shoulder. www.physsportsmed.com/issues/2000/09-00sandor.htm
5. Wilson CH: Exercise for arthritis. In Basmajian JV (ed): Therapeutic Exercise, 4th ed. Baltimore, Williams & Wilkins, 1984, pp 529–545.
6. Lennard TA (ed): Pain Procedures in Clinical Practice, 2nd ed. Philadelphia, Hanley & Belfus, 2000.
7. Robinson R: Fight Against Contractures. www.mdausa.org/publications/Quest/q34contrc.html.
8. Countering Contractures. www.adbiomech.com/o14-1.html

104 Deep Vein Thrombosis

Ricardo Knight, MD, PT

Synonyms

Venous
thromboembolism (VTE)

Blood clot

Thrombophlebitis

Phlebothrombosis

ICD-9 Code

451.1
Phlebitis and
thrombophlebitis, of
deep vessels of lower
extremities

Definition

A deep vein
thrombosis (DVT)
occurs when a fibrin
clot abnormally
occludes a vein in the
deep venous system.
The circumstances
that are necessary for
DVTs to develop are
classically described
by Virchow's triad,
which includes
venous stasis, intimal
injury, and hyper-
coagulopathy. The
risk of developing a
DVT varies according
to specific characteristics of the patient, the surgical procedure, or the
medical condition (Table 1).

TABLE 1. Risk Factors for DVT		
Patient Factors	**Diseases**	**Procedures**
Age > 40	Thrombophilia	Pelvic surgery
Obesity	• Antithrombin III,	Lower limb
Varicose veins	protein C, protein	orthopedic
Immobility	S deficiency	surgery
Pregnancy	• Antiphospholipid	Neurosurgery
High dose	antibody, lupus	
estrogen	anticoagulant	
therapy	Malignancy	
Previous DVT	Major medical illness	
	Trauma	
	Spinal cord injury	
	Paralysis	

Surgical patients can be placed in categories according to their risk for
developing a venous thromboembolism (VTE)[1] (Table 2), with orthopedic
surgery patients carrying the highest risk.[2] It is believed that orthopedic
procedures carry such a high risk of VTE development because the
mechanical destruction of bone marrow during most orthopedic procedures
causes intravasation of marrow cells, cell fragments, and elevations of
plasma tissue factor (TF).[3] Tissue factor is a potent trigger of blood
clotting[4] and is found in high concentration in bone marrow and the
adventitia surrounding the major blood vessels and the brain, putting
neurosurgical patients at great risk for developing VTE. After
neurosurgery the incidence of VTE has been reported to be as high as
50%.[5] Risk factors that increase the rates of VTE in neurosurgery patients
include intracranial surgery, malignant tumors, the duration of surgery,
and the presence of paresis or paralysis of the lower limbs.[6] Patients can
remain in this postsurgical hypercoagulable state for weeks after surgery.[7]

In addition to surgical patients, victims of orthopedic and neurologic
trauma are at great risk for developing DVT, especially if long bone
fractures or paralysis is involved. Patients who suffered spinal cord injury

TABLE 2.   Risk Categories of Venous Thromboembolism in Surgical Patients without Prophylaxis

Risk Category	Calf DVT	Proximal DVT	Fatal PE
High Major orthopedic surgery of the lower limb Major general surgery in patients > 40 years with cancer or recent DVT or PE Multiple trauma Thrombophilia	40%–80%	10%–30%	1%–5%

Moderate
General surgery in patients > 40 years that lasts 30 minutes
   or more without additional risk factors
General surgery in patients < 40 years receiving estrogen or
   with a history of DVT or PE
Emergency cesarean section in women > 35 years
	10%–40%	2%–10%	0.1%–0.8%

Low
Minor surgery (i.e., < 30 minutes in patients > 40 years without
   additional risk factors)
Uncomplicated surgery in patients < 40 years without additional
   risk factors
	< 10%	< 1%	< 0.01%

Modified from Bounameaux H: Integrating pharmacologic and mechanical prophylaxis of venous thromboembolism. Thromb Haemost 1999;82(2):931–993.

are in high jeopardy of VTE because of stasis and hypercogulability. Other conditions that may predispose one to VTE are malignancy, previous history of VTE, stroke, irritable bowel syndrome, and congestive heart failure.

Pregnancy, prolonged immobility, advanced age, and certain hereditary conditions also predispose to development of VTE. Hereditary conditions include patients with deficiencies in protein C and protein S and familial thrombophilia. Acquired deficiencies of the natural anticoagulant system include antibodies directed against antiphospholipid. The frequency of thromboembolism increases with age; this may be related to a heterozygous factor V Leiden mutation.[9]

Symptoms

Venous thrombosis often occurs asymptomatically. If this is not the case, a pulmonary embolus is typically the first symptom. Other symptoms of VTE may include lower extremity edema, fever, extremity warmth, and pain. It must be kept in mind that symptoms can only serve as a trigger for further diagnostic inquiry as they cannot, by themselves, rule in or out VTE.

Physical Examination

The classic signs of DVT are tenderness, swelling, warmth, and a positive Homans' sign; unfortunately, these same symptoms are present in many other clinical conditions. A Homans' sign (Fig. 1) is elicited by applying a dorsiflexion force at the foot, with the knee extended, and simultaneously palpating the mid-calf with the fingertips of the other hand. The patient will report pain or discomfort in a positive

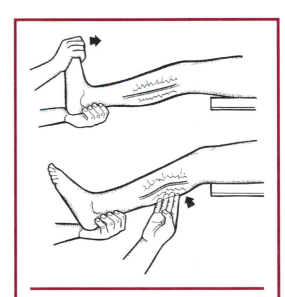

FIGURE 1.   *Top,* Homans' sign for deep vein thrombosis. *Bottom,* Tenderness elicited by deep palpation of the calf muscle indicates deep vein thrombosis.

test. Significant asymmetric calf edema is an important sign and can be determined by taking the circumferential measurement of the calf 10 cm below the tibial tuberosity. A 3-cm difference in calf girth is considered a significant clinical difference. As with symptoms, physical examination is not very sensitive or specific; in more than 50% percent of the instances in which there was a verified DVT, there was a normal physical exam.

Functional Limitations

A DVT rarely causes functional compromise, except calf pain during walking. Absolute bed rest is generally not indicated, but patients should suspend their lower extremity exercise program until they are fully anticoagulated.

Diagnostic Studies

Venography is the "gold standard" for the diagnosis of DVT and is the only test that can reliably detect DVT isolated to calf veins, the iliac veins, and the inferior vena cava (Figs. 2 and 3). The drawbacks to venography are its technical complexity, the requirement for the use of contrast dye, and the risk of allergic reaction.

Real-time, B-mode venous ultrasonography is the procedure of choice for the investigation of patients with a suspected DVT. Venous ultrasound allows direct visualization of the vein lumen; inability to compress that lumen is the main criterion for a positive test. Other adjunctive findings include vein distention, absence of flow, echogenic signals within the vessel lumen, and visualization of filling defects by color Doppler. Visualization of calf veins by ultrasound is technically more difficult and less reliable than diagnosing venous thrombus in the area between the trifurcation of the popliteal vein and the femoral vein in the groin. Other non-invasive diagnostic methods include Doppler ultrasound; impedance plethysmography; and ^{125}I fibrinogen scanning, which looks for the presence or absence of fibrin accretion.

D-dimer assay has recently emerged as a method to help predict the presence of VTE. D-dimer is a degradation product of the cross-linked fibrin blood clot, and as such is typically elevated in patients with VTE. D-dimer levels may also be elevated in a variety of non-thrombotic disorders, including recent major surgery, hemorrhage, trauma, malignancy, or sepsis. Due to its high sensitivity (but low specificity) of the D-dimer assay, is a good tool for excluding VTE if the test is negative.

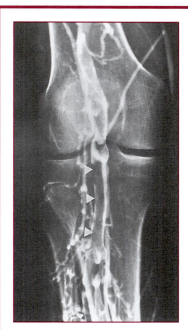
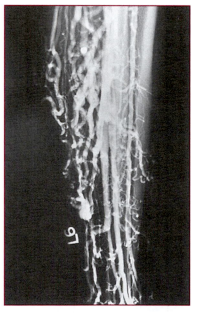

FIGURE 2 (Left). Acute deep venous thrombosis (DVT) of popliteal vein. Note the intraluminal filling defect (arrowheads) and "tram-tracking" of contrast around the thrombus.

FIGURE 3 (Right). Chronic lower-extremity deep venous thrombosis (DVT) with abundant collaterals. (From Katz DS, Math KR, Groskin SA: Radiology Secrets. Philadelphia, Hanley & Belfus, 1998, p 527, with permission.)

The first step in the diagnostic approach is the determination of risk. Patients can be separated by clinical criteria into high, moderate, and low risk categories. A nine-point clinical criteria scoring system has been developed (see Table 2)[10] to determine a patient's pre-test probability for DVT, and can be a useful adjunct to non-invasive testing.[11] All symptomatic patients suspected of having a DVT should, at the very least, undergo venous ultrasound imaging of the proximal venous system. Patients at moderate or high risk should have the ultrasound repeated in 1 week, or they could be ruled out on the basis of a negative D-dimer. If the D-dimer is positive, a followup ultrasound in 1 week is indicated.

Differential Diagnosis

Claudication   Ruptured Baker's cysts

Cellulitis   Hematoma

Lymphedema

Treatment

Initial

Nowhere in medicine is the aphorism "an ounce of prevention is worth a pound of cure" more appropriate than when considering the prevention of DVT. Choosing the most appropriate prophylactic method depends on the clinical scenario and the risk-benefit profile for the particular patient. Unfractionated (UFH) low-dose subcutaneous heparin (5000 U q8 to 12hr), while appropriate for most medical patients, has been slowly replaced by low-molecular weight heparin (LMWH) as the agent of choice in many clinical situations. Large meta-analyses comparing LMWHs to UFH in general and orthopedic surgery[12] have shown LMWH as safe and more efficacious than UFH. Antiplatelet agents such as aspirin also reduce the risk of VTE in some patients; however, the evidence is not overwhelming for using with more than low risk patients. Low dose warfarin is better than aspirin or placebo in patients with hip fractures but may not be satisfactory in preventing VTE after elective hip and knee surgery.

Mechanical VTE prophylaxis can be achieved with intermittent pneumatic leg compression (IPC), intermittent pneumatic foot compression (IPFC), or graduated compression stockings. IPC provides increase in peak-flow velocity and flow in the common femoral vein and is better than placebo in preventing DVT. IPFC is a high-pressure system that exerts a compression limited to the foot. These devices are best for patients who underwent lower extremity orthopedic surgery and could not be fitted with the IPC devices. The IPFC devices offer no advantage over LMWH in the prevention of DVTs, except for a lower rate of bleeding complications. Graded compression elastic stockings work by increasing venous blood flow velocity. Knee-length stockings are sized to fit, and they deliver graduated pressure of 40 mm Hg at the ankle, 36 mm HG at the lower calf, and 21 mm Hg at the upper calf.

The optimal duration of pharmacologic prophylaxis also varies with individual risk and clinical situation. Current standard of care is to stop prophylaxis 7 to 10 days after a surgical procedure, or in medical patients, when the patient is ambulating freely. Following major orthopedic surgery, prolongation of prophylaxis to 4 to 6 weeks is most advantageous. In patients with spinal cord injuries, prophylaxis is best maintained for 6 to 10 weeks.

The goals of treatment are to prevent local extension of thrombosus, embolization, and recurrent thrombosis. The cornerstone of medical treatment of DVT is anticoagulation therapy. Evidence for its efficacy comes from a study that showed death in 26% of patients who had clinically suspected PE and did not receive anticoagulation, compared with no deaths in the treatment group.[13]

Treatment of established DVT is usually initiated with heparin or LMWH. The early establishment of a therapeutic-range activated prothrombin time (aPTT) is essential. Many medical centers have adopted some kind of weight-adjusted nomogram to increase the likelihood of obtaining a therapeutic anticoagulation effect early. The nomogram that has been found to achieve the most rapid target aPTT acquisition is one in which the initial bolus of 80 U/kg is followed by an infusion rate of 18 U/kg/hr. Activated prothrombin time should be checked every 4 to 6 hours until a therapeutic range of 1.5 is achieved.

The duration of heparin treatment ranges between 4 to 10 days. Patients with large iliofemoral vein thrombosis or major PE require a 7- to 10-day course of heparin, with a delay in the initiation of warfarin until the aPTT is in the therapeutic range. Studies demonstrate that a 4- to 5-day course of heparin with warfarin administered within 24 hours of heparin initiation in patients without major PE of large proximal clots was as effective as 9 to 10 days of heparin.

LMWH are fragments of unfractionated heparin produced by either chemical or enzymatic depolymerization. LMWH display improved bioavailability, dose-independent clearance, and a more predictable dose response when compared with unfractionated heparin. These agents can, therefore, usually be given once or twice daily subcutaneously in weight-adjusted doses without laboratory monitoring.

The FDA has approved three LMWHs—ardeparin (Normiflo), dalteparin (Fragmin), and enoxaparin (Levonox)—for perioperative VTE prophylaxis (Table 3). Enoxaparin can be used for the inpatient with DVT with or without PE and outpatient treatment of DVT without PE.

Unmonitored outpatient therapy with LMWH is thought to be as safe and effective as in-hospital intravenous unfractionated heparin in patients with proximal DVT.[14] As with patients receiving unfractionated heparin, those treated with LMWH should begin taking warfarin within 24 to 48 hours. LMWH can be discontinued after a minimum of 5 days, provided that the INR has been therapeutic for 2 consecutive days.

Thrombolytic therapy has a limited role in the treatment of DVT. It has been suggested that pharmacologic lysis of a DVT could prevent post-thrombotic syndrome if complete lysis could be achieved before valve destruction occurs. However, thrombolysis, whether given systemically or via catheter, is expensive, the risk of bleeding complications is higher, and the evidence of additional benefit is not convincing. Thrombolysis should be reserved for patients with massive iliofemoral thrombosis or unstable cardiac or pulmonary disease with no contraindications to thrombolytic therapy.

After initial treatment with heparin, long-term anticoagulation therapy to prevent recurrent DVT is needed. An INR goal of 2 to 3 is generally considered effective in preventing recurrent DVT and is associated with a lower risk of bleeding than with higher INR levels. Treatment duration ranges between 3 and 6 months—the short duration is reserved for those who had some risk factor (e.g., immobility for surgery). Patients who wear compression stockings for 1 year after initial DVT have a lower incidence of post-thrombotic syndrome.

TABLE 3. FDA-Approved Uses of Low Molecular Weight Heparins

Name	FDA-Approved Indications	Dosage
Dalteparin (Fragmin)	DVT prophylaxis	5000 IU SC daily
Enoxaparin (Levonox)	1. DVT prophylaxis following knee surgery	1. 30 mg SC q12h
	2. DVT prophylaxis following hip surgery	2. 30 mg SC q12h or 40 mg SC daily
	3. DVT prophylaxis following abdominal surgery	3. 40 mg SC daily
	4. Inpatient treatment of acute DVT with or without PE.	4. 1mg/kg SC q12h or 1.5 mg/kg SC daily
	5. Outpatient treatment of acute DVT without PE	5. 1 mg/kg SC q12h
Ardeparin (Normiflo)	DVT prophylaxis following knee arthroplasty	50 anti-Xa U per kg of body weight every 12 hours

Untreated calf vein thrombosis does not commonly result in clinically important PE unless the thrombus extends into the proximal venous segments, which occurs in about one quarter of the cases. It is safe to monitor calf thrombi with serial venous ultrasound or impedance plethysmography and to initiate therapy only if the thrombus extends into the popliteal or more proximal veins. Treatment of superficial venous thrombosis is usually not indicated.

Pregnant women with DVT are classically treated with unfractionated heparin for 5 days, followed by adjusted-dose subcutaneous heparin every 12 hours until delivery. Warfarin is contraindicated during pregnancy but is safe for mother and nursing child after delivery.

Rehabilitation

There is no strict contraindication against therapeutic exercises and ambulatory activities following a DVT, but it is recommended that these activities be suspended until the patient is in the therapeutic range for heparin or has been on LMWH for 24 hours.

On the other hand, physical and occupational therapy ordered immediately after high risk surgical procedures can greatly improve a patient's postoperative mobility and lessen the chance of developing a DVT.

Procedures

Vena cava filters are indicated in patients with DVT who have a high risk of bleeding or who suffered a PE or recurrent PE despite adequate anticoagulation. Caval interruption has been found to be effective in preventing subsequent PE; however, this is counterbalanced by the increased incidence of recurrent DVT. Patients who have significant but temporary contraindications to the use of anticoagulants who receive caval interruption devices should begin taking anticoagulation medication as soon as possible.

Surgery

Surgical removal of acute DVT by thrombectomy or embolectomy is rarely used and should only be considered in patients with massive thrombosis and compromised arterial circulation who do not respond to or who have an absolute contraindication to thrombolytic therapy.

Potential Disease Complications

If untreated, proximal DVT is linked with a 10% immediate risk of fatal PE and approximately 20% higher risk of developing a severe post-thrombotic syndrome (PTS) 5 to 10 years later[15] (Fig. 4). There are two predominant patterns of DVT: an ascending pattern, with DVT arising in the calf veins, and a descending pattern, with DVT occurring initially in the iliac and/or common femoral vein. The descending pattern more commonly results in pulmonary embolus. PTS is a condition characterized by chronic edema and debilitating pain and can lead to ulceration; infection; or in rare cases, amputation. Heparin use and the wearing of graduated compression stockings have been associated with a lower risk of PTS development.

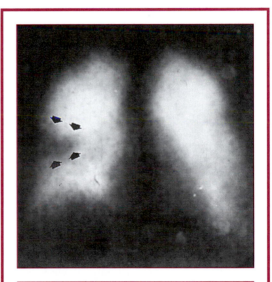

FIGURE 4. Frontal image from subsequent perfusion lung scan shows a corresponding peripheral, pleural-based area of absent perfusion in the right mid-lung. The ventilation study showed diminished ventilation in this area, consistent with pulmonary embolus with infarction, and multiple unmatched perfusion defects were seen in the left lung, indicating that the probability of pulmonary embolism is high. (From Katz DS, Math KR, Groskin SA: Radiology Secrets. Philadephia, Hanley & Belfus, 1998, p 55, with permission.)

Potential Treatment Complications

All pharmacologic anticoagulation agents alter the hemostatic mechanisms to some extent by decreasing blood coagulation or platelet function, and all carry a risk of bleeding. Both unfractionated heparin and LMWH are associated with similar increased risk of bleeding complications. Heparin induced thrombocytopenia (HIT) is a potential complication of heparin use and is seen slightly less commonly with LMWH than with unfractionated heparin because of LMWH's lower affinity for platelet binding. A diagnosis of HIT is made when there is a 50% reduction in platelet count or with the presence of antiplatelet antibodies. Once the diagnosis is made, all heparins are contraindicated. Skin necrosis is a rare complication of warfarin use, and it can be prevented if high dose warfarin is delayed until the aPTT is therapeutic with heparin.

Complications from caval interruption include problems related to the deployment of the device and include hemorrhage, hematomas, femoral artery injury, femoral nerve injury, infections, and site pain. Other potential complications are PE from embolization of the device itself or from failure of the device to capture an emboli. A clot-laden caval interruption device can impede venous flow and lead to lower extremity venous stasis and edema.

Osteoporosis and risk of bone fracture are associated with long-term use of unfractionated heparin[16]; the risk may be less with LMWH .

Contraindications to the use of warfarin include advanced liver disease, alcoholism, poor compliance with follow-up, poorly controlled hypertension, major bleeding, and pregnancy.[18]

References

1. Clagett GP, et al: Prevention of venous thromboembolism. Chest 1998;114(5): 531s–560s.
2. Pineo GF, Hull RD: Prophylaxis of Venous Thromboembolism Following Orthopedic Surgery: Mechanical and Pharmacological Approaches and the need for Extended Prophylaxis. Thromb Haemost 1999;82(2):918–924.
3. Giercksky, K, et al: Circulating tissue thromboplastin during hip surgery. Eur Surg Res 1979;11:296–300.
4. Camerer E, Kolsto AB, Prydz H: Cector the biology of tissue factor the principal initiator of blood coagulation. Thromb Res 1996;81:1–14.
5. Joffe, SN: Incidence of postoperative deep vein thrombosis in neurosurgical patients. J Neurosurg 1975;42:201–203.
6. Flinn W, Sandager G, Silva M: Prospective surveillance for perioperative venous thrombosis: experience in 2643 patients. Arch Surg 1996;131:472–480.
7. Dahl OE, et al: Increased activation of coagulation and formation of late deep venous thrombosis following discontinuation of thromboprophylaxis after hip replacement surgery. Thromb Res 1995;80(4):299–306.
8. Bounameaux H: Integrating pharmacologic and mechanical prophylaxis of venous thromboembolism. Thromb Haemost 1999;82(2):931–937.
9. Ridher P, et al: Age-specific incidence rates of venous thromboembolim among heterozygous carriers of factor V leiden mutation. Ann Intern Med 1997;126:528–531.
10. Anderson DR, Wells PS: Improvements in the diagnostic approach for patients with suspected deep vein thrombosis or pulmonary embolism. Thromb Haemost 1999;82(2):878–886.
11. Wells PS, et al: A simple clinical model for the diagnosis of deep-vein thrombosis combined with impedance plethysmography: potential for an improvement in the diagnostic process. J Intern Med 1998;243(1):15–23.
12. Nurmohamed M, et al: Low-molecular-weight heparin versus standard heparin in general and Orthopaedic surgery: a meta-analysis. Lancet 1992;340:152–156.
13. Barritt DW, Johnson SC: Anticoagulation drugs in the treatment of pulmonary embolism trial. Lancet 1960;1:1309–1312.
14. Siragusa S, et al: Low-molecular-weight heparins and unfractionated heparin in the treatment of patients with acure venous thromboembolism: Results of a meta-analysis. Am J Med 1996;100:269–277.
15. Bounameaux H, et al: Differential inhibition of thrombin activity and thrombin generation by a synthetic direct thrombin inhibitor (napsagatran, Ro 46-6240) and unfractionated heparin in patients with deep vein thrombosis. ADVENT Investigators. Thromb Haemost 1999;81(4):498–501.
16. Dahlman T: Osteoporotic fractures and the recurrence during pregnancy and puerperium in 94 women undergoing thromboprophylaxis with heparin. Am J Obster Gynecol 1983;168:1265–1270.
17. Monreal M, et al: Comparison of subcutaneous unfractionated heparin with a low molecular weight heparin (fragmin) in patients with thromboembolism and contraindications to coumadin. Thromb Haemost 1894;71:7–11.
18. Hoppenfeld S: Physical Examination of the Spine and Extremities. Norwalk, CT, Appleton & Lange, 1976.

105 Dementia

Melvyn L. Hecht, MD

Definition

Dementia is an acquired, persistent impairment of intellectual function with compromise in at least three of the following spheres of mental activity: language, memory, and visuospatial skills; emotion or personality; and cognition.[1]

Dementia represents several disorders with similar effects on mental activity. Of these, Alzheimer's dementia accounts for approximately 70% to 90% of cases, multi-infarct dementia for 15% , and the remaining 1% to 5% are represented by Parkinson's dementia, Creuztfeldt-Jacob disease, Huntington's disease, Pick's disease, Lewy body dementia, and progressive supranuclear palsy. Dementia can be divided into cortical and subcortical types. Alzheimer's dementia is typical of the cortical dementias, whereas Parkinson's disease represents the subcortical type (Table 1).

Alzheimer's disease is the most common dementia for people age 65 years and older. It is estimated that 4.5 million people currently suffer with the disorder. It affects approximately 5% of the population at age 65, with a prevalence reaching 35% at age 85.

The etiology of Alzheimer's disease is still not clearly known; however, the pathologic agent of this disease is amyloid plaques in the brain. Age is the most important risk factor. Other risk factors include a positive family history, estrogen deficiency in postmenopausal women, severe head trauma, and the presence of a genetic factor called the Apo-E-4 allele. Screening for this gene is still controversial since there are no clear disease prevention therapies.

Functional limitations depend on the stage of diagnosis and the underlying cause of the dementia. In Alzheimer's patients, functional limitations slowly progress with time–memory loss through a continuum to a vegetative status. In Parkinson's dementia, the functional limitation of the motor disease progresses more rapidly. In multi-infarct dementia the tendency is for step-wise progression, with cognitive and motor functioning losses worsening after new brain injury, followed by periods of stability.

The cortical dementias are mostly characterized, in early stages, by memory problems. The subcortical dementias show motor findings early in the clinical course.

TABLE 1. Clinical Differentiation among the Dementias

	Cortical*	Subcortical†	Corticosubcortical‡	Multifocal§
Alzheimer's	X			
Frontotemporal lobar	X			
Alcoholic encephalopathy	X			
Frontotemporal	X			
Parkinson's		X		
Hungtington's chorea		X		
Progressive supranuclear palsy		X		
Vascular encephalopathy			X	
Lewy body disease			X	
Creutzfeldt-Jacob disease				X

* Cortical dementias predominantly present with memory impairment, poor judgment, and aphasic syndromes.
† Subcortical dementias present with slowness and rigidity of thinking and perseveration of responses.
‡ Corticosubcortical dementias present with more rapid losses than cortical dementias and often with behavioral symptoms.
§ Multifocal dementias present with loss of cognitive symptoms and rapid loss of neurologic function.

Symptoms

Symptoms of dementia are often insidious, with memory loss the most common early sign. Patients and families often allow these losses to continue for extended periods before having the problem assessed.

The memory symptoms most often described are inability to remember names, appointments, or recent important family gatherings. More important symptoms are wandering, especially getting lost in familiar areas. Occasionally, the patient will present with behavioral problems, such as aggression and sexual disinhibition.

The diagnosis of Alzheimer's dementia is one of exclusion. History taking is extremely important, especially in defining onset of symptoms, disease progression, and to rule out focal neurologic symptoms. By definition, there is a requirement that the patient have *impairment of both short- and long-term memory* in addition to abnormalities in at least one of the areas of mental function: abstract thinking, judgment, language, praxis, visual recognition, constructional abilities, or personality. These disturbances must be sufficiently severe to interfere with work, social activities, or relationships with others.[1]

These symptoms are present by definition for at least six months and with a clear sensorium.

Physical Examination

On neurologic examination, focal findings such as unilateral weakness of a cranial or peripheral nerve group, painful neuropathic changes, or paresthesias are especially important to rule out cerebrovascular disease or tumors. Usually, there are no physical or neurologic findings and the disorder is diagnosed by history and findings on the Mini-Mental Status Exam.[2] Occasionally, patient, structured neuropsychologic tests, including the geriatric depression scale, are necessary to rule out depression and ischemic disease. Since the dementing disorders are exclusionary, the following should be evaluated during the mental status examination: state of consciousness, orientation, memory (long and short term), language, visuospatial functions, calculations, insight, judgment, mood, and affect.

The examination for all dementias is similar to that of the workup of Alzheimer's dementia. The significant findings between the various dementing disorders will be based on the neurologic exam. For example, in Lewy body dementia, findings including tremor and rigidity are often present. In supranuclear palsy, ocular findings with abnormal gaze may be present.

Functional Limitations

The functional implications of dementia range from none to vegetation and coma. Most commonly, inability to dress and feed oneself is found in residents of nursing homes. In the outpatient setting, disorders of gait and toileting are often causes for visits to the clinician.

The functional limitations are characterized by loss of learning; inability to manage complex tasks; and difficulties with problem solving, navigating familiar routes, and driving. The patient may have difficulty finding the right words, especially with stress. Abnormal behaviors, such as incontinence, can limit the patient's ability to lead normal day-to-day activities.

Diagnostic Studies

Since the diagnosis of dementing disorders is usually made by exclusion, a recent review of diagnostic guidelines attempts to highlight areas of agreement.[3] Laboratory tests generally recommended are CBC, electrolytes, calcium, glucose, BUN, liver function, thyroid function, serum B_{12}, and syphilis serology.

Other diagnostic tests, including CT/MRI/SPECT scanning, should be left to targeted populations with confusing physical or mental status findings. Note that HIV screening may be included among the targeted, special populations to be tested. EEG is usually not used, except in patients with a history consistent with a seizure disorder.

Neuropsychologic testing is useful in discriminating Alzheimer's disease from vascular dementia. It is especially helpful to rule out depression as a secondary complication of the disease.

Differential Diagnosis

Delirium	Multiple sclerosis
Neoplasm	Medication side effects[4]
Trauma	Depression
Toxins (e.g., alcoholism, heavy metals)	Normal pressure hydrocephalus
Infection	

Treatment

Initial

Treatment is mostly symptom based. In Alzheimer's type dementia, three drugs have been approved for the treatment of memory loss and cognitive decline. All three drugs—tacrine, donepezil, and rivastigmine—work by increasing the brain's supply of acetylcholine. Tacrine is administered four times a day, starting at 10 mg, and based on tolerance and liver function monitoring, up to a maximum dose of 120 mg. Donepezil is given once a day in 5 or 10 mg dosing, with a slight benefit to the 10 mg dose. Rivastigmine is given twice a day, usually at 3 mg, but can be titrated to 6 mg twice a day.

It is important to note that none of these drugs will cure Alzheimer's disease but only slow its progression. All drugs have similar side effect profiles, with the exception of tacrine, which has the potential for liver toxicity. The common side effects are nausea, diarrhea, and insomnia.

Other pharmacologic interventions, including the use of antioxidants, anti-inflammatory agents, and estrogen replacement therapy, are still under investigation and not proven to slow or inhibit disease progression.

Treatment of abnormal behaviors with anti-psychotics, anxiolytics, and anti-depressants can be useful in certain circumstances. Depression is especially common, and consideration for use of anti-depressants early in the disease is important. The management of behavior needs to be balanced with the high side effect profile of these drugs.

After a relationship has been established with the clinician, but early in the treatment, the patient and family should be counseled about living wills, health care proxy, and guardianship. An excellent resource for this information is local chapters of the Alzheimer's Association.

Rehabilitation

The rehabilitation of the patient with dementia calls for a coordinated effort with the clinician, therapists, and family. Obviously, the patient should participate as much as he or she can in the decision making process and treatment plan. Therapists and family members who are working with patients who have dementia should be well versed in the use of diversionary tactics and visual, tactile, and auditory instructions. The environment needs to be homelike, with visual aids such as family portraits and other familiar objects. Use of appropriate lighting to prevent "sun downing" is critical.

The rehabilitation of patients with dementia is complicated by their cognitive status. While there is no specific literature on the recovery of patients with Alzheimer's and other dementias, several factors aid in their rehabilitation. These factors include motivation/socialization, reality orientation, and cognitive training.[5] For motivation training, the team often looks for early success, such as recognition of the patient's room. In reality orientation, opportunities are taken as often as possible to orient the patient to time and place. In cognitive training, patients are given techniques to aid memory (e.g., using cue cards to recite the name of objects).

Repeated measures of functional abilities that are relevant to the patient's environment as well as the adaptation of the environment to the patient's abilities are all essential elements of the rehabilitation process.[6] Careful assessment of the patient's function; the setting of realistic goals; and prevention of secondary disabilities such as urinary incontinence, depression, and weight loss, as well as complications of immobility such as skin breakdown, are all key to successful management of the patient with dementia.

Physical therapy interventions focus on gait and mobility. As dementia progresses, impairment in gait becomes problematic. This impairment can be complicated by degenerative joint changes and orthopedic injuries. The physical therapist needs to provide a good deal of repetition with respect to the exercise program. Techniques should be individualized to the level of cognition and abnormal behaviors.

Occupational therapy is especially important in the rehabilitation of the patient with dementia. The primary focus in this area includes dressing, toileting, and cognition. The occupational therapist is a key member of the treatment team, responsible for structuring activities such as reminiscence, reality orientation, and other group-based therapies. The speech and language pathologist evaluates and guides decisions regarding feeding/swallowing.

Most data on the effectiveness of rehabilitation come from studies of geriatric assessment units, and results to date have been both positive and negative.[7] In addition to functional goals, focus on improvement of medical conditions and reduction of polypharmacy is vital. Certainly, rehabilitation of the patient with dementia needs further research focus to improve techniques.

Procedures

The only procedural intervention currently performed is shunting for normal pressure hydrocephalus. Results are mixed but can be dramatic in patients diagnosed early with this disorder.

Surgery

Surgical considerations in patients with dementia need to be evaluated in view of the patient's difficulty in cooperating with the recovery and rehabilitation process. However, surgical decisions are assessed using the same guidelines currently published for the general population.

Potential Disease Complications

Complications observed in Alzheimer's disease and related dementias become progressively more devastating with advancement of the disease. Three of the most significant complications are depression, loss of cognitive function, and loss of motor function.

Depression can be a significant issue, especially early during the disease process, a period of time when patient recognize their deficits. Untreated and undiagnosed depression can produce worsening cognitive function, increased confusion, and social isolation.

Loss of cognitive function brings the loss of independence. Driving should be discouraged and discontinued. Patients who have been found wandering will require 24-hour supervision to prevent injury.

The most devastating physical complications result from the loss of motor function. These include falls, resulting in fracture; aspiration, causing pneumonia; and contractures, which eventually can lead to skin breakdown.

Potential Treatment Complications

Postsurgical patients often have worsening of their cognitive abilities requiring, on average, 6 weeks to return to baseline functioning. Use of anti-psychotics needs to be monitored for extrapyramidal signs.

References
1. Cummings JL, Benson D, Frank: Dementia: A Clinical Approach, 2nd ed. Boston, MA, Butterworth-Heinemann, 1992.
2. Agency for Healthcare Policy and Research: Alzheimer's Disease: Diagnosis, Treatment. Baltimore, MD, Agency for Healthcare Policy and Research, 1996.
3. Massoud F, Devi G, Mordosey JT, et al: The role of routine laboratory studies and neuroimaging in the diagnosis of dementia: A clinicopathological study. J Am Geriatr Soc 2000;48(10):1204–1216.
4. Costa PT Jr, Williams TF, et al: Recognition and initial assessment of Alzheimer's disease and related dementias. Washington, DC, AHCPR Publication, 1996.
5. Williams T, Franklin: Rehabilitation in the Aging. New York, Raven Press, 1984.
6. Kane RL: Essentials of Clinical Geriatrics. New York, McGraw-Hill, 1999.
7. Rubenstein LZ, et al: Impact of geriatric evaluation and management programs on defined outcomes. JAm Geriatr Soc 1991;39(Suppl):8–16.

106 Diabetic and Peripheral Vascular Foot Disease

Timothy R. Dillingham, MD

Synonyms

Vascular claudication

Poor circulation

Arterial insufficiency

ICD-9 Codes

250.7
Diabetes with peripheral circulatory disorders

440.20
Atherosclerosis of the extremities, unspecified

440.21
Atherosclerosis of the extremities with intermittent claudication

440.22
Atherosclerosis of the extremities with rest pain

440.23
Atherosclerosis of the extremities with ulceration

440.24
Atherosclerosis of the extremities with gangrene

707.10
Ulcer of lower limb, unspecified

707.13
Ulcer of ankle

707.14
Ulcer of heel and midfoot

707.15
Ulcer of other part of foot

707.9
Chronic ulcer of unspecified site

Definition

The incidence of lower limb amputations due to vascular disease increased in the United States by approximately 20% during the last decade and disproportionately afflicts minorities.[1] Persons with diabetes mellitus and peripheral vascular disease should be identified and prophylactic foot education and preventative care instituted to reduce the risk of limb loss.[2]

Atherosclerosis is a vascular disease that can involve the peripheral arterial system. It is estimated that up to 12% of the population older than 66 years suffer from this problem.[3] Risk factors that predispose a person to develop peripheral vascular disease (PVD) or accelerate its progression include high plasma cholesterol and lipoproteins, smoking, hypertension, diabetes, a sedentary lifestyle, and a positive family history.[3]

Diabetes mellitus is a multisystem disease that causes two conditions that place the foot at high risk for amputation: polyneuropathy and PVD. Diabetes affects about 13 million Americans,[3] and is on the rise in the United States, particularly in African American and Hispanic populations.[4] Persons with diabetes are up to 25 times more likely than nondiabetic persons to sustain a lower limb amputation, underscoring the need to prevent foot ulcers and subsequent limb loss.[5] Multidisciplinary clinics that identify and manage patients with at-risk feet have demonstrated impressive reductions of 44% to 85% in the incidence of foot ulcers and lower limb amputations.[3] Minor foot trauma in a person with poor underlying circulation and reduced sensation can lead to skin ulceration. Skin ulcers can fail to heal and progress such that an amputation becomes necessary. This sequence of events can often be prevented before it starts.

Symptoms

The patient with a diabetic foot may demonstrate no symptoms, as peripheral neuropathy can mask painful ulcers, foot collapse due to Charcot's joints, or ischemic skin.

Persons with PVD present with claudication pain when walking due to insufficient arterial blood supply to meet the demand of exercising muscles. Pain with vascular claudication is typically in the calf and worsened with ambulation. Patients with spinal claudication due to spinal stenosis can have similar leg or calf pain with walking, but must bend at the waist or sit to relieve the symptoms.

Physical Examination

The history and physical examination are key elements in the identification and management of persons with a foot at risk for amputation. In addition to a standard physical examination, special areas must be highlighted:

TABLE 1. Risk Factors for Foot Ulceration in Diabetic Patients

Neuropathy	Thick mycotic nails
Sensorimotor (abnormal protective sensation)	Deformities secondary to Charcot's arthropathy
Autonomic (dry, cracked skin)	Previous ulcers or amputation
Vascular disease	Soft tissue atrophy and loss of
Abnormal plantar pressure (elevated in neuropathy, even in absence of deformity)	fat pad under metatarsal heads
	Poor hygiene
Abnormal gait in elderly living alone	Inappropriate footwear
Degenerative joint diseases of hip and knee	Blind or partially sighted
	Elevated activity profile
Muscle weakness	Lack of education/poor
Heel cord tightness	Foot deformities
Pronation, supination deformities of the foot	Claw toes
	Hammer toes
	Hallux valgus
Toe contractures	Hallux rigidus

From Pandian G, Hamid F, Hammond MC: Rehabilitation of the patient with PVD and diabetic foot problems. In Delisa J, Gans BM (eds): Rehabilitation Medicine: Principles and Practice. Philadelphia, Lippincott-Raven, 1998, pp 1517–1544.

1. Inspect for ulcerations, cracked skin, or trophic skin changes (thin, shiny, hairless).[3]

2. Evaluate for any foot deformities that predispose it to abnormal stress distribution. These include collapsed foot arches due to Charcot's joints, high arched feet due to intrinsic muscle atrophy from polyneuropathy, or changes in stress distribution from previous toe or ray amputations.

3. Assess distal pulses, particularly dorsalis pedis and posterior tibial. Absent or weak pulses suggest the need for further testing for vascular integrity.

4. Assess sensation since persons with loss of protective sensation are at risk for skin ulceration.

5. Probe any ulcers. If bone is reached, this identifies persons with osteomyelitis, and other special bone imaging is unnecessary.[6]

Table 1 describes history and physical examination findings that place the limb at risk.[3]

Functional Limitations

Persons with diabetes can develop peripheral polyneuropathy with loss of position sense and weakness. These can lead to gait instability and falls. Persons with PVD are often limited in community ambulation and vocational activities due to pain from claudication. Ambulation may be precluded owing to non-healing foot ulcers.

Diagnostic Studies

There are many non-invasive and invasive tests for PVD that are beyond the scope of this discussion. Angiography can identify surgically remediable lesions.

In the outpatient setting, ankle brachial index (ABI) testing is convenient, easy to perform, and provides objective assessment of lower limb vascular status. The ABI is measured by inflating a blood pressure cuff around the ankle at rest and then slowly deflating the cuff until the arterial blood flow is detected distal to the cuff with continuous-wave Doppler. This number is used along with the brachial pressure to produce a ratio (ankle pressure:brachial pressure = ABI). An index of 0.9 or greater is normal, 0.7 to 0.9 indicates mild disease, 0.4 to 0.6 reflects moderate to severe disease, and less than 0.4 indicates severe disease.[3] Measuring systolic pressure in the foot also provides a measure of arterial integrity.

Transcutaneous oximetry ($TcPO_2$) is the best method for assessing cutaneous ischemia.[3] $TcPO_2$ pressures of greater than 40 mm Hg are normal, 20 to 40 mm Hg indicate moderate disease, and potential for healing a skin ulcer is less likely. With pressures less than 20 mm Hg, severe skin ischemia is present and this bodes poorly for skin healing.

Systolic blood pressure measurements in the foot are also helpful in quantifying the severity of ischemia. Persons with ischemic ulcers and ankle systolic pressures of less than 40 to 60mm Hg are considered to have severe ischemia. Persons with persistently recurring ischemic rest pain and ankle systolic pressures of 50 mm Hg or less are severely involved. Frank ulceration and gangrene of the foot or toes with an ankle pressure of less than 50 mm Hg reflects severe limb ischemia.[3]

If a person complains of numbness in the legs or feet or has low back pain, electrodiagnostic testing (EMG and nerve conduction studies) should be used to identify whether peripheral polyneuropathy is present or whether lumbosacral radiculopathy is responsible for these symptoms.

Differential Diagnoses

Radiculopathy

Peripheral neuropathy

Lumbar spinal stenosis

Plantar fasciitis

Treatment

Initial

Meticulous attention to the feet by both patient and physician, as well as detailed patient education, are the mainstays of preventative foot care. Table 2 is an educational list for clinicians and patients.[3] Deformities should prompt the clinician to consider custom shoe inserts to distribute pressures evenly over the foot. Extra depth shoes may be necessary to accommodate hammer toes. Tennis or running shoes are an inexpensive alternative for persons without foot deformities. However, if there are any aberrations in foot bony architecture, custom footwear with molded sole inserts is desirable. Management of risk factors, particularly the discontinuance of smoking, may slow PVD. Patients should be encouraged to routinely visit a podiatrist for nail care and general foot care.

Early treatment of skin infections with antibiotics is warranted, along with minimizing or eliminating weight bearing during healing. Debridement with dressing changes or whirlpool is sometimes necessary. Deep infections into bone or infections that extend along fascial planes require debridement. If pedal osteomyelitis is suspected, a 10-week course of oral antibiotic therapy guided by cultures obtained during debridement is an effective clinical approach.[7] Other wound care measures such as total contact casting can assist with the resolution of plantar surface ulcers.

Rehabilitation

Rehabilitation may include referral to a physical therapist or other health care provider for patient education regarding proper footwear. An orthotist or pedorthist may assist with shoe orthotics and custom modifications, such as a rocker bottom sole. Patients may need to use an assistive device (e.g., walker) to walk without excessive weight on a foot with an ulcer and/or to improve balance. Formal exercises may be prescribed in some instances. Exercise to just beyond the point of discomfort followed by rest can increase exercise capacity for persons with claudication.[3] Exercise, however, is contraindicated in the presence of an ischemic ulcer or rest pain.[3]

TABLE 2. Foot Care Instructions

1. Wash your feet every day with a mild soap and warm water. Check the water temperature with your elbow. Use a soft wash cloth to clean.

2. Dry them with a soft towel by blotting or patting; dry thoroughly between the toes.

3. Inspect daily for redness, blisters, or cuts; change in temperature (hot or cool); and swelling or loss of feeling. If you cannot see to do this yourself, have another member of the family inspect your feet or use a mirror.

4. Clean dirt out from under the toenails; never use a knife or anything sharp. An orange stick or nail file should be used. Cut toenails straight across. Use sandpaper or a fine emery board to rub down corns and calluses after soaking.

5. Never use corn remedies. Corn pads should be used only on doctor's advice.

6. Do not use inserts or pads without medical advice. Do not wear shoes without socks.

7. Use a lotion on feet and legs daily; do not use between the toes.

8. Never walk barefooted at home or on hot surfaces such as beaches or swimming pools.

9. Protect your feet with warm cotton or woolen socks in cold weather.

10. Inspect shoes daily for cracks in the soles, wrinkles in the lining, and bunching up of construction material. Wear shoes that fit properly with plenty of room for toes.

11. Avoid pointed or open-toed shoes. Sandals or thongs also may cause problems.

12. New shoes should always be broken in slowly. Start by wearing them for 1 hour on the first day, increasing by 1 hour each day. Gradually build up to a full day.

13. Wear leather or canvas shoes that permit moisture to evaporate and absorb perspiration better. Allow time for footwear to air and dry between wearing.

14. Remove shoes whenever possible. Take frequent rest periods during the day and elevate your feet. Change your shoes every 5 hours.

15. Purchase shoes in the afternoon, when feet are the largest due to swelling.

16. Never use hot water bottles, compresses, heating pads, or lamps near your feet.

17. Avoid elastic socks, garters, girdles, and socks that have holes, mends, seams, or edges. Do not tie your stockings.

18. To avoid nerve pressure injury, do not cross legs while sitting.

19. Loosen bed clothing at the bottom of the bed to reduce pressure on the toes.

20. Do not smoke.

21. Have your physician examine your feet at each visit.

22. Be sure that anyone caring for your feet knows that you are a diabetic. This includes the shoe salesman.

23. REMEMBER—THE FEET YOU SAVE ARE YOURS!

Reprinted with permission from the Dallas Medical Journal 1994;80:502. Dallas County Medical Society.

Procedures

Debridement of ulcers is important in the healing process and should be performed by someone who is experienced in the care of these wounds.

Surgery

An acute painful, pale, pulseless limb should be evaluated emergently because this indicates acute arterial compromise. Likewise, gangrene or an ulcer extending to bone should receive prompt surgical consultation. Sharp debridement for a necrotic wound is often necessary to remove devitalized tissue and promote healing of ulcers.

Vascular bypass procedures may be necessary to provide enough oxygenated arterial blood to a limb to heal open sores, improve symptoms of claudication, or save an extremity at risk for amputation.

Potential Disease Complications

Complications include ischemic pain from arterial insufficiency (claudication or rest pain), non-healing or slow-to-heal foot ulcers, cellulitis and deeper wound infections in the foot, amputation of the lower limb, and Charcot's joints and bone fractures in the foot due to diabetic polyneuropathy.

Potential Treatment Complications

Infection of arterial bypass grafts and infection of foot ulcers after debridement are possible complications.

References

1. Dillingham TR, Pezzin LE, MacKenzie EJ: Racial differences in the incidence of limb loss secondary to peripheral vascular disease: A population-based study (unpublished observations).
2. Sanders L: Diabetes Mellitus: Prevention of amputation. J Am Podiatr Med Assoc 1994;84(7):322–328.
3. Pandian G, Hamid F, Hammond MC: Rehabilitation of the patient with PVD and diabetic foot problems. In Delisa J, Gans BM (eds): Rehabilitation Medicine: Principles and Practice. Philadelphia, Lippincott-Raven, 1998, pp 1517–1544.
4. Harris MI: Diabetes in America: Epidemiology and scope of the problem. Diabetes Care 1998;21(Suppl 3):C11–C14.
5. Lavery LA, Ashry HR, van Houtum W, et al: Variation in the incidence and proportion of diabetes-related amputations in minorities. Diabetes Care 1996;19(1):48–52.
6. Grayson M, Gibbons G, Balough K, et al: Probing to bone in infected pedal ulcers:A clinical sign of underlying osteomyelitis in diabetic patients. JAMA 1995;273(9):721–723.
7. Eckman M, Greenfield S, Mackey W, et al: Foot infections in diabetic patients: Decision and cost-effectiveness analyses. JAMA 1995;273(9):712–720.

107 Dysphagia

Jeffrey B. Palmer, MD

Synonyms

Swallowing disorder

Swallowing impairment

Deglutition disorder

ICD-9 Codes

530.11
Reflux esophagitis

530.3
Stricture and stenosis of the esophagus (compression of the esophagus, obstruction of the esophagus)

530.5
Dyskinesia of the esophagus (difficulty in performing voluntary esophageal movements)

530.81
Esophageal reflux (regurgitation of the contents of the stomach into the esophagus, without inflammation)

787.2
Dysphagia (difficulty in swallowing)

Definition

Dysphagia generally refers to any difficulty with swallowing, including occult or asymptomatic impairments. It is a common problem, affecting one third to one half of all stroke patients and about one sixth of elderly individuals. It is common in head and neck cancer, degenerative disorders of the nervous system, gastroesophageal reflux disease, and inflammatory muscle disease. Dysphagia is classified according to the location of the problem as *oropharyngeal* (localized to the oral cavity and/or pharynx, not just the oropharynx, per se), or *esophageal*. It may also be classified as *mechanical* (due to a structural lesion of the foodway) or *functional* (caused by a physiologic abnormality of foodway function) (Table 1).[1]

Sudden onset is suggestive of stroke. Concomitant limb weakness suggests a neurologic or neuromuscular disorder. Medication-induced dysphagia is commonly overlooked. Medications that impair level of consciousness (such as sedatives or tranquilizers), have anticholinergic effects (tricyclics, propantheline), or can damage mucous membranes (NSAID's, aspirin, quinidine) may also cause dysphagia.[2]

TABLE 1. Selected Causes of Oral and Pharyngeal Dysphagia

Neurologic Disorders and Stroke	Structural Lesions
Cerebral infarction	Thyromegaly
Brainstem infarction	Cervical hyperostosis
Intracranial hemorrhage	Congenital web
Parkinson's disease	Zenker's diverticulum
Multiple sclerosis	Caustic ingestion
Amyotrophic lateral sclerosis	Neoplasm
Poliomyelitis	Post ablative surgery
Myasthenia gravis	Radiation fibrosis
Dementias	

Connective Tissue Diseases	Psychiatric Disorders
Polymyositis	Psychogenic dysphagia
Muscular dystrophy	

Symptoms

The most common symptoms of dysphagia are coughing or choking during eating, or the sensation of food sticking in the throat or chest.[1]

TABLE 2. Symptoms and Signs of Dysphagia
Oral or Pharyngeal Dysphagia
Coughing or choking with swallowing
Difficulty initiating swallowing
Sensation of food sticking in the throat
Drooling
Unexplained weight loss
Change in dietary habits
Recurrent pneumonia
Change in voice or speech
Nasal regurgitation
Dehydration
Esophageal Dysphagia
Sensation of food sticking in the chest or throat
Oral or pharyngeal regurgitation
Drooling
Unexplained weight loss
Change in dietary habits
Recurrent pneumonia
Dehydration

Some of the many symptoms and signs of dysphagia are listed in Table 2. A history of drooling, significant weight loss, or recurrent pneumonia suggests that the dysphagia is severe. The history is most useful for identifying esophageal dysphagia; the complaint of food sticking in the chest is usually associated with an esophageal disorder. In contrast, the complaint of food sticking in the throat has little localizing value and is often caused by an esophageal disorder. Coughing and choking during swallowing suggest an oropharyngeal origin and may be elicited by *aspiration* (penetration of material through the vocal folds and into the trachea) (Fig. 1). However, some patients have impaired cough reflexes, resulting in *silent* aspiration (without cough).[3] Pain on swallowing (odynophagia) may occur transiently in pharyngitis, but persistent pain is unusual and is suggestive of neoplasia. Heartburn is a non-specific complaint and is usually not associated with swallowing but occurs after meals.

Heartburn may occur in gastroesophageal reflux disease (GERD), but a more specific symptom of GERD is regurgitation of sour or bitter-tasting material into the throat after eating.

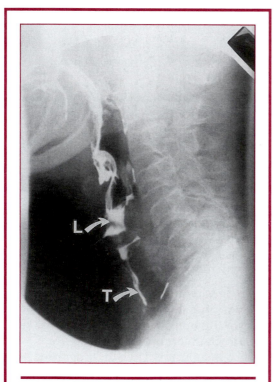

FIGURE 1. Lateral radiograph demonstrating laryngeal penetration *(L)* and tracheal aspiration *(T).* (From Lennard TA: Pain Procedures in Clinical Practice, 2nd ed. Philadelphia, Hanley and Belfus, 2000, p 60, with permission.)

Physical Examination

An examination of the oral cavity and neck may identify structural abnormalities, weakness, or sensory deficits. The finding of dysarthria (abnormal articulation of speech) or dysphonia (abnormal voice quality) is often associated with oropharyngeal dysphagia. However, the examination is primarily useful for finding evidence of underlying neurologic, neuromuscular, or connective tissue disease. The examination should always include trial swallows of water. During the swallow, there should be prompt elevation of the hyoid bone and larynx. Changes in voice quality or spontaneous coughing after swallowing suggest the presence of pharyngeal dysfunction. The history and physical examination are limited in their ability to detect and characterize dysphagia, so instrumental studies are usually necessary.

Neurologic examination is important in the evaluation of dysphagic individuals because neurologic disorders commonly cause dysphagia. Disorders of either upper or lower motor neuron (UMN or LMN) may produce dysphagia. The findings of atrophy and/or fasciculations of the tongue or palate suggest LMN dysfunction of the brainstem motor nuclei. In contrast to the prevailing wisdom, the gag reflex is not strongly predictive of the ability to swallow. It may be absent in normal individuals and normal in individuals with severe dysphagia and aspiration.

Functional Limitations

Functional limitations depend on the nature and severity of the dysphagia. Many individuals modify their diets to eliminate foods that are difficult to swallow. Some require inordinate amounts of time to consume a meal. In severe cases, tube feeding is necessary. These alterations in the ability to eat a meal may have a profound effect on psychologic and social function. Interaction with family and friends often centers on mealtime—family dinners, "going out" for a drink or for dinner, "coming over" for a snack or for dessert. Difficulty in eating a meal may disrupt relationships and result in social isolation. Some patients may require supervision during meals or feel unsafe when eating alone, causing further disruption of social and vocational function.

Diagnostic Studies

Since the mechanics of swallowing are largely invisible to the naked eye, diagnostic studies are commonly needed. The *sine qua non* for diagnosis of oropharyngeal swallowing disorders is the videofluorographic swallowing study (*VFSS*). In this test, the patient eats and drinks a variety of solids and liquids combined with barium while images are recorded with videofluorography (x-ray videotaping). The VFSS is usually performed jointly by a physician (physiatrist or radiologist) and a speech-language pathologist. A unique benefit of the VFSS is that therapeutic techniques (such as modifying food consistency, body position, or respiration) can be tested and their effects on swallowing observed during the study. A routine barium swallow is normally sufficient if the problem is clearly esophageal.

If a VFSS cannot be performed, *fiberoptic laryngoscopy* is sometimes used to visualize the pharynx and larynx during eating, but this test neglects essential aspects of swallowing, such as opening of the upper esophageal sphincter. In cases of esophageal dysphagia, *esophagoscopy* is often necessary to detect mucosal lesions or masses. Biopsy is indicated when mucosal abnormalities are detected.

Manometry is useful for detecting and characterizing motor disorders of the esophagus. EMG is indicated when neuromuscular disease is suspected and is useful for detecting LMN dysfunction of the larynx and pharynx.

Differential Diagnosis

Myocardial ischemia
Globus sensation
Heartburn due to gastroesophageal reflux disease
Indirect aspiration (aspiration of refluxed gastric contents)

Treatment

Initial

The treatment of dysphagia depends on its causes and mechanism. Common treatments are listed in Table 3.

TABLE 3. Principal Treatments for Selected Disorders Affecting Swallowing

Problems	Principal Treatments
Amyotrophic lateral sclerosis	Dietary modification Compensatory maneuvers Counseling and Advance Directives
Carcinoma of esophagus	Esophagectomy
Gastroesophageal reflux disease	Dietary modification No eating at bedtime Pharmacological therapy Smoking cessation
Parkinson's disease, polymyositis, myasthenia gravis	Pharmacological treatment of underlying disease (Dietary modification, compensatory maneuvers, and dysphagia therapy only if necessary)
Esophageal stricture or web	Dilatation
Stroke, multiple sclerosis	Dietary modification Compensatory maneuvers Dysphagia therapy

Whenever possible, initial treatment should be directed at the underlying disease process (e.g., medications such as levodopa for Parkinson's disease or steroids for polymyositis). Esophageal dysphagia necessitates evaluation and treatment by a gastroenterologist. When no therapy exists for the underlying disease or the therapy is ineffective or contraindicated, rehabilitative strategies are appropriate.

Rehabilitation

Many patients benefit from structured swallowing therapy provided by a speech-language pathologist, including instruction and supervision regarding diet, compensatory maneuvers, and exercise. The goals of therapy include reducing aspiration, improving the ability to eat and drink, and optimizing nutritional status. Therapy is individualized according to the patient's specific anatomic and structural abnormalities and the initial responses to treatment trials observed at the bedside or during the VFSS.[6] A fundamental principle of rehabilitation is that the best therapy for any activity is the activity itself; swallowing is generally the best therapy for swallowing disorders, so the rehabilitation evaluation is directed at identifying circumstances for safe and effective swallowing for each patient.

Diet modification is a common treatment for dysphagia.[7] Patients vary in ability to swallow thin and thick liquids, and that determination is usually best made by VFSS. Usually, a patient can receive adequate oral hydration with either thin liquids (e.g., water or apple juice) or thick liquids (e.g., apricot nectar, tomato juice). Rarely, a patient may be limited to pudding consistency if thin and thick liquids are freely aspirated. Most patients with significant dysphagia are unable to safely eat meats or similarly tough foods and require a mechanical soft diet. A pureed diet is recommended for patients who exhibit oral preparatory phase difficulties, pocket food in the buccal recesses (between the teeth and the cheek), or significant pharyngeal retention with chewed solid foods. Maintaining oral feeding often requires compensatory techniques to reduce aspiration or improve pharyngeal clearance. A variety of behavioral techniques are utilized, including modifications of posture, head position, and respiration, as well as specific swallow maneuvers.[8]

Exercise therapy for dysphagia is indicated when the problem is related to weakness of the muscles of swallowing. The choice of exercises must be individualized depending on the physiologic assessment. The full range of exercises is beyond the scope of this chapter, but the following examples illustrate the principles: (1) in tongue weakness, the muscles that protrude and lateralize the tongue tip are strengthened by manual resistive exercise; (2) strengthening the anterior suprahyoid muscles is useful when the upper esophageal sphincter opens poorly (flexing the neck against gravity while lying supine can strengthen these muscles); and (3) vocal fold adduction exercises may be useful in cases of aspiration due to weakness of these muscles (these exercises are done on a daily basis whenever possible).

Procedures

VFSS functions as both a diagnostic and therapeutic procedure for dysphagia, especially for the oropharyngeal type, since it can be used to test the effectiveness of modifying food consistency and other compensatory techniques.[9] Endoscopy with dilatation of the esophagus is often indicated in cases of partial esophageal obstruction due to structure or web.

Surgery

Surgery is rarely indicated in the care of patients with oral or pharyngeal dysphagia. The most common procedure for pharyngeal dysphagia is cricopharyngeal myotomy, during which the upper esophageal sphincter is disrupted to reduce the resistance of the pharyngeal outflow tract. However, the effectiveness of myotomy is highly controversial.[10] Esophagectomy may be necessary in the case of esophageal cancer or obstructive strictures. Feeding gastrostomy (usually *percutaneous endoscopic gastrostomy* or [*PEG*]) is indicated when the severity of the dysphagia makes it impossible to obtain adequate alimentation and/or hydration orally, although intravenous hydration or nasogastric tube feedings may be sufficient on a time-limited basis.[11] Orogastric tube feedings have been used successfully by patients who have absent gag reflexes and can tolerate intermittent oral catheterization.

Potential Disease Complications

Severe dysphagia may result in aspiration pneumonia,[12] airway obstruction, bronchiectasis, dehydration, or starvation[13] and is potentially fatal. Severe dysphagia often causes social isolation because of the inability to consume a meal in the usual manner. This may lead to depression, sometimes severe. Suicide has been reported.

Potential Treatment Complications

The VFSS is safe and is very well tolerated. Prescribing a modified diet often means substituting thick for thin liquids. Some patients find these unpalatable and reduce fluid intake to the point of dehydration and malnutrition. Failure to re-evaluate patients in a timely manner may lead to unnecessary prolongation of dietary restrictions, increasing the risk of malnutrition and adverse psychologic effects of dysphagia. Dilatation of the esophagus or sphincters may result in perforation, but this complication is uncommon. PEG may have direct or indirect sequelae. Direct sequelae, such as pain, infection, and obstruction of the feeding tube, are common. PEG tube feeding may promote aspiration pneumonia in individuals with severe gastroesophageal reflux disease.

References
1. Palmer JB, Drennan JC, Baba M: Evaluation and treatment of swallowing impairments. Am Fam Physician 2000;61:2453–2462.
2. Buchholz DW: Oropharyngeal dysphagia due to iatrogenic neurological dysfunction. Dysphagia 1995;10:248–254.
3. Smith CH, Logemann JA, Colangelo LA, et al: Incidence and patient characteristics associated with silent aspiration in the acute care setting [see comments]. Dysphagia 1999;14:1–7.
4. Palmer JB: Evaluation of swallowing disorders. In Grabois M, Garrison SJ, Hart KA, Lehmkuhl DL (eds): Physical Medicine Rehabilitation: The Complete Approach. Malden, MA, Blackwell Science, 1999, pp 277–290.
5. Palmer JB, Kuhlemeier KV, Tippett DC, Lynch C: A protocol for the videofluorographic swallowing study. Dysphagia 1993;8:209–214.
6. Ott DJ, Hodge RG, Pikna LA, et al:. Modified barium swallow: Clinical and radiographic correlation and relation to feeding recommendations [see comments]. Dysphagia 1996;11:187–190.
7. Bisch EM, Logemann JA, Rademaker AW, et al: Pharyngeal effects of bolus volume, viscosity, and temperature in patients with dysphagia resulting from neurologic impairment and in normal subjects. J Speech Lang Hear Res 1994;37:1041–1059.
8. Logemann JA: Behavioral management for oropharyngeal dysphagia. Folia Phoniatr Logop 1999;51:199–212.
9. Palmer JB, Carden E: The role of radiology in the rehabilitation of swallowing. In Jones B (ed): Normal and Abnormal Swallowing: Imaging in Diagnosis and Therapy. New York, Springer-Verlag, in press.
10. Jacobs JR, Logemann J, Pajak TF, et al: Failure of cricopharyngeal myotomy to improve dysphagia following head and neck cancer surgery. Arch Otolaryngol Head Neck Surg 1999;125:942–946.
11. Britton JE, Lipscomb G, Mohr PD, et al: The use of percutaneous endoscopic gastrostomy (PEG) feeding tubes in patients with neurological disease. J Neurol 1997;244:431–434.
12. Ding R, Logemann JA: Pneumonia in stroke patients: A retrospective study. Dysphagia 2000;15:51–57.
13. Finestone HM, Greene-Finestone LS, Wilson ES, Teasell RW: Malnutrition in stroke patients on the rehabilitation service and at follow-up: Prevalence and predictors. Arch Phys Med Rehabil 1995;76:310–316.

108 Enteropathic Arthritides

Karen Atkinson, MD, MPH

Synonyms

Bowel-associated
arthritis

Reactive arthritis

Seronegative
spondyloarthropathy

ICD-9 Codes

711.0
Pyogenic arthritis
  arthritis or polyarthritis
    (due to):
  coliform [Escherichia
    coli]
  Hemophilus influenzae
    [H. influenzae]
  pneumococcal
  Pseudomonas
  staphylococcal
  streptococcal

711.1
Arthropathy associated
with Reiter's disease and
nonspecific urethritis

711.9
Unspecified infective
arthritis

713.1
Arthropathy associated
with gastrointestinal
conditions other than
infections

Definition

The term enteropathic arthritis is used to describe arthritis that is associated with pathology of the bowel. This category includes the arthritis seen in association with infection (Reiter's syndrome), inflammatory bowel disease (IBD), Whipple's disease, intestinal bypass surgery, and celiac disease (gluten-sensitive enteropathy).[1]

Reiter's syndrome (reactive arthritis) usually occurs in young to middle age adults after genitourinary (*Chlamydia*) or gastrointestinal (typically, *Salmonella*, *Shigella*, *Campylobacter*, or *Yersinia*) infection. Men are affected more often in cases that occur after genitourinary infection, but the sex distribution is equal in cases occurring after gastrointestinal infection. The term was originally used to describe patients with the classic triad of nongonococcal urethritis, arthritis, and conjunctivitis. Peripheral joint arthritis occurs in 90% of patients with Reiter's syndrome, whereas axial involvement (spondylitis or sacroiliitis) affects fewer than 50% of patients.[1,2]

Arthritis associated with inflammatory bowel disease also typically affects young to middle age adults. The sex distribution is equal. Peripheral arthritis occurs in 10% to 20% of patients and axial disease in 10% of patients.[1,2]

Whipple's disease, intestinal bypass and celiac disease all can have associated arthritis. Typically, the joint involvement occurs in a symmetric peripheral polyarticular pattern that resembles rheumatoid arthritis. Whipple's disease can have axial involvement (spondylitis or sacroiliitis) in 8% to 20% of cases.[3]

Symptoms

Constitutional symptoms are common to all forms of enteropathic arthritis. Patients can experience fever, malaise, weight loss, and fatigue. Morning stiffness of greater than 30 to 60 minutes indicates inflammatory disease. Location of stiffness may occur in the hands or other peripheral joints or in the back of patients with axial involvement. Other symptoms vary according to the type of enteropathic arthritis.[2-7]

IBD-associated (Crohn's and Ulcerative Colitis) Arthritis

Patients experience pain and swelling in joints that can be transient or migratory but recurrent. Lower extremity joints are affected more frequently than those of the upper extremity. Patients with dactylitis complain of diffusely swollen digits. Active bowel inflammation leads to diarrhea and/or bloody stools. Peripheral arthritis flares with the bowel; axial involvement does not correlate with active bowel disease and can be asymptomatic. Heel or foot pain occurs secondary to enthesitis, which is inflammation at the site of tendon or ligamentous insertion onto bone. Patients with spondylitis or sacroiliitis describe back or buttock pain. Painful oral ulcer may be described. Red or violet bumps (erythema nodosum) can develop; they are painful and most commonly located over the shins. Ulcerating lesions (pyoderma gangrenosum) are less common. Red eyes indicate conjunctivitis or iritis. In iritis (anterior uveitis), the patient experiences pain and decreased vision.

Reiter's Syndrome

Patients experience painful, swollen joints. The minority of patients report preceding diarrhea, even upon direct questioning. Arthritis involves lower extremity joints more often than upper extremity joints. Heel or foot pain occurs secondary to enthesitis. As in IBD, back or buttock pain occurs with spondylitis and sacroiliitis. Some form of skin involvement occurs in almost 50% of patients. Lesions include rash over the palms and soles (keratoderma blennorrhagicum), penile lesions (circinate balanitis), and nail changes (onycholysis but not nail pitting). About 15% of patients develop oral ulcers. Urogenital symptoms include penile or vaginal discharge and ulcers. As in IBD-associated arthritis, eye symptoms including redness, pain, and/or decreased vision. Symptoms of left-sided heart failure or heart block (syncope) can result from aortic root/valve inflammation.

Whipple's Disease

Whipple's disease is characterized by fever, diarrhea, foul smelling or floating stools (steatorrhea), and profound weight loss. Patients with Whipple's disease complain of migratory arthralgias or transient episodes of swollen joints. Swollen glands may be a feature. If pleural effusions are present, patients may experience chest pain or shortness of breath. Complaints of double vision (ocular palsies) or mental status changes accompany nervous system involvement.

Intestinal Bypass

Patients complain of painful, swollen joints. Cutaneous vasculitis causes rash in some patients.

Celiac Disease

Patients with gluten-sensitive enteropathy can also develop joint aches or swelling, which usually affects the large joints. Only 50% of patients have diarrhea. Patients with associated dermatitis herpetiformis complain of burning and itching of the skin.

Physical Examination

Physical examination findings vary according to the etiology of enteropathic arthritis .[2-7]

IBD-associated Arthritis

Patients with inflammatory bowel disease usually have a monoarticular (one joint) or oligoarticular (two to four joints) asymmetric arthritis involving the peripheral joints. The knees, ankles, and feet are most commonly affected. Large effusions occur, especially in the knee. Limited lumbar mobility secondary to spondylitis is documented with an abnormal Schober's maneuver (Fig. 1). To perform this maneuver the clinician makes a mark at the level of the posterior superior iliac spines (dimples of the pelvis) and another mark 10 cm above the first mark with the patient standing. The patient is then asked to bend forward, attempting to touch his or her toes. The distance between the two marks is re-measured. With normal lumbar motion, the distance between the two points increases by at least 5 cm. Maneuvers such as pelvic distraction or compression to elicit pain associated with sacroiliitis lack specificity. Thickening of the Achilles tendon or pain at the

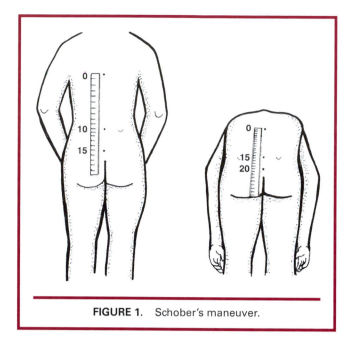

FIGURE 1. Schober's maneuver.

insertion site of the Achilles or plantar fascia on the calcaneous is found in patients with enthesitis. Examination of the skin may reveal red or violet subcutaneous nodules (erythema nodosum) or painful ulcers with irregular borders (pyoderma gangrenosum). Conjunctivitis causes a red/injected eye. Pericorneal injection, corneal clouding, and miosis suggest anterior uveitis (usually iritis with sparing of the ciliary body). Slit-lamp examination will reveal cells in the anterior chamber.

Reiter's Syndrome

Like inflammatory bowel disease, Reiter's syndrome causes a monoarticular or oligoarticular asymmetric peripheral arthritis that usually affects the lower limbs. Enthesitis, dactylitis, conjunctivitis, and uveitis also occur, and evaluation of these is as previously described. Urogenital evaluation may reveal a mucoid discharge secondary to inflammation (urethritis or cervicitis). Fifty percent of patients will have some skin manifestation. Keratoderma blennorrhagicum and circinate balanitis each occur in about 25% of patients with Reiter's syndrome. Keratoderma blennorrhagicum is a papulosquamous lesion that appears identical to psoriasis but is usually limited to the palms and soles. Circinate balanitis occurs on the shaft or glans and appears different in men who are circumcised (dry, plaque-like lesions resembling keratoderma) versus uncircumcised (shallow, serpiginous penile ulcers surrounding the meatus). Nail changes include onycholysis and hyperkeratosis. Lack of pitting may distinguish this from psoriatic changes. Pyoderma gangrenosum can occur. Oral or genital ulcers can be found and are often painless. Aortitis and valve insufficiency can cause a murmur.

Whipple's Disease

The arthritis of Whipple's disease is typically a symmetric, peripheral polyarthritis (greater than four joints). Lymphadenopathy may be noted. Pleural effusions can occur and are detected during pulmonary examination. Neurologic exam may demonstrate ocular palsies or encephalopathy.

Intestinal Bypass

Patients who have undergone intestinal bypass can develop a symmetric, peripheral non-deforming polyarthritis. Lesions that can be found on the skin include vesiculopustular lesions, erythema nodosum, urticaria, or ecchymosis.

Celiac Disease

Joint exam reveals a symmetric peripheral polyarthritis. Dermatitis herpetiformis can be associated with this disorder and appear as urtcarial wheals, vesicles, bullae, or erythema that occur symmetrically on limbs or the trunk.

Functional Limitations

Functional limitations depend on the location and severity of joint involvement. The criteria for the assessment of functional status that have been established for rheumatoid arthritis (see Chapter 134) are also applied to patients with psoriatic arthritis. These criteria are based on activities of daily living, including self-care (dressing, feeding, bathing, grooming, and toileting); vocational (work, school, and homemaking); and avocational activities (recreational and/or leisure).[8] Visual impairment can result from inflammatory eye disease.

Diagnostic Studies

Laboratory testing in all of these diseases may reveal anemia and an elevated sedimentation rate. Rheumatoid factor and ANA are usually negative. Synovial fluid is inflammatory (greater than 2000 WBC) with negative cultures and no crystals when examined under polarized microscopy. HLA-B27 is highly associated with Reiter's syndrome, occurring in 81% of patients. There is no increased frequency of HLA-B27 in patients with inflammatory bowel disease alone, but 50% of IBD patients with spondylitis are B27 positive.[1]

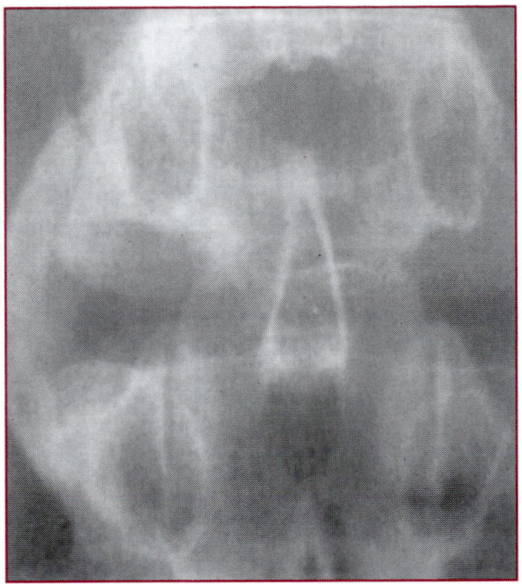

Radiographic evaluation of the axial skeleton may confirm spondylitis or sacroiliitis. In IBD, sacroiliitis is usually symmetric, and syndesmophytes usually insert marginally on the vertebral body—findings which are indistinguishable from ankylosing spondylitis (Fig. 2). Asymmetric sacroiliitis is found in Reiter's syndrome. Peripheral joints in both IBD and Reiter's syndrome may show erosion, but adjacent bone proliferation may distinguish these changes from rheumatoid arthritis. In patients with a history suggestive of enthesitis, calcaneal films will often show proliferative bone formation at the tendon/ligamentous insertion site.[4] There are usually no radiographic changes in patients with Whipple's disease, intestinal bypass, or celiac disease.

FIGURE 2. Radiograph of spine showing a large "jug-handle" syndesmophyte. (From West SG: Rheumatology Secrets. Philadelphia, Hanley & Belfus, 1997, with permission.)

Other tests should be directed toward the underlying illness or symptom. In patients without confirmed IBD, evaluation of the bowel with endoscopy or colonoscopy and biopsy is indicated. Skin biopsy may be helpful when clinical findings are not typical or are in question. Patients with ocular symptoms should be referred for ophthalmologic (slit-lamp) examination.

In patients with suspected Reiter's syndrome, cervical/uretheral smears should be performed to rule out gonorrhea and to evaluate for *Chlamydia*. Stool samples from patients who report preceding or concurrent diarrhea should also be sent. If aortitis and/or aortic insufficiency are suspected, electrocardiogram and echocardiogram are indicated.

The diagnosis of Whipple's disease may be confirmed with characteristic PAS-staining deposits on small bowel biopsy or lymph node or synovial biopsy. Diagnosis is also now possible using PCR for *T. whippelii* on blood or tissue samples.

Celiac disease can be diagnosed by small bowel biopsy. Antibody tests are now available, including antigliadin and endomysial antibodies. A presumptive diagnosis can be made if symptoms resolve on a gluten-free diet.

Differential Diagnosis

Other spondyloarthropathies
   Psoriatic arthritis
   Ankylosing spondylitis
Rheumatoid arthritis

Treatment

Initial

The treatment of IBD-associated arthritis and the arthritis of Reiter's syndrome is generally the same as for other spondyloarthropathies.[5,9] Nonsteroidal anti-inflammatory drugs (NSAIDs) are effective in many patients. COX-2 specific anti-inflammatories may reduce the incidence of gastrointestinal symptoms in patients who have a history of bleeding or who are intolerant of traditional NSAIDs.

For patients with inadequate response or progressive, erosive disease, disease modifying drugs (DMARDs) should be initiated. Antimalarials, IM gold, sulfasalazine, azathioprine, methotrexate, and cyclosporin A have all been shown to be effective. As with the treatment of other inflammatory arthritides, combination therapy can be effective, though controlled data supporting this approach are unavailable. Corticosteroids can be very useful and can be administered systemically as a bridge to therapy with DMARDs or intra-articularly for monoarticular or oligoarticular involvement. Antibiotic treatment targeting the precipitating infection does not improve Reiter's syndrome, but should be administered if a microbe is isolated to prevent spread of infection.

Patients with Whipple's disease can achieve remission with long-term (greater or equal to 1 year) of antibiotic treatment with tetracyclines.[5]

The arthritis associated with intestinal bypass is sometimes controlled with NSAIDs or glucocorticoids. Resolution of the arthritis can be achieved with normalization of gut anatomy.[5]

In patients with celiac disease, the arthritis responds to a gluten-free diet.[4]

Rehabilitation

Approaches to rehabilitation are identical to those in rheumatoid and other inflammatory arthritis. The role of occupational and physical therapy may be different in early or established disease and end-stage disease. In early disease, occupational therapy is directed toward patient education about how to use the joints to minimize joint stress when performing activities of daily living. Splints may be used to provide joint rest and reduce inflammation. Splints may also allow functional use of joints that would otherwise be limited by pain; however, not all clinicians advocate this use. Paraffin baths can provide relief of pain and stiffness in the small joints of the hands. In end-stage disease, the occupational therapist plays an important role, providing aids and adaptive devices such as raised toilet seats, special chairs and beds, special grips, and other devices that can assist in self-care.

Physical therapy can be very helpful in reducing joint inflammation and pain. The therapist may employ a variety of techniques, including the application of heat or cold, transcutaneous nerve stimulation, and iontophoresis. Water exercise (hydrotherapy) is used to increase muscle strength without joint overuse. In patients with foot involvement such as dactylitis, a high toe box or extra-depth shoe may provide decreased pain and a more normal gait. Shoe inserts are often used in Achilles tendonitis and plantar fasciitis. For patients with axial involvement, the goal of therapy is maintaining a normal upright posture through stretching of paravertebral musculature and correcting the tendency toward kyphotic posture. In end-stage disease, the goals of therapy are reducing joint inflammation, loosening fixed position of joints, improving the function of damaged joints, and improving strength and general condition. Local immobilization may be utilized to reduce inflammation and pain. Non-fixed contractures may be prevented or improved with periods of splinting combined with goal-oriented exercise. Muscle strength and overall conditioning may be improved by static, range of motion, and relaxation exercises. In recent years, aerobic exercises and weight-training have been used without detrimental effect to the joints. These dynamic exercises are more effective in increasing muscle strength, range of motion, and physical capacity. The motivation and encouragement provided by the therapist should not be underestimated.

Procedures

For monoarticular or oligoarticular involvement, local steroid injection may be used when oral medications fail to control joint inflammation.

Surgery

Joint replacement, tendon repair, or synovectomy may be required. Reversal of intestinal bypass is curative in patients with this disorder.

Potential Disease Complications

For patients with IBD-associated arthritis and Reiter's syndrome, progressive damage to joints, including ankylosis, results in loss of function. Ruptured tendons can occur secondary to chronic enthesitis. Visual loss may occur secondary to chronic or poorly controlled inflammatory eye disease. Patients with inflammatory bowel disease, especially Crohn's, may develop secondary amyloidosis.

Potential Treatment Complications

Side effects vary according to the drug used (Table 1).[10]

TABLE 1. Toxicities of Medications Used in the Treatment of Enteropathic Arthritis

Medication	Side Effects	Medication	Side Effects
NSAIDs	Dyspepsia, ulcer, or bleeding Renal insufficiency Hepatotoxicity Rash Inhibited platelet function	Gold	Myelosuppression Proteinuria or hematuria Oral ulcers Rash Pruritis
COX-2 inhibitors	Same as traditional NSAIDs but GI side effects occur less often No platelet effect	Sulfasalazine	Myelosuppression Hemolysis (G6PD deficient patients Hepatotoxicity Photosensitivity/rash Dyspepsia/diarrhea Headaches Oligospermia
Glucocorticoids	Increased appetite/weight gain/cushingoid habitus Acne Fluid retention Hypertention Diabetes Glaucoma/cataracts Atherosclerosis Avascular necrosis Osteoporosis Impaired wound healing Increased susceptibility to infection	Azathioprine	Myelosuppression Hepatotoxicity Pancreatitis (rarely) Lymphoproliferative disorders (long-term risk)
		Methotrexate	Hepatic fibrosis/cirrhosis Pneumonitis Myelosuppression Mucositis Dyspepsia Alopecia
Antimalarials	Dyspepsia Macular damage Abnormal skin pigmentation Neuromyopathy Rash	Cyclosporin A	Renal insufficiency Hypertension Anemia

References

1. Taurog JD: Seronegative spondyloarthropathies: epidemiology, pathology and pathogenesis, In Klippel JH (e): Primer on the Rheumatic Diseases, 11th ed. Arthritis Foundation, 1997, pp 180–183.
2. Gladman DD: Clinical aspects of the spondyloarthropathies. Am J Med Sci 1998;316:234–238.
3. Dobbins WO: Whipple's disease: An historical perspective. QJM 1985;56:523–531.
4. Veys EM, Hielants H: Enteropathic arthropathies. In Klippel JH, Dieppe PA (eds): Rheumatolog, 2nd ed. London, Mosby, 1998, pp 24.1–24.8.
5. Wollheim FA: Enteropathic arthritis. In Kelley WN, Ruddy S, Harris ED Jr, Sledge CB, (eds): Textbook of Rheumatology, 5th ed. Philadelphia, W.B. Saunders, 1997, pp 1006–1014.
6. Arnett FC: Reactive arthritis (Reiter's syndrome) and enteropathic arthritis. In Klippel JH (ed): Primer on the Rheumatic Diseases, 11th ed. Arthritis Foundation, 1997, pp 184–188.
7. Leirisalo-Repo M, Repo H: Gut and spondyloarthropathies. Rheum Dis Clin North Am 1992;18:23–35.
8. Hochberg MC, Chang RW, Dwosh I, et al: The American College of Rheumatology 1991 Revised Criteria for the classification of global functional status in rheumatoid arthritis. Arthritis Rheum 1992;35:493–502.
9. Haslock I: Ankylosing spondylitis: Management. In Klippel JH, Dieppe PA (eds): Rheumatolog, 2nd ed. London, Mosby, 1998, pp 19.1–19.10.
10. Cash JM, Klippel JH: Drug therapy: second-line drug therapy for rheumatoid arthritis. N Engl J Med 1994;330(19):1368–1375.

109 Fibromyalgia

Joanne Borg-Stein, MD

Synonym

Fibrositis

ICD-9 Code

729.1
Myalgia and myositis,
unspecified

Definition

Fibromyalgia is a syndrome defined by chronic widespread pain of at least 6 months duration.

According to the currently accepted 1990 American College of Rheumatology criteria, a patient must experience pain

- In the axial skeleton
- Above and below the waist
- To palpation in at least 11 of 18 paired tender points throughout the body

The majority of patients (80%) with fibromyalgia are women.

Symptoms

The symptoms of fibromyalgia are widespread pain, fatigue, sleep disturbance, and myalgias.

Commonly associated syndromes are migraine, irritable bowel syndrome, interstitial cystitis, depression, anxiety, and temporomandibular dysfunction.

Physical Examination

The general medical and neurologic examinations should be normal. The 18 paired tender points should be palpated with approximately 4 kg/cm^2 of pressure. This is just enough pressure to blanch the fingernail of the clinician. The patient will experience pain at these locations (Fig. 1).

In addition, a comprehensive musculoskeletal examination should be performed to rule out superimposed pain generators such as bursitis, tendinitis, radiculopathy, and myofascial trigger points.

Functional Limitations

Patients are limited by both pain and fatigue. Patients also report cognitive dysfunction with difficulty in concentration, organization, and motivation; this has been termed "fibro fog." Approximately 25% of patients with fibromyalgia report themselves as disabled and are collecting some form of disability payments. Individuals are more likely to become disabled if they

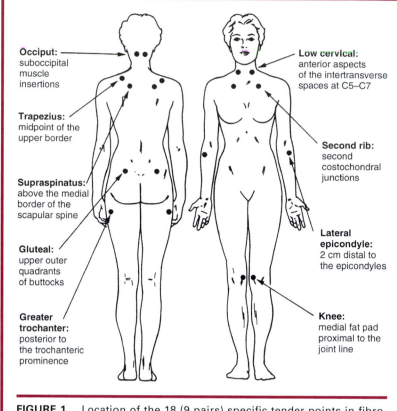

Occiput: suboccipital muscle insertions

Trapezius: midpoint of the upper border

Supraspinatus: above the medial border of the scapular spine

Gluteal: upper outer quadrants of buttocks

Greater trochanter: posterior to the trochanteric prominence

Low cervical: anterior aspects of the intertransverse spaces at C5–C7

Second rib: second costochondral junctions

Lateral epicondyle: 2 cm distal to the epicondyles

Knee: medial fat pad proximal to the joint line

FIGURE 1. Location of the 18 (9 pairs) specific tender points in fibromyalgia patients. (From Freundlich B, Leventhal L: The fibromyalgia syndrome. In Schumacher HR Jr, Klippel JH, Koopman WJ (eds): Primer on the Rheumatic Diseases, 10th ed. Atlanta, Arthritis Foundation, 1993, pp 247–249, with permission.)

report higher pain scores, work at a job that requires heavy physical labor, have poor coping strategies and feel helpless, or are involved in litigation.[2,3]

Diagnostic Studies

Fibromyalgia is a clinical diagnosis. In order to exclude other diagnoses, it may be appropriate to include basic laboratory tests (e.g., complete blood count, thyroid function studies, and erythrocyte sedimentation rate). Primary sleep disorders may need to be identified by sleep studies. Radiographs and/or magnetic resonance imaging (MRI) may be indicated if osteoarthritis, radiculopathy, spinal stenosis, or intrinsic joint pathology is suspected.

Electrodiagnostic studies may be useful if an entrapment neuropathy or radiculopathy is suspected.

Differential Diagnosis:

Thyroid myopathy   Mood disturbances
Metabolic myopathy   Somatoform pain disorders

Treatment

Initial

Initial treatment includes patient education, pharmacologic treatment, gentle exercise, and relaxation training. Patient education includes individual and group classes that review the symptoms of fibromyalgia, reassure as to the generally benign course, and outline the treatment path.[4]

Pharmacologic management aims to normalize sleep patterns and diminish pain. Low dose tricyclic antidepressants at bedtime (i.e., 10 to 25 mg amitriptyline) in combination with low dose selective serotonin reuptake inhibitors (i.e., fluoxetine 20 mg qam) is an excellent combination. This combination generally works better than either medication alone.

Pain may be relieved with simple analgesics such as acetaminophen or a nonsteroidal anti-inflammatory drug (NSAID). Tramadol is the next-line agent. Opioids are rarely necessary.

Adjunctive non-pharmacologic pain control methods include acupuncture, massage, and biofeedback.

Associated depression and anxiety often need psychopharmacologic treatment as well.

Rehabilitation

Physical therapy is utilized to educate the patient on a stretching, gentle strengthening, and cardiovascular fitness program. This can improve fitness and function and decrease pain. Occupational therapy is incorporated to review ergonomics of occupational activities at the worksite and activities of daily living are reviewed. Task simplification, pacing, and maximization of function are emphasized.[5,6]

Mental health professionals can be helpful in the rehabilitative phase to educate patients in a mind-body stress reduction program. This provides the patient with positive coping strategies for living with chronic pain.[7]

Procedures

Myofascial trigger points may be injected with local anesthetic to decrease local pain (Fig. 2).

If patients have concurrent bursitis, tendinitis, or nerve entrapment, then therapeutic injections may be performed to treat these specific diagnoses.

Acupuncture can be utilized for treatment of pain and fatigue. Preliminary studies suggest that the benefit may last up to several months.[8]

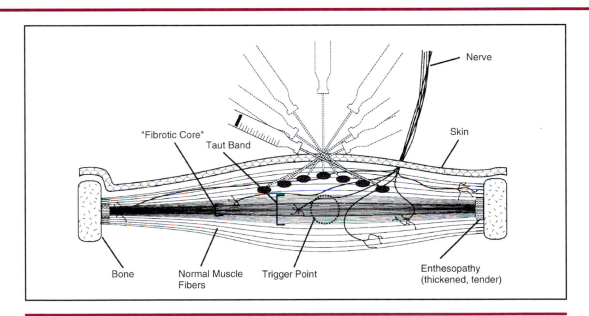

FIGURE 2. Under sterile conditions, using a 25- or 27-gauge (⅝- to 1½-inch) needle, trigger points can be injected with 1 to 2 cc of local anesthetic. Larger volumes can be injected in increments as the needle penetrates the muscle at different levels. Caution should be used not to inject a large volume into one area (0.1 cc to 0.2 cc is ideal) as this may cause muscle damage. This can be done using a short acting anesthetic (e.g., 1% lidocaine) or a combination of a short acting and longer acting anesthetic (e.g., 1% lidocaine mixed with 0.25% bupivacaine). In the case of allergy to the "—caine" group, saline can be used instead. A vapocoolant such as ethyl chloride can be used immediately prior to the injection to diminish the pain from the needle prick. (From Lennard TA: Pain Procedures in Clinical Practice, 2nd ed. Philadelphia, Hanley & Belfus, 2000, with permission.)

Surgery

There is no surgery indicated for fibromyalgia.

Potential Disease Complications

Failure to make the diagnosis early may lead to delay in treatment, deconditioning, and expensive unnecessary medical testing and procedures. Chronic, intractable pain may occur despite treatment.

Potential Treatment Complications

Tricyclic antidepressant medications can be associated with anticholinergic side effects such as urinary retention, sedation, constipation, and weight gain. Selective serotonin reuptake inhibitor medications may be associated with sexual dysfunction, gastrointestinal intolerance, and anorexia. Tramadol can cause gastrointestinal symptoms and may lower the seizure threshold. Thus it should not be used in someone with a known seizure history. Overly aggressive exercise programs may transiently increase pain in some patients. Local injections may result in local pain, ecchymosis, intravascular injection, or pneumothorax if improperly executed.

References
1. Goldenberg DL: Fibromyalgia syndrome a decade later, what have we learned? Arch Intern Med 1999;159:777–785.
2. Goldenberg DL, Mossey CJ, et al: A model to assess severity and impact of fibromyalgia. J Rheumatol 1995;22(12): 2313–2318.
3. Bennett RM: Fibromyalgia and the disability dilemma. Arthritis Rheum 1996;19(10):1627–1633.
4. Bennett RM: Multidisciplinary group programs to treat fibromyalgia patients. Rheum Dis Clin North Am 1996;22(2): 351–367.
5. Gowans SE, deHueck A, et al: A randomized, controlled trial of exercise and education for individuals with fibromyalgia. Arthritis Care Research 1999;12(2):120–128.
6. Rosen NB: Physical medicine and rehabilitation approaches to the management of myofascial pain and fibromyalgia syndromes. Bailliere's Clinical Rheumatology 1994;8(4):881–916.
7. Kaplan KH, Goldenberg DL, et al: The impact of a meditation-based stress reduction program on fibromyalgia. General Hospital Psychiatry 1993;15:284–289.
8. Berman BM, Exxo J, et al: Is acupuncture effective in the treatment of fibromyalgia? J Fam Pract 1999;48(3):213–218.

110 Headaches

Elizabeth Loder, MD

Synonyms

General
Benign headaches
Nonmalignant
  headache disorder

Migraine
Sick headache
Vascular headache

Cluster
Suicide headache
Alarm clock headache
Histamine cephalgia
Migrainous neuralgia
Autonomic cephalgia

Tension-type
Ordinary headache
Muscle contraction
  headache
Tension headache

ICD-9 Codes

307.81
Tension headache

346.9
Migraine, unspecified

784.0
Headache

Definition

The three major primary headache disorders are migraine, tension-type, and cluster headache.[1] While all three syndromes are characterized by chronic, recurrent, and potentially disabling headaches, specific diagnosis is important because of differing natural history and treatment.

The benign headache disorders are classified according to criteria developed by the International Headache Society (IHS) in 1988[2]; these will be periodically revised.[1] Diagnosis remains clinical, based on patient history and an examination that rules out secondary causes of headache (not covered in this chapter). The IHS criteria were developed for research purposes and lack sensitivity when used in the clinical setting.

Migraine

Migraine is subclassified as migraine without aura (replaces older term of "common migraine") (Table 1) and migraine with aura (replaces older term of "classic migraine") (Table 2). Twenty percent of patients have preceding *aura*, which consists of focal neurologic signs or symptoms that begin gradually and fade away within 30 to 60 minutes as the headache begins.

TABLE 1. Diagnostic Criteria for Migraine without Aura

A. At least five attacks fulfilling B-D.

B. Headache attacks lasting 4–72 hours (untreated or unsuccessfully treated).

C. Headache has at least two of the following characteristics:
1. Unilateral location.
2. Pulsating quality.
3. Moderate or severe intensity (inhibits or prohibits daily activities).
4. Aggravation by walking stairs or similar routine physical activity.

D. During headache at least one of the following:
1. Nausea and/or vomiting.
2. Photophobia and phonophobia.

E. At least one of the following:
1. History physical, and neurologic examinations do not suggest one of the disorders listed in groups 5–11.
2. History and/or physical and/or neurologic examinations do suggest such disorder, but it is ruled out by appropriate investigations.
3. Such disorder is present, but migraine attacks do not occur for the first time in close temporal relation to the disorder.

From Lipton RB, Newman LC: Migraine. In Kanner R (ed): Pain Management Secrets. Philadelphia, Hanley & Belfus, 1997, pp 42–43.

A. At least two attacks fulfilling B.

B. At least three of the following four characteristics:
  1. One or more fully reversible aura symptoms indicating focal cerebral cortical and/or brainstem dysfunction.
  2. At least one aura symptom develops gradually over more than 4 minutes, or two or more symptoms occur in succession.
  3. No aura symptom lasts more than 60 minutes. If more than one aura symptom is present, accepted duration is proportionally increased.
  4. Headache follows aura with a free interval of less than 60 minutes. (It may also begin before or simultaneously with the aura.)

C. At least one of the following:
  1. History, physical, and neurologic examinations do not suggest one of the disorders listed in groups 5–11.
  2. History and/or physical and/or neurologic examinations do suggest such disorder, but it is ruled out by appropriate investigations.
  3. Such disorder is present, but migraine attacks do not occur for the first time in close temporal relation to the disorder.

From Lipton RB, Newman LC: Migraine. In Kanner R (ed): Pain Management Secrets. Philadelphia, Hanley & Belfus, 1997, pp 42–43.

Cluster

The following are characteristics of cluster headaches:

- 1 headache every other day, up to eight headaches per day, lasting 15 to 180 minutes untreated or unsuccessfully treated
- Always unilateral, behind eye
- Steady, severe pain
- Must have at least one associated autonomic sign on side of pain
    Conjunctival injection
    Lacrimation
    Rhinorrhea
    Ptosis
    Meiosis

Cluster headache is subclassified as episodic cluster headache or chronic cluster headache. In episodic cluster headache, attacks generally occur daily for a period of from 2 weeks to 3 months, then remit for months or years. In chronic cluster headache, there are no headache-free periods, or they are less than 2 weeks in duration.

Patients with cluster headache usually describe alcohol intolerance and generally note intense restlessness during the headache.

Tension-type

The following are characteristics of tension-type headaches:

- Headaches lasting 30 minutes to 7 days
- Bilateral
- Mild to moderate in intensity
- Pressing or squeezing
- Not worse with physical activity
- No associated nausea, vomiting, photophobia or phonophobia (on the rare occasion that these symptoms are present, they are much milder than seen with migraines)

Tension-type headache is subclassified as episodic tension-type headache, which occurs less than 15 days per month, and chronic tension-type headache, with attacks occurring 15 or more days per month for at least 6 months.

Patients with tension-type headache typically do not report symptoms beyond the headache. If multiple associated symptoms are reported, a diagnosis of migraine should be re-examined.

Symptoms

In addition to the aforementioned symptoms that are required for diagnosis, many patients with migraine report *prodromal* symptoms, such as yawning; neck and shoulder muscle discomfort; excessive salivation; and changes in appetite, mood, sleep, gastrointestinal function, and urination.

Postdromal symptoms in migraine include fatigue, exercise intolerance, and neck and shoulder muscle discomfort.

Physical Examination

The primary headache disorders are diagnosed by history; there are currently no laboratory, genetic, or imaging markers that confirm the diagnosis. The major purpose of physical and neurologic examination is to *rule out* the presence of secondary headache disorders. Accordingly, the most important parts of the physical examination are funduscopic examination to exclude papilledema and neurologic examination to exclude other abnormalities that might increase suspicion of a malignancy, collagen vascular disease, or infectious cause for headaches.[3]

Interictally, the physical and neurologic examinations will be normal in primary headache disorders, or if another disorder is identified it must not be causally related to the primary headache.

If the patient is examined during a headache attack, the following points should be specifically noted:

- Patients experiencing migraine lie quietly, avoid movement, and may appear pale and diaphoretic. They typically display marked photophobia and phonophobia.
- Patients experiencing cluster headache are physically restless. Head banging and agitation are common. Autonomic signs should be documented to confirm the diagnosis. Between attacks, persistent ptosis and conjunctival injection may occasionally be seen.
- Patients experiencing tension-type headache may appear uncomfortable, but are not incapacitated.
- Neck, shoulder, and jaw tightness is common in patients with prolonged headache of all types and does not necessarily represent the underlying cause of the headache. In most cases, these muscular complaints will improve with appropriate treatment of the headache and do not need to be treated separately. There is no evidence that, as a group, patients with tension-type headache have abnormally elevated muscle tension. In fact, patients with migraine have routinely been shown to have higher muscle tension than patients with tension-type headache. While biofeedback-assisted muscle relaxation is clearly of benefit in migraine and tension-type headache, it may exert its effect through mechanisms other than muscle relaxation.

Functional Limitations

Quality of life surveys and other data suggest that patients with primary headache disorders are more functionally impaired than is commonly appreciated. Obviously, acute attacks of migraine and cluster headache prohibit function and generally require bed rest if untreated. Visual aura can render driving or other hazardous activities dangerous or even impossible. Tension-type headache does not generally prohibit activities, but may inhibit them. Patients commonly report feeling that they are not functioning at "full capacity."

In many cases, severely affected patients report that fear and anxiety about possible attacks lead them to avoid, cancel, or decline work, social, and academic opportunities. The depression that can occur as a result of poorly controlled headaches also may lead to impaired function. The functional limitations imposed on many patients by nonspecific sedative treatments for migraine or by prophylactic treatments, which can cause fatigue, exercise intolerance, weight gain, and depression, are underappreciated.[4]

Diagnostic Studies

The primary headache disorders are clinical diagnoses. Imaging studies or laboratory tests are done to rule out secondary headache disorders, not to rule in primary disorders.

Differential Diagnosis

Migraine
Seizure disorder
Sinus infection
Early subarachnoid hemorrhage
Collagen-vascular disorders
Meningitis
Space-occupying central nervous
system lesion
Post-traumatic headache

Cluster
Trigeminal neuralgia
Cavernous sinus thrombosis
Central nervous system or ENT tumor
Orbital cellulites or fracture
Subarachnoid hemorrhage
Dental abscess

Tension type
Mild or "forme fruste" migraine attack
Temporomandibular disorder
Space-occupying central nervous system lesion

Treatment

Initial

Headache treatment consists of nonpharmacologic measures, lifestyle changes, and abortive treatment of acute attacks.[5] Prophylactic treatment, in which daily medication is given to decrease the frequency and severity of headache episodes, is reserved for patients who do not get acceptable relief from abortive therapy or have more than two headache attacks a week. While there is some overlap in treatment options among the various headache disorders, there are also important differences. In particular, cluster headache is often erroneously treated for years with migraine medication, to little or no avail.

Migraine

Lifestyle modification
Regular and adequate sleep
Avoidance of excess caffeine
Avoidance of missed meals
Avoidance of alcohol (not a trigger for all migraine patients)
Regular aerobic exercise
Although commonly advised, there is no scientific evidence that avoidance of chocolate, dairy products, or the myriad of other dietary factors anecdotally implicated in migraine is helpful for the majority of patients with migraine; several studies have exonerated various dietary factors (e.g., chocolate) as a cause of migraine; in the absence of scientific evidence to the contrary, it does not seem wise to promote food anxieties.

Nonpharmacologic treatment
Biofeedback-assisted relaxation (thermal or EMG)
Acupuncture (weak evidence of benefit)
Physical therapy *not* shown to be useful (one trial compared physical therapy with medication for migraine to medication alone—no benefit was seen with the addition of physical therapy); if used, it should be short term and focus on development of an aerobic or other exercise program rather than on passive modalities.

Abortive therapy
NSAIDs, with or without caffeine
Isometheptene compounds (Midrin)
Opioids, with or without aspirin or acetaminophen
Barbiturate-containing compounds (e.g., Fiorinal, Fioricet, Esgic, Phrenelin)
Ergots (Cafergot, Wigraine, DHE)
Triptans (sumatriptan, rizatriptan, zolmitriptan, naratriptan, frovatriptan, eletriptan)

Prophylactic therapy

NSAIDs

Beta blockers (except those with sympathomimetic activity)

Tricyclic antidepressants

Sodium valproate

Methysergide

Calcium channel antagonists

Riboflavin (vitamin B_2)

Selective serotonin reuptake inhibitors (weak evidence of benefit)

Cluster

Lifestyle modification

Alcohol avoidance

Stress reduction

Nonpharmacologic therapy

100% oxygen—10 to 12 liters at headache onset via nonrebreather mask for 10–15 minutes aborts headache in 80% of patients

Abortive therapy

Generally must be parenteral, since headaches are short and onset sudden; options include:

Oxygen, as previously described

Sumatriptan 6 mg subcutaneously

Dihydroergotamine 1 mg subcutaneously

Parenteral opioids

Prophylactic therapy

Lithium carbonate 300 mg po tid

Verapamil (high doses required)

Methysergide

Steroids

Sodium valproate (benefit unclear)

Topiramate (benefit unclear)

Tension-type

Lifestyle modification

Regular and adequate sleep

Aerobic exercise

Nonpharmacologic therapy

Biofeedback (thermal or EMG)

Physical therapy focusing on stretching, strengthening, development of exercise program rather than passive modalities

Acute therapy

NSAIDs

Isometheptene combinations (Midrin)

Potentially sedative or habit-forming opioid or barbiturate-containing compounds should generally be avoided

Prophylactic therapy

NSAIDs

Tricyclic antidepressants

Sodium valproate

Rehabilitation

Patients whose headaches are refractory to currently available treatments suffer significant disability. Secondary depression and medication overuse may develop, along with family dysfunction and poor work performance. The development of *chronic pain syndrome* (see Chapter 101), in which patients develop disability out of proportion to the underlying disease, with associated behavioral abnormalities, requires interdisciplinary treatment for best results. The treatment philosophy, which must be accepted by the patient and family, shifts from cure to management. Medication reduction, increased "up" time and regular physical exercise, involvement in hobbies or return to work, and psychologic intervention all help return the patient to some semblance of normal living, despite the persistence of headache. Specialized headache treatment programs employing an interdisciplinary approach can be located by contacting the

American Council for Headache Education at (800)255-ACHE. Inpatient treatment may be necessary for patients with severe medication overuse, who require special tapering from narcotic or barbiturate drugs, or who have associated medical or psychiatric morbidity that precludes outpatient treatment. Only a handful of such programs exist in the United States; they can be located by contacting the Commission on the Accreditation of Rehabilitation Facilities (CARF).

Procedures

Botulinum toxin injections into the pericranial musculature are currently under investigation for the treatment of both migraine and tension-type headache. Headaches associated with significant pericranial muscle spasm may benefit from localized trigger-point injections.

Surgery

Ablative surgical procedures on the fifth cranial nerve are employed in cases of refractory cluster headache. Radiofrequency, cryotherapy, and alcohol techniques are all employed. Many women with migraine contemplate oophorectomy, in the belief that elimination of hormonal cycling may eliminate migraine. In fact, abrupt surgical menopause seems to worsen, not improve, migraine, and this procedure should be discouraged.

Potential Disease Complications

Inadequately managed headaches can directly or indirectly lead to depression, suicide, analgesic nephropathy, withdrawal seizures, addiction and dependence syndromes, unemployment, divorce, and poor progress in school and the workplace.

Potential Treatment Complications

The usual complications from injections include an allergic reaction to the medication, and infection.

Potential complications from surgery include anesthesia dolorosa, dry eye, and facial anesthesia or weakness. Multiple reactions to medications are possible, and the clinician should be aware of the side-effect profile for any medications prescribed.

References

1. Stewart WF, Lipton RB, Celentano DD, Reed ML: Prevalence of migraine headache in the United States: Relation to age, income, race and other sociodemographic factors. J Am Med Assoc 1992;267:64–69.
2. Headache Classification Committee of the International Headache Society: Classification and diagnostic criteria for headache disorders, cranial neuralgias and facial pain. Cephalalgia 1988;8(Suppl 7):1–96.
3. Lance JW, Goadsby PJ: Mechanisms and Management of Headache, 6th ed, Boston, Butterworth Heinemann, 1998.
4. Loder E, Tietjen GE, Marcus DA: Evaluation and management issues in migraine. J Clin Outcomes Management 1999;6:58–74.
5. Silberstein SD, for the US Headache Consortium: Practice parameter: Evidence-based guidelines for migraine headache (an evidence-based review): Report of the Quality Standards Subcommittee of the American Academy of Neurology. Neurology 2000;55:754–762.

111 Heterotopic Ossification

Philip J. Blount, MD
William L. Bockenek, MD

Synonyms

Myositis ossificans

Ossifying fibromyopathy

Neurogenic heterotopic ossification

Periarticular ossification

Heterotopic ossification in paraplegia

Neurogenic ossifying fibromyositis

Neurogenic osteoma

ICD-9 Codes

728.1
Muscular calcification and ossification

728.10
Calcification and ossification, unspecified
  Massive calcification (paraplegic)

728.11
Progressive myositis ossificans

728.12
Traumatic myositis ossificans
  Myositis ossificans (circumscripta)

728.13
Postoperative heterotopic calcification

733.99
Other and unspecified disorders on bone and cartilage
  Hyptertrophy of bone

Definition

Heterotopic ossification (HO) is the formation of bone in non-skeletal tissue. Its etiology is unknown. HO is commonly seen in patients with traumatic brain injury (TBI), spinal cord injury (SCI), cerebral vascular accident (CVA), burns, trauma, and total joint arthroplasty. This condition has been appreciated in patients with central nervous system pathology since 1918 and in trauma patients since 1883. The term neurogenic heterotopic ossification has been commonly utilized for HO in patients with TBI, SCI, and CVA.[1,2]

Heterotopic ossification is the formation of mature, lamellar bone in non-skeletal tissue, usually occurring in soft tissue surrounding joints. The bone formation in HO differs from other disorders of calcium deposition in that HO results in encapsulated bone between muscle planes, not intra-articular or connected to periosteum.[3]

The incidence rate reported in the literature varies from 11% to 75% in patients with severe TBI and SCI. Lower rates have been reported in CVA patients. In the TBI and SCI population, studies have shown a 33% rate of loss of motion in those diagnosed with HO and 10% to 16% progressing to complete joint ankylosis.[1,5]

HO is both more common and more extensive in patients with severe spasticity. Increased spasticity and lower level of limb function not only increases the risk of developing HO, but also increases the rate of recurrence after surgical resection.[2] When ectopic bone is discovered in paraplegic patients, it is never found above the level of injury. HO is rarely seen in flaccid limbs. Interestingly, HO has not been reported with cerebral palsy or in children with anoxic brain injury.[1]

The pathogenic mechanisms of HO are still being investigated. Whether genetic factors or local phenomena (tissue hypoxia, venous insufficiency, edema, etc.) are triggering factors responsible, the final common pathway is inflammation and increased blood flow in the tissues. Bone matrix is laid down by osteoblasts believed to be transformed from perivascular undifferentiated mesenchymal cells. Mineralization and true bone formation are usually completed by 6 to 18 months. The extent of bone formation has been described in Brooker's

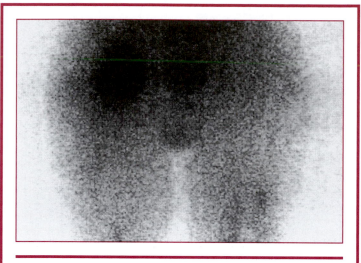

FIGURE 1. Radiograph of Brooker class IV HO of the right hip.

classification[1,4,6,7] for heterotopic ossification of the hip:

- Class I: Islands of bone with soft tissue
- Class II: Bone spurs from the pelvis or proximal femur, leaving at least 1 cm between bone surfaces
- Class III: Bone spurs from the pelvis or proximal femur, reducing the space between opposing surfaces to < 1 cm
- Class IV: Apparent bone ankylosis of the hip (Fig. 1)

It is important to note that only classes III and IV are generally clinically significant.

Symptoms

Several trends can be recognized in neurogenic HO. The most common symptom is pain (often absent in SCI). However, individuals demonstrate great variability in initial manifestation of symptomatology and degree of involvement. Symptoms range in their onset from 2 weeks, to 12 months after the inciting event and include warmth, redness, swelling, low-grade fever, pain, and tenderness.[1,4,8,9]

Physical Examination

Individuals vary in their time of onset, location, and degree of involvement of HO. Therefore, joints should be examined as frequently as possible to assess range of motion and assist in early diagnosis. The clinician should also inspect each joint for erythema and palpate the joints for point tenderness or masses. The most common physical finding is decreased range of motion of the joint.

It is important to note that distal joints of the hands and feet are almost never involved. Involvement of lower limb joints (hips and knees) is more common than that of upper limb joints (shoulder and elbow).[2]

In neurogenic HO secondary to TBI or SCI, the hip is the most common joint affected. Ossification usually occurs inferomedially to the joint and is usually associated with adductor spasticity. Several cases describe HO in other joints, including the elbow (variable ossification), the shoulder (internal rotator spasticity), and the knee (anteromedial involvement).

Functional Limitations

The loss of range of motion secondary to HO inhibits optimal rehabilitative efforts; interferes with hygiene, transfers, daily activities; and can ultimately cause catastrophic complications such as nerve entrapment, joint ankylosis, and even spinal cord compression.[9]

Diagnostic Studies

Three-phase bone scan is the current "gold standard" for early detection of HO. It is possible to discover increased metabolic activity as early as 2 to 4 weeks after injury. This procedure involves intravenous injection of 99mTc-labeled polyphosphate, which is known to accumulate in areas of active bone growth activity. The three phases are as follows (Fig. 2):[2,9]

Phase 1: Dynamic blood flow occurring immediately after injection

Phase 2: Immediate static scan detects areas of blood flow after injection

Phase 3: Static phase involving a repeat bone scan after several hours

A disadvantage of three-phase bone scanning is its lack of specificity and difficulty differentiating bone tumor, metastasis, or osteomyelitis from HO.

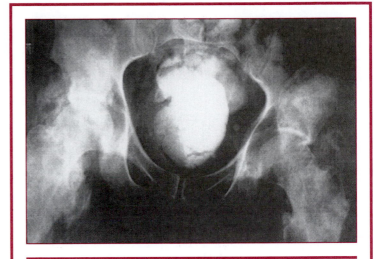

FIGURE 2. Three-phase bone scan showing increased activity at the right hip juxta-articular ossification site.

Radiographs are readily available and economical but may not show calcification for 7 to 10 days after clinical signs and symptoms have developed (see Fig. 1). HO has been described in three stages with variable time frames when examined radiologically:

1. Early: Increased activity on bone scan, no radiologic evidence
2. Intermediate: Radiographically appearing immature bone
3. Mature: Well developed, mature appearing bone

Both mature and immature bone can co-exist. It is not uncommon for mature ossification to radiographically obscure immature bone. Therefore, radiographically determining maturity of HO is often unreliable.[1,2]

CT scanning is rarely utilized in the early phases of HO. However, CT has proven especially helpful in preoperative planning for resection in order to establish relationships of bone to muscle and neurovascular bundles.[2]

A useful and widely used laboratory test for monitoring HO activities is the alkaline phosphatase (ALP) level. ALP has been shown to be elevated during the active bone formation of HO (normal range is 38 to 126 IU). ALP levels rise as early as 2 weeks post injury, reaching a peak around 10 weeks. Levels have been recorded up to 5000 IU and can remain elevated for months to years.[11] Some investigators have suggested using ALP not only as a screen for HO, but also a measure to begin empiric treatment. The specificity of ALP elevation is low. It is therefore recommended that three-phase bone scan be used to confirm suspected HO in cases of elevated ALP. (See Fig. 3.)[10]

Ultrasound and angiography are rarely utilized for HO diagnosis. Cases have been reported in which ultrasound has been used to help differentiate HO from primary bone tumor, hematoma, or abscess. Similarly, angiography has been used to differentiate traumatic myositis ossificans from tumor.[2]

Serum and urinary calcium, frequently a nonspecific response to trauma, does not provide any information regarding the ongoing ossification process and therefore is not used for HO diagnosis and monitoring. Also nonspecific and abandoned are analysis of urinary hydroxyproline and proteins from bone, connective tissue, and muscle.[2]

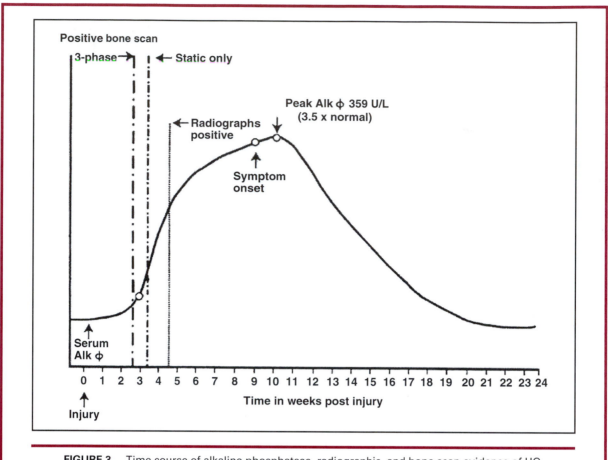

FIGURE 3. Time course of alkaline phosphatase, radiographic, and bone scan evidence of HO.

Differential Diagnosis

Deep vein thrombosis	Spasticity	Gout
Cellulitis/infection	Tumoral calcinosis	Pseudogout
Acute arthritis	Secondary hyperparathyroidism	Para-articular chondroma
Superficial thrombophlebitis	Hypervitaminosis D	Calcinosis circumscripta
Contracture		

Treatment

Initial

Nonsurgical strategies for treatment of HO include mobilization of the joint, medications to decrease inflammation or to decrease bone formation, and prophylactic low-dose radiation. Spasticity and patient pain can be barriers to providing proper range of motion. Both should be managed appropriately to ensure mobilization occurs. Non-steroidal anti-inflammatory medications (NSAIDs) can be used not only for patient comfort, but also to reduce bone formation by inhibiting prostaglandin synthetase. Studies have shown indomethacin and ibuprofen have been effective in total hip replacements for the prophylactic prevention of HO.[1,2,8,12,13]

Although failing to demonstrate promise in neurogenic HO, NSAIDs, such as indomethacin, have had success in preventing HO in the population with total joint arthroplasty. NSAIDs inhibit arachadonic acid metabolism, thereby inhibiting prostaglandin production, reducing inflammation, and slowing bone metabolism. Indomethacin, the most widely used, is started on postoperative day one with the usual prophylactic dose of 25 mg three times a day for 3 weeks and continued for up to 2 months.[1,2,6]

Etidronate disodium (EHDP), a bisphosphonate, is structurally similar to inorganic pyrophosphate and is shown to delay the aggregation of apatite crystals into large, calcified clusters in patients with TBI and SCI.[1,2,5] The recommended prophylactic treatment for HO in SCI is 20 mg/kg/day for 2 weeks, then 10mg/kg/day for 10 weeks. The current treatment recommendation for established HO is 300 mg IV daily for 3 days followed by 20 mg/kg/day for 6 months in spinal cord patients.[14] For TBI, it has been suggested to treat with 20 mg/kg/day for 3 months followed by 10 mg/kg/day for 3 months.[5]

Rehabilitation

Comprehensive physical and occupational therapy can be considered preventative, and a first line treatment modality. Several studies have shown that early range-of-motion exercises are beneficial in the prevention and treatment of HO. Controversy exists that joint manipulation may increase the inflammatory response, thereby increasing HO production. There has been no objective evidence to show this to be true.[1] Joint manipulation may not alter bone formation, but it can prevent soft tissue contractures and maintain functional range of motion. As physical therapy is often difficult secondary to pain or spasticity, forceful manipulation under anesthesia has been tried but is not a standard treatment modality. Range of motion is still considered the mainstay of HO prevention.[1,8]

Procedures

Radiation therapy has been shown to help prevent HO after total hip arthroplasty and after resection of mature HO. It is the only therapy for HO to date that acts locally. Studies report that doses of 1000 cGy in fractionated doses of 200 cGy/day for 5 days significantly lowered the incidence of HO after total hip arthroplasty[15]. Radiation therapy has also been used successfully following HO resection in neuromuscular disorders to help prevent recurrence.[1,6]

Surgery

Surgical resection of HO is considered only in refractory cases not satisfactorily relieved with conservative methods. Indications for surgery include joint immobility causing difficulty in patient positioning, hygiene, ambulation, or daily activities; ankylosed joints resulting in pressure sores or skin breakdown; and conditions in which HO contributes to peripheral neuropathy. Careful preoperative planning, often requiring 3D CT scanning, is needed to assess the relationship between HO and neurovascular structures at risk. Cautious dissection, good visibility, hemostasis, neurovasular bundle isolation, and adequate bone mass exposure all reduce risk of morbidity associated with hemorrhage, sepsis, or re-ankylosis. Normally, only a wedge resection of the amount of bone needed for functional range is required. Controversy exists as to the timing of the procedure as bone maturity is difficult to assess. It has been shown that immature HO has a greater incidence of recurrence. Three-phase bone scan and ALP levels are used to monitor bone maturity. It is not uncommon for surgery to be delayed for up to 2 years in TBI or SCI. Radiation therapy and NSAIDs are often used to prevent recurrence postoperatively.[1,2]

Potential Disease Complications

After the inflammatory response and HO deposition, loss of normal joint range of motion and secondary soft tissue contractures form and involve surrounding skin, muscles, ligaments, and neurovascular bundles. The resulting restrictive position predisposes the patient to the development of pressure sores and subsequent infections. Direct pressure or chronic spasticity can cause nerve ischemia and compression, resulting in peripheral neuropathy.[1] The loss of motion also encourages osteoporosis and subsequent pathologic fracture during patient transfer or lifting. Case reports also cite spinal cord compression and even osteosarcoma as complications of HO.[16,17]

Potential Treatment Complications

Analgesics, NSAIDs, and COX-2 inhibitors have well-known side effects that most commonly affect the gastric, hepatic, and renal systems. There is also the theoretical risk of defective bone-prosthesis union and poor bone healing in orthopedic populations while using NSAIDs for the purpose of HO prevention.[2,12]

Generally, EHDP is a safe method of prevention and treatment of HO, with only mild GI side effects of nausea and diarrhea occurring. It is not uncommon for the dosage to be split into two daily doses to alleviate these problems. EHDP carries with it the potential risk of bone fracture when used for prolonged periods, although this requires further study. A "rebound ossification" secondary to prolonged osteoclast inhibition upon withdrawal of EHDP has also been postulated.[5,12,14]

The use of radiation therapy does not disrupt wound healing, provided this area is not in the radiation field. Radiation therapy is rarely associated with malignancy. In orthopedic populations following total hip arthroplasty, there have been increased rates of trochanteric non-union with high-dose fractionated and single-dose protocols.[12,15]

Surgical complications, hemorrhage, sepsis, wound infection, re-ankylosis, and HO recurrence are not uncommon and carry high morbidity. The distorted anatomy in HO makes dissection visibility difficult, endangering neurovascular structures. Postoperative blood loss requiring transfusion is not uncommon despite good surgical hemostasis.[2,12]

References

1. Botte MJ, Keenan ME, Abrams RA, et al: Heterotopic ossification in neuromuscular disorders. Orthopedics 1997;20(4):335–341.
2. Buschbacher R: Heterotopic ossification: A review. Critical Reviews in PM&R 1992;4(3,4):199–213.
3. Venier L, Ditunno J: Heterotopic ossification in the paraplegic patient. Arch Phys Med Rehabil 1971;52:475.
4. Garland DE: Clinical observations on fractures and heterotopic ossification in the spinal cord and traumatic brain injured populations. Clin Orthop 1988;233:86–101.
5. Speilman G, Gennarelli TA, Ragers CR: Disodium etidronate: its role in preventing heterotopic ossification in severe head injury. Arch Phys Med Rehabil 1983;64: 539.
6. Puzas JE, Miller MD, Rosier RN: Pathologic bone formation. Clin Orthop 1989;245:269–281.
7. Brooker A: Ectopic ossification following total hip replacement, incidence and a method of classification. J Bone Joint Surg 1973;55A:1629.
8. Stover L, Hataway CG, Ziger HE: Heterotopic ossification in spinal cord injured patients. Arch Phys Med Rehabil 1975;56:199.
9. Johns JS, Cifu DX, Keyser-Marcus L, et al: Impact of clinically significant heterotopic ossification on functional outcome after traumatic brain injury. J Head Trauma Rehabil 1999;14(3): 269–276.
10. Garland DE: A clinical perspective on common forms of acquired heterotopic ossification. Clin Orthop 1991;13:263.
11. Furman R, Nicholas JJ, Jivoff L: Elevation of the serum alkaline phosphatase coincident with ectopic bone formation in paraplegic patients. J Bone Joint Surg 1970;52A:1131.
12. Ellerin B: Current therapy in the management of heterotopic ossification of the elbow. A review with case studies. Am J Phys Med Rehabil 1999;78:259–271.
13. Moore D: Indomethacin versus radiation therapy for prophylaxis against heterotopic ossification in acetabular fractures. A randomized, prospective study. J Bone Joint Surg 1998;80B:259.
14. Banovac K: The effect of etidronate on late development of heterotopic ossification after spinal cord injury. J Spinal Cord Med 2000;23(1):40–44.
15. Conventry MB, Scanlon PW: The use of radiation to discourage ectopic bone. A nine-year study in surgery about the hip. J Bone Joint Surg 1981;63A:201.
16. Aboulafia A: Osteosarcoma arising from HO after an electrical burn. J Bone Joint Surg 1999;81A:564.
17. Yamamoto Y: Spinal cord compression by HO associated with pseudohypoparathyroidism. J Int Res 1997;25:364–368.

112 Lymphedema

Atul T. Patel, MD

Definition

Lymphedema is the functional overload of the lymphatic system in which the lymphatic volume exceeds transport capabilities. This results in the accumulation of lymphatic fluid in the interstitial tissue that causes swelling, most often in the arms or legs and occasionally in other parts of the body. Primary lymphedema can be due to missing or hypoplastic lymphatic vessels or impaired lymph vessels. Most forms of primary lymphedema present after puberty (lymphedema praecox) with lower extremity swelling. The incidence is 1.15 per 100,000,[1] and it generally occurs in girls. Usually the leg is affected.

Secondary lymphedema or acquired lymphedema can develop as a result of damage to the lymphatic vessels and/or lymph nodes. Possible causes of acquired lymphedema are surgery, radiation treatment, infection, cancer, and trauma. Worldwide the most common cause of lymphedema is filariasis, whereas in the Western world treatment for breast cancer is the most common cause. Hence, in the United States women are primarily affected. The overall incidence of lymphedema after breast cancer treatment is 10% to 25%[2]; however, the rate is directly related to the extent of axillary surgery and radiation treatment. One study reported lymphedema in 19% of the patients who were treated with modified mastectomy and no radiation versus an incidence of 44% in those who underwent radical mastectomy and radiation treatment.[3]

Symptoms

The symtoms of lymphedema are the sensation of fullness in the affected limb or body part and the skin feeling tight, pain in the affected limb or body part, decreased flexibility/range of motion of affected joints, swelling, thickening of the skin (hyperkeratosis), and dry skin.

Physical Examination

In addition to a general physical examination, the history should guide one to an appropriate focused examination of the affected body area. This should include the assessment of the skin and lymph nodes and palpation for masses. The main feature is the observation of skin changes in the affected body part. The skin is usually thickened with signs of hyperkeratosis. Lymphedema can present at the following different stages of severity[4,5]:

Stage I (acute)—Pitting edema that is worse with a limb held in a dependent position or at the end of the day.

Stage II (chronic)—Non-pitting edema with a spongy consistency to the soft tissue. This marks fibrosis and the beginning of hardening of the limbs and increasing size.

Stage III (elephantiasis)—At this point, the swelling is also irreversible and usually the affected area is very large. The tissue is fibrotic and noncompliant to pressure.

Functional Limitations

Patients may have difficulty fitting into clothing in one specific area or have difficulty wearing items such as a wristwatch, bracelet, or ring if the involved limb is an upper extremity. Patients may also have functional limitations in activities of daily living (e.g., grooming, feeding, toileting, bathing, and dressing) if the upper limb is involved and mobility if the lower limb is involved.

Diagnostic Studies

The diagnosis of lymphedema is mainly clinical, based on history, physical examination, and exclusion of other possibilities. In cases of primary lymphedema and in cases with unclear causes of secondary lymphedema, further diagnostic testing may be necessary. In most cases of lymphedema postbreast cancer treatment, diagnostic testing is not necessary; however, diagnostic workup may be considered when other important co-morbidities need to be excluded, such as deep vein thrombosis or recurrent metastatic malignancy.

There is a lack of sensitive methods for investigation of lymphedema. Currently, lymphoscintigraphy (isotope lymphography) is considered the best for identifying edema of lymphatic origin. Radiolabelled colloid or protein is injected into the distal aspect of the limb and tracer uptake is monitored by a gamma camera. The path of the tracer can help in the evaluation of lymphatic function.[6] Lymphangiography is still the best method of assessing the anatomy of the lymphatics, but it offers little information about the lymphatic function. It also is technically difficult and can result in complications.[7]

Computed tomography (CT) and magnetic resonance imaging (MRI) detect a characteristic "honeycomb" pattern in the subcutaneous tissue not observed with other forms of edema. These tests assess the soft tissues and can help in differentiating fibrosis from metastasis.[8] Doppler ultrasound can also be of help in assessing for deep venous thrombosis.

Differential Diagnosis

Venous edema

Lipoedema or lipodystrophy

Treatment

Initial

Lymphedema is considered a long-term or lifelong condition, and the treatment is considered more as management of the condition rather than a cure. There is controversy regarding the optimal treatment program, and hence there are several approaches in use currently.

Initial treatment depends on the cause of lymphedema. This includes treatment complications of cancer, recurrence of cancer, deep venous thrombosis, cellulitis, and edema from other causes. If the patient has signs and symptoms of cellulitis, then this needs to be treated with antibiotics. Often treatment of the infection reduces some of the swelling and discoloration in the skin. Once the infection is under control or if infection has been ruled out, then treatment consists of edema management and will depend on the severity of the lymphedema. Management consists of manual lymphatic drainage; bandaging; proper skin care and diet; compression garments including sleeves, stockings, and devices that provide for the compression; training the patient to do self lymphatic drainage and bandaging; and exercise programs to improve patient fitness and function.

Medication use has limited value. Antibiotics are used if infection is suspected. Benzopyrones have been demonstrated to be of some help in reducing the inflammation and fibrosis and possibly in improving lymph flow.[9] Diuretics are not effective in lymphedema treatment.[10]

Patient education is crucial in the prevention of infections and further complications of lymphedema. This includes instruction on proper skin hygiene, avoidance of trauma to the affected area, use of appropriate techniques to maintain lymphedema control, and recognition of the signs and symptoms of infection. Proper diet and weight management are also important.

Rehabilitation

The goals of rehabilitation measures are to help drain away the lymph and reduce the swelling, to improve joint mobility and posture, and optimize function. The treatment program involves multiple modalities, an interdisciplinary approach, and often a protracted course of treatment. This needs to be communicated to the patient. Physical/occupational therapists or nurses trained in manual physiotherapeutic techniques usually perform the decongestive lymphatic treatment.

To monitor progress, the affected area, usually a limb, is measured. There are several methods, but the most common techniques involve multiple circumferential and volumetric measurement.[11]

The treatments consist of elevation of the affected limb, massage therapy, exercises, and external compression. There are no data on the efficacy of elevation in the treatment of lymphedema, and the mechanism of action is unclear. Hence, it can only be considered as an adjunct to therapy.

There are several different programs/methods that have been described as "complex physical therapy" (CPT), "complex lymphedema therapy" (CLT), "complex decongestive therapy" (CDT) or "decongestive lymphatic therapy" (DLT). These consist of a combination of manual lymph drainage, compression wrapping, compression pumping, and exercise. Massage treatment consists of facilitating normal lymphatic function in more proximal areas to allow for "decongestion" of affected areas. Compression is provided with bandage wraps or minimally elastic garments. These are usually applied after the massage treatment and are often used in the maintenance phase of therapy. These garments are available in both custom-made and prefabricated varieties. Customized garments may be needed for patients who are difficult to fit. Pressures ranging from 30 mm Hg to 60 mm Hg are used routinely. Pneumatic compression pumps are commonly used and consist of single- or multiple-chamber devices. There does not appear to be a great advantage over the compression garments other than a possible quicker response.[12]

Exercise is based on an initial evaluation of the patient and tailored accordingly. It consists of a combination of self-massage, flexibility, aerobic, and strengthening exercises. The exercise prescription for each patient will depend on age, lifestyle, level of physical fitness, and response to the exercise. The patients may need to be monitored initially to make sure that worsening edema does not develop. The goal, again, is to optimize function.

A critical review of the effectiveness of these treatments revealed that compression garments appear to reduce limb size after 6 months of use and that combinations of treatments including massage, pneumatic pump, and compression garments showed promising results.[13]

Procedures

Invasive procedures are not typically done in treating lymphedema.

Surgery

This is usually reserved for the few patients in whom rehabilitative measures have failed and the size of the limb interferes with mobility and function. Surgery consists of attempts to restore physiologic lymphatic function or excision of excess lymphedematous tissue. The former involves lymphatic-venous anastomoses or dermal flaps. Various degrees of success have been reported, and objective evaluations are scant.

Potential Disease Complications

Patients with lymphedema may experience dry skin, acute inflammatory episodes (infective and non-infective), fungal infections, hyperkeratosis, callosities, corns, chronic and acute pain, depression, decreased social interaction, and impaired sexual function.

Potential Treatment Complications

Possible complications are contact dermatitis from the use compression garments or compressive pump devices, entrapment neuropathies due to wrapping or the use of compressive garments, swelling elsewhere due to aggressive attempts at draining the lymph from the affected area, and risk of skin breakdown.

References
1. Smeltzer DM, Sticker GB, Schirger A: Primary lymphedema in children and adolescents: A follow-up study and review. Pediatrics 1985;76:206–217.
2. Petrek JA, Lerner R: Lymphedema. In Harris JR, Lippman ME, Morrow M, Osborne K (eds): Diseases of the Breast, 2nd ed. Philadelphia, Lippincott Williams & Wilkins, 2000, pp 103–140.
3. Schunemann H, Willich N: Lymphoedema of the arm after treatment of cancer of the breast. A study of 5868 cases. Detsch Med Wschr 1997;122:536–541.
4. Brennan MJ: Lymphedema following the surgical treatment of breast cancer: A review of pathophysiology and treatment. J Pain Symptom Manage 1992;7:110–116.
5. Davis S: Lymphedema following breast cancer treatment. Radiologic Technology 1998;70:42–56.
6. Case TC, Witte CL, Witte MH, et al: Magnetic resonance imaging in human lymphedema: Comparison with lymphangioscintigraphy. Magn Reson Imaging 1992;10:549–558.
7. Ter S, Alavi A, Kim CK, et al: Lymphoscintigraphy, a reliable test for the diagnosis of lymphedema. Clin Nucl Med 1993;18:646–654.
8. Dixon AK, Wheeler TK, Lomas DJ, et al: Computed tomography or magnetic resonance imaging for axillary symptoms following treatment of breast carcinoma? A randomized trial. Clin Radiol 1993;48:481–488.
9. Casley-Smith JR, Morgan RG, Pillar NB: Treatment of lymphedema of the arms and legs with 5,6-benzo[a]pyrene. N Engl J Med 1993;329:1158–1163.
10. Mortimer PS: Therapy approaches for lymphedema. Angiology 1997;48:87–91.
11. Gerber LH: A review of measures of lymphedema. Cancer 1998;83(Suppl):2803–2804.
12. Dini D, Del Mastro L, Gazzo A, et al: The role of pneumatic compression in the treatment of postmastectomy lymphedema. A randomized phase III study. Ann Oncol 1998;9:187–190.
13. Megens A, Harris SR: Physical therapist management of lymphedema following treatment for breast cancer: A critical review of its effectiveness. Phys Ther 1998;78:1302–1311.

113 Metabolic Bone Disease

Cynthia C. Su, MD

Definition

Metabolic bone disease[1] describes a large set of disorders that result in the formation of abnormal bone. Abnormal increased bone turnover is indicated by increased serum alkaline phosphatase (ALP) in most of the disorders. These disease processes may affect the absorption and utilization of calcium and vitamin D from the gut, the creation of bone matrix, the mineralization and hardening of the matrix, and the regulation of bone resorption and reformation. There may be associated pathology of other organ systems, including the kidneys, parathyroid gland, intestines, pancreas, skin, and blood.

Disorders of bone metabolism encompass three general subsets of defective bone formation: *osteomalacia*, *osteosclerosis*, and *osteoporosis*. Osteoporosis, which occurs diffusely with age, is the unbalanced remodeling of bone that results in decreased bone mass per volume. The osteoporotic bone is characteristically brittle and prone to fractures. In contrast, osteomalacia describes the production of soft, under-calcified bones that are prone to bowing and eventual fractures. The composition of osteomalacic bone has a decreased ratio of inorganic minerals to organic bone tissue. Rickets is a subtype of osteomalacia that affects growth plates in children. Paget's disease is an example of focal osteoporosis and osteosclerosis—the increase of bone mass with accelerated, disorganized remodeling. Osteoporosis is discussed in Chapter 122, but Paget's disease of bone and the various causes of osteomalacia are covered in this chapter.

Symptoms

Most persons with Paget's disease are asymptomatic, and the diagnosis is made incidentally by elevated serum alkaline phosphatase or on x-ray during the evaluation of other unrelated complaints. Paget's disease produces expanded, hypervascular changes in all or parts of one or more bones, usually the pelvis, femur, skull, vertebrae, and tibia. Patients may complain of focal or diffuse bone pain, arthritic pain, weakness of the hips and knees, and back pain.[2] Because pagetic bone is hypervascular and may stretch peripheral nerves and soft tissue, there may be an uncomfortable sensation of warmth over the tibia or femur. Paget's of the skull may be an uncomfortable sensation of warmth over the head. Paget's of the skull may present with complaints of disfigurement due to asymmetric bony bossing.

Skull involvement may also cause hearing loss due to auditory nerve entrapment or stretch, or from labyrinth hypertrophy.

Osteomalacia secondary to senile hypovitaminosis D may be asymptomatic until patients present with a femoral fracture after a fall. They may complain of pain without history of trauma. Associated muscle pain and weakness are common complaints. Rickets is often characterized by pain, thin bones, bowing of the long bones, poor dentition, and short stature. Primary hyperparathyroidism, characterized by hypercalcemia, causes muscle weakness, physical and mental fatigue, polyuria, and polydipsia. The increased serum calcium may result in kidney stone formation with the presenting symptoms of flank pain, hematuria, or dysuria. The rare hypercalcemic crisis produces signs and symptoms of severe dehydration, altered mental status, and cardiac arrhythmia. In renal osteodystrophy or osteomalacia due to renal tubular acidosis, patients' symptoms are associated with their primary kidney disease. Symptoms of decreased endurance and weakness are hard to distinguish from hypercalcemia or dialysis.

History may suggest the cause of the osteomalacia. Pertinent information includes history of dietary intake of calcium and vitamin D, history of gastrointestinal malabsorption syndromes (e.g., sprue, chronic diarrhea), bulimia or anorexia, renal insufficiency, cancer, or family history of hyperparathyroidism or osteomalacia. Because Paget's disease may be inherited or related to viral exposure, family history and exposure to measles should be noted.[3,4]

Physical Examination

Physical examination includes a musculoskeletal survey, with abnormal skull shape or long bone curvatures, scoliosis, areas of focal warmth or tenderness, strength, and range of motion noted. Hypertrophy of the costochondral junction (rachitic rosary), may be found on physical and x-ray examination. Osteomalacia and rickets produce a waddling gait because of proximal muscle weakness and hip pain. Hearing and cranial nerve testing and palpation of the distal pulses are indicated to exclude neurovascular entrapment by pagetic bone. Eye examination may reveal band keratopathy suggestive of prolonged hypercalcemia. Dental exam may reveal defects in enamel associated with rickets or bulimia. Alopecia and epidermoid cysts may be associated with vitamin D-dependent rickets type II. Examination of the neck and abdomen for masses should be performed to find subtle signs of nephrocalcinosis or parathyroid or other glandular enlargements.

Functional Limitations

Because of the skeletal malformations, abnormal body mechanics develop and the functional transfers and gait may be altered. For example, bowing of the tibia of one leg may result in leg-length discrepancy. To swing the longer leg forward during gait, the patient may compensate by leaning his or her torso to the contralateral side and raising the hip of the longer leg (hip hiking) or by swinging his or her leg out to the side first in an arc (circumduction). The compensated gait uses more energy and requires asymmetric body movements that result in overuse of the hip and back muscles. Tibial and femoral deformities also alter the angle of the knee, causing abnormal increased wear and osteoarthritis of the knee. Muscles shorten across acute joint angles and are overly stretched across obtuse angles. Muscles have a range of optimal length for strength, and deviations from that length cause the muscles to be weaker and less able to maintain joint stability and therefore are more prone to injury.

Pain may also limit strength and movement. Pain may be the result of metabolic bone disease, strain of muscles compensating for abnormal body mechanics, or osteoarthritis. Pain causes changes in body mechanics because of guarding. Patients may limit their activity and find a significant reduction in activities of daily living.

Diagnostic Studies

Paget's disease and the various types of osteomalacia are diagnosed by laboratory studies and radiologic imaging, correlated with pertinent history and physical examination. Serum ALP is often found to be elevated incidentally during routine testing. Because ALP can be high in liver disease, finding an elevated serum bone-specific ALP confirms the bony source. Basic metabolic panel, calcium, and phosphorus levels also should be checked to assess the function of electrolyte homeostasis and to differentiate between the different causes of metabolic bone disease.

Paget's disease is characterized by increased serum ALP and urine hydroxyproline. These values may be monitored to assess the effectiveness of treatment. The degree of ALP elevation may suggest the extent of disease. Higher values suggest more sites, and skull involvement usually produces the highest values. Total body bone scans are sensitive to areas of increased bone turnover but are non-specific. Plain radiographs of the involved pelvis and skull will show disorganized focal areas of increased bone density and porosity (Fig. 1). The plain x-ray of the involved bone also demonstrates typical cortical expansion and coarsening of trabeculae. A radiograph of a bowed long bone, such as the tibia, will reveal increased bone density and possibly microfractures of the convex surfaces. Bone biopsies generally are not necessary, but serve to confirm the diagnosis. The areas noted to be involved on clinical presentation usually do not increase over time. Worsening of pain or development of new sites may warrant biopsy to rule out metastatic bone disease or sarcomatous transformation.

Evaluation of osteomalacia also involves checking the levels of calcium, phosphorus, magnesium, parathyroid hormone (PTH), and vitamin D (1,25-[OH]$_2$-D3 and 25-[OH]-D3). *Primary hyperparathyroidism is characterized by elevated calcium and parathyroid hormone and low phosphorus levels.* Rickets causes low calcium and high ALP and PTH, but the level of vitamin D distinguishes the different types. Renal tubular acidosis and chronic renal failure cause secondary hyperparathyroidism characterized by renal calcium and phosphate wasting (increased urine concentration of calcium and phosphorus) and altered vitamin D metabolism. Oncogenic osteomalacia causes low serum phosphorus, high urine phosphorus, variable serum calcium, and low vitamin D levels.[5] The presence of progressive weight loss and anemia in a patient with a pathologic fracture and risk factors for cancer should prompt a thorough search for a primary

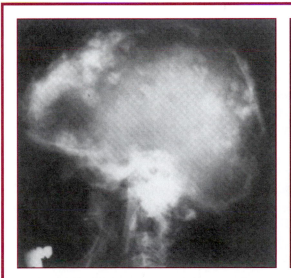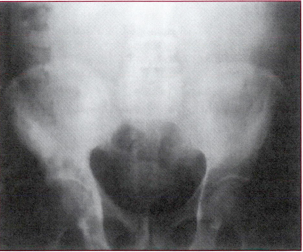

FIGURE 1. Skull radiograph showing a thickened cranium with regions of dense sclerosis and osteopenia resulting in a "cotton-wool" appearance. Pelvic radiograph showing right hemipelvic loss of normal trabeculation, sclerosis, and cortical thickening, along with sclerosis of the iliopectineal line. (From West SG: Rheumatology Secrets. Philadelphia, Hanley & Belfus, 1997, with permission.)

tumor by physical examination and appropriate radiologic imaging (CT, MRI, mammogram) and the ruling out of bone metastasis.[6]

Osteomalacia is hard to distinguish from osteoporosis in plain film, but the findings of bilateral symmetric pseudofractures in adults (Fig. 2) and laboratory data diagnosing the cause of osteomalacia are sufficient evidence. Plain film findings of osteitis fibrosa cystica in hyperparathyroidism include subperiosteal lucency of the distal phalanges, cysts of the long bones, and tapering of the distal clavicles. The skull film has a characteristic "salt and pepper" appearance.

Iliac bone biopsy with tetracycline labeling distinguishes between osteoporosis and osteomalacia when there is insufficient clinical, laboratory, and radiologic evidence to make a clear diagnosis. Biopsy of pathologic fractures may reveal cancer as a cause.

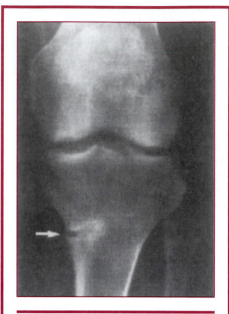

FIGURE 2. Pseudofractures (*arrows*) in osteomalacia involving the knee. (From West SG: Rheumatology Secrets. Philadelphia, Hanley & Belfus, 1997, with permission.)

Differential Diagnosis

Polymyalgia rheumatica	Bone metastasis
Rheumatoid arthritis	Osteoarthritis
Myositis	Ankylosing spondylitis
Myopathy	Gout
Osteosarcoma	Pseudogout
Benign giant cell tumor	Other metabolic bone diseases
Osteoporosis	

Treatment

Initial

In Paget's disease, the goal of pharmacologic treatment is to slow progression of the disease, reduce pain, and reduce the risk of fractures and neurovascular complications. The asymptomatic patient with involvement of bone carrying low risk of complications (sacrum, iliac crest, ribs, or scapula) may not need pharmacologic therapy. However, medications are indicated for bone pain, arthritis, neurologic complications, and prior to orthopedic surgery. Medication is also indicated for asymptomatic patients with involvement of the spine, skull base, femur, and tibia.[7] Anti-resorptive options include bisphosphonates and calcitonin. Bisphosphonates are the therapy of choice to decrease osteoclastic activity by binding to bone and inhibiting mineral resorption and to decrease osteoclastic recruitment and survival. Six-month oral treatment with etidronate (400 mg/day) or alendronate (40 mg/day) may be tried. Calcitonin is less effective in reducing bone resorption, but improves pain. Available formulations include salmon calcitonin 50 to 100 IU, intramuscularly or subcutaneously, or intranasal calcitonin, 200 to 400 IU.[6] Nonsteroidal anti-inflammatory drugs and acetaminophen may also be used in conjunction with anti-resorptive therapy.

The underlying cause of osteomalacia should be treated (Table 1). Neck exploration and parathyroidectomy are curative in primary hyperparathyroidism. Medical management of non-surgical candidates includes a moderate calcium diet and avoidance of thiazide diuretics. Follow-up serum values should be evaluated twice yearly.

Tumor-induced osteomalacia may respond to treatment of the cancer. Life-threatening hypercalcemia should be treated with intravenous hydration, loop diuretics, and intravenous pamidronate.

Avoidance of gluten in celiac sprue and counseling for anorexia and bulimia improve osteomalacia. Supplementation of vitamin D and phosphorus is indicated in deficiencies. Limiting phosphorus intake or the use of phosphorus binding agents may help in renal osteodystrophy. Stopping medications, such as phenytoin, rifampin, aluminum, or bisphosphonates, is also indicated.

Rehabilitation

The goals of rehabilitation are pain management, strengthening, improved balance, and maintenance and improvement of gait and functional transfers.

TABLE 1. Differential Causes and Treatment of Osteomalacia

Cause	Defect	Treatment

Nutritional
  Dietary restriction
  Anorexia/bulimia
  Gastrectomy
  Total parenteral nutrition
	Decreased intake of calcium, phosphorus,
	  vitamin D
		Supplement

Decreased absorption
  Celiac sprue
	Gluten sensitivity causes intestinal changes
	  and affects absorption
		Avoid gluten

1,25(OH)$_2$D deficiency	Vitamin deficiency or defect in conversion to active form	Supplement vitamin D
Cholestyramine	Binds vitamin D in the gut	Stop drug
Aluminum antacid	Binds phosphorus	Stop drug
Liver disease	Interferes with vitamin D to 25(OH)D conversion	Supplement 25(OH)D

Phenytoin, phenobarbital,
  rifampin, alcohol
	Interferes with vitamin D to 25(OH)D conversion
	  by competing for cytochrome P$_{450}$
		Stop drug and supplement
		  Supplement 25(OH) D and
		  stop drug

Skin
  Increased melanin
  Decreased sun exposure
	Decreased production of vitamin D$_3$	Supplement vitamin D$_3$ or
		  hydroxylated vitamin D
		  forms

Vitamin D-dependent
  rickets, type I
	Autosomal recessive lack of renal 25-vitamin D
	  1αhydroxylase to convert 25(OH)D to 1,25(OH)$_2$D
		Supplement 1,25(OH)$_2$D

Vitamin D-dependent
  rickets, type II
	Defect in 1,25(OH)$_2$D receptor, causing decreased bone
	  mineralization and decreased calcium absorption
		Supplement 1,25(OH)$_2$D
		  and calcium 3 g/day

Hypophosphatemic
  vitamin D-resistant rickets
	Proximal renal phosphate wasting	Phosphorus 0.6 g qid
		  High dose vitamin D

Tumor induced	Renal phosphate wasting
	Decreased kidney production of 1,25(OH)$_2$D
		Resect tumor
		  Supplement 1,25(OH)$_2$D
		  and phosphorus

Fanconi's syndrome Renal tubular acidosis II Cadmium, lead, mercury	Renal phosphate wasting Decreased kidney production of 1,25(OH)$_2$D	Supplement 1,25(OH)$_2$D and phosphorus
Renal tubular acidosis I	Renal calcium wasting	Bicarbonate, calcium
Aluminum, fluoride, bisphosphonates	Interferes with bone mineralization	Stop drugs

Hypophosphatasia	Rare genetic defect in tissue non-specific alkaline
	  phosphatase resulting in accumulation of
	  phosphorus/phosphocompounds that interfere
	  with mineralization
		Do *not* supplement
		  Symptomatic treatment;
		  dentures, intramedullary
		  rodding for fractures

Physical and occupational therapists can instruct and monitor the patient during exercises and give feedback about the patient's progress and any new developing symptoms, such as pain or dyspnea, to the physician, who may alter therapies or perform further medical evaluations. The nutritionist provides instruction on diets that optimize bone formation, caloric management, and protein intake. The orthotist provides bracing and adaptive equipment. Vigilant supervision by the rehabilitation team is necessary because of the fragility of osteomalacic bone.

Modalities in pain management include the use of cold packs to reduce inflammation. Transcutaneous nerve stimulation and electrical bone stimulator may also be effective in providing analgesia. *Ultrasound is relatively contraindicated because of the possibility of occult fractures.* Active stretching and progressive resistive exercise as tolerated maintain and improve strength and help joint stability. Weight bearing promotes bone formation, but excessive weight bearing may worsen long bone bowing or cause fractures. Balance exercises reduce the risk of falls and subsequent fractures. Persons with moderate-to-severe kyphoscoliosis associated with rickets may receive instruction in pulmonary rehabilitation and endurance training during respiratory therapy, PT, or OT, separately or in co-treatment. Bracing of the spine or extremities and the use of a cane, walker, or reacher can be suggested by the team and provided by the orthotist or therapists.

Excessive weight bearing and aggressive passive range of motion should be avoided to prevent fractures. Cardiac precautions may be warranted if there is a history of arrhythmia, cardiomyopathy, or hypertension associated with hyperparathyroidism. Endurance may be limited because of associated disease processes, as in renal osteodystrophy and renal failure.

Procedures

Procedures are generally not indicated for metabolic bone disease.

Surgery

Total joint replacement may become necessary in Paget's disease complicated by osteoarthritis. Osteotomy of the femur or tibia may be needed to correct severe bowing in rickets and Paget's disease. Intramedullary rodding stabilizes pathologic long bone fractures. Parathyroidectomy is curative in most cases of primary hyperparathyroidism. Tumor resection may improve the bone disease of cancer. Peripheral nerve decompression may be warranted in Paget's disease.

Potential Disease Complications

Possible complications include, pain, gout, pseudogout, osteoarthritis, fracture, hematoma (Paget's), and myopathy. Other complications include entrapment neuropathy (hearing loss, facial drop, foot drop), vascular compromise, congestive heart failure, cardiac arrhythmia, nephrolithiasis, nephrocalcinosis, heterotopic calcification of soft tissue, and digitalis sensitivity.

Potential Treatment Complications

Bisphosphonates may result in gastritis or peptic ulcer, osteomalacia, and flu-like symptoms (pamidronate). Calcitonin can produce nausea and flushing. Phosphate binding agents can cause aluminum toxicity, hypercalcemia, and heterotopic soft tissue ossification. Nephrolithiasis is a side effect of phosphorus supplementation. Orthopedic procedures can result in excessive blood loss (Paget's), peri-prosthetic fracture, non-union, or prosthetic loosening secondary to increased bone resorption.[9] Overly aggressive physical or occupational therapy can result in fractures.

References

1. Favus MJ (ed): Primer on the Metabolic Bone Diseases and Disorders of Mineral Metabolism, 3rd ed. Philadelphia, Lippincott-Raven, 1996.
2. Reginato AJ, Falasca GF, Pappu R, et al: Musculoskeletal manifestations of osteomalacia: Report of 26 cases and literature review. Semin Arthritis Rheum 1999;28:287–304.
3. Hocking L, Slee F, Haslam SI, et al: Familial Paget's disease of bone: Patterns of inheritance and frequency of linkage to chromosome 18q. Bone 2000;26:577–580.
4. Kurihara N, Reddy SV, Menaa C, et al: Osteoclasts expressing the measles virus nucleocapsid gene display a pagetic phenotype. J Clin Invest 2000;105:607–614.
5. Huang QL, Feig DS, Blackstein ME: Development of tertiary hyperparathyroidism after phosphate supplementation in oncogenic osteomalacia. J Endocrinol Invest 2000;23:263–267.
6. Sundaram M, McCarthy EF: Oncogenic osteomalacia. Skeletal Radiol 2000;29:117–124.
7. Delmas PD, Meunier PJ: The management of Paget's disease of bone. N Engl J Med 1997;336:558–566.
8. Roux C, Dougados M: Treatment of patients with Paget's disease of bone. Drugs 1999;58:823–830.
9. Lewallen DG: Hip arthroplasty in patients with Paget's disease. Clin Orthop 1999;369:243–250.

114 Motor Neuron Disease

Lisa S. Krivickas, MD

Synonyms

Amyotrophic lateral sclerosis (ALS or Lou Gehrig's disease)

Progressive muscular atrophy (PMA)

Progressive lateral sclerosis (PLS)

Progressive bulbar palsy (PBP)

Adult spinal muscular atrophy (SMA)

Spinobulbar muscular atrophy (Kennedy's disease)

ICD-9 Codes

335.1   Spinal muscular atrophy

335.10   Spinal muscular atrophy, unspecified

335.11   Kugelberg-Welander disease
  Spinal muscular atrophy familial juvenile

335.19   Other
  Adult spinal muscular atrophy

335.2   Motor neuron disease

335.20   Amyotrophic lateral sclerosis
  Motor neuron disease (bulbar) (mixed type)

335.21   Progressive muscular atrophy
  Duchenne-Aran muscular atrophy
  Progressive muscular atrophy (pure)

335.22   Progressive bulbar palsy

335.23   Pseudobulbar palsy

335.24   Primary lateral sclerosis

335.29 Other

Definition

The term *motor neuron disease (MND)* refers to a progressive neuromuscular disorder in which upper and/or lower motor neurons degenerate. The most common form of MND is amyotrophic lateral sclerosis (ALS), which is the primary focus of this chapter. Management principles for other forms of MND are similar. To meet diagnostic criteria for ALS, an individual must have both upper and lower motor neuron dysfunction. If only lower motor neuron dysfunction is present, the disease is called *progressive muscular atrophy (PMA);* if only upper motor neuron dysfunction is present, it is called *progressive lateral sclerosis (PLS)*. If only bulbar dysfunction is present, the disease is called *progressive bulbar palsy (PBP)*. Most patients initially diagnosed as having PMA, PLS, or PBP eventually develop full-blown ALS. Those whose condition does not convert to ALS have a slower rate of disease progression.

Most cases of ALS are idiopathic. However, 5% to 10% of patients have a familial form transmitted in an autosomal dominant fashion. In approximately 15% of these familial cases, mutations in superoxide dismutase (SOD1) can be identified. Other rare forms of inherited adult MND are Kennedy's disease (x-linked recessive) and adult spinal muscular atrophy (SMA) (autosomal recessive), which both present with only lower motor neuron dysfunction.

ALS rapidly produces skeletal muscle weakness, eventually leading to the requirement for ventilatory support or death from respiratory failure. The onset of weakness may be in any limb, the bulbar muscles, or the respiratory muscles. The extraocular muscles and bowel and bladder function are generally spared. Mean survival without tracheostomy is 3 years from symptom onset, but the range may be from less than 1 year to more than 20 years. The mean age of onset is in the mid 50s, but adults of any age may develop ALS. The cause of the disease is unknown, but leading theories concerning pathogenesis implicate glutamate excitotoxicity and oxidative stress.

Symptoms

Patients with upper motor neuron (UMN) dysfunction may present with spasticity, loss of dexterity, stiffness, weakness due to spasticity, and loss of voluntary motor control.

Patients with lower motor neuron (LMN) dysfunction may present with weakness, fasciculations, muscle atrophy, and muscle cramps. Patients with bulbar dysfunction may present with dysarthria, dysphagia, sialorrhea (drooling), aspiration, and pseudobulbar affect (laughter or crying disconcordant with mood).

Respiratory failure and constitutional symptoms (e.g., weight loss, generalized fatigue) may also be present.

Physical Examination

The physical examination of a patient with suspected or diagnosed MND should emphasize the neurologic, musculoskeletal, and cardiorespiratory systems. On neurologic examination, the clinician looks for evidence of upper and lower motor neuron dysfunction. The mental status, non-motor cranial nerve function, sensory examination, and cerebellar examinations should be normal. The "gold standard" used to diagnose upper motor neuron pathology is the presence of pathologic reflexes—the Babinski sign, Hoffmann sign, and brisk jaw jerk. Evidence of lower motor neuron pathology includes muscle weakness, atrophy, hypotonia, hyporeflexia, and fasciculations. Atrophy often appears first in the hand intrinsic muscles. Although fasciculations are not a necessary criterion for the diagnosis of ALS, the clinician should question the diagnosis when none are observed. The tongue should be examined for fasciculations and atrophy, and tongue strength and range of motion should be assessed. The musculoskeletal exam should focus on assessing range of motion and evaluating painful joints or soft tissue structures. Because patients develop progressive respiratory failure, the cardiorespiratory system should be assessed at each visit. Forced vital capacity (FVC) can be measured with a handheld spirometer in the office setting.

Functional Limitations

The majority of functional limitations that develop in patients with ALS are the direct or indirect result of muscle weakness. As the disease progresses, patients develop impaired mobility and difficulties with performing even the most basic activities of daily living, such as feeding themselves. Bulbar muscle weakness produces dysarthria and dysphagia; eventually, some patients become anarthric and unable to swallow even their own saliva. Reactive depression, generalized fatigue, and musculoskeletal pain may further limit function.

Diagnostic Studies

The diagnosis of ALS is based on appropriate physical examination and electrodiagnostic findings and the use of neuroimaging and clinical laboratory studies to exclude other conditions that may mimic ALS. *All patients should undergo electrodiagnostic testing.* The revised El Escorial Criteria are currently used to diagnose ALS.[1] They classify the certainty level of the diagnosis as falling into one of five categories: definite, probable, probable with laboratory support, possible, and suspected. The motor system is divided into 4 regions: bulbar, cervical, thoracic, and lumbosacral. Clinical evidence of UMN and LMN pathology is sought in each region. The certainty level of diagnosis depends on how many regions reveal UMN and/or LMN pathology. Electrophysiologic findings can be used both to confirm LMN dysfunction in clinically affected regions and to detect LMN dysfunction in clinically uninvolved regions.

Imaging studies are used to exclude possibilities other than MND from the differential diagnosis. Magnetic resonance imaging (MRI) is the primary imaging modality used in evaluation of patients with suspected ALS. Almost all patients should have an MRI of the cervical spine to exclude cord compression, a syrinx, or other spinal cord pathology. The location of symptoms will dictate whether other regions of the spinal cord should be imaged. In those presenting with bulbar symptoms, a brain MRI should be performed to exclude stroke, tumor, syringobulbia, etc.

TABLE 1. Suggested Laboratory Studies

Hematology
  Complete blood count
  Erythrocyte sedimentation rate
Chemistry
  Electrolytes, BUN, creatinine
  Glucose
  Hemoglobin A_{1C}
  Calcium
  Phosphorous
  Magnesium
  Creatine kinase
  Liver function tests
  Serum lead level
  Urine heavy metal screen
  B_{12}
  Folate
Endocrine
  T_4, TSH
Immunology
  Serum immunoelectrophoresis
  Urine assay for Bence Jones proteins
  Antinuclear antibody (ANA)
  Rheumatoid factor
  GM1 antibody panel
Microbiology
  Lyme titre
  VDRL
Optional
  HIV test—if risk factors present
  Anti-Hu antibody—if suspicion of malignancy

From Carter GT, Krivickas LS: Adult motor neuron disease. In Kirshblum S, Campagnolo D, DeLisa JA (eds): Spinal Cord Injury Medicine. Philadelphia, Lippincott, Williams & Wilkins, 2001.

In most neuromuscular clinics, a routine panel of laboratory tests is administered to all patients suspected of having ALS. A suggested set of such tests is provided in Table 1. The rationale behind performing this extensive battery of tests is to assess the general health of the patient and exclude treatable conditions. The differential diagnosis, developed after the history and physical exam, may suggest that more specialized testing be performed. Table 2 lists additional tests that may be warranted when the presentation is with the PMA, PLS, or PBP phenotype. When there is a family history of MND, SOD1 testing may be considered.

Differential Diagnosis

The differential diagnosis differs depending on whether the presentation is primarily LMN, UMN, bulbar or mixed LMN and UMN.

LMN Only

Polio/Post-polio syndrome

Benign monomelic amyotrophy

Hexosaminidase A deficiency

Polyradiculopathy

Multifocal motor neuropathy with conduction block

Chronic inflammatory demyelinating polyneuropathy

Motor neuropathy or neuronopathy

Lambert-Eaton syndrome

Plexopathy

Benign fasciculations

UMN Only

Multiple sclerosis   Familial spastic paraparesis
Adrenoleukodystrophy   Myelopathy
Subacute combined systems degeneration   Syringomyelia

Bulbar

Myasthenia gravis   Stroke
Multiple sclerosis   Syringobulbia
Foramen magnum tumor   Head and neck cancer
Brainstem glioma   Polymyositis

UMN and LMN

Cervical myelopathy with radiculopathy   Spinal cord tumor or arteriovenous malformation
Syringomyelia   Lyme disease

TABLE 2. Specialized Laboratory Testing

Phenotype	Test	Diagnosis Excluded
PMA	DNA test—CAG repeat on X chromosome	Kennedy's disease
	DNA test—SMN gene mutation	SMA
	Hexosaminidase A	Hexosaminidase A deficiency (heterozygous Tay-Sachs disease)
	Voltage gated Ca++ channel antibody test	Lambert-Eaton myasthenic syndrome
	CSF examination	Polyradiculopathy—infectious or neoplastic
PLS	Very long chain fatty acids	Adrenoleukodystrophy
	HTLV-1 antibodies	HTLV-1 myelopathy (tropical spastic paraparesis)
	Parathyroid hormone	Hyperparathyroid myelopathy
	CSF examination	Multiple sclerosis
PBP	Acetylcholine receptor antibodies	Myasthenia gravis
	DNA test—CAG repeat on X chromosome	Kennedy's disease
	CSF examination	Multiple sclerosis

From Carter GT, Krivickas LS: Adult motor neuron disease. In Kirshblum S, Campagnolo D, DeLisa JA (eds): Spinal Cord Injury Medicine. Philadelphia, Lippincott, Williams & Wilkins, 2001.

Treatment

Initial

Although there is not a cure for ALS, significant research advances are being made in an attempt to identify drugs that will slow disease progression. Offering patients pharmacologic treatment for their disease has psychologic benefits that may outweigh the actual slowing of disease progression that currently can be achieved. Riluzole (Rilutek) is the only drug approved by the FDA specifically for treatment of ALS. However, many neuromuscular experts recommend that their patients also take a combination of antioxidant vitamins and creatine.

Riluzole was approved by the FDA for treatment of ALS in 1995 after the completion of two clinical trials that showed that the drug slowed disease progression.[2,3] Median survival benefit was 60 days. Unfortunately, no functional benefit was derived, as strength declined at a similar rate in those taking riluzole and placebo. The recommended dose of riluzole is 50 mg bid. The most common adverse side effects are fatigue, nausea, and elevation of hepatic enzymes. Riluzole is contraindicated in those with hepatic enzymes greater than 5 times the upper limit of normal.

Because oxidative stress is one of the proposed pathogenic factors in ALS, many clinicians recommend a variety of antioxidants; vitamin E, vitamin C, and coenzyme Q10 are the most frequently used. Two recent studies have generated interest in using creatine to improve strength and slow disease progression in patients with ALS.[4,5] No double-blind, placebo-controlled trials have proven the efficacy of these treatments. Safe recommended daily dose ranges are 1000 to 3000 mg vitamin C, 400 to 800 IU vitamin E, 60 to 240 mg coenzyme Q10, and 3–5 g creatine. Creatine is contraindicated in those with renal disease.

Recent ALS clinical trials have tested a number of growth factors, glutamate antagonists, calcium channel blockers, and amino acids. Trials of neurotrophic factors, antioxidants, glutamate antagonists, and creatine are ongoing. A cocktail approach to slowing disease progression may be the ideal treatment strategy.

A number of drugs are useful for treating symptoms such as spasticity, pain, sialorrhea, pseudobulbar affect, depression, and anxiety, as described in the following:

Spasticity

Spasticity requires treatment only if it interferes with function. Non-pharmacologic management involves teaching patients stretching exercises and positioning techniques that decrease muscle tone. Baclofen (Lioresal) is the most effective pharmacologic agent, followed by tizanidine (Zanaflex). Diazepam (Valium) should be avoided because it may suppress respiration, and dantrolene (Dantrium) is not recommended because it causes excessive muscle weakness. In general, pharmacologic management of spasticity is less successful in ALS than in multiple sclerosis or spinal cord injury because the lower motor neuron component of ALS makes patients extremely susceptible to the development of excessive weakness. (See Chapter 136.)

Sialorrhea

Patients with bulbar dysfunction experience sialorrhea because they have difficulty with swallowing and managing the oral secretions that they normally produce. A variety of anticholinergic drugs may be used to dry the mouth. Tricyclic antidepressants (TCAs) are often tried first but may not be tolerated because of adverse side effects (e.g., dry mouth, somnolence, urinary retention). One benefit of the TCAs is that they may treat other ALS-related symptoms such as pseudobulbar affect, insomnia, and pain. TCAs are contraindicated in patients with cardiac arrhythmia or conduction disorder. When TCAs are not tolerated, a scopalamine patch (Transderm-Scōp) or glycopyrrolate (Robinul) may be helpful.

Pseudobulbar Affect

Pseudobulbar affect, also sometimes called "emotional incontinence," refers to the patient's inability to accurately portray emotions he or she is experiencing. Patients laugh or cry when they are experiencing sadness or happiness, respectively. They also may have an exaggerated response to situationally appropriate feelings. Amitriptyline (Elavil), a combination of dextromethorphan (Robitussin, Organidin NR, Humibid) and quinidine, or fluvoxamine (Luvox) may help blunt the intensity of these inappropriate or exaggerated reactions.

Anxiety/Depression

Reactive depression and anxiety are both normal responses to a diagnosis of ALS.[6] Patients and their families may benefit from individual counseling and participation in ALS support groups. Anxiety may be treated with benzodiazepines as long as the patient does not have significant reduction of vital capacity. Undetected hypoventilation may produce or contribute to pre-existing feelings of anxiety. Depression should be treated pharmacologically because not treating it may have a significant negative impact on the quality of life remaining. Selective serotonin reuptake inhibitors are good first choices because of their minimal side effects. However, the TCAs may be preferred if they are also needed to treat other symptoms, such as sialorrhea or pseudobulbar affect.

Pain

Acetaminophen; nonsteroidal anti-inflammatory drugs; and, if necessary, opioids should be used to alleviate musculoskeletal pain. The major concerns with opiate use are respiratory depression and constipation. The respiratory depression may be acceptable in the late stages of the disease; in fact, morphine is a good way to relieve air hunger in the terminal stage.

Rehabilitation

Skeletal muscle weakness is the primary impairment in ALS and causes the majority of the clinical problems. In the early stages of ALS, patients often inquire about the role of exercise in preventing or forestalling the development of weakness. Later in the disease, rehabilitation strategies must be used to maintain function and compensate for muscle weakness.

Three forms of exercise training are relevant to patients with ALS: *flexibility*, *strengthening*, and *aerobic* exercise. Flexibility training helps prevent the development of painful contractures and non-pharmacologically decreases spasticity and painful muscle spasms. Traditionally, clinicians have been reluctant to recommend strengthening exercises because they fear that overuse weakness will occur, accelerating disability. This philosophy promotes the development of disuse weakness and muscle deconditioning, which may compound the weakness produced by ALS itself. The literature supporting the development of overwork weakness in neuromuscular patients is anecdotal, and overuse weakness has not been demonstrated in any controlled prospective studies.

Studies of patients with more slowly progressive neuromuscular diseases suggest that a moderate resistance strengthening program can strengthen muscles that are only mildly affected by the disease process.[7,8] High-resistance eccentric exercise should be avoided because it may produce muscle damage. Motivated ALS patients can begin or continue with a strengthening program to maximize the strength of unaffected or mildly affected muscles in an attempt to delay impaired function. Weight training should be performed with a weight that the individual can comfortably lift 20 times. If an exercise regimen consistently produces muscle soreness or fatigue lasting longer than 30 minutes after exercise, it is too strenuous. Aerobic exercise helps maintain cardiorespiratory fitness. Given the lack of any apparent contraindication, aerobic exercise training is recommended for patients with ALS as long as it can be performed safely without a risk of falling or injury. In addition to the physical benefits, strengthening and aerobic exercise may have a beneficial effect on mood, psychologic well-being, appetite, and sleep.

As ALS progresses, the rehabilitation focus shifts from exercise to maintaining independent mobility and function for as long as possible. Interventions include the use of assistive devices such as canes, walkers, braces, hand splints, wheelchairs, and scooters; home equipment such as dressing aids, adapted utensils, grab bars, raised toilet seats, shower benches, and lifts; home modifications such as ramps and wide doorways; and automobile adaptations such as hand controls. A multidisciplinary team that includes physiatrists, physical therapists, occupational therapists, and orthotists best provides these rehabilitation interventions.

Patients commonly develop musculoskeletal pain syndromes such as adhesive capsulitis, low back pain, and neck pain due to muscle weakness and inability to change positions. Measures to prevent adhesive capsulitis include range-of-motion exercises and supporting the arm as much as possible rather than allowing it to dangle at the side. Low back pain can be triggered by an uncomfortable seating system. Preventive measures include a lumbar support for the wheelchair, a good cushion on a solid seat, encouraging frequent weight shifts, and a reclining-back or tilt-in-space wheelchair. Neck pain associated with head drop is one of the most difficult musculoskeletal pain issues to remedy. A variety of cervical collars may be tried. A head support on the wheelchair or a reclining lounge chair may be more comfortable than a collar.

Adequate swallowing function is necessary to maintain the nutritional status of the patient with ALS (unless he or she has a feeding tube). If nutritional status is not properly maintained, patients tend to use muscle as fuel and thus lose muscle mass and strength earlier than they otherwise would. Swallowing dysfunction may also precipitate aspiration pneumonia and/or respiratory failure. Early signs and symptoms of dysphagia are drooling, a wet voice, coughing during or after drinking thin liquids, nasal regurgitation, and requiring an excessive amount of time to complete meals. Patients should be referred to a speech therapist when the first signs of dysphagia develop. Those with mild swallowing difficulties can be taught compensatory techniques to reduce the risk of aspiration and choking.[9] Recommendations may be given concerning modification of food consistencies. The development of aspiration pneumonia, loss of more than 10% of body weight, or requiring an excessive amount of time to eat such that quality of life is impaired are all indications for feeding tube placement.

Early or mild dysarthria may be managed by having a speech therapist teach patients adaptive strategies such as overarticulation and slowing speaking rate. In patients with hypernasal speech caused by palatal weakness and primarily lower motor neuron dysfunction, a palatal lift and/or augmentation prosthesis often improve speech clarity.[10] As dysarthria worsens, patients will require alternative forms of communication. Writing is a good alternative while hand function is intact. For those unable to write, low-technology interventions include the use of letter or word boards. Higher-technology solutions are augmentative communication devices that may have a voice synthesizer. As long as a patient has one muscle somewhere in the body that he or she can voluntarily activate (including the extraocular muscles), he or she should be able to operate a communication device. High-technology solutions to communication problems are not suitable for all patients. Systems must be flexible so that the method of access can be modified as weakness progresses.

Respiratory failure is the primary cause of death in ALS. In the absence of underlying intrinsic pulmonary disease, the respiratory failure in ALS is purely mechanical. Because of muscle weakness, the lungs do not inflate fully on inspiration. Most patients with ALS remain asymptomatic until the FVC is less than 50% of predicted. Pulmonary function tests, particularly FVC, should be monitored every few months, depending on rate of disease progression. The earliest symptoms of respiratory failure are caused by nocturnal hypoventilation and include poor sleep with frequent awakening, nightmares, early morning headaches, and excessive daytime fatigue and sleepiness. Another early sign of respiratory muscle weakness is a weak cough and difficulty with clearing secretions.

The management of respiratory failure in ALS involves preventing infection when possible and providing mechanical ventilatory assistance. All patients with ALS should receive a pneumococcal vaccination and a yearly influenza vaccination. If the expiratory muscles are too weak to generate an adequate cough, patients can be helped by either manually assisted coughing or the In-Exsufflator (J.H. Emerson Co., Cambridge, Mass).[11] Providing patients with supplemental oxygen can relieve symptoms of air hunger and dyspnea but also may suppress respiratory drive, exacerbate alveolar hypoventilation, and ultimately lead to CO_2 narcosis and respiratory arrest.[12] Supplemental oxygen is recommended only for patients with concomitant pulmonary disease or as a comfort measure for those who decline assisted ventilation. Discussion concerning the possibility of respiratory failure should be initiated soon after the diagnosis of ALS so that patients and their families can learn about their choices and, ideally, make a decision about ventilator use in a non-crisis situation. Non-invasive respiratory muscle aids are not a permanent solution to respiratory failure but do provide many patients with additional time to make a decision concerning tracheostomy. Ultimately, fewer than 5% of ALS patients choose long-term ventilatory support via tracheostomy.[13]

Non-invasive positive-pressure ventilation (NIPPV) can be delivered through a variety of oral or nasal masks and interfaces using bilevel positive airway pressure (BiPAP) machines or portable volume-cycled ventilators. BiPAP is the most commonly used form of NIPPV. Recent studies suggest that use of NIPPV may prolong survival and slow the decline of FVC.[14,15] NIPPV is introduced when the FVC falls to 50% of predicted, or earlier if the patient is symptomatic. Initially, NIPPV is used only at night. As FVC continues to decline, ventilator use extends into the day for varying periods and eventually becomes continuous.

Procedures

Gastrostomy tube: A percutaneous endoscopic gastrostomy (PEG) tube is recommended when a feeding tube is needed. The timing of PEG tube placement is critical. The morbidity and mortality of the procedure increase when the FVC is less than 50% of predicted.[17] Studies have suggested longer survival in patients who choose PEG tube placement when compared with patients who refuse PEG.[18,19]

Surgery

Management of sialorrhea: Transtympanic neurectomy, salivary duct ligation, and parotid gland irradiation have been used to decrease saliva production but are associated with high failure and complication rates.[16]

Tracheostomy: This is best performed on a planned basis when patients choose long-term ventilatory support. However, it is more commonly performed in a crisis situation. A cuffless tracheostomy tube or a tube with a deflated cuff is preferred.

Potential Disease Complications

Potential disease complications include progressive weakness, joint contractures, musculoskeletal pain syndromes, dysphagia, aspiration, dysarthria, progressive respiratory failure, depression, and death.

Potential Treatment Complications

Treatment complications include drug reactions (e.g., to riluzole, TCAs) and PEG tube malfunction or infection. Complications of long term ventilation via tracheostomy may include tracheomalacia, loss of extraocular movements, totally locked-in state, and dementia.

References
1. World Federation of Neurology Research Group on Motor Neuron Diseases: El Escorial revisited: Revised criteria for the diagnosis of amyotrophic lateral sclerosis. 1998.
2. Bensimon G, Lacomblez L, Meininger V, Group ARS: A controlled trial of riluzole in amyotrophic lateral sclerosis. N Engl J Med 1994;330:585–591.
3. Lacomblez L, Bensimon G, Leigh PN, et al: Dose-ranging study of riluzole in amyotrophic lateral sclerosis. Lancet 1996;347:1425–1431.
4. Klivenyi P, Ferrante RJ, Matthews RT, et al: Neuroprotective effects of creatine in a transgenic animal model of amyotrophic lateral sclerosis. Nature Med 1999; 5:347–350.
5. Tarnopolsky M, Martin J: Creatine monohydrate increases strength in patients with neuromuscular disease. Neurology 1999;52:854–857.
6. Ganzini L, Johnston WS, Hoffman WF: Correlates of suffering in amyotrophic lateral sclerosis. Neurology 1999;52:1434–1440.
7. Lindeman E, Leffers P, Spaans F, et al: Strength training in patients with myotonic dystrophy and hereditary motor and sensory neuropathy: A randomized clinical trial. Arch Phys Med Rehabil 1995;76:612–620.
8. Aitkens SG, McCrory MA, Kilmer DD, Bernauer EM: Moderate resistance exercise program: Its effect in slowly progressive neuromuscular disease. Arch Phys Med Rehabil 1993;74:711–715.
9. Strand EA, Miller RM, Yorkston KM, Hillel AD: Management of oral-pharyngeal dysphagia symptoms in amyotrophic lateral sclerosis. Dysphagia 1996;11:129–139.
10. Esposito S, Mitsumoto H, Shanks M: Use of palatal lift and palatal augmentation prostheses to improve dysarthria in patients with amyotrophic lateral sclerosis: a case series. J Prosthetic Dentistry 2000;83:90–98.
11. Bach J: Respiratory muscle aids for the prevention of morbidity and mortality. Semin Neurology 1995;15:72–83.
12. Gay P, Edmonds L: Severe hypercapnia after low flow oxygen therapy in patients with neuromuscular disease and diaphragmatic dysfunction. Mayo Clinic Proceedings 1995;70:327–330.
13. Moss A, Casey P, Stocking C, et al: Home ventilation for amyotrophic lateral sclerosis patients: Outcomes, costs, and patient, family, and physician attitudes. Neurology 1993;43:438–443.
14. Kleopa KA, Sherman M, Neal B, et al: Bipap improves survival and rate of pulmonary function decline in patients with ALS. J Neurolog Sci 1999;164:82–88.
15. Aboussouan LS, Khan SU, Meeker DP, et al: Effect of noninvasive positive pressure ventilation on survival in amyotrophic lateral sclerosis. Ann Intern Med 1997;127:450–453.
16. Yorkston KM, Miller RM, Strand EA: Management of speech and swallowing in degenerative diseases. Tucson, Communication Skill Builders, 1995, p 253.
17. Miller R, Rosenberg J, Gelinas D, et al: Practice parameter: the care of the patient with amyotrophic lateral sclerosis (an evidence based review). Neurology 1999;52:1311–1323.
18. Mathus-Vliegen L, Louwerse L, Merkus M, et al: Percutaneous endoscopic gastrostomy in patients with amyotrophic lateral sclerosis and impaired pulmonary function. Gastrointest Endosc 1994;40:463–469.
19. Mazzini L, Corra T, Zaccala M, et al: Percutaneous endoscopic gastrostomy and enteral nutrition in amyotrophic lateral sclerosis. J Neurol 1995;242:695–698.

115 Movement Disorders

Kenneth H. Silver, MD

Synonyms

Extrapyramidal disease

Hypokinesias

Hyperkinesias

Dyskinesias

ICD-9 Codes

307.2   Tics

307.20   Tic disorder, unspecified

307.22   Chronic motor tic disorder

307.23   Gilles de la Tourette's disorder

332   Parkinson's disease

332.0   Parkinsonism or Parkinson's disease: primary, idiopathic

332.1   Secondary Parkinsonism
   Parkinsonism due to drugs

333.0   Other degenerative diseases of the basal ganglia
   Progressive supranuclear ophthalmoplegia
   Shy-Drager syndrome

333.1   Essential and other specified forms of tremor

333.2   Myoclonus

333.4   Huntington's chorea

333.5   Other choreas

333.6   Idiopathic torsion dystonia

333.84   Organic writers' cramp

781.0   Abnormal involuntary movements: abnormal head movements, spasms, fasciculation, tremor

Definition

Involuntary movement disorders can usually be classified as those characterized by either too little (hypokinetic) or too much movement (hyperkinetic). Hypokinetic problems include Parkinson's disease (PD), progressive supranuclear palsy, olivopontocerebellar degeneration, multisystem atrophy (Shy-Drager syndrome), and nigral-striatal degeneration. Hyperkinetic disorders include Parkinsonian and non-Parkinsonian tremor, tics, Gilles de la Tourette's syndrome, dystonia, dyskinesias (including tardive dyskinesias), hemifacial spasm, athetosis, chorea (including Huntington's disease), hemiballismus, myoclonus, and asterixis.

Symptoms

Parkinsonian patients commonly show a resting tremor; slowness of movement or bradykinesia; and a form of increased muscular tone, called *rigidity* (see Chapter 123 for more details). Other common features include a reduction in movements of facial expression resulting in "masked facies," stooped posture, and reduction of the amplitude of movements (hypometria). Also seen are changes in speech to a soft monotone (hypophonia) and small, less legible handwriting (micrographia). Walking becomes slower, stride length is reduced, and pivoting is replaced with a series of small steps (turning "en bloc"). The following syndromes typically present with the listed features in addition to the characteristic symptoms of Parkinson's disease (tremor and rigidity):

1. Shy-Drager's syndrome: autonomic failure with prominent postural hypotension.
2. Progressive supranuclear palsy (PSP): reduction in vertical gaze and slowing of eye movements.
3. Vascular parkinsonism: early dementia with brisk tendon reflexes.
4. Multiple head trauma-"Parkinsonism pugilistica": early dementia with brisk tendon reflexes.
5. Olivopontocerebellar degeneration (OPCA): prominent intention tremor and ataxia.[1]

Tremors, the most common form of involuntary movement disorders, are characterized by rhythmic oscillations of a body part. Tremors can be classified as to the situation in which they are most prominent. First, is the tremor most pronounced at rest or with movement? Tremors with movement are subdivided into those occurring: (1) with maintained posture (postural or static tremor, tested by holding arms out in front of them); (2) with movement from point to point (kinetic or intentional tremor, tested by performing finger-to-nose); or (3) only with a specific type of movement (task-specific tremor). *Tremors that are at their worst at rest are exclusively associated with Parkinson's disease or other parkinsonian states* (such as those produced by neuroleptics).[2,3]

Tics are sustained non-rhythmic muscle contractions that are rapid and stereotyped, often occurring in the same extremity or body part during times of stress. Usually the muscles of the face and neck are involved, with movement of a rotational sort away from the body's midline. They are commonly familial and often seen in otherwise normal children between ages of 5 and 10 and usually disappear by the end of adolescence. Tourette's syndrome is characterized by motor and vocal tics lasting for more than 1 year and may involve involuntary use of obscenities and obscene gestures, although such behavior may be mild and transient and occurs only in a minority of afflicted persons.

Dystonias are slow, sustained contractions of muscles that frequently cause twisting movements or abnormal postures. The disorder resembles athetosis but shows a more sustained static contraction. When rapid movements are involved they are usually repetitive and continuous. Dystonia often increases with emotional or physical stress, anxiety, pain, or fatigue and disappears with sleep. The dystonias are further classified as focal, segmental, or multifocal, based on the distribution of muscles affected. Symptoms of hemifacial spasm usually begin in the orbicularis oculi and later involve other muscles innervated by cranial nerve VII.[4]

Tardive dyskinesia is a condition characterized by involuntary, choreiform movements of the face and tongue associated with chronic neuroleptic medication use. Common movements include chewing, sucking, mouthing, licking, "fly-catching movements," puckering, or smacking (buccal-lingual-masticatory syndrome). Choreiform movements of the trunk and extremities can also occur along with dystonic movements of the neck and trunk.

Athetosis is characterized by involuntary, slow, writhing, and repetitious movements. They are slower than choreiform movements and less sustained than dystonia. Athetosis may be seen alone or in combination with other movement disorders and itself leads to bizarre but characteristic postures. Any part of the body can be affected, but it is usually the face and distal upper extremities that are involved. Chorea presents as nonstereotyped, unpredictable, and jerky movements that interfere with purposeful motion. The movements are rapid, erratic, and complex and can be seen in any or all body parts but usually involve the oral structures, causing abnormal speech and respiratory patterns. Hemiballismus is an uncommon disorder consisting of extremely violent flinging of the arms and legs on one side of the body.

Myoclonus is one of the most common involuntary movement disorders of central nervous system origin. It is characterized by sudden, jerky, irregular contractions of a muscle or groups of muscles. It can be subdivided into myoclonus that is stimulus sensitive (reflex myoclonus)—appearing with volitional movement, muscle stretch, or superficial stimuli such as touch—or non-stimulus sensitive myoclonus, which occurs at rest (spontaneous myoclonus). Myoclonic movements can be either irregular or periodic.

Physical Examination

A complete general history and physical are key to ruling out treatable causes of the presenting movement disorder, such as infectious (encephalitis), medication side effect (such as in tardive dyskinesia), genetic (Tourette's syndrome), or endocrinologic (tremor-associated thyrotoxicosis).

A good neurologic examination of patients suspected of having a movement disorder helps to identify an underlying causative condition such as stroke(s) (e.g., cerebrovascular-based Parkinson's disease, hemiballismus, or ataxia), tumor, brain trauma, or even peripheral nerve injury–associated focal dystonias. Other aspects of physical examination focus on characterizing the type of abnormal movements by detailing their body distribution (limb, trunk, head, face or widespread), their quality (tremor, writhing, explosive, rigidity), their frequency (rapid and repetitive or slow and sustained), and their general quantity or lack thereof (hyperactive or hypoactive).

Functional Limitations

Functional limitations depend on the severity of the movement disorder. Some tremors and tics may be more a cosmetic and psychologic concern, whereas severe postural disturbance in PD, or stroke-induced ataxia can clearly impair standing and ambulating in the former and upper extremity use in the later. In PD, postural changes, such as stooping, with the development of permanent kyphosis can occur after years of disease. Depression and social isolation are commonly seen in Parkinson's patients. Many physical activities require additional effort to perform. This leads to declining efficiency at work and, in many cases, abandoning many forms of leisure activities. Manual dexterity is invariably impaired as Parkinson's worsens, affecting many daily activities such as dressing, cutting food, writing, and handling small objects such as coins.[5]

In cervical dystonia (torticollis) social stigmatization is a major concern, as well as functional impairments, which can include driving, reading, or activities that involve looking down and using the hands. In another focal dystonia, writer's or occupational cramp, the symptoms present in a certain posture or position; for instance, a patient may be able to write at a blackboard but not seated at a desk. With lingual involvement in oromandibular dystonia, the tongue has abnormal movements during speaking or deglutition. The result of such dystonias is impairment of speech and eating. In Huntington's chorea, along with the choreiform movement, progressive dementia and emotional/behavioral abnormalities are seen. As the disease progresses, the presentation becomes less choreiform and more parkinsonian and dystonic (i.e., restricted motions, immobility, and unsteadiness of gait). Intellectual impairment and psychosis invariably occur and progress rapidly to become the most disabling features.[6]

Diagnostic Studies

In most cases of movement disorders, such as Parkinson's, tardive dyskinesia, essential tremor, and dystonia, the diagnosis is made on the grounds of clinical examination and history, with no one specific test pathognomonic for the disease. However, underlying causes of many of the movement disorders, such as stroke, traumatic brain injury, tumor, infection, and metabolic/endocrinologic disease, should be worked up with appropriate tests including head and spinal magnetic resonance imaging/computed tomography (MRI/CT) and cerebrospinal and blood serum analysis. Electrodiagnostic tests (EMG and nerve conduction studies) may be useful in some case, such as focal dystonias, to rule out co-existing or causative peripheral nerve entrapment. Electroencephalography (EEG) is often helpful to distinguish focal seizures from myoclonus or other repetitive movement presentations. Further tests may be necessary to confirm or exclude other diagnoses, such as human immunodeficiency virus (HIV) related diseases, central nervous system infection, toxic exposures, or psychiatric illnesses.

Differential Diagnosis

Seizures

Psychiatric illness

Spasticity/spasms

Treatment

Initial

Treatment is highly dependent on which specific category of movement disorder is present. Typically, pharmacologic treatment is initiated when the symptoms become severe enough to cause discomfort or disability.

L-Dopa given in combination with carbidopa-levodopa (Sinemet) is the most effective medication for the relief of Parkinson's disease, but is usually not the first medication given to a newly diagnosed patient. Patients will develop loss of L-Dopa efficacy usually within 3 to 5 years after beginning the medication, so that an effort is made to manage early PD with other medications. A guiding principle is to start L-Dopa treatment in patients with symptoms that interfere with the performance of daily life functions despite of other treatment. Anticholinergic drugs such as trihexyphenidyl (Artane) are widely used to treat early PD patients, with tremor as their primary symptom. Amantadine (Symmetrel) is another useful medication in early Parkinson's disease. Although its usefulness in early PD is controversial, the monoamine oxidase inhibitor deprenyl or selegiline (Eldepryl) is widely given to newly diagnosed patients. Within 1 to 2 years most patients will have sufficient enough difficulties with movement and daily activities to require L-dopa. Gradually over the years the patient's frequency of dosing will increase and the total dose needed will increase, along with the need for other supplemental medications. The two most useful are bromocriptine (Parlodel) and pergolide (Permax).[1]

Propranolol is the most useful medication in treating essential tremor (the most common symptomatic tremor), task-specific tremor, and action tremor. Other beta-blockers have fewer side effects but are less effective. The anti-convulsant primidone and the benzodiazepine clonazepam are also effective antitremor drugs.[3] Tics can be managed with neuroleptics; pimozide and haloperidol are generally effective but sedation limits their use. Other medications shown to be of use include benzodiazepines, clonazepam, clonidine, reserpine, and calcium channel blockers. Anticholinergic medications, such as trihexyphenidyl and benztropine, are the most effective oral agents for both generalized and focal dystonias. Baclofen, carbamazepine, and clonazepam are sometimes helpful. Focal dystonias are now commonly treated with botulinum toxin injections.[7] (See Procedures section.) The atypical neuroleptics clozapine and risperidone are useful to control psychosis in tardive dyskinesia patients without worsening symptoms. Benzodiazepines, such as clonazepam, are the most useful medications for suppression of the movements. Dopamine depletion with reserpine can improve symptoms but is commonly associated with hypotension and depression. The response to drug therapy has been poor in patients with ataxia, with many agents touted as useful (propranolol, isoniazid, carbamazepine, clonazepam, tryptophan, buspirone, thyroid stimulating hormone [TSH]) but none with demonstrated efficacy. A number of drugs have been used to treat myoclonus and can be effective in some situations. These include diazepam, clonazepam, and valproate. Tryptophan was once considered useful but is no longer prescribed because of an uncommon, severe side effect—the eosinophilia-myalgia syndrome.[8]

Rehabilitation

In general, the Parkinson patient needs to be counseled to maintain a reasonable level of activity at all costs as physical exertion becomes more difficult and the risk of deconditioning increases. Exercises focus on proper body alignment (upright posture) and postural reflexes (response to dynamic balance challenges), as well as limb range of motion and strengthening of proximal musculature to assist in stairclimbing and coming to stand. Exercises are also aimed at restoring diminished reciprocal limb motions and increasing step length. The tendency to freeze can be reduced with visual targets, such as markers on the floor, counting, or marching rhythmically. The difficulty in arising from sitting surfaces can be addressed with elevated sitting surfaces (chair, toilet) and strategically placed grab rails/bars (bed, bathtub). Although wheeled walkers are useful in assisting ambulation, particularly by preventing backwards instability, patients with significant postural deficits may prefer more stable devices , such as a supermarket shopping cart or walking behind a wheelchair. Adaptive equipment is provided when deficits in upper extremity control limit efficient and safe function.[9]

In tremor, measures to reduce or alleviate anxiety (e.g., biofeedback, relaxation exercises) are useful, as are strategies to control oscillation excursion with weights or other mechanical compensations.[10] Lifestyle changes may include restricting caffeine intake or other stimulants that may temporarily augment symptoms. In addition, alcohol consumption may lead to transient improvement for many with essential tremor.

Stretching exercises may be important for maintaining or recovering range of motion for affected joints in a dystonic limb. Certain types of occupational-based focal limb dystonias (e.g., writer's or musician's cramp) may be treated with muscle reeducation techniques, including biofeedback. A regular program of stretching exercises may assist affected individuals in regaining full range of motion after a botulinum toxin injection has weakened a dystonic muscle. Some patients use so-called "sensory tricks" to temporarily relieve their symptoms. These commonly involve touching or stroking a particular spot on the skin. In addition, in some patients, certain types of braces may provide the same stimulation and be equally effective.[4]

Ataxic patients may benefit from rehabilitation to help learn compensatory techniques for performing basic self-care and occupational activities, and for assessing the benefits of weighted bracelets or similar devices to damp the oscillations. Gait training and education in the use of assistive devices for walking can prevent falls and enhance mobility in the ataxic individual. In disorders involving athetosis, ballismus, or Huntington's disease, careful weighting of the extremities can help at times. Rehabilitation techniques involving improving co-activation and trunk stability, rhythmical stabilization, and traditional relaxation techniques including biofeedback have been mentioned as reasonable strategies. Some have suggested value in oral desensitization when hyper-reactivity to sensory stimuli exists for reducing excessive facial movements in tardive dyskinesia, but other rehabilitation strategies are not of proven utility.

Procedures

Botulinum toxin injections are beneficial in numerous hyperkinetic movement disorders including focal dystonias and tremor. Trigger point injections may provide relief in painful muscles associated with focal dystonias (e.g., cervical torticollis).

The muscles selected for botulinum toxin injection are based on understanding the primary clinical patterns of spasticity or dystonia.

Direct injection via palpation technique may be appropriate for superficial muscles, while EMG or electrical stimulation guidance is commonly used to identify deeper muscles. Each muscle is injected in one or more sites, the number being a function of the size of the muscle. Dosage is variable, but typically does not exceed 400 units total body dose for a three-month period. Botulinum toxin A is reconstituted in the vial with perservative-free normal saline, at varying dilutions depending on the muscle size: very small muscles needing 20 units per 0.1 ml, average size muscle 10 units per 0.1 ml, and large muscles 5 units or less per 0.1 ml.

The skin is cleansed with an alcohol swab and allowed to dry. When utilizing EMG or E-stim guidance, a specialized needle with an exposed tip connected by wire to the recording or stimulating device is needed. Needles are typically 37 mm in length and 27 gauge; larger or smaller needles are often needed depending on muscle size and depth. In adults, pre-anesthesizing the skin is usually unnecessary; in children, local anesthetic creams are helpful. When injecting botulinum toxin, aspirating the syringe to prevent injection into a blood vessel is standard technique. Prior to the injection, informed consent is obtained.

Surgery

Deep brain stimulation, thalamotomy, and pallidotomy have been used with success in some patients with Parkinson's disease as well as other movement disorders (e.g. dystonia and tremor).

Additionally, peripheral destructive procedures such as myectomy, rhizotomy, and peripheral nerve denervation are occasionally performed on individuals with dystonic limbs who have proven refractory to more conventional management.

Potential Disease Complications

Many of the movement disorders, particularly Parkinson's disease, are progressive and can result in the following: muscle weakness and immobility, severe limb contractures, aspiration of food and respiratory compromise, social isolation and depression, and intellectual impairment and dementia.

Potential Treatment Complications

Anti-Parkinson medications may have numerous side effects including nausea and other gastrointestinal symptoms, drowsiness, confusion, hallucinations, or psychosis. Similar adverse medication effects are described with other agents used to suppress unwanted movements. Botulinum toxin is generally well tolerated, but can cause transient unwanted weakness in target or adjacent muscles, including dysphagia. Risks associated with surgical approaches to central nervous system structures are considerable and need to be properly weighed prior to selecting these options.

References
1. Weiner W, Lang A: Movement Disorders. New York, Futura, !989.
2. Elbe R, Koller W: Tremor. Baltimore, Johns Hopkins Press, 1990.
3. Hallett M: Classification and treatment of tremor. JAMA 1991;266:1115.
4. Pentland B: Parkinsonism and dystonia. In Greenwood R, Barnes M, McMillan T, Ward C (eds): Neurological Rehabilitation. London, Churchhill Livingstone, 1993.
5. Duvaisin R: Parkinson's Disease: A Guide for Patients and Families. New York, Raven Press, 1991.
6. Ranen N, Peyser C, Folstein S: A Physician's Guide to the Management of Huntington's Disease. New York, Huntington's Disease Society of America, 1993.
7. Jankovic J, Hallett M: Therapy with Botulinum Toxin. New York, Marcel Dekker, 1994.
8. Johnson R, Griffen J (eds): Current Therapy in Neurologic Disease. St. Louis, Mosby, 1993.
9. Turnbull G (ed): Physical Therapy Management of Parkinson's Disease. New York, Churchill-Livingstone, 1992.
10. Scott S: Movement disorders, including tremors. In DeLisa JA (ed): Rehabilitation Medicine, Principles and Practice. Philadelphia, J.B. Lippincott, 1988, p 463–475.
11. WE MOVE website. Available at www.wemove.org/mov. (accessed 2000).

116 Multiple Sclerosis

Bertram Greenspun, DO

Definition

Multiple sclerosis (MS) is defined clinically as a disorder characterized by *distinct episodes of neurologic deficits, separated in time, and attributable to white matter lesions that are separated in space* (Table 1).[1]

Approximately 400,000 people in the United States have been diagnosed with MS. Symptoms usually begin during young adulthood, with a peak onset at age 24. Women are affected almost twice as often as men. Caucasians are affected at twice the rate of African-Americans.[2]

Clinical types of MS are as follows[3]:

1. Relapsing-remitting MS with periods of neurologic impairment interspersed with periods of stability; present in 80% of patients.[4]

2. Primarily-progressive MS with a relentless progression of neurologic involvement.

3. Secondary-progressive MS with the worsening of neurologic involvement occurring later in the course of the disease.

4. Progressive-relapsing MS, which is progressive from the outset with clear acute relapses; continuing progression is seen during the periods between relapses.

Irreversible disability occurs sooner in patients whose course is progressive from the start than in those with the relapsing-remitting type.[5]

In general, females have a better prognosis than males; usually the younger the individual is early in the disease, the better the prognosis. The onset with sensory symptoms as opposed to motor symptoms is better

TABLE 1. Diagnostic Criteria for Multiple Sclerosis (MS)

Possible MS
1. History of relapsing and remitting without prior documentation
2. Only one site of involvement in CNS by physical examination, laboratory, or imaging studies
3. No other diagnostic explanation

Probable MS
1. Two documented attacks with clinical, laboratory, or imaging evidence of at least one lesion
2. One documented attack with clinical, laboratory, or imaging evidence of two separate lesions

Definite MS
Two attacks separated by at least one month with clinical, laboratory, or imaging evidence of at least two lesions

From Braddom RL (ed): Physical Medicine and Rehabilitation. Philadelphia, WB Saunders, 1996, p 1104.

prognostically, and the relapsing course is better than the progressive course. A low relapsing rate in the first few years is better than a high relapsing rate in the first few years.

With the use of MRI, immunohistochemistry and microscopy, MS has been shown to be a disease with inflammatory myelin destruction and axonal pathology.[6]

Symptoms

Patients with MS may manifest multiple symptoms (Table 2). Visual loss due to optic neuritis may be the initial presentation. Scotomata is both a symptom and a sign and is characterized by an isolated area of varying size and shape in the visual field in which vision is absent or depressed. Dyschromatopsia (imperfect color vision) will often be persistent. Taking a careful history regarding any past visual changes is important.

TABLE 2. Symptoms of Multiple Sclerosis	
Anosmia	Malaise
Balance problems*	Numbness*
Bladder abnormalities	Nystagmus
Bowel dysfunction	Oscillopsia
Cognitive disturbances	Pain
Deafness	Paresthesias
Depression	Seizures
Diploplia*	Sexual dysfunction
Dizziness	Sleep problems
Dysarthria	Spasticity
Dysesthesias	Speech dysfunction
Dysphagia	Tinnitus
Euphoria	Visual loss*
Fatigue*	Weakness*
Incoordination	Weight loss
Intention tremor	

* Frequent, early, and common symptoms.

MS is often the cause of a rapidly progressive paraparesis, a sensory level in the trunk, sphincter disturbances, and bilateral toe extensor signs.

It is also important to assess for signs of depression that may be associated with MS, particularly as it progresses. Speech and swallowing problems should be noted. Swallowing problems occur when cranial nerves VII, IX, X, or XII are involved. Urinary tract infection (UTI) is common at some time with MS and may be associated with urinary frequency, incontinence, and burning. Fever may also be present.

Patients with MS are often intolerant to heat, and symptoms may be exacerbated in hot weather or warm environments.

Physical Examination[2,4,5,9,10]

Findings may involve the optic nerves, brainstem, cerebellum, and spinal cord.

A complete neurologic examination is essential, including a careful ophthalmologic examination. Ophthalmologic findings may include abducting nystagmus that is irregular in amplitude and rhythm, which is suggestive of involvement of the medial longitudinal fasciculus. Loss of smooth pursuit may be a subtle finding and can best be observed if one utilizes a slow rate of pursuit. Optic neuritis may result in a scotomata involving the macula and blind spots. A negative scotomata is a scotomata that is not ordinarily perceived but is detected only on examination of the visual field. As expected, a positive scotomata is a scotomata that is perceived as a black spot within the field of vision. A variety of field defects may occur, and there may be edema of the optic nerve head. Demyelination in the course of the third nerve through the brainstem may result in permanent enlargement of the pupil.

Sensory testing may reveal dissociated pin and temperature findings during an acute relapse; vibratory and proprioceptive abnormalities may be subtle but persistent findings, and they may be localized.

Patients may also experience slurred speech. The most prominent speech problems involve difficulty in controlling the loudness and harshness of speech. Defective articulation is commonly present as well.

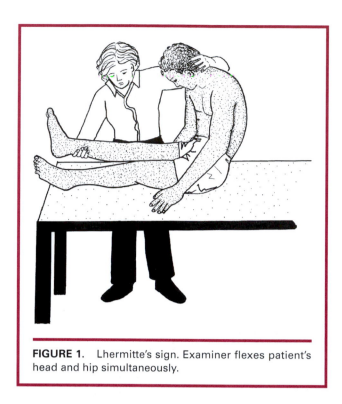

FIGURE 1. Lhermitte's sign. Examiner flexes patient's head and hip simultaneously.

Deep tendon reflexes may be asymmetric and should be tested in more than one position to ascertain whether they are consistent; absent or decreased reflexes can be important segmental signs. Hyperactive reflexes are common early in the course of the disease, whereas an absent reflex is unusual. Asymmetry in the plantar response is a strong sign of corticospinal tract involvement. If the plantar response is very hyperactive, there may be a triple flexion reflex. The abdominal reflex is commonly lost early in the course of the disease when the corticospinal tract is involved.

Facial myokymia (continuous involuntary quivering in the facial muscles) may be present. Weakness noted on a manual muscle examination is a common early finding; clinically, this weakness may be seen as dragging of a leg or poor control of a lower extremity. The patient may also present with spastic or ataxic gait. The Lhermitte sign, which involves passive flexion of the neck that induces a tingling, electric like feeling down the shoulders and back and less often into the anterior thighs, is frequently seen in MS (Fig. 1). Another common group of findings includes varying degrees of spastic ataxia and sensory changes in the extremities, indicating spinal damage.

Functional Limitations

Balance problems and/or dizziness may cause difficulty with mobility and result in falls. There may be hesitancy to leave home for fear of being injured.

Bladder and bowel incontinence may cause embarrassment and lead to the use of a diaper or catheter. Urinary frequency may result in the individual continually looking for access to a bathroom when outside the home or may discourage the patient from leaving home. Bowel incontinence is more likely to result in a hesitancy to leave the home. Depression can result in patients becoming unable to function with people or even to take care of themselves.

The lack of energy, weakness, or fatigue can limit activities of daily living and mobility.

Nystagmus, loss of vision, and decreased balance and strength can put the patient at risk for falls and subsequent injury.

Seizure disorders, if unable to be adequately controlled, can cause patients to lose their jobs.

Sleep difficulty, depending on the degree, can affect daily activities, mood, mobility, alertness, cognitive ability, energy, etc. Sexual dysfunction can lead to difficulty with relationships. Spasticity often leads to mobility problems and difficulty in daily activities. Intolerance to heat can result in exacerbations and resultant limitations.

Diagnostic Studies

Diagnostic imaging studies in the form of computerized tomography (CT) and magnetic resonance imaging (MRI) are most valuable in the evaluation of MS.

CT can detect low density demyelinating lesions (thought to indicate active disease) in patients with MS. However, these changes are not specific for MS. A double dose of contrast given 1 hour prior to the CT is the most sensitive use of CT.

MRI is estimated to have a sensitivity 10 times that of CT in detecting MS lesions. *MRI has been found to be the most useful test in the diagnosis of MS*. With gadolinium administration, lesions that brighten indicate an area of blood-brain barrier breakdown. MRI has set the standard for determining how well therapy is working and determines disease activity, burden, and type.

MRI spectroscopy complements conventional MRI. It quantifies the chemical pathology within lesions as well as in normal appearing white matter.[11]

There is some evidence that the measurement of the ventricular diameter by transcranial sonography can be helpful in serial followup evaluation of the patient with MS.[12]

Somatosensory evoked potentials (SEPs) go through the spinal cord, brainstem, and cerebral hemispheres. Lower extremity stimulation is used to evaluate the entire spinal cord and can detect asymptomatic lesions (see ref 8, p 330).

Oligoclonal banding in cerebrospinal fluid is positive in approximately 50% of patients with suspected MS and almost 90% of patients with clinically definite MS.

Neuropsychologic testing is not specific or sensitive but may be helpful in following the course of the disease. It is estimated that 60% of patients with MS have abnormal findings.

Urodynamic and electrophysiologic testing may show evidence of a neuropathic bladder but is not specific for MS.

Differential Diagnosis

Acute disseminated encephalomyelitis
    Cerebrovascular disease
        Primary cerebralvasculitis
        Systemic lupus erythematosus
        Polyarteritis nodosa
        Familial cavernous hemangiomata
        Eales disease with neurological involvement
    Inflammatory central nervous system disease
        Behçet's
        Lyme disease
        Neurosarcoidosis
        Neurobrucellosis
        Sjögren's syndrome
        Migratory sensory neuritis

Metastatic and remote effects of cancer
    Multiple metastases
    Paraneoplastic syndromes
Vitamin B_{12} deficiency
Myasthenia gravis
HTLV-1-associated myelopathy
Acquired immunodeficiency syndrome myelopathy
Other human immunodeficiency virus syndromes
Herpes zoster myelitis
Arachnoiditis
Chronic fatigue syndrome
Adult onset leukodystrophy

Treatment

Initial

Patient and family education is of paramount importance in treating patients with MS. General good health habits should be reinforced, particularly as the patient becomes more disabled. These include adequate but not excessive dietary intake; hygiene; and home, work, and recreation issues. Patients with MS may be candidates early on for a parking permit for disabled persons. Both the patient and family should monitor for signs of depression.

For relapses, intravenous methylprednisolone can be used for 5 days. Then oral prednisone can be used. There is some evidence that early use of methylprednisolone and prednisone delays the recurrence rate of relapse for 2 years.[16] One regimen recommends a bolus of 500 mg daily for 3 to 5 days followed by high doses of prednisone (e.g., 80 mg daily for 4 days, followed by 60, 40, 20, 10, and 5 mg each for 4 days, and then four doses of 5 mg on alternate days).[7,9,20] On the other hand, there is a suggestion that use of prednisone might increase the risk of recurrent disease activity.[14]

Seven alternate-day plasma exchanges resulted in good improvement in about 40% of patients who had not responded to corticosteroids.[18]

Determining optimal treatment after initial findings that indicate possible MS remains difficult.[19]

In relapsing MS, the use of interferon beta-1b appears to decrease the frequency of relapses by 30%.[20] Interferon beta-1a, interferon beta-1b, and glatiramer acetate appear to reduce the development of new gadolinium-enhancing lesions on MRI with varying results. There has been no established long-term (beyond 5 years) benefit. There is also no definite information concerning timing with these agents.[4] A recent study suggests that starting treatment with interferon beta-1a with the initial demyelinating event benefits patients.[21]

Medications for spasticity include baclofen, which is the first drug of choice; diazepam; dantrolene; clonidine; and tizanidine. Baclofen is started at 5 mg twice a day (bid) and gradually increased to 80 mg/day. Many patients with MS require and can tolerate higher doses. Diazepam can be used in adults at dosages from 2 to 10 mg, 3 or 4 times daily. Dantrolene may be prescribed for adults starting at 25 mg daily and increasing gradually as high as 100 mg, 2 to 4 times daily. Clonidine can be initiated at 0.1 mg bid and gradually increased to 2.4 mg daily as the maximal dose. Tizanidine can be started at 4 mg and gradually increased, if needed for benefit, to 4 mg, 3 times daily (36 mg/day should not be exceeded). Orthostatic hypotension and sedation are the main side effects.[20] Botulinum toxin injections can be useful with specific spastic muscles.

Pain is no longer believed to be rare in MS and can vary greatly in character and intensity. Some medications that may be helpful include tricyclic antidepressants, baclofen, and phenytoin. Gabapentin is a relatively newer agent and has been reportedly helpful for pain relief. There is no known technique to improve sensory deficits, and it is important for the patient to be made aware of any sensory deficits for self-protection.

Bladder dysfunction with difficulty in storing and/or emptying is common. Once the problem has been determined, appropriate medication or techniques can be utilized. If the patient is unable to void, an intermittent catheterization program can be instituted with either the patient or some support person(s) who has been taught appropriate catheterization. If the findings indicate that there is low residual volume due to an irritative type pathology, anticholinergics may be effective. An indwelling catheter should be avoided, if at all possible, but consideration must be given to its use if all other measures fail.

Constipation may occur for a variety of reasons, and a consistent bowel routine is required to prevent impaction. Measures include appropriate fluid intake and use of fiber, oral osmotic agents, or glycerin suppositories. Diarrhea is much less common.

Sexual dysfunction is common and may be present along with bowel and bladder problems. The most common problem for the male is inability to get or maintain an erection, as well as difficulty with ejaculating, decreased genital sensation, and a decrease in desire. Females commonly report fatigue, impaired genital sensation, and changes in orgasm or desire for sex. Vaginal lubrication may be another problem. It is important to encourage partners to try different techniques and devices, to provide them with information, to make specific suggestions, and to provide therapy when needed.[7,8]

Cognitive and/or affective impairment should be evaluated. A neuropsychologist can commonly be helpful in these situations. With significant cognitive problems there may be difficulty in complying with a rehabilitation program. If there is concomitant depression, tricyclic antidepressants may be helpful, if the side effects are tolerable. Fluoxetine has been found to be effective.[13] Frank dementia is rare. There may be problems with recalling intentions, processing new or complex information and doing two things at once. Frontal lobe involvement may cause problems with initiating activities, planning, and working independently. Impulsivity may be seen, and inhibition of inappropriate activities may be impaired. It is not yet proven that cognitive rehabilitation therapy is effective. Compensatory strategies such as lists, associations, and cueing may be helpful if practiced conscientiously to the point in which they become almost automatic. Structure in the patient's life is important.

Rehabilitation

Deconditioning can be addressed with a general conditioning program to improve strength without causing undue fatigue or increasing the core body temperature. Some types of equipment that can be used are stationary bicycles, cool therapeutic pools (84 degrees Fahrenheit or less), and upper extremity ergometers. Progressive resistive exercises also can be used. It was found that aerobic exercise significantly improved depression and quality of life measures in patients with MS.[24] Functionally range of motion exercises , carefully performed strengthening activities, gait and transfer training, balance activities, bracing when indicated, and the use of assistive devices such as walkers and canes may all be helpful . For the individual with greater mobility impairment, wheelchairs or motorized scooters may eventually be required. It is important to emphasize safety and appropriate equipment for the patient with increasing disability.

Spasticity is common in MS. It can be useful for functioning when it involves the lower extremity extensor muscles and may aid in standing, transferring, and walking—in which case it should not be treated unless it causes other intolerable problems. When spasticity becomes a problem, treatment can include medication (see the previous section); rehabilitation therapies; and attempts to eliminate the sensory stimuli, such as bowel or bladder distention and pressure ulcers, that can increase or cause spasticity. Procedures that may be required in an attempt to cope with spasticity are described in the next section.

Decreased balance and coordination are common in MS. These may be associated with tremor and dysmetria, with involvement in the cerebellum and its connections as well as the brainstem and the dorsal columns. In its worse form, incoordination can reduce or totally prevent standing, walking, sitting, and the ability to perform activities of daily living. Therapy techniques include compensatory strategies, attempts to stabilize affected body parts, relaxation therapy, and balance and coordination work. Weights can help increase stabilization, but one must be aware of the fatigue factor as well as weakness that may be present when they are used. Coordination and balance activities require much effort on the part of the patient since they must be precise and prolonged. Falls may be a result of the problems with balance and strength. None of the evaluation procedures to predict falls in the older adult has proved worthwhile in the MS population. A description of prior falls should be obtained and may help to establish a program to prevent future falls. For example, if the patient has fallen forward while reaching for an object, training can be initiated to increase the safety of the individual in reaching forward. The patient should be trained on how to get up from a fall. Any caregiver needs to know how to help the patient get up after a fall. Previously mentioned bracing may be helpful in preventing falls. Another measure that may help is to try to increase the strength in the lower extremities, if feasible. Transfer techniques are important because the person with the ability to transfer has a much greater degree of independence than someone needing help with this basic activity. In addition, if the caregiver is somewhat frail and unable to help, the patient may then need to be in an assisted living situation instead of being at home. Again, any caregiver who will be assisting with transfers has to be trained.

Diminished self care assessment is important. There are many evaluation scales that can be utilized that give a quantitative value.[22] Instructing the caregiver(s) in the activities that require assistance and those that do not is important. The occupational therapist can help the patient with upper extremity contractures and incoordination and can provide low vision aids and teach energy conservation, work simplification, and ergometric techniques. There is a host of adaptive equipment that is available to the patient in need. Some people are psychologically hesitant to use adaptive equipment and need to be approached with care. There may be a need for instruction in pacing; scheduling certain activities when patients are at their best; and compensatory techniques for memory loss, delayed processing, and other cognitive difficulties.

Dysarthria and/or swallowing dysfunction can be addressed by a speech pathologist. With severe involvement, to the point that the patient cannot be understood, various types of communication aids are available. Problems with swallowing can be dealt with by downgrading the consistency of the food, taking smaller bites, and eating the largest meal early in the day if fatigue is believed to be a causative factor. Another alternative is to eat several small meals during the day.

Procedures

Intramuscular botulinum toxin can be effective in dealing with specific spastic muscles (see Chapter 136).

Nerve blocks and motor point blocks can also be utilized in the localized treatment of spasticity.

In the presence of intractable spasticity, an implantable pump for the administration of baclofen may be helpful. This can be particularly useful in decreasing severe spinal spasticity and in improving function. As a last resort, the use of intraspinal alcohol or phenol injections may be used in patients who have lost most of their function and have severe disabling spasticity.

Surgery

Rarely, surgical procedures may be needed to deal with severe spasticity that has not improved with non-surgical therapy. Such procedures can include dorsal root section; dorsal column stimulation; dorsal root entry zone lesions; Bischof's myelotomy; or as a last resort, cordectomy.[9]

With disabling, high amplitude, cerebellar-outflow tremors, there may be some improvement after continued contralateral thalamic stimulation or ablative thalamotomy.[4]

Potential Disease Complications

Simply stated, the complications of the disease are the progression of MS to the point that patients may become completely dependent on caregivers, unable to do anything for themselves, and experience severe pain and spasticity as well as worsening cognitive dysfunction. MS is rarely the direct cause of death. Respiratory failure from cervical myelopathy or extensive cerebral and brain stem demyelination occasionally caused death. Pneumonia, pulmonary emboli, aspiration,urosepsis, and decubiti cause 50% of the deaths. Most of the other causes of death in patients with MS are the same as those in the general population (e.g., cancer, heart disease, cerebrovascular disease and trauma). Suicide is estimated to be two to seven times higher in MS patients than in the general population.

Potential Treatment Complications

Corticosteroids (prednisone and methylprednisolone) may mask signs of infection, and result in glaucoma, immunosupression, edema, osteoporosis, cataracts, avascular necrosis, myopathic problems, and myriad other potential side effects.[26]

The most common side effects of interferon beta-1b and beta-1a include flu-like symptoms and injection site reactions. Antibodies to the agents may result from continued use.[27]

In the case of baclofen, it is important not to abruptly withdraw the medication because of the potential for hallucinations and/or seizures. Weakness, drowsiness, dizziness, and fatigue can occur.

The major side effect of dantrolene is hepatotoxicity. Orthostatic hypotension and sedation are the main side effects of tizanidine.[20]

References

1. Cotran RS, Kumar V, Robbins SL: Pathologic Basis of Disease, 5th ed. Philadelphia, W.B. Saunders, 1994, p 1326.
2. Goetz CG, Pappert EJ: Textbook of Clinical Neurology. Philadelphia, W.B. Saunders, 1999, pp 973–977.
3. Lublin FD, Reingold SC: National Multiple Sclerosis Society (USA) Advisory Committee on Clinical Trials of New Agents in MS: Defining the clinical course of multiple sclerosis: Results of an international survey. Neurology 1996;46:907–911.
4. Noseworthy JH, Lucchinetti C, Rodriguez M, et al: Multiple Sclerosis N Engl J Med 2000;343:938-52.
5. Confavreux C, Vukusic S, Moreau T, et al: Relapses and progression of disability in multiple sclerosis. N Engl J Med 2000;343:1430–1438.
6. Ransohoff R: A fundamentally new view of multiple sclerosis. Int J of MS Care 2000; 2(2):2–8.
7. Adams RD, Victor M, Ropper AH: Principles of Neurology, 6th ed. New York, McGraw-Hill, 1997, pp 909–913.
8. DeLisa JA, Gans BM (eds): Rehabilitation Medicine, 2nd ed. Philadelphia, J.B. Lippincott, 1993, p 863.
9. Paty DW, Ebers GC: Multiple Sclerosis. Philadelphia, F.A. Davis, 1998, pp 79–80.
10. Kurtzke JF: Rating neurologic impairment in multiple sclerosis: An expanded disability status scale (EDSS). Neurology 1983;33:1444–1452.
11. Vollmer T: Use of MRI technology in determining prognosis and tracking therapeutic benefit in multiple sclerosis. Int J MS Care 2000;2(2):4–14.
12. Berg D, Maurer M, Warmuth-Metz M, et al: The correlation between ventricular diameter measured by transcranial sonography and clinical disability and cognitive dysfunction in patients with multiple sclerosis. Arch Neurol 2000;57:1289–1292.
13. Shafey H: The effect of fluoxetine in depression associated with multiple sclerosis [Letters].Clin J Psych 1990;37:147–148.
14. Beck RW: The Optic Neuritis Treatment Trial: Three-year follow-up results. Arch Ophthalmol 1995;113:136–137.
15. Krupp LB, Alvarez LA, Larocca NG, et al: Fatigue in multiple sclerosis. Arch Neurol 1988;45 435–437.
16. Beck RW, Cleary PA, Anderson MM Jr, et a: A randomized, controlled trial of corticosteroids in the treatment of acute optic neuritis. N Engl J Med 1992;326:581–588.
17. LaBan MM, Martin T, Pechur J, et al: Physical and occupational therapy in the treatment of patients with multiple sclerosis. Phys Med Rehabil Clin N Am 1998;9:603–614.
18. Weinshenker BG, O'Brien PC, Petterson TM, et al: A randomized trial of plasma exchange in acute central nervous system inflammatory demyelinating disease. Ann Neurol 1999;46:878–886.
19. Comi G, Filippi M, Barkhof F, et al: Interferon beta 1a (Rebif) in patients with acute neurological syndromes suggestive of multiple sclerosis: a multi-center, randomized, double-blind, placebo-controlled study. Neurology 2000;54(Suppl3):A85–A86.
20. The IFNB Multiple Sclerosis Study Group, University of British Columbia MS/MRI Analysis Group: Interferon B-1b in the treatment of multiple sclerosis: Final outcome of the randomized controlled trial. Neurology 1995;45:1277–1285.
21. Jacobs LD, Beck RW, Simon JH, et al: Intramuscular interferon beta 1a therapy initiated during a first demyelinating event in multiple sclerosis. N Engl J Med 2000;343:898–904.
22. Pizzorno JE, Murray MT (eds): Textbook of Natural Medicine, 2nd ed. Edinburgh and London, Churchill Livingstone, 1999, pp 1415–1423.
23. Drug Facts and Comparisons 2001, 35th ed. Saint Louis, Facts and Comparisons, 2001, pp 1106–1107.
24. Frontera WR, Dawson DM, Slovik DM: Exercise in Rehabilitation Medicine. Champaign, IL, Human Kinetics, 1999, p 354.
25. Trombly CA: Occupational therapy for physical dysfunction. Baltimore, Williams & Wilkins, 1995, p 744.
26. Drug facts and comparisons 2001 (pocket version). Saint Louis, Facts and Comparisons, 2000, pp 124–126.
27. Rosenblum D, Saffir M: Therapeutic and symptomatic treatment of multiple sclerosis. Phys Med & Rehabil Clin N Am Multiple Sclerosis 1998:9:590.

117 Myofascial Pain and Dysfunction Syndrome

Howard J. Hoffberg, MD
Norman B. Rosen, MD

Synonyms

Myofascial pain
syndrome

Trigger points syndrome

Soft tissue syndrome

Tension myalgia

Somatic dysfunction

(Myo)fibrositis

Myofascitis

Localized fibromyalgia

Muscular rheumatism

ICD-9 Codes

729.1
Myalgia and myositis,
unspecified

847
Sprains and strains of
other and unspecified
parts of the back

847.0
Neck

847.1
Thoracic

847.2
Lumbar

847.3
Sacrum

847.4
Coccyx

847.9
Unspecified site of back

Definition

Although the term *myofascial pain syndrome* is generally considered by many to be a single muscle syndrome, more often, multiple muscles in a myotatic unit are involved, resulting in a clinical syndrome that includes a combination of several overlapping trigger-point referral patterns. (The *myotatic unit* refers to a group of muscles that move, stabilize, or retard motion at any joint.) This results in reduced muscle (and joint) range of motion, weakness, and muscular imbalance. The resultant tissue dysfunction may or may not be associated with pain.

Therefore, a better term than myofascial pain syndrome is *myofascial pain and dysfunction syndrome*, which takes into consideration *both* the pain *and* the associated tissue dysfunction (i.e., weakness and tightness of the muscle with reflex neurologic and vascular compensations).

Myofascial pain originates in the muscles and their fascial linings and is often associated with a trigger point(s). A *trigger point* is a localized area of tenderness and hyperirritability in the muscle, tendons, ligaments, and/or periosteum and is associated with a characteristic referral pattern. In muscles, there may be a taut band ("fibrositic nodule"), palpation of which may result in a "jump" sign. This latter finding has been variably reported as either a local snapping response of the taut band, a brief muscular contraction resulting in joint motion after snapping of the taut band, or a startle response of the patient in response to snapping. All three phenomena may occur. This local twitch response may occur more readily after needling of the trigger point.

Referral patterns include sensory disturbances (e.g., pain, dysesthesias, and tenderness) *both* locally and elsewhere. Trigger points can also cause referred motor, autonomic (including cutaneous hyperemia) and/or visceral symptoms. Trigger points may be active (i.e., have clinical manifestations of pain), or latent (i.e., insufficiently irritable to cause a clinical pain complaint but associated with a localized region of tenderness or a taut band). Trigger points must be differentiated from *tender points* (commonly found with fibromyalgia), in which there is no taut band or referral pattern. Both trigger and tender points are tender; however, whereas myofascial pain and dysfunction syndrome occurs equally in men and women, fibromyalgia occurs much more commonly in women. Fibromyalgia also differs in that it is a systemic condition characterized by generalized myalgias, easy fatigability, sleep disturbance, and headaches and is often associated with gastrointestinal, genitourologic and psychologic dysfunction. It is postulated that this is a result of a centrally mediated pain mechanism, resulting in a lowered pain threshold that can be modulated by imbalances of neurotransmitters superimposed on a hereditary susceptibility for reduced energy capacity in the muscle mitochondria.

Postulated mechanisms for myofascial pain include an energy imbalance due to sustained vasoconstriction of the myofascial tissues (sympathetic dysfunction), resulting in reduced oxygen tension, a build up of metabolic waste products, and the release of nociceptive chemicals (serotonin, bradykinin, substance P, CRP-related peptides, and histamine), which can sensitize pain fibers locally.

Both peripheral and central sensitization can occur through alterations of the wide dynamic range neurons. Reflex shortening of myofascial fibers may lead to the development of the taut band, possibly as the result of local changes in calcium transport. The twitch response is considered to be a local spinal reflex. Other theories have implicated the proprioceptive muscle afferents in the spindles and tendons (mediated through the gamma system), which may be sensitized by acute or chronic overload. Recent research has focused on neuromuscular junction and endplate dysfunction that causes altered acetylcholine release, which may excessively activate muscle fibers, causing premature fatigue and resulting in myalgia. The characteristic referral patterns may be related to nociceptive sensory overload of the segmental dorsal root ganglion and dorsal horn of the spinal cord, resulting in overflow on a dermatomal, sclerotomal, myotomal, radicular, or autonomic pattern.

It is important to note that *myofascial pain and dysfunction syndrome always occurs secondary to some other factor or condition* (e.g., cervical radiculopathy). However, once developed, the trigger points can persist as an independent and autonomous pain (and dysfunction) generators. If the condition is ineffectively treated, the trigger points may spread dysfunction to contiguous muscles, causing a very confusing clinical picture. Additionally, unrecognized (and therefore untreated) precipitating factors can cause the condition to become chronic.

Symptoms

The hallmark of myofascial pain and dysfunction syndrome is muscle pain with activities and stretching, which may be described as local aching and stiffness (or generalized, if multifocal involvement is present). Sometimes a history of direct trauma is reported, but more often, indirect factors including overload (eccentric greater than concentric), overwork, repetitive stress, or postural aberrations are present. The condition may be exacerbated by physical or emotional stress or by changes in temperature and/or barometric pressure. In addition, it may be precipitated (and perpetuated) by a combination of physical, psychologic, nutritional, metabolic, and/or endocrinologic factors, including anemia, vitamin C, electrolyte, sex hormone, or thyroid abnormalities. Characteristic referral patterns include headaches, paresthesias, and radiating symptoms.

Physical Examination

Posture is evaluated including stance, scoliosis, and any right-to-left asymmetries. Range of motion of all affected limbs, jaw, and spine, with observation of barriers during passive motion associated with pain or joint subluxations are important. Strength testing may reveal subtle weakness and muscular imbalances. Soft tissue palpation that includes superficial and deep tissue texture and using 3 pounds of force, observing for taut bands, twitch response or jump sign, and reproducibility of the patient's symptoms. The neurologic exam is usually normal, but patients may report non-dermatomal sensory disturbances.

Functional Limitations

Patients often present with impaired strength, endurance, and flexibility, resulting in impairments of mobility, activities of daily living, work performance, recreation, sex, and sleep.

Diagnostic Studies

The diagnosis of myofascial pain and dysfunction syndrome is based on clinical findings, but testing may be performed to exclude other causes of symptoms or explore the various perpetuating (and precipitating) factors (e.g., MRI to evaluate whether a cervical radiculopathy is present).

Differential Diagnosis

If Localized

May mimic peripheral neurologic dysfunction
  Complex regional pain syndrome (reflex sympathetic dystrophy)
  Migraine headaches
  Spinal radiculopathies
  Entrapment neuropathies (thoracic outlet syndrome, carpal tunnel syndrome, ulnar nerve entrapment at the elbow, or sciatic nerve involvement)

May mimic musculoskeletal dysfunction
  Muscular strain, muscle tears
  Ligamentous sprains, joint instability
  Bursitis, tendinitis
  Shoulder impingement
  Craniofacial (tempomandibular) dysfunction, muscle contraction (tension) headaches
  Costalchondritis
  Epicondylitis
  Enthesopathies
  Periostitis
  Patellofemoral syndrome
  Spinal facet syndrome or pelvic girdle dysfunction

If Multifocal or Widespread

Tender points
  Fibromyalgia (multiple subsets)
  Polymyalgia rheumatica
  Poor sleep
  Polymyositis

Diffuse pain
  Central pain sensitization
  Central disinhibition syndromes
  Somatization disorders
  Psychogenic rheumatism

Treatment

Initial

Treatment is conservative. Patients should be reassured about the benign nature of their presentations. Relative rest, analgesics and/or NSAIDs, combined with a home exercise program (consisting of stretching and correction of postural abnormalities) are recommended. Ice, followed by gentle stretching may be used to achieve peripheral desensitization and reduce muscle spasm. Adjunctive medications may include the use of stronger analgesics, psychotropics, muscle relaxants, hypnotics, antihistamines, or topical medications. Narcotics should be avoided as much as possible because of the serious potential for dependence.

Rehabilitation

Physical medicine modalities often are performed by physical and occupational therapists and include superficial and deep heat (ultrasound), electrical stimulation, and vapocoolant spray. Manual medicine techniques include massage; passive range of motion; "myofascial releases"; and static contraction, followed by stretch, soft tissue, and joint mobilization. The common goal of these techniques is to promote vasodilation and restore flexibility by stretching the dysfunctional tissue, thereby decreasing the sensitivity of the stretch reflex.

Rehabilitation efforts should emphasize a daily exercise program that includes stretching, strengthening, postural awareness, dynamic stabilization, work hardening, and aerobic conditioning (endurance training) to achieve optimal range of motion, strength, and musculoskeletal balance. The treatment goals should focus on rapid restoration of function. Emphasis should be placed on patient education including instruction in techniques of energy conservation, ergonomics, and pacing. The patient should be informed that recurring symptoms may occur and that formal treatment may need to be resumed.

In refractory or chronic cases, considerations should be made for further diagnostic evaluation for co-existing and/or evolving pathology. Adaptive equipment including elastic supports may also be considered. An interdisciplinary multimodal approach (e.g., chronic pain program) is strongly recommended in resistant or dysfunctional patients, with attention given to psychosocial factors that may be contributing to the presentation, including stress, secondary gain, and disability neurosis. This may require formal counseling (including family) for pain coping strategies, relaxation training (including biofeedback), and behavioral modification.

Procedures

Trigger point injections using local anesthetics, saline, steroids (used judiciously), and serapin (herbal) into involved muscles, followed by passive stretch, are more effective when used in combination with other treatment approaches that promote maximum flexibility and strength (Figs. 1–3). Dry needling may be helpful in some cases.

Some clinicians recommend pre-injection blocks with local anesthetics into the myotomal paraspinals of the affected muscles. More recently, botulinum toxin injections (20 to 100 units of botulinum toxin A injected in selected trigger points every 3 to 6 months) followed by ice and electrical stimulation has been performed.

Acupuncture points often overlap with trigger points and may also be useful.

Surgery

Surgery is not recommended for the treatment of this condition unless it is done to correct an underlying disease process (e.g., cervical radiculopathy).

Potential Disease Complications

Inadequate treatment may result in a physical deconditioning syndrome, including impaired posture, flexibility, strength, and endurance. This may lead to chronic intractable pain. Obesity, insomnia, medication dependency, and overuse of other medical care because of misdiagnosis (including unnecessary surgery in some cases) may occur.

Emotional and spiritual decompensation may also occur, resulting in depression, anger, anxiety, and fear of activities (kinesiophobia). Psychologic dependency may ultimately result in a chronic pain syndrome and prolonged disability.

Potential Treatment Complications

Trigger point injections may cause postinjection soreness; vasovagal and allergic reactions; and transient nerve blocks with weakness, bleeding, infection, and pneumothorax. Analgesics, NSAIDs, and COX-2 inhibitors have well-known side effects that most commonly affect the gastric, hepatic, and renal systems. Excessive sedation and dependency with narcotics, hypnotics, and muscle relaxants.

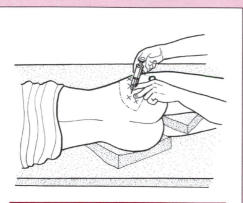

FIGURE 1. Ask the patient to point with one finger to the area of most intense pain. Then palpate for a taut band. Once localized, under sterile conditions, using a 27-gauge 2-inch needle, inject approximately 0.5 cc of a local anesthetic (e.g., 1% lidocaine) into the muscle at this site (gluteus minimus is shown). This should be accompanied by needling of the entire taut band to mechanically break up the abnormal and sensitized tender tissue. It is generally not advisable to inject local steroids into the muscle. This may be repeated in several areas during a single procedure visit. Additionally, this procedure may need to be repeated on several occasions, depending on the patient's symptoms and reported relief from the treatment. Postinjection care may include spray and stretch with a vapocoolant by the clinician and avoidance of aggressive use of the injected muscles by the patient. Heat or ice may be used depending on the patient's preference.

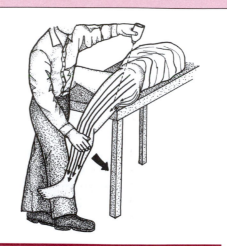

FIGURE 2. Passive stretch of the gluteus minimus performed by the clinician using vapocoolant spray. The stream of spray covers the injected region and the referred area of pain.

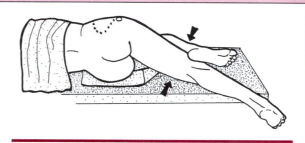

FIGURE 3. Passive stretch of the gluteus minimus performed by the patient. This position can be held for 30 seconds and then repeated 5 times.

References
1. Cailliet R: Soft Tissue Pain and Disability. Philadelphia, F.A. Davis, 1977.
2. Greenman P: Principles of Manual Medicine. Baltimore, Williams & Wilkins, 1996.
3. Lennard TA: Pain Procedures in Clinical Practice. Philadelphia, Hanley & Belfus, 2000.
4. Rosen NB, Hoffberg HJ: Conservative management of low back pain. Phys Med Clin North Am 1998;9:2:435–472.
5. Rosen NB: Physical medicine and rehabilitation approaches to the myofascial pain and fibromyalgia syndromes. Clin Rheumatol 1994;8:881–911.
6. Rosen NB: The myofascial pain syndromes. Phys Med Rehab Clin North Am 1993;4:41–63.
7. Rosen NB: Myofascial pain—the great mimicker and potentiator or muscle pain syndromes. Maryland Med J 1993;42:3:261–266.
8. Snider R: Essentials of Musculoskeletal Care. Rosemont, IL, American Academy of Orthopedic Surgeons, 1997.
9. Travell J, Simons D: Myofascial Pain and Dysfunction: The Trigger Point Manual. Baltimore, Williams & Wilkins, 1992 (vol 2), 1999 (vol 1).

118 Myopathies

Erik Ensrud, MD

Synonym

Muscular dystrophies

ICD-9 Codes

359.0
Congenital hereditary
muscular distrophy

359.1
Hereditary progressive
muscular dystrophy

359.2
Myotonic disorders

359.4
Toxic myopathy

359.5
Endocrine myopathy

359.6
Inflammatory myopathy
in other diseases

359.8
Other myopathies

359.9
Myopathy, unspecified

710.3
Dermatomyositis

710.4
Polymyositis

Definition

A myopathy is an abnormality of muscle that can arise from a variety of etiologies (Table 1). Depending on the particular etiology, myopathies can have acute, subacute, or chronic presentations.

Muscular Dystrophies

These are inherited disorders of muscle due to abnormal muscle proteins that are characterized by progressive course and early onset (Table 2).

Congenital Myopathies

These are a group of slowly progressive or non-progressive myopathies that usually present in the neonatal period. Each of these disorders has a characteristic muscle finding on muscle biopsy. They include central core myopathy, nemaline myopathy, myotubular (centronuclear) myopathy, and congenital fiber disproportion (see Table 1).

Metabolic Myopathies

Metabolic myopathies are muscle disorders resulting from inherited defects in intracellular energy production. They may present as cramps and myoglobinuria, as part of a diffuse neurologic syndrome often involving the central nervous system, and as a typical proximal myopathy. Patients with cramps and myoglobinuria often have disorders in the glycogen or lipid metabolism pathways. They may be asymptomatic at rest but develop symptoms after exercise (Tables 1 and 3).

TABLE 1. Myopathic Disorders

Inflammatory Myopathies
  Polymyositis
  Dermatomyositis
  Inclusion body myositis
  Viral
Muscular dystrophies
  X-linked
  Limb-girdle
  Congenital
  Facioscapulohumeral
  Scapuloperoneal
  Distal (Welander type)
Myotonic syndromes
  Myotonic dystrophy
  Inherited
  Schwartz-Jampel
  Drug-induced
Congenital myopathies
  Central core disease
  Nemaline myopathy
  Myotubular
  Fiber-type disproportion
  Other
Metabolic myopathies
  Glycogenoses
  Mitochondrial
  Periodic paralysis
Endocrine myopathies
  Thyroid
  Parathyroid
  Adrenal/steroid
  Pituitary
Drug-induced/toxic

From Dumitru D: Electrodiagnostic Medicine. Philadelphia, Hanley & Belfus, 1995, p 1054.

TABLE 2. Muscular Dystrophies

Disorder	Inheritance*
Duchenne's muscular dystrophy	X-linked recessive
Becker's muscular dystrophy	X-linked recessive
Facioscapulohumeral dystrophy	Autosomal dominant
Scapuloperoneal dystrophy	Autosomal dominant
Limb-girdle dystrophy	Autosomal recessive/dominant
Oculopharyngeal dystrophy	Autosomal dominant
Distal myopathy/muscular dystrophy	Autosomal dominant/recessive
Congenital muscular dystrophy	Autosomal recessive/sporadic
Myotonic dystrophy	Autosomal dominant

* Major forms of inheritance are noted, although several variations are also possible.
(From Dumitru D: Electrodiagnostic Medicine. Philadelphia, Hanley & Belfus, 1995, p 1067.)

Inflammatory Myopathies

Inflammatory myopathies are acquired myopathies associated with an immunologic or infectious attack. They include the immune-mediated myopathies polymyositis and dermatomyositis. They present with an acute or subacute course that is almost always associated with an elevated serum creatine kinase (CK) level. Parasites, bacteria, or viruses may cause infectious myopathies (Table 4).

Atrophic Myopathies

Atrophic myopathies usually present with clinical evidence of a myopathy, with or without elevated serum CK levels. They include drug-induced myopathies and endocrine myopathies. Drug-induced myopathies include those caused by colchicine; azidothymidine (AZT); cholesterol-lowering agents including the statins; alcohol; chloroquine; hydroxychloroquine; corticosterioids; and pentazocine (Table 5). Endocrine myopathies include both hyperthyroid and hypothyroid myopathies, as well as hyperparathyroidism.

Myotonic Myopathies

A number of disorders are associated with clinical and/or electrical myotonia. There are two major categories of myotonic dystrophies—congenital and adult. Individuals with myotonic dystrophy may not notice any problems until reaching adolescence or early adult life. The first symptom may be difficulty releasing an object. Progressive weakness generally leads to death

TABLE 3. Glycogen Storage Disorders

Type	Associated Name	Enzyme Deficiency	Clinical Features	EDM
I	von Gierke's disease	Glucose-6-phosphate	—	—
II	Pompe's disease	Acid maltase (α1,4-glucosidase)	Infantile: profound weakness; fatal Childhood/adult: limb girdle weakness	MI, CRD, BSAPP, myotonia
III	Cori-Forbes disease	Debranching (amylo-1,6-glucosidase)	Infantile: hypotonia Adult: limb girdle weakness	Rare MI, CRD, and rare fasciculations, BSAPP
IV	Andersen's disease	Branching (amylo-1,4–1,6-transglucosidase)	Infantile: muscle wasting	Rare MI, BSAPP
V	McArcle's disease	Mycophosphorylase	Infantile: profound weakness Adult: exercise intolerance, cramps, fatigue	Rare MI, occasional CRD, electrically silent cramps, decrement of CMAP to 20 Hz, rare BSAPP
VI	—	Liver phosphorylase	—	—
VII	Tauri's disease	Phosphofructokinase	Childhood: cramps, fatigue, exercise intolerance	See McArdle's disease

EDM = electrodiagnostic medicine findings; MI = membrane instability referring to positive sharp waves and fibrillation potentials; CRD = complex repetitive discharge; BSAPP = brief small abundant polyphasic potentials.
(From Dumitru D: Electrodiagnostic Medicine. Philadelphia, Hanley & Belfus, 1995, p 1093.)

occurring in the fifth or sixth decade of life, due to cardiopulmonary compromise (Table 6).

Symptoms

The primary symptom in myopathies is muscle weakness. Nearly all myopathies affect the proximal muscles to the greatest extent. The weakness is constant, although symptoms may flucuate with the effects of fatigue. The earliest symptoms are often related to weakness of the hip and proximal leg muscles. Patients will have difficulty rising from a deep chair or sofa, often requiring the support of their arms. They can have difficulty rising from the floor or a bathtub. Compensating for leg extensor weakness by bracing the legs with the hands while rising to a standing position is known as Gowers' maneuver. Walking up stairs may be difficult due to quadriceps weakness. Walking down stairs may be difficult due to hip extensor weakness. Proximal upper extremity weakness can present as fatigue or inability with overhead tasks, such as hairbrushing, brushing teeth, and lifting objects to elevated shelves.

Distal extremity weakness may be present and can be the primary symptom in hereditary distal myopathies and inclusion body myopathy.[1] This can manifest as ankle instability and difficulty with manual tasks, such as turning doorknobs and opening jars. The weakness preferentially affects certain distal muscle groups, as contrasted with polyneuropathy.

Pain can be associated with inflammatory and metabolic myopathies, usually those that have a high serum CK level. A small proportion of patients with muscular dystrophy may experience cramps and myalgias. The pain usually has an aching, dull, and crampy quality. Patients may use terms such as "soreness," "aching," "cramps," "spasms," and "fatigue." The pain is usually poorly localized. They normally do not complain of numbness or paresthesias. Exercise-induced pain suggests an inherited metabolic myopathy. Frank exercise-induced weakness that develops over a short period suggests a neuromuscular junction disorder.

FIGURE 4. Inflammatory Myopathies

Polymyositis
 I. Simple*
 II. Associated with systemic autoimmune disorders
   A. Crohn's disease
   B. Sarcoidosis
   C. Behçet's disease
   D. Psoriasis
   E. Lyme disease
   F. Myasthenia gravis
   G. Discoid lupus
   H. Ankylosing spondylitis
   I. Hashimoto's disease
   J. Kawasaki's disease
   K. Agammaglobulinemia
   L. IgA deficiency
 III. Associated with viruses/bacteria/parasites
   A. Viral myositis
     1. Acute form
       a. Benign myositis   Associated virus   Influenza types A, B, C (rare)   Adenovirus 2
       b. Rhabdomyolysis   Influenza A & B   Coxsackie virus B5   Echo 9   Adenovirus 21   Herpes simples
     2. Chronic form
       Dermatomyositis-like Echo syndrome associated with agammaglobulinemia
     3. Human immunodeficiency virus (HIV) associated
   B. Parasites
     1. Protozoans
       a. Toxoplasmosis
       b. Sarcocystis
       c. Trypanosomiasis (Chagas disease)
     2. Cestodes (tapeworms)
       a. Cystircercosis
       b. Hydatidosis
       c. Coneurosis
       d. Sparganosis
     3. Nematodes (unsegmented roundworms)
       a. Trichinosis
       b. Visceral/cutaneous larva migrans
       c. Dracunculiasis

Dermatomyositis
 Simple
 Associated with connective tissue disorders
 Associated with malignancies

Inclusion Body Myositis

Other
 Polymyalgia rheumatica   Sarcoid myopathy
 Eosinophilic polymyositis   Vasculitis
 Focal myositis

* Simple is used to describe polymyositis uncomplicated by other disease or organism, or drug factors.
(From Dumitru D: Electrodiagnostic Medicine. Philadelphia, Hanley & Belfus, 1995, p 1055.)

TABLE 5. Drug- and Toxin-induced Disorders of Muscle

Disorder	Drug/Toxin	Clinical Features	Serum CK	EDM Findings
Focal myopathy (IM injection)	Antibiotics Pentazocine Heroin	Localized region of muscle induration, atrophied, and contracted. If deltoid affected, arm may be slightly abducted at rest	Normal or slightly elevated	BSAPP; variable degree of positive sharp waves and fibrillation potentials depending on amount of muscle damage; abnormalities localized to injection site only
Acute/subacute painful proximal myopathy	Clofibrate EACA Emetine Heroin	Muscle cramping and pain; tendency for proximal or more generalized weakness; deep tendon reflexes OK or slightly reduced	Markedly elevated	BSAPP; positive sharp waves and fibrillation potentials may be prominent
	Vincrinstine	Muscle pain, weakness, and atrophy present in a proximal distribution; deep tendon reflexes may be diminished or absent	Unclear	Not clearly known; detailed studies required
Hypokalemia	Diuretics Purgatives Licorice Amphotericin B Alcohol	Fluctuating weakness; diminished or absent deep tendon reflexes	Moderately to markedly elevated	BSAPP; variable degree of fibrillation potentials and positive sharp waves depending on the degree of muscle injury
Inflammatory myopathy	D-penicillamine Procainamide Levodopa Phenytoin Penicillin Cimetidine Contaminated L-tryptophan	Proximal muscle weakness and pain	Markedly elevated	BSAPP; positive sharp waves and fibrillation potentials; complex repetitive discharges
Acute rhabdomyolysis	Heroin Amphetamines Alcohol Diazepam Barbiturates Amphotericin B Isoniazid	Profound muscle pain, swelling, cramps, areflexia, possible quadriparesis, myoglobinuria, acute renal failure	Markedly elevated	BSAPP; significant degrees of fibrillation potentials positive and sharp waves

EDM = electrodiagnostic medicine; BSAPP = brief small abundant polyphasic motor unit action potentials; IM = intramuscular; EACA = epsilon aminocaproic acid.
Modified from Argov and Mastaglia; Lane and Mastaglia; Mastaglia; and Victor.

Physical Examination

The evaluation should start with observation of the undressed patient, with the clinician assessing for muscle atrophy. The most important part of the exam is muscle strength testing, which should be thorough and involve proximal and distal muscles in all extremities, as well as facial muscles and neck flexors/extensors. Hip girdle muscles are best isolated for strength testing while the patient is in the supine and prone positions. The tasks of walking, arising from a chair (or floor in pediatric patients), and stepping onto a low stool are often helpful in evaluating leg weakness.[2] Examination of the shoulder may reveal winging of the scapula, a characteristic finding in fascioscapulohumeral muscular dystrophy (FSH). Facial weakness and temporalis muscle wasting are also present in FSH.

Range of motion at joints should be examined because contractures may have marked functional effects. Reflexes should be normal or decreased proportional to muscle weakness in myopathies. Sensory testing is usually normal.

Functional Limitations

The most common functional limitations are related to the prominent symptom of proximal weakness, which can have a marked effect on transfers, ascending and descending stairs, and ambulation. In severe myopathies, patients may be restricted to wheelchair mobility. Proximal upper extremity weakness can interfere with activities of daily living such as dressing, grooming, and cooking. Fatigue is common secondary to the increased effort required with weakened muscles. Respiratory insufficiency requiring ventilation can result in difficulty with daily activities and increased fatigue. The dysphagia involved in some myopathies may make eating time-consuming and difficult.

TABLE 6. Myotonic Disorders

Disorder	Pattern of Inheritance
Myotonic dystrophy	Autosomal dominant
Myotonia congenita	
Thomsen's disease	Autosomal dominant
Recessive (Becker) type	Autosomal recessive
Myotonia fluctuans	Autosomal dominant
Paramyotonia congenita	Autosomal dominant
Periodic paralysis	
Hypokalemic	Autosomal dominant
Normo/hyperkalemic	Autosomal dominant
Chondrodystrophic myotonia (Schwartz-Jampel syndrome)	Autosomal recessive
Acquired myotonia (Drug-induced)	
Aromatic carboxylic acid intoxication (2,4-D, 9-AC)	
20,25 diazocholesterol	
Clofibrate	

Modified from Harper PS: Myotonic disorders. In Engel AG, Banker BQ (eds): Myology. New York, McGraw-Hill, 1986, pp 1267–1296.

Diagnostic Studies

The serum CK is the most commonly ordered test in the evaluation of a myopathy. It is important to note that a CK of less than 1000 may be normal and that there have been variations in normal ranges related to race. A survey of 1500 hospital employees without myopathy found the following upper limits of normal (97.5 percentile): black men, 520 U/liter; black women and non–black men, 345 U/liter; and non–black women, 145 U/liter.[3,4]

Serum CK is usually elevated in inflammatory myopathies (although it can be normal), muscular dystrophies, and metabolic myopathies. It is often normal in congenital myopathies, Emery-Dreifuss muscular dystrophy, fascioscapular muscular dystrophy, and atrophic myopathies.

Exercise, especially if very strenuous or in a sedentary individual, can cause marked CK elevation which peaks 12 to 18 hours after the activity but may remain elevated days later (~ 50% reduction every 2 days after initial peak). Patients should be advised to abstain from strenuous exercise for five days before serum CK testing. CK may be elevated as much as 10 times normal in motor neuron disease.

Nerve conduction studies are important to perform in cases of suspected myopathy. The sensory studies should be normal in myopathies. Motor nerve conduction studies are usually normal, except distal compound muscle action potentials may be reduced. Exceptions include patients with inclusion body myositis (30% have a sensory or sensorimotor polyneuropathy); sarcoidosis; and co-existent neuropathies, such as diabetic polyneuropathy.

The needle EMG exam can be very helpful in the evaluation of myopathies. Primarily, the size of motor units is decreased by the dysfunction or loss of individual muscle fibers, leading to motor unit action potentials (MUAPs) that characteristically have decreased duration, decreased amplitude, and increased phases.[5] These findings contrast with the neuropathic MUAP findings of increased amplitude and increased duration. In addition, denervating potentials (fibrillations and positive sharp waves) occur in many myopathic disorders. It is important to sample both proximal and distal muscles, with the paraspinal muscles (most proximal) often being high-yield.

Muscle biopsy is often useful in the diagnosis of myopathy. The selection of muscle to biopsy is important because a muscle that is end-stage is likely to show only fibrotic replacement of muscle tissue and an unaffected muscle may be normal. In an acute myopathy, it is best to select a muscle for biopsy that is clinically weak, and in a chronic myopathy to select a muscle that is only mildly weak. The muscle selected should not have been sampled by needle EMG, which may result in temporary inflammation. The pathologist to investigate possible etiologies performs specific histochemical stains and electron microscopy on the specimen.

Genetic testing has become routine in the evaluation of muscular dystrophies and may be useful in the evaluation of chronic myopathies of unknown etiology. A helpful resource is the journal *Neuromuscular Disorders*, which each month includes a list of all known genetic muscle disorders.[6]

Differential Diagnosis

Motor neuron disease
    Amyotrophic lateral sclerosis (ALS)
    Late-onset spinal muscular atrophy

Neuromuscular junction disorders
    Myasthenia gravis
    Lambert-Eaton myasthenic syndrome

Motor neuropathies
    Demyelinating motor neuropathies such as multifocal motor neuropathy diabetic amyotrophy

Spinal stenosis/myelopathy

Parkinson's disease

Polio/post-polio syndrome

Treatment

Initial

Patients should be informed that they should not exert themselves to the point of exhaustion. Referral to the Muscular Dystrophy Association (MDA) is very helpful for patient education and support.

Steroids are often effective in the treatment of inflammatory myopathies (as are other immunosuppressants) and have been shown to slow progression in some muscular dystrophies. Pain can be treated with NSAIDs/COX-2 inhibitors and analgesics.

Rehabilitation

Physical and occupational therapy are often necessary for gait training and stretching. Assistive devices such as canes, walkers, and wheelchairs, as indicated in a particular patient, can minimize disability. Assistive devices should be utilized preferably after training with a physical therapist. Bracing may be helpful for foot drop.

Adaptive equipment may be prescribed to assist a patient with daily activities. Home adaptations such as tub bars, entrance ramps, and lowered beds may be of great assistance to patients with proximal muscle weakness.

Exercise can help to maintain joint range of motion. High resistance exercise has been shown to have deleterious effect in neuromuscular disease, leading to the consensus that moderate exercise not to the point of exhaustion is preferable.[7]

Procedures

Assisted ventilation, including negative pressure ventilation, non-invasive positive pressure ventilation (i.e., BiPAP), and invasive positive pressure ventilation (i.e., endotracheal tube or tracheostomy) may be indicated for patients with insufficient ventilation. Feeding tubes may be necessary for patients with dysphagia due to severe bulbar myopathy.

Surgery

Patients with muscular dystrophies may require contracture release and spine stabilization surgeries.

Potential Disease Complications

Severe myopathies, including muscular dystrophies, can cause restrictive pulmonary disease due to chest wall muscle weakness and scoliosis.[8] Assisted ventilation, including negative pressure ventilation, non-invasive positive pressure ventilation (i.e., BiPAP), and invasive positive pressure ventilation (endotracheal tube or tracheostomy), may be indicated. Decreased mobility can result from proximal lower and upper extremity weakness. Contractures can be caused by disuse and fibrosis, as well as scoliosis due to paraspinal muscle weakness. Cardiac involvement can be present in myotonic dystrophy, Emery-Dreifuss muscular dystrophy, and inflammatory myopathies.

Potential Treatment Complications

Immunosuppresion may have associated side effects. Steroid use and decreased mobility may lead to osteoporosis and the subsequent risk of pathologic fractures. NSAIDs and analgesics have well known side effects. COX-2 inhibitors may have fewer gastric complications.

References
1. Barohn RJ, Amato AA: Distal Myopathies. Sem Neurol 1999;19:45–58.
2. Brooke MH: Proximal, distal, and generalized weakness. In Neurology in Clinical Practice [online]. Available at: www.nicp.com. Accessed Jan 8, 2001.
3. Harris EK, Wong ET, Shaw ST: Statistical criteria for separate reference intervals; race and gender groups in creatinine kinase. Clin Chem 1991;37:1580–1582.
4. Henderson AT, McQueen MJ, Patten RL, et al: Testing for creatinine kinase-2 in Ontario: Reference ranges and assay types. Clin Chem 1991;38:1365–1370.
5. Preston DC, Shapiro BE: Electromyography and Neuromuscular Disorders. Boston, Butterworth-Heinemann, 1998.
6. Neuromuscular disorders. Elsevier Science B.V.
7. Kilmer DD, McCrory MA, Wright NC, et al: The effect of a high resistance exercise program in slowly progressive neuro-muscular disease. Arch Phys Med Rehabil 1994;75:560–563.
8. Nelson MR: Rehabilitation concerns in myopathies. In Braddom RL (ed): Physical Medicine and Rehabilitation. Philadelphia, W.B. Saunders, 1996, pp 1003–1026.

119 Neural Tube Defects

Walton O. Schalick III, MD, PhD

Synonyms

Spinal dysraphism

Spina bifida
(aperta/cystica/
manifesta, occulta)

Hydrocele spinalis

Schistorachis

Lipomyelomeningocele

Myelomeningocele
("myelo")

Myelocystomeningocele

Meningomyelocele
(Fig. 1)

Anencephaly

Iniencephaly

Craniorachischisis

Encephalocele

ICD-9 Codes

740.0
Anencephalus

740.1
Craniorachischisis

740.2
Iniencephaly

741.0
Spina bifida, with
hydrocephalus

741.9
Spina bifida, without
mention of
hydrocephalus

742.0
Encephalocele

742.9
Unspecified anomaly of
brain, spinal cord, and
nervous system

V54.8
Orthopedic aftercare:
changes, check or removal
of casts, splint (external)

Definition

Neural tube defects (NTDs) encompass a spectrum of disorders characterized by failure of closure of the neural tube (26 days of postovulatory age) or re-opening of a closed tube during embryologic development (28 to 56 days of postovulatory age). Anatomically these lesions involve varying degrees of protrusion of the membranes and cord elements through a vertebral defect.

NTDs (spina bifida and anencephaly) have an incidence of 1 per 1000 pregnancies (roughly 4000 pregnancies per year—one third of which are lost to spontaneous or elective abortion) in the United States.[1] Survival into adulthood (third decade of life) for those who have had surgical repair of the NTD now exceeds 65%.

Tethered cord syndrome may be an initial presentation of a patient without a prior diagnosis of NTD or a patient with a known but previously stable NTD.[2,3]

Adults with NTDs have a bimodal distribution as either nonambulators or community ambulators.[4] Nearly all children with lumbosacral myelomenigoceles have a type II Arnold-Chiari malformation that results in hydrocephalus (Figs. 1 and 2). These often require shunts.[5,6] Cognitive limitations are thought to be postnatally acquired (often secondary to hydrocephalus) and may significantly add to the physical impairments.

Patients with NTDs almost always have a significant latex allergy.[7] Consequently, non-latex examination gloves should be used.

Symptoms

The spectrum of NTDs is rather large, ranging from asymptomatic to incompatible with life. In general, the symptoms depend on the anatomic extent and the neurologic level of the lesion.[8]

Neurologic

Presenting symptoms of Chiari II malformations (brainstem compression and hydrocephalus) include neck pain, visual disturbance, facial numbness, respiratory compromise, and painless joint swelling. Symptoms of a later onset Chiari II malformation include swallowing difficulties, sleep related periodic breathing, stridor, and central sleep apnea.

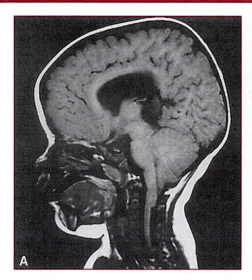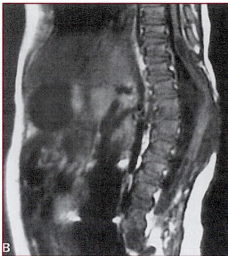

FIGURE 1. *A,* Unenhanced midsagittal T1-weighted MRI in a 6-month old boy with type II Arnold-Chiari malformation. Note "herniation" or downward displacement of the cerebellar tonsils through the foramen magnum to the level of C2 and the associated obstructive hydrocephalus. *B,* Unenhanced midsagittal T1-weighted MRI lumbosacral spine: extensive thoracolumbar myelomeningocele associated with the Arnold-Chiari malformation in *A.* Note the dorsal kyphosis, absence of posterior elements of the vertebrae and the malformed spinal cord at the level of the defect. A small syrinx in the cord is present above the defect. (From Rolak LA: Neurology Secrets, 3rd ed. Philadelphia, Hanley & Belfus, 2001, with permission.)

New leg weakness and atrophy is the most common presentation in adults with Chiari hydrosyringomyelia complex (commonly called a syrinx), but they may present with headache, neck pain, or pain/temperature sensory loss.

Tethered cord syndrome presents with new or progressive weakness and spasticity, deteriorating gait, change of bowel/bladder function and back or leg pain. Progressive scoliosis or foot deformity may also be noted. Tethered cord syndrome often presents with significant pain, but the neurologic signs and musculoskeletal deformities (especially lordoscoliosis and contractures) may be subtle. A change in urodynamic studies may be the first clue.

Close monitoring of shunt function is necessary as neuropsychological functioning may be improved with shunt placement or repair. Seizures, headache, neck pain, and fever may all herald a shunt malfunction or infection. Prolonged, untreated hydrocephalus may result in diminished intelligence.

Epilepsy is an active issue in approximately 9% of adult patients with NTDs.

Dermatologic

As with any spinal cord injury, patients need constant monitoring for skin breakdown, with the focus of concentration particularly on the ischium, sacrum, and heel, depending on ambulatory status.

Reproductive

Fertility of male patients may be impaired by the association of NTDs with cryptorchidism and complications of NTD management.

In women with NTDs, fertility is often not impaired, necessitating vigilant prenatal care if pregnancy is desired. Men and women with NTDs may have an increased risk of having a child with an NTD (in women it is about 4%). For all women, the value of folic acid supplements (400 mcg daily when considering pregnancy) is solidly supported.[9] Recent advances in *in utero* repair of NTDs remain experimental.[10]

Orthopedic

Scoliosis occurs in as many as 60% of cases, depending on the motor level affected. Degenerative hip, knee, and ankle osteoarthritis is increasingly common in this adult population, and a recent study reported a 70% prevalence of joint deformities or contractures in the adult NTD population.[11]

Osteoporosis, especially in patients with impaired mobility of their lower extremities (osteoporosis of immobility), can also lead to fractures as heraldic events. Routine screening for pain, history of trauma, and assessment of adequate transfer techniques and positioning are necessary to monitor for these sequelae.

Nutritional

Obesity is a common consequence of the impairments of NTDs and may be a cause for deteriorating mobility, particularly in adolescents. The impact of NTDs on eating disorders, particularly in young adult women, is slowly being recognized.[12]

Gastrointestinal

Swallowing difficulties have been noted as a symptom of late onset Chiari II deformity. Bowel incontinence, diarrhea, constipation, and megacolon are all attendant upon the degree of bowel control and completeness of management. Assistance with bowel management is typical of adults with NTDs.

Urologic

Urologic care is often intensively followed during childhood, but some studies indicate that adult-based risk categories exist and need to be followed aggressively into adulthood as well; these include patients with elevated creatinine and hydronephrosis.[13] In a retrospective study of 695 adults with NTDs, renal failure secondary to urinary tract complications was the primary cause of death.[14,15] Tethered cord syndrome may be associated with refractory urologic symptoms, requiring more intensive follow-up.[2]

Psychosocial

NTDs have been associated with the psychosocial sequelae of delayed or prolonged adolescence with its attendant exploratory behaviors.[16]

Physical Examination

The physical examination of a patient with an NTD should be consistent with a spinal cord injury at the level affected, including weakness, loss of sensation, and chronic upper motor neuron signs (e.g., spasticity, weakness, fatigability, and increased proprioceptive reflexes). A thorough musculoskeletal examination should be performed that evaluates range of motion at the joints and assesses for any co-existing pathology (e.g., rotator cuff injury at the shoulder due to overuse of the arms for mobility purposes).

A patient with a spinal tuft of hair or dimple, particularly in the lumbosacral region, and paralysis below the skin finding may have a previously undiagnosed or misdiagnosed NTD.

Findings in Chiari II malformation may include Charcot joint, neck pain with flexion or Valsalva maneuver, and decreased pain and temperature sensitivity.

Some patients, treated for hydrocephalus as children, may still have ventriculoperitoneal (VP) shunts (roughly 90% of children with myelomeningocele have them). Shunt obstruction and infection should always be considered when evaluating a patient with altered neurologic signs or headache; a neurosurgical referral for shunt tapping/culture may be useful.

Skin should be monitored for breakdown, and the nutritional status should be assessed.

Functional Limitations

As with any spinal cord injury, the functional limitations depend on the level affected. Common limitations include impaired ambulation and difficulty with daily activities, such as snow shoveling, carrying groceries, vacuuming, etc. Work activities may be limited due to mobility and cognitive issues. Ongoing seizure activity may also limit employment and socialization outside the home. Similarly, incontinence of bowel and/or bladder can also limit these activities.

Diagnostic Studies

Imaging and laboratory studies are generally performed to evaluate a variety of co-existing problems in the patient with a history of NTD (e.g., new fractures).

MRI is the study of choice for evaluating hydrocephalus and tethered cord syndrome. In a patient with prior surgery for tethered cord syndrome and new onset of similar symptoms, a spinal MRI for evidence of retethering is warranted. When an occult lumbosacral dysraphism is suspected in a young adult, conventional three-plane MRI is still preferable compared to fast screening two-plane MRI.[17] Urologic studies have also been shown to help elucidate tethered cord syndrome.[2,14]

Routine annual serum creatinine and renal ultrasound may be used as screening tools throughout adulthood. In the patient with a neurogenic bladder, standard spinal cord management and vigilance for symptomatic infections are appropriate (e.g., following for urinary tract infections or renal impairment or calcifications).

Evaluation for altered urologic status or new-onset back pain in pre-menopausal women should include a workup for pregnancy.

Additionally, standard screens (e.g., screening for bladder cancer) for adults with spinal cord injuries should be considered for patients with NTDs.[13] This may be especially important as longevity increases, given evidence that older patients with NTDs have less frequent care.

For women with NTDs, routine health maintenance should be pursued even more aggressively, as it is often neglected. Thus breast exams, Pap smears, and discussions of contraception and sexually transmitted diseases are requisite.

New, rapid techniques for evaluating latex allergies are emerging, but standbys include quantitative IgE determination.[7]

Differential Diagnosis

Multiple Sclerosis	Tumor
Spinal cord infarction	Progressive spastic paraparesis

Treatment

Initial

Clinicians caring for adult patients with NTDs usually inherit the results of initial treatment that patients received as children.[18] Occult tethered cord syndrome is an exception, during which neurosurgical consultation is advised.[3,19] However, it is important to note that surgery for this condition remains controversial.

In the adult stage, the focus is on prevention, both with respect to sequelae of the disease and to the natural effects of aging. Contractures and fractures should be prevented, while cardiovascular fitness should be maximized and obesity minimized.[11,12] Vocational rehabilitation and its success are dependent on cognitive abilities. Management of appropriate referrals and services maximizes potential. Specific medical issues should be addressed appropriately (e.g., skin breakdown). Refer to the other chapters in this text for management of specific problems (e.g., osteoporosis).

Counseling and monitoring of caloric intake with diet and energy expenditure are advised for obesity.

A sensitive balance is necessary in counseling family members of young adults with NTDs, as the nature and degree of family involvement and encouragement alter the functional outcome of such patients.[20] Similarly, familial counseling is requisite to assist in ongoing stressors, both verbalized and non-verbalized.[21] The educational transition requires a thorough review of plans and needs. Although young adults with NTDs generally fare better than those with cerebral palsy or other complex prenatal conditions, strong guidance and assessment are necessary. Multidisciplinary cooperation is the cornerstone to all care of the patient with NTDs, but this dictum is especially true in the psychosocial/educational arena.[22]

As with most people, those with NTDs often have a strong interest in sexual activity, however, they require more dialogue with their health care providers, particularly in the transitional periods of adolescence and young adulthood.[23] Sildenafil (Viagra) has been used successfully in male patients with NTDs and impotence.[24]

Rehabilitation

Physical and occupational therapy referrals can be immensely helpful to the patient with NTD. The focus of supervised therapy can encompass a number of goals, including evaluating mobility issues, such as wheelchair equipment, braces, crutches, etc. Residua of foot conditions (including club feet, calcaneovalgus, and vertical talus deformities) may need to be addressed with therapy, orthotics, or surgery. Therapy can include improving range of motion at the joints and general strengthening exercises. Night splints can be used to help improve ankle flexion contractures; however, it is important to carefully monitor the skin. Adaptive equipment (e.g., reacher, hand controls for the car) may be recommended by skilled therapists.

New braces can be fabricated with the help of a skilled orthotist. Wheelchair options should be explored with a reputable vendor.

General conditioning is important for overall good health, but also to prevent obesity and maintain mobility as the patient ages. Supervised therapy can be instrumental in providing someone with an appropriate home exercise program to achieve these goals.

Vocational counseling may also be beneficial to assist job entry or retention. Cognitive issues as well as mobility may limit employment options. Ergonomic adaptive equipment and goal-oriented vocational training can markedly improve a patient's chances of becoming gainfully employed.

Procedures

Botulinum toxin or phenol injections may be considered for assisting in spasticity management (refer to Chapter 136).

Surgery

Potentially useful surgical procedures include primary closure of the NTD; tenotomy, tendon transfer, muscle release, and club foot repair; spinal fusion; tethered cord release; osteotomy; cervical decompression; and cystoplasty. Although management of adult tethered spinal cord is controversial, early surgery is suggested.[3,19]

Potential Disease Complications

As noted previously, tethered cord syndrome, whether operated on or not, and Chiari II malformations are complications of NTDs. In addition to the symptoms already discussed, the sequelae of NTDs include skin breakdown, dysfunctional swallowing and changing bowel control, infertility, scoliosis, osteoporosis, obesity, urinary tract infections, and psychosocial concerns.

Potential Treatment Complications

The possible complications depend on the individual treatments administered. A cautionary reminder is to the well documented association of NTDs with latex allergies. Education for both patients and health care providers should be emphasized to minimize exposure.[6]

References

1. Botto LD, et al: Neural-tube defects. N Engl J Med 1999;341:1509–1519.
2. Giddens JL, Radomski SB, Hirschberg ED, et al: Urodynamic findings in adults with the tethered cord syndrome. J Urol 1999;161:1249–254.
3. Iskandar BJ, et al: Congenital tethered spinal cord syndrome in adults. J Neurosurg 1998;88:958–961.
4. Stillwell A, Menelaus MB: Walking ability in mature patients with spina bifida. J Pediatr Orthop 1983;3:184–90.
5. Mataro M, Poca MA, Sahuquillo J, et al: Cognitive changes after cerebrospinal fluid shunting in young adults with spina bifida and assumed arrested hydrocephalus. J Neurol Neurosurg Psychiatry 2000;68:615–621.
6. McDonnell GV, McCann JP: Link between the CSF shunt and achievement in adults with spina bifida. J Neurol Neurosurg Psychiatry 2000;68:800.
7. Niggemann B, Wahn U: A new dipstick test (Allergodip) for in vitro diagnosis of latex allergy—validation in patients with spina bifida. Pediatr Allergy Immunol 2000;11:56–59.
8. Pang D (ed): Spinal dysraphism. Neurosurg Clin North Am 1995;6:1–417.
9. Berry RJ, et al: Prevention of neural-tube defects with folic acid in China. N Engl J Med 1999;341:1485–1490.
10. Bruner JP, et al: Fetal surgery for myelomeningocele and the incidence of shunt-dependent hydrocephalus. JAMA 1999;282:1819–1825.
11. McDonnell GV, McCann JP: Issues of medical management in adults with spina bifida. Childs Nerv Syst 2000;16:222–227.
12. Gross SM, Ireys HT, Knisman SL: Young women with physical disabilities: Risk factors of symptoms of eating disorders. J Dev Behav Pediatr 2000;21:87–96.
13. Game X, Villers A, Malavaud B, Sarramon J: Bladder cancer arising in a spina bifida patient. Urology 1999;54:923.
14. Persun ML, Ginsberg PC, Harmon JD, Harkaway RC: Role of urologic evaluation in the adult spina bifida patient. Urol Int 1999;62:205–208.
15. Singhal B, Mathew KM: Factors affecting mortality and morbidity in adult spina bifida. Eur J Pediatr Surg 1999;9(Suppl 1):31–32.
16. Fiorenino L, Datta D, Gentle S, et al: Transition from school to adult life for physically disabled young people. Arch Dis Child 1998;79:306–311.
17. Santiago Medina L, al-Orfali M, Zurakowski D, et al: Occult lumbosacral dysraphism in children and young adults: Diagnostic performance of fast screening and conventional MR imaging. Radiology 1999;211:767–771.
18. Alderson JD: Adult spina bifida. Anaesthesia 2000;55:697–698.
19. Craig JJ, Gray WJ, McCann JP: The Chiari/hydrosyringomyelia complex presenting in adults with myelomeningocele: An indication for early intervention. Spinal Cord 1999;37:275–278.
20. Loomis JW, Javornisky JG, Monahan JJ, et al: Relations between family environment and adjustment outcomes in young adults with spina bifida. Dev Med Child Neurol 1997;39:620–627.
21. Monsen RB: Mothers' experiences of living worried when parenting children with spina bifida. J Pediatr Nurs 1999;14:157–163.
22. Kaufman BA, et al: Disbanding a multidisciplinary clinic: Effects on the health care of myelomeningocele patients. Pediatr Neurosurg 1994;21:36–44.
23. Sawyer SM, Roberts KV: Sexual and reproductive health in young people with spina bifida. Dev Med Child Neurol 1999; 41:671–675.
24. Palmer JS, Kaplan WE, Firlit CF: Erectile dysfunction in spina bifida is treatable. Lancet 1999;354:125–126.

120 Neurogenic Bladder

Ayal M. Kaynan, MD
Inder Perkash, MD

Synonyms

None

ICD-9 Codes

344.61
Cauda equina syndrome
with neurogenic bladder

596.4
Atony of bladder

596.51
Hypertonicity of bladder

596.52
Low bladder compliance

596.53
Paralysis of bladder

596.54
Neurogenic bladder NOS

596.55
Detrusor sphincter
dyssynergia

596.59
Other functional disorder
of bladder

596.9
Unspecified disorder of
bladder

Definition

The term *neurogenic bladder* describes a process of dysfunctional voiding as the result of neurologic injury. In one way or another, this type of injury can interfere with urine storage at low bladder pressures or with controlled coordinated urinary voiding. Approximately 91,000 patients are discharged from hospital care annually in the United States for paralysis and hereditary or degenerative neurologic disease.[1] Because control of bladder function is at multiple levels throughout the central nervous system and subject to multiple pathophysiologic processes, voiding dysfunction results in most of these patients.

Symptoms

The symptoms of neurogenic bladder run a wide spectrum of presentation and include urinary incontinence, urinary retention, suprapubic or pelvic pain, incomplete voiding, paroxysmal hypertension with diaphoresis (autonomic dysreflexia), urinary tract infection, and occult deterioration in renal function. The symptoms vary according to the pathophysiology and are detailed later. To understand the pathophysiologies, the clinician must have a thorough understanding of the relevant anatomy.

The micturition reflex center has been localized to the pontine mesencephalic reticular formation in the brainstem.[2,3] Efferent axons from the pontine micturition center travel down the spinal cord in the reticulospinal tract to the detrusor motor nuclei located in the S2, S3, and S4 segments in the sacral gray matter (vertebral levels T12 to L2).[4]

Parasympathetic nerves take their origin from nuclei at the intermediolateral gray column of the spinal cord at S2, S3, and S4, and travel via the pelvic nerve and pelvic plexus to ganglia in the bladder wall. Acetylcholine is released from the postganglionic nerves, which in turn excite muscarinic receptors.

Preganglionic sympathetic neurons originate in the intermediolateral gray column of the spinal cord from spinal segments T10 to L2. These nerves course to the sympathetic chain ganglion and ultimately through the pelvic plexus to the bladder neck, which constitutes the internal (smooth muscle, involuntary) urethral sphincter, as well as the fundus of the bladder. Receptors at the bladder neck are primarily alpha-adrenergic,[6] stimulation of which results in closure of the internal sphincter during urinary storage, and in men, during ejaculation, as well. In contrast to the bladder neck, the fundus of the bladder is populated with beta-adrenergic receptors, which contribute to bladder relaxation (and therefore urinary storage) during sympathetic activation.

The external urethral sphincter (striated muscle, voluntary) surrounds the membranous urethra and extends up and around the distal part of the prostatic urethra. The pudendal nerves, which innervate the external sphincter, take their origin from the somatic motor nuclei in the anterior gray matter of the sacral cord (conus, S2 to S4); however, it is the S2 spinal segment that provides the principal motor contribution.[7] The toe plantar flexors also have S1 and S2 innervation. Thus, the preservation of toe plantar flexors following spinal cord injury suggests that the external urethral sphincter is intact.

Cortical lesions (lesions above the pontine micturition center) result in loss of voluntary inhibition of the micturition reflex, though the reflex is coordinated. The result is a hyperreflexic bladder with coordinated (synergic) sphincter function.[9] In the absence of outflow obstruction (e.g., urethral stricture, benign prostatic hyperplasia, large uterine leiomyoma, fecal impaction), complete bladder evacuation with incontinence is the outcome.

All lesions from the pons to spinal cord level S2 result in loss of cortical inhibition and loss of coordinated sphincter activity during reflex voiding. Reflex arcs in this arrangement, without inhibitory or coordinated control from higher centers, result in a hyperreflexic bladder with dyssynergic sphincter function (*detrusor-sphincter dyssynergia* [*DSD*]), which often results in incomplete voiding, high bladder pressures, and ureteral reflux.[10] Urinary retention from functional obstruction occurs; overflow incontinence may occur.

Complete spinal cord lesions above T5–T6 result in *autonomic dysreflexia*, in which the bladder is allowed to fill to excess. This is virtually always seen in conjunction with DSD.[11] It results from loss of cortical and medullary inhibitory reflexes modulating sympathetic activity of the splanchnic bed (T5 to T8). Accentuated visceral activity (e.g., full bladder, fecal impaction), which causes sympathetically mediated vasoconstriction, is normally inhibited by secondary output from the medulla and is countered by vasodilation in the splanchnic bed through the greater splanchnic nerve. Without the proper inhibitory reflexes or control of the splanchnic bed to redistribute circulating blood volume, blood pressure rises sharply. With the carotid bodies and vagal nerves intact, bradycardia results. The full syndrome is characterized by paroxysmal and extreme elevation in blood pressure, facial flushing, perspiration, goose pimples, headache, and bradycardia.

Spinal cord lesions at S2 or below result in lower motor neuron injury to the bladder and external sphincter. The effect on the bladder is predictable: areflexia. Because the parasympathetic ganglia reside in or near the bladder wall, bladder tone is generally maintained. Bladder compliance therefore tends to decrease with time as a result of neural decentralization (and/or infection related fibrosis).[12] The results on the bladder neck and external sphincter are not as intuitive. Although an atonic synergic sphincter system might be expected, the external sphincter usually retains some fixed tone, though not under voluntary control, and the bladder neck is often competent, but non-relaxing. Even though bladder pressures are generally low during filling/storage, obstructive physiology is often the case during voiding.[13] Overflow incontinence is typical.

In the acute phase of injury, most CNS lesions result in a temporarily areflexic bladder.[14,15] This phase, termed CNS shock, is variable and can last weeks to months.

The specific patterns of voiding dysfunction seen with the most common neurologic abnormalities in the chronic phase are detailed in Table 1 and Figure 1.

Confounding medical problems such as diabetes, and many cardiovascular drugs (Table 2) will profoundly affect upon bladder function. Patients who catheterize themselves intermittently should be asked about the size of catheter used and whether there is any resistance or trauma during catheterization—clues to the presence of a urethral stricture. Patterns of voiding should be elicited, and changes in voiding habits should be scrutinized. Patients with suprasacral spinal cord

TABLE 1 Patterns of Voiding Dysfunction in Chronic Neurologic Disease

Neurologic Disorder	Detrusor Activity	Striated Sphincter	Comments
Suprapontine	**Hyperreflexic**	**Synergic**	
Brain tumor			DSD may occur in those with spinal cord damage; voluntary control may be impaired
Cerebral palsy			
Cerebrovascular accident			Voluntary control may be impaired
Delayed CNS maturation			Persistence of uninhibited bladder beyond age 2–3 years; enuresis later
Dementia			Voluntary control is impaired
Parkinson's disease			Detrusor contractility and voluntary control may be impaired
Pernicious anemia			Bladder compliance may be decreased
Shy-Drager syndrome			Bladder neck remains open; bladder compliance may be decreased
Pons–S1	**Hyperreflexic**	**Dyssynergic**	
Anterior spinal cord			Bladder compliance may be decreased
Ischemia			
Multiple sclerosis			
Myelodysplasia			
Trauma			
Below S1	**Areflexic**	**Fixed Tone**	
Acute transverse myelitis			Bladder neck may be closed but non-relaxing
Diabetes			
Guillain-Barré syndrome			
Herniated intervertebral disk			
Myelodysplasia			Decreased bladder compliance may develop; bladder neck may be open
Poliomyelitis			
Radical pelvic surgery			Bladder neck is open
Tabes dorsalis a			Bladder neck may be closed but non-relaxing
Trauma			

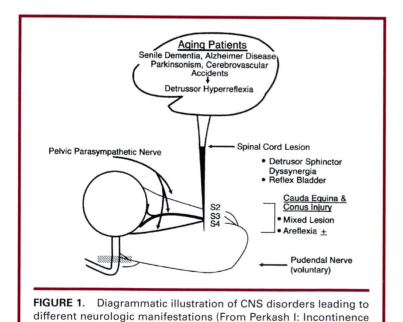

FIGURE 1. Diagrammatic illustration of CNS disorders leading to different neurologic manifestations (From Perkash I: Incontinence in patients with spinal cord injuries. In O'Donnell P (ed): Geriatric Urology. Boston, Little, Brown, 1994, pp 321–325, with permission.)

injury, for example, often give a history of intermittent stream coinciding with spasticity of their lower extremities, a strong clue to DSD. Approximately 50% of men ultimately have benign prostatic hyperplasia. Thus, even in the case of stable neurologic disease, these men may develop difficulty voiding from progressive outflow obstruction. Typical symptoms include nocturia, decreased force of stream, hesitancy, and postvoid dribbling. However, patients with outflow obstruction frequently have irritative voiding symptoms as well. It is important to learn whether there has been evidence of symptomatic infection: back pain, suprapubic pain, fevers, dysuria, urgency, frequency, or hematuria. These symptoms are

TABLE 2. Pharmacological Action on the Bladder

Drug	Indication	Mechanism	Side Effects/Cautions
Cholinergics Bethanechol	Areflexic bladder	Muscarinic receptor agonists	Bronchospasm, miosis

Anticholinergics
  Hyoscyamine
  Oxybutynin
  Tolterodine
	Hyperreflexic bladder	Muscarinic receptor antagonists	Constipation, dry mouth, tachycardia

Sympathomimetics
  Norepinephrine
  Pseudoephedrine
	Open bladder neck	Alpha receptor agonists	Arrhythmia, hypertension, coronary vasospasm, excitability, tremors

Antiadrenergics
  Phenoxybenzamine
  Phentolamine
  Terazosin
  Doxazosin
  Tamsulosin
	Smooth sphincter dys-synergia (competent, non-relaxing bladder neck)	Alpha receptor antagonists	Orthostatic hypotension, dizziness, rhinitis, retrograde ejaculation

Tricyclic antidepressants
  Amitriptyline
  Imipramine
	Hyperreflexic bladder with stress incontinence	Anticholinergic and sympathomimetic properties	Myocardial infarction, tachycardia, stroke, seizures, blood dyscrasias, dry mouth, drowsiness, constipation, blurred vision

Benzodiazepines Chlordiazepoxide	Extremity spasticity with detrusor-sphincter dyssynergia*	GABA channel activator, centrally acting muscle relaxant	Dizziness, drowsiness, extra-pyramidal effects, ataxia, agranulocytosis
Baclofen	Extremity spasticity with detrusor-sphincter dyssynergia*	GABA-b channel activator?, exact mechanism unknown; centrally acting muscle relaxant	CNS depression, cardiovascular collapse, respiratory failure, seizures, dizziness, weakness, hypotonia, constipation, blurred vision*
Dantrolene	Extremity spasticity with detrusor-sphincter dyssynergia	Direct muscle relaxant via Ca^{++} sequestration in the sarcoplasmic reticulum	Hepatic dysfunction, seizures, pleural effusion, incoordination, dizziness, nausea, vomiting, abdominal pain
Botulinum toxin	Detrusor-sphincter dyssynergia	Inhibits release of acetylcholine	Repeat injections necessary

* Note that Baclofen is also administered intrathecally via an implanted pump in these patients, and adverse effects are primarily limited to the CNS. Bladder contractility may also be reduced. No significant change in DSD.

not specific and can reflect many of the processes discussed. Their presence must therefore be interpreted according to context.

Physical Examination

General considerations include the level of disability and the capability to use upper and lower extremities. The neurologic exam should focus on the strength and dexterity of the upper extremities and the tone and reflexes of the lower extremities. Perianal sensation should be tested for evidence of sacral sparing.

The genitalia are examined for condition of the penis, whether it is circumcised, its size, and adequacy of the meatus. Attention should be given to the presence of meatal erosion. In women, it is important to note the appearance of the urethral meatus—this structure erodes quite readily with longstanding catheterization. Pelvic exam will identify confounding factors to voiding dysfunction, such as uterine prolapse or leiomyoma. Rectal exam should yield information on anal tone, size of prostate, and any presence of fecal impaction. Voluntary contraction of the anal sphincter indicates control over the perineal muscles, and in the presence of quadriplegia, it indicates an incomplete central cord type lesion. To determine voluntary contraction, the clinician places a finger in the patient's anal canal. The bulbocavernosus reflex should be tested. Because deep tendon reflexes at the patella reflect status of the spinal cord at L4, hyperreflexia at the knee almost certainly indicates increased tone at the pelvic diaphragm and thus DSD. Spasticity of the toe flexors reflects upper motor neuron damage to S2, and it therefore predicts spasticity of the external urinary sphincter (DSD). For patients with spinal cord injury, the return of reflexes heralds the conclusion of spinal cord shock. Acute phase physiology then switches to chronic physiology.

The first and most important determination with regard to bladder function should be the establishment of good bladder evacuation. The abdomen must be examined therefore for bladder palpability following a trial of voiding. Either a bladder ultrasound scan or urinary catheterization should be performed to determine the postvoid residual.

Functional Limitations

Functional limitations are typically due to incontinence and include social rejection and isolation. Incontinence may also affect a patient's ability to work, participate in recreational activities, and sustain interpersonal relationships.

Diagnostic Studies

All patients with neural injury should have blood chemistries drawn at baseline and periodically during followup for BUN and creatinine. Renal and bladder ultrasound should be performed to assess the status of the urinary tract, including size, shape, and echogenicity of the kidneys; presence of hydronephrosis and/or hydroureter; presence of renal or bladder stones; change in hydronephrosis during and after voiding; and completeness of the void. If vesicoureteral reflux or urethral strictures are suspected, a voiding cystourethrogram may be performed.

If renal stones are suspected, a non-contrast CT (renal stone protocol) is an excellent tool for identification of the size and location of the stones. When dealing with renal stones, it is sometimes important to assess calyceal or ureteral anatomy, or differential renal function, in which case an intravenous urogram (IVU) may be performed. Finer qualitative assessment of differential renal function may be performed by Tc^{99}-MAG3 nuclear renal scan. When there is suspicion for compromise of renal function, this test may be useful.

Transrectal linear array ultrasonography may be performed to assess prostate size, the presence of a prominent median prostatic lobe, the presence of a ledge at the bladder neck,[27] and proximal urethral/bladder neck strictures.

Cystoscopy is an excellent tool for studying bladder and urethral anatomy: it quickly identifies the presence of a urethral stricture (though it may not determine its length or depth), provides an assessment of internal prostatic size; provides indirect evidence of high intravesical pressures (bladder trabeculation), and readily demonstrates bladder stones. Cytoscopy is essential in the assessment of hematuria (more than 5 rbc/hpf on two or more urine specimens). While hematuria in neurally injured patients is commonly related to infection or traumatic catheterization, the use of catheters, particularly indwelling catheters, places these patients at significantly higher risk for bladder cancer.[28] It has been suggested therefore that these patients undergo surveillance cystoscopy annually, particularly if they have other risk factors for bladder cancer, such as smoking or a family history with bladder cancer. No test is as sensitive for the detection of bladder tumors. Note that cystoscopy does not provide functional information: the best single test for bladder function is urodynamics.

Formal urodynamic testing, including cystometrogram (CMG) and electromyography (EMG), is crucial to the proper documentation of bladder and outlet function. The test is subject to inherent errors in technique, interpretation, and patient cooperation, however, and the astute clinician must interpret the results in light of the entire clinical scenario. Properly performed, it will elucidate and quantify postvoid residual of urine, bladder capacity, bladder compliance, bladder pressures during filling and voiding, and external sphincteric coordination. In conjunction with videofluoroscopic monitoring, ureteral reflux, bladder position, and internal and external sphincteric function may be visualized. Urodynamics should be performed at baseline for all patients with neurologic disease. Because of CNS shock in the acute phase of injury, it is best to perform urodynamics after shock resolves—upon return of distal reflexes. Figure 2 illustrates a normal voiding pattern. Figure 3 illustrates the urodynamic findings of an areflexic bladder. Figure 4A shows detrusor-sphincter dyssynergia. The sonographic correlate of detrusor-sphincter dyssynergia is shown in Figure 4B (non-relaxation of the external urethral sphincter is demonstrated).

Differential Diagnosis

The diseases listed in Table 1 are the most common causes of neurogenic bladder.

Treatment

Initial

The priorities of bladder management relate first to preservation of renal function and abolition of infection and secondly to social concerns. Overflow incontinence, ureteral reflux, or high bladder pressures in the presence of renal insufficiency or active infection must be managed aggressively by ensuring proper egress for urine. A source for persistent infection such as urinary lithiasis must be sought, and if found, eliminated. High bladder pressure (more than 40 cmH$_2$O) alone ultimately results in deterioration of renal function and should therefore be addressed actively, even if renal function is normal.[29]

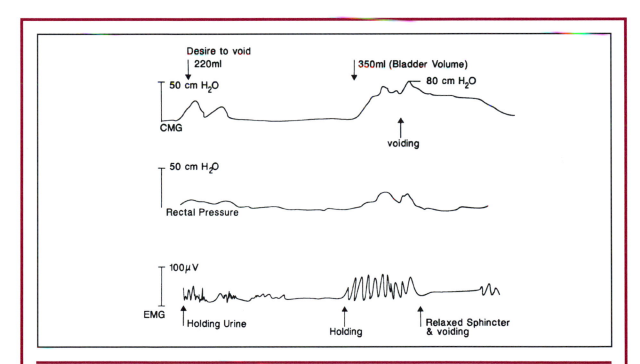

FIGURE 2. Urodynamic study consisting of simultaneous cystometrogram (CMG), rectal pressure, and EMG of the external urethral sphincter. During Bladder filling, the desire to void is usually expressed between 300 and 400 ml. When the normal person is asked to hold urine, the external urethral sphincter contracts and the bladder relaxes. When asked, this person voided voluntarily at a filling volume of approximately 350 ml: the external urethral sphincter relaxed just prior to voiding, indicating a normal study.

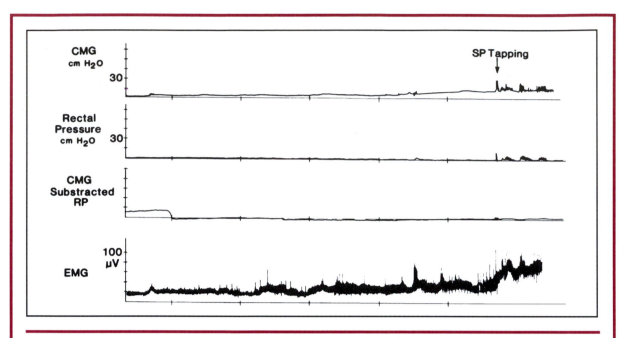

FIGURE 3. Urodynamic study demonstrating an areflexic bladder in a patient with spinal cord injury. There is minimal increase in EMG activity during filling of the bladder. There is no bladder contraction, even after tapping suprapubically, indicating overdistention areflexia or a lower motor neuron lesion.

Patients at risk for degenerative neurogenic bladders, particularly those with (or at risk for) sensory neuropathies (e.g., diabetics, phenytoin users), should be placed on a timed voiding schedule to prevent overdistention and progression to bladder areflexia. A 24-hour voiding diary, including fluid intake, time and quantity voided, and postvoid residual (by catheterization), should be recorded periodically. These patients should void every 6 hours, void again immediately following the first void, and adjust their fluid intake and voiding frequency according to the voiding diary. Patients with diabetes should be careful to maintain good glycemic control, not only for global prevention of related degenerative disease but also to prevent osmotic diuresis.

Most neurogenic injuries to the bladder are associated with impaired bowel function. Fecal impaction and obstipation not only place the patient at risk for colon perforation, they may also cause mechanical obstruction to the passage of urine. Further, many of the medications used to reduce bladder contractility, particularly the anticholinergics, exacerbate bowel motile dysfunction. It is important therefore that these patients be routinely placed on high fiber diets, stool softeners (e.g., docusate 100 mg po tid), laxatives (e.g., psyllium 1 packet po qd), and suppositories (e.g., bisacodyl 10 mg pr qd) and undergo digital stimulation either daily or qod. Digital stimulation is best performed following a meal in order to take advantage of the gastrocolic reflex.

Crede's method (suprapubic pressure) alone can lead to high intravesical pressures and even vesicoureteral reflux. Such pressure, or persistent tapping of the suprapubic region for 2 minutes at a time, should only be performed when methods to relieve bladder outlet obstruction have been ensured. This should not be performed in patients with active detrusor-sphincter dyssynergia because it will only exacerbate already high bladder pressures, and urine will not be completely evacuated.

Acute Phase/CNS Shock

This phase usually lasts days to weeks but sometimes persists for months. The bladder is areflexic during this period, and adequate bladder drainage should be secured to prevent the areflexic bladder from developing overdistention and atony. Indwelling continuous Foley catheter (14 Fr) is

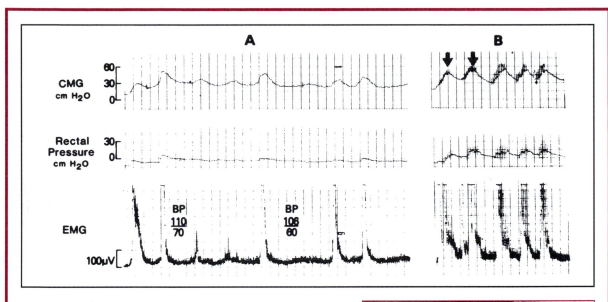

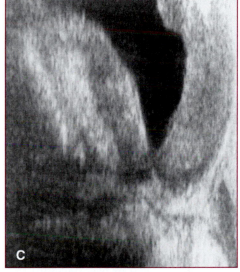

FIGURE 4. *A* and *B*, Detrusor-sphincter dyssynergia in a patient with spinal cord injury: each bladder contraction (CMG) is accompanied by a marked increase in EMG activity of the external urethral sphincter. *C*, Ultrasound cystourethrogram during an attempted void in a patient with spinal cord injury with detrusor-sphincter dyssynergia. The passage of urine is abruptly stopped by closure of the external urethral sphincter, and the posterior urethra is dilated.

the easiest way to ensure bladder drainage. Alternatively, intermittent catheterization may be performed, and when used from the onset, reduces the incidence of infection and stone disease.[30]

Catheterization is performed every 4 to 6 hours and fluid is restricted to 2 liters per day, if possible. The frequency of catheterization should be adjusted so that residuals are no more than 300 to 400 cc. For patients with a hyperreflexic bladder, long-term intermittent catheterization requires mitigation of the detrusor reflex with anticholinergic medication to reduce bladder pressures to safe levels (less than 40 cmH$_2$O), and to achieve continence between catheterizations.

Autonomic Dysreflexia

The control of widespread sympathetic activity below the spinal lesion is the key factor in the management of autonomic dysreflexia, and prevention is the first concern. Noxious stimuli such as overdistention of the bladder should be reversed immediately by catheter drainage. Local instillation of 25 to 50 cc of 0.25% tetracaine via the Foley catheter or suprapubic tube may provide topical anesthesia of the vesical mucosa and reduce triggering impulses to the spinal cord. Consideration of procedures for patients at risk (spinal lesions above T6) should include spinal anesthesia, use of ganglion blockers, and use of adrenergic blockers.

In the acute episode, if reversal of the noxious stimulus fails to control symptoms, administration of nifedipine 30 mg po is usually adequate to reduce blood pressure.[41] Note that normal blood pressure for a patient with spinal cord injury is less than 100 mm Hg systolic. If nifedipine fails, hydralazine 5 mg IV, or 5 to 20 mg IM, may be administered and repeated every 5 minutes as necessary to maintain a low blood pressure. Other useful drugs include alpha-blockers, such as prazosin, guanethidine, clonidine, and anticholinergics, such as oxybutynin or tolterudine. For long-term management of subacute autonomic dysreflexia, clonidine 0.1 to 0.3 mg po bid is useful. Note that the chronic form of this syndrome is often related to active DSD, and methods aimed at controlling this phenomenon, such as transurethral sphincterotomy, may alleviate the patient of autonomic dysreflexia.[11]

Urinary Tract Infections

For those who have had indwelling Foley catheters for an extended period (more than several days) and require catheter removal or exchange, antibiotics should be administered prophylactically before, during, and after removal of the existing catheter. Gentamicin 80 mg IM once just prior to removal of the catheter is appropriate for most patients with stable renal function (even if function is impaired) and has both gram-positive and gram-negative coverage. Those with prosthetics, aortic stenosis, or other risk factors for seeding should have co-administration of ampicillin 1 g IV for enterococcus coverage. Alternatively, amoxicillin/clavulanic acid 750 mg or ciprofloxacin 500 mg may be given po bid pericatheter removal. In addition, the bladder should be irrigated gently via the catheter with 50 ml of normal saline containing 120 ug/ml Neosporin and 60 ug/ml polymixin B. Irrigation is continued while the catheter is being pulled through the urethra. This method has been shown to significantly reduce urinary tract infection related to catheter changes.[42,43]

Attention to hygiene is paramount in the prevention of urinary tract infections in the spinal cord injured population. Those who wear condom catheters should change the catheter once a day. Leg bags should be routinely disinfected with 6% Clorox solution or bleach (most cost-efficient) and then washed well with running water. Wheelchair seat cushions should be changed and cleaned, and the patient should take a shower daily to reduce colony counts at the perineum. Patients who demonstrate recurrent infections should be considered for suppressive treatment. Nitrofurantoin 50 to 100 mg po twice a day is sufficient. Methenamine hippurate 1 g po tid and ascorbic acid 500 mg po qd acidify the urine and are good for UTI prophylaxis.[44]

Rehabilitation

Supervised physical or occupational therapy is not typically indicated in neurogenic bladder except in cases where patients need training or assistance in self-catheterization. Rehabilitation nurses may also be involved in this educational process.

Procedures

Another alternative to long-term management of these bladders is placement of a suprapubic catheter. This is preferable to chronic transurethral catheterization because it eliminates the risk of urethral or meatal erosion and is less often the cause of epididymitis/orchitis. Urinary tract infections, however, are just as likely, and these catheters require changing once a month. They are best placed either in the operating room under cystoscopic guidance, or better, via suprapubic incision to ascertain that the catheter ultimately resides as superiorly as possible, far from the bladder neck. This helps to prevent irritation at the bladder neck, which often causes reflex bladder contractions, particularly if the catheter balloon (also in an indwelling Foley catheter) drops down into the posterior urethra (Fig. 5).

For patients with hyperreflexic bladders, electrical stimulation through peripheral patch electrodes or implantation of a sacral nerve root stimulator may be of some benefit. The treatment is dependent on intact sacral reflex and works by inhibition of the pudendal-pelvic nerve reflex. Patients must be able to voluntarily (or Valsalva) empty their bladders when the device is turned off or be capable of

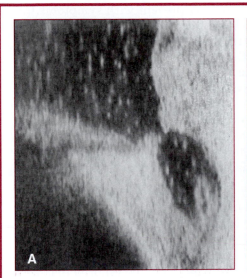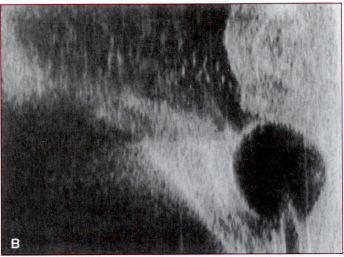

FIGURE 5. *A,* Linear array ultrasound–voiding cystourethrogram shows a contracted bladder neck and dilated prostatic urethra. *B,* The balloon of the urethral Foley is lodged in the prostatic urethra. This occurs uncommonly; however, it may lead to inadequate bladder drainage and, in patients with lesions above T6, autonomic dysreflexia.

performing self-intermittent catheterization. Its effectiveness varies: the majority have no benefit and approximately one third have a 30% decrease in urinary frequency.[38] It should be noted that studies reported are primarily in able-bodied populations with idiopathic detrusor hyperreflexia.[39]

Surgery

Transurethral sphincterotomy has been used in suprasacral lesions in the past and has fallen into disfavor because of intraoperative and delayed bleeding potential. Use of the sapphire-tip contact Nd:YAG laser[31] and other laser energy sources yield virtually no intraoperative bleeding and are capable of vaporizing the obstructive tissue very efficiently. This procedure results in global incontinence postoperatively and requires the use of an external condom catheter.

There are rare circumstances in which bladder management has aggravated renal function, evidenced by recurrent ascending urinary tract infections or a bladder that is too contracted to store sufficient volumes. Some patients find it socially unacceptable to be incontinent and are willing to perform self-intermittent catheterization, but the body habitus precludes them from this. In such cases, there are certain reconstructive options that should be considered. Cystectomy and either incontinent diversion (uretero-ileal conduit) or continent diversion (uretero-ileocecal conduit) may be performed. Patients must have reasonably good renal function to qualify for continent diversion, lest they suffer from electrolyte and metabolic disturbances.[36]

The most common reconstructive alternative is an ileovesical conduit. The bladder is augmented by a segment of ileum that acts as a conduit to the skin where a stoma is fashioned. The ureters remain in their native locations. Bladder pressure is reduced because the system is opened, and continence is dependent on a hyperactive sphincter.

For bladders that have low pressures and good compliance but leak through fixed sphincters, the Mitrofanoff and bladder neck closure may be an excellent option. Spina bifida patients with conus lesions might be good candidates for this procedure. Egress through the bladder neck is eliminated, and the appendix is interposed between the bladder and the umbilicus where it is opened. In the common event that the bladder has poor compliance, an ileal bladder augmentation will raise bladder volume and lower bladder pressure. Patients would then catheterize their augmented bladders via the umbilicus.

Patients with spinal cord injury who have a UTI commonly may not present with symptoms.[4] Fevers, chills, back pain, suprapubic pain, dysuria, frequency, and testicular swelling in the setting of positive urine cultures should be regarded as a urinary tract infection. Patients without overt symptoms of pyelonephritis, prostatitis, epididymitis/orchitis, or cystitis are more difficult to diagnose, particularly if they have an indwelling catheter or are being managed by intermittent catheterization. Those using catheters are virtually always colonized with bacteria,[45] and the injudicious use of antibiotics will only select out resistant strains. Factors indicating a need for treatment include presence of urinary lithiasis, as these are most often related to infection (struvite, magnesium ammonium phosphate), and pyuria (8 to 10 WBCs per high power field, or 100 WBCs/ml) in the setting of bacteriuria (more than 10,000 CFU per ml).[4] Urine pH should be checked periodically: pH greater than 7 is invariably associated with infection from urea-splitting organisms, which may lead to struvite stone formation.

Patients with DSD or urinary retention of any kind should have their bladders drained expeditiously with a fresh Foley catheter during the course of their treatment to ascertain good egress of infected urine. If prostatitis is suspected, transurethral insertion of a Foley catheter is absolutely contraindicated, and drainage should be ensured suprapubically. Fluoroquinolones are an excellent first choice for most urinary tract infections; therapy may then be tailored to culture and sensitivity when results return. Three to five days is sufficient for cystitis. Pyelonephritis requires 2 to 3 weeks of therapy. Epididymitis requires at least 3 weeks of therapy, and prostatitis often requires 6 weeks.

Potential Disease Complications

Urinary tract infections (Table 2), kidney stones, and autonomic dysreflexia are common disease complications associated with neurogenic bladder. Social isolation due to incontinence may lead to depression.

Potential Treatment Complications

Stoma care is a source of great consternation for many who have it because of frequent appliance leaks and skin irritation. Also, the stoma must be situated properly on the abdomen according to patient habitus and positioning in the wheelchair. It should be recognized that bladder augmentations of any kind are susceptible to perforations and life-threatening infections (as much as 10%). These patients have a 3% chance of small bowel obstruction from adhesions during their lifetime.[37] Chronic indwelling Foley catheters carry the potential for urinary infection, meatal erosion, epididymitis/orchitis, and urethral fistula. In women, the urethra becomes patulous in time and incontinent with or without a catheter. Finally, with time and repeat infections, indwelling catheters put patients at risk for developing squamous cell cancer of the bladder. While the incidence is low, gross hematuria should be evaluated with great suspicion in these patients because this disease is often advanced at time of discovery and is quite fatal.[32]

References
1. Clinical classifications for health policy research: Hospital inpatient statistics, 1995. Table 1: Statistics for 1995 HCUP-3 nationwide inpatient sample, by expanded CCHPR diagnosis (prinicipal diagnosis only), section 6: Diseases of the nervous system and sense organs. http://www.ahcpr.gov/hcup/his95/table1b.htm#6
2. Bradley WE, Timm GW, Scott FB: Innervation of the detrusor muscle and urethra. Urol Clin North Am 1974;1:3.
3. Denny-Brown D, Robertson EG: On the physiology of micturition. Brain 1933;56:149.
4. Perkash I: Long-term urologic management of the patient with spinal cord injury. Urol Clin North Am 1993;3:423–434.
5. Igawa Y: Discussion: Functional role of M(1), M(2), and M(3) muscarinic receptors in overactive bladder. Urol 2000;55(Suppl 5A):47–49.
6. Gosling JA, Dixon JS: The structure and innervation of smooth muscle in the wall of the bladder neck and proximal urethra. Br J Urol 1975;47:549.
7. Perkash I: Management of neurogenic dysfunction of the bladder. Xxx 2000; xxx.
8. deGroat WC, Ryall RW: Reflexes to sacral parasympathetic concerned with micturition in the cat. J Physiol 1969;200:87.
9. Khan A, Hertanu J, Yang WC, et al: Predictive correlation of urodynamic dysfunction and brain injury after cerebrovascular accident. J Urol 1981;126:86–88.

10. deGroat WC, Steers WD: Autonomic regulation of the urinary bladder and sexual organs. In Loewy AD, Spyer KM (eds): Central Regulation of Autonomic Functions, 1st ed. Oxford, Oxford University Press, 1990, p 313–314.
11. Perkash I: Pressor response during cystomanometry in spinal injury patients complicated with detrusor-sphincter dyssynergia. J Urol 1979;121:778–782.
12. Fam B, Yalla SV: Vesicourethral dysfunction in spinal cord injury and its management. Semin Neurol 1988;8:150.
13. Wein AJ: Neuromuscular dysfunction of the lower urinary tract and its treatment. In Walsh PC, Retik AB, Vaughan ED, et al (eds): Campbell's Urology, 7th ed. Philadelphia, W.B. Saunders, 1998, p 955.
14. Burney TL, Senapti M, Desai S, et al: Acute cerebrovascular accident and lower urinary tract dysfunction: A prospective correlation of the site of brain injury with urodynamic findings. J Urol 1996;156:1748–1750.
15. Borrie MJ, Campbell A, Caradoc-Davies TH, et al: Urinary incontinence after stroke: A prospective study. Age Ageing 1986;177:15.
16. Berger Y, Salinas J, Blaivas J: Urodynamic differentiation of Parkinson disease and the Shy-Drager syndrome. Neurourol Urodynam 1990;9:117.
17. Wein AJ, Barrett DM: Etiologic possibilities for increased pelvic floor electromyography activity during bladder filling. J Urol 1982;127:949.
18. Wein AJ: Neuromuscular dysfunction of the lower urinary tract and its treatment. In Walsh PC, Retik AB, Vaughan ED, et al (eds): Campbell's Urology, 7th ed. Philadelphia, W.B. Saunders, 1998, p 957.
19. Blaivas JG, Kaplan SA: Urologic dysfunction in patients with multiple sclerosis. Semin Urol 1988;8:159.
20. Mayo ME, Chetner MP: Lower urinary tract dysfunction in multiple sclerosis. Urology 1992;39:67.
21. Giddens JL, Radomski SB, Hirshberg ED, et al: Urodynamic findings in adults with the tethered cord syndrome. J Urol 1999;161:1249–1254.
22. Wheeler JS, Culken DJ, Ottara RJ, et al: Bladder dysfunction and neurosyphilis. J Urol 1986;136:903.
23. Frimodt-Moller C: Diabetes Cystopathy: A Clinical study on the frequency of bladder dysfunction in diabetics. Dan Med Bull 1976;23:267.
24. Appell RA. Voiding dysfunction and lumbar disc disorders. Prob Urol 1993;7:35–40.
25. Leveckis J, Boucher NR, Parys BT, et al: Bladder and erectile dysfunction before and after rectal surgery for cancer. Br J Urol 1995;76:752–756.
26. Khan Z, Bhola A: Urinary incontinence after transurethral resection of prostate in myasthenia gravis patients. Urol 1989;34:168.
27. Perkash I, Friedland GW: Posterior ledge at the bladder neck: crucial diagnostic role of ultrasonography. Urol Radiol 1986;8:175–183.
28. West DA, Cummings JM, Longo WE: Role of chronic catheterization in the development of bladder cancer in patients with spinal cord injury. Urol 1999;53:292–297.
29. Flood HD, Ritchey ML, Bloom DA, et al: Outcome of reflux in children with myelodysplasia managed by bladder pressure monitoring. J Urol 1994;152:1574–1577.
30. Guttman L, Frankel H: Value of intermittent catheterization in early management of traumatic paraplegia and teraplegia. Paraplegia 1966;4:63.
31. Perkash I: Contact laser sphincterotomy: further experience and longer follow-up. Spinal Cord 1996;34:227–233.
32. Serretta V, Pomara G, Piazza F, et al: Pure squamous cell carcinoma of the bladder in western countries. Report on 19 consecutive cases. Eur Urol 2000;37:85–89.
33. Gillberg PG, Sundquist S, Nilvebrant L: Comparison of the in vitro and in vivo profiles of tolterodine with those of subtype-selective muscarinic receptor antagonists. Eur J Pharmacol 1998;349:285-292.
34. Drutz HP, Apell RA, Gleason D, et al: Clinical efficacy and safety of tolterodine compared to oxybutynin and placebo in patients with overactive bladder. Int Urogynecol J Pelvic Floor Dysfunct 1999:10:283–289.
35. Perkash I: Management of neurogenic bladder dysfunctions following acute traumatic cervical central cord syndrome (incomplete tetraplegia). Paraplegia 1977;15: 21–37.
36. McDougal WS: Use of intestinal segments and urinary diversion. In Walsh PC, Retik AB, Vaughan ED, et al (eds): Campbell's Urology, 7th ed. Philadelphia, W.B. Saunders, 1998, p 1346.
37. Rink RC, Adams MCL: Augmentation cystoplasty. In Walsh PC, Retik AB, Vaughan ED, et al (eds): Campbell's Urology, 7th ed. Philadelphia, W.B. Saunders, 1998, pp 3167–3189.
38. Ohlsson BL, Fall M, Frankenberg-Sommars D: Effects of external and direct pudendal nerve maximal electrical stimulation in the treatment of the uninhibited overactive bladder. Br J Urol 1989;64:374.
39. Jonas U, Fowler CJ, Chancellor MB, et al: Efficacy of sacral nerve stimulation for urinary retention: Results 18 months after implantation. J Urol 2001;165:15–19.
40. Gasparini ME, Schmidt RA, Tanagho EA: Selective sacral rhizotomy in the management of the reflex neuropathic bladder: A report on 17 patients with long-term followup. J Urol 1992;148:1207–1210.
41. Messerli FH, Grossman E: The use of sublingual nifedipine: a continuing concern. Arch Intern Med 1999;159: 2259–2260.
42. Rhame FS, Perkash I: Urinary tract infections occurring in recent spinal cord injury patients on intermittent catheterization. J Urol 1979;122:669–673.
43. Pearman JW: Prevention of urinary tract infections following spinal cord injury. Paraplegia 1971;9:95.
44. Banovac K, Wade N, Gonzalez F, et al. Decreased incidence of urinary tract infections in patients with spinal cord injury: effect of methenamine. J Am Paraplegia Soc 1991;14:52–54.
45. Brisset L, Vernet-Garnier V, Carquin J, et al: In vivo and in vitro analysis of the ability of urinary catheter to microbial colonization. Pathol Biol 1996;44: 397–404.

121 Osteoarthritis

Andrew D. Shiller, MD

Synonyms

Degenerative joint
disease (DJD)

ICD-9 Codes

715.0
Osteoarthrosis,
generalized

715.1
Osteoarthrosis, localized,
primary

715.2
Osteoarthrosis, localized,
secondary

715.3
Osteoarthrosis, localized,
not specified whether
primary or secondary

715.9
Osteoarthrosis,
unspecified whether
generalized or localized

716.1
Traumatic arthropathy

716.9
Arthropathy, unspecified

Definition

Osteoarthritis (OA) is the most common form of chronic arthritis and is characterized by degeneration of the articular cartilage. It is one of the most common causes of chronic disability among older persons in the United States. The typical patient with OA is middle-aged or elderly.

OA is a localized, rather than systemic, disease. Joint involvement is usually asymmetric, with a predilection for weight-bearing joints. Common sites of involvement are the hip, knee, distal and proximal interphalangeal joints, and facet joints of the spine. Less common sites of involvement are the ankle, wrist, and shoulder. Inflammation and joint effusion are present in some cases.

Risk factors for OA include advanced age, obesity, and participation in activities that predispose toward repetitive microfractures.[1] Epidemiologic data also suggest increased risk of OA in persons with low levels of vitamins D and C and estrogen deficiency.[2] Other causative factors include inflammatory arthritis (rheumatoid arthritis or spondyloarthropathies), metabolic joint disease (hemochromatosis, acromegaly, gout, pseudogout), trauma, and congenital structural abnormalities.

The mechanisms of cartilage degeneration, pain, and functional loss in OA are not completely understood. Progression of disease and disability results from a complex interaction among biochemical, biomechanical, neuromuscular, and psychosocial variables (Fig. 1).

Symptoms

The most common symptoms of OA are joint stiffness and activity-related pain. In early disease, pain is usually gradual in onset, mild in intensity, brought on by joint usage, and relieved with rest. Pain is typically self-limited or intermittent. Pain at rest or at night suggests severe disease or another diagnosis. Stiffness tends to be most pronounced in the morning and after periods of inactivity. Patients with advanced disease may describe a sense of grinding or locking with joint motion, and buckling or instability of joints during demanding tasks. Spasm of periarticular muscles may be prominent and painful. Patients may complain of fatigue if biomechanical changes lead to increased energy requirements for activities of daily living. Overuse of alternative muscle groups can lead to development of pain syndromes in other parts of the musculoskeletal

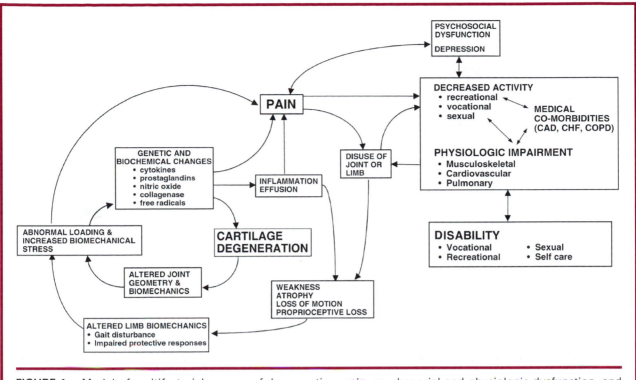

FIGURE 1. Model of multifactorial process of degeneration, pain, psychosocial and physiologic dysfunction, and diability that may occur in osteoarthritis.

system. For example, the lurching gait often associated with severe hip degeneration can result in back pain, or discomfort due to misalignment in the knee.

Some symptoms are specific to involved joints. For instance, hip pain often radiates to the groin, thigh, or knee. Spinal disease may cause neck or back pain. If spinal osteophytes compress nerve roots, radicular symptoms such as pain, weakness, or numbness may result. Erosive OA may be associated with painful inflammation and loss of dexterity in the hands.

Nerve impingement due to spinal disease can result in pain, weakness, or sensory loss in the related dermatome or myotome.

Physical Examination

Joint examination: Involved joints may show evidence of tenderness, bony enlargement, or misalignment. Inflammation occurs in some cases, and is suggested by mild to moderate warmth, soft-tissue swelling, or joint effusion. A hot, erythematous, markedly swollen joint suggests septic arthritis or superimposed crystal disease, such as gout or pseudogout. In OA, range of motion may be limited due to osteophytes, joint surface irregularity, periarticular muscle spasm, or chronic disuse. Range-of-motion testing may elicit pain and crepitus. Locking during range of motion suggests loose bodies or floating cartilage fragments in the joint. Joint contracture can result from holding a joint in slight flexion, which is less painful for inflamed or swollen joints. There may be secondary abnormalities in joints above or below the primarily involved joint.

Neuromuscular examination: Periarticular muscle atrophy and weakness may be present as previously described. It is notable that manual muscle testing is typically unreliable in the lower extremities due to the high baseline strength of these muscle groups. On the other hand, knee extensor strength can be assessed by asking the patient to rise one-legged from a chair. The Trendelenburg test (see page 191) can elicit weakness in hip abductors. A careful neurologic examination should be performed to ensure that pain is not a result of nerve impingement or neuropathic process.

Functional Limitations

Functional limitations will depend on the joints involved. Patients with disease in the hips and knees can suffer from reduced walking speed and efficiency; difficulty climbing stairs; trouble with transferring in and out of cars, chairs, or toilet facilities; and problems with lower body dressing and grooming. Degeneration in the shoulders or hands can limit vocational and recreational activities, grooming, eating, and other activities of daily living. Spinal degeneration can result in limitations with all mobility.

Diagnostic Studies

Plain radiographs are important in confirming the diagnosis of OA. The classic findings include asymmetric joint space narrowing, osteophytes at joint margins, cortical sclerosis, and subchondral cyst formation. There is a well-demonstrated discordance between x-ray findings and symptoms in OA. Asymptomatic individuals may have significant radiographic disease, and severe pain and dysfunction can occur in the setting of limited radiologic changes. Magnetic resonance imaging (MRI) is typically not needed for diagnosis of OA, but can be helpful in ruling out early osteonecrosis if OA is not evident on plain x-rays of painful joints.

Routine laboratory tests are usually normal in OA. Joint fluid analysis can be helpful in ruling out crystal deposition disease (gout, pseudogout), inflammatory arthritis, or infectious arthritis and should be pursued in patients with significant joint inflammation. In osteoarthritis, synovial fluid leukocyte counts are typically less than 2000 cells/mm^3. A markedly elevated erythrocyte sedimentation rate raises suspicion for polymyalgia rheumatica, other inflammatory disorder, malignancy, or occult infection.

Differential Diagnosis

Neoplasm	Soft tissue infection	Radiculopathy
Deep venous thrombosis	Bursitis	Neuropathy
Osteomyelitis	Tendinitis	Polymyalgia rheumatica
Occult fracture	Ligamentous injury	Inflammatory arthritis
Aseptic necrosis	Overuse injury	Crystal arthritis (gout, pseudogout)

Treatment

Initial

The management of osteoarthritis involves attention to four important principles: avoiding drug toxicity, limiting physical disability, relieving pain and other symptoms, and maximizing physical function and psychosocial adjustment.

No intervention has been shown conclusively to alter disease progression in OA. A number of interventions have been demonstrated to reduce pain and stiffness and improve functional status.

Acetaminophen and nonsteroidal anti-inflammatory drugs (NSAIDs) are typically first-line agents and useful in reducing pain. They are best used in conjunction with nonpharmacologic interventions as well. Clinical trials have not shown benefit of NSAIDs over acetaminophen.[3,4] However, clinical experience and a series of blinded n-of-1 crossover trials suggest that some individuals seem to respond better to NSAIDs than acetaminophen.[5]

A quantitative systematic review of 86 trials evaluating the efficacy of topical NSAIDs in osteoarthritis and tendinitis found them significantly more effective than placebo.[6] However, no one topical NSAID seems to be better than the others.[7]

Topical capsaicin cream has also been shown to reduce pain in joints affected by OA. This derivative of cayenne pepper causes exuberant release and depletion of substance P, which is involved in pain transmission. Limited data from controlled trials have shown improvements with capsaicin.[8] It is worthwhile to caution patients that they may experience increased pain while beginning therapy with capsaicin.

Recent attention has focused on the use chondroitin or glucosamine. Chondroitin and glucosamine are naturally occurring substrates for the synthesis of articular cartilage. To date, there have been no large-scale randomized controlled trials of these compounds in humans with OA. Small controlled studies have shown that glucosamine affords pain relief that is similar in magnitude to that of NSAIDS.[9] Recent meta-analyses of both chondroitin and glucosamine found moderate to large reduction in symptoms of pain and immobility.[10] Studies that have evaluated time course of improvement have shown a delay of up to 1 month in onset of pain relief after treatment begins. The benefit has persisted for several weeks or months after glucosamine is discontinued. Patients considering the use of glucosamine or chondroitin should be cautioned that no long-term trials have evaluated their safety and that these products are not subject to regulation regarding purity or accuracy of labeling.

To prevent side effects, a prudent approach to systemic analgesic use involves acetaminophen to a maximum dosage of 4 g/day in patients with normal hepatic function. Patients who continue to have pain or those at low risk for toxicity should be given NSAIDs. Topical capsaicin or NSAIDs may also help reduce the use of systemic NSAIDs.

Patients with osteoarthritis should be screened for depression and treated appropriately with nonpharmacologic and pharmacologic interventions. Nonpharmacologic interventions are also important and effective in promoting wellness and reducing disability. Multifactorial self-management programs improve self-efficacy by providing experiential skills in disease management, physiologic self-regulation, emotional hygiene and interpersonal communication. Studies have demonstrated reduced pain, improvements in health behavior, and reduction in utilization of health care resources in patients with chronic pain and arthritis.[11-14] Group-based self-management programs are often available through a local chapter of the Arthritis Foundation and may overlap significantly in content with typical hospital-based behavioral medicine programs.

Rehabilitation

A comprehensive rehabilitative approach addresses prevention and treatment of pain and disability through counseling; education, encouraging weight loss; exercise; adaptive equipment; and superficial modalities, such as heat and cold.

A physical therapist can guide and encourage a stretching program that can ease the stiffness associated with sleep or prolonged immobility and prevent or reduce impairment in range of motion. Patients should be educated in appropriate positioning during extended inactivity or sleep. Appropriate use of heat before stretching can help loosen tight periarticular muscles, and application of ice packs after exercise can reduce the need for analgesic medications. Treatment time with the therapist should focus on education in the use of these interventions, rather than passive treatment. Gait and transfer training can improve functional mobility in patients with limitations in range of motion or strength. Finally, a therapist-guided program of aerobic and resistance exercise can safely decrease pain, prevent disability, and promote general conditioning.

Occupational therapy can provide training in energy conservation techniques to reduce fatigue in patients with reduced activity tolerance. In the setting of significant functional impairments, the therapist can provide assistive devices that help with feeding, grooming, dressing, and other activities of daily living.

Aerobic and resistive exercise provide important theoretical benefits, some of which are supported by clinical trials.[15] Static or dynamic strengthening exercises can maintain or improve periarticular muscle strength, thereby reversing or preventing biomechanical abnormalities and their contribution to joint dysfunction and degeneration. Aerobic exercise improves activity tolerance, increases pain threshold, and can have positive effects on mood and motivation for participation in other activities. There is evidence that exercise can also improve proprioception,[16] thus improving biomechanics and protective responses. A warm, shallow swimming pool is used as a setting for exercise in some rehabilitation centers. The warmth and buoyancy can contribute to improved range of motion and decreased impact during aerobic exercise.

Clinical trials have demonstrated the effectiveness of structured exercise programs in reducing pain and disability due to osteoarthritis of the hip and knee.[17,18] Compared with patients who received health education, patients assigned to aerobic and resistance exercise programs had fewer self-reported disabilities, less pain, and greater knee flexion strength. The greatest effect was seen after the initial 3 months of supervised exercise.[19]

Adaptive equipment, such as a cane or walker, can reduce hip or knee loading, thereby reducing pain. It may also prevent falls in patients with impaired balance. Proper training in the use of a cane is important, since it reduces joint loading in the contralateral hip but amplifies forces in the ipsilateral hip.

Orthotics, bracing, or taping can mitigate abnormal joint loading and localized stress-concentration. In subjects with degeneration in the medial compartment of the knee, pilot studies have shown that valgus knee bracing and heel wedges can increase medial compartment joint space and redistribute loading to the lateral articular surfaces. Reliable clinical trials have not been performed to demonstrate whether this approach decreases pain and increases function.

There are no consistent data from clinical trials supporting the use of therapeutic cold, heat, or ultrasound. Clinical experience suggests that cold and heat can be helpful in decreasing pain and increasing mobility. Limited data support the use of acupuncture to reduce pain.[20,21] The use of transcutaneous electrical nerve stimulation (TENS) is supported by a few small, short-term trials.

Procedures

In randomized trials, intra-articular corticosteroids provided slightly improved pain relief compared to placebo injection of saline, though the effects typically last for only 1 to 3 weeks.[22]

The use of intra-articular hyaluronic acid (HA) is supported by theoretical considerations and limited data from controlled studies. Intra-articular HA injection is also referred to as viscosupplementation.

Clinical trials of HA injections have focused on patients with knee OA and have shown mixed results. Several studies show that subjects receiving HA injection to the knee experienced greater and longer-lasting pain relief as well as improved walking distance when compared to intra-articular injection of placebo saline.[23] Side effects included local inflammation and increased pain at the injection site. There is no evidence that HA injection in humans alters biologic processes or progression of cartilage damage. No clear dose-response trial has been published to determine ideal number of injections or dosage.[24] A typical course of treatment involves weekly injection for 3 to 5 weeks, and is typically repeated 2 to 4 times per year.

Surgery

In patients for whom pain and loss of mobility are disabling despite conservative management, orthopedic consultation should be obtained to assess risks and benefits of surgery.

Arthroscopic lavage and removal of loose bodies or osteophytes may be helpful in some patients who fail conservative therapy. Osteotomy has been used with some success to correct biomechanics and unload areas of high stress. Fusion may be helpful in situations when joint replacement is not appropriate.

In the past few decades, joint replacement surgery has provided tremendous improvements in quality of life for people with severe osteoarthritis (see Chapters 56 and 74). In older patients who experience functional limitations due to OA, hip replacement surgery has been shown to be cost-effective. A recent systematic review of hip replacement surgery trials concluded that in 70% of subjects, pain and function scores were rated good or excellent at 10 years post-operatively.[25] Observational studies have suggested that better outcomes are associated with the following patient characteristics: age 45 to 75 years; weight less than 70 kg; good social support; higher educational level; and less preoperative morbidity.[26] A small percentage of patients require revision due to persistent or recurrent pain, which is most often a result of aseptic loosening of the prosthetic joint. Similar results have been achieved in total knee replacement. In older patients with medical co-morbidities, early inpatient rehabilitation after hip or knee arthroplasty has been shown to reduce hospital stays and cost of care.[27]

Potential Disease Complications

Potential complications include pain; immobility; loss of capacity to perform occupational, recreational and social roles; and loss of self-care skills.

Potential Treatment Complications

Analgesics, NSAIDs, and COX-2 inhibitors have well-known side effects that most commonly affect the gastric, hepatic, and renal systems. It is notable that gastrointestinal (GI) bleeding from NSAID-induced ulcers commonly occurs without pain or abdominal discomfort as a warning sign. Risk for GI toxicity is dose-dependent and increases with prolonged usage, concurrent medical illness, and advanced age. Unfortunately, OA is a chronic disease that requires long-term treatment and is most common in older patients, who are at risk for GI complications. Potential benefit of NSAIDs in individual patients must be weighed against the increased risk of GI toxicity.

Acetaminophen carries the risk of hepatitis, and topical NSAIDs/capsaicin may produce local irritation. The possible side effects of glucosamine/chondroitin are unknown. Intra-articular steroids or HA can result in infection and local irritation and pain.

The risk factors of joint replacement surgery are bleeding, prosthetic failure, infection, pain, venous thrombosis, pulmonary embolism, and complications of general anesthesia.

References

1. Delisa J, Lane NE, Block DA, et al: Long distance running, bone density, and osteoarthritis. JAMA 1986;225:1147–1152.
2. Felson DT: Preventing hip and knee osteoarthritis. Bulletin Rheum Dis 1998;47(7):1–4.
3. Bradley JD, Brandt KD, Katz BP, et al: Comparison of an anti-inflammatory dose of ibuprofen, an analgesic dose of ibuprofen, and acetaminophen in the treatment of patients with osteoarthritis of the knee. N Engl J Med 1991;325:87–91.
4. Williams HJ, Ward JR, Egger MJ, et al: Comparison of naproxen and acetaminophen in a 2-year study of treatment of osteoarthritis of the knee. Arthritis Rheum 1993;36:1196–1206.
5. March L, Irwig L, Schwarz J, et al: N-of-1 trials comparing non-steroidal anti-inflammatory drug with paracetamol in osteoarthritis. BMJ 1993;309:1041–1046.
6. Moore RA, Tramer MR, Carroll D, et al: Quantitative systematic review of topically applied non-steroidal anti-inflammatory drugs. BMJ 1998;316:333–338.
7. Dickson DJ: A double-blind evaluation of topical piroxicam gel with oral ibuprofen in osteoarthritis of the knee. Curr Ther Res Clin Exp 1991;49:199–207.
8. Zhang WY, Po ALW: The effectiveness of topically applied capsaicin: A meta-analysis. Eur J Clin Pharmacol 1994;46:517–522.
9. Delafuente JC: Glucosamine in the treatment of osteoarthritis. Rheumatic Disease Clin North Am 2000;26(1):1–11.
10. McAlindon TE, LaValley MP, Gulin JP, Felson DT. Glucosamine and chondroitin for treatment of osteoarthritis: A systematic quality assessment and meta-analysis. JAMA 2000;283(11):1469–1475.
11. Caudill M, et al: Decreased clinic use by chronic pain patients: Response to behavioral medicine intervention. Clin J Pain 1991;7(4):305–310.
12. Lorig K, Mazonson PD, Holman HR: Evidence suggesting that health education for self-management in patient with chronic arthritis has sustained health benefits while reducing health care costs. Arthritis Rheum 1993;36:439–446.

13. Lorig KR, et al: Evidence suggesting that a chronic disease self-management program can improve health status while reducing hospitalization: A randomized trial. Medical Care 1999. 37(1):5–14.
14. Sobel, D: Rethinking medicine: Improving health outcomes with cost-effective psychological interventions. Psychosomatic Med 1995;57:234–244.
15. Minor MA: Exercise in the treatment of osteoarthritis. Rheumatic Disease Clini North Am 199925(2):397–415.
16. Hurley MV: The role of muscle weakness in the pathogenesis of osteoarthritis. Rheumatic Disease Clin North Am 1999;25(2):283–298.
17. Puett DW, Griffin MR: Published trials of nonmedicinal and noninvasive therapies for hip and knee osteoarthritis. Ann Intern Med 1994;121(2):133–140.
18. Kovar PA, Allegrante JP, MacKenzie R, et al: Supervised fitness walking in patients with osteoarthritis of the knee. A randomized, controlled trial. Ann Intern Med 1992;116:529–534.
19. Ettinger WH Jr, Burns R, Messier SP, et al: A randomized trial comparing aerobic exercise and resistance exercise with a health education program in older adults with knee osteoarthritis: The Fitness Arthritis and Seniors Trial (FAST). JAMA 1997;277:25–31.
20. Ernst E: Acupuncture as a symptomatic treatment of osteoarthritis: A systematic review. Scand J Rheumatology 1997;26(6):444–447.
21. Berman BM, Singh BB, Lao L, et al: A randomized trial of acupuncture as an adjunctive therapy in osteoarthritis of the knee. Rheumatology 1999;38(4):346–354.
22. Creamer P: Intra-articular corticosteroid treatment in osteoarthritis. Curr Opin Rheumatology 1999;11(5):417–421.
23. Huskisson EC, Donnelly S: Hyaluronic acid in the treatment of osteoarthritis of the knee. Rheumatology 1999;38:602–7.
24. Simon LS: Viscosupplementation therapy with intra-articular hyaluronic acid: Fact or fantasy. Rheumatic Disease Clin North Am 1999;25(2):345–357.
25. Faulkner A, Kennedy LG, Baxter K, et al: Effectiveness of hip prostheses in primary total hip replacement: A critical review of evidence and an economic model. Health Technol Assess 1998;2:1–33.
26. Young NL, Cheah D, Waddell JP, et al. Patient characteristics that affect the outcome of total hip arthroplasty: a review. Can J Surg 1998;41:188–195.
27. Munin MC, Rudy TE, Glynn NW, et al: Early inpatient rehabilitation after elective hip and knee arthroplasty. JAMA 1998;279(11):847–852.

122 Osteoporosis

David M. Slovik, MD

Definition

Osteoporosis is a systemic skeletal disease characterized by low bone mass and microarchitectural deterioration of bone tissue, with a consequent increase in bone fragility and susceptibility to fracture. Bone has a normal ratio of mineral to matrix.

Osteoporosis can also be defined according to World Health Organization criteria based on bone density measurements:

 a. Normal: A value for bone mineral density (BMD) or bone mineral content (BMC) that is not more than 1 standard deviation (SD) below the young adult mean value.

 b. Low bone mass (osteopenia): A value for BMD or BMC that lies between 1 and 2.5 SD below the young adult mean value.

 c. Osteoporosis: A value for BMD or BMC that is more than 2.5 SD below the young adult mean value.

 d. Severe osteoporosis (or established osteoporosis): A value for BMD or BMC more than 2.5 SD below the young adult mean value in the presence of one or more fragility fractures.

A *fragility fracture* is one that occurs without any trauma, after falling from a height of less than 12 inches, or after abrupt deceleration from a speed slower than a run.

Osteoporosis is the most common metabolic bone disease. The National Osteoporosis Foundation estimates that 10 million Americans have osteoporosis and another 18 million have decreased bone mass, putting them at increased risk for osteoporosis and fractures (Table 1). Of the 10 million, 8 million are women and 2 million are men. Annually in the United States more than 1.5 million fractures

TABLE 1.   Common Causes of Osteoporosis

Age-related: postmeno-
   pausal, senile

Endocrine-related
   Hypogonadism
   Hyperthyroidism
   Hyperparathyroidism
   Adrenal-cortical hormone
      excess
   Diabetes mellitus, type II

Genetics
   Osteogenesis
      imperfecta
   Ehlers-Danlos syndrome
   Homocystinuria

Immobilization

Hematologic disorders
   Multiple myeloma
   Systemic mastocytosis
   Thalassemia

Drug-related
   Glucocorticoids
   Thyroid hormone
      excess
   Cyclosporine
   Anti-convulsant drugs

Miscellaneous
   Rheumatoid arthritis

TABLE 2. Risk Factors for Osteoporosis

- Advanced age
- Female
- Small-boned, thin women
- Caucasian and Asian women
- Estrogen deficiency
- Personal history of fracture as adult
- Fracture in first-degree family members
- Inactivity
- Low calcium intake
- Cigarette smoking
- Alcoholism
- Medications such as glucocorticoids, excessive thyroid hormone, cyclosporine, antiseizure drugs

attributable to osteoporosis occur, including approximately 700,000 vertebral, 300,000 hip, and 250,000 wrist fractures. The annual cost of caring for osteoporotic-related fractures in the United States is in excess of $13 billion. In addition, there is a 10% to 20% excess mortality within the first year after a hip fracture.

Osteomalacia refers to a group of disorders characterized by an abnormality in bone mineralization. The ratio of mineral to matrix is diminished as a result of an excess of unmineralized osteoid.

Symptoms

Osteoporosis is a silent disease until a fracture occurs. Pain and deformity are usually present at the site of fracture. Vertebral fractures often occur with little trauma, such as coughing, lifting, or bending over. Acute back pain may be related to a vertebral compression fracture with pain localized to the fracture site or in a radicular distribution. New back pain or chronic back pain in a patient with osteoporosis and prior vertebral fractures may be related to new fractures, muscle spasm, or other causes.

With vertebral fractures there may be a gradual loss of height and the development of a kyphosis. Breathing may be difficult, and bloating—a sensation of fullness and dyspepsia may develop because of less room in the abdominal cavity.

Physical Examination

In evaluating patients with osteoporosis, it is important to diagnose treatable and reversible causes and to assess the risk factors for developing osteoporosis and osteoporotic fractures. Table 2 lists risk factors for osteoporosis.

The physical examination should focus on findings suggestive of secondary causes of osteoporosis (e.g., hyperthyroidism and Cushing's syndrome). One should also examine areas previously involved with fractures (e.g., back, hip, and wrist) to assess for deformity and limitation of function. A baseline measurement of height should be obtained and re-evaluated at subsequent visits.

Functional Limitations

Functional limitations will be related to the type of fracture and the long-term consequences and disabilities related to it. With vertebral fractures, the functional limitation may initially be related to the acute pain and inability to move. The chronic limitations may be related to loss of height, chronic back pain, difficulty moving, abdominal distention, and difficulty breathing. The functional limitations after a hip fracture are related to the decreased functional mobility, often the need for long-term use of assistive devices, the lack of independence, and the long-term need for assistive care.

Fifty percent of people with a hip fracture will permanently need an assistive device for ambulation, and two-thirds will lose some of their ability to perform ordinary daily activities.

Wrist fractures usually heal completely, but some people end up with chronic pain, deformity, and functional limitations.

Diagnostic Studies

Bone density measurements are the standard for assessing risk, diagnosing, and following patients with osteoporosis. Available techniques include single photon absorptiometry (SPA), dual-energy x-ray absorptiometry (DXA), quantitative computed tomography (QCT), and quantitative ultrasound (QUS). DXA, although not as sensitive as QCT for detecting early trabecular bone loss, is now the method of choice for measuring bone mineral density because of its good precision, low radiation dose, and fast examination time.

Bone mineral density (BMD) testing should only be performed if the results will influence a treatment decision. The National Osteoporosis Foundation suggests BMD testing in the following circumstances: (1) all post-menopausal women younger than 65 years who have one or more additional risk factors for osteoporosis (besides menopause); (2) all women 65 and older, regardless of additional risk factors; (3) postmenopausal women who present with fractures; (4) women who are considering therapy for osteoporosis, if BMD testing would facilitate the decision; and (5) women who have been receiving hormone replacement therapy for prolonged periods.[1]

BMD testing should also be obtained in patients receiving chronic glucocorticoid therapy, those with primary hyperparathyroidism, those with conditions placing them at high risk for osteoporosis, and to assess the response to treatment programs.

BMD is reported by T- and Z- scores (Table 3).

The T-score is the best measurement for risk assessment and can help confirm a diagnosis of osteoporosis. The lower the T-score the higher the risk for subsequent fractures. However, the score will not predict who will fracture since other factors come into play (e.g., fall velocity, type of fall, direction of fall, and protective padding).

TABLE 3.   BMD Reporting
T-score: Standard deviations (SDs) above or below peak bone mass in young, normal, sex-matched adults
Z-sore: Standard deviations (SDs) above or below age- and sex-matched adults

Specific laboratory testing should be obtained to help in the differential diagnosis of osteoporosis and to rule out osteomalacia. The general laboratory tests include a complete blood count, chemistry profile including liver and kidney tests, serum and urine protein electrophoresis, and thyroid-stimulating hormone. A 24-hour urine calcium and creatinine is also helpful. In some patients, especially elderly individuals suspected of having vitamin D deficiency, a serum 25-hydroxy vitamin D level should be obtained. A parathyroid hormone level should be obtained in suspected cases of primary or secondary hyperparathyroidism. Blood and urine tests are usually normal in uncomplicated cases of osteoporosis. After a fracture the alkaline phosphatase may be elevated. Biochemical markers of bone turnover, including urine N-telopeptide, may be helpful in selective patients to assess for bone turnover and whether someone is responding to treatment.

Differential Diagnosis

Common causes of osteoporosis are listed in Table 1.

Treatment

Initial

The initial approach to the prevention and treatment of osteoporosis involves non-pharmacologic intervention and, in appropriate patients, the use of various pharmacologic agents (Table 4). Treatment guidelines are in Table 5.

TABLE 4.   Treatment Options
Nonpharmacologic
Calcium
Vitamin D
Exercise
Fall prevention
Pharmacologic agents
Hormone-replacement therapy
Selective estrogen receptor modulators
Raloxifene
Bisphosphonates
Alendronate
Risedronate
Calcitonin

TABLE 5. Treatment Guidelines

Early menopausal women
  Hormone-replacement therapy (first
    choice)
  Raloxifene 60 mg/day
  Alendronate 5 mg/day or 35 mg once
    weekly
  Risedronate 5 mg/day

Late menopausal women
  Alendronate 10 mg/day or 70 mg
    once weekly (first choice)
  Risedronate 5 mg/day
  Raloxifene 60 mg/day
  Calcitonin (nasal spray) once daily
  Hormone replacement therapy

Calcium: Epidemiologic studies suggest that long-standing dietary calcium deficiency can result in lower bone mass. The average dietary calcium intake in postmenopausal women is less than 500 mg per day. Several studies have shown that calcium supplementation, especially in the elderly, may slow bone loss and reduce vertebral and nonvertebral fracture rates.[2] A total calcium intake of 1200 to 1500 mg per day is recommended for postmenopausal women. This can be achieved by consumption of foods that have a high calcium content, such as milk and dairy products, especially yogurt. Calcium supplementation is often required, especially in elderly individuals.

Vitamin D: Vitamin D deficiency is common in postmenopausal women with hip fracture and in elderly subjects, especially those who are chronically ill, housebound, institutionalized, and poorly nourished.[3] A dose of 400 to 800 IU per day (1to 2 multivitamins) should be sufficient in preventing vitamin D deficiency.

Exercise: There is increasing evidence that exercise is beneficial to bone in helping achieve peak bone mass and preserving bone later in life.[4] Bone adapts to physical and mechanical loads placed on it by altering its mass and strength. This occurs either by the direct impact from the weight-bearing activity or by the action of muscle attached to bone. Exercising can also help strengthen back muscles, improve balance, lessen the likelihood of falling, and give one a sense of well-being.[5] Back extension exercises and abdominal strengthening exercises are helpful. However, acute stresses to the back must be avoided to lessen the likelihood of fracturing. A proper exercise program should be established. Older postmenopausal women and even the frail elderly can tolerate and potentially show improvements in muscle strength and BMD in response to strength training and resistive exercise programs.

Fall prevention: Many factors can lead to falls, including poor vision, frailty, medication (especially hypotensive agents and psychotropic agents), and balance disturbances.[6] Each area needs to be assessed appropriately. Other prevention measures include the following:

Keeping room free from clutter	Having good lighting
Avoiding slippery floors	Placing grab bars in the bathroom
Being aware of thresholds	Using a portable telephone
Wearing supportive shoes	Having personal alarm activator
Tacking down rugs	Having someone check regularly

Hormone replacement therapy (HRT): HRT can be used in the short-term management of postmenopausal women with symptoms of estrogen deficiency, including hot flashes, memory deficits, urinary frequency, and vaginal dryness. Long-term HRT can slow bone loss and lower the incidence of fractures and may lessen the likelihood of heart disease, although recent studies have questioned this.[7] Estrogens may exert a protective effect against heart disease, acting both by favorably affecting lipoproteins (increasing HDL and lowering LDL) and by a direct vascular effect.

Long-term estrogen therapy has been shown to increase the incidence of cancer of the endometrium and probably gallbladder disease. In addition, studies have shown that there may be a small increase in the incidence of breast cancer with long-term hormone replacement therapy.

Women who have had a hysterectomy should be given estrogen alone. A progestin should be added to the estrogen regimen if the uterus is still present. The following two regimens of estrogen and progesterone together are commonly used:

1. Continuous estrogen plus cyclic progestin (e.g., medroxyprogesterone 5 mg orally or the equivalent for 10 to 14 days per month)

2. Continuous estrogen plus continuous progestin (e.g., medroxyprogesterone 2.5 mg orally per day or the equivalent)

Anti-estrogens (selective estrogen receptor modulators [SERMs]): SERMs are synthetic compounds that have both estrogen-antagonistic and estrogen-agonistic properties. Raloxifene (Evista) is approved by the FDA for the prevention and treatment of osteoporosis at an oral dose of 60 mg daily. Raloxifene reduces new vertebral fractures by 40% to 50% but not the risk of nonspine fractures.[8] Raloxifene acts as an anti-estrogen on breast tissue and has been reported to reduce the risk of invasive breast cancer.[9] Raloxifene does not produce uterine hypertrophy. Although it may have beneficial effects on serum lipoproteins, it is not clear whether it has any beneficial effect on cardiac disease. Raloxifene has no beneficial effects on menopausal symptoms and may increase the risk of deep vein thrombosis to a degree similar to estrogen.

Bisphosphonates: The bisphosphonates are a group of compounds related chemically to pyrophosphate. They are characterized by a P-C-P structure. Changes in the side chains affect the potency of the bisphosphonates. They are potent inhibitors of osteoclastic bone resorption. Alendronate is approved by the FDA for the prevention and treatment of postmenopausal osteoporosis. Alendronate is also approved for the treatment of glucocorticoid-induced osteoporosis[10] and osteoporosis in men.[11] The dose in postmenopausal women for *prevention* is 5 mg per day or 35 mg once weekly and for *treatment* 10 mg per day or 70 mg once weekly. Alendronate significantly increases bone mineral density at various sites. In addition, there is a significant decrease in the incidence of vertebral, hip, and wrist fractures, as well as painful vertebral fractures, hospitalization days, and other measurements of functional impairment.[12]

Risedronate is approved by the FDA for the prevention and treatment of postmenopausal osteoporosis with an oral dose of 5 mg daily. Studies have shown an increase in bone mineral density at various sites along with a decrease in vertebral and non-vertebral fractures.[13] Risedronate is also approved for the prevention and treatment of glucocorticoid-induced osteoporosis.

The bisphosphonates are very poorly absorbed and must be given on an empty stomach to maximize their absorption. Alendronate and risedronate must be taken at least 30 minutes before the first food, beverage, or medication with a full glass of plain water, and patients should avoid lying down for at least 30 minutes to avoid the potential side effect of esophagitis; patients with a history of reflux should not be given these medications.

Calcitonin: For more than 15 years, synthetic salmon calcitonin given parenterally by injection has been approved for the treatment of postmenopausal osteoporosis. Several years ago the nasal spray of calcitonin was approved in a dose of 200 units (one spray) daily. A reduction in new vertebral fractures has been reported but no effect on nonvertebral fractures. Occasional nasal irritation or headache may be seen with the nasal spray.

Rehabilitation

Rehabilitation efforts in osteoporosis can commence long before a fracture. Either a physical or occupational therapist can be involved in assessing the patient's home to make sure it is safe and to decrease the risk of falls. Specialized equipment, such as grab bars for the bathroom and handheld reachers for high cupboards, can be very helpful. Educating patients about keeping the floors clear of clutter and throw rugs is important. Small pets also can be a hazard underfoot.

Therapists can assess whether the patient would be safer ambulating with an assistive device (e.g., cane or walker) in the home and community. It is important that all assistive devices are appropriately prescribed and fitted for the patient.

Finally, therapists can instruct patients about how to exercise to improve strength, flexibility, and balance. All of these activities can help prevent falls, and weight-bearing strengthening exercises may also improve bone density.

In patients with a hip fracture or other disabling fracture, a multidisciplinary coordinated team approach involving the physician, therapists, and other rehabilitation specialists (e.g., nurse) is necessary for the patient to regain maximal function and lead a productive life. The initial rehabilitation program also involves pain control, bowel and bladder care, and maintaining skin integrity. The therapists, in addition to working on a program involving bed mobility, transfers, gait activities, safety precautions, and activities of daily living, must be cognizant of the medical problems in each patient. After an acute rehabilitation stay, some patients may need an additional stay in a transitional setting on their way to eventually getting home or else require long-term placement. For those able to go home, the team needs to teach the patient a home exercise program, order appropriate equipment, and arrange for continued therapy, either at home or in an outpatient setting.

Procedures

Other than surgery, procedures are generally not needed in the management of osteoporosis. Two procedures—vertebroplasty and kyphoplasty—to stabilize vertebral fractures and alleviate pain are under investigation.

Surgery

Surgical repair and stabilization is the preferred treatment for hip fracture and some other fractures.

Potential Disease Complications

As bone density decreases, the risk for sustaining a fracture increases. Osteoporosis is asymptomatic until a fracture occurs. Thereafter, all complications are related to the problems from these fractures; to the surgery, if required; and the recuperative period.

After vertebral fractures, acute pain may limit mobility. Bed rest and narcotic analgesics may be necessary. Severe constipation and urinary retention may ensue. Chronically, patients may suffer from severe back pain and have respiratory problems, abdominal distention, bloating, and constipation. Many patients who wear a back brace complain about the discomfort and difficulty in using it.

Potential Treatment Complications

The complications related to treatment can be related either to the surgical repair of the fracture and the recuperative phase or to medications used to prevent or treat osteoporosis.

Most osteoporotic fractures occur in older patients and result in loss of function and loss of independence and the need for long-term care. Since surgery is required to repair a hip fracture, complications from surgery, anesthesia, bed rest, and pain medications (often narcotics) are common. Pneumonia, phlebitis, urinary tract infection, constipation, and respiratory problems also are frequent.

Complications from drug therapy for osteoporosis include (1) potential increase in breast cancer, endometrial cancer (in those using only estrogen), and clotting from hormone-replacement therapyl; (2) hot flashes and increase in clotting from raloxifene; (3) upper gastrointestinal symptoms and esophagitis from alendronate and residronate; and (4) running nose and headache from calcitonin.

References

1. National Osteoporosis Foundation, et al: Physician's Guide to Prevention and Treatment of Osteoporosis. Excerpta Medica, 1998.
2. Dawson-Hughes B, Harris SS, Krall EA, Dallal GE: Effect of calcium and vitamin D supplementation on bone density in men and women 65 years of age or older. N Engl J Med 1997;337:670–676.
3. Leboff MS, Kohlmeier L, Hurwitz S, et al: Occult vitamin D deficiency in postmenopausal US women with acute hip fracture. JAMA 1999;281:1505–1511.
4. Slovik DM: Osteoporosis. In Frontera WF, Dawson D, Slovik DM (eds): Exercise in Rehabilitation Medicine. Human Kinetics, 1999, pp 313–348.
5. Nelson ME, Wernick S: Strong Women, Strong Bones. New York, G.P. Putnam, 2000.
6. Greenspan SL, Myers, ER, Kiel DP, et al: Fall direction, bone mineral density, and function: Risk factors for hip fracture in frail nursing home elderly. Am J Med 1998;104:539–545.
7. Hulley S, Grady D, Bush T, et al (for the Heart and Estrogen/Progestin Replacement Study (HERS) Research Group): Randomized trial of estrogen plus progestin for secondary prevention of coronary heart disease in postmenopausal women. JAMA 1998;280:605–613.
8. Ettinger B, Black DM, Mitlak BH, et al)for The Multiple Outcomes of Raloxifene Evaluation (MORE) Investigators): Reduction of vertebral fracture risk in postmenopausal women with osteoporosis treated with raloxifene: results from a 3-year randomized clinical trial. JAMA 1999;282:637–645.
9. Cummings SR, Eckert S, Krueger KA, et al: The effect of raloxifene on risk of breast cancer in postmenopausal women: results from the MORE randomized trial. JAMA 1999;281:2189–2197.
10. Saag KG, Emkey R, Schnitzer TJ, et al (for the Glucocorticoid Induced Osteoporosis Intervention Study Group): Alendronate for the prevention and treatment of glucocorticoid-induced osteoporosis. N Engl J Med 1998;339:292–299.
11. Orwoll E, Ettinger M, Weiss S, et al: Alendronate for the treatment of osteoporosis in men. N Engl J Med 2000;343:604–610.
12. Black DM, Cummings SR, Karpf DB, et al: Randomized trial of effect of alendronate on risk of fracture in women with existing vertebral fractures. Lancet 1996;348:1535–1541.
13. Harris ST, Watts NB, Genant HK, et al (for the Vertebral Efficacy with Risedronate Therapy (VERT) Study Group): Effects of risedronate treatment on vertebral and non-vertebral fractures in women with postmenopausal osteoporosis: a randomized, controlled trial. JAMA 1999;282:1344–1352.

123 Parkinson's Disease

Nutan Sharma, MD, PhD

Synonyms

Shaking palsy

Paralysis agitans

Idiopathic parkinsonism

ICD-9 Codes

332.0
Parkinsonism, primary

332.1
Parkinsonism, secondary

333.0
Supranuclear palsy

333.90
Extrapyramidal disease

781.0
Abnormal involuntary movements (tremor)

781.2
Gait abnormality

784.5
Other speech disturbance (dysarthria)

Definition

Parkinson's disease (PD) is a chronic, progressive neurodegenerative disease that is characterized, pathologically, by preferential degeneration of dopaminergic neurons in the substantia nigra pars compacta and the presence of cytoplasmic inclusions known as Lewy bodies.

PD has a prevalence of 110 per 100,000. Men have a slightly increased, age-adjusted incidence of PD. The average age of onset is 62 years. Clinically, the disease progresses slowly over the course of 10 to 15 years. Thus, depending on the age of onset, individuals may die from other causes unrelated to PD or from infection due to immobility at the end stages of PD.

Symptoms

Pain is a part of PD and may be the presenting complaint. An aching pain in the initially affected limb may first be attributed to bursitis or arthritis. Subsequent treatment with antiparkinson medication, resulting in improved mobility and pain relief, reveals that the pain is due to PD. Additional symptoms, seen early in the course of PD, include a resting tremor and a sensation of stiffness. The resting tremor is suppressed by either purposeful movement or sleep and exacerbated by anxiety. The sensation of stiffness occurs in the affected arm or leg and may be accompanied by the perception that one is slow with movement.

As the disease progresses, there is marked difficulty in both initiating and terminating movement. There is difficulty in arising from a seated position, particularly when one is seated in a sofa or chair without arm rests. Handwriting becomes smaller and more difficult to read. Friends and family members often complain that the patient's speech is more difficult to understand, particularly on the telephone. The symptom of a softer voice with a decline in enunciation is known as *hypophonia*.

Depression may be noted at any time during the course of the illness.

Physical Examination

The most common initial manifestations of PD are *rest tremor* and *bradykinesia*. Less common presenting complaints include hypophonia, gait difficulty, and fatigue. It is not uncommon for one of these features to be present for months or even years before others develop.

The most distinctive clinical feature is the rest tremor. It is typically present in a single upper extremity early in the course of the disease. As the disease progresses, the rest tremor may spread to both the ipsilateral lower limb as well as the contralateral limbs. Examination of motor tone reveals cogwheel rigidity in the affected limb. Strength, however, remains unaffected.

Additional features that must be evaluated in an examination include rapid, repetitive limb movements and gait. Examination of repetitive movements of the fingers or entire hand will reveal bradykinesia in the affected limb. Examination of gait will reveal decreased arm swing on the affected side, smaller steps, and an inability to pivot turn. Typically, patients make several steps to complete a turn because of some degree of postural instability. Neither deep tendon reflexes nor sensation are affected in PD.

In advanced PD, loss of postural reflexes becomes evident. Individuals are unable to maintain their balance when turning. Other manifestations of advanced PD include freezing episodes and dysphagia.

Mood and affect should be assessed for depression.

Working memory capacity has been shown to be decreased, as tested by short-term recall testing. There also appears to be a deficit in the ability to maintain attention. But keep in mind that this is different from the inability of Alzheimer's patients to maintain attention. In PD, it seems as if patients are slower to learn new things and have more difficulty in maintaining the new information than controls. However, PD patients are still able to learn new information, whereas Alzheimer's patients are unable to do so. PD patients do show difficulty with tests associated with frontal lobe function (e.g., Wisconsin Card Sorting Test, Stroop test).

Functional Limitations

Functional limitations depend on which symptoms are most prominent in a particular patient. Early in the course of PD, the sole limitation may be in one's ability to write legibly. Affected individuals are still able to perform activities of daily living, although they may prefer to use the unaffected limb for tasks such as shaving and dressing. Although the rest tremor may result in a feeling of self-consciousness or embarrassment, it does not affect one's independence, as it is suppressed with purposeful movement.

As the disease progresses, difficulty with standing and gait develops. Individuals will require more time to stand and initiate gait. They also develop postural instability with a tendency to retropulse. Thus, patients have difficulty climbing stairs and walking safely and quickly.

In end stage PD, limitations include difficulty swallowing and severe abnormalities of gait that require both devices and one to two persons for assistance. At this stage, help is necessary for all activities of daily living as well.

Diagnostic Studies

Parkinson's disease is a clinical diagnosis. Conventional laboratory investigations do not contribute to the diagnosis or management of PD. Computed tomography (CT) and magnetic resonance imaging (MRI) scans of the brain do not reveal any consistent abnormalities. Positron emission tomography (PET), using 6-[^{18}F]-fluorolevodopa, reveals reduced accumulation of radioisotope in the striata. There is greater loss contralateral to the side that is most affected clinically. These findings are consistent with the reduction of dopamine that occurs in PD. However, PET remains an experimental, rather than a diagnostic, tool.

TABLE 1. Classes of Antiparkinson Medications

Drug Class	Specific Agents	Mechanism of Action	Effective for	Side Effects
Anti-cholinergic	Benztropine	Muscarinic receptor blocker	Tremor, rigidity	Dry mouth, constipation, urinary retention, confusion, hallucinations, impaired concentration
Anti-viral	Amantadine	Promotes synthesis and release of dopamine	Tremor, rigidity, akinesia	Leg edema, livedo reticularis, confusion, hallucinations
Dopamine replacement	Levodopa	Converted to dopamine	Tremor, rigidity, akinesia, freezing	Nausea, diarrhea, confusion, hallucinations
Dopamine agonist (D1 and D2)	Bromocriptine, pergolide	Dopamine analog that binds to D1 and D2 receptors	Rigidity, akinesia	Leg edema, nausea, confusion, hallucinations
Dopamine agonist (D2)	Ropinirole, pramipexole	Dopamine analog that binds to D2 receptors	Rigidity, akinesia	Leg edema, sleep attacks, nausea, confusion, hallucinations
MAO B inhibitor	Selegiline	Inhibits the metabolism of dopamine	Mild amelioration of "wearing off" from levodopa	Nausea, hallucinations, confusion
COMT inhibitor	Entacapone	Inhibits the metabolism of dopamine	Mild amelioration of "wearing off" from levodopa	Dyskinesia, nausea, diarrhea

Differential Diagnosis

Parkinson's plus syndromes
   Multiple system atrophy
   Progressive supranuclear palsy
   Corticobasal degeneration
Intention tremor
Essential tremor

Treatment

Initial

The decision to initiate medical treatment is based on the degree of disability and discomfort that the patient is experiencing. Six classes of drugs are used to treat PD (Table 1). The selection of a particular drug depends on the patient's main complaint, which is usually either a rest tremor or bradykinesia.

Anticholinergic agents are the oldest class of medications used in PD. They are most effective in reducing the rest tremor and rigidity associated with PD. However, the side effects associated with anticholinergic agents typically limit their usefulness. In the periphery, anticholinergic agents may cause dry mouth, constipation, urinary retention, and visual blurring. In the central nervous system, the use of anticholinergic agents may cause difficulty with concentration, confusion, and hallucinations.

Amantadine is also used in the treatment of PD. Amantadine produces a limited improvement in akinesia, rigidity, and tremor. Common side effects include lower extremity edema, confusion, and hallucinations.

Dopamine replacement remains the cornerstone of antiparkinsonian therapy. Levodopa is the natural precursor to dopamine and is converted to dopamine by the enzyme aromatic-L-amino-acid decarboxylase. To ensure that adequate levels of levodopa reach the central nervous system, levodopa is administered simultaneously with a peripheral decarboxylase inhibitor. In the United States, the most commonly used peripheral decarboxylase inhibitor is carbidopa. Levodopa is most effective in reducing tremor, rigidity, and akinesia. The most common side effects, seen with the onset of treatment, are nausea, abdominal cramping, and diarrhea. Long-term treatment with levodopa is associated with three types of complications: hourly fluctuations in motor state; dyskinesias and a variety of psychiatric complaints, including hallucinations; and confusion.

Dopamine agonists, which directly stimulate dopamine receptors, are also used in the treatment of PD. These agents can be used either as an adjunct to levodopa therapy or as monotherapy. The older dopamine agonists, which are relatively non-specific and exert their effects at both D1 and D2 receptors, are bromocriptine and pergolide. In comparison with the side effects seen with levodopa, there is a lower frequency of dyskinesias and a higher frequency of confusion and hallucinations with both the older and newer dopamine agonists. The newer dopamine agonists, pramipexole and ropinirole, are more specific for D2 receptors. These newer agents have been reported to cause excessive lethargy and sleep attacks.[1a] All dopamine agonists can cause orthostatic hypotension, particularly when they are first introduced. It is best to start with a small dose of medication at bedtime and then slowly increase the total daily dosage.

Inhibitors of dopamine metabolism are also used in the medical treatment of PD. Selegiline inhibits monoamine oxidase B (MAO B), which metabolizes dopamine in the central nervous system. Thus, inhibitors of MAO B are thought to improve an individual's response to levodopa by alleviating the motor fluctuations that are seen with long-term levodopa treatment. Another agent that inhibits the metabolism of dopamine is entacapone. Entacapone inhibits catechol-O-methyl transferase (COMT) in the periphery. Entacapone is administered in conjunction with levodopa and, by inhibiting peripheral COMT activity, increases the amount of levodopa that reaches the central nervous system. The benefits of entacapone treatment include a reduction in total daily levodopa dosage and an improvement in the length of time of maximum mobility.[2]

Many PD patients have been treated for depression safely and effectively with selective serotonin reuptake inhibitors (SSRIs) such as fluoxetine or paroexetine. Tricyclic antidepressants can be used, although their anticholinergic properties may limit their effectiveness.

Gastrointestinal complications also occur in PD. Dysphagia is typically due to poor control of the muscles of both mastication and the oropharynx. Soft food is easier to eat, and antiparkinsonian medication improves swallowing. Constipation is a common complaint. Treatment includes increasing physical activity; discontinuing anticholinergic drugs; and consuming a diet consisting of adequate fluid intake, fruit, vegetables, fiber, and lactulose (10 to 20 g daily).

Rehabilitation

The clinical pathology seen in PD reveals that patients tend to become more passive, less active, and less motivated as the disease progresses. The benefits of physical and occupational therapy are thus more far reaching than a simple improvement in motor function. The physical benefits include improving muscle strength and tone as well as maintaining an adequate range of motion in the joints. The psychologic benefits include enlisting the patient as an active participant in treatment and providing a sense of mastery over the effects of PD. Both physical and occupational therapy focus on mobility, the use of adaptive equipment, and safety in both the home and community.

Speech therapy plays a critical role for PD patients who suffer from communication difficulties. Although dysarthria is difficult to treat, hypophonia can be overcome with training. Swallow evaluation and therapy are also helpful in the treatment of dysphagia, which occurs as PD progresses.

Procedures

Feeding tubes are sometimes used in individuals who have severe end stage PD. Some patients elect hospice care, without artificial feeding at that point. Individuals who do get feeding tubes may need to have their medication doses adjusted (e.g., Sinemet [carbidopa/levodopa is the generic name] will now bypass the esophagus and have a shortened time to onset of action).

Surgical

Although a large number of medications are available for the treatment of early and moderately advanced PD, they are of limited efficacy in those with advanced PD. Several surgical procedures are currently available for those with advanced PD.[3] As these procedures are currently under intense investigation, the recommendations included in this chapter will continue to evolve over the next several years.

Thalamotomy consists of introducing a lesion in the ventral intermediate (Vim) nucleus of the thalamus. Thalamotomy has been reported to produce a reduction in tremor of the contralateral limb in 80% of the patients who were treated.[4] No improvements have been reported in bradykinesia, gait, or speech abnormalities. Thalamotomy is recommended in PD patients with an asymmetric, severe, medically intractable tremor.

Unilateral pallidotomy consists of introducing a lesion in the globus pallidus. The most striking benefits are a reduction in contralateral drug-induced dyskinesias, contralateral tremor, bradykinesia. and rigidity.[5,6] Unilateral pallidotomy is recommended in PD patients with bradykinesia, rigidity, and tremor who experience significant drug-induced dyskinesia despite optimal medical therapy. Little data are available regarding the cognitive effects of unilateral pallidotomy. Thus, neuropsychologic evaluation is recommended in all patients both prior to and following surgery.

Deep brain stimulation (DBS) consists of high-frequency electrical stimulation in one of the following locations: Vim nucleus of the thalamus, the globus pallidus, or the subthalamic nucleus. DBS requires surgery, in which the source of electrical stimulation is placed subcutaneously in the chest wall and the leads to which it is attached are placed in one of the locations previously listed. The advantage of DBS is that the degree of electrical stimulation can be easily adjusted, externally, once the DBS unit is in place. In contrast, both thalamotomy and pallidotomy result in permanent, fixed lesions in the brain. DBS of the Vim nucleus of the thalamus is effective in the treatment of a severe and disabling tremor that is unresponsive to medical therapy. DBS of the globus pallidus results in a marked reduction in dyskinesia. There are also improvements in bradykinesia, speech, gait, rigidity, and tremor. DBS of the subthalamic nucleus also results in marked improvement in tremor, akinesia, gait, and postural stability. Comprehensive studies on the effects of DBS of the subthalamic nucleus are limited, and the procedure is still considered to be under investigation.

Surgical treatment for medication-resistant PD is rapidly becoming an important therapeutic option. In carefully selected cases, thalamotomy and DBS of the thalamus can safely and effectively control contralateral tremor. Unilateral pallidotomy has been demonstrated to be an effective treatment of severe dyskinesias. DBS of the subthalamic nucleus appears promising for the treatment of akinesia, although its use remains under investigation.

Potential Disease Complications

Depression occurs in at least 30% of PD cases.[7] It may be difficult to distinguish true depression from the apathy associated with PD. The crucial factor is whether the patient has a true disturbance of mood, with loss of interest; sleep disturbance; and sometimes, suicidal thoughts. The reasons for depression in PD are a subject of debate. There is a suspicion that the pathology of PD itself may predispose patients to depression. Regardless of the cause, recognition and treatment of depression may have a significant impact on the overall disability caused by the illness.

Potential Treatment Complications

The motor complications seen with treatment are divided into two categories: fluctuations ("off" state) and levodopa-induced dyskinesias. The "off" state consists of a return of the signs and symptoms of PD: bradykinesia, tremor, and rigidity. Patients may also experience anxiety, dysphoria, or panic during an "off" state.

The development of levodopa-induced dyskinesias appears to be related to the degree of dopamine receptor supersensitivity. As PD progresses, there is an increasing loss of dopamine receptors. This results in an increased sensitivity of the remaining dopamine receptors to dopamine itself. Thus, there is a greater chance of developing dyskinesias at a given dose of levodopa. Treatment options include lowering each dose of levodopa but increasing the frequency with which it is taken; adding or increasing the dose of a dopamine agonist while decreasing the dose of levodopa; and adding amantadine, which has been shown to be an antidyskinetic agent in some patients.[8]

References
1. Tanner CM, Hubble JP, Chan P: Epidemiology and genetics of Parkinson's disease. In Watts RL, Koller WC (eds): Movement Disorders. New York, McGraw-Hill, 1997, pp 137–152.
1a. Frucht S, Rogers JD, Greene PE, et al: Falling asleep at the wheel: Motor vehicle mishaps in persons taking pramipexole and ropinirole. Neurology 1999;52:1908–1910.
2. Parkinson Study Group: The COMT inhibitor entacapone increases on time in levodopa treated Parkinson's disease patients with motor fluctuations. Ann Neurol 1997;42:747–755.
3. Hallett M, Litvan I, and the Task Force on Surgery for Parkinson's Disease: Evaluation of surgery for Parkinson's disease: A report of the therapeutics and technology assessment subcommittee of the American Academy of Neurology. Neurology 1999;53:1910–1921.
4. Jankovic J, Cardoso F, Grossman RG, Hamilton WJ: Outcome after stereotactic thalamotomy for parkinsonian, essential, and other types of tremor. Neurosurgery 1995;37:680–687.
5. Fazzini E, Dogali M, Sterio D, et al: Stereotactic pallidotomy for Parkinson's disease: A long-term follow-up of unilateral pallidotomy. Neurology 1997;48:1273–1277.
6. Lang AE, Lozano AM, Montgomery E, et al: Posteroventral medial pallidotomy in advanced Parkinson's disease. N Engl J Med 1997;337:1036–1042.
7. Dooneief G, Chen J, Mirabello E, et al: An estimate of the incidence of depression in idiopathic Parkinson's disease. Arch Neurol 1992;49:305–307.
8. Metman LV, Del Dotto P, van den Munckhof P, et al: Amantadine as treatment for dyskinesias and motor fluctuations in Parkinson's disease. Neurology 1998;50:1323–1326.

124 Peripheral Neuropathies

Seward B. Rutkove, MD

Definition

Peripheral neuropathies are a collection of disorders characterized by the generalized dysfunction of nerves. This group of diseases is heterogeneous, including those that predominantly affect the nerve axon (axonal), others that predominantly affect the myelin sheath (demyelinating), and still others that involve both parts of the nerve simultaneously (mixed) (Figs. 1 and 2). In addition, some peripheral neuropathies only affect small, unmyelinated fibers whereas others predominantly involve only large myelinated ones.

Peripheral neuropathy is quite common, with one study suggesting a prevalence of about 3.5%.[1] Peripheral neuropathy may be due to many different causes (Table 1). Diabetes mellitus is a common cause of peripheral neuropathy; one study demonstrated clinical peripheral neuropathy affecting 8.3% of individuals as compared with a control population

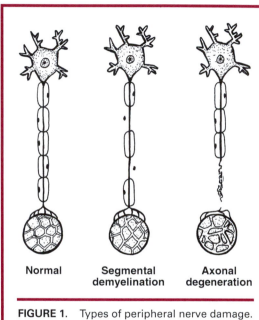

FIGURE 1. Types of peripheral nerve damage.

Normal | Segmental demyelination | Axonal degeneration

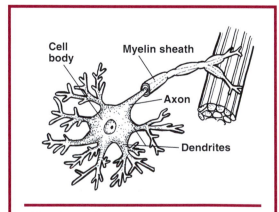

FIGURE 2. Schematic representation of a motor nerve extending from a cell body to the muscle it innervates.

Cell body | Myelin sheath | Axon | Dendrites

TABLE 1. Specific Disorders of Peripheral Nerves

I. **Uniform demyelination:** Mixed sensory motor polyneuropathy
  Hereditary motor sensory neuropathies
    HMSN I: Hypertrophic Charcot-Marie-Tooth disease
    HMSN II: Hypertrophic neuropathy of infancy (Dejerine-Sottas syndrome)
    HMSN IV: Hypertrophic neuropathy associated with phytanic acid excess (Refsum's syndrome)
  Metachromatic leukodystrophy
  Galactosylceramide lipodosis (globoid cell leukodystrophy; Krabbe's disease)
  Adrenoleukodystrophy and adrenomyeloneuropathy
  Tangier's disease
  Cerebrotendinous xanthomatosis (cholestanolosis)
  Cockayne's syndrome

II. **Segmental demyelination:** Motor greater than sensory polyneuropathy
  Acute inflammatory demyelinating polyradiculo-neuropathy (Guillain-Barré syndrome)
  Chronic inflammatory demyelinating polyneuropathy
  Multifocal neuropathy with motor conduction block (motor neuropathy with multifocal conduction block)
  Leprosy (Hansen's disease)
  Diphtheritic neuropathy
  Peripheral nerve disease associated with HIV infection
    Distal symmetric polyneuropathy (primary axonal loss)
    Inflammatory demyelinating polyneuropathy (primary demyelination with some axonal loss)
    Mononeuropathy multiplex (mixed: axonal loss and demyelination to varying degrees)
    Progressive polyradiculopathy (primary axonal loss)
  Lyme disease peripheral neuropathy
  Arsenic neuropathy
  Hereditary neuropathy with susceptibility to pressure palsies
  Osteosclerotic myeloma (POEMS syndrome)
  Monoclonal gammopathy of undetermined significance
  Acromegaly
  Sjögren's syndrome
  Angiofollicular lymph node hyperplasia (Castleman's disease)
  Gamma chain disease
  Hypothyroid neuropathy
  Lymphoma
  Marinesco-Sjögren-Garland syndrome
  Post-portacaval anastomosis

II. **Segmental demyelination:** Motor greater than sensory polyneuropathy (*Cont.*)
  Progressive external ophthalmoplegia
  Systemic lupus erythematosus
  Ulcerative colitis
  Waldenström's macroglobulinemia
  Medications

III. **Axonal loss:** Motor greater than sensory polyneuropathy
  Porphyria
  AIDP: Acute axonal form (acute axonal Guillain-Barré syndrome)
  HMSN II (Charcot-Marie-Tooth disease; neuronal form)
  HMSN V (spastic paraplegia)
  Lead neuropathy
  Hypoglycemia and hyperinsulinemia
  Remote effects of carcinoma
  Cryoglobulinemic neuropathy
  Hexacarbon neuropathy (n-hexane/methyl n-butyl ketone)
  Medications

IV. **Axonal loss:** Sensory neuropathy and neuronopathy
  Friedreich's ataxia
  Spinocerebellar degenerations
  Vitamin E deficiency
  Abetalipoproteinemia (Bassen-Kornzweig disease)
  Thalidomide
  Idiopathic sensory neuropathy and neuronopathy
  AIDP: Fisher variant (Miller-Fisher syndrome)
  Remote effects of carcinoma and lymphoma
  Hereditary sensory autonomic neuropathies
    HSAN type I
    HSAN type II
    HSAN Type III (Riley-Day syndrome: familial dysautonomia)
    HSAN type IV
    HSAN type V
  Ataxia-telangiectasia
  Cis-Platinum
  Crohn's disease (granulomatous colitis)
  Gluten-induced enteropathy (non-tropical sprue neuropathy)
  Paraproteinemia
  Primary biliary cirrhosis
  Pyridoxine neuropathy
  Sjögren's syndrome
  Vinyl benzene (styrene)

From Dumitru D: Electrodiagnostic Medicine. Philadelphia, Hanley & Belfus, 1995, pp 741–742.

in whom 2.1% of individuals were affected.[2] After 10 years, 41.9% of the diabetic patients had developed peripheral neuropathy as compared with 6% of the control subjects.

Symptoms

Patients with peripheral neuropathy present with a number of specific sensory complaints that occur most commonly in the feet first. These include decreased sensation often associated with pain, tingling (paresthesias), and burning. Some patients, usually with more advanced disease,

TABLE 2. Toxins Producing Peripheral Nerve Degeneration

I. **Industrial Chemicals**
   A. **Affects peripheral nervous system preferentially**
      Lead
      Acrylamide
      Organophosphates
      Thallium
   B. **Some affects on central nervous system**
      Carbon disulfide
      Methyl mercury
      Methylbromide
   C. **Large amounts required**
      Arsenic
      Trichloroethylene
      Tetrachloroethane
      2,4-D (Dichlorophenoxyacetic acid)
      Pentachlorophenol
      DDT
   D. **Some effects on other than nervous tissue**
      Carbon tetrachloride
      Carbon monoxide

II. **Pharmaceutical Substances**

Arsenic	Nitrofurantoin
Arsenic-based chemicals	Phenytoin
Clioquinol	Sulfonamides
Disulfiram	Thalidomide
Gold	Thallium
Hydralazine	Vincristine
Isoniazid	

Modified from Gilliatt RW: Recent advances in the pathophysiology of nerve conduction. In Desmedt JE (ed): New developments in electromyography and clinical neurophysiology. Basel, Karger, 1973, pp 2–18.

will note thinning of the feet and some weakness, especially with the development of partial foot drop. Walking difficulties usually also develop once sensation is significantly impaired. Sensory symptoms in the hand (again, paresthesias and reduced tactile sensation) usually develop once an axonal peripheral neuropathy has progressed up to about the level of the knees. In patients with generalized demyelinating peripheral neuropathies, more diffuse symptoms of weakness and sensory loss are often present, although distally predominant paresthesias often occur.

The history should include a detailed past medical history, review of systems, and any prior exposure to toxins (Table 2).

Physical Examination

The physical examination demonstrates distinct abnormalities corresponding to the form of peripheral neuropathy present. Most commonly, patients present with a sensorimotor axonal peripheral neuropathy. In this situation, decreased sensation to pinprick, vibration, light touch, and temperature may be identified distally in the lower extremities, with normalization of the exam more proximally. Some weakness of toe or foot extension and flexion may also be apparent. Deep tendon reflexes will be hypoactive distally (e.g., ankle jerks decreased relative to the knees). In patients with acquired demyelinating peripheral neuropathy, the examination may demonstrate marked generalized weakness with only mild sensory findings, usually including decreased joint position sense. In this disorder, deep tendon reflexes may be reduced or absent diffusely. Patients with hereditary demyelinating polyneuropathies may demonstrate distal muscle atrophy in the feet and lower legs. Such patients may develop a pes cavus foot deformity, in which the forefoot is shortened and has a very high arch. A "champagne bottle" appearance to the legs may also be present. As any peripheral neuropathy progresses, lower extremity sensory loss may lead to gait unsteadiness and upper extremity sensory loss may produce decreased hand dexterity.

Functional Limitations

Patients with peripheral neuropathy face a number of potential functional limitations. In individuals with a distal axonal peripheral neuropathy, limitations usually include problems with gait and unsteadiness, especially as the neuropathy progresses. If pain is a prominent symptom, then the activities of daily living may be compromised to some extent; pain may also be prominent at night, interfering with sleep. In those patients with very advanced axonal peripheral neuropathy or demyelinating forms, such as hereditary Charcot-Marie-Tooth disease, weakness can produce major functional limitations, restricting the patient's walking ability and in some cases leading to dyspnea and nocturnal hypoventilation. In patients with some chronic forms of demyelinating polyneuropathy, weakness of both proximal and distal muscles can become severe, limiting the patient from performing many activities of daily living. Sensory deficits can limit one's ability to button shirts, zip pants, turn a key in a lock, tie shoelaces, type on the computer, and so on.

Diagnostic Studies

Electrodiagnostic studies (including electromyography and nerve conduction studies) remain the most important first tests in the evaluation of polyneuropathy.[3] Nerve conduction studies assist in determining whether the peripheral neuropathy is mainly demyelinating, axonal or mixed (Figs. 1 and 2).[4] Likewise, nerve conduction studies will help determine the severity of the process as well. Although needle electromyography (EMG) plays a more limited role in the diagnosis of peripheral neuropathy, a gradient of reinnervation, in which distal muscles are most abnormal and proximal muscles less affected, helps determine the degree of motor involvement. In addition, needle EMG may assist in determining whether a superimposed problem, such as polyradiculopathy, is also contributing.

Generally, a number of serologic tests are also performed to identify the cause of the peripheral neuropathy. These are outlined in Table 3.

Additional work-up is occasionally necessary. For example, quantitative sensory testing can help delineate the degree of sensory loss and the extent to which specific modalities are affected. In this technique, patients are asked to determine whether they can feel certain sensations generated by a probe touching the skin. By utilizing certain algorithms, the clinician can obtain an accurate assessment of the severity of sensory deficit and the modalities affected. This form of testing can be especially helpful in small-fiber peripheral neuropathies, as standard electrodiagnostic testing may be normal. Autonomic testing may also be helpful (such as tilt table testing and heart rate variability to deep breathing) in delineating the involvement of the autonomic nervous system in the neuropathic process. Sural nerve biopsy can be useful in determining the etiology of the polyneuropathy for some difficult-to-diagnosis conditions such as amyloid neuropathy as well as some other unusual forms of peripheral neuropathy. Occasionally, muscle biopsy may also be helpful in this regard as well, as vasculitic abnormalities or amyloid can also be identified. Lumbar puncture may be helpful in determining whether an acquired demyelinating peripheral neuropathy is present by the identification of a very elevated cerebrospinal fluid protein and normal white cell count (so-called albuminocytologic dissociation). Recently, the analysis of cutaneous sensory fibers through the use of skin biopsy has also been introduced to help identify the presence of small fiber peripheral neuropathies.[5]

Differential Diagnosis

Myelopathy	Lumbar stenosis
Lumbosacral polyradiculopathy	Mononeuropathy mulitplex

TABLE 3. Serologic Testing in Peripheral Neuropathy

Baseline testing
- Vitamin B_{12}
- Thyroid stimulating hormone
- RPR (or VDRL)
- Serum glucose
- Serum hemoglobin A1c
- Anti-nuclear antibody
- Erythrocyte sedimentation rate
- Serum protein electrophoresis
- Urine protein electrophoresis

Some additional tests, depending on clinical suspicion
- Serum protein immunophoresis
- 24-hour urine for heavy metals
- 24-hour urine for porphyrins
- HIV testing
- Anti-Ro, anti-La antibodies (Sjögren's syndrome)
- Anti-Hu antibody (paraneoplastic neuropathy)
- Additional antibody testing in certain demyelinating disorders
    - Anti-myelin associated glycoprotein
    - Anti-sulfatide antibody
- Genetic testing (for disorders such as familial amyloidosis, Charcot-Marie-Tooth disease)

Treatment

Initial

If a cause of the axonal peripheral neuropathy is known or identified (which generally is achieved only about 70% of the time), treatment geared toward the underlying disorder itself might help slow progression of the polyneuropathy. For example, improved glucose control can help improve neuronal function in diabetic neuropathy.[6] Likewise, in patients with a neuropathy secondary to toxin exposure, such as alcoholic neuropathy, decreased exposure to the toxin may, of course, be helpful.

In patients with axonal peripheral neuropathies, treatment is usually symptom-based with efforts toward reducing pain and dysesthesias. A number of drugs have proven to be useful in this regard.[7] The tricyclic antidepressants remain most effective (generally nortriptyline or amitriptyline, starting with 10 mg at bedtime and increasing as needed until improvement occurs). Gabapentin (starting at dose of 100 to 300 mg tid) has also gained wide acceptance in the treatment of this disorder over the past several years.[8] Other medications, including carbamazepine; diphenylhydantoin; and more recently, topiramate, have been used as well. Application of capsaicin ointment to the feet can also occasionally be helpful. Finally, in patients in whom these measures prove of limited value, the use of long-acting narcotic agents may be necessary.

In patients with certain forms of demyelinating peripheral neuropathy (such as chronic inflammatory demyelinating polyradiculoneuropathy [CIDP]), immunosuppressive or immunomodulating therapies can make a dramatic difference in the patients' symptoms and level of function. Drugs including corticosteroids, azathioprine, cyclosporin, and cyclophosphamide can be used.[9] Intravenous immunoglobulin (IVIG) and plasmapheresis are also widely used in this group of disorders.

Finally, in all patients with distal sensory loss due to peripheral neuropathy, regular podiatric care is extremely important in helping to prevent the development of serious foot complications, such as ulcerations.[10,11]

Rehabilitation

Physical therapy may be recommended to work on strength, and balance and to improve mobility. In patients with moderate to severe peripheral neuropathy, gait training may consist of balance exercises and/or use of an assistive device, such as a cane or walker. Either a physical or occupational therapist can review falls precautions (e.g., avoiding throw rugs in the home, using a chair in the bath or shower). Some patients may benefit from a short leg brace (ankle foot orthosis commonly called an AFO); however, in patients with compromised sensation monitoring the skin to prevent breakdown when a brace is used is critical. Patients can be taught to self-monitor their skin using a long handled mirror to check the bottom of their feet.

Custom shoes (e.g., extra depth and width) may be beneficial, as can custom shoe orthotics.

In patients with more advanced peripheral neuropathy, evaluation by an occupational therapist may be helpful in maximizing the function of the hands and arms. The occupational therapist can provide the patient with information regarding adaptive equipment such as elastic shoelaces, wide grip handles for cookware and utensils, shoehorns, etc.

If pain is an issue, both physical and occupational therapists can assist with modalities that may help to alleviate the pain. These may include instruction on using transcutaneous electrical nerve stimulation (TENS), paraffin baths, etc. It is important to caution the patient with impaired sensation not to use any heat or ice that may cause burns or frostbite. Individuals with impaired vascular status also should be advised not to use ice due to its vasoconstrictive properties.

Procedures

Patients with peripheral neuropathy are generally at increased risk of developing superimposed compressive neuropathies, such as carpal tunnel syndrome. Treatment with local corticosteroid injections can be helpful for this problem (see Chapter 34).

Surgery

Surgery may be necessary for some associated conditions, including severe carpal tunnel syndrome, but is usually more relevant for patients who develop infections of the distal lower extremities and require amputations. Other, less severe distal leg problems may also develop and require orthopedic or podiatric surgery.

Potential Disease Complications

A number of potential foot complications can occur, including persistent, intractable pain; skin ulcerations; and foot trauma, possibly leading to amputations. Serious trauma secondary to increased gait unsteadiness is another potential problem. Finally, depression due to immobility and persistent pain also often plays a role in patients with more advanced peripheral neuropathy.

Potential Treatment Complications

The tricyclic antidepressants and other pain medications all have the potential side effect of drowsiness. Dry mouth, constipation, and urinary retention also occur commonly with the tricyclic antidepressants. The anti-seizure medications, especially carbamazepine, have the potential of causing severe ataxia at higher doses. Rarely, a life-threatening idiosyncratic reaction to diphenylhydantoin characterized by skin defoliation and necrosis can occur (Stevens-Johnson syndrome). With narcotic use, addiction remains a significant concern.

Treatment for the autoimmune peripheral neuropathies poses significant risk, given the inherent toxicity of the medications used. Patients using immunosuppressive medications are at increased risk of infection, malignancy, anemia, and multiple other side effects (e.g., liver toxicity with azathioprine, renal failure with intravenous immunoglobulin, hemorrhagic cystitis with cyclophosphamide).

Skin breakdown may occur with improper bracing.

References

1. The Italian General Practitioner Study Group: Chronic symmetric symptomatic polyneuropathy in the elderly: A field screening investigation in two Italian regions. Neurology 1995;1995:1832–1836.
2. Partanen J, Niskanen L, Lehtinen J, et al: Natural history of peripheral neuropathy in patients with non-insulin dependent diabetes mellitus. N Engl J Med 1995;333:89–94.
3. Dyck P, Dyck P, Grant I, Fealey R: Ten steps in characterizing and diagnosing patients with peripheral neuropathy. Neurology 1996;47:10–17.
4. Albers J: Clinical neurophysiology of generalized polyneuropathy. J Clin Neurophys 1993;10:149–166.
5. Hermann D, Griffin F, Hauer P, et al: Epidermal nerve fiber density and sural nerve morphometry in peripheral neuropathies. Neurology 1999;53:1634–1640.
6. Troni W, Carta Q, Cantello R, et al: Peripheral nerve function and metabolic control in diabetes mellitus. Ann Neurol 1984;16:178–183.
7. Sindrup S, Jensen T: Pharmacologic treatment of pain in polyneuropathy. Neurology 2000;55:915–920.
8. Backonja M, Beydoun A, Edwards KR, et al: Gabapentin for the symptomatic treatment of painful neuropathy in patients with diabetes mellitus: A randomized controlled trial [see comments]. Jama 1998;280:1831–1836.
9. Barnett MH, Pollard JD, Davies L, McLeod JG: Cyclosporin A in resistant chronic inflammatory demyelinating polyradiculoneuropathy. Muscle Nerve 1998;21:454–460.
10. Hahn A, Bolton C, Zochodne D, Feasby T: Intravenous immunoglobulin treatment in chronic inflammatory demyelinating polyneuropathy. Brain 1996;119:1067–1077.
11. Hahn A, Bolton C, Pillay N, et al: Plasma-exchange therapy in chronic inflammatory demyelinating polyneuropathy. Brain 1996;119:1055–1066.

125 Plexopathy—Brachial

Lester S. Duplechan, MD

Synonyms

Neuralgic amyotrophy

Brachial neuritis

Acute shoulder neuritis

Acute brachial radiculitis

Parsonage-Turner syndrome

Obstetric brachial plexus palsy (OBPP)

ICD-9 Codes

353.0
Brachial plexus lesions

353.5
Neuralgic amyotrophy

723.4
Brachial neuritis or radiculitis NOS

767.6
Birth trauma

Definition

Brachial plexus lesions have been described in the literature over several decades. Spillane described a syndrome of abrupt shoulder pain followed by atrophy and weakness in British soldiers in 1943.[1] These patients had severe shoulder pain, usually during the convalescence of an illness. Proximal shoulder weakness, particularly involving the serratus anterior, deltoid, and scalenes muscles shortly followed the resolution of the pain.[2] Further reports by Turner and Parsonage describe variants of the observed "brachial neuritis," which they termed "neuralgic amyotrophy."[3]

TABLE 1.	Neuralgic Amytrophy[1,4]
Incidence	1.64 per 1000,000 population
Male:Female	2.4:1
Age of onset	3 months–74 years
Antecedent or associated illness	About 45% of patients
Mode of onset	Rapid onset pain/paralysis (paresis)
Initial symptom	Pain in 95% of patients
Weakness	Confined to single peripheral nerve: 10% of patients. Single nerves commonly affected: radial; long thoracic; axillary; suprascapular
Sensory deficit	Noted in about 67% of patients; most common: axillary and lateral antebrachial cutaneous
Laterality	Unilateral: 66% (right side 54%), bilateral: 34%
Laboratory	Normal
Electrodiagnosis	Abnormal: helps to localize and follow disease progress

From Dumitru D, Amato A, Zwarts M: Electrodiagnostic Medicine, 2nd ed. Philadelphia, Hanley & Belfus, 2002, with permission.

More recent literature may suggest that neuralgic amyotrophy could be a manifestation of a mononeuritis multiplex[4–6] (Table 1).

Post-traumatic brachial plexus lesions can be classified etiologically as either open or closed. Open lesions are most commonly due to stab wounds and less commonly secondary to gunshot wounds.

Closed injuries are most likely due to traction injuries. The mechanism of traction can give a clue to the possible site of the lesion. A widening of the angle between the neck and the shoulder causes traction of the plexus.[7] Normally, the scalenes muscles proximally and the soft tissues more

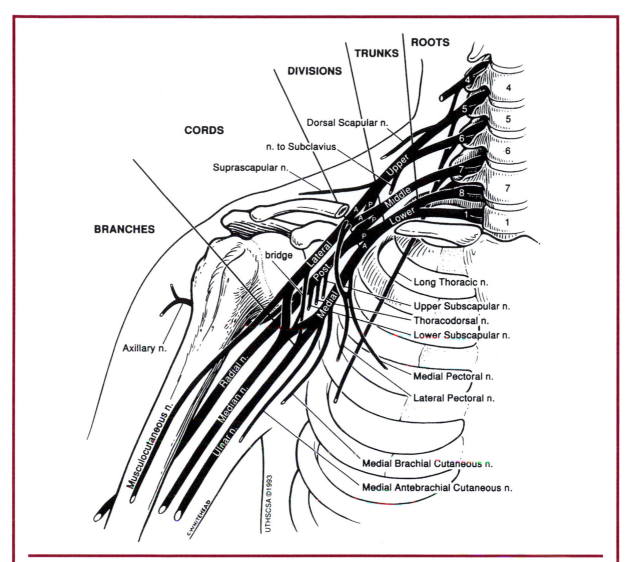

FIGURE 1. The brachial plexus. The clinician must be able to visualize and reproduce this figure when performing an electrodiagnostic medicine consultation so as to examine an appropriate number of muscles and nerves to localize a lesion. (From Dumitru D, Amato A, Zwarts M: Electrodiagnostic Medicine, 2nd ed. Philadelphia, Hanley & Belfus, 2002, with permission.)

distally are helpful in resisting traction of the nervous structures. Traction on the shoulder with the arm in the neutral or anatomic position causes injury to C5 and C6; with the arm in mid-abduction, C7, and with the arm fully abducted, the damage occurs at C8–T1. Obstetric brachial plexus palsy (OBPP), occurs more commonly in large weight infants as a result of position and shoulder dystocia. Breech presentation of the normal weight infant is also a significant risk factor.[8] The most common palsy in the obstetric group is a C5–C6 or upper trunk variety, often presenting with the "waiter's tip" posture.

Plexus Anatomy

The brachial plexus is normally formed from the ventral rami of C5–T1 spinal nerves (Fig. 1). This structure allows for the formation of peripheral nerves, which supply the upper extremity and shoulder girdle.

In approximately 10% of cases there is a significant contribution of axons from the C4 level. A smaller percentage of patients have contribution of T2 axons. The former situation is referred to as a pre-fixed brachial plexus, and the latter, a post-fixed plexus.

Symptoms

The most consistent symptom in brachial neuritis or amyotrophy is the abrupt onset of severe pain, followed by proximal shoulder weakness.[9] Sensory deficit is usually restricted to the axillary distribution along the lateral aspect of the shoulder but may occur in the dermatomal distribution of any affected nerve.

The site of the lesion can also greatly influence the symptoms. Preganglionic lesions occur at the level of the rootlets proximal to the dorsal root ganglion. Patients with these lesions have loss of sensation and motor weakness; however, sensory conduction studies are unaffected since the sensory axons are in continuity with their cell bodies in the dorsal root ganglion. Preganglionic lesions tend to be due to high energy trauma and are therefore more severe, lending to a worse prognosis for recovery.

Postganglionic lesions may occur at many sites—both supraclavicular and infraclavicular. Sensory nerve conduction studies are abnormal in postganglionic lesions.

Physical Examination

Observation should be performed to determine any skin or hair changes, warmth/coldness, muscle atrophy, or fasciculations. Muscle bulk, flexibility, and tone should be noted as well.

Upper extremity symmetry in arm swing during gait or abnormal guarding gestures with dressing, handshake, etc., should also be documented.

Physical examination typically reveals impaired active range of motion in the shoulder girdle, with noted scapular and deltoid atrophy in many cases. Sensation is most typically lost in the axillary nerve distribution in patients with neuralgic amyotrophy, but may be absent or decreased in any peripheral nerve distribution. Tinel's phenomenon should be attempted along the course of the nerve in question and marked. A preganglionic lesion or avulsion may not have a Tinel's sign, which may suggest a poor prognosis for spontaneous recovery.

Functional Limitations

Proximal weakness typically affects most activities of daily living, including those requiring shoulder abduction, flexion, extension, and external rotation and elbow flexion. Activities that can be significantly affected include bathing, dressing, feeding, and grooming. These impairments may lead to disabilities in both occupational and recreational activities, including driving, lifting, and typing.

Diagnostic Studies

Electrodiagnostic testing is valuable in determining the level of the injury, in addition to the degree of neuropathy (Table 2). Conventional motor conduction studies across the site of the lesion 1 to 2 weeks following the injury can determine whether the lesion is due to demyelination or axonopathy. The loss of motor conduction distal to the proposed site of injury is suggestive of axon loss and therefore a poorer prognosis.[10] Needle electrodiagnostic studies may be of great assistance in determining both the site of the injury as well as the severity. The presence of fibrillation potentials and positive waves on EMG of muscles innervated prior to the formation of the brachial plexus may place the injury site at the level of the spinal nerve. Similarly, a lack of EMG findings

TABLE 2. Brachial Plexus: Key Upper Extremity Neural Innervation Pathways

Muscle	Root	Trunk	Division	Cord	Peripheral Nerve
Spinal nerve origin					
Rhomboid major/minor	(C4)–C5				Dorsal scapular
Serratus anterior	C5,C6,(C7)				Long thoracic
Trunk Origin					
Supraspinatus	C5,C6	Upper			Suprascapular
Infraspinatus	C5,C6	Upper			Suprascapular
Cord origin					
Pectoralis major	C5,C6,C7	Upper/middle	Anterior	Lateral	Lateral pectoral
Pectoralis major/minor	C8,T1	Lower	Anterior	Medial	Medial pectoral
Latissimus dorsi	C6,C7,C8	Upper/middle	Posterior	Posterior	Thoracodorsal
Teres major	C5,C6,C7	Upper/middle	Posterior	Posterior	Lower subscapular
Peripheral nerve branch origin					
Biceps brachii	C5,C6	Upper	Anterior	Lateral	Musculocutaneous
Deltoid	C5,C6	Upper	Posterior	Posterior	Axillary
Triceps	(C6),C7,C8	(Upper)/middle/lower	Posterior	Posterior	Radial
Anconeus	C7,C8	Middle/lower	Posterior	Posterior	Radial
Brachioradialis	C5,C6	Upper	Posterior	Posterior	Radial
Extensor carpi radialis	C6,C7	Upper/middle	Posterior	Posterior	Radial
Extensor digitorum	C7,C8	Middle/lower	Posterior	Posterior	Radial
Extensor indicis	C7,C8	Middle/lower	Posterior	Posterior	Radial
Pronator teres	C6,C7	Middle/lower	Anterior	Lateral	Median
Flexor carpi radialis	C6,C7,(C8)	Upper/middle/lower	Anterior	Lateral/medial	Median
Flexor pollicis longus	(C7),C8,T1	Middle/lower	Anterior	Lateral/medial	Median
Pronator quadratus	C8,T1	Lower	Anterior	Medial	Median
Abductor pollicis brevis	C8,T1	Lower	Anterior	Medial	Median
Opponens pollicis	C8,T1	Lower	Anterior	Medial	Median
Flexor carpi ulnaris	C7,C8,T1	Middle/lower	Anterior	Lateral/medial	Ulnar
Flexor digitorum profundus (III and IV)	C7,C8,T1	Middle/lower	Anterior	Lateral/medial	Ulnar
Abductor digiti minimi	C8,T1	Lower	Anterior	Medial	Ulnar
First dorsal interosseous	C8,T1	Lower	Anterior	Medial	Ulnar

Commonly examined muscles with a needle electrode during the electrodiagnostic medicine examination. Spinal levels in parentheses are occasionally present. The clinician must be able to reproduce this table from memory prior to attempting to diagnose brachial plexus lesions. (From Dumitru D, Amato A, Zwarts M: Electrodiagnostic Medicine, 2nd ed. Philadelphia, Hanley & Belfus, 2002, with permission.)

in the diaphragm, serratus anterior, and dorsal scapular innervated muscles suggests that the injury site is distal to the spinal nerve.

Serologic testing is normal, without elevation of sedimentation rate or white blood cell count. CSF examination is normal as well.

Plain films are helpful in determining whether clavicular, humeral, or transverse process fractures are involved, particularly in post-traumatic cases. Plain film examination of the chest or fluoroscopic evaluation of the diaphragm is necessary to assist in determination of phrenic nerve involvement, which may suggest a level I or II injury (spinal nerve).[11]

Magnetic resonance imaging (MRI) of the cervical spine and axilla assists in the determination of cord and rootlet damage. MRI with and without contrast may assist in determining whether root avulsion has occurred.

Differential Diagnosis[4,9]

Mononeuritis multiplex	Poliomyelitis
Adhesive capsulitis	Amyotrophic lateral sclerosis
Cervical radiculopathy	Herpes zoster
Rotator cuff tear	Tumors of the spinal cord
Impingement syndrome	

Treatment

Initial

Pain is the most disabling symptom in the acute phase of rehabilitation. The neuropathic pain produced by a peripheral mononeuropathy or polyneuropathy is described as severe, with predominating continuous dysesthesias. The treatment of neuropathic pain has been detailed in extensive investigations of postherpetic neuralgia and diabetic neuropathy. Tricyclic antidepressants (amitriptyline, desipramine, and nortriptyline) remain the first line medications in the treatment of continuous dysesthetic pain. Amitriptyline potentiates serotonergic and noradrenergic descending inhibition of the superficial layers of the dorsal horn. The use of tricyclic antidepressants has been shown to reduce continuous neuropathic pain from moderate or severe to mild in 50% to 67% of patients.[12] A reasonable starting dose is 25 mg/day, with increases by 10 to 25 mg every 7 to 10 days. Elderly patients may begin with 10 mg/day dosage secondary to anticholinergic effects.

Gabapentin, an anticonvulsant, has also shown promise in treating continuous dysesthetic pain, similar to that of amitriptyline without a significant increase in side effect profile. Topical agents such as capsaicin and lidocaine patches are used as adjuvants to first and second line agents. Investigations with the use of opioids have revealed a significant reduction of pain; however, complete pain relief is uncommon. The ceiling effect observed with opioid medication renders a small therapeutic window. The conversion from short- to long-acting opioids early in the treatment course is most appropriate in achieving adequate pain control.

Psychologic evaluation and counseling are necessary and beneficial in assisting the patient with full participation in his or her own rehabilitation. In addition, the patient is encouraged to discuss his or her fears and concerns as part of appropriate coping mechanisms.

The prognosis is poor if there is no spontaneous recovery of motor or sensory function within 6 months from the injury date. The lack of a Tinel's phenomenon along the course of the nerve is an early indication of a severe axonopathy. A repeat needle electrodiagnostic study at 8 to 12 weeks should allow the clinician to estimate a percentage of motor units present (if any), or the possibility of regenerating axons in the muscles just distal to the injury site. Patients with severe motor and sensory deficit with little to no functional or objective improvement at 3 months of rehabilitation should have an expedited surgical opinion (since the potential for a good outcome is significantly reduced after 6 months).[13]

Rehabilitation

Passive joint range of motion and sensorimotor re-education are important aspects of early physical therapy. Desensitization techniques, performed with an occupational or physical therapist, facilitate appropriate sensory input along damaged axons. A reduced pain threshold leads to continuous dysesthetic discharges, in addition to allodynia (pain in response to a normally non-noxious stimulus). Patients are initially introduced to tactile stimulation of coarse objects and progressively are able to distinguish and manipulate fine objects. Once pain is reduced to manageable levels, muscle re-education with strengthening exercises are initiated.

Splinting of the shoulder and upper extremity may be static or dynamic, with the goals of protection and enchanced upper extremity function. A balance must be struck in preventing further gravitational traction along the neurologic structures, while allowing for frequent range of motion to prevent contractures. Although not yet clinically proven, electrical stimulation is widely used in conjunction with motor retraining to assist in reduction of muscle atrophy and strengthening.

Procedures

Peripheral nerve blocks are sometimes useful in peripheral mononeuropathies, particularly as a diagnostic tool in the determination of the nerve affected. Blocks with local anesthetics are temporary and rarely helpful long term. The use of alcohol and other long-lasting denervating agents has not demonstrated effectiveness in brachial plexopathies.

Surgery

Penetrating and high velocity blunt injuries require an early assessment of the degree of damage rendered by a knife or high velocity missile. The vascular surgeon may explore the plexus during the evaluation and treatment of suspected vascular damage immediately following the injury. This early assessment may assist in the determination of the site of injury (infraclavicular or supraclavicular), as well as provide valuable information regarding possible loss of nerve continuity (neurotmesis).

The reconstructive surgeon should be involved in the consideration of possible microneural reconstruction.

Grade I (first degree), or neurapraxic, lesions will regenerate, and good recovery can be expected if a comprehensive conservative treatment program is started early following the injury.

Grade II [second to fourth degree) injuries may also benefit from conservative care during the initial postinjury phase. Frequent functional re-evaluation of the patient is critical during the conservative treatment program. Early determination of the lack of progressive recovery should indicate surgical exploration. The initial rehabilitation period should not extend for longer than 5 months without proof of progressive recovery, since the optimal period for direct repair is within 6 months following an injury.[13]

Potential Disease Complications

Scarring and fibrosis of neural elements following severe injuries lead to loss of sensory and motor function in the affected nerve distributions. Joint and musculotendinous contractures may restrict normal function of the entire upper extremity. Causalgia may occur weeks to months after a partial nerve injury to a somatic nerve or plexus. Patients often have significant pain and depression.

Potential Treatment Complications

Possible side effects of medications utilized in the treatment of neuropathic pain are well known and documented.

Tricyclic antidepressives have the potential for cardiotoxicity, sedation, and anticholinergic side effects. Amitriptyline has the highest incidence of side serious effects among the tricylcic antidepressants and must be used with caution in the elderly. Urinary retention may occur in men, particularly if they have pre-existing prostate problems.

Anticonvulsants (carbamazepine) may cause sedation, diplopia, nausea, leukopenia, thrombocytopenia, and hepatotoxicity. Complete blood count and liver function tests should be performed prior to initiating therapy and should be obtained periodically for safety.

In opioid medications, a ceiling effect may be reached—whereby increased dose levels cause significant side effects without improving the analgesia. Meperidine and morphine have active metabolites that may accumulate quickly in persons with altered renal function; propoxyphene is not well tolerated by patients with renal or hepatic disease, in addition to inhibiting carbamazepine metabolism.

Vascular and nerve injury may result from surgical repair or exploration.

References

1. Spillane JD: Localised neuritis of the shoulder girdle. Lancet 1943;532–535.
2. Dixon GJ, Dick TBS, et al: Acute brachial radiculitis, course and prognosis. Lancet 1945;707–708.
3. Turner JW, Parsonage MJ, et al: Neuralgic amyotrophy (paralytic brachial neuritis) with special reference to prognosis. Lancet 1957;209–212.
4. Tsairis P, Dyck PJ, et al: Natural history of brachial plexus neuropathy. Arch Neurol 1972;27:109–117.
5. England JD: The variations of neuralgic amyotrophy. Muscle Nerve 1999;22:435–436.
6. Lahrmann H, Grisold W, et al. Neuralgic amyotrophy with phrenic nerve involvement. Muscle Nerve 1999;22:437–442.
7. Coene LNJEM: Mechanisms of brachial plexus lesions. Clin Neurol Neurosurg 1993;95(Suppl):S23–S29.
8. Eng GD, Binder H, et al: Obstetrical brachial plexus palsy (OBPP) outcome with conservative management. Muscle Nerve 1996;19:884–891.
9. McCarty EC, Tsairis P, et al: Brachial neuritis. Clin Orthop Rel Res 1999;368:37–43.
10. Parry GJ: Electodiagnostic studies in the evaluation of peripheral nerve and brachial plexus injuries. Neurol Clin 1992;10(4):921–934.
11. Dumitru D. Brachial Plexopathies and Proximal Mononeuropathies in Electrodiagnostic Medicine. Philadelphia, Hanley & Belfus, 1995.
12. Watson CPN: The treatment of neuropathic pain: Antidepressants and opioids. Clin J Pain 2000;16:S49–S55.
13. Millesi H: Trauma involving the brachial plexus. In Omer G, Spinner M, Van Beck A (eds): Management of Peripheral Nerve Problems, 2nd ed. Philadelphia, W.B. Saunders, 1998.

126 Plexopathy—Lumbosacral

Alice Fann, MD

Definition

Lumbosacral plexopathy is an injury to one or more nerves that branch from the lumbosacral plexus. The lumbar plexus is formed primarily by the anastomosis of the L1 to L4 nerve roots (Fig. 1). Like the brachial plexus, these nerve roots divide into dorsal and ventral rami as they exit through the intervertebral foramina. The dorsal rami innervate the muscles of the back and supply its cutaneous sensation. The ventral rami for the lumbar plexus supply the motor and sensory nerves to the anterior and medial sides of the thigh and the skin on the medial side of the leg and foot. The undivided anterior primary rami of the lumbar sacral nerves also carry postganglionic sympathetic fibers that are mainly responsible for vasoregulation in the lower extremity. The branches of the lumbar plexus include the iliohypogastric, ilioinguinal, genitofemoral, femoral, lateral femoral cutaneous, and obturator nerves.[1]

The sacral plexus innervates the muscles of the buttocks, posterior thigh, and leg below the knee and the skin of the posterior thigh and leg, lateral leg, foot, and perineum. It is formed from the lumbosacral trunk and the ventral rami of S1 to S3 (or S4) nerve roots (Fig 2). The anterior primary rami of S2 and S3 nerve roots carry parasympathetic fibers that mainly control the urinary bladder and anal sphincters. The triangular sacral plexus lies on the anterior surface of the sacrum, in the immediate vicinity of the sacroiliac joint and lateral to the cervix or prostate.[1,2] The branches of the sacral plexus include the superior gluteal, inferior gluteal, sciatic (tibial and common peroneal divisions), pudendal, and posterior cutaneous nerves of the thigh.

Surgical procedures, trauma, labor and delivery, and complications of treatment for pelvic tumors can cause lumbosacral plexopathies. Injury to the lumbosacral plexus may occur during surgery of the abdominal or perineal areas that uses a modified lithotomy position, in which the legs are placed in skis and the hips are abducted, flexed, and externally rotated.[3] Diabetic, alcoholic, thin, and elderly patients are at increased risk for this injury. Clinically detectable injury to the lumbosacral plexus occurs in up to 10% of hip replacement procedures, and subclinical injury (detected electromyographically) takes place in up to 70% of such operations.[4] Trauma is the most common cause of retroperitoneal hemorrhage, which can injure the lumbosacral plexus; in patients receiving anticoagulant therapy or with acquired or congenital coagulopathies, hemorrhage may occur with no precipitating injury.[2,5]

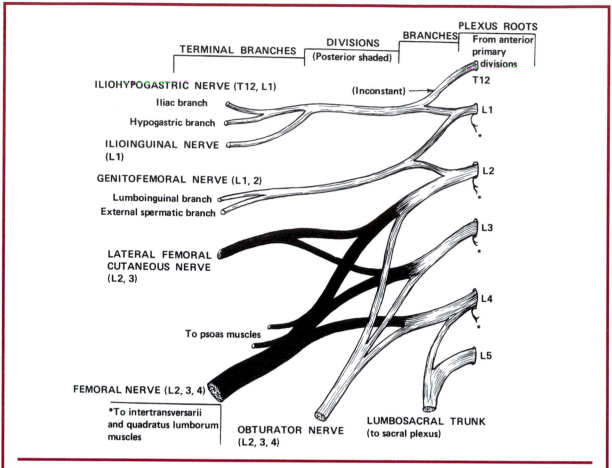

FIGURE 1. The lumbar plexus and its peripheral terminal branches. The shaded portions represent the posterior divisions of the ventral primary rami; those not shaded are either the ventral primary rami or their anterior branches. In this diagram the nerve to the psoas major arises from the femoral nerve, as opposed to directly from the spinal nerve region. (From de Groot J, Chusid JG: Correlative Neuroanatomy, 21st ed. Norwalk, CT, Appleton & Lange, 1991, with permission.)

The lumbosacral plexus may be damaged by traction due to distortion of the pelvis.[6] The injury in traumatic pelvic fractures may be overlooked and not discovered until after the patient is out of intensive care.[7,8] Because static radiographs do not demonstrate the full extent of the initial fracture displacement of the pelvic bones, the clinician cannot correlate or predict plexus injury from the severity of the fracture dislocation as seen on the radiographs.[8,9] Most of these injuries are associated with injury to the sacroiliac area,[8] where the lumbosacral plexus lies in close proximity to the joint.

The lumbosacral plexus may be compressed as a complication of labor and delivery. During the second stage of labor, direct pressure of the fetal head may compress the lumbosacral plexus against the rim of the pelvis, resulting in nerve injury.[10]

The treatment of pelvic malignancies and tumors can damage the lumbosacral plexus. Pelvic radiation therapy may cause a delayed lumbosacral plexopathy that can occur 3 months to 22 years after completion of treatment,[11] with the median amount of time from completion of treatment to onset of symptoms being about 5 years.[12] Chemotherapeutic agents delivered by catheters in the internal or external iliac arteries for treatment of pelvic or lower extremity tumors have resulted in lumbosacral plexopathies.[13] Cisplatin, 5-fluorouracil, mitomycin-C and bleomycin have been implicated in the majority of these plexopathies.

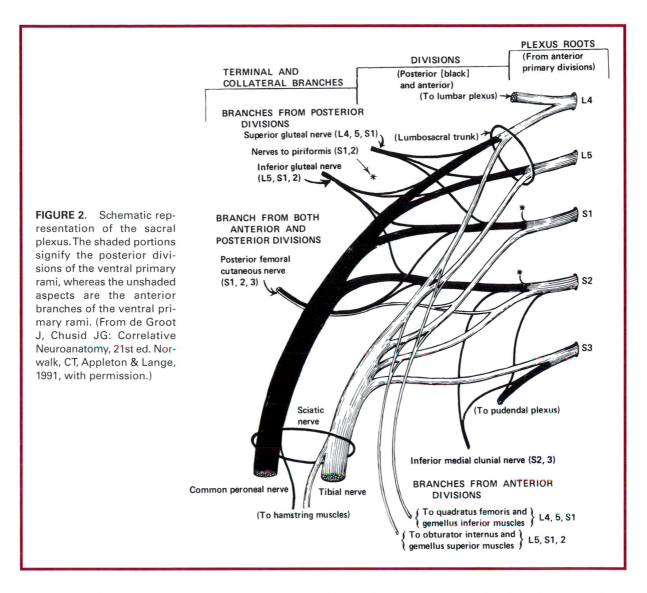

FIGURE 2. Schematic representation of the sacral plexus. The shaded portions signify the posterior divisions of the ventral primary rami, whereas the unshaded aspects are the anterior branches of the ventral primary rami. (From de Groot J, Chusid JG: Correlative Neuroanatomy, 21st ed. Norwalk, CT, Appleton & Lange, 1991, with permission.)

Another lumbosacral plexus disorder is an idiopathic syndrome consisting of pain (often severe), followed by weakness and loss of deep tendon reflexes. The area of pain reflects the affected part of the plexus. Recovery from pain usually occurs before recovery from weakness. Weakness may persist for years, and recovery is often incomplete, with maximum recovery usually occurring in 2 years.[14,15] Diabetic amyotrophy is another spontaneous lumbosacral plexopathy characterized by weakness and atrophy of the pelvic and femoral muscles with relative sparing of the distal muscles.[16] It has an insidious, slowly progressive course and usually occurs in middle age or in elderly patients with mild or previously undiscovered or recently diagnosed diabetes mellitus. The femoral, obturator, and gluteal nerves are the most commonly affected.[17]

Symptoms

The plexopathies may vary in their manifestations. A plexopathy affecting the upper roots, or lumbar plexus, will present with changes potentially in the femoral and obturator nerve distributions. These changes may include weakness of the hip flexors, knee extensors, and hip adductors and sensory changes on the anterolateral thigh. A plexopathy affecting the lower roots, or sacral plexus, will potentially present with changes in the gluteal and sciatic nerve distributions. Weakness may be observed in hip extension, hip abduction, knee flexion, dorsiflexion, and plantar flexion accompanied by changes in sensation on the posterior thigh, anterolateral and posterior leg, and dorsal and plantar surfaces of the foot. The etiology and nature of the injury determines whether the patient complains of pain. With a plexopathy due to a retroperitoneal hemorrhage, the patient typically has acute or subacute onset of pain in the groin with radiation to the buttocks and thigh; this pain increases with hip extension and decreases with hip flexion and external rotation. Symptoms of autonomic dysfunction such as impotence, incontinence, or sweating disturbances, although less common, may be present.

Trauma is the most common cause of retroperitoneal hemorrhage, which can injure the lumbosacral plexus; however, in patients receiving anticoagulant therapy or with acquired or congenital coagulopathies, hemorrhage may occur with no precipitating injury.[2,5] Ischemia, rather than compression, is thought to be the primary cause of this plexopathy. The patient typically has acute or subacute onset of pain in the groin with radiation to the buttocks and thigh.

Physical Examination

Evaluation for a lumbosacral plexopathy includes a neurologic examination, in which weakness, sensory loss, and reflex asymmetry (decreased or absent in affected areas) in the lower extremity are assessed. The sensory examination should include careful attention for changes over the distributions of both dermatomal and cutaneous nerves. Neurologic changes should be consistent with a pattern involving more than one nerve or nerve root of the lumbosacral plexus without diffuse changes that would suggest a peripheral neuropathy. Nerve-root stretch signs may be present if a mass or aneurysm is causing the plexopathy. The patient may also have edema in one lower extremity if the plexopathy is due to a pelvic mass.

In suspected cases of retroperitoneal hemorrhage, pain increases with hip extension and decreases with hip flexion and external rotation.

Functional Limitations

Functional limitations depend on which parts of the lumbosacral plexus are affected. The patient will usually present with mobility difficulties such as performing transfers, standing, and walking. These mobility problems may interfere with activities of daily living, including dressing, bathing, cooking, and cleaning. Vocational activities may also be affected. The initial complaint may be lack of progression back to independent activities after undergoing surgery or when recovering from pelvic trauma. Although less common, impotence, incontinence, or sweating disturbances may be present due to autonomic dysfunction.

Diagnostic Studies

Electrodiagnostic Testing

The preferred method for diagnosing a lumbosacral plexus injury, especially for determination of the location, pathophysiology of the injury, and the prognosis, remain *electrodiagnostic studies*. Results from electrodiagnostic testing will vary according to the type of injury. With denervating injuries, there should be electromyographic evidence of denervation and/or reinnervation in more than a single root or peripheral nerve distribution, and the paraspinal musculature should be spared. Plexopathies due to conduction block may be difficult to demonstrate with electrodiagnostic testing. Differentiation of lumbosacral plexopathies from single- or multiple-level radiculopathies must be made. With single- or multi-level radiculopathies compared with lumbosacral plexopathies, the paraspinal musculature should show evidence of denervation; sensory nerve conduction studies (NCS) should be normal and symmetric compared with the unaffected side. Electrodiagnostic studies will also help identify affected muscles, which may not be readily apparent on clinical exam. NCS can reveal loss of amplitude of the compound motor and sensory nerve action potentials when there is axonal loss distal to the dorsal root ganglion. Sensory and motor NCS should be compared with the unaffected side. When distal motor NCS are normal, late responses such as H-reflexes and F waves may be useful to detect a proximal lesion in the plexus. Prognosis will depend on the underlying cause and severity of the initial lesion.

Vascular Studies

If vascular compromise is considered as a cause of the plexopathy, then appropriate vascular studies of the aorta and iliac vessels should be completed. The lumbosacral plexus receives its major blood supply from the internal iliac artery and its branches, specifically the lateral sacral, iliolumbar, and superior gluteal arteries.[13,18,19] Injury or disease involving these vessels or the common iliac artery and aorta from which they are derived may result in malfunction of the plexus. Patients with occlusion of the aorta may present with signs and symptoms of a plexus injury before the symptoms of arterial insufficiency.[20] In cases precipitated by vascular surgery, interruption of the pelvic circulation is the primary cause of the plexopathy.[19]

Imaging Studies

The lumbosacral plexus, sciatic nerve, obturator nerve, lumbosacral trunk, and femoral nerve may all be directly visualized on CT scans. The pudendal and obturator nerves (in the obturator foramen) can be observed by using vascular markers. Other nerves such as the iliohypogastric, ilioinguinal, genitofemoral, and lateral femoral cutaneous nerves are difficult to visualize.[21] CT scans can differentiate between plexopathies caused by space-occupying lesions and those with no masses. Pelvic masses observed on CT originate most often from visceral or non-visceral pelvic neoplasms.[22] Pelvic malignancies that are either primary or metastatic can damage the lumbosacral plexus.[12,23] The tumors damage the plexus by either directly invading it or compressing it against the bony pelvis. The plexus may also be affected by tumors that arise from its nerve cell components, including plexiform neurofibromatosis, ependymomas, and schwannomas.[24] CT scans, along with abdominal ultrasound, may be used to diagnose a retroperitoneal hemorrhage that is affecting the plexus.

Using spin-echo techniques and phased array coils, the MRI provides a higher contrast resolution for the sacral plexus than do CT scans. However, because nerves and muscles have similar signal intensities, contrast is low with T1-weighted images. With increasing T2-weighted images there is an increase in the nerve signal intensity. The contrast resolution is further enhanced by the fact that the sacral plexus lies in fat between the sacrum and piriformis muscle.[25]

Other Tests

Entrapment of the ilioinguinal and iliohypogastric nerves may occur as a complication of inguinal herniorrhaphy, appendectomy, Pfannenstiel procedure, or needle suspension of the bladder.[26,27] The diagnosis should be confirmed with a temporary nerve block, and, if complete pain relief is obtained with the block, the nerves should be explored.[27]

Differential Diagnosis

Spinal cord injury

Cauda equina injury

Lumbosacral nerve root injury

Anterior horn cell diseases

Myopathies

Occlusion of the aorta

Treatment

Initial

Initial treatment is based on the presenting symptoms and etiology of the plexopathy. If the cause is treatable, the patient should be referred to the appropriate medical or surgical specialty. The initial rehabilitation goals include joint protection, preservation of range of motion, edema control, and pain amelioration (if pain is present). Compressive stockings, leg elevation, and intermittent compression devices may control edema. Anticonvulsant (e.g., gabapentin) and tricyclic antidepressant (e.g., amitriptyline) medications may most effectively treat pain. Opioids and nonsteroidal anti-inflammatory drugs may also provide some relief, but NSAIDs should not be used in cases caused by hemorrhage.

Rehabilitation

Rehabilitation efforts depend on what neurologic and functional deficits are present. The usual goal of therapy for a lumbosacral plexopathy is restoration of mobility, especially normalizing gait. Therefore, physical therapy will focus on strengthening exercises and flexibility and conditioning exercises, when appropriate. The patient may need an assistive device such as a walker, cane, or brace. Occupational therapy should be considered if mobility deficits interfere with daily activities.

The patient should be educated about energy conservation techniques and care of insensate areas. If present, edema can be controlled with compressive stockings, leg elevation, and intermittent compression devices. Transcutaneous electrical nerve stimulation (TENS) may also provide effective pain control.

Procedures

More invasive treatments for pain amelioration include sympathetic nerve blocks and chemoneurolysis, but these have low success rates.

Surgery

Surgical intervention may be indicated based on the etiology of the injury.

Potential Disease Complications

Potential disease complications include joint contractures, injury due to fall, skin breakdown if insensate on weight-bearing areas, permanent weakness, permanent loss of sensation, bowel and bladder incontinence, and sexual dysfunction.

Potential Treatment Complications

Treatment complications may include increased weakness if the rehabilitation program is too aggressive; skin breakdown due to braces; side effects of anticonvulsants, including dizziness, somnolence, ataxia, and gastrointestinal irritation; and side effects of tricyclic antidepressants, including dry mouth, urinary retention, and AV conduction block; side effects of opioids, including dependence, dizziness, somnolence, and constipation. Analgesics, NSAIDs, and COX-2 inhibitors have well-known side effects that most commonly affect the gastric, hepatic, and renal systems.

References

1. Jenkins DB: Hollinshead's Functional Anatomy of the Limbs and Back, 6th ed. Philadelphia, W.B. Saunders, 1991.
2. Chad DA, Bradley WG: Lumbosacral plexopathy. Semin Neurol 1987;7:97–107.
3. Flanagan WF, Webster GD, Brown MW, Massey EW: Lumbosacral plexus stretch injury following the use of the modified lithotomy position. J Urol 1985;134:567–568.
4. Solheim LF, Hagen R: Femoral and sciatic neuropathies after total hip arthroplasty. Acta Orthop Scand 1980;51:531–534.
5. Rajashekhar TP, Herbison GJ. Lumbosacral plexopathy caused by retroperitoneal hemorrhage: Report of two cases. Arch Phys Med Rehabil 1974;55:91–93.
6. Weis EB Jr. Subtle neurological injuries in pelvic fractures. J Trauma 1984, 24:983-985.
7. Conway RR, Hubbell SL: Electromyographic abnormalities in neurologic injury associated with pelvic fracture: Case report and review of the literature. Arch Phys Med Rehabil 1988;69:539–541.
8. Huittinen VM: Nerve injury in vertical pelvic fractures. Acta Chir Scand 1972;138:571–575.
9. Birchard JD, Pichora DR, Brown PM: External iliac artery and lumbosacral plexus injury secondary to an open book fracture of the pelvis: Report of a case. J Trauma 1990;30:906–908.
10. Feasby TE, Burton SR, Hahn AF: Obstetrical lumbosacral plexus injury. Muscle Nerve 1992;15:937–940.
11. Georgiou A, Grigsby PW, Perez CA: Radiation induced lumbosacral plexopathy in gynecologic tumors: Clinical findings and dosimetric analysis. Int J Radiat Oncol Biol Phys 1993;26:479–482.
12. Thomas JE, Cascino TL, Earle JD. Differential Diagnosis between radiation and tumor plexopathy of the pelvis. Neurology 1985, 35:1-7.
13. Castellanos AM, Glass JP, Yung WK. Regional nerve injury after intra-arterial chemotherapy. Neurology May 1987;37:834–837.
14. Awerbuch GI, Nigro MA, Sandyk R, Levin JR: Relapsing lumbosacral plexus neuropathy: Report of two cases. Eur Neurol 1991;31:348–351.
15. Thomson AJ. Idiopathic lumbosacral plexus neuropathy in two children. Dev Med Child Neurol Mar 1993, 35, 258-260.
16. Chokroverty S, Reyes MG, Rubino FA, Tonaki H: The syndrome of diabetic amyotrophy. Ann Neurol 1977;2:181–194.
17. Raff MC, Asbury AK: Ischemic mononeuropathy and mononeuropathy multiplex in diabetes mellitus. N Engl J Med 1968;279:17–21.
18. Cifu DX, Irani KD: Ischemic lumbosacral plexopathy in acute vascular compromise: Case report. Paraplegia 1991;29:70–75.
19. Gloviczki P, Cross SA, et al: Ischemic injury to the spinal cord or lumbosacral plexus after aorto-iliac reconstruction. Am J Surg 1991;162:131–136.
20. Larson WL, Wald JJ: Foot drop as a harbinger of aortic occlusion. Muscle Nerve 1995;18:899–903.
21. Dietemann JL, Sick H, Wolfram-Gabel R, et al: Anatomy and computed tomography of the normal lumbosacral plexus. Neuroradiology 1987;29:58–68.
22. Vock P, Mattle H, Studer M, Mumenthaler M. Lumbosacral plexus lesions: correlation of clinical signs and computed tomography. J Neurol Neurosurg Psychiatry 1988, 51:72-79.
23. Jaeckle KA, Young DF, Foley KM: The natural history of lumbosacral plexopathy in cancer. Neurology 1985;35:8–15.
24. Gierada DS, Erickson SJ, Haughton VM, et al: MR imaging of the sacral plexus: Normal findings. Am J Radiol 1993;160:1059–1065.
25. Gierada DS, Erickson SJ: MR imaging of the sacral plexus: Abnormal findings. Am J Radiol 1993;160:1067–1071.
26. Seid AS, Amos E: Entrapment neuropathy in laparoscopic herniorrhaphy. Surg Endosc 1994;8:1050–1053.
27. Starling JR, Harms BA. Diagnosis and treatment of genitofemoral and ilioinguinal neuralgia. World J Surg 1989, 13:585-591.

127 Post-Polio Syndrome

Julie K. Silver, MD
Dorothy D. Aiello, PT

Synonyms

Late effects of polio

Post-polio sequelae

ICD-9 Code

138
Late effects of acute
poliomyelitis

Definition

Polio is a disease caused by an RNA virus that has been eradicated from the United States (with the exception of vaccine related cases) since 1979. During the first half of the 20th century, however, there were major epidemics throughout the United States, and although accurate statistics are difficult to obtain, there may be as many as 1.5 million polio survivors currently living in this country. There are many more millions of survivors worldwide, many of whom are children. In the United States, there are several historic reasons for the difficulty in tracking the number of survivors, including the fact that in the past, polio was thought to be either "paralytic" or "non-paralytic." We are beginning to appreciate that people who might have had a very mild episode of polio (perhaps clinically unappreciable—and therefore not classified as paralytic polio) may indeed have suffered some paralysis and may be at risk for post-polio syndrome (PPS).[1]

Post-polio syndrome is a neurologic disorder that is defined by a collection of symptoms that occur in polio survivors who experienced injury to their central nervous system (generally the anterior horn cells in the spinal cord) during their initial infection with the poliovirus. The symptoms of PPS typically occur many years after the initial episode, and the hallmark is *new weakness*. The new weakness may occur in muscles known to be previously affected or in muscles that were thought to be "normal." The majority of known paralytic polio survivors are reported to be affected (approximately 60%).[2] Although new weakness is the most defining symptom of PPS, other symptoms may include new muscle atrophy, pain, swallowing or breathing problems, cold intolerance, and fatigue.[3]

PPS is a diagnosis of exclusion and should fit specific criteria (Table 1).

The cause of PPS is uncertain. There is evidence to suggest that attrition of motor neurons is partially

TABLE 1.	PPS Criteria
1. History of old polio—preferably with recent electrodiagnostic findings consistent with remote anterior horn cell disease.[1]	
2. A period of at least partial recovery from the initial illness and then a long stable period (more than 10 to 20 years).	
3. New symptoms consistent with post-polio syndrome that are not attributable to any other medical condition(s).	

responsible.[4] An abnormality in acetylcholine transmission at the neuromuscular junction has also been suspected.[5] Metabolic factors may play a role.[6] Both the overuse of some muscles leading to attrition of surviving neurons and the disuse of other muscles likely also contribute to new weakness.

Normal motor neurons (Fig. 1) are lost in acute polio, and collateral sprouting of existing motor neurons occurs (Figs. 2A and 2B). Sprouts reinnervate denervated muscle fibers, resulting in larger-than-normal motor units (Fig. 2C). The burden on each of these remaining motor neurons is greater than under normal conditions because there are fewer motor units. As part of the aging process, there is gradual

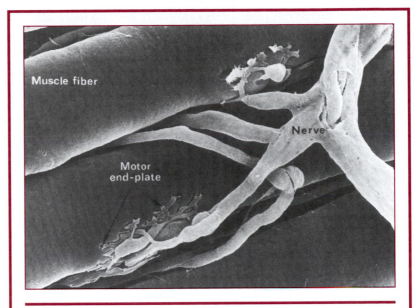

FIGURE 1. Normal neuromuscular junction. Note the nerve branching into several terminal axons, each innervating one muscle fiber. (From Fawcett DW: Bloom and Fawcett: A Textbook of Histology. Philadelphia, W.B. Saunders, 1986, with permission.)

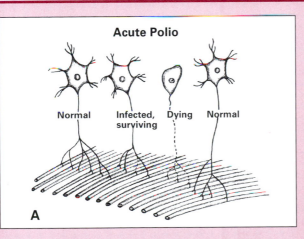

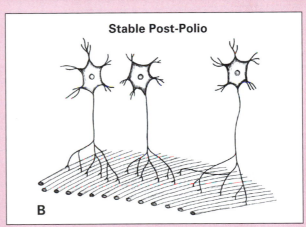

FIGURE 2. Polio neuromuscular junction. A, In acute polio, some neurons die, others are affected but survive, and still others are unaffected. B, In the stable post-polio period, the surviving neurons cover more territory than they did before the polio. C, In post-polio syndrome, there is attrition of surviving axons and neurons.

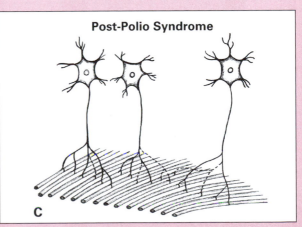

loss of some motor neurons.[7] Polio survivors may be more affected by this loss of motor neurons because they have fewer neurons.

Symptoms

Weakness

As stated earlier, the hallmark of PPS is new weakness. Patients may report that they once were able to go up and down stairs using only one railing but now they need two railings, or they may say that it has become more difficult or even impossible to lift a gallon of milk. They may give a history of falling as a result of knee buckling or tripping due to increased difficulty with clearing their foot. Some patients may report that a limb or muscle looks smaller than it once did, which indicates new atrophy. It is important to glean from the history whether an individual has paresthesias, numbness, back or neck pain, or bowel and bladder symptoms that would all point to another etiology (e.g., myelopathy or radiculopathy). Also, a history of progressive weakness over weeks to months may suggest an alternative diagnosis as well (e.g., thyroid myopathy, amyotrophic lateral sclerosis).

Fatigue

Fatigue is the most common complaint, affecting 87% of polio survivors.[8] Typically, polio survivors report that they feel refreshed in the morning, but feel exhausted later in the day. They may complain that they "hit a wall" or "a curtain comes down." Generally, this fatigue improves with rest. For individuals who are tired first thing in the morning, an alternative diagnosis, such as depression or a sleep disorder, may be present.

Pain

Pain associated with PPS presents as an aching, burning, or cramping in the muscles. Often, the pain is more prominent at the end of the day. Polio survivors are also susceptible to other types of pain resulting from muscle imbalance and stress. Pain may be due to a variety of factors including osteoarthritis that may occur earlier or more severely because of a lack of strong muscles to support the joints, upper extremity neuropathies, etc.

Respiratory Problems

New breathing problems are not uncommon in polio survivors, particularly those who had initial involvement of their respiratory muscles. The most common presentation is new weakness of the respiratory muscles, causing *restrictive* lung disease that is associated with *chronic alveolar hypoventilation*. This restriction is worse in obese patients because of the excess weight over the thoracic cage and abdominal cavity. Patients may complain of shortness of breath, dyspnea on exertion, and/or chronic respiratory infections. Sleep-disordered breathing is also common in polio survivors, and patients may present only with a history of fatigue.

Swallowing Problems

New swallowing problems occur most commonly in patients who had "bulbar" polio that affected the swallowing muscles during the initial infection. Patients may complain of choking, gagging, or coughing or just have vague complaints that they do not feel as comfortable eating as they once did.

Cold Intolerance

Cold intolerance often affects one or more limbs. Most often, limbs that were noticeably paralyzed are affected, but patients may complain of a general inability to thermoregulate. Cold intolerance may be exacerbated by other medical conditions such as peripheral vascular disease.

Physical Examination

The musculoskeletal and neurologic examination should be consistent with a lower motor neuron disease process with absent or diminished reflexes, decreased muscle tone, and asymmetric atrophy and weakness/paralysis of the limb(s) and/or trunk. Sensation should be spared. Fasciculations should be noted and if pronounced and diffuse, an alternative diagnosis should be considered (e.g., amyotrophic lateral sclerosis). Since median and ulnar neuropathies are common in polio survivors, it is important to note sensory deficits and asymmetric muscle atrophy in the hands.[3,9,10] In some individuals, the findings on physical examination may be quite subtle.

Biomechanical abnormalities should also be assessed. These can include lower extremity contractures due to muscle weakness (particularly at the hip and ankle), joint abnormalities (e.g., genu recurvatum at the knee due to weak quadriceps muscles), and loss of joint range of motion without apparent contributing weakness (common in the cervical spine and shoulders). Scoliosis and kyphosis may be present due to muscle imbalance.

When following established testing protocols, manual muscle testing is a useful measure of strength. Since this patient population tends to use compensatory movements, proper stabilization and testing through the range are critical components of manual muscle testing. Proper positioning is also essential for assessing grip and pinch strength with a dynamometer and a pinch gauge.

Specific areas that the patient reports as painful should be evaluated (e.g., rotator cuff pathology in someone who complains of shoulder pain).[11] Gait and seated posture should be assessed since poor posture and biomechanical imbalances can contribute to painful sequelae.

With respect to fatigue, it is important to note the patient's mood and affect, assessing for depression. Blood pressure can be measured to determine whether orthostatic changes that may occur with anemia have taken place. Capillary refill with compression of the digits can be useful. Assessment of any underlying thyroid or respiratory conditions or chronic infections can help to rule out alternative causes of fatigue.

Patients who complain of decreased endurance or shortness of breath should be evaluated in the same manner as any patient with respiratory complaints; this includes vital signs and a baseline pulse oximetry, if available. Pulmonary and cardiac auscultation are also important.

Swallowing problems are best assessed by a clinician who specializes in treating these disorders since they nearly always require technical examinations with specialized equipment to visualize the pharynx and larynx. Cold intolerance should be assessed by noting the temperature and color of the extremities. Assessing peripheral pulses and edema is also important.

Functional Limitations

A recent study showed that polio survivors lose strength at a rate greater than that associated with normal aging in both upper and lower extremity musculature.[12] New weakness can greatly affect mobility, including walking and transfers. New weakness can also affect the patient's ability to perform daily activities, such as gardening, grocery shopping, and even going to get the mail—which can significantly alter their level of independence. New leg weakness may also increase fall risk.

Fatigue may be purely muscular or may affect cognition in terms of memory and concentration.[13] Post-polio fatigue, which typically occurs most profoundly in the afternoon, may affect an individual's ability to work full time. The need for a break or a nap may markedly limit what patients can accomplish during the day, and an early bedtime may limit social activities, resulting in social isolation. Poor sleep associated with anxiety/depression, sleep apnea, or periodic limb movement disorder may also contribute to fatigue and cognitive dysfunction.

Many polio survivors function well despite pain.[14] However, there are some people who have such severe pain that they curtail their activities, particularly activities that exacerbate their symptoms, such as walking and lifting.

New breathing problems may limit patients' ability to do their usual activities, particularly activities that require some physical endurance, such as walking. Reduction of activity can have the negative effect of contributing to muscular deconditioning that can cause even-greater breathing problems and decreased endurance. New swallowing problems, if severe, may cause social isolation or on the other hand may cause patients to feel as though they cannot be left alone when eating. Many people limit exposure to cold, such as avoiding going outside during cold weather. Some people may even choose to live in a warmer climate for comfort reasons. Others may turn up the furnace to accommodate for their cold intolerance.

Diagnostic Studies

Weakness

Initial testing should focus on new weakness since it generally is the primary feature of PPS. Electrodiagnostic studies (EMG and nerve conduction studies) are recommended to rule out other neuromuscular diseases and to help establish a previous history of polio. Although a history of polio can't be proven by electrodiagnostic studies, there are some classic findings such as very large motor unit action potentials that, if present, make the diagnosis much more likely and, if absent, essentially rule out the diagnosis.

If clinically appropriate to establish the correct diagnosis, imaging of the spine (e.g., magnetic resonance imaging [MRI] or computed tomography [CT] with or without myelography) can help to evaluate whether a myelopathy or radiculopathy is present. Useful laboratory studies may include thyroid function studies to rule out thyroid myopathy and muscle enzymes, which can be mildly elevated in PPS.

Fatigue

Patients presenting with fatigue should have a work up for anemia, thyroid dysfunction, depression, and sleep disorders. Sleep disorders are common in polio survivors and are often present as sleep apnea.[15] There should be a very low threshold for ordering a sleep study in a polio survivor complaining of fatigue.

Chronic conditions such as congestive heart failure, diabetes, and chronic infections can also contribute to fatigue and should lead to appropriate work ups. Cancer and other serious alternative diagnoses should be ruled out. Respiratory etiology should also be considered (see the following Respiratory Problems discussion).

Pain

Pain can be a result of many different causes and should be thoroughly investigated. Post-polio pain is diagnosed by history and physical examination. However, diagnostic studies can be contemplated to rule out other conditions. If suspected, upper extremity neuropathies such as carpal tunnel syndrome should be considered and ruled out with electrodiagnostic studies. Plain x-rays can help to diagnose osteoarthritis, spinal stenosis, etc. MRI and CT scans are used to rule out alternative diagnoses.

Respiratory Problems

Respiratory problems often present as chronic alveolar hypoventilation and can be initially evaluated with baseline pulmonary function tests. Chest x-ray and laboratory studies (e.g., arterial blood gas) may also be useful. Pulse oximetry (at rest, during exercise, and while sleeping) may provide additional information. Again, sleep studies are recommended for polio survivors with complaints of fatigue or difficulty with breathing.

Swallowing Problems

Swallowing disorders can be diagnosed with a variety of different imaging studies—most commonly the *modified barium swallow* or the *functional endoscopic evaluation of swallowing*.

Cold Intolerance

Cold intolerance is likely a result of a variety of factors including alterations in the sympathetic nervous system and the paralysis of muscles in the extremities that are important to help maintain dynamic blood flow. Diagnostic studies are generally not performed for this symptom, except to rule out other conditions (e.g., peripheral vascular disease).

Differential Diagnosis

Weakness
- Myopathy
- Amyotrophic lateral sclerosis
- Myelopathy (e.g., due to spinal stenosis, spinal tumors)
- Radiculopathy
- Peripheral neuropathy
- Deconditioning
- Multiple sclerosis
- Myasthenia gravis
- Parkinson's disease
- Adult spinal muscular atrophy

Fatigue
- Sleep disorder
- Depression
- Thyroid dysfunction
- Anemia
- Deconditioning
- Cancer
- Chronic infections
- Respiratory dysfunction
- Cardiac dysfunction
- Chronic systemic disease (e.g., systemic lupus erythematosus, diabetes)
- Fibromyalgia
- Medication side effect

Pain
- Tendinitis
- Bursitis
- Osteoarthritis
- Radiculopathy
- Peripheral neuropathy
- Fibromyalgia
- Myofascial pain syndrome

Respiratory problems
- Cardiac disease
- Chronic obstructive pulmonary disease
- Asthma
- Anemia
- Deconditioning

Swallowing problems
- Gastroesophageal reflux disease
- Benign or malignant lesion
- Stricture

Cold intolerance
- Peripheral vascular disease

Treatment

Initial

Weakness

Currently, there are no medications that significantly improve strength in polio survivors. Pyridostigmine, which is generally gradually increased to a dose of 60 mg tid, has been used with mixed results to improve strength.[16,17]

Fatigue

Fatigue is managed by treating any medical conditions that may be contributing to it. It is particularly important to address sleep disorders in polio survivors who have documented sleep apnea and/or periodic limb movement disorders.[18] Proper sleep hygiene is important (e.g., regular bedtimes, avoidance of caffeine late in the day). Underlying depression can be treated with medications or counseling or both. Additionally, encouraging patients to pace themselves, take rest breaks during the day, and avoid alcohol can be helpful.

In patients with chronic debilitating fatigue, methylphenidate hydrochloride and bromocriptine have been tried with mixed results. More recently, modafinil has been used for treating fatigue pharmacologically.[19,20] The starting dose is usually 200 mg po every morning and may be increased to 400 mg.

Pain

Pain is generally relieved when the underlying medical condition is addressed (e.g., carpal tunnel syndrome, arthritis). If medications are considered, nonsteroidal anti-inflammatory drugs (NSAIDs) including cyclooxygenase- (COX-) 2 inhibitors can be tried as can non-narcotic analgesics. Post-polio myalgias can be treated and have been reported to respond to low-dose tricyclic antidepressants. However, keep in mind that these may exacerbate some sleep disorders.

Respiratory Problems

Respiratory problems, particularly sleep apnea, is often treated with significant improvement in symptoms with continuous positive airway pressure (CPAP) or bilevel positive airway pressure (BiPAP) at night. Oxygen can exacerbate chronic alveolar hypoventilation and should be used with caution.

Swallowing Problems

Swallowing problems are generally amenable to conservative treatment with a speech and language pathologist. Occasionally, surgical intervention is helpful. In rare instances, an alternative to oral feeding is required.

Cold Intolerance

Cold intolerance is treated symptomatically with layered clothing and thermal undergarments.

Rehabilitation

Rehabilitation should focus on patient education, therapeutic exercise, and addressing adaptive equipment needs. Patient education will include knowledge of the diagnosis and appropriate precautions, pacing, falls precautions, postural education, ergonomics, pain management, a home exercise program, and home safety. Home safety may include a home visit because recommending home modifications can markedly improve how safe people are in their homes.[21,22]

The exercise program should be individualized and address flexibility, strength, and conditioning. A non-fatiguing protocol should be used for muscle groups affected by polio. The conditioning program should be done gradually, with protocols similar to a walking program; it should work the individual's less involved muscle groups. Cross-training is a crucial exercise principle for this group because of muscle fatigability.

Evaluating equipment needs should include the consideration of orthotic evaluation, walking aids, scooter/power wheelchair, chairlift, and driving adaptations. Orthotic evaluation should be very comprehensive and may include both upper and lower extremity orthoses. For example, wrist splints may be prescribed for carpal tunnel syndrome and elbow pads for ulnar neuropathy. There are a variety of bracing options and materials; consider light-weight options such as carbon fiber and Kevlar, for this population.[23]

A physical, occupational, or respiratory therapist skilled in treating respiratory disorders may be helpful in teaching the patient some breathing and postural techniques. Additionally, knowledgeable therapists can help patients to conserve energy that can decrease respiratory demands.

Speech and language pathologists can assist with swallowing difficulties by teaching the patient techniques to assist with swallowing and prevent choking and aspiration. Also, the therapist can make recommendations regarding which foods or liquids to avoid. For safety, family members may be instructed in the Heimlich maneuver.

Procedures

Occasionally, therapeutic procedures are recommended based on specific symptoms. For instance, a wide variety of musculsokeletal conditions that are commonly found in polio survivors may be treated with injections (e.g., rotator cuff injury, carpal tunnel syndrome, cervical myofascial pain syndrome).

Surgery

Surgery may be recommended for a variety of orthopedic conditions such as joint replacements and carpal tunnel release. In some instances, individuals with severe swallowing problems are occasionally candidates for surgery or feeding tube placement.

Potential Disease Complications

PPS is characterized by slow progression of symptoms. One of the most significant complications of post-polio syndrome is falling with subsequent injury. Of 233 polio survivors surveyed, 64% reported falling at least once within the last year.[24] This same study also correlated falls in polio survivors with a high incidence of fractures; 82 of 233 surveyed (35%) reported that they had a history of at least one fracture due to a fall. Because of osteopenia/osteoporosis in paralyzed limbs, polio survivors may be more susceptible to injuries.[25] Polio survivors will often report a decrease in functional ability after a serious fall.

Progressive respiratory compromise can also notably change functional status by decreasing endurance. Supplemental oxygen use may even become necessary for an individual who has never needed it before.

Difficulty with swallowing can lead to aspiration pneumonia or malnutrition; these are serious and potentially life-threatening complications.

Potential Treatment Complications

There are three categories of treatment complications. Complications are related to medication side effects, falls, and inappropriate intervention.

Analgesics, NSAIDs, and COX-2 inhibitors have well-known side effects that most commonly affect the gastric, hepatic, and renal systems. Pyridostigmine's side effects are generally dose related and can be recalled by the anacronym SLUD (increased *s*alivation, *l*acrimation, *u*rination and *d*efecation). Respiratory secretions may also be increased with this medication. Tricyclic anti-depressants have cholinergic side effects—the most serious of which is the possibility of acute urinary retention in men (generally men with underlying prostate problems are at risk). Modafinil's side effects include headache, nausea and nervousness. Modafinil may increase the circulating levels of diazepam, phenytoin, and propanolol.

In physical therapy, caution should be used when altering an individual's gait and movement patterns. During gait, a tight gastrocnemius can aid in creating a plantarflexion moment that will produce an extension moment at the knee that will aid a weak quadriceps. If the gastrocnemius is stretched before addressing bracing, the individual may be at increased risk for knee buckling. Heavy and/or inappropriate bracing or mobility devices may hinder mobility and can lead to falls.

Inappropriate interventions may adversely affect a polio survivor. Overly aggressive exercise programs are thought to increase the risk for further weakness and may also result in disabling musculoskeletal injuries.

The bedrest associated with some surgeries seems to pose a significant recuperative problem for polio survivors. Postoperative rehabilitation is often necessary. Also, anecdotally, polio survivors have been reported to have difficulty with general anesthesia and may require larger-than-usual doses of postoperative pain medication. Careful consideration should be given to weighing the risks and benefits of surgery for this population.

References

1. Halstead LS, Silver JK: Nonparalytic polio and postpolio syndrome. Am J Phys Med Rehabil 2000;79:13–18.
2. Gawne AC, Halstead LS: Post-polio syndrome: Pathophysiology and clinical management. Crit Rev Phys Rehabil Med 1995;7(2):147–188.
3. Silver JK: Post-Polio: A Guide for Polio Survivors and their Families. New Haven, CT: Yale University Press, 2001.
4. Dalakas MC: Pathogenetic mechanisms of post-polio syndrome: Morphological, electrophysiological, virological, and immunological correlations. Ann N Y Acad Sci 1995;753:167–185.
5. Maselli RA, Wollmann R, Roos R: Function and ultra-structure of the neuromuscular junction in post-polio syndrome. Ann N Y Acad Sci 1995;753:129–137.
6. Grimby G, Tolback A, Muller U, Larsson L: Fatigue of chronically overused motor units in prior polio patients. Muscle Nerve 1996;June 19:728–737.
7. Halstead LS: Managing Post-Polio: A Guide to Living Well with Post-Polio Syndrome. Washington, DC, NRH Press, 1998.
8. Halstead LS, Rossi CD: New Problems in old polio patients: result of survey of 539 polio survivors. Orthopedics 1985;8:845–850.
9. Werner R, Waring W, Davidoff G: Risk factors for median mononeuropathy of the wrist in postpoliomyelitis patients. Arch Phys Med Rehabil 1989;70(6):464–467.
10. Veerendrakumar M, Taly AB, Nagaraja D: Ulnar nerve palsy due to axillary crutch. Neurol India 2001;49(1):67–70.
11. Klein MG, Whyte J, Keenan MA, et al: The relation between lower extremity strength and shoulder overuse symptoms: A model based on polio survivors. Arch Phys Med Rehabil 2000;81:789–795.
12. Klein MG, Whyte J, Keenan MA, et al: Changes in strength over time among polio survivors. Arch Phys Med Rehabil 2000;81:1059–1064.
13. Bruno RL, Zimmerman JR: Word finding difficulty as a post-polio sequalae. Am J Phys Med Rehabil 2000;79(4): 343–348.
14. Widar M, Ahlstrom G: Pain in persons with post-polio: The Swedish version of the multidimensional pain inventory (MPI). Scand J Caring S 1999;13:33–40.
15. Dean AC, Graham BA, Dalakas M, Sato S: Sleep apnea in patients with postpolio syndrome. Ann Neurol 1998;43(5): 661–664.
16. Seivert BP, Speier JL, Canine JK: Pyridostigmine effect on strength, endurance and fatigue in post-polio patients [abstract]. Arch Phys Med Rehabil 1994;75:1049.
17. Trojan DA, Collet JP, Shapiro S, et al: A multicenter, randomized, double-blind trial of pyridostigmine in post-polio syndrome. Neurology 1999;53:1225–1233.
18. Hsu AA, Staata BA: "Post-polio" sequelae and sleep-related disordered breathing. Mayo Clin Proc 1998;73(3):216–224.
19. Kingshott RN, et al: Randomized, double-blind, placebo-controlled crossover trial of modafinil in the treatment of residual excessive daytime sleepiness in the sleep apnea/hypopnea syndrome. Am J Respir Crit Care Med 2001;163(4): 918–923.
20. Mitler MM, Harsh J, Hiroshkowitz M, Guilleminault C: Long-term efficacy and safety of modafinil (Provigil) for the treatment of excessive daytime sleepiness associated with narcolepsy. Sleep Med 2000;1(3):231–243.
21. Salkeld G, et al: The cost effectiveness of a home hazard reduction program to reduce falls among older persons. Aust N Z J Public Health 2000;24(3):265–271.
22. Cumming RG, et al: Home visits by an occupational therapist for assessment and modification of environmental hazards: A randomized trial of falls prevention. J Am Geriatr Soc 1999;47(12):1397–1402.
23. Silver JK, Aiello DD, Drillio RC: Light weight carbon fiber and Kevlar floor reaction AFO in two polio survivors with new weakness [abstract]. Arch Phys Med Rehab, 1999;80:1180.
24. Silver JK, Aiello DD: Risk of falls in survivors of poliomyelitis [abstract]. Arch Phys Med Rehabil 2000;81:1272.
25. Silver JK: Aging, comorbidities, and secondary disabilities in polio survivors. In Halstead LS (ed): Managing Post-Polio: A Guide to Living Well with Post-Polio Syndrome. Washington, DC, NRH Press, 1998.

128 Post-Concussion Syndrome

Mel B. Glenn, MD

Definition

Post-concussion syndrome (PCS) is a set of signs and symptoms commonly seen following concussion, though many of the symptoms may be related to events other than the cerebral insult. There may be a lag of days or weeks between the concussion and the patient's first complaints, and some related phenomenon, such as depression or anxiety, may not become apparent until months after the initial injury. Although these symptoms can be seen with any severity of injury, the "syndrome" is usually discussed in the context of mild traumatic brain injury (TBI). This chapter addresses some of the more common sequelae following mild TBI.

The term concussion is generally used to refer to an event that results in a mild TBI. The following is one common definition of mild TBI:

A traumatically induced physiological disruption of brain function, manifested by *at least* one of the following: (1) any period of loss of consciousness; (2) any loss of memory for events immediately before or after the accident; (3) any alteration in mental state at the time of the accident (e.g., feeling dazed, disoriented, or confused); and (4) focal neurologic deficit(s) which may or may not be transient; but where the severity of injury does not exceed the following: loss of consciousness of approximately 30 minutes or less; after 30 minutes, an initial Glasgow Coma Scale of 13–15; and posttraumatic amnesia not greater than 24 hours.[1]

Concussion can be graded according to criteria established by the American Academy of Neurology for the purpose of managing concussion after sports injury[2] (Table 1). Grade 1 and 2 concussions are characterized by only transient confusion with no loss of consciousness (LOC). If confusion or concussion symptoms resolve within 15 minutes, the concussion is considered Grade 1. If they last more than 15 minutes, it is a Grade 2 concussion. If there is any loss of consciousness, the concussion is considered Grade 3.

Symptoms

The patient with PCS may present with headache, dizziness (vertigo) and poor balance, forgetfulness, poor concentration, slowed thinking, fatigue and poor energy, insomnia, depression, anxiety, irritability, sensitivity to noise, and sensitivity to light.[3–6]

TABLE 1. When to Return to Play After Removal from Contest

Grade of Concussion	Time Until Return to Play*
Multiple Grade I concussion	1 week
Grade 2 concussion	1 week
Multiple Grade 2 concussions	2 weeks
Grade 3—brief loss of consciousness (seconds)	1 week
Grade 3—prolonged loss of consciousness (minutes)	2 weeks
Multiple Grade 3 concussions	1 month or longer, based on clinical decision of evaluating physician

* Only after being asymptomatic with normal neurologic assessment at rest and with exercise.

The etiology of the symptoms of PCS is often multifactorial, and much of it still not well understood. The usual inciting factors are mild TBI with residual impairment of attention and memory; whiplash or other soft tissue injury to the head and neck; and, at times, disruption of the vestibular apparatus. Problems with attention, forgetfulness, and fatigue commonly coupled with the development of headaches, insomnia, and vertigo may lead to considerable anxiety and depression and a "shaken sense of self."[7] In the small-but-significant percentage of patients who develop a persistent post-concussion syndrome (PPCS), these symptoms often exacerbate each other,[4] further exacerbating the neuropsychologic impairment, which may then be slow to improve even as the underlying brain injury continues to recover.[7,8]

Cognitive

The patient should be questioned about the inciting event with regard to whether there was a LOC, loss of memory, alteration in mental status, or focal neurologic findings. A patient's subjective feeling of being dazed or confused may or may not reflect actual brain injury. It is common for a person to feel dazed due to the emotional shock experienced after an accident. There is often limited or no documentation of the details of the patient's mental status immediately following the accident, and a clinician must do his or her best to reconstruct the situation based largely on the history given by the patient. The observations of others may help to clarify whether the patient was responding slowly or otherwise appeared confused. Emergency medical records should be obtained whenever possible. The clinician's history of the events surrounding the initial accident should also include exploration of other associated injuries, seizure, vomiting, and drug or alcohol intoxication. A pre-injury social, psychologic, vocational, and educational history should be obtained, including any history of learning disability or attention deficit disorder.

Headaches

Tension, musculoskeletal, vascular, and mixed headaches are the most common types seen after concussion.[5,9–11] The patient should be questioned with respect to severity, quality, location and radiation, date of onset, duration, frequency, and exacerbating or ameliorating factors.

Vestibular

Vertigo can be caused by cupulolithiasis or canalithiasis (benign paroxysmal positional vertigo [BPPV]), perilymph fistula, endolymphatic hydrops, or labyrinthine concussion, or it may be cervicogenic. Perilymph fistula, endolymphatic hydrops, and labyrinthine concussion are usually associated with hearing loss and tinnitus, as well. Non-vertiginous dizziness is not usually directly related to concussion; medication-induced dizziness (e.g., by NSAIDs and antidepressants) and other causes should be considered, including psychogenic dizziness.[12]

Physical Examination

The examination of the individual with PCS will often elicit problems with attention and memory on mental status evaluation. Mini-mental status testing may be normal; more extensive evaluation and perhaps neuropsychologic testing, including reaction time[13] and continuous performance tasks, may be necessary to reveal the deficits. Findings more severe than would be expected for a mild TBI indicate that there are likely to be other contributing factors. Medications, anxiety, depression, insomnia, pain, and either conscious or unconscious symptom augmentation can all exacerbate or cause problems with attention and memory.[6,7] Assessment of mood and affect may reveal evidence of depression and anxiety.

Examination of the head and neck often elicits restriction of motion, tender points, or trigger points radiating to the head.[10,14]

During acute vertigo, nystagmus should be present. As adaptation begins to occur, nystagmus may only be seen with certain maneuvers (e.g., following 20 horizontal head shakes). When BPPV is the cause, the Hallpike-Dix maneuver is usually positive. This maneuver is performed with the patient in the sitting position on a flat surface with the head rotated 45 degrees to either side. The patient is quickly lowered from the sitting to lying position, until the head, still rotated, is extended over the edge of the examining table. Vertigo is experienced and nystagmus is seen after a lag of up to 30 seconds.[12] Patients with vertigo may have difficulty with tandem walk, hopping, and other maneuvers involving movement of the head and eye-body coordination.

Some patients complain of a feeling of visual disorientation or blurred vision. The symptoms can be related to a need for changes in refraction or can be related to vestibular, attentional, or psychologic problems. Commonly, nothing will be found on routine examination. The sense of smell may be affected by damage to branches of the olfactory nerve as they pass through the cribiform plate or focal cortical contusion.[14] *Neurologic examination is usually otherwise normal.*

Functional Limitations

The extent to which post-concussion disorders interfere with function varies with the extent of the associated pathology but also depends on the psychologic reaction to the post-concussion impairments. Patients with pre-existing social, psychologic, and vocational difficulties; individuals older than 40 years; patients with previous concussion; or patients with pre-existing learning disabilities or attentional disorders are more susceptible to PCS.[6,15]

The most common consequences of PCS are limitations in home and community living skills and/or social, academic, or vocational disability. Patients may be forgetful and inattentive; have difficulty following conversations; and may find crowded, noisy environments difficult to tolerate. Headaches are often exacerbated by attentional demands and other stresses. Vertigo causes difficulty tolerating motion, including, for some, moving vehicles.

Diagnostic Studies

If not done acutely, CT scan of the head should be obtained shortly after injury to rule out intracranial hematoma in all patients with mild head injury who have had any question of loss of consciousness and who also have any of the following: focal neurologic findings, headache, vomiting, age older than 60 years, drug or alcohol intoxication, anterograde amnesia, physical evidence of trauma above the clavicles, or seizures.[16] Although definitive criteria have not been established for those who have had no LOC, it is probably wise to obtain a CT scan or MRI on anyone who continues to have significant problems with headaches, lethargy, confusion or anterograde memory loss; who has focal neurologic findings; and who did not have any neuroimaging acutely. Functional neuroimaging has not yet been studied thoroughly enough to be used routinely following mild TBI. [17]

Cervical spine x-rays should be performed on patients with significant neck pain shortly after the accident to assess for fracture or subluxation.

Neuropsychologic evaluation should be performed if forgetfulness and attention deficits persist, particularly when rehabilitation therapies are to be pursued. Testing can provide the patient and the treatment team with a more thorough understanding of the patient's neuropsychologic strengths and weaknesses and in some instances can assist with understanding the interplay between neurocognitive and other psychologic contributions to cognitive disturbance. Tests for assessing malingering and symptom magnification can be incorporated when necessary.

A sleep study (polysomnography) is indicated, largely to rule out sleep apnea, when excessive daytime sleepiness does not improve despite the absence of sedating medications and despite apparently adequate sleep. The threshold for obtaining polysomnography should be lower for obese patients and/or those who snore prominently.

When vestibular complaints are prominent or are not improving in the early months following the injury, a thorough vestibular evaluation, including electronystagmography, is indicated. Audiologic evaluations should be done when hearing loss is suspected or when tinnitus persists.[12]

Ophthalmology or optometry evaluation should be considered when visual symptoms are present.

Differential Diagnosis

Depressive disorders

Anxiety disorders

Somatoform disorder

Whiplash injury with headache
(myofascial pain syndrome)

Sleep apnea

Early progressive dementia

Malingering and symptom magnification

Treatment

Initial

Treatment will depend on the specific constellation of symptoms and their severity. In general, if the patient is seen in the first few weeks following the injury, the major emphasis should be placed on caring for acute problems such as vertigo, headache, neck pain, and insomnia and on educating the patient and significant others. Explanations should integrate the physical, cognitive, and psychologic dimensions of the symptoms in as clear and simple a manner as possible. This is no small task, given the diversity of symptoms, possible etiologies, and the limited understanding of post-concussion disorders at this time. The patient's experience, including the psychologic reactions, should be validated and normalized.[7] The patient should be told that improvement is to be expected; after milder concussions, reasonable reassurance should be given that a good recovery is likely without dismissing what the patient is experiencing. Establishing a reasonable expectation for recovery can be helpful in preventing persistent post-concussion syndrome.[18] Anticipating the psychologic reactions to post-concussion symptoms that occur in some patients allows patients to recognize these reactions if and when they begin, and leaves the door open for them to seek psychologic help. Follow-up should be planned and more extensive counseling provided at the first signs of significant distress or if substantial improvement is not seen within 3 months without apparent psychologic turmoil. Patients with significant symptoms should be instructed to take time off from work, school, or other taxing activities since the stresses of attempting to perform under these circumstances can exacerbate the symptoms.[15] Clinicians working with sports injuries should familiarize themselves with the American Academy of Neurology guidelines for the management of concussion in sports.[2] (See Potential Disease Complications.)

Acute vertigo may require a few days of bed rest.[12] The management of acute neck pain is described in Chapter 5.

Rehabilitation

Cognitive

If symptoms persist, patients may benefit from speech and/or occupational therapy to learn strategies for managing problems with arousal, attention, memory, and organization. The timing of therapies depends on the severity of the disability and the pace of recovery, which can often be determined within the first 3 months after injury. There is no published data on the timing of these interventions, and there are no specific guidelines available. Therapies should address the specific functional tasks that the individual faces on a daily basis and may need to include community outings. Foam earplugs or sunglasses can be tried for patients sensitive to noise and light, respectively.[14] Paper or electronic memory aids may be helpful. Psychostimulant[19] or dopaminergic drug therapy may be useful for reducing the extent of attention deficits.

Psychological

As previously noted, if symptoms persist beyond a few months, psychologic counseling is almost always indicated. Some individuals benefit from learning relaxation techniques and sleep hygiene. Educating the patient and significant others should continue to emphasize the interaction between the cognitive, psychologic, and physical sequelae. It is important that the treatment team communicate on a regular basis for treatment planning and to ensure that all clinicians approach these issues from a common framework so that mixed messages are not delivered to the patient. Support groups are often useful as well and offer an opportunity for further education about the symptoms. Family counseling should be offered when there is evidence of significant stress on family members or problematic family dynamics.

Depression and anxiety can also be addressed pharmacologically. It is usually best to begin with non-sedating, non-anticholinergic agents such as the selective serotonin reuptake inhibitors (e.g., paroxetine 20 to 60 mg/day or venlafaxine 75 to 300 mg/day) to avoid further exacerbation of neuropsychologic problems. Sedating agents such as trazodone (50 to 300 mg hs) or mirtazepine (15 to 60 mg hs) may be necessary for those with significant insomnia.[5,19]

Headaches

The etiology of post-traumatic headache is probably multifactorial.[5,8–11,14,15] Addressing problems with attention, sleep disorders, and psychologic stresses may reduce the tension component of headaches. When myofascial pain originating in the neck, upper back, or temporomandibular (TMJ) joints contributes, physical therapy, including stretching and strengthening exercises, postural retraining, environmental modification, trigger point massage, modalities, and/or massage should be tried (see Chapters 5 and 9). However, headaches often persist despite these interventions. Trigger point injections can be helpful, as can pharmacologic approaches. Patients with TMJ problems can be treated with myofascial techniques, mouthguards, and exercises (see Chapter 9). Headaches with an apparent vascular component may respond to some NSAIDs or vasoconstrictive agents commonly used to abort migraine headaches (e.g., sumatriptan) or those used for prophylaxis, such as some beta-blockers (e.g., propranolol), calcium-channel blockers (e.g., verapamil), antidepressants, anticonvulsants (particularly valproic acid), and serotonin antagonists (e.g., cyproheptadine). Tension headaches may respond to some of these agents as well, though not to calcium-channel blockers. Injection and ablative techniques can be considered for occipital neuralgia that does not respond to more conservative approaches.[5,20,21]

Vestibular

When vestibular symptoms persist, vestibular rehabilitation may both encourage central nervous system accommodation under controlled circumstances and assist the patient in learning compensatory strategies. Positioning maneuvers may bring relief from BPPV by displacing calcium debris. Suppressive medications can interfere with central accommodation and result in rebound vertigo and should be used judiciously, if at all.[12] Cervicogenic dizziness can be treated by addressing the underlying cervical musculoskeletal problems (see Chapter 7).

Vocational

The extent to which an employer or academic institution is supportive following a mild TBI can be crucial to successful return to work or school. Vocational counselors can facilitate communication between the patient and the workplace. Therapies should attempt to simulate workplace tasks. A gradual return to work can ease the transition.[7]

Potential Disease Complications

As previously noted, PPCS is a possible outcome of PCS. Patients with PPCS may present primarily as having a chronic pain problem or chronic depression.

Individuals who sustain a second concussion while still symptomatic from another recent concussion are susceptible to cerebral edema and dangerous increases in incracranial pressure (second impact syndrome). Multiple concussions, even after apparent clinical recovery from earlier episodes, can result in cumulative brain injury. Thus, caution must be exercised by those responsible for returning athletes to play.[22]

Potential Treatment Complications

Those treating the patient with post-concussive syndrome may contribute to the persistence of symptoms by either overemphasizing the role of brain injury in causing symptoms with other etiologies or, conversely, by overemphasizing psychologic factors when brain injury and other physiologic variables are more prominent.[7,15] There is often a fine line to be walked, and each patient must be approached individually in this regard, though there is little data available to guide the clinician.

Some of the complications related to medications can appear paradoxic: the frequent use of analgesics (NSAIDs and acetaminophen) can occasionally cause rebound headaches, as can the too frequent use of ergotamine. Although generally well tolerated, psychostimulants, dopaminergic agents, and antidepressants can lead to sedation, worsening attention, agitation, or psychosis. There is a myriad of other complications possible from the use of the medications previously mentioned.

References

1. Mild Traumatic Brain Injury Committee of the Head Injury Interdisciplinary Special Interest Group of the American Congress of Rehabilitation Medicine: Definition of mild traumatic brain injury. J Head Trauma Rehabil 1993;8(3): 86–87.
2. Quality Standards Subcommittee of the American Academy of Neurology: Practice parameter: The management of concussion in sports (summary statement). Neurology 1997;48:581–585.
3. Alves W, Macciocchi SN, Barth JT: Postconcussive symptoms after uncomplicated mild head injury. J Head Trauma Rehabil 1993;8(3):48–59.
4. Cicerone KD, Kalmar K: Persistent postconcussion syndrome: The structure of subjective complaints after mild traumatic brain injury. J Head Trauma Rehabil 1995;10(3):1–17.
5. Hines ME: Posttraumatic headaches. In Varney NR, Roberts RJ (eds): The Evaluation and Treatment of Mild Traumatic Brain Injury. Mahwah, NJ, Lawrence Erlbaum Associates, 1999, pp 375–410.
6. Mittenberg W, Strauman S: Diagnosis of mild head injury and the postconcussion syndrome. J Head Trauma Rehabil 2000;15(2):783–791.
7. Kay T: Neuropsychological treatment of mild traumatic brain injury. J Head Trauma Rehabil 1993;8(3):74–85.
8. Martelli MF, Grayson RL, Zasler ND: Posttraumatic headache: Neuropsychological and psychological effects and treatment implications. J Head Trauma Rehabil 1999;14(1):49–69.
9. Packard RC: Epidemiology and pathogenesis of posttraumatic headache. J Head Trauma Rehabil 1999;14(1):9–21.
10. Zafonte RD, Horn LJ: Clinical assessment of posttraumatic headaches. J Head Trauma Rehabil 1999;14(1):22–33.
11. Zasler ND: Mild traumatic brain injury: Medical assessment and intervention. J Head Trauma Rehabil 1993;8(3):13–29.

12. Tusa RJ, Brown SB: Neuro-otologic trauma and dizziness. In Rizzo M, Tranel D (eds): Head Injury and Postconcussive Syndrome. New York, Churchill Livingstone, 1996, pp 177–200.
13. Bleiberg J, Halpern EL, Reeves D, Daniel JC: Future directions for the neuropsychological assessment of sports concussion. J Head Trauma Rehabil 1998;13(2):36–44.
14. Zasler ND: Neuromedical diagnosis and management of post-concussive disorders. Phys Med Rehabil State Art Rev 1992;6:33–67.
15. Alexander MP: Minor traumatic brain injury: A review of physiogenesis and psychogenesis. Semin Clin Neuropsychiatry 1997;2:177–187.
16. Haydel MJ, Preston CA, Mills TJ, et al: Indications for computed tomography in patients with minor head injury. N Engl J Med 2000;343:100–105.
17. Herscovitch P: Functional brain imaging—basic principles and application to head trauma. In Rizzo M, Tranel D (eds): Head Injury and Postconcussive Syndrome. New York, Churchill Livingstone, 1996, pp 89–118.
18. Mittenberg W, Tremont G, Zielinski RE, et al: Cognitive-behavioral prevention of postconcussion syndrome. Arch Clin Neuropsych 1996;11:139–145.
19. Gualtieri TC: The pharmacologic treatment of mild brain injury. In Varney NR, Roberts RJ (eds): The Evaluation and Treatment of Mild Traumatic Brain Injury. Mahwah, NJ, Lawrence Erlbaum Associates, 1999, pp 411–419.
20. Barcellos S, Rizzo M: Post-traumatic headaches. In Rizzo M, Tranel D (eds): Head Injury and Postconcussive Syndrome. New York, Churchill Livingstone, 1996, pp 139–175.
21. Bell KR, Kraus EE, Zasler ND: Medical management of posttraumatic headaches: pharmacological and physical treatment. J Head Trauma Rehabil 1999;14(1):34–48.
22. Kelly JP, Rosenberg J: Diagnosis and management of concussion in sports. Neurology 1997;48:575–580.

129 Psoriatic Arthritis

Karen Atkinson, MD, MPH

Synonyms

Inflammatory arthritis associated with psoriasis

Spondyloarthropathy associated with psoriasis

Seronegative spondyloarthropathy

ICD-9 Code

696.0
Psoriatic arthropathy

Definition

Psoriatic arthritis is an inflammatory arthritis occurring in approximately 5% to 7% of patients with psoriasis.[1] No diagnostic criteria exist for this disease, but patients generally present with an inflammatory arthritis, negative rheumatoid factor, and psoriatic skin disease. Unlike rheumatoid arthritis, there is an equal sex distribution. The onset of arthritis, however, can coincide with or precede the onset of skin disease.

Several patterns or subgroups of psoriatic arthritis are recognized[2]:

1. Symmetric arthritis similar to rheumatoid arthritis
2. Inflammatory arthritis confined to the distal interphalangeal (DIP) joints of the hands and feet
3. Arthritis mutilans
4. Spondyloarthropathy (spondylitis and sacroiliitis)
5. Oligoarticular arthritis

Symptoms

Patients report a variety of constitutional, joint, eye, and skin symptoms.[2–6]

General

Morning stiffness is a prominent feature of psoriatic arthritis. Unlike the brief (5 to 10 minutes) of stiffness that occurs in patients with osteoarthritis, the morning stiffness in psoriatic arthritis is greater than 30 to 60 minutes and often lasts for hours. Fatigue and generalized malaise are also common complaints.

Joint

Patients present with joint pain and swelling. Patients may also complain of loss of joint function, which may be due to joint inflammation or structural damage. A Baker's cyst can develop and cause pain and/or swelling of the popliteal fossa. If the cyst ruptures, it causes pain, swelling, and erythema of the calf. Back pain and stiffness can be prominent features of the history. Enthesitis, inflammation at the site of tendon or ligamentous insertion onto bone, is common in psoriatic arthritis. Achilles enthesitis results in pain at the heel, and plantar fasciitis causes plantar foot pain that is typically most intense upon rising in the morning.

Eye

Patients with conjunctivitis complain of red eyes. Iritis causes deep pain and tearing. As in rheumatoid arthritis, patients can have keratoconjunctivitis sicca (dry eyes) and relate a feeling of foreign body sensation, burning, and/or discharge.

Skin

Psoriasis is present in 90% of patients at the time of diagnosis of psoriatic arthritis. The arthritis, however, may precede the onset of skin disease.

TABLE 1. Joint Involvement

Pattern or Subgroup	Clinical Features
Symmetric polyarthritis (RA-like)	Small joints of hands and feet/wrists/ankles/elbows/knees (may include DIP joint, distinguishing it from RA) Seronegative
Distal interphalangeal (DIP) involvement	Inflammatory changes in the DIP joints High association with psoriatic nail changes (onycholysis and pitting)
Arthritis mutilans	Severe resorptive arthritis resulting in floppy or flail digits Shortening of the digits with skin folds that can be extended by the clinician (telescoping)
Spondyloarthropathy	Spondylitis Sacroiliitis Enthesitis
Oligoarthritis	Large joint (e.g., knee) One or two small joints of hands/feet Dactylitis (sausage digit)

Physical Examination

All joints should be examined for swelling, warmth, effusion, range of motion, and deformity. Psoriatic arthritis can present in several different clinical patterns (see Table 1).[2,3] Any joint can be involved. If patients do not relate a history of psoriasis, the examiner should do a careful examination of the scalp, flexural regions, and nails (onycholysis, pitting, and/or hyperkeratosis).

In the hands, DIP joint involvement occurs and is associated with psoriatic nail changes. Dactylitis is the result of digital joint and tendon sheath inflammation and causes a diffusely swollen (sausage) digit. Inflammation of the Achilles tendon and/or its insertion site on the calcaneus can cause tenderness and/or thickening.

Patients with conjunctivitis will have red, injected sclera. Iritis causes pericorneal erythema (ciliary flush) and miosis.

Functional Limitations

Functional limitations depend on the location and severity of joint involvement. The criteria for the assessment of functional status that have been established for rheumatoid arthritis are also applied to patients with psoriatic arthritis (see Chapter 134). These criteria are based on activities of daily living, including self-care (dressing, feeding, bathing, grooming, and toileting) and vocational (work, school, and homemaking) and avocational (recreational and/or leisure) activities.[6]

Diagnostic Studies

Laboratory studies may reveal anemia of chronic disease and an elevated sedimentation rate. Joint fluid is inflammatory (greater than 2000 WBC) with negative cultures and crystal examination. Rheumatoid factor (RF) is usually negative. In patients with positive RF, the co-existence of psoriasis and rheumatoid arthritis must be considered, especially if the pattern is a symmetric polyarthritis. In the spondylitic form, 25% of patients are HLA-B27 positive.[5]

Radiographs can assist in the evaluation of both axial and peripheral involvement.[3,7] Spine films may show syndesmophytes, though they often spare the thoracolumbar junction and are "chunky," helping to distinguish them from the changes of ankylosing spondylitis. Cervical spine views may show erosion of the odontoid and atlantoaxial subluxation. Radiologic evaluation of peripheral joints can help to distinguish this form of arthritis from rheumatoid arthritis. Psoriatic changes include DIP involvement, osteolysis (metacarpals and phalanges), joint ankylosis, periostitis, and pencil-in-cup deformity. Bony proliferation may be found in the pelvis and calcaneous, corresponding to enthesitis.

Differential Diagnosis

Other spondyloarthropathies
  Enteropathic arthritis
  Ankylosing spondylitis

Rheumatoid arthritis

Crystal-induced arthritis (especially with DIP involvement)
  Gout
  Pseudogout

Treatment

Initial

The approach to treatment is generally the same as for other spondyloarthropathies.[8,9] Nonsteroidal anti-inflammatory drugs (NSAIDs) are effective in many patients. COX-2 specific anti-inflammatories may reduce the incidence of gastrointestinal symptoms in patients who have a history of bleeding or who are intolerant of traditional NSAIDs. For patients with inadequate response or progressive, erosive disease, disease modifying drugs (DMARDs) should be initiated. Antimalarials, intramuscular gold, sulfasalazine, azathioprine, methotrexate, and cyclosporin A have all been shown to be effective. As with the treatment of other inflammatory arthridities, combination therapy can be effective. Biologic agents such as anti-TNF antibodies are currently being studied.[10] Corticosteroids can be very useful and can be administered systemically as a bridge to therapy with DMARDs or intra-articularly for monoarticular or oligoarticular involvement.

Photochemotherapy (PUVA) used by the dermatologist for skin disease can sometimes improve peripheral joint involvement but does not affect axial disease.[5]

Rehabilitation

Approaches to rehabilitation are identical to those in rheumatoid and other inflammatory arthritis. The role of occupational and physical therapy may be different in early or established disease and end stage disease. In early disease, occupational therapy is directed toward patient education about how to minimize joint stress when performing activities of daily living. Splints may be employed to provide joint rest and reduce inflammation. Splints may also allow functional use of joints that would otherwise be limited by pain. Paraffin baths can provide relief of pain and stiffness in the small joints of the hands. In end stage disease, the occupational therapist plays an important role, providing aids and adaptive devices, such as raised toilet seats, special chairs and beds, and special grips, that can assist in self-care.

Physical therapy can be very helpful in reducing joint inflammation and pain. The therapist may employ a variety of techniques, including the application of heat or cold, transcutaneous nerve stimulation, and iontophoresis. Water exercise (hydrotherapy) is used to increase muscle strength without joint overuse. In patients with foot involvement, such as dactylitis, a high toe box or extra-depth shoe may provide decreased pain and a more normal gait. Shoe inserts are often used in Achilles tendinitis and plantar fasciitis. For patients with axial involvement, the goal of therapy is maintaining a normal upright posture through stretching of paravertebral musculature and correcting the tendency toward kyphotic posture. In end stage disease, the goals of therapy are reducing joint inflammation, loosening fixed position of joints, improving the function of damaged joints, and improving strength and general condition. Local immobilization may be utilized to reduce inflammation and pain. Non-fixed contractures may be prevented or improved with periods of splinting combined with goal-oriented exercise. Muscle strength and overall conditioning may be improved by static, range-of-motion, and relaxation exercises. In recent years, aerobic and dynamic strengthening exercises have been used without detrimental effect to the joints. These dynamic exercises are more effective in increasing muscle strength, range of motion, and physical capacity.[11] The motivation and encouragement provided by the therapist should not be underestimated.

Procedures

For monoarticular or oligoarticular involvement, local steroid injection may be used when NSAIDs fail to control joint inflammation.

Surgery

Orthopedic intervention including joint replacement, tendon repair, and synovectomy may be indicated. Patients with suspected or confirmed cervical spine involvement will need special consideration/handling by anaesthesiology during intubation.

Potential Disease Complications

Psoriatic arthritis can lead to progressive damage to joints, including ankylosis, resulting in lack of function. Ankylosis of the spine, together with osteoporosis, increases the susceptibility to fracture. Ruptured tendons result secondary to chronic enthesitis. Inflammatory eye disease sometimes results in visual loss.

Potential Treatment Complications

Side effects vary according to the drug used (Table 2). [12]

TABLE 2. Toxicities of Medications Used in Psoriatic Arthritis

Medication	Side Effects	Medication	Side Effects
NSAIDs		Sulfasalazine	Myelosuppression
Traditional	Dyspepsia, ulcer, or bleeding		Hemolysis (G6PD deficient patients)
	Renal insufficiency		
	Hepatotoxicity		Hepatotoxicity
	Rash		Photosensitivity/rash
			Dyspepsia/diarrhea
COX-2 inhibitors	Same as traditional NSAIDs but GI side effects occur less often		Headaches
	No platelet effect		Oligospermia
Glucocorticoids	Increased appetite/weight gain	Azathioprine	Myelosuppression
	Cushingoid habitus		Hepatotoxicity
	Acne		Pancreatitis (rarely)
	Fluid retention		Lymphoproliferative disorders (long-term risk)
	Hypertension		
	Diabetes		
	Glaucoma/cataracts		
	Atherosclerosis		
	Avascular necrosis		
	Osteoporosis		
	Impaired wound healing		
	Increased susceptibility to infection		
Antimalarials	Dyspepsia	Methotrexate	Hepatic fibrosis/cirrhosis
	Hemolysis (G6PD deficient patients)		Pneumonitis
	Macular damage		Myelosuppression
	Abnormal skin pigmentation		Mucositis
	Neuromyopathy		Dyspepsia
	Rash		Alopecia
Gold	Myelosuppression	Cyclosporin A	Renal insufficiency
	Proteinuria or hematuria		Hypertension
	Oral ulcers		Anemia
	Rash		
	Pruritus		

References

1. Espinoza LR, Cuellar MI, Silveira LH: Psoriatic arthritis. Curr Opin Rheumatol 1992;4:470–478.
2. Pitzalis C, Pipitone N: Psoriatic arthritis. J R Soc Med 2000;93(8)412–415.
3. Helliwell PS, Wright V: Psoriatic arthritis: Clinical features. In Klippel JH, Dieppe PA (eds): Rheumatolog, 2nd ed. London, Mosby, 1998, pp 21.1–21.8.
4. Moll JMH, Wright V: Psoriatic arthritis. Semin Arthritis Rheum 1973;3:55–78.
5. Boumpas DT, Tassiulas IO: Psoriatic arthritis. In Klippel JH (ed): Primer on the Rheumatic Diseases, 11th ed. Arthritis Foundation, 1997, pp 175–179.
6. Hochberg MC, Chang RW, Dwosh I, et al: The American College of Rheumatology 1991 Revised Criteria for the classification of global functional status in rheumatoid arthritis. Arthritis Rheum 1992;35:493–502.
7. Resnick D, Niwayama G: Psoriatic arthritis. In Resnick D, Niwayama G (eds): Diagnsis of bone and joint disorders, vol 2. Philadelphia, W.B. Saunders, 1981, pp 1103–1129.
8. Gladman DD: Psoriatic arthritis: Recent advances in pathogenesis and treatment. Rheum Dis Clin North Am 1992;18:247–256.
9. Haslock I: Ankylosing spondylitis: Management. In Klippel JH, Dieppe PA (eds): Rheumatology, 2nd ed. London, Mosby, 1998, pp 19.1–19.10.
10. Mease PJ, Goffe BS, Metz J, et al: Etanercept in the treatment of psoriatic arthritis and psoriasis: A randomized trial. Lancet 2000;356:385–390.
11. van den Ende CH, Breedveld FC, le Cessie S, et al: Effect of invasive exercise on patients with active rheumatoid arthritis: A randomized clinical trial 2000;59(8):615–621.
12. Cash JM, Klippel JH: Drug therapy: Second-line drug therapy for rheumatoid arthritis. N Engl J Med 1994;330(19):1368–1375.

130 Pressure Ulcers

Christopher R. Rehm, MD
Hilary Siebens, MD

Synonyms

Pressure sores

Bed sores

Decubitus ulcers

ICD-9 Code

707.0
Decubitus ulcer, pressure ulcer

Definition

A pressure ulcer is an unrelieved pressure over a defined area, usually over a bony prominence, resulting in ischemia, cell death, and tissue necrosis.[1] Due to the variety of locations in which pressure ulcers develop and the multiple precipitating circumstances that cause them, the term *pressure ulcer* is preferred over *decubitus ulcer*. The most common locations for pressure ulcers to develop are the sacrum, ischial tuberosities, greater trochanters, heels, and lateral malleoli.[2] To facilitate consistent communication between health care providers, pressure ulcers are staged or graded using standardized systems. The following is the staging system recommended in the Agency for Health Care Policy and Research (AHCPR) guidelines for treating pressure ulcers.[3] A recent review of the literature found no significant changes or advances in the approach to treating pressure ulcers since the AHCPR guidelines were published in 1994.[4]

Stage 1: Nonblanchable erythema of intact skin, the heralding lesion of skin ulceration. In individuals with darker skin, discoloration of the skin, warmth, edema, induration, or hardness may also be indicators.

Stage II: Partial thickness skin loss involving epidermis, dermis, or both. The ulcer is superficial and presents clinically as an abrasion, blister, or shallow crater.

Stage III: Full thickness skin loss involving damage to or necrosis of subcutaneous tissue that may extend down to, but not through, underlying fascia. The ulcer presents clinically as a deep crater with or without undermining of adjacent tissue.

Stage IV: Full thickness skin loss with extensive destruction; tissue necrosis; or damage to muscle, bone, or supporting structures (i.e., tendon, joint capsule). Undermining and sinus tracts also may be associated with stage IV pressure ulcers.

The incidence of pressure ulcers among patients in acute care hospitals ranges from 1% to 5%, with a prevalence of 3% to 14%. The prevalence of pressure ulcers on admission to skilled nursing facilities ranges between 15% to 25%.[5]

Symptoms

Pressure ulcers can cause pain and discomfort in people with intact sensation; however, these ulcers can be painless in patients with spinal cord injuries. Most commonly, patients suffer from osteomyelitis, bacteremia, and cellulitis in association with pressure ulcers.[3] In non-healing pressure ulcers, osteomyelitis can occur up to one third of the time.[6] With these complications, patients can suffer from fever, malaise, and chills. The wound may be draining and or foul smelling. It is also important to assess the patient for symptoms of depression, alcohol or drug abuse, and polypharmacy because these are common in patients with pressure ulcers.

Physical Examination

The critical first step in evaluating for a pressure ulcer is to thoroughly examine the skin surfaces. If an ulcer is found, prior to staging, all necrotic tissue must be removed. Once appropriate debriding is completed, a detailed exam of the area is used to establish proper staging. Included in the description should be the length, width, and depth and presence or absence of sinus tracts, undermining, exudates, granulation tissue, and epithelialization. Often a photograph is taken or a drawing is done in the chart to compare with subsequent exams.

On the general exam, evaluating overall strength, muscle tone, and spasticity as well as range of motion and presence of contractures is important. Abnormalities in these areas can contribute to both the development and the persistence of pressure ulcers. In addition, assessment of the individual, including overall physical health, co-morbid conditions, nutritional status, pain level, and psychosocial health, is equally important. Proper staging combined with the overall assessment forms the basis for instituting a treatment plan and monitoring progress.[3]

Once a patient develops a pressure ulcer, the ulcer must be examined regularly to monitor treatment progress. At the minimum, weekly assessments should be performed to ensure that the treatment plan is having the desired effect.

Functional Limitations

The functional limitations of a patient depend in large part on the location of the pressure ulcer and the primary diagnosis. For example, a wheelchair dependent spinal cord patient with an ischial pressure ulcer will lose independence with mobility because treatment requires minimal, if any, time spent in the seated position. Less obvious is a hemiplegic patient who always rolls and pivots to one side to get out of bed. If he or she has a greater trochanter pressure ulcer on the side that is aggravated by the pressure, shear, and friction of getting out of bed, he or she will either be limited in being able to independently get out of bed, or a new technique must be explored.

Sometimes a pressure ulcer can give clues to the patient's mood and activity level. For example, the typical pressure ulcer in someone with a spinal cord injury who uses a wheelchair would be ischial due to the seated position during wheelchair use. However, if that same individual came in with a trochanteric pressure ulcer, presumably from lying in bed, the clinician would question whether the patient is depressed and not getting up and about.

The pressure ulcer and its location will impact a patient's ability to participate in therapy and wear appropriate bracing or orthotics, affect his or her independence with mobility and transfers, and alter his or her performance of activities of daily living and instrumental activities of daily living. Pressure relief, minimizing shear and friction, and required dressing changes can significantly alter a patient's functional status.

Diagnostic Studies

It is well accepted that malnutrition is linked to both the development of pressure ulcers and their ability to heal. Diagnostically, a nutritional assessment that indicates malnutrition is a serum albumin level of less than 3.5, total lymphocyte count of less than 1800/mm, or body weight decreased by more than 15% since the prior assessment. A nutritional assessment should be repeated every 12 weeks.[3]

Once a patient has a pressure ulcer, determining whether bacterial infection, underlying osteomyelitis, related abscess, or sinus tracts are hindering the healing process becomes important. If bacterial infection is a consideration, obtaining either a needle aspiration of fluid or a biopsy of ulcer tissue is the proper way to determine active wound infection.[7] Plain films, computerized tomography, bone scan (with or without a white blood cell scan), and MRI can all be used to better assess the underlying and surrounding tissue and bones for possible associated complications. The proper imaging for each patient will depend on the history and desired focus of the study.

Differential Diagnosis

Ischemic ulcer

Surgical wound dehiscence

Abscess

Abrasion

Treatment

Initial

Prevention

The key to caring for patients with pressure ulcers is attempting to prevent the ulcers from forming. Impaired mobility, incontinence, poor nutritional status, and altered level of consciousness can all increase a patient's risk of developing a pressure ulcer. In the wheelchair dependent population, broken wheelchairs or poor seating systems can contribute to pressure ulcers. One tool to help clinicians assess a patient's risk of developing pressure ulcers is the Braden Scale. This scale helps stratify patients into groups at different levels of risk for pressure ulcers. The scale is composed of six subscales (activity, mobility, sensory perception, nutrition, moisture, and friction and shear). All subscales are rated from 1 (least favorable) to 4 (most favorable), except for the friction/shear subscale, which is rated from 1 to 3. Possible scores range from 6 to 23, with lower scores predicting higher risk of a pressure ulcer forming. Using Braden scores, patients can be divided in groups: high risk, less than 12; moderate risk, 13 to 15; low risk, greater than 16. Risk assessment can then be used to help the clinician prescribe preventative measures to decrease the incidence of pressure ulcers.[8]

At-risk patients should have a detailed skin inspection at least daily to monitor for signs of impending pressure ulcer development. Prior to developing a stage I ulcer, the concerning area may show redness that resolves within 20 minutes of eliminating the pressure. If pressure is not relieved from this area, it may progress to a stage I pressure ulcer. Persistent pressure in this area will cause progression to a stage II, stage III, and ultimately to a stage IV ulcer.

In addition to monitoring areas over bony prominences, the clinician must check skin underneath braces, prostheses, splints, and serial casts for evidence of skin breakdown.

Treatment

Once a pressure ulcer develops, therapy must focus on medically treating the ulcer while at the same time addressing the factors that led to ulcer formation. Treatment is generally divided into four components: (1) debriding necrotic tissue as needed (sharp, mechanical, enzymatic, or autolytic debridement); (2) cleaning the wound initially and with each dressing change (normal saline is recommended—avoid skin cleansers or antiseptic agents); (3) preventing infection and diagnosing and treating an infection if one occurs; and (4) dressing the ulcer to keep the ulcer bed moist and the surrounding tissue dry.[3]

In addition, positioning in both the lying and seated positions should be evaluated. Patients should be positioned to keep pressure off of the ulcer area. Immobile patients in bed should be turned on a scheduled basis, at least every 2 hours. If necessary, pillows or foam wedges can be used to help patients maintain a position that keeps the ulcer area pressure free. Multiple mattresses and overlays are available, depending on the patient, extent and location of the pressure ulcer, and goals of therapy. Sitting should be avoided if pressure cannot be relieved from the ulcer area in the sitting position. Special seating and cushions are available to help distribute weight off of a pressure ulcer. Cushions can be divided into four categories: foam, viscoelastic foam, gel, and fluid flotation. Which cushion is best for a patient depends on pressure evaluation, lifestyle, postural stability, continence, and cost.[9] Pressure relief maneuvers should be done every 20 to 30 minutes while the patient is in the sitting position to keep ischial tuberosity pressure ulcers from forming.

Within 1 to 2 weeks of the initiation of treatment, partial thickness pressure ulcers should show signs of healing. Full thickness ulcers should show reduction in size after 2 to 4 weeks of treatment.[10] If the ulcer is not healing, the different aspects of the treatment plan previously outlined should be reviewed. In addition, adjuvant therapy (electrical stimulation) and the possible need for surgical intervention for stage III and IV ulcers that are recalcitrant to standard therapy should be considered. Electrical stimulation has been shown in multiple studies to improve the rate and degree of healing when used in addition to standard interventions on recalcitrant ulcers.[11] When treating a pressure ulcer, the clinician should always keep in mind that the main precipitating factors are pressure, shearing forces, friction, and moisture and therefore focus treatment on minimizing these factors.[9]

Treating the pressure ulcer directly without evaluating and treating the overall status of the patient will decrease the individual's ability to heal the pressure ulcer. The co-morbid conditions shown to delay ulcer healing are peripheral vascular disease, diabetes mellitus, immune deficiencies, collagen vascular diseases, malignancies, psychosis, and depression.[12] Identifying and treating these conditions in patients with pressure ulcers are important.

If malnutrition is a factor, aggressive nutritional supplementation or support should be instituted to place the patient into a positive nitrogen balance. Nutritional support should occur only if it is consistent with the patient's wishes and is likely to change the patient's prognosis. Also, supplemental vitamins should be given if deficiencies are suspected by exam or confirmed by lab evaluation. Supplement vitamin C and zinc should be prescribed if deficiencies are detected. If deficiencies are suspected, the clinician can institute high potency vitamin and mineral supplementation. Individual supplements up to 10 times the RDA for a particular water-soluble vitamin can be provided if found to be deficient.[3]

Pain should also be addressed and treated appropriately. Some pain may be eliminated or controlled by covering the wound and using appropriate positioning. If the pain persists, provide analgesia (i.e., acetaminophen, NSAIDs/COX-2 inhibitors, or narcotic medications) as needed during manipulations of the wound and for chronic wound pain.[10]

Rehabilitation

Rehabilitation is crucial to treating pressure ulcers for several reasons. Patients commonly develop pressure ulcers due to poor mobility. General strengthening, conditioning, and use of assistive devices can improve a patient's mobility. Increasing mobility can decrease the chances of developing a pressure ulcer. Moreover, prescribing properly fitting wheelchairs and appropriate seat cushions for spinal cord injury patients decreases risk. Spasticity and contracture management also impacts the development of pressure ulcers (see Chapters 103 and 136). Education, an important component of rehabilitation, ensures that the patient knows the importance of weight shifting, pressure relief, and skin monitoring. In particular, spinal cord injury patients should be taught both the techniques and importance of pressure relief, starting early in their hospital course.

In patients who undergo operative repair of a pressure ulcer, the postoperative rehabilitative course should begin with graduated, progressive weight bearing on the operative site. Start with 15 minutes, check the skin afterward for erythema, and progress daily as tolerated. If the patient's postoperative wound is slow to heal or if complicating factors exist, start weight bearing at 6 weeks instead of 4 weeks.[13]

Procedures

Debriding necrotic tissue from the wound is essential for healing to occur. Debridement can be accomplished by several different approaches. Sharp debridement is performed by a qualified clinician who uses a scalpel either at the bedside or in surgery. Mechanical debridement is commonly done with wet to dry dressings changed twice a day. Autolytic debridement is done by allowing the enzymes in the wound to dissolve the necrotic tissue by covering the wound with a moisture retentitive dressing. Lastly, enzymatic debridement uses exogenous enzymes in commercial preparations, such as Santyl or Accuzyme, to dissolve the necrotic tissue.[14]

Surgery

A variety of surgical options are available to close stage III and IV pressure ulcers that do not heal by conservative means. Possible surgeries are as follows: direct closure, split or full thickness skin grafts, skin flaps, musculocutaneous flaps, and free flaps. The type of surgical repair depends on the location of the ulcer, the primary diagnosis of the patient, co-morbid conditions, and the goals of treatment.

Potential Disease Complications

The following complications are associated with pressure ulcers: bacteremia, osteomyelitis, cellulitis, amyloidosis, endocarditis, heterotopic bone formation, maggot infestation, meningitis, perineal-urethral fistula, pseudoaneurysm, septic arthritis, sinus tract or abscess, and squamous cell carcinoma in the ulcer.[3]

Potential Treatment Complications

Pressure relief to the area of the ulcer may lead to another pressure ulcer forming in a different location. Increased pain may occur with dressing changes and sharp or mechanical debridement. Surgical complications of infection, bleeding, and wound dehiscence are possible. Medication side effects from NSAIDs (including COX-2 inhibitors), acetaminophen, and narcotics are well known and include gastric, renal, and liver toxicities. Drug dependency is an issue with narcotics.

References

1. National Pressure Ulcer Advisory Panel: Pressure ulcers: Incidence, economics, risk assessment. Consensus Development Conference Statement. West Dundee, IL, S-N Publications, 1989.
2. Agris J, Spira M: Clinical Symposia: Pressure ulcers: Prevention and treatment. 1979;31(5):1–32.
3. Bergstrom N, et al: Treatment of Pressure Ulcers. Clinical Practice Guideline No. 14. AHCPR Publication No. 95-0642. Rockville, MD, Agency for Health Care Policy and Research, Public Health Service, U.S. Department of Health and Human Services, 1994.
4. Cervo FA, Cruz AC, Posillico JA: Pressure ulcers: Analysis of guidelines for treatment and management. Geriatrics 2000;55:55–60.
5. The National Pressure Ulcer Advisory Panel: Pressure ulcers prevalence, cost and risk assessment: Consensus development conference statement. Decubitus 1989;2(2):4–8.
6. Sugarman M, Hawes S, Musher DM, et al: Osteomyelitis beneath pressure sores. Archi Intern Med 1983;143:683–688.
7. Garner JS, Jarvis WR, Emori TG, et al: CDC definitions for nosocomial infections, 1988. American J Infect Control 1988;16(3):128–140.
9. Kanj LF, Wilking SVB, Phillips TJ: Continuing medical education: Pressure ulcers. J Am Acad Dermatol 1998;38(4):517–536.
10. Van Rijswijk L, Braden BJ: Pressure ulcer patient and wound assessment: An AHCPR Clinical Practice Guideline update. Ostomy/Wound Management 1999;45(Suppl 1A):56S–67S.
11. Paralyzed Veterans of America/Consortium for Spinal Cord Medicine: Pressure Ulcer Prevention and Treatment Following Spinal Cord Injury: A Clinical Practice Guideline for Health-Care Professionals. Paralyzed Veterans of America, 2000.
12. Lazarus GS, Cooper DM, Knighton DR, et al: Definitions and guidelines for assessment of wounds and evaluation of healing. Arch Dermatol 1994;130:489–493.
13. Schryvers OI, Miroslaw FS, et al: Surgical treatment of pressure ulcers: 20-year experience. Arch Phys Med Rehabil 2000;81:1556–1562.
14. Ratliff CR, et al: Lippincott's Primary Care Practice: Pressure ulcer assessment and management. 1999;3(2):242–258.

131 Pulmonary Outpatient Rehabilitation

Rosemarie Filart, MD
John Bach, MD

Definition

Pulmonary rehabilitation has been defined as "the art of medical practice wherein an individually tailored, multidisciplinary program is formulated through which accurate diagnosis, therapy, emotional support, and education stabilize or reverse both the physiopathology and psychopathology of pulmonary diseases in an attempt to return the patient to the highest possible functional capacity allowed by his or her pulmonary handicap and overall life situation."[1,2] This definition becomes more comprehensive when expanded to include the evaluation for specialized equipment and physical medicine interventions to maximize lung and general functioning.

Program goals include reversing the cycle of dyspnea and deconditioning, optimizing airway secretion management and respiratory muscle function, reducing frequency of hospitalizations and pulmonary complications, addressing psychosocial factors to facilitate rehabilitation and community integration, and improving daily function.[1–4] Candidates for outpatient pulmonary rehabilitation include pediatric and adult individuals who can benefit from the aforementioned program goals, have pulmonary dysfunction that limits their functional goals, and whose conditions are medically stable for outpatient management.

In developing a prescription for an outpatient pulmonary rehabilitation program, it is essential to delineate the etiology of the pulmonary dysfunction. Clinical patient profiles of pulmonary dysfunction can be categorized into two types, based on the major impairment: (1) predominantly oxygenation impairment (i.e., primarily lung or airways disease) and (2) predominately ventilatory impairment (i.e., disorders with reduced respiratory muscle force). Patients with predominant oxygenation impairment often have hypoxia with a normal carbon dioxide level. Patients with predominant ventilatory impairment retain carbon dioxide. With this pulmonary dysfunction classification scheme, a clinician can better generate a focused outpatient pulmonary rehabilitation prescription. Subsequently, this chapter outlines treatment based on this classification. Conditions associated with predominant oxygenation impairment are listed in Table 1. When there is an equal overlap of impairments, a prescription is written to reflect modifications of both types of treatments.[8]

TABLE 1.

Conditions with predominant oxygenation impairment[8,17,18]
  Chronic obstructive pulmonary disease
  Asthma
  Emphysema and emphysema following lung
    volume reduction surgery
  Cystic fibrosis
  Bronchiectasis
  Some restrictive diseases (e.g., pulmonary
    fibrosis, primary parenchymal disease)

Conditions with predominant ventilatory impairment[8,17]
  Neuromuscular diseases and myopathies:
    Duchenne muscular dystrophy
    Becker muscular dystrophy
    Limb-girdle muscular dystrophy
    Emery-Dreifuss muscular dystrophy
    Facioscapulohumeral muscular dystrophy
    Congenital, autosomal recessive, myotonic
      muscular dystrophy
    Generalized non-dystrophic myopathies
    Congenital, metabolic, inflammatory
      myopathies
    Myasthenia gravis
    Mixed connective tissue disease
      myopathies
  Neurological disorders:
    Amyotrophic lateral sclerosis
    Spinal cord dysfunction
    Spinal muscular atrophies
    Motor neuron diseases
    Poliomyelitis
    Hereditary sensory motor neuropathies
    Phrenic nerve neuropathies, Guillain-Barré
      syndrome
    Multiple sclerosis
    Friedreich's ataxia
    Myelopathies
    Botulism
  Sleep disordered breathing:
    Obesity hypoventilation
    Central and congenital hypoventilation
      syndromes
    Hypoventilation associated with diabetic
      microangiopathy
    Down syndrome
    Familial dysautonomia
  Musculoskeletal:
    Thoracic wall deformities
    Kyphoscoliosis
    Ankylosing spondylitis
    Osteogenesis imperfecta
    Rigid spine syndrome
    Spondyloepiphyseal dysplasia
      congenita
  Restrictive lung diseases:
    Diseases of the pleura and chest wall
    Tuberculosis
    Milroy's disease

The prevalence of chronic obstructive pulmonary disease (COPD) in the adult population is approximately 4% to 6% in men and 1% to 3% in women. In the 1996 National Health Interview Survey, approximately 14 million adults had chronic bronchitis.[5–8]

Potential outcomes of an outpatient pulmonary rehabilitation program include decreased morbidity, decreased symptoms, improved quality of life, increased functional activity, improved neuropsychologic condition, decreased rate of respiratory complications and hospitalizations, increased ability to work, and effective use of assistive respiratory technology.

Overall, pulmonary rehabilitation outpatient management is centered on improving the functional status and quality of life of patients with disabling respiratory conditions through an interdisciplinary team approach involving the patient and health care professionals through physical medicine and rehabilitation interventions. In addition, respiratory morbidity and mortality can often be prevented. Each prescription is individual-specific and is adjusted according to the patient's progress.

Symptoms

Psychosocial disturbances may present as symptoms of anxiety, fatigue, depression, headaches, daytime hypersomnolence, and difficulty with concentration.[9] Ambulatory patients complain of dyspnea and impaired exercise tolerance. Specific symptoms commonly seen among patients according to impairment are listed below:

Predominant Oxygenation Impairment

Patients may have symptoms of dyspnea, sputum production, coughing, wheezing, chest pains that vary with the respiratory cycle, weight loss, orthopnea, sleep disturbances, and low endurance. A constellation of allergy symptoms may also be seen. Associated symptoms may include fever and hemoptysis, as in patients with bronchiectasis.

Predominant Ventilatory Impairment

Patients may have symptoms of exertional dyspnea, weight loss, sleep disturbances, and low endurance. For patients who use a wheelchair or scooter, minimal symptoms are common, and usually these patients only complain of anxiety or inability to fall asleep—a harbinger of respiratory failure.

Physical Examination

Predominant Oxygenation Impairment

For predominant lung or airways disease, the physical examination depends on the underlying medical disorder (see Table 1). For patients with COPD, the exam may reveal plentiful sputum production, auxiliary respiratory muscle use, and "barrel" chest. Auscultation reveals wheezes, rales, and/or hyperresonant lung sounds. Evaluation using pulse oximetry during rest and exercise will reveal oxygenation impairment with activity.[8]

Predominant Ventilatory Impairment

For disorders with reduced respiratory muscle force, the physical examination depends on the underlying medical disorder (see Table 1). Patients may have increased respiratory rate, shallow breathing, purely diaphragmatic or paradoxic breathing, nasal flaring, peribuccale or generalized cyanosis, flushing or pallor, drooling, difficulty with controlling airway secretions, dysphagia, and nasality of speech. Body habitus may reveal weak bulbar or respiratory muscles with notable increased respiratory rate and shallow breathing.[8]

Functional Limitations

In determining a patient's specific functional limitations due to pulmonary dysfunction, it is necessary to identify the patient's goals and the baseline level of functioning. Overall, chronic respiratory dysfunction may result in difficulty with controlling secretions and decreased social interaction. Tolerance and intensity of mobility and daily activities from the patient's baseline activity level are decreased. Examples of activities affected may include home chores, yard work, walking, shopping, work duties, recreational pursuits, stairclimbing, and sexual activity. It is important to note that many patients with neurologic, neuromuscular, and myopathic impairments who require the use of respiratory muscle aids may have only the use of finger and facial movements.

Diagnostic Studies

Before placing a patient in an outpatient pulmonary rehabilitation program, diagnostic testing should identify whether the patient has a predominantly ventilatory or oxygenation impairment. In addition to the patient's clinical presentation, pulmonary function tests can differentiate between the two impairments. With predominant oxygenation impairment, patients have at least one of the following: a respiratory limitation to exercise at 75% of predicted maximum oxygen consumption; irreversible airway obstruction with a forced expiratory volume in 1 second (FEV_1) of less than 2000 ml or an FEV_1 to forced vital capacity ratio (FEV_1/FVC ratio) of less than 60%; or pulmonary vascular disease with carbon monoxide diffusion capacity of less than 80% of predicted. With predominant ventilatory impairment, patients have at least one of the following: hypercapnia; a respiratory limitation to exercise at 75% of predicted maximum oxygen consumption; or restrictive lung disease with low vital capacity (VC), normal to high FEV_1/FVC ratio, and low lung volume measurements (i.e., total lung capacity [TLC], low functional residual capacity [FRC], and residual volume [RV]. Additionally, patients with this predominant ventilatory impairment, as well as with neuromuscular disease, thoracic wall deformity, and/or accessory muscle weakness have decreased maximum inspiratory and expiratory pressures, which correlate with inspiratory and expiratory muscle strength.[8]

Predominant Oxygenation Impairment

Active patients who are still able to walk several blocks but who have noted yearly decreases in exercise tolerance or who have recently begun to require ongoing medical attention for pulmonary symptoms or complications are ideal candidates for outpatient pulmonary rehabilitation. All patients undergo a 3-, 6-, or 12-minute walk test. The patient is instructed to gradually increase walking speed and duration on subsequent walking exercise and tests.[10–12]

Clinical exercise testing can best determine the extent of the patient's functional impairment due to pulmonary disease. It can diagnose and measure functional reserve and the capacity to perform exercise, the factors that limit exercise, and the reasons for exercise-related symptoms.[12–14] Clinical exercise testing permits the clinician to determine whether the primary disability is pulmonary, cardiac, or from exercise induced bronchospasm.[14] The latter two diagnoses and even the presence of purely restrictive pulmonary syndromes are commonly mistaken for COPD. When performed both before and after the rehabilitation program, clinical exercise testing documents patient progress.

Vital signs, electrocardiography, oxygen consumption, carbon dioxide production, respiratory quotient, ventilatory equivalent, minute ventilation, and metabolic rate are monitored during clinical exercise testing, which is done using a treadmill, stationary bicycle, or upper extremity ergometry. A clinical exercise test advances until oxygen consumption fails to increase, maximum allowable heart rate for age is reached; or electrocardiographic changes, chest pain, severe dyspnea, or fatigue occurs. Oximetry is performed to determine the need for supplemental oxygen therapy during reconditioning exercise (Sao_2 less than 90% to 95%) or on a long term basis (Po_2 less than 60 mm Hg). When metabolic energy cost studies are not available, maximum exercise tolerance may be estimated from pulmonary function data.[12–15]

Predominant Ventilatory Impairment

Progress among patients with predominant ventilatory impairment is initially evaluated and re-evaluated utilizing a spirometry test for VC in sitting and supine positions and maximum insufflation capacity, unassisted and assisted peak cough flows (PCFs) via peak flow meter, end-tidal carbon dioxide measurements, and pulse oximetry.[4,9,16] Supine VC provides an early indication of ventilatory dysfunction. When the VC is less than 2000 ml or about 50% of normal and PCFs are less than 300 L/min, the patient is trained to perform maximal insufflation techniques, such as air stacking. Air stacking can be achieved by holding with a closed glottis serially delivered volumes of air. These techniques along with manually or mechanically assisted coughing are aimed at maintaining adequate airway secretion clearance, and preventing atelectasis and pneumonia. PCF less than 270 L/min indicates initiation of the oximetry, a respiratory aid protocol. PCF of greater than 160 L/min is the minimum needed for adequate airway secretion clearance and hence can indicate the removal of a tracheostomy tube. Pulse oximetry can aid in diagnosing and monitoring severity of impairment. Symptoms of nocturnal hypoventilation, end-tidal CO_2 greater than 45 mm Hg, or daytime or nocturnal oxygen desaturations warrant a nocturnal trial of non-invasive positive airway pressure ventilation.[8]

Differential Diagnosis

Deconditioning	Pulmonary infection
Cardiac dysfunction	Obesity

Treatment

Initial

The main treatment for pulmonary rehabilitation is summarized in Table 2. The patient and caregivers are educated on preventive care measures. Smoking cessation is emphasized to reduce chronic phlegm production and decrease the rate of annual loss of FEV_1 to the level of non-smokers.[19] Avoidance of atmospheric or vocational pollutants and other aggravating factors such as pollen, aerosols, excessive humidity, stress, large meals, and ill contacts with respiratory infections are suggested. Adhering to medications as prescribed and reporting any problems with medications to the clinician are encouraged. Recommended vaccinations include annual influenza vaccinations and the pneumococcal vaccinations, provided there are no contraindications.[20,21] Nutritional counseling reinforces good nutrition with adequate caloric intake, carbohydrate balance, and adequate hydration.[14,22,23]

TABLE 2. Pulmonary Rehabilitation[1,2,7,8,11,13,14,36]

Basic outpatient pulmonary rehabilitation program
  Initial assessment of:
    Respiratory disease process
    Underlying medical disorder
    General medical condition
    Functional status
    Patient goals

Select treatment goals

Interdisciplinary team management
  Medication optimization
  Adjustment of supplemental oxygen therapy
  Airway secretion elimination techniques and devices
  Smoking cessation program
  Exercise program
    Ventilatory muscle training
    Endurance and strength training
  Breathing retraining
  Alternative breathing techniques
  Energy conservation techniques
  Therapeutic modalities
  Adaptive devices and mobility equipment
  Psychosocial counseling
  Nutritional counseling
  Patient and caregiver education

Maintenance program

Medical therapy involves optimal pharmacologic management of reversible bronchospasm when present, including the use of bronchodilators such as anticholinergics, methylxanthine derivatives, sympathomimetics, and combination medications (Table 3). An improvement in FEV_1 greater than 20% is significant with bronchodilator use. Inhaled adrenergics and anticholinergics appear to benefit many patients despite little objective evidence of improvement. Training for proper administration of nebulizers or inhalers is important to promote optimal medication deposition and to prevent inefficient use. Other medications such as expectorants, mucolytics, corticosteroids, antibiotics, and disodium cromoglycate are used along with humidification and bronchial toilet, as warranted, to prepare the patient for optimum participation in the therapeutic exercise program.

TABLE 3. Commonly Prescribed Medications

Category	Representative Types	Main Respiratory Clinical Effects	Main Side Effects
Bronchodilator	Anticholinergics, sympathomimetics, methylxanthine derivatives, combinations	Relief of bronchospasm by relaxing bronchial smooth muscle	See under specific medicines
Anticholinergics	Ipratropium	Relief of bronchospasm by relaxing bronchial smooth muscle	Headache, dry mouth, dizziness, dyspnea, GI disturbances
		Relief of bronchospasm	Tachycardia, palpitations, GI distress, nervousness, dry mouth, tremor

From Physician's Desk Reference, 55th ed. Medical Economics; 2001.

Early medical attention for upper or lower respiratory tract infections is important. Broad-spectrum antibiotics and glucocorticoids should be considered. Among patients with severely limiting myopathies, oxygen saturations of less than 95% portend respiratory decline. This is most commonly secondary to mucus plugging. Hence, in such patients, it is necessary to initiate techniques to mobilize and remove secretions.

For treatment and preventive care, respiratory secretion management is emphasized. This involves training in the techniques of chest percussion, postural drainage, and with huffing ventilatory and airway secretion clearance devices. Additionally, autogenic drainage is a technique of breathing low tidal volumes between the functional residual capacity and residual volume, followed by taking increasingly larger tidal volumes and forced expirations to mobilize and evacuate mucus. Positive expiratory pressure (PEEP) breathing techniques theoretically mobilize secretions by coughing or forced expirations with alveolar pressure and volume pushing behind mucous plugs. Flutter breathing with a flutter device applied to the mouth utilizes two mucus-evacuating techniques: PEEP and oscillation.

Devices that provide mechanical vibration or oscillation to the thorax include the Hayek Oscillator (Breasy Medical Equipment Inc., Stamford, CT), THAIRapy System (American Biosystems, Inc., St. Paul, Minn); and intrapulmonary percussive ventilation, which provides aerosolized medications as high flow percussive mini-bursts or air delivered to the airways (Percussionaire Corp, Sandpoint, Idaho). A mechanical insufflation-exsufflation (MI-E) device is used mostly among ventilatory impaired patients. It provides a 10 L/sec of expiratory flow directly to airways through the mouth or tracheostomy (Cough Assist, JH Emerson Co., Cambridge, Mass). Manual assisted coughing can be useful and can be combined with MI-E.[8]

Predominant Oxygenation Impairment

Home oxygen therapy is used for oxygenation impaired patients with lung disease if the P_{O_2} is less than 60 mm Hg and when it remains so for more than 2 months following an acute exacerbation. This type of therapy decreases reactive pulmonary hypertension and polycythemia, improves cognition, prolongs survival, and may decrease hospitalizations. Transtracheal oxygen delivery avoids waste around the nose and mouth, *avoids* the "dead space" of the nasopharynx, and prevents discomfort and drying associated with nasal cannulas and face masks. High altitude travel may require ½ L/minute of additional supplemental oxygen.

Predominant Ventilatory Impairment

Abdominal binders are useful for tetraplegic and thoracic level paraplegic spinal cord patients.[8] The clinical effect is seen with increased diaphragmatic excursion and vital capacity.

For sleep disordered breathing, continuous pressure airway pressure or bilevel positive airway pressure can be used. For the latter, the greater the pulse pressure difference (i.e., the difference between the inspiratory positive airway pressure [IPAP] and the expiratory positive airway pressure [EPAP]), the greater the inspiratory muscle assistance. Modifications are made for mask discomfort and air leakage. Portable volume ventilators are alternatively utilized for those who necessitate greater inspiratory muscle assistance, such as for a morbidly obese patient or for any patient with neuromuscular disease who is able to perform air stacking.[8]

Psychosocial counseling addresses symptoms of depression, anxiety, and stress as well as social impediments of good progress. The goal is to break the influence of these psychosocial issues on the cycle of respiratory decline.[9]

Rehabilitation

An outpatient pulmonary rehabilitation program incorporates physical medicine interventions, evaluation for respiratory equipment, and rehabilitation with an interdisciplinary team approach with the patient, medical and nursing staff, respiratory therapists, physical therapists,

TABLE 4. Types of Exercise[1,2,7,8,13,14,17,33,36]

Type of Exercise	Example
Ventilatory muscle training	*Inspiratory resistive exercise:* maximum sustained ventilation, inspiratory resistive loading, inspiratory threshold loading, sustained hyperpnea
Strength training	*Upper extremity exercise:* pulleys, elastic bands, supervised circuit training, weight-lifting with low resistance Lower extremity exercise: supervised circuit training, weightlifting with low resistance
Endurance training	*Upper extremity exercise:* unsupported upper extremity activities ranging from activities of daily living to athletic activities, supervised arm cycling, low impact aerobics, pool therapy *Lower extremity exercise:* incremental treadmill program, supervised walking, cycling and stairclimbing program, low impact aerobics, pool therapy

occupational therapists, speech therapists, social workers, and a nutritionist. In addition, psychology or psychiatry services, recreational therapists, and vocational rehabilitation may be integrated as part of the team.

Exercise training for endurance, strength, and functional specific activities is prescribed (Table 4). The progress is monitored, and modifications to the prescription are made. Scheduling re-evaluations of the prescription depends on each patient, with the early stages of the program and any acute medical issues affecting the need for possible prescription modifications. Frequency, duration, intensity, and specificity are general exercise components. Frequency of exercise is generally advised 3 to 5 times a week to see a training effect.[14]

Predominant Oxygenation Impairment

Carefully prescribed exercise provides the greatest benefits for reducing dyspnea and respiratory rate, and increasing exercise tolerance, maximum oxygen consumption, 6- and 12-minute walk distance and speed, activities of daily living, work output, mechanical efficiency, and possibly gas exchange.[32–36] Anxiety and depression are also significantly decreased, and cognition and sense of well being are improved.[9]

Low intensity training can be prescribed based on objective and/or subjective measures. Objective measures involve calculating the maximal oxygen consumption and/or maximum heart rate. If an open circuit spirometry and metabolic cart are available, specific target intensity may be 50% of peak rate of oxygen uptake (VO_2 peak). Heart rate parameters may be most useful for patients with cardiac conditions. Several formulas are used. One is the desired exercise intensity multiplied by the maximum predicted heart rate. Hence, if the desired exercise intensity is defined as 60% of maximum predicted HR, then

$$\text{Target HR} = 0.60 \times [\text{HRmax} = 220 - \text{age}].$$

Another is the Karvonen formula. For the target HR range for 50% to 85%:

$$\text{HR reserve} = [\text{HRmax} - \text{HR rest}) \times 0.50] + \text{HR rest}; [\text{HRmax} - \text{HR rest}) \times 0.85] + \text{HR rest}$$

Initial targets can be 50% (range: 50% to 80%) of either objective measure.[14]

When objective measures are not applicable, as in the case of patients taking negative chronotropic medications (e.g., beta-blockers or calcium channel blockers) and heart transplant patients, subjective measures may be more predictive of exercise tolerance. In addition, since patients are often limited by exertional dyspnea, subjective measures may be more desirable.[14]

Subjective measures of exercise tolerance, such as the Borg's rating of perceived exertion (RPE) scale or dyspnea rating scales, allow patients to guide the program based on their symptoms alone. The Borg's RPE scale form 6 to 20 is linearly related to heart rate. This is illustrated by multiplying the chosen scale number by 10 to obtain the estimated predicted HR. For example, when the patient chooses the number 10 on the scale to describe exertion symptoms, then HR is estimated using the following equation:

$$10 \times 10 = 100 \ (\pm 10)$$

The original Borg scale uses this method.[14,27]

Training specificity is determined by the patient's goal for daily activities and occupational pursuits. Daily activities in mobility and exercise programs are tailored accordingly. Depending on the patient's form of mobility and baseline level of function, specific mobility and endurance exercise programs can include walking, stairclimbing, aerobic exercise, stationary bicycling, and pool activities. For mobility, work, and recreational pursuits, assistive devices to improve daily activities may include wheelchair, walker, or cane. Strength training increases function in daily activities, mobility, and specific occupational related tasks. Intermingled with endurance, strength and task specific training are energy conservation techniques that provide the patient with more energy efficient methods to perform daily activities.[8]

Review of the training program is made with the patient and caregiver. A plan is agreed on and is flexible to change, according to patient toleration. The patient is made responsible for a progressive program to reinforce adherence and independence.

Increased endurance for exercise can occur independently of changes in ventilatory muscle endurance. Respiratory muscle trainers are often added to daily training programs.[28] Their use results in significant improvements in respiratory muscle endurance. However, there are no reported improvements in strength or decreased occurrence of pulmonary exacerbations or respiratory failure.

Breathing retraining exercises are used with the goals of modifying the breathing pattern, strengthening respiratory muscles, and improving the cough mechanism. Pursed lip and diaphragmatic breathing decrease the respiratory rate, coordinate the breathing pattern, and tend to prevent collapse of smaller bronchi. Air shifting is performed several times per hour. It involves a deep inspiration that is held with the glottis closed for 5 seconds. The air shifts to lesser-ventilated areas of the lung and may help prevent microatelectasis. The subsequent expiration is via pursed lips. Pursed lip breathing aids in relaxation, as well. Other relaxation exercises, such as Jacobson exercises and biofeedback, can be used to decrease tension and anxiety.[29]

For hypercapnic patients, interspersing periods of respiratory muscle rest with exercise of specific respiratory muscle groups is a principle of pulmonary rehabilitation. Rest can be achieved by overnight use of nasal bi-level positive airway pressure (BiPAP).[30,31] Improved daytime gases, increased VC, decreased fatigue, and increased well being have been reported in such programs.

Following the acute rehabilitation period, continued surveillance and attention to abstinence from smoking, bronchial hygiene (Table 5), breathing retraining, physical reconditioning, oxygen therapy, and airway secretion mobilization have been shown to reduce hospital admissions, length of hospital stays, and cost.[37,38] The benefits of pulmonary rehabilitation on exercise performance and quality of life are greatest during the first year and last up to 5 years.[7,35,36,39–42]

TABLE 5. Pulmonary Hygiene Options[13,11,43]

Inhalers
  Bronchodilators
  Inhaled steroids
  Leukotriene inhibitors
  Mucolytics
Methods of Airway Secretions Elimination
  Oral, nasal, or transtracheal suctioning
  Chest percussion and postural drainage
  Positive expiratory pressure breathing
  Flutter mucus clearance devices
  Mechanical vibration devices to the chest wall
  Intrapulmonary percussive ventilation with aerosolized
    medications
  Mechanical insufflation-exsufflation applications
  Autogenic drainage
  Manual assisted cough
  Abdominal binder

Predominant Ventilatory Impairment

Ninety percent of episodes of acute respiratory failure are caused by ineffective coughing during otherwise benign upper respiratory tract infections; therefore, when assisted PCFs have decreased to less than 270 L/min, patients are prescribed oximeters and trained in air stacking consecutively delivered volumes of air provided via the mouth and nasal interfaces from a manual resuscitator (Ambu bag) to improve cough flows. They are also taught manually assisted coughing (abdominal thrusts timed to glottic opening following maximal lung insufflation). They are introduced to mechanical insufflation-exsufflation (Cough Assist, JH Emerson Co., Cambridge, Mass) provided at +35 to +50 to –35 to –50 cm H_2O pressure drops, with abdominal thrusts applied during exsufflations. Patients must have rapid (less than 2-hour) access to portable volume ventilators, Cough Assists and various mouthpieces and nasal interfaces when they develop respiratory tract infections.

Patients and care providers are instructed to use continuous oxygen saturation (SaO_2) monitoring at the first sign of upper respiratory tract infection. Any decreases in SaO_2 less than 95% indicate either hypoventilation or the presence of airway mucus accumulation that must be cleared to prevent atelectasis, pneumonia, and respiratory failure. They are also told to use SaO_2 monitoring whenever fatigued, short of breath, or ill. They are instructed to use manually and mechanically assisted coughing, as needed, to maintain normal SaO_2 at all times.

When symptomatic or nocturnal SaO_2 means are less than 95% and a trial of nocturnal nasal intermittent positive pressure ventilation (IPPV) relieves desaturation and improves symptoms, patients are encouraged to continue to use nocturnal nasal IPPV. Most young patients use non-invasive IPPV for the first time to assist lung ventilation during chest infections and need it continuously during these episodes without requiring hospitalization.[16] Although inherent muscle weakness may progress, patients may be maintained on non-invasive IPPV continuously without ever requiring hospitalization.

Procedures

There are no procedures routinely utilized during an outpatient pulmonary rehabilitation program.

Surgery

Surgical interventions are not a routine part of an outpatient pulmonary rehabilitation program. Candidates for lung transplantation and post-lung transplantation patients may be prescribed an inpatient and outpatient pulmonary rehabilitation program, depending on the patient's goal and medical stability.[24,25] Among patients with pulmonary dysfunction who have significant nutritional deficiencies by oral intake, alternative routes for nutrition, such as a percutaneous gastrostomy tube, are considered.

Predominant Oxygenation Impairment

Lung volume reduction surgery (LVRS) is performed for patients with severely functionally limiting emphysema with the goals of improving gas exchange, exercise capacity, lung function, and quality of life. Candidates for LVRS as well as post-LVRS patients may be prescribed an inpatient and outpatient pulmonary rehabilitation program, depending on the patient's goals and medical stability.[26]

Predominant Ventilatory Impairment

Tracheostomy is needed only when there is a significant risk of aspiration pneumonia such as in severe cases of bulbar dysfunction in which the assisted peak cough flow is less than 160 L/min.[8]

Potential Disease Complications

Potential disease complications play a significant role in the outpatient pulmonary rehabilitation prescription. In generating a prescription, it is important to be informed of the patient's specific pulmonary diagnosis and potential complications to better delineate program specifics and predict patient outcome. Hence, this section expounds on general concepts. Complications of chronic respiratory disease depend on respiratory muscle dysfunction, neuromuscular and musculoskeletal conditions, nutritional deficits, psychosocial issues, and co-morbidities.

Predominant Oxygenation Impairment

Patients with primarily oxygenation impairment due to lung or airways disease often have intermittent exacerbations with episodes of acute respiratory failure. These often require acute hospitalization and invasive management. They are largely caused by inability to mobilize peripherally trapped airway secretions. There are many secretion mobilization systems to help mobilize airway secretions, but there is no clear evidence that one system works better than any others. The best strategy for a patient with lung disease at high risk of acute respiratory failure is to administer and monitor compliance with antibiotics, bronchodilators, oxygen, mucolytics, and other medications; to supplement airway secretion mobilization efforts; and to use chest percussion and postural drainage, huffing, and other inexpensive mobilization techniques such as active cycle of breathing and the use of positive expiratory pressure masks, flutter valves, or the more expensive high frequency chest wall or airway oscillation methods.[43]

Predominant Ventilatory Impairment

The evaluation for long-term airway protection with a tracheostomy is a common clinical scenario. Only a small number of conditions progress to requiring a tracheostomy. For those with high risk for aspiration pneumonia from severe bulbar dysfunction, tracheotomy can be warranted. Once aspiration of saliva causes the SaO_2 baseline to decrease to less than 95%, there is a high risk of aspiration pneumonia, and tracheostomy is warranted. Although this only occurs for patients with advanced bulbar amyotrophic lateral sclerosis; children with type 1 spinal muscular atrophy without sufficient home care; occasionally, a patient with facioscapulohumeral muscular dystrophy; and a few others, tracheostomy is considered whenever maximum assisted peak cough flows decrease to less than 160 L/m.[44]

Potential Treatment Complications

Potential treatment complications can result from patient co-morbidities, such as concomitant cardiac or atherosclerotic peripheral vascular disease, and pharmacologic treatment. Routine evaluation of a patient's medication profile by the treating clinician is necessary during the outpatient pulmonary rehabilitation program. When an outpatient pulmonary rehabilitation prescription is specific for each individual, potential treatment complications may be preventable. Each individual's progress through the daily activities, mobility, and exercise programs is followed-up and the prescription modified accordingly. Precautions toward each individual's co-morbidities are stated with each prescription. For example, if a patient has a history of or potential for supplemental oxygenation, oxygen saturation parameters are written with both rest and activity requirements in mind. Cardiac precautions are defined based on the maximum and minimum heart rate and blood pressure ranges tolerable for activities.

References

1. Hodgkin J, Farrell M, Gibson S, et al: Pulmonary rehabilitation. Official ATS statement. Am Rev Respir Dis 1981;124:663–666.
2. American Thoracic Society: Medical section of the American Lung Association, pulmonary rehabilitation 1999, official ATS statement. Am J Resp Crit Care Med 1999;159:1666–1682.
3. American College of Chest Physicians and American Association of Cardiovascular and Pulmonary Rehabilitation. Pulmonary rehabilitation: Joint ACCP/AACVPR evidence-based guidelines [Special report]. Chest 1997;112:5.
4. Bach JR. Rehabilitation of the patient with respiratory dysfunction. In DeLisa JA, Gans BM (eds): Rehabilitation Medicine: Principles and Practice, 3rd ed. Philadelphia, Lippincott-Raven, 1998, pp 1359–1383.
5. Higgins MW, Thom T: Incidence, prevalence, and mortality: Intra- and intercountry differences. In Hensley MJ, Saunders NA (eds): Clinical Epidemiology of Chronic Obstructive Pulmonary Disease. New York, Marcel Dekker, 1989, pp 23–43.
6. Feinleib M, Rosenberg HM, Collins JG, et al: Trends in COPD morbidity and mortality in the United States. Am Rev Respir Dis 1989;140:S9–S18.
7. Verbrugge LM, Patrick DL. Seven chronic conditions: Their impact on US adults' activity levels and use of medical services. Am J Public Health 1995;85:173–182.
8. National Center for Health Statistics: Current estimates from the National Health Interview Survey, 1993. Vital and health statistics, series 10, No. 190 USDHHS (PHS), 95-1518.
9. Smoller JW, et al: Panic anxiety, dyspnea, and respiratory disease: Theoretical and clinical considerations. Am J Respir Crit Care Med 1996;154:6–17.
10. Guyatt GH, Thompson PJ, Berman LB, et al: How should we measure function in patients with chronic heart and lung disease? J Chron Dis 1985;38:517–524.
11. American Association of Cardiovascular and Pulmonary Rehabilitation. Guidelines for Pulmonary Rehabilitation Programs, 2nd ed. Champaign, IL, Human Kinetics, 1998.
12. American College of Sports Medicine: Guidelines for Exercise Testing and Prescription, 5th ed. Philadelphia, Williams & Wilkins, 1995.
13. Jones NL: Current concepts: new tests to assess lung function. N Engl J Med 1975;293:541–544.
14. Jones NL, Campbell EJM: Clinical Exercise Testing, 2nd ed. Philadelphia, W.B. Saunders, 1982, p 158.
15. Carlson DJ, Ries AL, Kaplan RM: Prediction of maximum exercise tolerance in patients with COPD. Chest 1991;100:307–311.
16. Bach JR, Ishikawa Y, Kim H: Prevention of pulmonary morbidity for patients with Duchenne muscular dystrophy. Chest 1997;112:1024–1028.
17. Balado D: Exercise Physiology: Energy, Nutrition, and Human Performance, 4th ed. Philadelphia, Williams & Wilkins, 1996.
18. Moy ML, et al: Health related quality of life improves following pulmonary rehabilitation and lung volume reduction surgery. Chest 1999;115(2):383–389.
19. Camilli AE, Burrows B, Knudson RJ, et al: Longitudinal changes in forced expiratory volume in one second in adults. Effects of smoking and smoking cessation. Am Rev Respir Dis 1987;135:794–799.
20. U.S. Department of Health and Human Services, Public Health Service. Prevention of pneumococcal disease: Recommendations of the Advisory Committee on Immunization Practices. 1997;46:RR-8.
21. U.S. Department of Health and Human Services, Public Health Service: Prevention and control of influenza: Recommendations of the Advisory Committee on Immunization Practices. 2000;49:RR-3.
22. Wilson DO, et al: Body weight in chronic obstructive pulmonary disease. Am Rev Respir Dis 1989;139:1435–1438.
23. Askanazi J, et al: Nutrition and the respiratory system. Crit Care Med 1982;10:163–172.
24. Palmer SM, Tapson VF: Pulmonary rehabilitation in the surgical patient. Lung transplantation and lung volume reduction surgery. Respir Car Clin N Am 1998;4(1):71–83.
25. Manzetti JD, et al: Exercise, education, and quality of life in lung transplant candidates. J Heart Lung Transplant 1994;13(2):297–305.
26. Criner GJ, et al: Prospective randomized trial comparing bilateral lung volume reduction surgery to pulmonary rehabilitation in severe chronic obstructive pulmonary disease. Am J Respir Crit Care Med 1999;160:2018–2027.
27. Noble BJ, Borg GAV, et al: A category-ratio perceived exertion scale: Relationship to blood and muscle lactates and heart rate. Med Sci Sports Exerc 1983;15:523–528.
28. Reina-Rosenbaum R, Bach JR, Penek J: The cost/benefits of outpatient based pulmonary rehabilitation. Arch Phys Med Rehabil 1997;78:240–244.
29. Kahn AU: Effectiveness of biofeedback and counter conditioning in the treatment of bronchial asthma. J Psychosom Res 1977;21:97–104.
30. Elliot MW, Mulvey D, Moxham J, et al: Domiciliary nocturnal nasal intermittent positive pressure ventilation in COPD: Mechanisms underlying changes in arterial blood gas tensions. Eur Respir J 1991;4:1044–1052.
31. Gay P, Hubmayr RD, Stroetz RW: Efficacy of nocturnal nasal positive pressure ventilation combined with oxygen therapy and oxygen monotherapy in patients with severe COPD. Am J Respir Care Med 1996;154:353–358.
32. Gozal D: Nocturnal ventilatory supports in patients with cystic fibrosis: Comparison with supplemental oxygen. Eur Respir J 1997;10:1999–2003.
33. Gimenez M, Servera E, Vergara P, et al: Endurance training in patients with chronic obstructive pulmonary disease: A comparison of high versus moderate intensity. Arch Phys Med Rehabil 2000;81:102–109.
34. Carter R, Nicotra B, Clark L, et al: Exercise conditioning in rehabilitation of patients with chronic obstructive pulmonary disease. Arch Phys Med Rehabil 1988;69:118–122.
35. Troosters T, et al: Short and long-term effects of outpatient rehabilitation in patients with chronic obstructive pulmonary disease: A randomized trial. Am J Med 2000;109:207–212.

36. Make B: Pulmonary rehabilitation and outcome measure. In Baum GL, Crapo JD, Celli BR Karlinsky JB (eds): Textbook of Pulmonary Diseases, 6th ed. Philadelphia, Lippincott-Raven, 1998, pp 987–1006.
37. Hudson LD, Tyler ML, Petty T: Hospitalization needs during an outpatient rehabilitation program for chronic airway obstruction. Chest 1976;70:606–610.
38. Roselle S, D'Amico FJ: The effect of home respiratory therapy on hospital re-admission rates of patients with chronic obstructive pulmonary disease. Respir Care 1990;35:1208–1213.
39. Holle RHO, Williams DV, Vandree JC, et al: Increased muscle efficiency and sustained benefits in an outpatient community hospital-based pulmonary rehabilitation program. Chest 1988;94:1161–1168.
40. Ilowite J, Niederman M, Fein A, et al: Can benefits seen in pulmonary rehabilitation be sustained long term? Chest 1991;100:182.
41. Mall RW, Medieros M: Objective evaluation of results of a pulmonary rehabilitation program in a community hospital. Chest 1988;94:1156–1160.
42. Vale F, Reardon J, ZuWallack R: Is improvement sustained following pulmonary rehabilitation? Chest 1991;100:56s.
43. Hardy KA: A review of airway clearance: New techniques, indications, and recommendations. Respir Care 1994;39:440–455.
44. Bach JR, Saporito LR: Criteria for extubation and tracheostomy tube removal for patients with ventilatory failure: A different approach to weaning. Chest 1996;110:1566–1571.

132 Reflex Sympathetic Dystrophy

Joseph Biundo, MD

Synonyms

Complex regional pain syndrome I and 2

Post-traumatic dystrophy

Sudeck's atrophy

Sudeck's syndrome

Osteodystrophy

Algoneurodystrophy

Post-traumatic osteoporosis

Shoulder hand syndrome

Sympathetically maintained pain

ICD-9 Codes

337.21
Reflex sympathetic dystrophy of the upper limb

337.22
Reflex sympathetic dystrophy of the lower limb

Definition

Reflex sympathetic dystrophy (RSD) is a complex constellation of findings in an extremity in which persistent, burning pain is present that usually follows a traumatic event in association with hyperactivity of the sympathetic nervous system with redness, pallor, edema (swelling), increased sweating of that involved area, and the development of localized osteoporosis.[1]

Many terms and definitions have evolved over the years since the first report of the syndrome in 1864 by Dr. Silas Weir Mitchell as a result of his study of Civil War gunshot wounds that caused nerve injuries. The term *causalgia,* a Greek word meaning burning pain, is used in connection with RSD; major causalgia describes RSD with nerve injury, and minor causalgia describes RSD without nerve injury.

In 1994 the terminology of RSD was changed by the International Association for the Study of Pain (IASP) to the term Complex Regional Pain Syndrome (CRPS). Type 1 follows trauma without known specific nerve injury, and Type 2 develops after injury to a specific nerve.[2] The following four criteria were established by IASP, all of which are required to be present to confirm a clinical diagnosis of CRPS:

1. An inciting noxious event (or nerve injury for type 2) resulting in immobilization of an extremity.
2. Disproportionate degree of pain, allodynia, and/or hyperalgesia.
3. Edema, alteration in blood flow, or abnormal sudomotor (sweating) activity in the region of pain.
4. Exclusion of underlying conditions that would otherwise account for these symptoms.

Emotional factors are often seen and may be misleading, particularly because RSD may be unrecognized. The diagnosis can be very difficult to make. For example, an incomplete picture of RSD is common, in which the patient may not have the full-blown classic case. Mild cases of RSD exist, as with most diseases, and the clinician must be able to recognize the mild, early, or partial cases. In some cases, severe pain is present but the sympathetic features are less overt. Some cases seem to have somewhat of an intermittent nature of swelling, burning pain, and extremity coolness. Different locations of RSD can occur at different times, presumably secondary to different injuries. Also, some cases occur without any known trauma, which often hinders diagnosis. RSD may present as frozen shoulder (shoulder-hand syndrome) or can be seen in the hand and arm that have been affected by a stroke.

RSD has been classified into three stages.[3] However, the disease does not always follow these stages, and like most diseases is a spectrum.

The Stages of RSD are as follows:

Stage One: Agonizing pain; pitting edema; redness; warmth, but coolness may begin; increased hair and nail growth; hyperhidrosis may begin; osteoporosis begins.

Stage Two: Pain, brawny edema, periarticular thickening, cyanosis or pallor, livedo reticularis, coolness, hyperhidrosis, increased osteoporosis, ridged nails.

Stage Three: Pallor; dry, cool skin; atrophic soft tissue (dystrophy); contracture; extensive osteoporosis.

Symptoms

Pain is the major symptom and is agonizing and burning.[4] The hand is the most common site of involvement, often with the adjacent wrist and forearm involved. The foot and ankle are also sites for RSD.[5] In addition, the knee has been reported to be affected by RSD.[6] The onset gradually begins days or even weeks after the initial injury, which may be an overt injury, such as a fracture, bruise, sprain, strain, laceration, and extremity surgery, or nerve injury.[7] However, pain may start within a few hours after the initial injury, and the injury in some cases is minor and overlooked. Basically, any injury that causes pain and immobilization can induce RSD. In most cases, the pain seems disproportionally severe compared to the degree of the injury. The pain may be described as being worse with use and pressure on the involved area. The patient usually stops using the involved limb because of the pain and tries to protect it from being touched. Swelling is usually obvious to the patient, and he or she may note color changes and coolness of the involved limb.

Physical Examination

On first seeing a patient with RSD, the initial clue to the diagnosis might be the characteristic arm position that is commonly observed. This repetitive position might be labeled the "RSD posture," in which the forearm is held rigidly against the chest wall, the wrist is held rigid, and the hand is flexed and immobilized. When someone comes near the hand, the patient quickly moves away, trying to avoid any contact with his or her hand or arm. Further observe for color changes of the skin, comparing the involved extremity with the uninvolved side. Pallor, a dusky appearance, or livedo reticularis can be seen. Generalized swelling is usually present and in the hand may involve the dorsal and volar aspects. Extension to the wrist and forearm may occur, encompassing articular and non-articular areas. Very gently, palpate the involved extremity for tenderness, which is usually exquisite. Pain can even occur with very light palpation or even by light rubbing of the skin, which is known as allodynia and is characteristic of RSD. Severe pain often limits a range of motion examination. Often the skin of the extremity with RSD is slightly cool. A comparison with the opposite side should be made to enhance accuracy of this assessment. In chronic cases of RSD, dystrophic skin changes, stiffness, and joint contractures may be seen. Although obtaining an accurate assessment of a limb involved with RSD may be difficult because of the pain, a finding of muscle weakness may help point to neurologic etiology, such as brachial plexopathy. Similarly, any alteration in deep tendon reflexes should be interpreted to help determine the lesion. Arterial pulses should be normal in RSD.

Differential Diagnosis

Cellulitis

Lymphedema

Occult or stress fracture

Acute synovitis

Septic arthritis

Septic tenosynovitis

Subclavian, axillary, or brachial venous thrombosis

Venous thrombosis of lower limb

Scleroderma

Plexitis, peripheral neuropathy

Functional Limitations

Profound, disabling pain is the major problem, and this pain is often difficult to treat. The severe pain leads to immobilization; inability to use the hand in many cases; and ultimately, loss of work. Workers compensation and disability issues are present in many cases of RSD. Most commonly, the upper limb is involved in RSD, particularly the hand; thus limitation in work activities, such as writing, typing, filing, and using machinery, may be present. The individual may also have difficulty using the affected hand in feeding, dressing, bathing, toileting, and other daily activities.

Diagnostic Studies

Plain x-rays of the involved extremity, such as a hand, may show patchy osteoporosis in addition to the soft tissue swelling, which is apparent without x-ray.[8] The osteoporosis tends to be more pronounced in chronic cases, especially when there is significant loss of function of the hand. Technetium-99 radionuclide bone scans are often positive in the involved RSD area and may be used to aid in the diagnosis.[9] Scintigraphy has proved to have a specificity of 86% and a sensitivity of 68% in RSD (Fig. 1).[10] However, a triple phase bone scan does not seem to add much to the diagnosis over the single delayed scans.

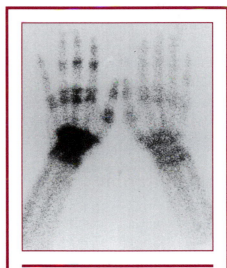

FIGURE 1. Bone scintiscan (3-hour delay) of a 30-year-old man with reflex sympathetic dystrophy of the left hand. Note diffuse increased isotope uptake at the wrist and proximal finger joints. The first two phases also displayed increased isotope uptake. (From Weinzweig J: Plastic Surgery Secrets. Philadelphia, Hanley & Belfus, 1999, p 459, with permission.)

Treatment

Initial

Many medications have been used over the years for the treatment of RSD with variable success.[7,11] The quicker the diagnosis is made and treatment initiated, the better the response. To treat RSD the clinician must be familiar with the various treatment options and when they might be utilized. Reduction of pain and swelling and mobilization of the involved limb are the main goals.

The mainstay of treatment in early RSD is a course of oral corticosteroids.[7,10,12] A practical regimen is to give oral prednisone, starting at about a dose of 1 mg/kg. The total dose, which often is about 60 to 70 mg per day, is prescribed in at least two to three divided doses. The prednisone is tapered daily or every other day by 10 mg over 1 to 2 weeks. This course may be repeated for lingering or recurrent symptoms.

Tricyclic anti-depressants may be of benefit for neurogenic pain and for their desired effect of nighttime sedation and muscle relaxation. Individuals with RSD, as with most patients with acute and chronic pain, suffer poor sleep and its consequences, which can lead to fatigue, depression, and worsening pain. A reasonable regimen would be to start with amitriptyline at a low dose of 10 mg at bedtime. This medication can be gradually increased to 50 to 100 mg at bedtime, using quality of sleep as a parameter for the adjustment. Mouth dryness and bladder or bowel dysfunction may occur as a result of the anticholenergic side effects of amitriptyline. Other tricyclic antidepressants, such as nortriptyline or trazodone, may be substituted when amitriptyline's side effects hinder achieving a suitable quality of sleep or improvement in pain. If maximal doses of amitriptyline can be achieved but do not help, it is unlikely that switching to another tricyclic antidepressant would be of benefit. However, the use of doxepin may be helpful because of its known soporific effects.

Favorable responses of pain relief and reversal of skin and soft tissue manifestations have been obtained with gabapentin.[13] A low starting dose of 300 mg at bedtime may be given. As needed, the dose may be gradually increased to a peak dose of 2400 mg to 3600 mg per day. Phenytoin and carbamazepine have been used to treat RSD in their usual doses.[14]

Because of the suspected role of the sympathetic nervous system in RSD, alpha adrenergic blockers have been used. Phenoxybenzamine may be started at a dose of 10 mg 2 to 3 times a day and increased every 2 days by 10 mg.[15] A total maximum dose may range from 40 to 120 mg per day. In one study, a total daily dose needed for relief was 80 mg. The main side effect is postural hypotension, which may limit the dose. Abdominal binders and stockings can be used for this problem. Prazosin at a dose of 1 to 8 mg per day can also be used. Nifedipine, a calcium channel blocker, has been reported to be of benefit in a dose of 10 to 30 mg 3 times daily.

Calcitonin at high doses, 400 IU per day IM for 2 weeks, has been used with some success in early RSD. Unpleasant side effects such as nausea, malaise, and flushes have limited its use. Topically, capsaicin has been advocated. It has the advantage of no systemic side effects or drug interactions, but must be used with caution to prevent mucosal irritation.

Other treatment options include NSAIDs/COX-2 inhibitors, bisphosphonates, mexiletine, and ketamine topically or as an intravenous infusion. An attempt should be made to limit the use of narcotics in RSD. A patient with RSD should be followed-up carefully, and alterations in the treatment regimen should be made as needed.

Rehabilitation

The vicious cycle of pain, immobility, edema, contractures, and atrophy, leading to more pain, has to be broken. Early mobilization is critical to a favorable outcome.[16] The main goal in therapy is to try to achieve movement in the entire limb, which is involved with RSD. Immobilization adds to the edema of the limb, contributes to the pain, and leads to contractures of the affected limb. Edema control should be sought with range of motion exercises to elevate the limb and provide venous and lymphatic drainage. Compressive (Isotoner) gloves may be tried, but the pain may limit use. Desensitization of the limb affected by this hyperactive sympathetic system can sometimes be achieved with contrast baths, alternating hot (100° F, 43° C) and cold (65° F, 18° C) water soaks for few minutes. This modality can easily be taught to the patient for home use. Transcutaneous electrical nerve stimulation (TENS) has been used with mixed results. Heat to an involved limb is to be avoided in the edematous, acute phase, but may help the contractures of chronic RSD in absence of inflammation. Paraffin baths or fluidotherapy are practical means for administering such modalities.

Procedures

Sympathetic blocks are a key element in controlling RSD.[3,17] Stellate ganglion blocks for upper limb and lumbar chain blocks for lower limb RSD can be done by trained anesthesiologists or physiatrists. They offer at times spectacular, instantaneous relief. Response to such blocks is in fact one of the diagnostic criteria for RSD. These injections may be repeated if improvement is satisfactory for a period of time. Bier block is another procedure which can be used, and has been reported to have a 57% improvement in one study.[3,11] It involves an intravenous infusion of a chemical into limb after gravitationally draining the venous bed; lidocaine, hydrocortisone and guanethidine have been used. Brachial plexus block may provide analgesia for upper limb RSD; low dose morphine has been used with reported success. Radiofrequency sympathectomy has been successful in sympathetic denervation of the upper limb.[11]

Surgery

When a chemical block is effective but short lasting, surgical sympathectomy has been advocated and is fairly successful. A neurosurgical dorsal root entry zone (DREZ) ablation, where available, is another option for chronic severe cases.[18]

Potential Disease Complications

RSD can lead to chronic profound disabling pain, which is difficult to treat. Hand edema and contractures may pose significant functional limitations and disability from work.

Potential Treatment Complication

Complications of therapy depend on the specific treatment utilized. A short course of corticosteroids should not lead to any significant endocrine disturbances. Sedation is a common side effect with tricyclics and antiepileptics. Orthostatic hypotension may be a limiting factor when using antihypertensive drugs. Analgesics, NSAIDs, and COX-2 inhibitors have well-known side effects that most commonly affect the gastric, hepatic, and renal systems. Potential complications from a stellate ganglion block are inadvertent arterial artery injection and seizures, and recurrent laryngeal nerve injury.[18] With a lumbar sympathetic block, a perforation of the aorta, vena cava, or kidney can occur. As always, the therapeutic benefits have to be weighed against potential side effects.

References

1. Ochoa JL, Verdugo RJ: The mythology of reflex sympathetic dystrophy and sympathetically maintained pains. Phys Med Rehabil Clin NA 1993;4:151–163.
2. Stanton-Hicks M, Janig W, Hassenbusch S, et al: Reflex sympathetic dystrophy: Changing concepts and taxonomy. Pain 1995; 63:127–133.
3. Schwartzman RJ, McLellan TL: Reflex sympathetic dystrophy: A review. Arch Neurol 1987;44:555–561.
4. Veldman P, Reynen HM, Arntz IE, Goris RJ: Signs and symptoms of reflex sympathetic dystrophy: Prospective study of 829 patients. Lancet 1993;342:1012–1016.
5. Anderson DJ, Falat LM: Complex regional pain syndrome of the lower extremity: A retrospective study of 33 patients. J Foot Ankle Surg 1999;38:381–387.
6. O'Brien SJ, Ngeow J, Gibney MA, et al: Reflex sympathetic dystrophy of the knee: Causes, diagnosis, and treatment. Am J Orthop Surg 1995:23:655–659.
7. Allen G, Galer BS, Schwartz L: Epidemiology of complex regional pain syndrome: A retrospective chart review of 134 patients. Pain 1999;80:539–544.
8. Kozin F, Genant HK, Bekerman C, McCarty DJ: The reflex sympathetic dystrophy syndrome: ll. Roentgenographic and scintigraphic evidence of bilaterality and of periarticular accentuation. Am J Med 1976;60:332–338.
9. Mackinnon SE, Holder LE: the use of three-phase radionuclide bone scanning in the diagnosis of reflex sympathetic dystrophy. J hand Surg 1984;9A:556–563.
10. Kozin F, Ryan LM, Carrera GF, et al: The reflex sympathetic dystrophy syndrome (RSDS) lll. Scintigraphic studies, further evidence for the therapeutic efficacy of systemic corticosteroids, and proposed diagnostic criteria. Am J Med 1981;70:23–30.
11. Babur H: Reflex sympathetic dystrophy. J Neurol Orthop Med Surg 1991;12:46–59.
12. Moat AG: Treatment of the shoulder-hand syndrome with corticosteroids. Ann Rheum Dis. 1974;33:120–123.
13. Malice GA, Mellick LB: Reflex sympathetic dystrophy treated with gabapentin. Arch Phys Med Rehabil 1997;78:98–105.
14. Kingly WS: A critical review of controlled clinical trials for peripheral neuropathic pain and complex regional pain syndromes. Pain 1997;73(2):123–139.
15. Ghostine SY, Comair YG, Turner DM, et al: Phenoxybenzamine in the treatment of causalgia: Report of 40 cases. J Neurosurg 1984;60:1263–1268.
16. Stanton-Hicks M, Baron R, Boas R, et al: Complex regional pain syndromes: Guidelines for therapy. Clin J Pain 1998;14:155–166.
17. Bonica JJ: Causalgia and other reflex sympathetic dystrophies. Post Grad Med 1973;53:143–148.
18. Payne R: Neuropathic pain syndromes, with special reference to causalgia and reflex sympathetic dystrophy. Clin J Pain 1986;2:59–73.

133 Repetitive Strain Injuries

Walter Panis, MD

Synonyms

Cumulative trauma disorders

Occupational "neuroses"

Pain in limb[1]

Upper extremity musculoskeletal disorders

ICD-9 Codes

None

Definition

Upper extremity repetitive strain injuries (RSIs) are an incompletely understood complex of symptoms without a currently known etiology, pathology, and treatment. Although sometimes known as cumulative trauma disorders (CTDs), there is no one traumatic event that can be identified. These injuries are typically seen in the workplace where repetitive movements are demanded in the completion of tasks (e.g., filing, typing, assembly work).

One needs to distinguish between repetitive strain, or cumulative trauma, as a mechanism of injury in recognizable entities such as carpal tunnel syndrome or medial and lateral epicondylitis and the use of the terms RSI/CTD as diagnostic groupings. For the purposes of this chapter, RSIs will be classified as *upper extremity musculoskeletal disorders that do not fit into another specific diagnostic category and occur due to repetitive use of the arm*. They are classified as occupational illnesses rather than injuries.[1,2]

There are two disparate groups that hold views as to the etiology of RSI. Ergonomists believe that the injuries are due to force, repetition, vibration, and abnormal postures. On the other side, epidemiologists attribute many of the symptoms to psychosocial and political issues. Therefore a discussion of RSI cannot take place without the recognition of the psychosocial and economic issues that are involved. Because of the paucity of findings in these individuals, the American Society of Surgery of the Hand does not classify these symptoms as being musculoskeletal in nature. Indeed, attempts at defining pathology by biopsy of muscles and tendons have not been successful. Treatments that should usually alleviate the symptoms of tendinitis or muscle pain often fail.

There is a close relationship between RSI, the dystonias that are associated with writer's cramp, and the overuse syndromes seen in musicians.[3] The central nervous system basis of many dystonias may indeed point to the central nervous system origin of this syndrome, although this is not clear.

It is also important to understand that whenever an individual with a musculoskeletal complaint is involved in a situation in which compensation is a factor (e.g., motor vehicle accident, worker's compensation claim), the injured party takes on the additional role of being a claimant. This can change the perception of both patient and caregiver in many aspects of the healing process. These issues are especially true in upper extremity problems, as it is known there is a longer disability from RSI than other workers' compensation claims.[3]

Symptoms

The primary symptom in RSI is arm or hand pain. Often the pain may be initiated with minimal exertion, such as gripping a door handle or carrying a purse. The symptoms usually begin in one region of a limb (e.g., wrist, elbow, or forearm) but can quickly spread to involve the entire arm and even the other arm.

Associated symptoms of paresthesias, numbness, and weakness may or may not be present, and if present, may cross dermatomal and peripheral nerve boundaries.

Patients often complain of night pain, resulting in poor sleep. Depression may result when pain and poor sleep efficiency are protracted. Assessment of sleep habits is important because sleep disruption is very common and needs to be addressed.

In taking a history, the clinician needs to get an accurate understanding of the patient's job and workplace. Not only is it important to understand the mechanics of the job, such as the desk and chair set up, placement of the computer keyboard and screen, or the size of the components that are being assembled and speed of assembly, but the patient's perception of the workplace is paramount. Dissatisfied workers are notorious for work related medical claims.

Moreover, delving into issues of personal habits and family life is essential in determining any "red flags" that may suggest negative factors contributing to ongoing complaints. These red flags include (1) poor work performance evaluation and/or worker dissatisfaction, (2) drug and alcohol abuse, (3) marital problems, (4) child care issues, (5) concomitant depression, (6) dysfunctional family, and (7) family history of chronic pain/disability.

Physical Examination

A diagnosis of RSI is one of exclusion. Typically there are no objective physical findings. On inspection, there is no evidence of muscular atrophy or fasciculation, which would be present in conjunction with a peripheral nerve injury. Deep tendon reflexes are normal and symmetric. Muscle strength testing is generally inconsistent depending on the patient's effort and pain level with exertion. Use of objective and reproducible strength tests are important. These include a hand or pinch dynamometer. Sensory testing is often difficult, and subjective abnormalities are quite common. However, the distribution of the sensory abnormalities does not typically follow anatomic guidelines. Provocative tests such as percussion over the median nerve at the wrist, the ulnar nerve at the cubital tunnel, or the radial nerve at the elbow may elicit pain or paresthesias but are not necessarily indicative of nerve injuries.

Functional Limitations

Patients may be limited in many, if not all, of their activities of daily living as well as their work related activities. For example, pain may prevent an individual from brushing his or her teeth, cooking a meal, driving a car, or using a computer at work. Pain may also limit sexual and recreational activities.

Diagnostic Studies

As previously noted, diagnostic testing is used to exclude other definitive conditions. Electrodiagnostic studies (EMG and nerve conduction studies) are often necessary to rule out a median nerve compression at the wrist or another peripheral nerve lesion. MRIs of the neck are often ordered, but care should be taken to explain to the patient prior to the exam that abnormalities found on the MRI (e.g., bulging discs, uncinate arthritis), although real, are often found in people without pain complaints and may not explain the current symptom complex.

Case managers and employers often advocate functional capacity evaluations (FCEs). Whether they add any benefit to the diagnosis and treatment plan is controversial.

Differential Diagnosis

Cervical radiculopathy	Compressive neuropathies
Myofascial pain syndrome	Tendinitis (e.g., medial epicondylitis)
Thoracic outlet syndrome	Osteoarthritis
Rotator cuff tendinitis	Fractures

Treatment

Initial

Initial treatment for RSI involves avoidance of repetitive activities, particularly those that cause pain. Carefully following work related restrictions can keep the patient at work, allowing him or her to continue to earn a living and maintain a working life style and eliminates worker's compensation payments for being out of work.

Icing the limb for 15 to 20 minutes two to three times daily in association with wrist or elbow splinting can decrease symptoms. Contrast baths may also be useful. Typically these are done using hot (but not scalding) water for 10 minutes and then immediately placing the limb in ice water for 1 minute. This can be repeated several times. Ice massage is often another effective treatment that patients can do at home or work. To do this, the patient freezes water in a paper cup, then tears off the top rim of the cup thereby exposing the ice, and massages the injured area for 5 to 10 minutes with the exposed ice.

Transcutaneous electrical nerve stimulation (TENS) may also be effective in controlling some pain symptoms.

NSAIDs/COX-2 inhibitors can be used for controlling pain and inflammation, if present. It is useful to try several different types of NSAIDs because patient responses can be very idiosyncratic. Restoration of sleep can be attempted with the use of low-dose tricyclic antidepressants (e.g., 10 to 50 mg of nortriptyline or amitriptyline). Anticonvulsant medications such as gabapentin and carbamazepine are also used for pain. Gabapentin is most often prescribed, and it has a dose range of 300 to 3600 mg per day (generally bid or tid). Patients need to be warned that their effective dose may not be reached quickly. If depression is present, appropriate treatment or referral to a specialist is indicated.

It is important to encourage physical activity as much as possible. This includes general aerobic conditioning as a method of increased a positive health perception. Of course, weight reduction, if needed, and smoking cessation are included in any plan to improve health.

Rehabilitation

Rehabilitative measures include the fabrication of splints as needed, massage, myofascial release, icing, and empirical iontophoresis or ultrasound. Adaptive equipment ranging from voice-activated software, foot mouse, and ergonomic keyboards to large handled tools, is available.

Referral to a physical therapist, occupational therapist, or hand therapist familiar with RSI is essential. The experienced therapist will lead the patient through a regimen of stretching and strengthening in conjunction with emphasizing posture control at work and home. Often, a therapist is capable of making an ergonomic assessment of the workplace to provide recommendations that can decrease or eliminate complaints. Today, the marketplace is full of many devices that can assist an individual with RSI. Voice-activated technology can allow many workers to continue to use computers effectively without their hands. Ergonomically designed computer keyboards, touch pads, a foot controlled mouse, and document holders are among the tools that can help decrease symptoms.

Therapists may also assist with fabricating splints, if needed. They can do "hands-on" treatments, such as massage and myofascial release techniques. They can perform spray and stretch techniques with a vapocoolant spray. Modalities such as iontophoresis, ultrasound, and paraffin baths can be used to decrease symptoms.

Progressive resistive exercise programs can be used, but worsening pain symptoms with exercise is often an issue. This can significantly limit patient participation and thus the strength gains that are possible with treatment. Additionally, this can limit the effectiveness of work hardening and work conditioning programs.

Individuals who are having difficulty returning to their previous level of work activity should be evaluated for alternative jobs. This can be with their current employer, or in some instances, a different vocation must be pursued. In the latter instance, a consultation with a vocational rehabilitation specialist is advised.

Procedures

Procedures are uncommon in RSI. However, in treating patients with such a non-definitive diagnosis and one in which treatment failures are frequent, trigger point injections, lateral epicondylar injections, carpal tunnel injections, etc. can be tried to see if symptoms improve.

Surgery

Surgery is not indicated for RSI.

Potential Disease Complications

The complications of not treating the illness include increasing disability in all aspects of life. Feeling incapable of using the arms and hands results in the inability to participate in home, work, and recreational activities. Depression and social isolation may result from prolonged periods of being out of work.

Potential Treatment Complications

Treatment complications stem from the medications used. Analgesics, NSAIDs, and COX-2 inhibitors have well-known side effects that most commonly affect the gastric, hepatic, and renal systems. Gabapentin can cause fatigue, ataxia, edema, or nausea. Tricyclic antidepressants have a high profile of fatigue, dizziness, dry mouth, and constipation.

References
1. Vender MI, Kasdan ML, Truppa KL: Upper extremity disorders: A literature review to determine work-relatedness. J Hand Surg 1995;20A:534–541.
2. Derebery VJ: Injuries and rehabilitation of the upper extremity. Phys Med Rehabil State Art Rev 1998;12: 77–18
3. Webster BS, Snook SH: The cost of compensable upper extremity cumulative trauma disorders, J Occup Med 1994;36:713–717.

134 Rheumatoid Arthritis

Karen Atkinson, MD, MPH

Synonyms

None

ICD-9 Code

714.0
Rheumatoid arthritis

Definition

Rheumatoid arthritis (RA) is a chronic inflammatory disorder that primarily affects joints but may also have prominent extra-articular features. The arthritis is classically symmetric and affects the peripheral joints. The prevalence of rheumatoid arthritis is approximately 1%, and it affects women about 2 to 2.5 times more often than men. Peak incidence of RA is in the third and fourth decades.[1] Classification criteria are available for RA and may be helpful in evaluating patients (Table 1). Many patients with early disease, however, will not fulfill these criteria.[2]

Symptoms

Rheumatoid arthritis is a systemic disease, and symptoms vary according to the system involved.[3–5]

General

Morning stiffness is a prominent feature of rheumatoid arthritis. Unlike the brief (5 to 10 minutes) of stiffness that occurs in patients with osteoarthritis, the morning stiffness in rheumatoid arthritis is greater than 30 to 60 minutes and often lasts for hours. Fatigue and generalized malaise are also common complaints.

Joint

Patients present with joint pain and swelling. Patients may also complain of loss of joint function, which may be due to joint inflammation or structural damage. A Baker's cyst can develop and cause pain and/or swelling of the popliteal fossa. If the cyst ruptures, it causes pain, swelling, and erythema of the calf. If the cricoarytenoid joint is involved, patients may complain of laryngeal pain, hoarseness, or difficulty in swallowing.

Eye

Up to one third of patients will complain of dry eyes (keratoconjunctivitis sicca). These patients may also complain of foreign body sensation, burning, and/or discharge. Patients with episcleritis will complain of red, painful eyes.

TABLE 1. Classification Criteria for Rheumatoid Arthritis

Criterion	Definition
Morning Stiffness	Morning stiffness in or around the joints lasting at least 1 hour before maximal improvement.
Arthritis of three or more joint areas	Soft tissue swelling or fluid in at least three joints observed by a clinician. The 14 possible joints include right or left PIP, MCP, wrist, elbow, knee, ankle, and MTP joints.
Arthritis of the hand joints	At least one area swollen in a wrist, MCP, or PIP joint.
Symmetric arthritis	Simultaneous involvement of the same joint areas on both sides of the body. Involvement of the small joint groups (MCPs, PIPs, and MTPs) is acceptable without absolute symmetry.
Rheumatoid nodules	Subcutaneous nodules occurring over bony prominences, extensor surfaces, or juxta-articular regions. These must be observed by a clinician.
Serum rheumatoid factor	Abnormal amounts of serum rheumatoid factor by any method for which the result has been positive in < 5% of normal control subjects.
Radiographic changes	Posteroanterior hand and wrist films that demonstrate erosion or unequivocal bony decalcification localized in or most marked adjacent to the involved joints.

* A patient is said to have rheumatoid arthritis if he or she satisfies at least four of the seven criteria. Criteria one through four must have been present for at least 6 weeks.

Skin

Patients may note small, painless subcutaneous nodules, mainly over the extensor surfaces. Rheumatoid vasculitis will cause rash that may lead to ulceration. Patients with vasculitis may also complain of discoloration around the fingertips (digital infarcts).

Neurologic

Numbness and tingling are common symptoms of nerve involvement. Nerves can be affected in several ways. Nerve entrapment results from joint inflammation. The most common site is at the wrist, where median nerve involvement causes carpal tunnel symptoms. Mononeuritis mutiplex is the result of vasculitis and presents as weakness or numbness/tingling in discrete nerve distributions (e.g., foot or wrist drop). Cervical spine instability may lead to myelopathy, causing sensory symptoms and weakness, most commonly in the upper extremities. This can occur in the absence of neck pain in patients with longstanding RA.

Cardiac

Patients may complain of chest pain and shortness of breath consistent with pericarditis; however, pericardial involvement is usually asymptomatic.

Pulmonary

Pleural inflammation or nodulosis may produce typical symptoms of pleurisy. Shortness of breath may occur secondary to pleural or interstitial disease.

Physical Examination

All joints should be examined for swelling, warmth, effusion, range of motion, and deformity. Rheumatoid arthritis is a symmetric polyarthritis (more than 4 joints involved). Fingers, feet, wrists, and knees are most commonly involved. The distal interphalangeal (DIP) joints are usually spared. Any joint can be affected. In rare cases, patients will present with monoarthritis (single joint involvement). Rheumatoid nodules are present in about 30% of patients and occur over bony prominences, extensor surfaces, or in juxta-articular regions.[3]

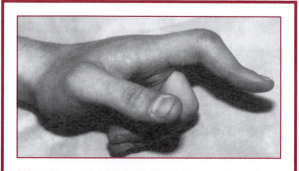

FIGURE 1. The boutonnière deformity, involving hyperextension of the DIP joint with flexion of the PIP joint, also is caused by a derangement of the extensor mechanism—typically a rupture of the central extensor tendon at its insertion in the middle phlanax. Early diagnosis and prolonged splinting of the PIP in extension are necessary for successful treatment of this difficult injury. (From Concannon MJ: Common Hand Problems in Primary Care. Philadelphia, Hanley & Belfus, 1999, p 151, with permission.)

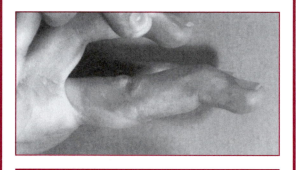

FIGURE 2. The swan neck deformity (recurvatum) involves hyperextension of the PIP joint with flexion of the DIP joint. This is caused by a derangement in the extensor mechanism, with a dorsal migration of the lateral bands. (From Concannon MJ: Common Hand Problems in Primary Care. Philadelphia, Hanley & Belfus, 1999, p 151, with permission.)

In the hands, early rheumatoid arthritis causes fusiform swelling at the proximal interphalangeal (PIP) joint. Chronic inflammation may lead to subluxation of the metacarpophalangeal (MCP) joints with ulnar deviation of the fingers. Damage to collateral ligaments at the PIP joints results in the classic boutonnière (PIP flexion and DIP hyperextension) and swan neck (PIP hyperextension and DIP flexion) deformities (Figs. 1 and 2).

Symmetric wrist swelling is usually present in RA. Subluxation results from synovitis and weakening of the ligaments and causes prominence of the ulnar styloid.

Inflammation of the synovial tendon sheath is called tenosynovitis. This may occur in the flexor or extensor tendons of the fingers. Examination will reveal passive motion as greater than active motion. Crepitus is often felt when the hands are placed over the tendon sheaths and the fingers are flexed and extended. If the patient has a trigger finger, placing one finger over the flexor tendon while flexing and extending the affected finger will allow palpation of a nodule.

Elbow involvement is common. In early disease, inflammation and effusion cause decreased extension. Effusions can be palpated in the dimple (para-olecranon groove) found on either side of the olecranon process. With chronic inflammation and erosion of the cartilage between the radius and ulna, loss of extension and flexion occurs. Rheumatoid nodules are often found over the extensor aspect of the proximal ulna. The olecranon bursa may be enlarged and filled with fluid and/or nodules.

The shoulder may be involved in RA. Effusions are best seen on the anterior aspect of the shoulder below the acromion. Evaluation of rotator cuff strength is important since inflammation of the rotator cuff may result in destruction. A ruptured biceps tendon will cause a bulge in the biceps when flexed against resistance.

The cervical spine may have decreased range of motion or pain with range of motion. Physical exam is not adequate to assess stability. Patients with suspected cervical instability should have a thorough neurologic exam. Patients with cord involvement may demonstrate paresthesias, weakness, or pathologic reflexes. Tingling paresthesias that descend the thoracolumbar spine upon flexion of the cervical spine are called L'hermitte's sign. (See page 602.)

The hip joint is deep, limiting evaluation for synovitis and effusion. An inflamed hip will cause groin pain upon active and passive range of motion. Patients may walk with an antalgic gait, rapidly taking weight off the affected leg. Pain in the hip region may also result from trochanteric bursitis. Applying pressure over the lateral hip region reproduces the pain from the trochanteric bursa. Lateral hip pain and lack of groin pain distinguish trochanteric bursitis from joint inflammation. Iliopsoas bursitis may result in an inguinal mass.

The knee is commonly involved in RA. Small effusions can be detected by looking for a "bulge" sign. To perform this maneuver, the patient should be lying down. With one hand, the clinician makes an upward stroke to depress the medial synovial pouch. A downward stroke on the lateral aspect of the knee will result in a bulge of the medial pouch if a small effusion is present. A ballotable patella (patellar tap) indicates a larger effusion. A Baker's cyst occurs as an extension of synovial fluid from the joint cavity (see Chapter 59). The cyst causes fullness in the popliteal fossa that can be seen when the client is standing with his or her back facing the clinician. Erythema and swelling of the calf may be seen if a Baker's cyst has ruptured. Evaluating for hemorrhage below the maleolli of the ankle (the "crescent" sign) can distinguish this from thrombophlebitis.

The ankle may have synovitis, effusion, or decreased range of motion. Involvement of the hindfoot (subtalar and talonavicular joints) may result in valgus deformity and flat foot. Metatarsophalangeal (MTP) involvement is common. Synovitis causes pain and fullness with palpation. Hallux valgus deformity is also common. Progressive disease causes dorsal dislocation of the MTP joints and claw toes.

Functional Limitations

Functional limitations depend on the location and severity of joint and extra-articular involvement. Criteria for the assessment of functional status have been established (Table 2) and are based on activities of daily living, including self-care (e.g., dressing, feeding, bathing, grooming, and toileting) and vocational (e.g., work, school, and homemaking) and avocational (e.g., recreational and/or leisure) activities.[6]

TABLE 2. Criteria for Classification of Functional Status in Rheumatoid Arthritis

Class I	Able to perform all activities of daily living (self-care, vocational, and avocational)
Class II	Able to perform self-care and vocational activities, but limited in avocational activities
Class III	Able to perform usual self-care activities, but limited in vocational and avocational activities
Class IV	Limited in all activities of daily living (self-care, vocational, and avocational)

Diagnostic Studies

Laboratory histologic findings and radiographic findings may be suggestive of rheumatoid arthritis, but no test is diagnostic of the disease (Figs. 3 and 4).[3,7] Rheumatoid factor is present in the serum of 85% of patients.[5] Normochromic, normocytic anemia consistent with chronic disease is often found, and the degree of anemia often correlates with disease activity. Acute phase reactants such as the erythrocyte sedimentation rate (ESR), C-reactive protein (CRP), erythrocyte and platelet count are elevated. Eosinophilia may be found in patients with extra-articular manifestations. Patients with Felty's syndrome (RA, splenomegaly, and leukopenia) exhibit low white blood cell counts and may have thrombocytopenia. A variant of Felty's syndrome has been described in which patients have large granular lymphocytes present in blood and bone marrow in addition to neutropenia. Liver function tests including serum glutamic oxaloacetic transaminase and alkaline phoshatase are often elevated in patients with active disease.

Evaluation of fluid taken from an affected joint will have an inflammatory cell count (greater than 2000 WBCs). Joint fluid should always be sent for culture to rule out infection and evaluated under a polarized microscope to exclude crystal disease. If pleurocardiocentesis or pericardiocentesis is necessary, the fluid has low complement, high protein and a predominance of lymphocytes. The glucose is characteristically extremely low or may even be absent.

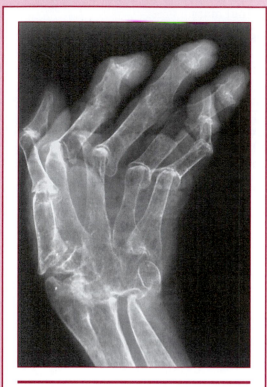

FIGURE 3. Advanced rheumatoid arthritis—hand and wrist. Bony ankylosis at the wrist, penciling of the distal ulna, and marked erosive changes at the metacarpophalangeal (MCP) joints with ulnar deviation of the fingers are classic RA findings. Also note the more severe involvement of the carpus and MCP joints; interphalangeal joints are typically less severely affected. (From Katz DS, et al: Radiology Secrets. Philadelphia, Hanley & Belfus, 1998, p 273, with permission.)

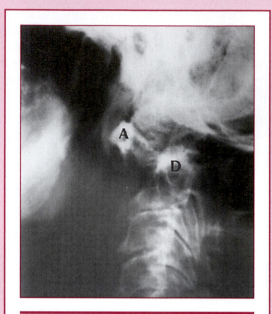

FIGURE 4. Atlantoaxial subluxation—RA. There is marked widening of the space between the anterior arch of the atlas (A) and the margin of the dens (D). (From Katz DS, et al: Radiology Secrets. Philadelphia, Hanley & Belfus, 1998, p 273, with permission.)

Characteristic changes on joint radiographs include periarticular osteopenia and/or marginal erosions. Early in the disease, however, joint films may be normal. Baseline hand and wrist films may aid in diagnosis and can be used to follow disease progression. Flexion and extension views of the cervical spine may demonstrate erosion of the odontoid and atlantoaxial subluxation. Pulmonary nodules or interstitial fibrosis can be seen on chest radiograph. Echocardiography often reveals a small pericardial effusion, valvular thickening, or aortic root dilatation, but these are most often asymptomatic. Electrocardiogram may reveal conduction abnormalities due to involvement of the cardiac conduction system by rheumatoid nodules.

Differential Diagnosis

Crystal-induced arthritis
   Gout
   Pseudogout

Spondyloarthropathies
   Psoriatic arthritis
   Ankylosing spondylitis
   Enteropathic arthritis

Treatment

Initial

Nonsteroidal anti-inflammatory drugs (NSAIDs) are effective in some patients. COX-2 specific anti-inflammatories may reduce the incidence of gastrointestinal symptoms in patients who have a history of bleeding or who are intolerant of traditional NSAIDs.

For patients with inadequate response to NSAIDs or poor prognostic indicators, disease modifying drugs (DMARDs) should be initiated. Poor prognostic factors include high titer rheumatoid factor, early presence of bony erosion, many affected joints, extra-articular involvement, and considerable degree of physical disability at disease onset.[8]

DMARDs that are prescribed include antimalarials, intramuscular gold, sulfasalazine, azathioprine, methotrexate, leflunomide, cyclosporine, and cyclophosphamide.[8,9] Biologic agents directed against tumor necrosis factor include etanercept and infliximab and are now available and approved for patients with disease refractory to traditional DMARDs.[10] Corticosteroids can be very useful and can be administered systemically as a bridge to therapy with DMARDs or intra-articularly for monoarticular or oligoarticular involvement.

Rehabilitation

The role of occupational and physical therapy may be different in early or established disease and end stage disease.[11,12] In early disease, occupational therapy is directed toward patient education about how to the use joints to minimize joint stress when performing activities of daily living. Splints may be used to provide joint rest and reduce inflammation. Splints may also allow functional use of joints that would otherwise be limited by pain. Not all clinicians advocate this use. Paraffin baths can provide relief of pain and stiffness in the small joints of the hands. In end stage disease, the occupational therapist plays an important role, providing aids and adaptive devices, such as raised toilet seats, special chairs and beds, and special grips, that can assist in self-care.

Physical therapy can be very helpful in reducing joint inflammation and pain. The therapist may employ a variety of techniques, including the application of heat or cold, transcutaneous nerve stimulation, and iontophoresis. Water exercise (hydrotherapy) is used to increase muscle strength without joint overuse. In patients with foot involvement, small alterations to footwear or inserts may provide decreased pain and a more normal gait. In end stage disease, the goals of therapy are reducing joint inflammation, loosening fixed position of joints, improving the function of damaged joints, and improving strength and general condition. Local immobilization may be utilized to reduce inflammation and pain. Non-fixed contractures may be prevented or improved with periods of splinting combined with goal-oriented exercise. Muscle strength and overall conditioning may be improved by static, range-of-motion, and relaxation exercises. In recent years, aerobic and weight-bearing exercises have been used without detrimental effect to the joints. These dynamic exercises are more effective in increasing muscle strength, range of motion, and physical capacity.[13] The motivation and encouragement provided by the therapist should not be underestimated.

Procedures

For monoarticular or oligoarticular involvement, local steroid injection may be used when oral medications fail to control joint inflammation.

Surgery

Orthopedic intervention including joint reconstruction or replacement (Fig. 5), tendon repair, and synovectomy may be indicated. Patients with suspected or confirmed cervical spine involvement will need special consideration/handling by anesthesiology during intubation (Fig. 6). Cervical spine stabilization is usually not performed unless the patient has neurologic symptoms.

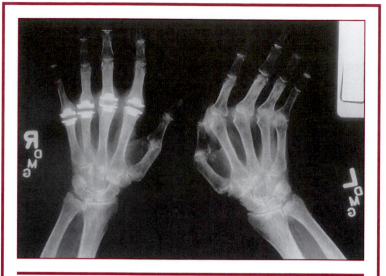

FIGURE 5. Hinged silicone prosthesis with grommets. Radiograph of implanted prostheses at the metacarpophalangeal joints of the index, middle, ring, and little fingers on the right hand. (From Weinzweig J: Plastic Surgery Secrets. Philadelphia, Hanley & Belfus, 1999, p 543, with permission.)

Potential Disease Complications

The most common complication is joint destruction and subsequent decreased functional use of affected joints. Neuropathy may occur due to entrapment, pressure, or deposition of amyloid. Cervical instability can lead to myelopathy. Irregular bony edges may result in tendon rupture. Nodules may break down and ulcerate. Skin ulcerations may also occur in pressure points in the immobilized patient. The kidneys and gastrointestinal tract may be sites of deposition in patients who develop secondary amyloidosis. Scleritis may result in scleromalacia.

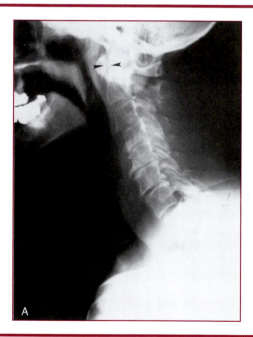

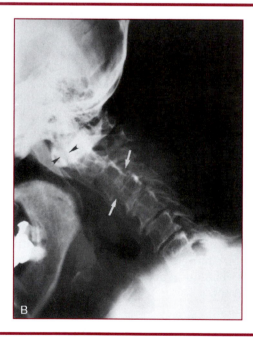

FIGURE 6. Subluxation of vertebrae in rheumatoid arthritis. The abnormal movement between vertebrae due to laxity of ligaments becomes more apparent in flexion of the cervical spine. Lateral flexion-extension views are requested if subluxation of cervical vertebrae is suspected. The x-ray in *A* is taken in the neutral position, and the one in *B* is taken in flexion. The black arrow heads mark the distance between the anterior surface of odontoid process and the posterior surface of the arch of atlas. This space is increased in flexion because of subluxation of the arch of atlas onthe second vertebra. The white arrows show anterior slippage of the third cervical vertebra on fourth. In a normal cervical spine, the posterior surface of vertebral bodies forms a smooth curve that is convex anteriorly (lordosis). This curve is disturbed and a step-like deformity is seen (white arrows) at the posteroinferior angle of upper vertebra and posterosuperior angle of lower vertebra in subluxation. (From Mehta AJ: Common Musculoskeletal Problems. Philadelphia, Hanley & Belfus, 1997, p 149, with permission.)

TABLE 3. Side Effects of Medications Used to Treat Patients with Rheumatoid Arthritis

Medication	Side Effects	Medication	Side Effects
NSAIDs		Sulfasalazine	Myelosuppression
Traditional	Dyspepsia, ulcer, or bleeding		Hemolysis (G6PD deficient patients)
	Renal insufficiency		Hepatotoxicity
	Hepatotoxicity		Photosensitivity/rash
	Rash		Dyspepsia/diarrhea
	Inhibit platelet function		Headaches
COX-2 inhibitors	Same as traditional NSAIDs but GI side effects occur less often		Oligospermia
	No platelet effect		
Glucocorticoids	Increased appetite/weight gain	Azathioprine	Myelosuppression
	Cushingoid habitus		Hepatotoxicity
	Acne		Pancreatitis (rarely)
	Fluid retention		Lymphoproliferative disorders (long-term risk)
	Hypertension		
	Diabetes		
	Glaucoma/cataracts		
	Atherosclerosis		
	Avascular necrosis		
	Osteoporosis		
	Impaired wound healing		
	Susceptibility to infection		
Antimalarials	Dyspepsia	Methotrexate	Hepatic fibrosis/cirrhosis
	Hemolysis (G6PD deficient patients)		Pneumonitis
	Macular damage		Myelosuppression
	Abnormal skin pigmentation		Mucositis
	Neuromyopathy		Dyspepsia
	Rash		Alopecia
			Increased rheumatoid nodules
Gold	Myelosupression	Leflunomide	Hepatic fibrosis/cirrhosis
	Proteinuria or hematuria		Myelosuppression
	Oral ulcers		Dyspepsia
	Rash		Alopecia
	Pruritis		
Etanercept	Injection site reaction	Infliximab	Infusion reaction
	Exacerbation of infection		Exacerbation of infection
Cyclosporin A	Renal insufficiency	Cyclophosphamide	Dyspepsia/diarrhea
	Hypertension		Myelosuppression
	Anemia		Alopecia
			Hemorrhagic cystitis
			Ovarian and testicular failure
			Teratogenicity
			Malignancy
			Opportunistic infection

Potential Treatment Complications

Side effects vary according to drug (Table 3).[9]

Overly aggressive physical or occupational therapy can cause increased joint inflammation and pain.

References

1. MacGregor AJ, Silman AJ: Rheumatoid arthritis: Classification and epidemiology. In Klippel JH, Dieppe PA (eds): Rheumatology, 2nded. London, Mosby, 1998, pp 5.2.2-6.
2. Arnet FC, Edworthy SM, Bloch DA, et al: The American Rheumatism Association 1987 revised criteria for the classification of rheumatoid arthritis. Arthritis Rheum 1988;31:315–324.
3. Fuchs HA, Sergent JS: Rheumatoid arthritis: The clinical picture. In Koopman (ed): Arthritis and Allied Conditions: A Textbook of Rheumatology, 13th ed. Baltimore, Williams & Wilkins, 1997, pp 1041–1070.
4. Gordon AG, Hastings DE: Rheumatoid arthritis: Clinical features of early, progressive and late disease. In Klippel JH, Dieppe PA (eds): Rheumatology. 2nd ed. London, Mosby, 1998, pp 5.3.1-14.
5. Anderson RJ: Rheumatoid arthritis: Clinical and laboratory features. In Klippel JH (ed): Primer on the Rheumatic Diseases, 11th ed. Arthritis Foundation, 1997, pp 161–167.
6. Hochberg MC, Chang RW, Dwosh I, et al: The American College of Rheumatology 1991 Revised Criteria for the classification of global functional status in rheumatoid arthritis. Arthritis Rheum 1992;35:493–502.
7. Matteson EL, Cohen MD, Doyt DL: Rheumatoid arthritis: Clinical features and systemic involvement. In Klippel JH, Dieppe PA (eds): Rheumatology, 2nd ed. London, Mosby 1998, pp 5.4.1-7.
8. Paget SA: Rheumatoid arthritis: Treatment. In Klippel JH (ed): Primer on the Rheumatic Diseases, 11th ed. Arthritis Foundation, 1997, pp 168–173.
9. Cash JM, Klippel JH: Drug therapy: second-line drug therapy for rheumatoid arthritis. N Engl J Med 1994;330(19):1368–1375.
10. Matteson EL: Current treatment strategies for rheumatoid arthritis. Mayo Clin Proc 2000;75(1):69–74.
11. van Riel PL, Wijnands MJH, van de Putte LBA: Rheumatoid arthritis: Evaluation and management of active inflammatory disease. In Klippel JH, Dieppe PA (eds): Rheumatology, 2nd ed. London, Mosby, 1998, pp 5.14.1-12.
12. Hazes JMW, Cats A:Rheumatoid arthritis: Management: end stage and complications. In Klippel JH, Dieppe PA (eds): Rheumatology, 2nd ed. London, Mosby, 1998, pp 5.15.1-10.
13. van den Ende CH, Breedveld FC, le Cessie S, et al: Effect of invasive exercise on patients with active rheumatoid arthritis: A randomized clinical trial. Ann Rheum Dis 2000;59(8): 615–621.

135 Scoliosis and Kyphosis

Mark A. Thomas, MD
Yumei Wang, MD

Definition

Scoliosis (Fig. 1) is a postural deformity of the spine resulting in a lateral (coronal) deviation, or curve. Scoliosis is commonly associated with rotation of the vertebral bodies located within the curve. It affects between 3% and 30% of the population, with its incidence increasing with age.[1] The scoliotic curve may be congenital, appearing during infancy (infantile scoliosis), or develop in childhood (juvenile scoliosis), adolescence (adolescent scoliosis), or adulthood (degenerative scoliosis). When the diagnosis of scoliosis is made in an adult patient, the curve should be defined as *adult onset* (usually degenerative) or *adult presenting* (most commonly an idiopathic adolescent curve that was not previously diagnosed). Scoliosis can result from congenital, degenerative, disease-related, or idiopathic causes. An idiopathic etiology of scoliosis is more common than scoliosis due to other causes, such as degenerative disc disease and spondylosis, congenital malformation of the vertebrae, tumor, neuromuscular disease, or connective tissue disease.

Kyphosis (Fig. 2) is defined as a sagittal deviation in spinal alignment, or backward curve exceeding normal values. Normal kyphosis in the thoracic spine varies between 20 and 40 degrees.[2-4] Pathologic kyphosis occurs in association with structural changes in the spine due to pathology such as osteoporotic compression fractures, tumor, or Scheuermann's disease (juvenile kyphosis). It is caused by the resulting wedge deformity of the vertebral bodies.

Symptoms

Scoliosis

The symptoms produced by scoliosis relate to the etiology, location, and severity of the curve. The curve itself often does not produce symptoms or complaints, particularly a curve that does not exceed 20 degrees. When scoliosis is severe, pain and cosmetic deformities occur. Deformity, such as humping of the back, asymmetric shoulder or hip height, or asymmetry of breast size or waist contour may produce psychosocial symptoms such as low self-esteem, anxiety, and depression. These may be the presenting complaints. Curves that exceed 60 degrees begin to affect other systems. They can produce shortness of breath due to restrictive lung disease;

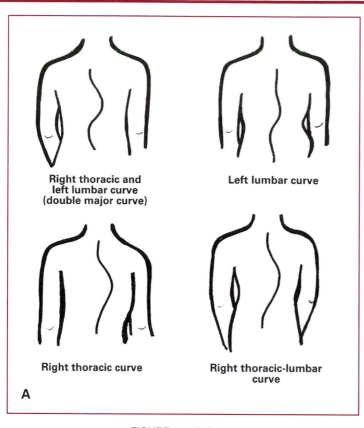

Right thoracic and
left lumbar curve
(double major curve)

Left lumbar curve

Right thoracic curve

Right thoracic-lumbar
curve

A

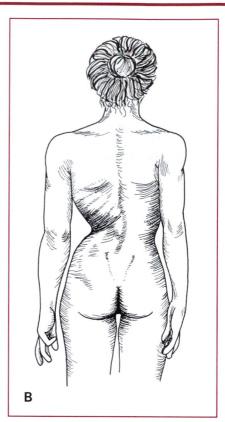

B

FIGURE 1. *A*, Examples of scoliosis curve patterns. *B*, Scoliosis.

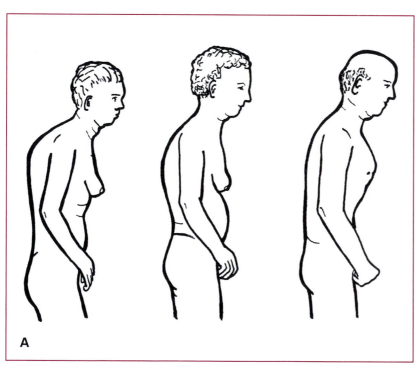

A

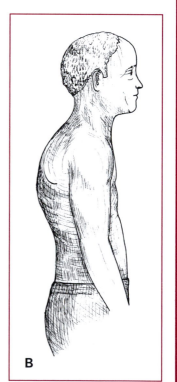

B

FIGURE 2. *A*, Kyphotic deformities. *B*, Kyphosis.

weakness, pain, paresthesia; or hypesthesia due to compression or impingement of nerve roots; and impaired activity tolerance due to increased energy costs for maintaining trunk stability. Severe lumbar curves commonly produce low back pain, whereas severe thoracic curvature often results in psychosocial symptoms.

Kyphosis

Complaints relate to the degree and location of the kyphos. Intermittent aching back pain and stiffness are the most usual presenting complaints and are most prominent at the apex of the kyphos. Pain and stiffness may be most severe when the patient is leaning forward. A compensatory increase in lumbar lordosis, with or without spondylolysis, may be present and associated with low back pain.[2,5–7] Cardiopulmonary compromise, though unusual, can also develop in severe cases, causing shortness of breath, fatigue, and poor activity tolerance.

Physical Examination

Scoliosis

Minor curves are difficult to detect on inspection of the patient. An easy way to detect a subtle thoracic or lumbar curve is to drop a plumb line from the occiput, or C7 spinous process, and inspect the spine for lateral deviations from this line. Have the patient bend forward, because the rotation associated with scoliosis is most easily seen in the forward flexed position. Asymmetry of the back contour in this position is due to vertebral body or rib rotation and may be quantified. A trunk rotation angle of 7 degrees roughly corresponds to a coronal curve of 20 degrees.

Subtle indicators that can be sought on physical examination include apparent (not actual) unequal breast size, asymmetry of the waist fold contour, or unequal iliac crest and shoulder height. Scoliosis should be suspected when café au lait spots (often associated with neurofibromatosis) or a leg-length discrepancy exceeding 2.2 cm is present.[8,9] Thorough serial assessments are advisable every 6 to 12 months. These assessments usually include x-rays and should focus on the degree of curvature, location and extent of the curve, degree of rotation, degree of skeletal maturity, correctibility of the curve, height, vital capacity, and expiratory pulmonary function tests.

Patients with degenerative scoliosis should be examined for neurologic deficits. Lower extremity strength, sensation, and reflexes should also be checked when the curvature exceeds 40 degrees or when the patient complains of weakness, paresthesias, or decreased sensation regardless of the etiology of the scoliosis.

A full evaluation of a scoliotic curve necessitates identification of the etiology of the curve for optimal treatment and prognostication. Curves may be idiopathic (juvenile, adolescent), functional (muscle spasm, posture), congenital (vertebral malformation), or degenerative or paralytic (motor unit disease). Scoliosis should be treated in the context of a patient's global status, and identifying underlying or idiopathic causes of the curve allows care to be provided within the context of the patient's overall health.

Kyphosis

Increased thoracic kyphos results in a forward displacement of the head and neck and a compensatory increase in lumbar lordosis. These are apparent on inspection. The rounding of the back will not fully correct with trunk extension in a prone position, but the degree to which the curve reverses should be noted. Thoracolumbar and lumbar kyphoses are less readily appreciated on inspection. The clinician should note any prominence of the spinous processes, which indicates lower spine kyphosis.[6,10–12] Associated scoliosis should be sought and will be present in about one third of patients.[13–15] Restricted trunk extension results from either deformity or pain. Tenderness to palpation may be elicited over the spinous processes. Tightness of the hamstring and pectoralis muscles is common.

A neurologic examination should be performed when the patient complains of weakness, sensory changes, or gait abnormalities. Vital capacity, peak flow, and other expiratory respiratory parameters should be performed when the kyphosis exceeds 40 to 50 degrees.

Functional Limitations

The functional limitations related to scoliosis and kyphosis result from the loss of spinal motion.[6] A kyphosis related restriction in upward gaze may affect driving and cause difficulty with lying prone or swimming in a prone position. Loss of shoulder range of motion, particularly forward flexion and abduction, may result from restricted scapular excursion over the thorax. This can interfere with overhead activities of daily living. Pain can result in limited sitting, standing, or walking tolerance.

The disruption of spinal balance that occurs will displace the center of gravity, particularly with severe kyphosis. This increases the energy costs for standing and ambulation. It can also impair balance. With severe deformity, cardiopulmonary compromise may decrease endurance. If the patient perceives cosmetic deformities as severe, social isolation can result.

Diagnostic Studies

Standing anteroposterior (AP) and lateral x-rays are useful in the evaluation of scoliosis and kyphosis. Bending or supine radiographs are not usually done but can help to determine the flexibility or correctability of the curve. X-rays can reveal congenital abnormalities of the vertebral body that cause spinal imbalance (block, bar, butterfly vertebrae), evidence of Scheuermann's disease (endplate fluting), or the lateral vertebral body wedging that is characteristic of idiopathic scoliosis.[16]

Measurement of the scoliotic curve on plain films is done by either the Cobb or Risser method. The most common measurement, the Cobb angle, is determined by the intersection of two lines drawn perpendicular to the vertebral endplates that represent the maximal deviation of the spine (Fig. 3).

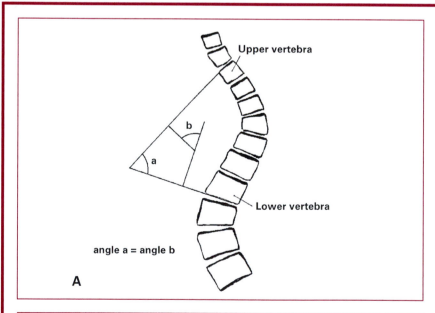
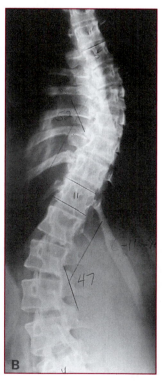

FIGURE 3. *A*, Measurement of idiopathic scoliosis using the Cobb angle. *B*, Idiopathic adolescent scoliosis. There is a primary thoracic dextroscoliosis (convexity to the right side) measuring 52° and a compensatory lumbar levoscoliosis (convexity to the left side) measuring 47°. (From Katz DS, et al: Radiology Secrets. Philadelphia, Hanley & Belfus, 1998, p 321, with permission.)

Plain films also allow assessment of vertebral body rotation and the growth centers in the ilium, vertebrae, and humerus. The degree of vertebral body rotation is gauged by the deviation from the midline of either the spinous process or pedicles. Rotation is graded 0 (no rotation) to 4 (rotation of 90 degrees or more). Epiphyseal closure can sometimes be assessed by plain films. Closure of the growth plates proceeds in a cephalad manner. Since vertebral growth plates are not consistently demonstrated on plain films, the iliac crest is a useful site for assessing spine growth status. This is Risser's sign, which is graded 0 (no mineralization) to 5 (fusion of the growth plate).

Magnetic resonance imaging (MRI), computerized tomography (CT), and nuclear medicine scans are indicated for specific purposes, such as identifying a neurofibroma or diastomatomyelia. If a neurologic deficit is present, MRI or CT should be performed to delineate the lesion. Electrodiagnostic studies are a useful adjunct to these tests for grading the severity of the lesion and prognostication. If surgery is being considered, preoperative MRI or CT myelogram is indicated. Bone scans are helpful to exclude discitis or tumor as the cause of pain or spinal deformity. Pulmonary function testing, particularly volume and expiratory studies, should be performed when curves exceed 60 degrees.

Differential Diagnosis

Lateral listhesis

Spondylolisthesis

Spondyloepiphyseal dysplasia tarda

Morquio's disease

Deformity resulting from other
　pathology (e.g., fracture, tumor)

Treatment

Initial

In all patients, regardless of age, it is important to identify curves that are likely to be progressive. Curves that are large (degree of curvature), closely packed (spanning a relatively small spinal segment), related to congenital vertebral body malformation, and very rotated or occur in the immature spine require more aggressive intervention. In general, scoliotic curves less than 20 degrees and kyphotic curves less than 40 degrees are observed through serial assessment. NSAIDs/COX-2 inhibitors or analgesics may be used for pain management. Transcutaneous electrical nerve stimulation (TENS) may also be used to manage pain.

If the scoliosis exceeds 20 degrees or the kyphosis exceeds 40 degrees, assess for bracing or surgery. The treatment goal for idiopathic curves is to limit progression of the scoliosis or kyphosis and maintain full activity, independence, and comfort. This is best done with patient education, exercise, and bracing.

Rehabilitation

Exercise is beneficial for general well-being, flexibility, and to improve posture. There is no clear evidence that exercise is a disease-modifying intervention for idiopathic scoliosis. Kyphosis may improve with cervicothoracic extension exercise; pelvic tilt to reduce lumbar lordosis; and stretching/strengthening exercise of the hamstring, hip flexor, and pectoralis muscles. Exercise, particularly spinal extension, abdominal strengthening, and hamstring stretch, is also helpful to reduce back pain.[6,13,17]

Bracing is an important part of the rehabilitation intervention. There is no consensus regarding recommended brace wear-time per day; recommendations range between 8 and 23 hours of daily wear. Some correction of the curvature may take place with conscientious use of the orthosis, although the goal of orthotic treatment is to reduce pain and limit progression of the curve. The most common brace selection is a body jacket thoracolumbosacral orthosis (TLSO) such as the

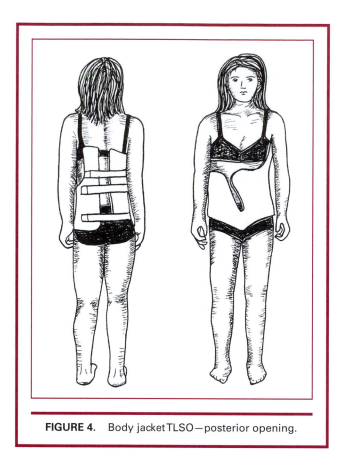

FIGURE 4. Body jacket TLSO—posterior opening.

Boston or Denver brace (Fig. 4). High thoracic and cervical curves and kyphotic curves may require a Milwaukee cervicothoracolumbosacral orthosis (CTLSO). Bracing for idiopathic curves in a growing child or adolescent is maintained until spinal growth centers fuse. When a TLSO body jacket or corset is used to decrease pain and improve posture for patients with degenerative scoliosis, wear time depends on symptoms.

For scoliosis associated with neuromuscular diseases, bracing is often withheld if the patient is ambulatory. When a body jacket is provided, an abdominal window is needed to allow respiratory excursion. Contoured or custom molded seating systems that align and support the trunk are useful. These allow the child, adolescent, or adult to maintain an upright posture while seated, improving head control and hand function.

Procedures

There are no invasive procedures indicated for the treatment of scoliosis or kyphosis.

Surgery

Surgical procedures attempt to restore spinal balance. The goal of surgery is to stabilize the spine through correction or control of the deformity. Improved cosmesis is a secondary goal. Restoring lumbar lordosis is important.[18,19] Indications for surgical correction of scoliosis or kyphosis include progressive deformity, instability, progressive or new neurologic deficit, and cardiopulmonary compromise. Surgical stabilization of the spine for scoliosis associated with neuromuscular disease is performed earlier than for curves due to other causes. Pain, even when refractory to conservative management, is a controversial indication for surgery. Inability to use a brace, and severe cosmetic deformity may be relative indications for surgery in specific instances.[4,6,20–23]

Scoliosis

Surgery addresses the coronal and rotational deformities by derotation and, less commonly, distraction. Any spinal instability is eliminated through compression or bony fusion.[23] Spine surgery may be complemented by rib resection in an attempt to improve appearance. The postoperative management of surgical patients varies according to the etiology of the curve, age of the patient, and specifics of the surgery. Some patients may be placed in a cast or body jacket to immobilize the operated segment until bony fusion occurs. Cotrel-Dubbousset instrumentation and its various modifications that derotate the spine commonly do not require fusion, immobilization, or rib resection. Other surgical procedures such as osteotomy or laminectomy are done as appropriate.

Kyphosis

Various surgical approaches have been used, but anterior plus posterior instrumentation with fusion currently provides the highest success rate for lasting correction and pain relief.[4,24,25]

Potential Disease Complications

Complications of scoliosis or kyphosis result from the structural and degenerative changes that occur in the spine, along with secondary tightness or restriction due to soft tissue shortening. An increased incidence of spondylosis, facet arthropathy, spondylolisthesis, and spondylolysis is associated with large curves and correlates with the angle and rotation at the curve apex.[26,27,28,29] Such degenerative changes related to the curve are the most common causes of pain, but scoliosis can also produce discogenic pain.[30]

Foraminal, recess, or canal stenosis can occur with resulting neurologic compromise.[31,32] Root entrapment usually occurs on the concave side of the curve (rarely both convex and concave sides). Cauda equina compression has also been reported.[31] Lumbar spinal stenosis due to scoliosis can sometimes be differentiated from other types of stenosis because the disease and symptoms are more structural than positional. Patients often will not report relief of symptoms when sitting.[16]

Restrictive lung disease may occur as a complication of scoliotic curves exceeding 40 degrees or kyphosis in excess of 50 degrees, and cor pulmonale can complicate severe kyphosis or scoliotic curves in excess of 110 degrees.[26]

Potential Treatment Complications

Most treatment complications relate to surgery or bracing. Reported complications of bracing include skin breakdown; dermatitis due to an allergy to the orthotic material; hyperhidrosis; cutaneous infection; gastroesophageal reflux disease (GERD); esophagitis; altered gastrointestinal motility; and psychosocial complications including low self-esteem, altered body image, and depression.

Surgery may cause vascular or neurologic injury, pseudarthrosis, infection, graft donor site pain, progressive pelvic obliquity, painful degenerative changes in the segment adjacent to the level of fusion, instability, hardware prominence or failure, and thromboembolism.[18,23,33] Hardware complications include slippage of anchoring hooks, bending or fracture of a rod, wire pull-out, and migration of the hardware. Progression of the curve is possible despite surgical fixation. In the growing adolescent the crankshaft phenomenon—progressive deformity resulting from continued growth of the anterior spine after posterior arthrodesis—may occur. This results in further loss of spinal balance, but is usually not problematic. The patient with degenerative scoliosis who has undergone otherwise successful surgery may continue to experience pain or restricted mobility.

Exercise related complications are less common but include overuse conditions of the soft tissues (tendinitis, bursitis, sprain, strain). Complications following NSAID therapy are possible, particularly in the gastric, renal, and hepatic systems.

References

1. Olgivie JW: Adult scoliosis: Evaluation and nonsurgical treatment. Instr Course Lect 1992;41:251–255.
2. Lowe TG: Scheuermann's disease. J Bone Joint Surg Am 1990;72:940–945.
3. Tribus CB: Scheuermann's kyphosis in adolescents and adults: Diagnosis and management. J Am Acad Orthop Surg 1998;6:36–43.
4. Esses SI: Textbook of Spinal Disorders. Philadelphia, J.B. Lippincott, 1995.
5. Sawark JF, Kramer A: Pediatric spinal deformity. Curr Opin Pediatr 1998;10:82–86.
6. Lonstein JE, Bradford DS, Winter RB, Ogilvie JW: Moe's Textbook of Scoliosis and Other Spinal Deformities, 3rd ed. Philadelphia, W.B. Saunders, 1995.
7. Olgivie JW, Sherman J: Spondylolysis in Scheuermann's disease. Spine 1987;12:251–253.
8. Kann P, Schulz G, Schehler B, Beyer J: Backache and osteoporosis in perimenopausal women. Med Klin 1993;88(1):9–15.
9. Papaiaonnou T, Stokes I, Kenwright J: Scoliosis associated with limb-length inequality. J Bone Joint Surg Am 1982;64(1):59–62.
10. Bradford DS: Kyphosis and postural roundback deformity in children and adolescents. Minn Med 1073;56:144.
11. Outland T: Juvenile dorsal kyphosis. Clin Orthop 1955;5:155.
12. Wassman K: Kyphosis juvenilis Scheuermann. Acta Orthop Scand 1951;21:65.
13. Ali RM, Green DW, Patel TC: Scheuermann's kyphosis. Curr Opin Pediatr 1999;11:70–75.
14. Sorenson KH: Scheuermann's kyphosis. In Clinical Appearance, Radiography, Aetiology and Prognosis. Copenhagen, Junksgaard, 1964.

15. Bradford DS, Moe JH, Montalvo FJ: Scheuermann's kyphosis and roundback deformity. Results of Milwaukee brace treatment. J Bone Joint Surg Am 1974;56A:740–758.
16. Grubb SA, Lipscomb HJ, Coonrad RW: Degenerative adult onset scoliosis. Spine 1988; 13(3):241–245.
17. Wenger DR, Frick SL: Scheuermann kyphosis. Spine 1999;24:2630–2638.
18. Manchesi DG, Aebi M: Pedicle fixation devices in the treatment of adult lumbar scoliosis. Spine 1992;17(8 Suppl): S304–S309.
19. Zubriggen C, Markwalder TM, Wyss S: Long-term results in patients treated with posterior instrumentation and fusion for degenerative scoliosis of the lumbar spine. Acta Neurochir (Wien) 1999;141(1):21–26.
20. Lowe TG: Double L-rod instrumentation in the treatment of severe kyphosis secondary to Scheuermann's disease. Spine 1988;13:1099–1103.
21. Lowe TG: Scheuermann's disease. Orthop Clin North Am 1999;30(3):475–487.
22. Otsuka NY, Hall JE, Mah JU: Posterior fusion for Scheuermann kyphosis. Clin Orthop 1990;251:134–239.
23. Grubb SA, Lipscomb HJ, Suh PB: Results of surgical treatment of painful adult scoliosis. Spine 1994;19(14):1619–1627.
24. Bradford DS, Ahmed KB, Moe JH, et al: The surgical management of patients with Scheuermann's disease. J Bone Joint Surg Am 1980;62:705–712.
25. Herndon WA, Emans JB, Micheli LJ, Hall JE: Combined anterior and posterior fusion for Scheuermann's kyphosis. Spine 1981;6(2):125–130.
26. Kita N: Ultrastructural studies of articular cartilaginous degeneration in the facet joints of spinal scoliosis. Nippon Seikeigeka Gakkai Zasshi 1994;68(4):184–195.
27. Richter DE, Nash CL Jr, Moskowitz RW, et al: Idiopathic adolescent scoliosis—a prototype of degenerative joint disease. The relation of biomechanic factors to osteophyte formation. Clin Orthop 1985;(193):221–229.
28. Hensiger RN, Green TL, Hunter L: Back pain and vertebral changes simulating Scheuermann's kyphosis. Spine 1982;6:341–342.
29. Tallroth K, Schlenzka D: Spinal stenosis subsequent to juvenile lumbar osteochondrosis. Skel Radiol 1990;19:203–205.
30. Grubb SA, Lipscomb HJ: Diagnostic findings in painful adult scoliosis. Spine 1992;17(5):518–527.
31. Bennini A: Root compression in lumbar scoliosis—clinical picture and treatment based on 13 personal cases. Neurochirugia (Stuttg) 1982;25(6):195–201.
32. Dick W: Surgical treatment of the degenerative lumbar spine in old age. Orthopade 1994;23(1):45–49.
33. Balderston RA, Albert TJ, McIntosh T, et al: Magnetic resonance imaging analysis of lumbar disc changes below scoliosis fusions. A prospective study. Spine 1998;23(1):54–58.

136 Spasticity

Joel Stein, MD

Synonyms

Increased muscle tone

Spastic dystonia

ICD-9 Code

728.85
Spasm of muscle

Definition

Spasticity is often defined as a velocity-dependent increase in muscle tone. This means that the faster the passive movement of the limb through its range, the greater the increase in muscle tone. The definition usually also includes clonus and flexor and extensor muscle spasms. Spasticity occurs in the context of an upper motor neuron (UMN) lesion (brain or spinal cord pathology) and in association with exaggerated deep tendon reflexes.

Symptoms

Spasticity reduces an individual's ability to move affected limbs actively or passively. Spasms may be a feature, and pain is present in some cases.

Physical Examination

Spasticity occurs in the presence of other signs and symptoms of UMN damage, including hyperreflexia, Babinski responses, reduced motor control, and other evidence of brain and/or spinal cord damage. Increased muscle tone in the absence of these findings should lead to consideration of alternative causes of increased muscle tone, such as dystonia, Parkinson's disease, paratonia associated with Alzheimer's disease, or pain-associated muscle spasm.

Contracture and spasticity commonly co-exist, though in some cases it may be difficult to determine how much contracture is present in an individual with severe spasticity. The "clasp-knife" phenomenon, seen more commonly in spasticity of spinal origin, is characterized by a relaxation of the involved muscle after spasticity has been overcome. The presence and severity of ankle clonus, withdrawal reflexes, and extensor spasms should be noted. The skin should be inspected because abnormal positioning due to spasticity may directly cause skin injury (e.g., maceration of the palm due to a clenched fist) or contribute to decubitus ulcer formation.

Functional Limitations

Functional limitations include difficulty with ambulation or brace usage, positioning in a wheelchair, urinary catheterization and/or hygiene, and interrupted sleep. Impaired sexual function may result from adductor muscle or other muscle spasms.

In some cases spasticity may interfere with volitional function; yet in others, it may serve as a partial substitute for voluntary muscle contraction. In the rehabilitation setting, patients who use their increased tone to help them ambulate are often noted to be "walking on their spasticity." A common example of substitution for voluntary muscle function is the hip and knee extensor spasticity seen after stroke, which may allow successful weight bearing through the weak leg and contribute to restored walking ability. Therefore, one must always be cognizant of this phenomenon, because overly aggressive treatment of spasticity may actually worsen an individual's ability to function.

Diagnostic Studies

Spasticity is a clinical diagnosis without any specific laboratory confirmation. Clinical measurement scales to quantify the severity of spasticity may be useful to monitor the efficacy of treatment. The most commonly used scales are the Ashworth scale (see page 787),[1] which measures resistance of the muscle to passive stretch, and the Spasm Frequency scale, which characterizes the frequency of muscle spasms.

Differential Diagnosis

Dystonia

Rigidity (e.g., Parkinson's disease)

Paratonia (e.g., Alzheimer's disease)

Severe muscle spasm (due to pain)

Contracture

Treatment

Initial

Pharmacotherapy with oral medications (Table 1) is most effective in spasticity of spinal origin, as occurs in spinal cord injury or many cases of multiple sclerosis. Oral medications are often less effective in spasticity resulting from stroke or traumatic brain injury. Medications commonly used include baclofen, benzodiazepines, tizanidine,[2,3] and dantrolene.[4] With the exception of dantrolene, these medications work centrally at the GABA-A receptors (benzodiazepines), GABA-B receptors (baclofen), and the alpha-adrenoreceptors (tizanidine). Dantrolene exerts its effects directly at the muscle, preventing calcium influx at the sarcoplasmic reticulum level and thereby reducing muscle force.

Rehabilitation

Stretching and passive range of motion are key elements of spasticity management, regardless of etiology. These activities serve to prevent contracture and to temporarily reduce increased muscle

TABLE 1. Commonly Used Oral Antispasticity Medications				
Medication	Starting Dose	Maximum Dose	Common Effects	Relative Contraindications
Baclofen	5–10 mg tid	20 mg qid*	Sedation, rare hepatotoxicity	Cognitive impairment
Diazepam (other benzodiazepines have similar effects)	2 mg bid	10 mg qid	Sedation	History of benzodiazepine or other substance abuse
Tizanidine	2 mg Tid	12 mg tid	Sedation, hypotension, hepatotoxicity	Cognitive impairment
Dantrolene	25 mg daily	10 mg qid	Weakness, hepatotoxicity, occasional sedation	Liver disease

* FDA approved only up to 80 mg/day, but many clinicians exceed this in patients who tolerate this medication well but do not respond to lower doses.

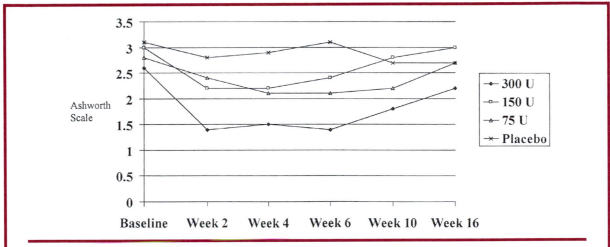

FIGURE 1. Wrist spasticity after botulinum toxin injection. (Adapted from Simpson DM, et al: Botulinum toxin type A in the treatment of upper extremity spasticity: A randomized, double-blind, placebo controlled study. Neurology 1996;46:1306–1310.)

tone. Splinting a spastic limb is another critical aspect of a comprehensive rehabilitation program for spasticity and can include pre-fabricated splints, low temperature thermoplastic custom splints, and plaster or fiberglass casts. Physical therapists can instruct the patient and caregivers regarding appropriate stretching techniques. Physical therapists with experience in casting can fabricate plaster or fiberglass casts or assist in selecting a prefabricated leg splint from a commercial vendor. If a sturdier device is needed (e.g., one that permits weight bearing through the device), an orthotist may be called upon to fabricate a custom brace. Occupational therapists can similarly provide instruction in stretching and splinting of the upper extremity. Most occupational therapists are trained in fabrication of custom hand splints.

Procedures

Injections for spasticity are an effective means of obtaining substantial reduction in spasticity in specific muscles with little risk of systemic side effects. Local anesthetic injections may be useful to assess the efficacy and benefits of more permanent injections. Intramuscular botulinum toxin type A injection provides local relief of spasticity for 3 to 4 months (Fig. 1).[5] Botulinum toxin type B is likely to prove effective as well,[6] although efficacy and dosing are not yet established. Perineural phenol injection may provide more long-term relief and may in some cases cause permanent reduction of spasticity.[7]

Botulinum toxin injections may use anatomic guidance for large, easily identified muscles (e.g., biceps brachii), but EMG or nerve stimulator guidance is necessary for smaller, harder to identify muscles (e.g., forearm muscles). Botulinum toxin type A doses for spasticity generally vary from 30–200 units per muscle, with larger muscles requiring higher doses. Dosage for spasticity management has not been established for type B. Type A is generally diluted to 100 units/cc with nonpreserved sterile saline, although more dilute concentrations are useful for small doses. After dilution, the toxin is drawn into a small syringe (1–3 cc), and a Teflon-coated injection needle is connected via a wire to either an EMG machine or a nerve stimulator. Given the limited motor control and muscle synergies seen in spasticity, nerve stimulator guidance often proves more useful than EMG guidance in distinguishing different muscles . With nerve stimulator guidance, the muscle is stimulated and the clinical response observed (e.g., finger flexion when the flexor digitorum profundus is stimulated). Toxin is then injected in small aliquots distributed in the muscle.

Early post-injection symptoms are unusual, and related more to the effects of an intramuscular injection than to the botulinum toxin itself. There are no specific activity restrictions necessary post-injection. Clinical effects are generally evident 24–72 hours after the injection.

Surgery

Neurosurgical intervention includes the placement of an intrathecal baclofen pump—a highly effective treatment for individuals with intractable bilateral lower extremity spasticity.[8,9] Alternative neurosurgical procedures useful in carefully selected patients include rhizotomy and myelotomy. Orthopedic surgery, including tendon lengthening, tenotomy, or joint fusion, can be used after failure of more conservative measures (e.g., stretching, casting, and blocks) to provide adequate control of spasticity and contracture.

Potential Disease Complications

Permanent loss of range of motion can result from inadequately controlled spasticity or insufficient stretching and splinting. Contractures can hinder seating; contribute to skin breakdown; and interfere with hygiene, ambulation, and transfers.

Potential Treatment Complications

As noted earlier, some individuals function better with a degree of spasticity because it can substitute for lost motor function. Therefore, overly aggressive treatment of spasticity may result in a decline in functional ability.

All centrally acting medications can cause significant sedation, which often determines the upper limit of the dose that can be tolerated. In individuals with pre-existing cognitive impairments (e.g., stroke, TBI), this maximally tolerated dose may be insufficient to control the symptoms of spasticity and may indicate the need to consider alternative therapies. Abrupt discontinuation of oral antispasticity medications is inadvisable, since seizures have been described after abrupt discontinuation of baclofen, and rebound spasticity is a concern with all of these medications.

Phenol poses some risk of painful dysesthesia if peripheral nerves with cutaneous sensory representation are injected. Botulinum toxin is generally very well tolerated in therapeutic doses but can cause transient (3 to 4 months) weakness of muscles adjacent to those targeted by treatment due to diffusion of toxin. Dysphagia has been described after injection of the sternocleidomastoid and other cervical muscles. Injection of excessive doses of botulinum toxin could lead to symptoms of systemic botulism, though this can be prevented by restricting injection to 6 units/kg of botulinum toxin type A or less within any 1-month period. Antibodies to botulinum toxin can develop after repeated injection—this causes lack of efficacy; however, allergic or anaphylactic reactions have not been reported.

Intrathecal baclofen pump treatment can result in iatrogenic meningitis or infection of the external surface of the pump. Catheter failures can result in need for surgical intervention. Both overdosage due to programming errors and severe withdrawal symptoms due to pump failure have been described.[10]

References
1. Ashworth B: Preliminary trial of carisoprodol in multiple sclerosis. Practitioner 1964;192:540–542.
2. Nance PW, Bugaresti J, Shellenberger K, et al: Efficacy and safety of tizanidine in the treatment of spasticity in patients with spinal cord injury. North American Tizanidine Study Group. Neurology 1994;44:S44–S45.
3. Smith C, Birnbaum G, Carter JL, et al: Tizanidine treatment of spasticity caused by multiple sclerosis: results of a double-blind, placebo-controlled trial. US Tizanidine Study Group. Neurology 1994;44:S34–S42.
4. Kita M, Goodkin DE: Drugs used to treat spasticity. Drugs 2000;59(3):487–495.
5. Simpson DM, et al: Botulinum toxin type A in the treatment of upper extremity spasticity: A randomized, double-blind, placebo controlled study. Neurology 1996;46:1306–1310.
6. Brashear A, Lew MF, Dykstra DD, et al: Safety and efficacy of NeuroBloc (botulinum toxin type B) in type A-responsive cervical dystonia. Neurology 1999;53(7):1439–1446.
7. Glenn MB, Whyte J: The Practical management of spasticity in children and adults. Philadelphia, Lea & Febiger, 1990.
8. Van Schaeybroeck P, Nuttin B, Lagae L, et al: Intrathecal baclofen for intractable cerebral spasticity: A prospective placebo-controlled, double-blind study. Neurosurgery 2000;46:603–609.
9. Meythaler JM, Guin-Renfroe S, Grabb P, Hadley MN: Long-term continuously infused intrathecal baclofen for spastic-dystonic hypertonia in traumatic brain injury: 1-year experience. Arch Phys Med Rehab 1999;80:13–19.
10. Reeves RK, Stolp-Smith KA, Christopherson MW: Hyperthermia, rhabdomyolysis, and disseminated intravascular coagulation associated with baclofen pump catheter failure. Arch Phys Med Rehab 1998;79:353–356.

137 Speech and Language Disorders

Jason H. Kortte, MS, CCC-SLP
Jeffrey B. Palmer, MD

Synonyms

Communication disorders

Motor speech disorders

Speech or language impairment

ICD-9 Codes

784.3
Aphasia

784.4
Voice disturbance

784.40
Voice disturbance, unspecified

784.41
Aphonia: loss of voice

784.49
Other: dysphonia

784.5
Other speech disturbance: dysarthria, dysphasia, slurred speech

784.69
Other, apraxia

Definition

Aphasia is a language processing disturbance that can involve the expression of language, the comprehension of language, or both. Aphasia is classified into specific syndromes according to the ability to produce, understand, and repeat language.[1] The ability to produce language is assessed in terms of fluency, which is defined as the rate of speech and the amount of effort in producing speech. Each syndrome of aphasia is associated with a particular set of language capabilities and disabilities. For example, an individual with Wernicke's aphasia produces fluent language but has impaired auditory comprehension and poor repetition skills. Aphasia can be manifested in other modalities of language as well (e.g., reading, writing, and gestures). See Table 1 for an overview of aphasia syndromes.

Apraxia of speech (AOS) is a motor speech disorder disrupting the motor programming of the volitional movements for speech.[2] AOS is characterized by difficulties positioning and sequentially moving muscles for the production of speech.

Dysarthria is a group of motor speech disorders resulting from damage to the central or peripheral nervous systems. These disorders may result from weakness, paralysis, and/or uncoordinated movements of the speech muscles and can impair articulation, respiration, and phonation (voice production). Dysarthria can be subdivided into different types depending on the speech characteristics and underlying pathophysiology.[3] In addition,

TABLE 1. Aphasia Syndromes

Type of Aphasia	Speech	Comprehension	Repetition
Broca's	Nonfluent	Intact	Poor
Wernicke's	Fluent	Poor	Poor
Conduction	Fluent	Intact	Poor
Transcortical motor	Nonfluent	Intact	Intact
Transcortical sensory	Fluent	Poor	Intact
Anomic	Fluent	Intact	Intact

Adapted from Damasio AR, Damasio H: Aphasia and the neuro basis of language. In Mesulam M (eds): Principles of Behavioral and Cognitive Neurology, 2nd ed. New York, Oxford University Press, 2000, pp 294–315.

dysarthria may be due to structural abnormalities, such as those found in cleft palate and postablative surgery. The extreme form of dysarthria is anarthria, in which the individual is entirely incapable of producing articulated speech.

Dysphonia is a term used to describe faulty or abnormal phonation (voice production). There are a variety of processes that may alter the structure or function of the vocal cords, including vocal abusive behaviors (excessive talking, screaming, smoking), trauma or surgery to laryngeal structures, neurogenic motor disturbances (resulting in paresis or paralysis), or diseases such as laryngeal cancer of reflux laryngitis. Dysphonia is distinguished from dysarthria in that the former involves only the sound of the voice, whereas the latter involves the overall sound of speech, including resonance and articulation.

Symptoms

Individuals with aphasia often complain of difficulty with speaking, reading, writing, or understanding speech. They will often report difficulty in finding the word they wish to say. Some aphasic individuals, however, are unaware of their deficits. Individuals with motor speech disorders (e.g., dysarthria, dysphonia, and AOS) have no difficulty finding the words they wish to say but complain of difficulty with making their speech intelligible. These individuals report no difficulties with reading, writing, or auditory comprehension.

Physical Examination

During the initial interaction with the patient, it is important to attend to the patient's speech intelligibility, vocal quality, language fluency and content, and comprehension. Deficits in these areas may warrant a referral to a speech-language pathologist for comprehensive evaluation. Typical findings are described in the following for the four main categories of speech and language disorders.

Aphasia

Findings of the speech-language examination present in aphasia may vary greatly, depending on the location and size of the lesion in the brain (see Table 1). One classic sign of aphasia is difficulty in comprehending spoken, gestural, or written language. Significant impairment can be characterized by difficulty with following simple commands, whereas more mild impairments may only be obvious during lengthy or complicated messages. Individuals who are aphasic may also have deficits in verbal expression (producing meaningful speech), which may manifest as a total loss of language, with the individual producing only jargon (multiple whole-word substitutions) or meaningless sounds. A person with less severe aphasia may be able to express basic wants and needs but have difficulty expressing complex ideas in conversation. The extent of impairment can vary for each modality of language and involve listening, reading, writing, recognizing numbers, and gesturing. Aphasia is *not* a result of decreased auditory or visual perceptual skills, disordered thought processes, impaired motor programming, or weakness/incoordination of speech musculature.[1]

Apraxia

The most common sign of AOS is a struggle to speak. This struggle is a direct result of the individual having difficulty in finding correct position of his or her articulators (i.e., lips, tongue). Speech is often halting and may contain sound substitutions, distortions, omissions, additions, and repetitions.[4] The individual is aware of his or her speech errors and will attempt to correct them with varying degrees of success. Severe forms of AOS may result in the inability to produce simple words. Interestingly, most individuals with AOS can produce common everyday phrases or sayings without error (e.g., "How are you?," "Have a nice day," or "Thank you."). A symptom that commonly coincides with AOS is non-verbal oral apraxia, which is the inability to imitate or follow

TABLE 2. Classification of Dysarthria

Type	Localization	Motor deficit
Flaccid	Lower motor neuron	Weakness hypotonia
Spastic	Bilateral upper motor neuron	Spasticity
Ataxia	Cerebellum	Incoordination, inaccurate range, timing, direction, slow rate
Hypokinetic	Extrapyramidal system (basal ganglia circuit)	Variable speed of repetitive movements, rigidity
Hyperkinetic	Extrapyramidal system	Involuntary movements
Mixed	Multiple motor systems (amyotrophic lateral sclerosis, multiple sclerosis)	Weakness, reduced rate and range of motion

Adapted from Duffy JR: Motor Speech Disorders: Substrates, Differential Diagnosis, and Management. St Louis, Mosby, 1995.

commands to perform volitional movements with the mouth or tongue.[2] AOS is not caused by muscle weakness or incoordination, nor is it the result of linguistic disturbances as seen in aphasia. It differs from dysarthria in that AOS is not a result of paresis/paralysis or the uncoordinated movements of speech muscles.

Dysarthria

In dysarthria, speech is often characterized as being "slurred"; the predominant errors are distortions of speech sounds. Dysarthria may also be characterized by changes in a person's rate, volume, and rhythm of speech. Depending on the pathophysiology, the findings will vary greatly. See Table 2 for an overview of dysarthria classification.

Dysphonia

Dysphonia is characterized by a reduction in voice quality. Vocal quality may vary by degrees of loudness, breathiness, hoarseness, or harshness. A common example of this symptom is the hoarse vocal quality of individuals with laryngitis. In the extreme form, aphonia, the individual is incapable of producing any voice but may be able to produce voiceless speech (e.g., whispering).

Functional Limitations

Functional limitations depend on the nature and severity of the communication impairment. Severe deficits may impair the person's ability to express daily wants and needs or understand simple directions. He or she may not be able to effectively interact with family members or health care workers. Less severe impairments may allow the individual to express and understand basic information but will impair higher level activities. These may include expressing and understanding complex and lengthy information to meet the person's vocational and/or social needs. Speech and language impairments may affect the individual's ability to read bills, newspapers, and environmental signs; use the telephone; participate in conversations; attend school; or obtain employment. Speech and language impairments may result in frustration and can cause disruptions in personal relationships, community and religious participation, and vocational functioning.

Diagnostic Studies

There are a variety of standardized instruments that can be administered by the speech-language pathologist or neuropsychologist to diagnose aphasia. The aim of these instruments is to identify the pattern of symptoms in order to classify the aphasic syndrome, which is critical for the development of individualized interventions. Similarly, there are structured assessments to diagnose dysphonia, apraxia, and dysarthria These in-depth assessments involve an oral-motor examination to identify the structure and function of oral musculature and to identify the patient's speech characteristics (i.e., rate, volume, intelligibility). To determine the etiology and pathophysiology of dysphonia, a referral to an otolaryngologist is warranted. *Laryngoscopy* may be necessary to evaluate both the structure and the function of the larynx. *Biopsy* is often indicated when mass lesions are seen. *Stroboscopic* examination of the larynx may reveal subtle abnormalities of the vocal fold motion. The *voice spectrogram* is sometimes useful for measuring voice features quantitatively.

Differential Diagnosis

Aphasia
   Confusion/delirium
   Schizophrenia
   Apraxia of speech
   Neurogenic stuttering
   Echolalia
   Palilalia
   Selective mutism
   Depression
   Abulia

Apraxia of speech
   Dysarthria
   Aphasia
   Neurogenic stuttering

Dysarthria
   Apraxia of speech
   Aphasia
   Depression
   Abulia

Dysphonia
   Acute and chronic laryngitis
   Laryngeal hyperfunction
      (abuse and misuse)
   Neurogenic disorders
   Psychogenic disorders (i.e.,
      conversion dysphonia)
   Spasmodic dysphonia
   Structural disorders of the larynx
      (congenital, traumatic, arthritic,
      neoplastic)

Treatment

Initial

Treatment of speech and language disorders usually requires referral to a speech-language pathologist. Initial treatment depends on the nature and severity of the disorder. The treatment plans for aphasia, apraxia of speech, dysarthria, and dysphonia not only vary greatly among each disorder, but also need to be individualized to meet the patient's communication needs. Initial intervention may include patient and family education regarding the communication impairment and effective compensatory strategies to facilitate communication.

Rehabilitation

To maximize a patient's communication skills, a speech-language pathologist can offer specific strategies, exercises, and activities to regain functional communication abilities.

Aphasia

Intervention for aphasia is largely based on the specific aphasia syndrome diagnosed. Common therapeutic activities to improve verbal expression may include naming tasks using hierarchical cueing techniques to improve language content and structure. Therapy may begin by having the patient produce automatic speech, such as stating the numbers and the days of the week. More difficult tasks may involve the individual naming objects and describing pictures. Written expression may be targeted through functional activities to improve spelling, such as writing or copying biographical information. Common activities to improve auditory comprehension involve following simple and/or complex commands and answering spoken questions correctly. Therapy to improve reading comprehension may involve the patient matching objects to written words, following written directions, or reading functional information (e.g., bills, medication labels, environmental signs).

It is important to teach the patient and family compensatory strategies to improve communication skills. Environmental modification and partner-facilitated approaches can dramatically improve communication success. These can include turning off the television to reduce distractions, speaking slowly, and using simple language.

Apraxia

Treatment of AOS involves techniques to elicit accurate voluntary speech production. The speech-language therapist incorporates multimodality cues such as modeling mouth and lip movements, using verbal cues to describe accurate tongue and lip placement, and intoning words and sentences.

Dysarthria

Dysarthria rehabilitation also varies depending on the specific type of dysarthria diagnosed. Approaches to treatment include medical intervention, oral prosthetic devices, and behavioral management.[2] For example, dysarthric individuals with Parkinson's disease may benefit from dopamine agonists. Palatal lifts and voice amplifiers are common prosthetics used to improve intelligibility. Treatment of severe expressive dysarthria and/or aphasia may include the development of an augmentative communication system in which the individual uses pictures, written words, or alphabet/pictograph boards to communicate wants and needs. Behavioral management involves muscle strengthening, improving breath support, and posture modification. The individual is trained to use compensatory techniques to decrease rate of speech and to "overarticulate." As with aphasia, the family is educated regarding strategies to maximize communication.

Dysphonia

Management of dysphonia is based on the underlying disorder and the pathophysiology. Vocal hygiene education and proper voicing techniques are used to improve vocal quality for individuals with vocal nodules due to laryngeal hyperfunction (vocal abuse). Techniques can be taught to achieve firmer vocal fold approximation in individuals with decreased vocal cord movement due to paresis. Laryngitis due to gastroesophageal reflux disease is treated with a vigorous antireflux regimen, including proton pump inhibitors.

Procedures

Injection of a paralyzed vocal cord with an absorbable gelatin sponge (Gelfoam) or polytef (Teflon) is sometimes performed to increase its mass and bring the medial edge of the cord closer to the midline. This permits the mobile contralateral vocal cord to contact it, thereby improving phonation. This solution is usually only temporary, however. For cases of spasmodic dysphonia, an injection of botulinum toxin into the affected muscles can result in improved voice by correcting the motion impairment of the vocal folds.[5]

Surgery

Surgery is sometimes needed for treatment of voice disorders. Individuals with mass lesions of the larynx may need surgical excision. For individuals with unilateral vocal cord paralysis, there are several surgical procedures designed to medialize the paralyzed cord. Implantation of a small device into the paralyzed hemilarynx can provide a lasting benefit in terms of improved voice quality. Surgical treatment of other speech and language disorders depends entirely on the etiology of the underlying disease process.

Structural lesions (e.g., cleft palate) or functional disorders (e.g., weakness of the palatal elevators) may cause inadequate seal of the velopharyngeal isthmus (the space between the soft palate and the posterior pharyngeal wall). In either case, a surgical procedure can sometimes provide improved speech quality by narrowing or closing the defect.

Potential Disease Complications

Individuals with severe speech and language disorders may suffer extreme psychosocial consequences, including isolation, unemployment, depression, alienation, ostracism, and inability to fulfill essential family roles.

Potential Treatment Complications

Injection or surgical implant of the larynx may result in complications including infection, hemorrhage, and local tissue trauma. Injected material may gradually slip out of place and lose effectiveness, but this rarely leads to serious sequelae. Botulinum toxin injection rarely causes airway obstruction if the vocal folds become immobilized in the medial position. Leakage of the toxin into adjacent muscles may worsen the voice disorder or produce dysphagia.

References

1. Damasio AR, Damasio H: Aphasia and the neuro basis of language. In Mesulam M (eds): Principles of Behavioral and Cognitive Neurology, 2nd ed. New York, Oxford University Press, 2000, pp 294–315.
2. Duffy JR: Motor Speech Disorders: Substrates, Differential diagnosis, and Management. St. Louis, Mosby, 1995.
3. Prater RJ, Swift RW: Manuel of Voice Therapy. Austin, Texas, Pro-ed, 1984.
4. Wertz RT, LaPointe LL, Rosenbek JC: Apraxia of Speech in Adults: The Disorder and Its Management. New York, Grune and Stratton, 1984.
5. Blitzer A, Brin MF, Fahn S, Lovelace R: Localized injections of botulinum toxin for the treatment of focal laryngeal dystonia (spastic dysphonia). Laryngoscope 1988;98:193–197.

138 Spinal Cord Injury (Cervical)

Michelle J. Alpert, MD

Synonyms

Tetraplegia

Quadriplegia

ICD-9 Codes

344.0
Quadriplegia and quadriparesis

344.00
Quadriplegia unspecified

344.01
C$_1$–C$_4$ complete

344.02
C$_1$–C$_4$ incomplete

344.03
C$_5$–C$_7$ complete

344.04
C$_5$–C$_7$ incomplete

344.09
Other

Definition

Cervical spinal cord injury is an impairment or loss of motor and/or sensory function in the cervical segments of the spinal cord due to damage of neural elements within the spinal canal. Tetraplegia results in impairment of function in the arms, trunk, legs, and pelvic organs.

A cervical spinal cord injury is either complete or incomplete; individuals with incomplete spinal cord injuries have a much better prognosis for recovery relative to complete injuries. A *complete* injury is defined as the absence of sensory and motor function in the lowest sacral segment (i.e., the absence of anal sensation on rectal examination and of voluntary external anal sphincter contraction). An *incomplete* injury is defined as the presence of sensory and/or motor function below the neurologic level of spinal cord injury and must include the lowest sacral segments (Table 1).[1]

It is important to note that many patients with cervical spinal cord injury suffer from sexual dysfunction and may have fertility issues as well. These are discussed in Chapter 139; however referral to specialists is appropriate in these cases.

TABLE 1. American Spinal Injury Association Impairment Scale

Grade	Category	Description
A	Complete	No sensory or motor function is preserved in the sacral segments S4–S5
B	Incomplete	Sensory but not motor function is preserved below the neurologic level and extends through the sacral segments S4–S5
C	Incomplete	Motor function is preserved below the neurologic level and the majority of key muscles below the neurologic level have a muscle grade less than 3
D	Incomplete	Motor function is preserved below the neurologic level and the majority of key muscles below the neurologic level have a muscle grade greater than or equal to 3
E	Normal	Sensory and motor function are normal

From Finklestein JA: Evaluation of spinal cord injury patients. Spine: State Art Rev 1999;13(3):471.

TABLE 2. University of Washington Classification of Chronic Spinal Cord Injury Pain

Pain Category (Major)	Pain Category (Specific)	Location	Related to Activity	Affected by Position	Worse with Light Touch
Neurogenic	Spinal cord pain	Below injury in area without normal sensation	±	−	±
	Transition zone pain	At level of injury and bilateral	−	−	+
	Radicular pain	At any dermatomal level, usually unilateral, usually radiates	+	+	−
	Visceral pain	In abdomen	−	−	−
Musculoskeletal	Mechanical spine pain	In back or neck, often bilateral	+	+	−
	Overuse pain	Often above injury in areas of normal sensation, in incomplete injury can be below	+	±	−

From Cardena DD: Current concepts of rehabilitation of spinal cord injury patients. Spine: State Art Rev 1999;13(3):583.

Symptoms

The patient with cervical spinal cord injury may present with new weakness/paralysis, spasticity, pain, cough/shortness of breath, bladder or bowel incontinence, and skin breakdown (Table 2).

Physical Examination

The physical examination of an individual with a cervical spinal cord injury should be consistent with an upper motor neuron process, consisting of both upper and lower extremity weakness or paralysis, increased muscle tone (spasticity), variable sensory loss, and increased muscle stretch reflexes.

New Weakness

Manual muscle testing of upper and lower extremities should be included in each examination, and any changes from previous assessments should be noted. Specific key muscle groups are tested to determine the motor level (Fig. 1). A muscle strength of 3 (active movement and full range of motion against gravity) is sufficient to classify the muscle as normal, as long as the next most rostral muscle is tested as 5 (normal active movement and full range of motion against resistance). The sensory level is determined by the dermatome chart. A motor and sensory level is recorded for each side. The neurologic level of injury is the most caudal segment of the spinal cord with normal motor and sensory function on both sides of the body, as determined by the motor and sensory examination.

Spasticity

The presence of increased resistance to passive movement and involuntary muscle spasms may indicate increased spasticity. This finding should be compared with previous exams because an increase in spasticity may indicate an underlying problem (e.g., urinary tract infection, pressure ulcer).

Pain

Range of motion at the shoulders, elbows, hips, knees, and ankles should also be assessed, as well as the presence of pain with resisted movement. Palpation for sites of tenderness is important and should be performed during joint motion and mobility assessment to detect articular abnormalities.

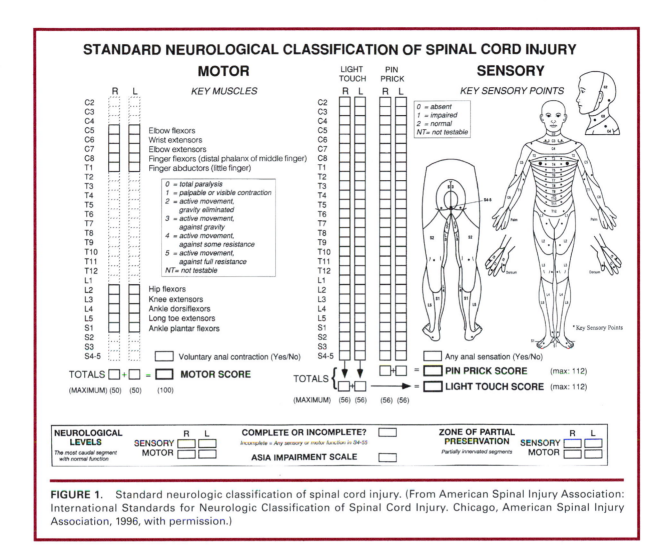

STANDARD NEUROLOGICAL CLASSIFICATION OF SPINAL CORD INJURY

FIGURE 1. Standard neurologic classification of spinal cord injury. (From American Spinal Injury Association: International Standards for Neurologic Classification of Spinal Cord Injury. Chicago, American Spinal Injury Association, 1996, with permission.)

Cough/Shortness of Breath

Physical examination should include vital signs, particularly temperature and respiratory rate. Auscultation should be performed to assess for rales, decreased breath sounds, or wheeze.

Skin Breakdown

Skin examination should be conducted in all pressure bearing areas (e.g., sacrum, heels, trochanters, ischial tuberosities).

Functional Limitations

New Weakness

Complaints of weakness will affect the patient's functional status. If upper extremity weakness predominates, the ability to perform self-care skills and transfers will be affected. If the injury is incomplete and ambulation with orthotics has been possible, increasing lower extremity weakness will contribute to an alteration in mobility. Both will contribute to a significant decline in the level of independence and potential loss of self-esteem.

Spasticity

Excessive spasticity can contribute to increased pain and interference with sleep. Flexor spasms can be so severe that patients are forced from their chair or may be unable to safely transfer.

Pain

Pain, whether musculoskeletal or neuropathic, may interfere with a patient's overall quality of life, leading to depression and anxiety and a subsequent inability to perform his or her daily routine.

Cough/Shortness of Breath

Any pulmonary impairment will affect endurance and ability to carry out activities of daily living, propel a wheelchair, etc.

Bowel and Bladder Incontinence

Bowel and bladder difficulties may lead to social isolation due to the fear of incontinence. Both may lead to skin breakdown and further functional limitations.

Skin Breakdown

Areas of skin breakdown will ultimately lead to decreased ability to sit or lie supine, thereby interfering with certain daily activities.

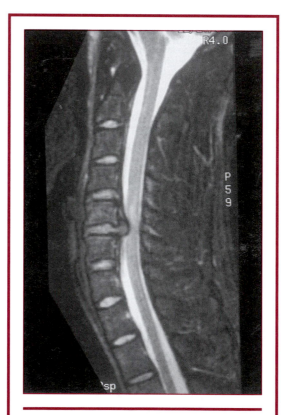

FIGURE 2. Midline sagittal T2 weighted MRI image of the cervical spine revealing a disc herniation at the C5–C6 level with thecal sac compression. (From Chapman JR, et al: Spine: State Art Rev 1999;13(3):442, with permission.)

Diagnostic Studies

If necessary, MRI is the diagnostic study of choice to confirm the presence of a cervical spinal cord injury, whether traumatic or non-traumatic (Fig. 2).

New Weakness

If neurologic decline is noted in a patient whose condition was previously stable, cervical spine radiographs are indicated to rule out spinal instability or new fracture. If the weakness is of a lower motor neuron quality and accompanied by tingling or burning pain, post-traumatic syringomyelia should be suspected and evaluated with MRI.[2]

Pain

Pain in cervical spinal cord injury may be multifactorial and is often diagnosed by characteristics reported in the history, including quality, location, onset, timing, relieving and exacerbating factors, and associated symptoms. Musculoskeletal pain is common and usually is related to overuse of the upper limbs to bear weight and propel a wheelchair. Radiographs of the shoulder are often indicated to evaluate the status of the rotator cuff or to rule out the presence of heterotopic ossification. Electrodiagnostic studies can be helpful to rule out carpal tunnel syndrome or other compressive mononeuropathies.[3] Neuropathic pain, often burning, aching, or tingling may be due to post-traumatic syringomyelia as previously described and warrants MRI of the cervical spine. Otherwise, secondary exacerbating factors such as depression, urinary tract infections, or new pressure sores need to be considered.

Cough/Shortness of Breath

Patients with quadriplegia who have baseline vital capacities of 1 to 2 L and peak cough flows of 3 to 5 L/sec should have oximeters at home to monitor their oxygen saturations, as needed. Patients who are at risk for pulmonary complications should have yearly measurements of forced vital capacity and repeat evaluations when new symptoms arise.[4]

Chest radiographs will show evidence of infiltrates and/or atelectasis. Sputum culture and gram stain will identify the involved pathogen(s) and help guide antibiotic therapy.

Bladder Incontinence

New urinary incontinence most likely is due to a urinary tract infection, confirmed by urinalysis and culture. Records of catheterization schedules, bladder volumes, and fluid intake are helpful to rule out overdistention and overflow as the causes of incontinence. Urodynamic studies are often helpful to further evaluate detrusor pressures and status of the external sphincter.

Bowel Incontinence

Bowel incontinence is usually the result of an inadequately regulated bowel program and subsequent impaction. A flat plate radiograph of the abdomen can demonstrate the presence of the fecal blockage. If antibiotics have recently been prescribed, a stool sample for the *Clostridium difficile* toxin should be sent.

Skin Breakdown

If a pressure ulcer appears to involve the bone, MRI or bone scan may be helpful to rule out the presence of osteomyelitis. Depending on the location of the ulcer, the efficacy of specific equipment will need to be assessed (e.g., the fit of lower extremity orthotics for ulcers on the feet and wheelchair seating and positioning for ulcers on the ischium or trochanters).

Differential Diagnosis

Post-traumatic syringomyelia   Peripheral polyneuropathy

Guillain-Barré syndrome   Spinal cord infarction

Amyotrophic lateral sclerosis

Treatment

Initial

New Weakness

Patients should be encouraged to comply with daily strengthening and conditioning programs to maintain endurance and muscle mass. Nutritional counseling can also help patients maintain general well being and stamina.[5]

Spasticity

If, despite compliance with a regular stretching and positioning program, spasticity is still painful or interferes with function, such as transfers, a trial of baclofen, up to doses of 40 mg po qid, is

TABLE 3. Common Antispasticity Medications

Drug	Oral Dose	Side Effects
Baclofen	Initial: 5 mg tid Maximum: 20 mg qid	Sedation, dizziness, ataxia, fatigue, lower seizure threshold
Tizanidine	Initial: 2 mg qhs Maximum: 36 mg in 3 or 4 divided doses	Drowsiness, tiredness, dry mouth, hallucinations, abnormal liver function tests
Dantrolene sodium	Initial: 25 mg qid Maximum: 100 mg qid	Dizziness, weakness, diarrhea, hypotension, hepatotoxicity with maximal dose
Diazepam	Initial: 2 mg bid Maximum: 20 mg tid	Sedation, depression, confusion
Clonidine	Initial: 0.1 mg bid Maximum: 0.1 mg bid	Orthostatic hypotension, drowsiness, dysrhythmias, dry mouth

From Cardenas DD: Current concepts of rehabilitation of spinal cord injury patients. Spine: State Art Rev 1999;13(3):583.

warranted (Table 3). If spasticity is still problematic, zanaflex can be added for synergistic effect. If the patient cannot tolerate oral medications or finds maximum dosages ineffective, referral for a trial of intrathecal baclofen should be considered.

Pain

Treatment of overuse syndromes of the upper extremity in the patient with tetraplegia should focus on decreasing the acute pain, dealing with the secondary disabilities (e.g., weakness, instability, stiffness) that may be causing the pain, and prevention. Acute musculoskeletal discomfort is often relieved with pharmacologic intervention such as nonsteroidal anti-inflammatories, acetaminophen, or muscle relaxants.

General measures of pain management center on prevention of complications and maintenance of good general physical health, including good nutrition and hydration as well as proper stretching and conditioning exercises. Also beneficial in pain management and treatment are reassurance, psychologic support, training in relaxation techniques, hypnosis, biofeedback, and other psychologic measures. Despite the lack of many clinical trials testing their efficacy and usefulness, tricyclic antidepressants are often initiated to treat refractory neuropathic pain. More recently, anticonvulsant medications such as gabapentin have fallen into favor (in doses up to 900 mg qid), with carbamazepine having been used for many years as well.[7]

Cough/Shortness of Breath

If cultures are all negative, viral respiratory infection may be the etiology of the patient's complaints, and only symptomatic therapy is warranted (e.g., fluids, cough suppressants). Weight control and smoking cessation are also important.

If chest x-ray and/or culture reveal evidence of bacterial pneumonia or tracheobronchitis, appropriate antibiotics are indicated. Nebulizers may also help promote bronchodilation and ease the work of breathing.

If oxygen desaturation is noted, supplemental oxygen and the use of manually and mechanically assisted cough may be necessary. Various types of non-invasive intermittent positive pressure ventilation are available, including continuous positive airway pressure (CPAP) and bilevel positive airway presure (BiPAP). These machines may need to be used temporarily until saturations and ventilation can be adequately maintained without assistance.[8]

Bladder Incontinence

Oral antibiotics will treat simple urinary tract infections. Anticholinergic therapy is warranted when urodynamics indicate a voiding pressure of more than 60 cm H_2O or a maximum filling pressure of more than 40 cm H_2O. Selective alpha-1 blockade is often added to reduce the simultaneous contraction of the external urethral sphincter.[9]

Bowel Incontinence

Bowel continence can often be established with a regular bowel program. Emptying of the bowel on a regularly scheduled basis and not allowing overdistention is the goal. A well lubricated suppository is inserted high into the rectum, next to the intestinal wall. Ten minutes after insertion, digital stimulation is performed by inserting a lubricated gloved finger or adaptive device into the rectum. The anal muscle is massaged in a circular motion until it relaxes. This digital stimulation may need to be repeated after 5 to 10 minutes until all stool is evacuated. The program is most effective after a meal or hot drink to stimulate peristalsis. The schedule must be frequent enough to avoid constipation and be convenient—either daily or every other day—as long as the timing is consistent. The importance of adequate dietary fiber and fluid intake to prevent constipation cannot be overemphasized.[10]

Skin Breakdown

Treatment of a pressure ulcer involves minimizing or eliminating pressure (see Chapter 130). Patients with sacral ulcers need to limit time in the supine position, and patients with ulcers on the ischium need to avoid sitting. Since adequate calories, vitamins, and minerals are essential for healing, protein supplements are often recommended in addition to vitamin C 500 mg bid and zinc sulfate 220 mg qd. Wet-to-dry dressings are often started for mechanical debridement of any devitalized tissue. Once the wound is clean, various dressings are available. Moisture occlusive or semiocclusive dressings are often the treatment of choice.[11]

Rehabilitation

New Weakness

Patients may benefit from skilled outpatient physical and occupational therapy to strengthen weak muscles, improve range of motion, and help minimize deconditioning. In the outpatient setting, emphasis is placed on fine motor skills and proper transfer technique.

Spasticity

A regular stretching and positioning program should be established to treat spasticity. Relaxation techniques, soft tissue massage, and biofeedback may be used to decrease the activation of spastic muscles. Serial casting is also beneficial to improve range-of-motion limitations.

Pain

Modalities such as ice, superficial heat, transcutaneous electrical nerve stimulation (TENS), or ultrasound are often helpful for acute musculoskeletal conditions. With an emphasis on prevention, patients should be instructed in proper body mechanics as well as energy conservation and joint and nerve protection techniques. Splinting can often be helpful to rest the involved joint.[12] For those who can use manual wheelchairs, wheelchair-push gloves should be worn for additional protection. If shoulder or wrist pain becomes severe enough, patients may need to change to a power wheelchair.[13]

Cough/Shortness of Breath

Wheelchair posture corrections for scoliosis or functional kyphosis should be emphasized as part of a respiratory health promotion plan (Fig. 3).

Regular resistive inspiratory muscle training has been shown to protect against respiratory infections, improve respiratory muscle strength, and decrease perceived difficulty with breathing in individuals with chronic cervical spinal cord injury.[14] Manually assisted cough methods can be taught to caregivers, and patients should be encouraged to use incentive spirometry regularly.

Procedures

Spasticity

If localized tone does not respond to regular stretching or other conservative measures, the use of nerve or motor point blocks with phenol may be used. Botulinum toxin injections to the muscle are

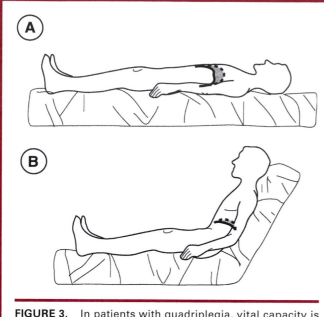

FIGURE 3. In patients with quadriplegia, vital capacity is decreased in the sitting position due to denervation of the phrenic nerve. Gravity holds the diaphragm down in the sitting position, thus causing diminished diaphragm excursion. (From Ökentenoglu BT, Benzel EC: Spine: State Art Rev 1999;13(3):456, with permission.)

another option. These procedures are typically performed in the biceps or hamstrings of patients with tetraplegia (e.g., when the excessive flexor tone presents functional impairment or pain [see Chapter 136]).

Shoulder pain due to subacromial bursitis is often responsive to local corticosteroid injections, as is the discomfort from carpal tunnel syndrome.

Surgery

New Weakness

Though controversial, surgical decompression of a syrinx by placement of a stent tube from the cavity to the subarachnoid or peritoneal space often leads to rapid improvement in many patients.

Spasticity

If muscle tone is severe diffusely and not controlled with maximum dosages of the aforementioned antispasticity medications, or if a patient is unable to tolerate the oral medications, the placement of an intrathecal baclofen pump should be considered. If the patient is amenable to the possibility of this invasive procedure, a test dose of intrathecal baclofen is necessary to evaluate the patient's response. These trials are usually performed by an anesthesiologist, with a physiatrist evaluating the status of the muscle tone before and after the injection.

Pain

Surgery is occasionally indicated to address pain that is not responsive to conservative measures (e.g., shoulder pain that interferes with transfers or other function may require surgical intervention).

Bladder Incontinence

In men who are able to wear an external condom catheter, external sphincterotomy is often indicated to treat refractory detrusor sphincter dyssynergia.[15]

Bowel Incontinence

If patients are good operative candidates, continue to have significant difficulty or complications with bowel care, and can demonstrate the ability to benefit from a colostomy, surgical intervention can be considered.[16]

Skin Breakdown

When pressure ulcers fail to close with conservative care, referral to plastic surgery for myocutaneous flap is indicated.

Potential Disease Complications

Complications of cervical spinal cord injury include progressive weakness, contracture, hydronephrosis, renal failure, osteomyelitis, and sepsis.

Potential Treatment Complications

Baclofen and tizanidine can cause sedation initially, though most patients will become tolerant to this side effect (see Table 3). If mental status changes persist, dose reduction is necessary. Liver function tests should be monitored regularly, and if increases in aspartate transaminase or alanine transaminase occur, dosage reduction or even complete discontinuation is necessary. This also applies to the anticonvulsant gabapentin. If carbamazepine is prescribed, white blood counts need to be monitored.

Tricyclic antidepressants and the medications used to control detrusor hyperreflexia have anticholinergic properties, leading to dry mouth and increased constipation.

Overaggressive therapy or exercise programs may lead to further overuse syndromes and more musculoskeletal pain. Excessive stretching of certain muscles (e.g., finger flexors and lumbar paraspinal musculature) can lead to functional deterioration. For example, the finger flexors often are left shortened to compensate for a weakened grasp, and increased tightness of the back musculature allows for added stability and balance with sitting.

References

1. American Spinal Injury Association: International Standards for Neurological and Functional Classification of Spinal Cord Injury. Chicago, American Spinal Injury Association, 1996.
2. Yarkony G (ed): Spinal Cord Injury: Management and Rehabilitation. Chicago, Aspen Publishers, 1994.
3. Bursell JP, et al: Electrodiagnosis in spinal cord injured persons with new weakness or sensory loss: Central and peripheral etiologies. Arch Phys Med Rehabil 1999;80:904–909.
4. Bach JR.:Noninvasive alternatives to tracheostomy for managing respiratory muscle dysfunction in spinal cord injury. Top Spinal Cord Inj Rehabil 1997;2(3):49–58.
5. Cassidy J: Nutritional health issues in people with high-level tetraplegia. Top Spinal Cord Inj Rehabil 1997;2(3):64–69.
6. Ditunno J, Formal C: Chronic spinal cord injury. N Engl J Med 1994;330(8):550–556.
7. Ragnarsson KT. Management of pain in persons with spinal cord injury. J Spinal Cord Med 1997;20;186–199.
8. Lanig IS, Peterson WP: The respiratory system in spinal cord injury. Phys Med and Rehabil Clin N Am 2000;11:29–43.
9. Rivas D, Abdill CK: Current management of detrusor sphincter dyssynergia. Top Spinal Cord Inj Rehabil 1996;1(3):1–17.
10. Chen D, Nussbaum S: The gastrointestinal system and bowel management following spinal cord injury. Phys Med Rehabil Clin N Am 2000;11(1):45–56.
11. Kirk P: Pressure ulcer management following spinal cord injury. Top Spinal Cord Inj Rehabil 1996;2(1):9–20.
12. Goldstein B: Musculoskeletal conditions after spinal cord injury. Phys Med Rehabil Clin N Am 2000;11(1):91–108.
13. Kirshblum S, et al: Musculoskeletal conditions in chronic spinal cord injury. Top Spinal Cord Inj Rehabil 1997;2(4):23–35.
14. Rutchik A, et al: Resistive inspiratory muscle training in subjects with chronic cervical spinal cord injury. Arch Phys Med Rehabil 1998;79:293–297.
15. Gray GJ, Yang, C: Surgical procedures of the bladder after spinal cord injury. Phys Med Rehabil Clin N Am 2000;11(1):57–72.
16. Stiens SA, et al: Neurogenic bowel dysfunction after spinal cord injury: Clinical evaluation and rehabilitative management. Arch Phys Med Rehabil 1997;78:S86–S102.

139 Spinal Cord Injury (Thoracic)

Shanker Nesathurai, MD
Jane Wierbicky, RN, BSN

Synonym

Paraplegia

ICD-9 Code

344.1
Paraplegia

Definition

Spinal cord injuries are a common cause of paralysis, particularly in young men (Table 1). Just more than one third of all spinal cord injuries (SCIs) occur at the thoracic level, most commonly at T12.[1] Compromise to the thoracic spinal cord typically results in paraplegia. Unlike paraplegia that results from compromise of the cauda equina associated with lumbar spine injuries, the clinical findings are consistent with upper motor neuron pathology. However, lower limb paralysis is not the only impairment. The thoracic spinal cord also segmentally innervates the intercostal muscles as well as the upper and lower abdominal muscles. The intercostal muscles are innervated by the T1 to T12 spinal segments. The upper abdominal muscles are innervated by the T8 to T10 spinal segments, whereas the T11 to T12 spinal segments innervate the lower abdominal muscles.[2]

A quantitative three-dimensional anatomy of the thoracic spine reveals three distinct zones: the cervical-thoracic transition zone, the middle region, and the thoracic-lumbar transition zone.[3,4] The T1 to T4 region is characterized by a narrowing of the vertebral end plate and spinal canal widths.[3] The middle thoracic region (T4 through T9) is notable for its relatively narrow end plate and small spinal canal. The rib articulations

TABLE 1. Demographic Comparison of Gunshot Spinal Cord Injury with Nonviolent Spinal Cord Trauma

	GS SCI (%)	Nonviolent Traumatic SCI (%)
Gender		
Male	95.1	79.1
Female	4.9	20.3
Ethnicity		
Caucasian	9.8	51.5
Non-Caucasian	91.2	48.5
Marital status		
Never married	70.7	38.9
Married	19.5	44.3
Not married	9.8	16.8
Employment status		
Employed	41.5	75.4
Unemployed	58.5	24.5
Mean age	27.1	42.2

Adapted from McKinley WO, Johns JS, Musgrove JJ: Clinical presentations, medical complications, and functional outcomes of individuals with gunshot wound–induced spinal cord injury. Am J Phys Med Rehabil 1999;78:102–107. In Lindsey RW, Gugala Z: Spine: State Art Rev 1999;13(3):530.

provide an increased level of protection at this level. An enlargement of the spinal canal characterizes the lower thoracic region (T10 through T12).[3] There is also less rigidity of the spine at the T11 and T12 segments because of the lack of ventral attachment to the ribs.[3] Therefore, there is an increased vulnerability to spinal cord injury at the lower thoracic levels. When compared to the cervical and lumbar spinal levels, the blood supply to the spinal cord is more tenuous in the thoracic spinal cord, and therefore such ischemia poses a greater threat to neurologic function in this area.[4]

Weakness, loss of sensation, and spasticity are the most common sequelae from a thoracic SCI. Issues commonly encountered in the outpatient clinic include pressure ulcer, urinary tract infection, dysreflexia, bowel irregularity, depression, sexual dysfunction, thrombosis, severe spasticity, heterotopic ossification (HO), contractures, osteoporosis, and pain.

Pressure ulcers are the most commonly encountered postinjury complication.[1] The human and economic costs of pressure ulcers are enormous. Excessive pressure, shearing, friction, and maceration can increase the risk of pressure ulcers. Other risk factors include spasticity, impaired sensation, immobility, poor nutrition, weight gain, and incontinence.[5]

Neurogenic bowel and bladder are also complications of thoracic SCI. Most patients with thoracic level SCI present with upper motor neuron bladder dysfunction. Low urinary volumes, high bladder pressures, bladder trabeculation, and diminished bladder compliance characterize upper motor neuron bladder dysfunction. Detrusor-sphincter dyssynergia—contraction of the bladder and sphincter—is common. Detrusor-sphincter dyssynergia can contribute to vesicoureteral reflux, which may result in hydronephrosis and subsequent chronic renal failure.

Sexual desire is not necessarily affected by SCI. However, associated depression, fears of inadequacy, and poor body image may consequently alter sexual desire. Sexual function (e.g., erection and ejaculation in men and lubrication in women) in patients with thoracic level injuries will be altered. In general, patients with more complete lesions have more impairment.

 Men with thoracic level lesions (with intact sacral reflexes) generally can achieve reflex erections with direct genital stimulation. However, many times, these reflex erections are of insufficient rigidity and duration for satisfactory vaginal penetration.[6]

SCI predisposes individuals to both deep vein thrombosis (DVT) and pulmonary embolism. According to one study, the risk of death resulting from pulmonary embolism for patients with acute SCI is 210 times greater than for a similar healthy population.[7] The risk decreases to 19.1 times of normal in postinjury years 2 to 5. The risk further decreases to 8.9 times of normal for those who survive for more than 5 years.[7] Etiology includes immobility as a result of paralysis and failure of the venous-muscle pump.

Osteoporosis among patients with spinal cord injuries is common. Immobilization and the lack of weight-loading activities are among the chief causes of osteoporosis. Other factors may include diet, lack of muscle traction on bone, and hormonal changes.[8] Osteoporosis in the lower extremities is the most common presentation in the individual with a thoracic level lesion. The loss of bone density develops in the acute stage of injury.[8] Patients with SCI are at significant risk for long bone fracture, and care must be taken to prevent fractures resulting from range-of-motion exercises and falls.

Individuals with spinal cord injuries above the T6 level are also susceptible to autonomic dysreflexia as a result of the disruption of the autonomic nervous system pathways.

The development of heterotopic ossification in the SCI population is most often seen in the first 6 months postinjury (see Chapter 111).[9]

Psychosocial adaptation subsequent to a SCI is a lifelong process. There is no single "classical" presentation of this phenomenon. Anger, hostility, anxiety, and depression often result from overwhelming losses confronting this population. Suicide is among the leading causes of death in these patients.

Autonomic dysreflexia, which results in elevated blood pressure, is usually precipitated by noxious stimuli below the level of the lesion. The major splanchnic outflow exists at the T6 through L2 levels.[10] The afferent impulses generated by the noxious stimuli ascend in the cord, stimulating sympathetic neurons in the intermediolateral gray matter and initiating sympathetic vasoconstrictor reflexes.[10] This massive sympathetic outflow is unopposed by higher cortical modulating centers because of the lesion in the spinal cord. Baroreceptors in the aorta and carotid arteries detect the increased pressure and vagal stimulation occurs, resulting in bradycardia.[11] Autonomic dysreflexia is considered a medical emergency, and prompt medical intervention is required. If untreated, autonomic dysreflexia can to lead to seizure, intracerebral hemorrhage, or even death.

Symptoms

The presenting symptoms of thoracic SCI are consistent with the alteration to the motor, sensory, and autonomic pathways. The chief symptoms include weakness or paralysis of the abdominal and lower extremity musculature, and loss of sensation in the lower limbs, thorax, and perineum. Altered bowel and bladder function and sexual dysfunction may also be expected. In the outpatient setting, the patient may complain of lower extremity spasticity, pain, and symptoms of autonomic dysreflexia (in patients with a thoracic cord lesion of T6 or higher). Patients with SCI are often insensate to the pain that accompanies deep venous thrombosis (DVT), and therefore both the clinician and patient should be attentive to objective signs such as edema, erythema, and increased tone. Heterotopic ossification may mimic DVT because the symptoms include swelling, decreased range of motion, erythema, increased spasticity, pain (if sensate), and low-grade fever.

Pain resulting from either abnormal mechanical forces or neuropathic etiology is common. Neuropathic pain resulting from central or peripheral nervous disruption may be described as burning or shooting.

Autonomic dysreflexia is characterized by elevated systolic and diastolic blood pressure, pounding headaches, nasal congestion, anxiety, visual disturbances, pallor below the level of injury, and sweating and flushing above the level of injury. In patients with an old, stable injury who are experiencing new or progressive symptoms (e.g., increasing weakness, loss of sensation), the clinician should consider the possibility of a syrinx.

Physical Examination

The diagnosis of a thoracic level SCI necessitates a thorough physical examination because of the multi-system complications that may ensue. The initial patient evaluation should also include the assessment of vital signs; respiratory function; skin integrity; bowel and bladder function; and the presence of spasticity, pain, and contractures. Pressure ulcers are more common over bony prominences such as the occiput, scapula, sacrum, calcaneus, and greater tuberosity.

On examination, new or progressive findings of weakness and/or loss of sensation should alert the clinician to consider imaging studies to rule out a syrinx.

Functional Limitations

Persons who suffer from thoracic SCI can have significantly different levels of disability, depending on their degree of paralysis and associated potential complications (e.g., contractures, spasticity). Typically, a patient with high thoracic paraplegia (i.e., T2 level) would have some component of truncal instability; as a result, the patient's wheelchair would require a "high back." In contrast, a person with low thoracic paraplegia generally has preservation of most of the intercostal muscles and could opt for a "low back" chair. Intercostal muscle impairment in patients with an SCI in the upper thoracic region may cause an impaired cough and a decreased ability to mobilize secretions. Bowel and bladder function may cause social embarrassment, leading to self-imposed social isolation. Sexual dysfunction may result in a loss of intimacy. The availability of partners is a concern for many patients since their disability and environmental and social barriers may preclude their involvement in some of the more typical dating activities. Depression is common in patients with SCI.

Diagnostic Studies

The diagnosis of thoracic SCI is often corroborated with magnetic resonance imaging (MRI). The stability of the injury is assessed by evaluating the anterior, middle, and posterior columns of the spinal cord. MRI is also the study of choice when a syrinx is suspected.

Urodynamic testing is commonly used to evaluate bladder function in the individual with spinal cord injury. Yearly renal evaluations often include a renal scan and ultrasound.

Patients with grade IV pressure ulcers may require a bone scan to detect osteomyelitis. The triple-phase bone scan is also used in the diagnosis of heterotopic ossification (see Chapter 111). Doppler surveillance studies are commonly performed to detect deep vein thrombosis in this highly susceptible population (see Chapter 104). Laboratory tests such as elevated serum alkaline phosphatase levels are used to assess for heterotopic ossification. In the postacute phase of SCI, renal function should be assessed with laboratory studies and renal ultrasound. If clinically indicated, urodynamic studies and urologic consultation can be considered. Routine colonoscopy and fecal occult testing may be appropriate for patients 50 years and older.[13] In patients susceptible to autonomic dysreflexia, appropriate precautions must be used during colonoscopy.

Differential Diagnosis

Amyotrophic lateral sclerosis

Post-traumatic syringomyelia

Guillain-Barré syndrome

Peripheral polyneuropathy

Spinal cord infarction

Treatment

Initial

Skin Management

The maintenance of skin integrity is an ever-present goal in patients with spinal cord injury. Pressure ulcer formation will lead to the development of scar tissue and an even greater likelihood of ulcer recurrence. Skin breakdown can be prevented by ensuring that seating and bedding surfaces are optimal. Seating surfaces should be re-evaluated on a regular basis. A cushion that may have been satisfactory previously may currently be worn out. Patients with substantial weight changes should have their seating systems re-evaluated.

Excessive pressure, shear forces, and moisture should be minimized. Patients are encouraged to perform daily skin examinations. Most paraplegic patients are able to independently perform pressure-relieving strategies, such as wheelchair push-ups. These techniques should be performed every 15 minutes to minimize excessive pressure. Patients are encouraged to minimize pressure by turning frequently when in bed and using a pressure-relieving mattress.

Patients who develop a pressure ulcer must eliminate pressure to that area until the wound is healed. A variety of debridement methods are available for removing necrotic debris from pressure ulcers. These methods include normal saline wet-to-dry gauze dressings, whirlpool therapy, irrigation, and chemical debridement agents (see Chapter 130).

Pain

In individuals who have pain, the specific condition should be addressed (e.g., tendinitis) The presentation of pain among the SCI population can be varied in nature: both neuropathic pain and pain resulting from abnormal mechanical stresses (e.g., tendinitis) are common. Analgesics and non-steroidal anti-inflammatory drugs (NSAIDs), including cyclooxygenase (COX–2) inhibitors, can be used to treat musculoskeletal causes of pain. Neuropathic pain generally is not responsive to analgesics; however, tricyclic antidepressants and antiseizure medications have been effective in its treatment.[14]

Bladder Management

Bladder management strategies should be individualized. In general, intermittent catheterization is the preferred treatment option. However, some patients are able to void with "reflexive maneuvers," such as bladder tapping or suprapubic pressure (e.g., Credé maneuver). Caution must be exercised before this approach is recommended to minimize the risk of vesicoureteral reflux.

A typical intermittent catheterization program requires bladder emptying 4 to 6 times per day. Urinary volumes should remain less than 500 cc. Most paraplegic patients have the manual dexterity to perform self-catheterization. However, some individuals, because of biologic and/or sociomedical factors, must use indwelling catheters (either suprapubic or urethral). Indwelling catheters are associated with a higher incidence of bladder stones and bladder carcinoma (both transitional cell and squamous).[15] In addition, in men, urethral catheters are associated with prostatitis, epididymitis, and urethral strictures.

The overriding goal of a bladder management program is to maintain socially acceptable continence and to minimize the long-term urologic sequelae of spinal cord injury. Detrusor-sphincter dyssynergia can be treated with medical interventions that decrease bladder tone (e.g., oxybutynin) or decrease sphincter tone (e.g., terazosin) (see Chapter 120).

Bowel Management

The patient with thoracic level injuries will most likely suffer from constipation; therefore, a bowel program is necessary. A reasonable goal for a bowel regimen is to achieve socially acceptable fecal continence, with bowel evacuations at least 3 times per week. A bowel regimen may include medications (Table 2). In addition, bowel evacuation is scheduled after a meal to capitalize on the intrinsic increase in peristalsis after meals (i.e., the gastrocolic reflex). Gentle digital stimulation of the rectum and insertion of a suppository can activate the rectocolic reflex to aid in bowel evacuation. Bowel care programs done on a raised toilet seat use the benefits of gravity. Digital stimulation (gently insertion of the finger) of the rectum and/or insertion of a suppository can activate the rectocolic reflex by stimulating peristalsis and promoting regular bowel movements. Glycerin and bisacodyl are colonic irritants that can be delivered via

TABLE 2. Oral Adjunctive Bowel Medications[13]

Medication	Brand	Mechanism of Action	Strength	Dose
Docusate sodium	Colace	Stool softener	100 mg (caps)	1–2 caps
Senna	Senokot	Colonic stimulant	187 mg (tabs)	ii qd
Bisacodyl	Dulcolax	Colonic irritant	5 mg (tabs)	ii qd
Psyllium powder	Metamucil	Bulk forming agent	3.4 mg per tsp	i tsp qd-tid
Metoclopra-mide	Reglan	Prokinetic agent	10 mg (tabs)	i tab qid

suppository, which can be a useful adjunctive agent in a bowel regimen. Enemas (Fleet, Soap Suds) should not be part of a regular bowel program; however, these agents are useful in providing a clear gut before a bowel program is begun or for treating fecal obstipation.[13] The administration of any enema can precipitate autonomic dysreflexia in susceptible patients.

Mental Health

In individuals suffering from depression or other psychologic sequelae, consultation with an appropriate mental health care professional is recommended, and continued follow-up should be encouraged, when appropriate.

Sexual and Reproductive Function

Many patients with SCI have numerous questions and fears regarding sexuality and sexual function. Treatment should address concerns related to body image, dating, and initiating and maintaining intimate relationships. Peer counselors can share their experiences, and their advice can be beneficial. Peer counselors may be located through local independent living centers or through local chapters of the National Spinal Cord Injury Association. In addition, mental health professionals (e.g., psychologists, psychiatrists, social workers) can be a valuable resource to the patient and rehabilitation team.

Several options available to men with erectile dysfunction include vacuum devices, oral medications (sildenafil), penile injection programs (papaverine), and surgically implanted prostheses. Ejaculatory dysfunction is also common. Ejaculation is a complex physiologic function that is primarily controlled by the sympathetic nervous system, with interaction between the nervous, circulatory, and endocrine systems.[16] Retrograde ejaculation into the bladder is not uncommon. Chronic SCI is also associated with poor semen quality and decreased spermatogenesis.[17] Elevated scrotal temperatures (from chronic sitting) and frequent urinary tract infections may negatively affect semen quality.

Women with thoracic level lesions may note changes in vaginal lubrication. However, at this level, women may achieve reflex lubrication, much like men achieve reflex erection.[16] Direct stimulation of the genital region may result in sufficient lubrication. A water-soluble lubricant is recommended for patients with complaints of decreased vaginal lubrication.

Orgasm for both men and women postinjury may be either non-existent, described as a primarily emotional event, or described as a pleasurable sensation in the pelvic region or sensory level with generalized muscle relaxation.[16]

Women with thoracic level SCI remain fertile. Contraceptive options include barrier methods (condoms, diaphragm) and oral contraceptives. However, a diaphragm requires hand dexterity, which may be unattainable in some patients. Intrauterine contraceptive devices are contraindicated because of the lack of sensation and the risk of developing pelvic inflammatory disease. Patients with SCI are at increased risk for the development of thromboembolism, and the administration of oral contraceptives further increases this risk.

The care of pregnant women with SCI has special challenges. Potential complications include premature labor, increased risk of urinary tract infection, autonomic dysreflexia, and constipation. Pregnant women with thoracic spinal cord injury levels above T10 will be unable to sense fetal movements and may require fetal monitoring.[18]

Deep Vein Thrombosis

The patient with SCI is often administered on prophylactic anticoagulant therapy during the initial weeks postinjury. The prophylactic use of thigh-high compression stockings and pneumatic compression boots is also recommended in the initial postinjury period (for more details on the prevention and treatment of deep vein thrombosis, see Chapter 104).

Spasticity Management

Spasticity should be treated when it results in significant pain, contributes to contractures, impairs hygiene, interferes with functional tasks, or obstructs nursing care. In the first instance, clinically significant spasticity should be treated by removing noxious stimuli that may be contributing to the condition, such as urinary tract infection, ingrown toenails, and tight clothing. Secondly, physical interventions such as daily stretching of muscles with terminal sustained stretch can be considered. If these are unsuccessful, medications such as tizanidine and baclofen can be prescribed.

Heterotopic Ossification

Treatment may include the administration of etidronate, which limits ossification, and physical therapy to maintain range of motion (see Chapter 136).

Osteoporosis

Supplementation with vitamin D is often recommended, although calcium supplementation remains controversial because of the associated risk of urinary calculi.[8] Others have investigated the use of alendronate and cyclical etidronate in the prevention of osteoporosis in this population (see Chapter 122).[8]

Autonomic Dysreflexia

To treat autonomic dysreflexia , it is necessary to remove the precipitating noxious stimulus. Patients should be placed in an upright position, if possible, to decrease blood pressure, and a search for a causative agent should be initiated. The majority of cases of autonomic dysreflexia are related to urinary tract irritation or bowel distention.[7] However, noxious stimuli such as ingrown toenails, pressure ulcer, and renal calculi are not uncommon. Vasodilating medications such as Nitropaste may be required to decrease the blood pressure while the clinician seeks the causative factor. (for more details on the treatment of dysreflexia, see page 631).[12]

Rehabilitation

Rehabilitation focuses on helping the patient to function at optimal levels. Thus, supervised physical and/or occupational therapy should address improving strength in all active muscle groups and range of motion in all joints. Mobility is a major issue that needs to be addressed both initially and then periodically as the patient's condition changes (e.g., women who become pregnant may require assistance with functional activities as the pregnancy progresses or a patient who could transfer independently and propel a manual wheelchair may require a power chair and assistance with transfers).

Adaptive equipment such as long-handled shoe horns, reachers, etc. can be recommended.

Passive interventions such as therapeutic heat and cold as well as transcutaneous electrical nerve stimulation (TENS) may be beneficial in the management of pain. However, particular caution must be used with therapeutic heat or cold modalities over insensate areas.

Physical interventions such as daily stretching of muscles with terminal sustained stretch can be considered a first-line rehabilitative treatment for spasticity. Positioning, as well as casting and splinting of the affected limbs, can minimize spasticity.

Procedures

A number of procedures can be used to address issues such as spasticity and pain. Interventional approaches for the treatment of spasticity include botulinum toxin injection, motor branch blocks, and peripheral nerve blocks (see Chapter 136). To decrease sphincter tone in men, botulinum toxin can be injected into the sphincter. This treatment in women is associated with an unacceptably high incidence of urinary incontinence.

A patient with dysreflexia caused by a bladder stone may require a urologic procedure for stone removal.

For men with ejaculatory dysfunction, retrieval of sperm for insemination has been successfully accomplished via electroejaculation and vibroejaculation methods. These procedures may result in dysreflexia and are performed under medical supervision.

Surgery

Pressure ulcers that do not heal with conservative methods may require surgical closure. Direct closure, skin grafts, musculocutaneous flaps, and skin flaps are among the surgical treatments available for wound closure. Mobilization after surgical closure must be done under close supervision, with careful monitoring of the surgical wound.

A variety of surgical procedures are used in patients who cannot be satisfactorily maintained on an intermittent catheterization program. Sphincter tone can be reduced with a sphincterotomy for men. Men must wear external collection devices after this procedure because it results in continuous incontinence. Sphincterotomies may occasionally require revision because of the development of fibrosis that obstructs outflow. Sphincterotomies may result in erectile dysfunction in some men.

Bladder augmentation is performed occasionally to increase bladder capacity. A piece of small bowel is interposed with the bladder tissue to increase vesical volume.

Patients with chronic dysreflexia resulting from persistent bowel management difficulties, such as frequent impaction, may be candidates for ileostomy or colostomy procedures. Patients with hemorrhoids aggravated by digital stimulation occasionally require surgical consult if the hemorrhoids are not relieved by more conservative methods (e.g., medicated suppositories or topical steroid creams).

Occasionally, men with erectile dysfunction that is not amenable to lesser invasive therapies may opt for an implantable penile prosthesis.

Surgical placement of an intrathecal morphine or baclofen pump may be beneficial for patients with severe pain or spasticity that is not responsive to non-invasive treatments.

Surgical interventions are indicated in some intractable cases of HO. Patients with functionally limited joint mobility or severe and chronic spasticity may benefit from surgical resection of the lesion.

Potential Disease Complications

Individuals with thoracic level SCIs are more likely to suffer from serious associated injuries than those with cervical or lumbosacral lesions. In one study, patients with thoracic cord injuries had a 46% occurrence of serious associated injuries such as hemothorax, pneumothorax, and intra-abdominal injuries compared with 12% of patients with cervical injuries and 22% of lumbar or caudal injuries.[19]

Thoracic SCI may be associated with a lower life expectancy.[1] The leading causes of death in people with paraplegia were septicemia, heart disease, suicide, pulmonary embolus, cancer, and pneumonia.

Complications arising from a thoracic level injury result from immobility, changing sensory patterns, and alterations in autonomic nervous system function.

Potential Treatment Complications

The anticholinergic side effects of tricyclic antidepressants, including dry mouth, blurred vision, and urinary retention, can pose additional difficulties for patient with spinal cord injury. Sphincterotomies, performed to alleviate detrusor-sphincter dyssenergia may result in urinary incontinence and occasionally sexual dysfunction in men. Voiding by the Credé maneuver may lead to vesicoureteral reflux. The long-term use of indwelling catheters, as stated previously, is associated with prostatitis, epididymitis, strictures, bladder stones, and bladder carcinoma.

Digital stimulation of the bowel can result in autonomic dysreflexia and hemorrhoids.

Medications used to treat autonomic dysreflexia can result in hypotension. The blood pressure must be closely monitored.

When the less invasive methods of treating spasticity are ineffective, botulinum toxin injections, motor branch blocks, or peripheral nerve blocks may be considered. Injections may result in bleeding or infection. Nerve blocks may result in dysesthesias and weakness. Patients with intrathecal baclofen pumps may experience drowsiness, weakness, catheter breakage, or infection.

References
1. 1999 Annual Report for the Model Spinal Cord Injury Care Systems. Birmingham, AL, National Spinal Cord Injury Statistical Center, 1999, p 98.
2. Nesathurai S, Gwardjan A: Clinical and functional evaluation. In Nesathurai S (ed): The Rehabilitation of People with Spinal Cord Injury. Malden, MA, Blackwell Science, 2000, pp 31–38.
3. Panjabi M, Koichiro T, Goel V, et al: Thoracic human vertebrae: Quantitative three-dimensional anatomy. Spine 1991;16:888–901.
4. Yashon D: Spinal Injury. New York, NY, Appleton-Century-Crofts, 1978, p 96.
5. Glover M: Pressure ulcers. In Nesathurai S (ed): The Rehabilitation of People with Spinal Cord Injury, 2nd ed. Malden, MA, Blackwell Science, 2000, pp 59–65.
6. Ducharme S, Gill K: Sexuality After Spinal Cord Injury. Baltimore, MD, Brookes, 1997.
7. Consortium for Spinal Cord Medicine: Clinical Practice Guidelines. Acute Management of Autonomic Dysreflexia: Adults with Spinal Cord Injury Presenting to Health-Care Facilities. Washington, DC, Paralyzed Veterans of America, 1997.
8. Pearson E, Nance P, Leslie W, et al. Cyclical etidronate: Its effects on bone density in patients with acute spinal cord injury. Arch Phys Med Rehabil 1997;78:269–272.
9. Garland, D. Heterotopic ossification. In Nesathurai S (ed): The Rehabilitation of People with Spinal Cord Injury, 2nd ed. Malden, MA, Blackwell Science, 2000, pp 81–83.
10. Consortium for Spinal Cord Medicine: Clinical Practice Guideline: Prevention of Thromboembolism in Spinal Cord Injury, 2nd ed. Washington, DC, Paralyzed Veterans of America, 1999.
11. Vapnek J: Autonomic Dysreflexia. Top Spinal Cord Inj Rehabil 1997;2(4):54–69.
12. DeSantis N: In Nesathurai S (ed): The Rehabilitation of People with Spinal Cord Injury, 2nd ed. Malden, MA, Blackwell Science, 2000, pp 71–74.
13. Bergman S: Bowel management. In Nesathurai S (ed): The Rehabilitation of People with Spinal Cord Injury, 2nd ed. Malden, MA, Blackwell Science, 2000, pp 53–58.
14. Roaf E: Aging and spinal cord injury. In Nesathurai S (ed): The Rehabilitation of People with Spinal Cord Injury, 2nd ed. Malden, MA, Blackwell Science, 2000, pp 95–101.
15. Nesathurai S: Bladder management. In Nesathurai S (ed): The Rehabilitation of People with Spinal Cord Injury, 2nd ed. Malden, MA, Blackwell Science, 2000, pp 45–52.
16. Ducharme S: In Nesathurai S (ed): The Rehabilitation of People with Spinal Cord Injury, 2nd ed. Malden, MA, Blackwell Science, 2000, pp 89–94.
17. Monga M, Bernie J, Rajasekaran M: Male infertility and erectile dysfunction in spinal cord injury: A review. Arch Phys Med Rehabil 1999;80:1331–1337.
18. Baker E, Cardenas D: Pregnancy in spinal cord injured women. Arch Phy Med Rehabil 1996;77:501–507.
19. Ducker T, Saul T: The poly-trauma and spinal cord injury. In Tator C (ed): Early Management of Acute Spinal Cord Injury. New York, 1982, pp 53–58.

140 Spinal Cord Injury (Lumbosacral)

Michelle J. Alpert, MD

Definition

Lumbar spinal cord injury refers to impairment or loss of motor and/or sensory function in the lumbar segments of the spinal cord secondary to the damage of neural elements within the spinal canal (the spinal cord ends at L1). With this level of injury, arm and trunk function are spared, but the legs and pelvic organs may be involved.

Conus medullaris syndrome results from an injury of the sacral cord and lumbar nerve roots within the spinal canal, which results in an areflexic bladder, bowel, and lower limbs. There may be preservation of some sacral reflexes (e.g., bulbocavernosus and micturition).

Cauda equina syndrome refers to injury to the lumbosacral nerve roots within the neural canal, resulting in an areflexic bladder, bowel, and lower limbs.

It is also important to note that individuals with lumbrosacral spinal cord injuries may have problems with sexual dysfunction and fertility. These issues are covered in more detail in Chapter 139; however, referral to a specialist is appropriate.

Symptoms

Patients with lumbosacral spinal injury may present with new weakness, spasticity, pain, bladder incontinence, bowel incontinence or constipation, and skin breakdown.

Physical Examination

The physical examination of an individual with a lumbosacral spinal injury will vary, depending on the exact level of the damage. For example, if injury occurs primarily to the lumbar spine, upper motor neuron weakness will predominate in the lower extremities, accompanied by increased muscle stretch reflexes and a variable degree of spasticity. Sensory loss is also variable, depending on the level of the injury. If the injury is more distal, affecting the sacral spine and/or some lumbar and/or sacral nerve roots, the clinical picture is more consistent with a lower motor neuron process—absent or diminished reflexes, decreased muscle tone in the lower extremities, and variable weakness in the lower extremities. Again, the sensory exam will vary.

TABLE 1. Spinal Level of Injury and Key Muscle Groups

Level	Muscle Group(s)
L2	Hip flexors (iliopsoas)
L3	Knee flexors (quadriceps)
L4	Ankle dorsiflexors (tibialis anterior)
L5	Long toe extensors (extensor hallucis longus)
S1	Ankle plantarflexors (gastrocnemius, soleus)

Modified from Finkelstein JA: Evaluation of spinal cord injury patients. Spine State Art Rev 1999;13(3):470.

The examination should include a thorough assessment of sacral reflexes, including anal tone, anocutaneous reflex, bulbocavernosus reflex, and the internal anal sphincter reflexes.

New Weakness

Manual muscle testing of all pertinent lower extremity muscles should be included in each examination, and any changes from previous evaluations should be noted. Specific key muscle groups are tested to determine the motor level (Table 1).

Spasticity

Passive range of motion in all planes of movement should be performed in the lower extremities to evaluate for the presence of spasticity and to rule out any joint limitations. Observation of the patient during functional activities (e.g., transfers) can help assess the degree of spasticity and its effect on the patient's abilities. Increases in spasticity may indicate other clinical pathology, such as a urinary tract infection.

Pain

During passive range of motion, the presence of pain with resisted movement can be detected at the shoulders, hips, knees, and ankles. Palpation for sites of tenderness (e.g., greater trochanters) should be performed during joint motion and mobility assessment.

Skin Breakdown

Skin examination should be conducted in all pressure bearing areas (e.g., sacrum, heels, trochanters, ischial tuberosities).

Functional Limitations

New Weakness

Increased weakness, whether localized or diffuse, will affect an individual's functional status, particularly mobility and ability to do self-care skills. Specific motor loss may affect an individual's ability to use previously prescribed lower extremity orthotics (e.g., new quadriceps weakness may lead to the need for long leg braces instead of short leg braces). Transfer technique may also need modification.

Spasticity

Increased spasticity may interfere with the safety of transfers or ability to ambulate. This increased tone may be painful and lead to difficulty with sleep. Intermittent spasms while the patient is wearing lower extremity orthotics can also contribute to skin breakdown.

Pain

Pain, whether nociceptive or neurogenic, may interfere with functional activities and reduce quality of life.

Bladder/Bowel Incontinence

Bowel and bladder irregularity can greatly affect an individual's daily routine and quality of life. Fear of incontinence may often lead to self-restriction of activity and social isolation.

Skin Breakdown

Areas of skin breakdown can lead to decreased ability to sit or lie supine, depending on their location, and thereby interfere with daily routines.

Diagnostic Studies

New Weakness

For further evaluation of neurologic decline, MRI of the spinal cord can reveal the presence of post-traumatic syringomyelia. Electrodiagnostic testing is useful to rule out lumbar myeloradiculopathy, especially quantitative needle electromyography of motor unit action potential amplitudes, F wave studies, and motor evoked potential central motor conduction times.[2]

Pain

Radiographs of the spine can help delineate conditions associated with neurologic change and/or spine pain, such as spine instability, instrumentation failure, degenerative changes, and neuropathic spinal arthropathy (Charcot's spine). CT scans may be necessary to further evaluate osseous and soft tissue changes. Radiographs of the lower extremity may help rule out the presence of occult fractures.[3]

Patients with paraplegia who are dependent on a wheelchair for mobility or who use crutches for ambulation commonly experience musculoskeletal pain at the shoulders or wrists, which usually is related to overuse of the upper limbs. Radiographs of the shoulder are often indicated to evaluate the status of the rotator cuff or to rule out the presence of other joint abnormalities. Electrodiagnostic studies can be helpful to rule out carpal tunnel syndrome or other compressive mononeuropathies.[4]

The so called "cauda equina pain"—described as symmetric burning and tingling discomfort affecting the sacral dermatomes of the "saddle region" (e.g., the buttocks, anus, genitals, and the soles of the feet)—can usually be diagnosed by history alone.[5]

Bladder Incontinence

Urinalysis is paramount to evaluate for infection as the cause of urinary incontinence. Urodynamic testing will enable determination of detrusor pressures and status of the external sphincter to guide a proper bladder program.

Bowel Incontinence/Constipation

A flat plate radiograph of the abdomen will help rule out impaction or obstruction as the source of bowel irregularity.

Skin Breakdown

If a pressure ulcer appears to involve the bone, MRI or bone scan may be helpful to rule out the presence of osteomyelitis. Depending on the location of the ulcer, the efficacy of specific equipment will need to be assessed (e.g., the fit of lower extremity orthotics for ulcers on the feet or wheelchair seating and positioning for ulcers on the ischium or trochanters).

Differential Diagnosis

Syringomyelia

Diabetic neuropathy or other polyneuropathy

Guillain-Barré syndrome

Amyotrophic lateral sclerosis

Normal pressure hydrocephalus

Treatment

Initial

New Weakness

All patients with spinal injuries should be encouraged to comply with a daily strengthening and conditioning program to maintain their endurance and muscle mass. Nutritional counseling is a beneficial adjunct to preventative health regimens.[6]

Spasticity

Before considering treatment for spasticity, it must be emphasized that spasticity may be helpful to the patient. Extensor tone may help stabilize lower limbs during stance or gait, just as flexor spasms can help leg positioning for lower body dressing.

The first step in spasticity management should be an attempt to discover factors that are increasing the severity of the spasms (if the lesion is not changing); for example, a urinary tract infection, new pressure sore, or other source of nociceptive input will markedly worsen the symptoms of spasticity. If after treatment of these secondary factors, the spasticity continues to interfere with function or causes excessive pain, pharmacologic therapy should be considered: Baclofen is the drug of choice. Tizanidine can be added if maximum dosages of baclofen do not produce the desired therapeutic effect.

Pain

Mechanical/musculoskeletal sources of pain, such as hamstring or groin muscle strains, may be alleviated by limited rest and by analgesics such as nonsteroidal anti-inflammatories. Lumbosacral corsets may be helpful to maintain posture, thereby providing some pain relief.

The treatment of neurogenic pain tends to be non-specific by trial and error and seldom results in complete elimination of the pain. Psychosocial factors such as depression and anxiety warrant treatment with counseling and/or antidepressants, given the relationship between these conditions and increased perception and complaints of pain. General physical health must also be optimized because functional disturbances of various organs, such as bladder overdistention, fecal impaction, and pressure sores, will exacerbate pain symptoms. First line pharmacologic agents for neuropathic pain are of the anticonvulsant class. Carbamazepine is the most widely studied drug (doses up to 400 mg tid), and gabapentin is now commonly used because of few reported side effects (doses up to 900 mg qid). Tricyclic antidepressants, such as amitriptyline, are often started at a dosage of 25 mg at night and increased to a maximum of 150 mg, depending on therapeutic effect. Only in rare cases of severe intractable pain and when other non-narcotic medications have failed are opioids prescribed.[8]

Bladder Incontinence

If urinary incontinence is the result of infection, appropriate antibiotics are prescribed. When increased detrusor pressures produce incontinence, an antispasmodic medication, such as oxybutynin or propantheline, is administered. If urodynamic studies confirm detrusor areflexia and competency of the sphincteric mechanism (the usual findings with conus medullaris and cauda equina syndromes), patients are taught to perform intermittent catheterization. This should be done every 4 to 6 hours to prevent overflow incontinence.[9]

Bowel Incontinence/Constipation

If impaction is present, prompt decompression of the bowel with manual disimpaction and provocation of the defecation reflex are necessary. To prevent recurrence, a regular bowel program must be followed; if injury is infrasacral, stool will need to be manually removed daily. If the injury is above the conus medullaris, the rectocolic reflex can be used to initiate defecation—digital stimulation with or without an appropriate chemical stimulus (e.g., suppository).

Skin Breakdown

Treatment of a pressure ulcer involves minimizing or eliminating pressure (see Chapter 130). Patients with sacral ulcers need to limit time in the supine position, and patients with ulcers on the ischium need to avoid sitting. The presence of heel ulcers warrants the need for appropriate resting splints to eliminate pressure on the calcaneus while the patient is lying supine. Since adequate calories, vitamins, and minerals are essential for healing, protein supplements are often recommended in addition to vitamin C 500 mg bid and zinc sulfate 220 mg qd. Wet-to-dry dressings are often started for mechanical debridement of any devitalized tissue. Once the wound is clean, various dressings are available. Moisture occlusive or semiocclusive dressings are often the treatment of choice.[10]

Rehabilitation

New Weakness

Outpatient physical therapy can address overall deconditioning and particular deficits in lower extremity strength. Once strength is regained, proper transfer technique and gait mechanics can be evaluated. An individualized home exercise program to maintain strength, range of motion, and endurance is mandatory.

If patients have adequate trunk balance and/or upper extremity strength, gait training with long leg braces can be attempted. Energy expenditure during ambulation will decrease with the presence of more functioning musculature in one or both lower extremities.

A knee-ankle-foot orthosis (KAFO) is usually required when the strength of the quadriceps is less than functional (less than 3/5). If hip and trunk strength is preserved but knee hyperextension and/or ankle instability/weakness persist, the patient may benefit from a trial of gait training with ankle-foot orthoses (AFOs).[11]

Periodic evaluations of lower extremity orthotics are necessary to monitor their fit, condition, and efficacy.

Spasticity

A daily stretching program is an integral component of any management program for spasticity. Regular range of motion exercises of the lower extremities helps prevent contractures.

Casting or splinting may improve the range of motion in the knees or ankles, allowing better positioning and fit of lower extremity braces. If ankle/knee strength is limited and increased tone exists (e.g., flexor tone at the knee, extensor tone at the ankle), resting splints may be beneficial to preserve range of motion and proper positioning.[12]

Pain

If pain is due to inflammation from overuse, modalities such as ice, superficial heat, transcutaneous electrical nerve stimulation (TENS), or ultrasound are often beneficial. Educational programs to prevent poor habits and to adhere to proper biomechanics are crucial components of the treatment program. Optimal posture in the wheelchair and bed should be emphasized, and a thorough assessment of the current back system, cushion, and entire seating system should be completed.

Procedures

Spasticity

If lower extremity tone continues to interfere with positioning, balance, ambulation, or hygiene, motor point or nerve blocks with phenol may help improve range of motion at particular joints (e.g., knees with hamstring block and ankle with posterior tibialis block). Intramuscular injections of botulinum toxin are another option.

Pain

Shoulder or hip pain due to subacromial or trochanteric bursitis, respectively, is often responsive to local corticosteroid injections, as is the discomfort from carpal tunnel syndrome.

Surgery

New Weakness

For treatment of syringomyelia, shunting—either syringopleural or syringoperitoneal—can yield gains, reversing neurologic decline.

Spasticity

If, despite maximum dosages of the aforementioned antispasticity medications, lower extremity muscle tone continues to be severe, painful, and/or bothersome or if a patient is unable to tolerate the oral medications, the placement of an intrathecal baclofen pump should be considered. If the patient is amenable to the possibility of this invasive procedure, a test dose of intrathecal baclofen is necessary to evaluate the patient's response. These trials are usually performed by an anesthesiologist, with a physiatrist evaluating the status of the muscle tone before and after the injection. If the trial confirms improved spasticity control with no adverse affects, referral to a neurosurgeon for definitive pump placement should be the next step.

Bladder Incontinence

If parasympathetic efferent neurons to the detrusor are intact, contraction of the detrusor can be produced by electrical stimulation. Intradural electrodes are placed on the sacral anterior nerve roots in the cauda equina and leads are tunneled subcutaneously to a radio-receiver under the skin of the abdomen and powered by a radio transmitter operated by the patient.[13]

If the sphincter fails to store urine because of denervation at the conal or cauda equina level, an artificial urinary sphincter device can be surgically placed.

Bowel Incontinence/Constipation

If patients are good operative candidates, continue to have significant difficulty or complications with bowel care, and can demonstrate the ability to benefit from a colostomy, surgical intervention can be considered.[14]

Skin Breakdown

When pressure ulcers fail to close with conservative care, referral to plastic surgery for myocutaneous flap is indicated.

Potential Disease Complications

Complications of lumbosacral spinal injury include progressive weakness, contracture, hydronephrosis, vesicoureteral reflux, renal failure, sepsis, toxic megacolon, colonic perforation, and osteomyelitis.

Potential Treatment Complications

Baclofen is generally well tolerated, with the major side effects being fatigue, dizziness, and gastrointestinal upset. Liver function tests need to be periodically monitored. Abrupt cessation of the drug should be avoided to reduce the risk of seizures, hallucinations, or palpitations. Tizanidine is also metabolized in the liver, and caution should be used in persons with liver disease. The principal side effects include lethargy and dry mouth.

Side effects of gabapentin, including dizziness and drowsiness, can be minimized by a slow upward titration from a low starting dose. The same slow titration is recommended for carbamazepine prescription to reduce possible dizziness, nausea, vomiting, and drowsiness. Bone marrow suppression can occur, as well as aplastic anemia or agranulocytosis, necessitating regular monitoring of complete blood counts.

Tricyclic antidepressants have anticholinergic properties, potentially leading to dry mouth and increased constipation, orthostatic hypotension, and urinary retention.

Overaggressive therapy programs may lead to further overuse syndromes and more musculoskeletal pain.

Potential complications of bladder functional neuromuscular stimulation systems, though rare, include infection of the implants and technical faults in the implanted equipment.

Postoperative complications of the artificial urinary sphincter device include urethral erosion and upper urinary tract deterioration.

References

1. American Spinal Injury Association: International Standards for Neurological and Functional Classification of Spinal Cord injury. Chicago, American Spinal Injury Association, 1996.
2. Little JW, et al: Neurologic recovery and neurologic decline after spinal cord injury. Phys Med Rehabil Clin N Am 2000;11(1): 73–89.
3. Young R, Woolsey R (eds): Diagnosis and Management of Disorders of the Spinal Cord. Philadelphia, W.B. Saunders, 1995.
4. Kirshblum S, et al: Musculoskeletal conditions in chronic spinal cord injury. Top Spinal Cord Inj Rehabil 1997;2(4):23–35.
5. Ragnarsson K: Management of pain in persons with spinal cord injury. J Spinal Cord Med 1997;20:186–199.
6. Cassidy J: Nutritional health issues in people with high-level tetraplegia. Top Spinal Cord Inj Rehabil 1997;2(3):65–69.
7. Goldstein B: Musculoskeletal conditions after spinal cord injury. Phys Med Rehabil Clin N Am 2000;11(1):91–108.
8. Bryce TN, Ragnarsson KT: Pain after spinal cord injury. Phys Med Rehabil Clin N Am 2000;11(1):157–168.
9. Young MN, et al: Intermittent catheterization, indwelling catheters, reflex voiding: A review of outcomes and management options in spinal cord injury. Top Spinal Cord Inj Rehabil 1996;1(3):45–54.
10. Kirk P: Pressure ulcer management following spinal cord injury. Top Spinal Cord Inj Rehabil 1996;2(1):9–20.
11. Atrice MB: Lower extremity orthotic management for the spinal-cord-injured client. Top Spinal Cord Inj Rehabil 2000;5(4):1–10.
12. Stein AB, et al: Evaluation and management of spasticity in spinal cord injury. Top Spinal Cord Inj Rehabil 1997;2(4):70–83.
13. Chae J, et al: Functional neuromuscular stimulation in spinal cord injury. Phys Med Rehabil Clin N Am 2000; 11(1):209–226.
14. Stiens SA, et al: Neurogenic bowel dysfunction after spinal cord injury: Clinical evaluation and rehabilitative management. Arch Phys Med Rehabil 1997;78:S86–S102.
15. Atrice MB: Lower extremity orthotic management for the spinal-cord-injured client. Top Spinal Cord Inj Rehabil 2000;5(4):1–10.

141 Stroke

Joel Stein, MD

Definition

Stroke is defined as an acquired injury of the brain caused by occlusion of a blood vessel or inadequate blood supply leading to an infarction, or a hemorrhage within the parenchyma of the brain. Stroke is the single largest cause of acquired disability in adults in the United States, with more than 600,000 strokes occurring each year and an estimated 4.5 million stroke survivors alive today.[1] While the death rate from stroke has fallen, the total number of strokes occurring each year in the United States has risen due to the aging of the population. Risk factors for stroke include age, sex, race, hypertension, smoking, diabetes, obesity, hypercholesterolemia, and a sedentary lifestyle. Hyperhomocysteinemia has recently been identified as a risk factor for stroke.[2] Risk factor modification includes smoking cessation, control of hypertension and diabetes, exercise, and weight loss if obesity is present.

Symptoms

Weakness, difficulty in speaking or swallowing, aphasia, cognitive disturbance, sensory loss, and visual disturbance are the most common presenting symptoms of stroke, and deficits in these areas often persist even after initial rehabilitation. Urinary urgency, increased muscle tone, fatigue, depression, and pain are symptoms that may present after a stroke has already occurred. Reflex sympathetic dystrophy (RSD, also known as regional complex pain syndrome type I) may occur after stroke, though most post-stroke pain results from mechanical (e.g., joint subluxation) or central etiologies (e.g., thalamic pain syndromes).

Physical Examination

A full neurologic examination is appropriate and includes mental status, cranial nerves, sensation, deep tendon reflexes (increased), abnormal reflexes (e.g., Babinski), motor strength and coordination, muscle tone (generally increased but may be decreased), and evaluation of functional mobility (sitting, transfers, and ambulation). The protean manifestations of stroke can cause many different combinations of abnormalities in these aspects of the neurologic exam. An assessment of mood and affect is important, given the high prevalence of post-stroke depression. Range of motion in affected limbs should be measured, as ankle plantar flexion contractures and upper limb contractures are common in hemiplegic stroke. Skin should be examined for any areas of breakdown. Limb swelling is common and should be noted. The fit and function of leg braces, upper extremity splints, slings, wheelchairs, and ambulatory aids should be assessed.

Functional Limitations

Difficulty in walking, performing activities of daily living, speaking, and swallowing are common manifestations of stroke. Cognitive impairments (e.g., memory, attention, visual spatial perception) and impaired communication due to aphasia and/or dysarthria may be present. Impaired sexual function should be identified; patients may not volunteer functional impairments in this area unless the clinician inquires.

As a result of the impairments just noted, many individuals may have difficulty or be unable to drive or use public transportation. Problems with communicating can lead to social isolation. Some individuals require ongoing supervision because of cognitive limitations. In severe cases, individuals with aphasia and/or cognitive impairments may not be able to live independently. Incontinence due to detrussor instability and urinary urgency can interfere with leaving the home and contribute to skin breakdown and social isolation.

Depression is quite common after stroke, affecting as many as 40% of stroke survivors, and should be identified as a treatable complication of stroke, rather than accepted as a consequence of functional loss.

Diagnostic Studies

In the acute setting, CT is often the first diagnostic test performed, due to the rapidity with which it can be obtained, its widespread availability, and its high sensitivity for cerebral hemorrhage. MRI provides greater anatomic resolution and avoids radiation exposure. With newer MRI sequences such as diffusion weighted imaging (DWI), abnormalities can be demonstrated at an earlier stage than with CT, providing important information for acute treatments such as thrombolysis.[3] Magnetic resonance angiography, non-invasive flow studies, Holter monitoring, and echocardiography are important studies to help determine the etiology of a stroke and determine the best treatment for prevention of recurrent stroke. In selected patients (particularly young individuals or those without typical risk factors), an evaluation for hypercoagulable states is indicated.

In patients with prior stroke, diagnostic studies are typically directed to complications of stroke, such as persistent dysphagia or urinary incontinence. Videofluoroscopic swallowing studies can be useful in swallowing disorders. Urodynamic studies may be useful in the assessment of urinary symptoms, particularly if initial treatment with anticholinergic medications is unsuccessful.

Differential Diagnosis

Hemiplegic migraine

Brain neoplasm

Postseizure (Todd's) paralysis

Multiple sclerosis

Treatment

Initial

When stroke is diagnosed within the first 3 hours, thrombolytic therapy has been shown to reduce disability.[4] In other cases, intravenous heparin is commonly used when an embolic etiology is suspected. Aspirin has been found to be effective when used in the acute setting. Long-term secondary prevention depends on the etiology of the stroke. Warfarin is commonly used for the prevention of embolic stroke, with the most extensive evidence for prevention of stroke in atrial fibrillation.[5] Antiplatelet agents, including aspirin, clopidogrel, ticlopidine, or combined aspirin/dipyridamole are used for prevention of small vessel stroke or when anticoagulation is desirable but contraindicated in comorbid conditions. Controversy continues regarding the best treatment for cryptogenic stroke (stroke of unknown etiology), intracranial stenosis, and other stroke etiologies. Risk factor modification, including treatment of hypertension, diabetes, hyperlipidemia, obesity, as well as smoking cessation and exercise should be addressed for all stroke survivors.

Treatment for cerebral hemorrhage is based, in part, on presumed etiology. For hypertensive hemorrhages, control of blood pressure with anti-hypertensive medications is the mainstay of treatment. For all causes of cerebral hemorrhage, avoidance of anticoagulants, antiplatelet medications, and alcohol is important.[6]

Medications useful in the management of stroke and its complications in the outpatient setting include anticholinergic medications for bladder detrussor instability (e.g., oxybutynin, tolterodine). Antispasticity medications include baclofen, tizanidine, and diazepam, though these are of limited efficacy in many cases (see Chapter 136). In cases of sexual dysfunction in men, sildenafil may be effective. Sildenafil's utility in women with post-stroke sexual dysfunction is unknown. Treatment with selective serotonin reuptake inhibitors (SSRIs) for post-stroke depression is widely employed, though a wide range of antidepressant medications can be effective. The use of psychostimulants, such as methylphenidate or dextroamphetamine may be useful for impaired attention. Anticonvulsants (e.g., gabapentin, carbamazepine) are used for central pain syndromes, though with variable benefit.

Rehabilitation

The rehabilitation program needs to be customized, based on the severity and nature of the impairments caused by the stroke. For individuals with moderate to severe stroke, a comprehensive multidisciplinary inpatient rehabilitation program in a rehabilitation hospital is often appropriate.[7] For these individuals, rehabilitation commonly continues through home care or outpatient services. Individuals with more isolated and less severe deficits may be discharged directly from the acute care hospital to home and participate in an outpatient rehabilitation program.[8]

Exercise

Therapeutic exercise programs are usually functionally oriented, with an emphasis on restoring functional mobility and ability to perform daily activities (Fig. 1). Instruction in compensatory techniques and family teaching are important in assisting individuals to return home. There is growing evidence of the impact of therapeutic exercise on cortical reorganization after stroke.[9] The optimal exercise program to facilitate recovery remains to be defined, however.

Dysphagia

Management of dysphagia may include modified diets (e.g., thickened liquids, pureed foods) and swallowing therapy (e.g., the use of compensatory strategies such as "tucking" the chin during swallowing). In more severe cases, the use of nasogastric or gastrostomy tube feedings may be necessary.

Communication

The rehabilitation of aphasia relies on extensive speech therapy as its mainstay, with selected patients benefiting from communication aids, such as a picture board. Speech therapy may provide significant benefit in patients with dysarthria, with improved intelligibility resulting. Severely dysarthic or anarthric patients may benefit from the use of computer based communication aids, including those with speech synthesis, as well as "low tech" solutions, such as spelling boards.

Cognition

Cognitive abilities are frequently affected by stroke, with alterations in memory, attention, insight, and problem solving among the most common. Neuropsychologic testing may be useful in defining the precise nature of these deficits and in helping to develop a remediation plan. Speech-language and occupational therapy approaches include both attempts at remediation and teaching compensatory techniques. Family education and training are important components of cognitive rehabilitation. Recognition and treatment of post-stroke depression is very important because depression can contribute to reduced cognitive performance after stroke.[10]

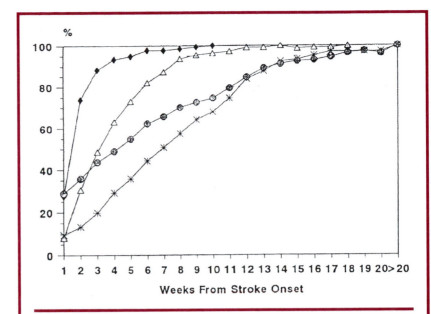

FIGURE 1. The time course of recovery after stroke is shown as the cumulative percentage of stroke survivors in each category who have reached their best daily activity function relative to initial functional disability. ◆ = Mild disability, △ = moderate disability, ● = severe disability, and * = very severe disability. (From Jorgensen HS, Nakayama H, Raaschou HO, et al: Outcome and time course of recovery in stroke: Part II: Time course of recovery. The Copenhagen Stroke Study. Arch Phys Med Rehabil 1995;76: 406–412, with permission.)

Bracing

Lower extremity bracing is frequently helpful in restoring mobility in hemiparetic stroke survivors. Most commonly, a plastic ankle foot orthosis (AFO) is utilized, although other braces are appropriate in selected circumstances. Bracing is helpful as a compensation for impaired ankle dorsiflexion, controlling ankle inversion and plantar flexor spasticity, and for providing some stabilization at the knee.

Ambulatory Aids, Wheelchairs

Due to hemiparesis, many stroke survivors require ambulatory aids, which may include a straight cane, four pronged ("quad") cane; hemi-walker; or, in some cases, a conventional walker. Wheelchairs are often needed for more severely impaired stroke survivors, or for longer distance travel in moderately impaired stroke survivors. A "hemi" wheelchair is lower to the ground and allows use of the non-paretic leg to assist with propulsion. Occasionally, a one-arm drive wheelchair is useful, as it allows control of both wheelchair wheels from one side. Active, non-ambulatory individuals may benefit from a power wheelchair.

Shoulder Subluxation

Shoulder subluxation commonly occurs in the setting of hemiplegia after stroke, although the presence of pain is highly variable. Supporting the arm by using arm boards and the selective use of slings is helpful in reducing subluxation. Electrical stimulation may have a beneficial effect as well.[11]

Splints

Splints for proper positioning of the hemiplegic arm and ankle/foot are important to prevent contracture. These are particularly important when spasticity is present.

Vocational Rehabilitation

Although stroke is predominantly a disease of older individuals, a significant portion of stroke survivors are of working age. Once daily activities have been mastered, vocational counseling may be useful to assist individuals who are seeking to return to work. Coordination with the rehabilitation team is important because retraining for certain job tasks may involve a multidisciplinary effort. Accommodations in the workplace may be necessary, and the Americans with Disabilities Act (ADA) may require the employer to provide reasonable accommodation for individuals with disabilities.

Procedures

Phenol or botulinum toxin blocks may be useful in the management of spasticity after stroke. These injections are described in greater detail in Chapter 136).

Surgery

Selected patients undergo craniotomy in the acute phase for evacuation of a large intracerebral hematoma or for severe swelling with increased intracranial pressure. Carotid endarterectomy in appropriately selected patients has been shown to reduce the risk of recurrent stroke.[12] In patients with chronic impairments from stroke, tendon lengthening procedures are occasionally needed for contractures.

Potential Disease Complications

Seizures can develop as an early or late complication of stroke, with strokes involving the cerebral cortex and hemorrhagic stroke carrying greater risk. The risk of deep venous thrombosis (DVT) is substantially elevated in hemiplegic stroke, and prophylactic treatment with subcutaneous heparin or low molecular weight heparin is advisable during the initial recovery phase.[13] The ideal duration of DVT prophylaxis post-stroke has not been established, though most in most cases it is discontinued after a period of several weeks. Stroke recurrence is a feared complication, and individuals with a history of stroke remain at increased risk for recurrent stroke despite risk factor reduction. Aspiration pneumonia can occur as a complication of dysphagia, though this risk tends to abate over time, except in the most severe cases.

Potential Treatment Complications

Both anticoagulants and antiplatelet medications can contribute to bleeding complications. Aspirin can cause gastritis. Ticlopidine has been associated with leukopenia and requires monitoring. Clopidogrel has been associated with thrombotic thrombocytopenic purpura (TTP).

Anticholinergic medications (e.g., oxybutynin, tolterodine) commonly cause dry mouth and may precipitate urinary retention. Antispasticity medications (e.g., baclofen, tizanidine, diazepam) can cause sedation and may exacerbate cognitive impairments. Sildenafil is known to be hazardous when used concurrently with nitrates and should be avoided in patients receiving these medications. SSRIs can cause gastrointestinal symptoms (especially nausea or anorexia), as well as interfere with libido and sexual function. Psychostimulants (e.g., methylphenidate, dextroamphetamine) can cause anorexia, insomnia, anxiety, or agitation and should be slowly titrated upwards for these reasons. Gabapentin is usually well tolerated, although occasional sedation has been reported. Carbamezapine may cause leukopenia.

References

1. American Heart Association: 2001 Heart and Stroke Statistical Update. Dallas, American Heart Association, 2000.
2. Bostom AG, Rosenberg IH, Silbershatz H, et al: Nonfasting plasma total homocysteine levels and stroke incidence in elderly persons: The Framingham Study. Ann Intern Med 1999;131(5):352–355.
3. Lansberg MG, Albers GW, Beaulieu C, Marks MP: Comparison of diffusion-weighted MRI and CT in acute stroke. Neurology 2000;54:1557–1561.
4. Anonymous: Tissue plasminogen activator for acute ischemic stroke. The National Institute of Neurological Disorders and Stroke rt-PA Stroke Study Group. N Engl J Med 1995;333:1581–1587.
5. The Boston Area Anticoagulation Trial for Atrial Fibrillation Investigators: The effect of low-dose warfarin on the risk of stroke in patients with nonrheumatic atrial fibrillation. N Engl J Med 1990;323:1505–1511.
6. Bronner LL, Kanter DS, Manson JE: Primary prevention of stroke. N Engl J Med 1995;333:1392–1400.
7. Kramer AM, Steiner JF, Schlenker RE, et al: Outcomes and costs after hip fracture and stroke: A comparison of rehabilitation settings. JAMA 1997;277(5):396–404.
8. Mayo NE, Wood-Dauphinee S, Cote R, et al: There's no place like home: An evaluation of early supported discharge for stroke. Stroke 2000;31:1016–1023.
9. Liepert J, Bauder H, Miltner WHR, et al: Treatment-induced cortical reorganization after stroke in humans. Stroke 2000;31:1210–1216.
10. Kimura M, Robinson RG, Kosier JT: Treatment of cognitive impairment after poststroke depression: A double-blind treatment trial. Stroke 2000;31:1482–1486.
11. Chantraine A, Baribeault A, Uebelhart D, Gremion G: Shoulder pain and dysfunction in hemiplegia: effects of functional electrical stimulation. Arch Phys Med Rehabil 1999;80:328–331.
12. Barnett HJ, Taylor DW, Eliasziw M, et al: Benefit of carotid endarterectomy in patients with symptomatic moderate or severe stenosis. North American Symptomatic Carotid Endarterectomy Trial Collaborators. N Engl J Med 1998;339:1415–1425.
13. Gresham G, Duncan PW, Stason WB (Post-Stroke Rehabilitation Guideline panel): Clinical Practice guideline No 16: Poststroke rehabilitation. Rockville, MD, U.S. Department of Health and Human Services, Agency for Health Care Policy and Research, 1995.

142 Stroke (Young)

Randie M. Black-Schaefer, MD

Definition

Four percent of strokes in the United States occur in adults younger than 45 years and an additional 26% percent in the 45 to 65 year old age group.[1] In persons younger than 30 years, more women suffer strokes than men; this trend reverses with advancing age. Strokes in young adults are particularly devastating events because they often occur in otherwise healthy seeming individuals who are in the prime of life and fully involved with family, community, and workplace responsibilities. Young adults also have high expectations of recovery and consequent difficulty adjusting to residual disability.

More than 60 different disorders that cause stroke in young adults have been identified and can be grouped into several broad categories: atherosclerotic disease accounts for approximately 20%, cardiac emboli another 20%, arteropathies 10%, coagulopathies 10%, and peripartum cerebrovascular accidents 5%. Another 20% may be related to mitral valve prolapse, migraine, and oral contraceptive use, and 15% remain unexplained after full evaluation. In a recent series, 2% of ischemic strokes in adults younger than 45 years were related to illegal drug use, mainly cocaine and heroin.[2,3] Approximately 75% of patients younger than 65 will survive 5 years or more following stroke.[1] Individual survival, of course, depends on the specific cause of the stroke and its treatment. Overall, the risk of recurrence in those who have suffered a first stroke is 5% per year.[4]

Symptoms

The presenting neurologic symptoms of stroke are the same in young as in elderly patients and have been reviewed in Chapter 141. The clinician caring for young adult stroke survivors in the outpatient setting is likely to encounter, in addition to neurologic residua of the stroke, a number of secondary symptoms that will require ongoing management. The most common of these are emotional effects, pain, increased muscle tone, bladder dysfunction, sexual dysfunction, and fatigue. These symptoms may also occur in older stroke patients; however, this chapter focuses on the impact they have on the young stroke survivor.

Emotional Effects

The common emotional consequences of stroke are depression, lability, and anxiety. Clinical depression occurs in approximately 40% of patients after stroke; it is more likely in severe strokes and in those affecting the left anterior circulation. Depression can be difficult to identify in aphasic patients who cannot respond reliably to questions about mood and in patients with motor aprosodia (loss of emotional tone in facial expression and voice) due to right hemispheric stroke. Patients tend to become more socially isolated following stroke because of language, cognitive, and/or physical deficits. Loss of social interaction and support increases the likelihood of depression. Stress related to marital role reversal after a stroke in one member of a couple is common, as is depression in caregivers.[5]

Neurologically mediated emotional lability, in which the patient has abrupt, difficult to control episodes of crying or laughing in response to mention of an emotionally meaningful topic, may be a source of embarrassment and distress to the patient and family. It may also complicate evaluation of the patient's true emotional state.

Patients may experience heightened anxiety chronically following stroke. In some cases, specific triggers of the anxiety, such as fear of falling while walking with a cane, or fear of being left alone, can be identified in the history.

Pain

Pain is a common problem following stroke in young patients. It usually affects the hemiparetic extremities and may be centrally or peripherally mediated. Shoulder pain occurs in up to 85% of stroke patients, usually during the first 6 to 12 months following stroke.[6] The history and exam should address its many potential causes (Table 1). In addition, younger individuals with partially

TABLE 1. Post-Stroke Shoulder Pain

Disorder	Inferior Subluxation	Rotator Cuff Tear	CRPS I (Shoulder/Hand)	Frozen Shoulder	Impingement Syndrome	Biceps Tendinitis
Exam	Acromio-humeral separation	Positive abduction test Positive drop arm test	Metacarpo-phalangeal compression test Skin color changes	External rotation less than 15 degrees Early scapular motion	Pain with abduction 70–90 degrees End range pain with forward flexion	Positive Yergason's test
	Flaccid	Flaccid or spastic	Flaccid or spastic	Spastic	Spastic	Flaccid or spastic
Diagnostic test	X-ray—standing Scapular plane view	X-ray Arthrogram Subacromial injection of lidocaine MRI	Triple phase bone scan Stellate ganglion block	Arthrogram	Subacromial injection of lidocaine	Tendon sheath injection of lidocaine
Treatment						
Initial	Analgesics, NSAIDs	Analgesics, NSAIDs	Oral cortico-steroids	Analgesics	Analgesics, NSAIDs	Analgesics, NSAIDs
Rehab	Hemi-Harris sling or wheelchair armboard	AAROM electrical stimulation/supraspinatus	AAROM, heat modalities	PROM manipulation	AAROM Scapular mobilization	AAROM
Procedures	None	Subacromial steroids, surgical repair Reduction of internal rotator tone	Stellate ganglion block	Subacromial or intra-articular steroids Debridement Reduction of internal rotator tone	Subacromial steroids Reduction of internal rotator tone	Tendon sheath injection of steroids

AAROM = active assisted range of motion; PROM = passive range of motion.
Adapted from Black-Schaffer RM, Kirsteins AE, Harvey RL: Stroke rehabilitation. 2. Co-morbidities and complications. Arch Phys Med Rehabil 1999;80:S8–S16.

recovered motor function may develop secondary sprains, tendinitis, skin breakdown, and nerve palsies in the paretic extremities, as they are pushed beyond their physiologic limits in the effort to resume normal activities. The normal arm and leg may suffer similar overuse injuries in the course of compensating for the weak side. Heavy use of assistive devices, including canes, walkers, braces, and splints, may contribute to these injuries.

Spasticity

Stiffness and heaviness of muscles and joints are common complaints of young stroke patients in the outpatient setting. These are often due to the evolution of muscle tone from the flaccid to the spastic state that occurs over the first several months following a stroke. Though occasionally helpful in allowing weight bearing on a leg with little voluntary motor return, spasticity more often complicates the patient 's efforts to resume normal motor function. In middle cerebral territory strokes, hypertonicity in the upper extremity typically occurs in a pattern of flexion, adduction, internal rotation, and pronation, involving variable combinations of the muscles subserving these movements. In the lower extremity the usual pattern is extensor with reduced knee flexion, increased plantarflexion and inversion of the ankle, and toe curling. This extensor pattern becomes apparent during gait and contributes to the slow speed and increased energy cost of hemiplegic gait. The reader is referred to Chapter 136 for further discussion of spasticity symptoms.

Joint stiffness may also be due to contracture, which is shortening of the muscles, ligaments, and tendons about a joint due to rheologic changes in the tissues. This is common in the finger joints of the affected hand. Frozen shoulder, with contracture of the glenohumeral joint capsule, also occurs.

Bladder Dysfunction

Chronically diminished bladder control with urge incontinence occurs commonly in younger stroke patients. The history should note chronicity and frequency of the problem; diurnal pattern; presence or absence of the sensation of needing to void; and whether there is a relationship to coughing, laughing, or straining. The patient should be queried about abdominal pain and pain on urination.

Sexual Dysfunction

Whether, and if so how, the physiology of sexual function changes as a result of stroke has not been scientifically established. Nonetheless, a majority of patients report diminished sexual function after their stroke. This may involve diminished libido and/or decreased erectile/ejaculatory function. Decreased libido correlates with the presence of depression; reduced physiologic sexual function correlates with medical co-morbidity. Neither clearly relates to size or location of stroke. A small number of patients report increased libido following stroke, and rarely, troublesome hypersexuality appears.[7,8] The history should note change in interest in and frequency of sexual activity, alteration in ability to achieve erection/ejaculation in males or lubrication/orgasm in females, and presence of depression or active medical co-morbidities that may influence sexual activity level. Medications should be reviewed for antihypertensives, antidepressants, and others that may hinder sexual function.

Fatigue

The complaints of increased fatigue and loss of stamina are common. Young adults who previously never needed naps, now do. Patients become fatigued, physically and mentally, with less effort than before the stroke.[9,10] Return to active work and family life may be limited by fatigue. The history should record the daily pattern of fatigue and sleep, including any symptoms of insomnia or sleep apnea. Medications should be reviewed to identify sedative agents. Depression and loss of physical conditioning may also affect energy levels.

Physical Examination

General

In the outpatient rehabilitation setting the exam of the younger patient after a stroke should include neurologic and functional status for evidence of improvement or deterioration.

Improved motor control in the affected leg may allow trimming back of a brace and progression in gait training to a less supportive assistive device. Worsening motor or sensory exam, on the other hand, may signal not only further cerebral events, but also intercurrent systemic illness, medication intolerance, new peripheral nerve injuries related to positioning or assistive devices, or worsening neuropathy.

Confrontation testing for visual fields and double sensory stimulation tests for visual and tactile neglect provide important information to the patient and clinician about suitability for community mobility, particularly driving. Clock drawing, line cancellation, and reading from a magazine can be quickly performed in the office and provide valuable information about neglect and attention. The Mini Mental State Examination is a rapid and helpful cognitive screen.[11]

The affected arm and leg should be inspected for skin breakdown. Maceration of the palm in a tightly flexed hand and friction marks on the dorsum of the foot and calf of patients using ankle/foot orthoses are common. It is particularly important to identify and treat these early in patients with diminished sensation.

Signs of unusual causative entities should be sought if the etiology of the stroke is unclear. These may include the skin laxity and hypermobility of Ehlers-Danlos syndrome; the unilateral ptosis, miosis, and anhydrosis (Horner's syndrome) associated with carotid dissection; multiple venipuncture marks, suggestive of intravenous drug abuse; livedo reticularis seen in Sneddon's syndrome; the vasculitic rash of connective tissue diseases, and the arachnodactyly and tall habitus of Marfan's syndrome.

Emotional Effects

Mood should be evaluated for signs of depression, lability, and anxiety. For patients with intact verbal function, the *DSM-IV* screening questions for major depression are a useful tool. In severely aphasic patients, the screen must, out of necessity, consider facial expression; gestures; posture; and the reports of caregivers regarding appetite, sleep, and mood. If the caregiver shows signs of depression, it may be helpful to identify this in the interview and offer a referral for further evaluation. Lability can often be elicited by discussing topics such as children or spouse. Physical exam signs of chronic anxiety may include hunched posture, fleeting eye contact, cold or moist hands, mild tachycardia, rapid and hypophonic speech, and ready startle reaction.

Pain

The exam should address appearance, tenderness, pain pattern, and range of motion of the painful regions and assess for signs of specific medical and musculoskeletal disorders. See Table 1 for helpful physical exam signs in the diagnosis of post-stroke shoulder pain.

Spasticity

Muscle tone at the shoulder adductors, elbow flexors and extensors, wrist and finger flexors, knee extensors, and ankle plantarflexors should be assessed and recorded at each visit using the Ashworth scale (Table 2). Pain

TABLE 2.	Modified Ashworth Scale for Measurement of Spasticity
0	No increase in muscle tone
1	Slight increase in muscle tone, manifested by a catch and release or by minimal resistance at the end of range of motion
1+	Slight increase in muscle tone, manifested by a catch, followed by minimal resistance throughout the remainder (less than half) of the ROM
2	More marked increase in muscle tone through most of the ROM, but affected part easily moved
3	Considerable increase in muscle tone, passive movement difficult
4	Affected part rigid in flexion or extension

encountered on range of motion should be recorded. Reflexes should be evaluated, assessing for sustained clonus, which at the ankle can compromise gait and in the wrist and finger flexors may be mistaken for seizure activity.

Bladder Dysfunction

Palpatory exam of the abdomen may reveal suprapubic tenderness, or an enlarged bladder indicative of retention with overflow incontinence.

Sexual Dysfunction

Full gynecologic and urologic exams will screen for infectious, traumatic, neoplastic, and hormonal causes of sexual dysfunction in young stroke survivors. The neurologic exam may reveal a neuropathy (manifested by decreased sensation in the feet/hands, decreased ankle and knee reflexes, and occasionally distal weakness) that may be affecting sexual function.

Fatigue

Idiopathic post-stroke fatigue is a diagnosis of exclusion. The exam must screen the patient for the many illnesses that cause fatigue. Among the more prominent of these in this population are Epstein-Barr viral disease, congestive heart failure, sleep apnea, anemia, dehydration, cerebral hypoperfusion, hypothyroidism, depression, malignancy, medications, and street drugs.

Functional Limitations

Driving

In most U.S. communities, the resumption of driving is a necessary step in returning to a normal lifestyle and avoiding social isolation. Once discharged home, young adult stroke patients are generally eager to resume driving. Many rehabilitation clinics offer written tests of driving ability. Even though these have not been shown to be adequate predictors of on-the-road performance, they serve a useful screening purpose. A number of factors have been shown to predict driving performance after stroke: right hemisphere location of stroke, visual perceptual deficits, reduced sustained and selective attention, impulsivity, poor judgment, and lack of organizational skills all correlate with poor performance behind the wheel. Aphasia, though it may negatively impact performance on written and road tests because of compromised processing of verbal instructions, does not always interfere with self-directed driving. Clinicians are often consulted about a patient's readiness to resume driving, and even though visual perception can be readily screened in an office setting, evaluation for impulsivity, judgment, and organizational ability is far more difficult. An on-the-road test performed either by a driving instructor or by the state licensing agency remains the "gold standard" for assessing driving ability.

Return to Work

The ability to perform valued work is central to self-esteem and an important goal for most young stroke patients. Between 11% and 81% of patients achieve this goal, with the wide range reported in this literature due to differing age ranges, definitions of work, and disability compensation systems. Factors predictive of success in returning to work include pure motor or no hemiparesis, good self-care and mobility function at completion of rehabilitation, no aphasia or apraxia, advanced education, and having a white collar job. Barriers to successful vocational rehabilitation, in addition to the reverse of factors just listed, include cognitive impairment, visual/perceptual impairment, and economic disincentives related to disability and retirement benefits. In the outpatient setting the rehabilitation clinician is often asked to certify that the young stroke patient is "medically cleared" to return to work. This may simply mean indicating that the patient has sufficient cardiovascular capacity to perform the job, but more often a detailed evaluation of the patient's cognitive and physical capacity as they relate to specific job tasks is desired. This assessment is complex and is ideally accomplished with the assistance of a coordinated multidisciplinary team, including physical, occupational, and speech therapist(s); neuropsychologist; and a vocational rehabilitation counselor.

Patients who are able to resume work after a stroke do so on average within the first 6 months. The 1990 Americans with Disabilities Act has had a positive impact on employers' responsiveness to the requests of stroke survivors for job accommodations, not only regarding physical access and equipment but also for personal assistance, schedule flexibility, and task modification.[12]

Parenting

The hemiparetic young adult stroke survivor who needs to return to parenting faces particular challenges in the performance of child bathing, dressing, feeding, and transporting tasks. Problem solving these tasks can be done with the assistance of other adult family members, home care occupational therapists, and/or hired child care assistants. Many helpful items of equipment are readily available, such as paper disposable diapers with easy to close tabs, microwaves for heating bottles, baby tub inserts, etc. Even when frequent assistance is needed, the patient should be encouraged to assume the supervisory role in child care.

Diagnostic Studies

Since the use of illicit drugs has been linked to strokes in younger individuals, ongoing screening in the outpatient setting for this may be indicated. For other diagnostic testing, see Chapter 141.

Differential Diagnosis

Hemiplegic migraine	Brain neoplasm
Postseizure (Todd's) paralysis	Multiple sclerosis

Treatment

Initial

The outpatient setting affords an excellent opportunity for the young stroke survivor and his or her clinician to review the etiology of the stroke, identify modifiable risk factors for recurrence, and jointly develop a plan to minimize these. The patient's motivation to comply with treatment for hypertension and diabetes; to develop a habit of compliance with newly prescribed anticoagulation therapy; and to quit smoking, avoid excessive alcohol intake, and turn away from the use of street drugs will be maximal in the months following the stroke. The remainder of this section will discuss specific treatments for the secondary symptoms previously detailed.

Emotional Effects

Post-stroke depression responds to antidepressant medications of several classes. The lower cardiac risk profile of selective serotonin reuptake inhibitors makes them an attractive option in patients with arrhythmias. They should be used with caution in patients with sexual dysfunction or significant spasticity, however. The sedative and urinary retentive properties of tricyclic antidepressants may be helpful for patients with concomitant sleep disturbance or urge incontinence. Family and community support, including local and national stroke support and education groups, are important resources for the young patient who is struggling with emotional adjustment to residual disability and altered lifestyle. Referral to a psychiatrist, psychologist, home care social worker, or psychiatric nurse is often helpful. Emotional lability may respond to selective serotonin reuptake inhibitors and usually diminishes over time. Management of anxiety in cognitively impaired young stroke patients should emphasize non-sedating anxiolytics such as buspirone, counseling, and environmental manipulation to reduce known triggers.

Pain

Measures for soft tissue based pain include non-narcotic analgesics and NSAIDs/COX-2 inhibitors. When narcotic relief is required, the fentanyl transdermal patch is a useful option. Neuropathic and central pain syndromes often respond to gabapentin. Tizanidine or gabapentin, both of which have analgesic effects independent of their muscle relaxant action, may help pain related to spasticity. See Table 1 for treatment options for the several varieties of post-stroke shoulder pain.

Spasticity

The management of muscle stiffness due to spasticity is discussed in detail in Chapter 136. Intercurrent infections, localized sores, stress, and anxiety can worsen spasticity and should be treated before adding other interventions. Sedation in this cognitively fragile population is to be avoided and limits dosage titration of all the available antispasticity agents. Tizanidine and gabapentin, because of their analgesic as well as antispasticity actions, are logical choices for painful spasticity. Selective serotonin reuptake inhibitors occasionally exacerbate spasticity.

Bladder Dysfunction

Frequent timed voiding, avoidance of evening fluid intake, use of padded clothing, and a commode or urinal by the bedside are helpful management strategies for the spastic neurogenic bladder post-stroke. External catheter drainage in males may be useful. Tricyclic antidepressants provide mild anticholinergic stimulation and can be used to increase bladder capacity in stroke patients, although the anticholinergics oxybutynin and tolterodine are first line agents.

Sexual Dysfunction

Treatment of depression (with medications such as bupropion, mirtazapine, or nefazodone, which do not hinder sexual function)[13] and of active concurrent medical illnesses can promote improved sexual functioning. Eliminating other medications that compromise ejaculatory or orgasmic function will obviously help as well. Treatment with testosterone to enhance libido and with sildenafil to improve erection, or estrogen to improve lubrication may be considered.

Fatigue

Efforts to ensure a normal sleep-wake cycle should be made. These include maintaining a consistent and appropriate bedtime, avoiding stimulant beverages late in the day, and taking hypnotics such as diphenhydramine or trazodone at bedtime, if needed. For the patient who sleeps well at night but remains easily fatigued during the day, a trial of methylphenidate or dextroamphetamine on arising and at noon may be considered. Loss of initiation due to frontal lobe disease may be perceived as fatigue and occasionally responds to amantadine. For the depressed patient with fatigue, a non-sedating antidepressant should be chosen. Short daytime naps in patients with normal nighttime sleep pattern should not be discouraged.

Rehabilitation

Emotional Effects

Neurologic and functional improvement are perhaps the best antidotes to post-stroke depression. A multidisciplinary stroke rehabilitation program that provides graded and progressive activities in many areas gives the patient the opportunity to make and to appreciate numerous improvements in parameters of mobility, self-care, language, and cognition. Therapists are skilled at providing encouragement and positive reinforcement for successes, large and small, in the targeted activities. The rehabilitation therapy environment, indeed, provides tremendous psychologic support to the patient, and it is common for depression first to become evident, or to worsen abruptly, at the time outpatient therapy finishes and this support system is withdrawn.

Pain

Rehabilitation treatment of pain syndromes is useful both in itself and because it allows close monitoring by a qualified therapist of the patient's symptoms and response to treatments. Soft tissue injuries often respond to stretching and strengthening, electrical stimulation of the affected muscles, and heat modalities (when sensation is adequate to allow their use). Transcutaneous electrical nerve stimulation (TENS) and functional electrical stimulation are often helpful in poorly defined shoulder pain, as are arm slings, such as the Harris hemi-sling, that promote optimal glenohumeral alignment.

Spasticity

Mild post-stroke spasticity in the heel cord and finger and wrist flexors can often be adequately controlled with a stretching program performed two to three times per day by the patient. For full discussion of rehabilitation measures for managing spasticity, see Chapter 136.

Bladder Dysfunction

Pelvic floor strengthening exercises are helpful for stress incontinence. There are no specific rehabilitation treatments for detrussor instability, although the patient's therapists are often in a position to observe and document the extent of the problem.

Fatigue

A tailored cardiovascular conditioning program is helpful to maximize the patient's aerobic capacity and physical stamina. Patients with significant physical impairment will benefit from a physical therapist's assistance in designing an adapted conditioning program, which may emphasize use of a stationary bicycle, arm ergometer, and therapeutic pool. Patients with limiting cardiovascular co-morbidities will require the clinician's input for heart rate and blood pressure guidelines.

Procedures

Emotional Effects

Electroconvulsive therapy may be indicated for refractory depression.

Spasticity

Muscle and nerve blocks with botulinum toxin and phenol can enhance gait pattern and hand function in young stroke survivors. See Chapter 136 for full discussion of these procedures.

Pain

Acupuncture can be beneficial for central pain syndromes, and subacromial bursa steroid injection will help approximately 50% of patients with post-stroke shoulder pain. Botulinum toxin and phenol injections provide relief when pain is due to spasticity in specific muscles.

Surgery

Pain

In post-stroke shoulder pain, surgical repair may be considered when rotator cuff tear can be established as the etiology, and surgical debridement may be required for severe, unremitting frozen shoulder.

Spasticity

Tendon lengthening, infrequently performed in elderly stroke patients because of limited life expectancy and medical risks, should be considered in younger patients when the pattern of hypertonicity has stabilized. It may allow improved gait in chronic equinovarus posturing due to spastic triceps surae and tibialis posterior or anterior muscles. Electrophysiologic evaluation of the extremity in a gait lab can provide useful information to supplement the physical exam and help ensure that the optimal muscles are targeted for surgical intervention.

Bladder Dysfunction

Bladder suspension surgery may be indicated for stress incontinence.

Potential Disease Complications

The spectrum of neurologic and medical complications of stroke is similar in young adults to that in older stroke patients. See Chapter 141.

Potential Treatment Complications

Complications of stroke treatment are similar in young and older adults. They are discussed in Chapter 141.

References

1. Weinfeld FD: National survey of stroke. Stroke 1981;1232 (pt 2 Suppl 1):I1–90.
2. Adams HP, Kappelle LJ, Biller J, et al: Ischemic stroke in young adults. Arch Neurol 1995;52:491–495.
3. Hart RG, Miller VT: Cerebral infarction in young adults: A practical approach. Stroke 1983;14: 110–114.
4. Sacco RL: Risk factors and outcomes for ischemic stroke. Neurology 1995;45(Suppl 1):S10–S14.
5. Dennis M, O'Rourke S, Lewis S, et al: Emotional outcomes after stroke: Factors associated with poor outcome. Neurol Neurosurg Psychiatry 2000;68:47.
6. Agency for Healthcare Policy and Research: Post-stroke Rehabilitation Clinical Practice Guideline. Rockville, MD, Agency for Healthcare Policy and Research, 1995: p.125.
7. Korpaelainen JT, Nieminen P, Myllyla VV: Sexual functioning among stroke patients and their spouses. Stroke 1999;30:715–719.
8. Carod J, Egido J, Gonzalez JL, et al: Poststroke sexual dysfunction and quality of life. Stroke 1999;30:2238–2239.
9. Sisson RA: Life after a stroke: Coping with change. Rehabil Nurs 1998;23:198–203.
10. Ingles JL, Eskes GA, Phillips SJ: Fatigue after stroke. Arch Phys Med Rehabil 1999;80:173–178.
11. Folstein MF, Folstein SE, McHugh PR: Mini-mental state: A practical method for grading the cognitive state of patients for the clinician. J Psychiat Res 1975;12:189–198.
12. Black-Schaffer RM, Lemieux L: Vocational outcome after stroke. Top Stroke Rehabil 1994;1:74–86.
13. Hirschfield RM: Care of the sexually active depressed patient. J Clin Psychiatry 1999;60(Suppl 17):32–35; discussion 46–48.

143 Systemic Lupus Erythematosus

Mahboob U. Rahman, MD, PhD

Synonyms

Lupus

Lupus Erythematosus

SLE

ICD-9 Code

710.0
Systemic lupus
erythematosus

Definition

Systemic lupus erythematosus (SLE) is an autoimmune multisystem disorder of unknown etiology with variable clinical and laboratory manifestations, course, and prognosis. The manifestations of SLE can vary from mild skin rashes and musculoskeletal symptoms to potentially life threatening involvement of major organ systems, including the kidneys, lungs, and heart, and the hematopoietic, gastrointestinal, and central nervous systems. Many other organs/systems can be involved alone or in combination. The characteristic laboratory manifestation is the presence of autoantibodies directed against the various components of the nucleus of a cell and thus termed as antinuclear antibodies (ANAs).

Although SLE is primarily a disease of young women of reproductive age, pediatric and geriatric cases are also encountered. The female-to-male ratio in the peak incidence group (15 to 40-year-olds) is approximately 5:1. The prevalence among the general population is approximately 1 in every 2000 persons, but it varies according to race, ethnicity, and socioeconomic background.

Classification criteria, which are essential for clinical trials and may provide a useful reference for clinical practice, have been proposed (see Table 1). Both the sensitivity and specificity of these criteria for the diagnosis of SLE is 95% (i.e., 5% of patients who have SLE will not meet these criteria, and 5% of patients who do not have SLE may meet these criteria for the diagnosis of SLE).

TABLE 1. American College of Rheumatology Criteria for the Classification of SLE*

1. Malar rash
2. Discoid rash
3. Photosensitivity
4. Oral ulcers
5. Arthritis
6. Serositis
7. Renal disorder (persistent proteinuria [more than 0.5 g/day] or cellular casts)
8. Neurologic disorder (seizures or psychosis)
9. Hematologic disorder (hemolytic anemia, leukopenia, lymphopenia, or thrombocytopenia)
10. Immunologic disorder (anti-DNA antibodies, anti-Sm antibodies, positive lupus erythematosus [LE] cell preparation)
11. Antinuclear antibody

* A patient may be classified as having SLE if 4 or more of the 11 criteria are present at any time.
Modified from reference 1.

The severity of the disease is also extremely variable, and a waxing and waning clinical course is common. The disease can be mild enough or can be controlled in most cases to allow for an essentially normal life with jobs and children. Pregnancy, however, can be complicated and requires close monitoring by a high risk obstetrician. Patients with SLE are at a much higher risk for developing atherosclerotic disease than is the general population.

Symptoms

The presentation varies widely according to the organ systems involved.[1,2] Most patients present with musculoskeletal and mucocutaneous symptoms, Raynaud's phenomenon, and chronic fatigue. The first noticeable symptom may be the classic "butterfly rash" across the nose. It is not uncommon to have a life threatening illness and severe disability due to involvement of major organ systems early in the course of the disease.

Pain, weakness, and generalized fatigue are all common symptoms of SLE (Table 2).

TABLE 2. Signs and Symptoms of SLE

Organ Systems	Signs/Symptoms
Constitutional	Fatigue, malaise, fever, anorexia, etc.
Skin and mucous membrane	Skin rashes (including the typical malar or "butterfly" rash, discoid and other rashes) Photosensitivity (develop skin rash and constitutional symptoms) Oral/nasal ulcerations (typically painless at the onset)

Musculoskeletal system	Joint pain
	    Polyarthralgia (symmetric joint pain)
	    Polyarthritis (symmetric joint pain with swelling, warmth, erythema, and morning stiffness)
	    Osteonecrosis (usually the ends of the long bones, and thus joint pain)
	Muscles
	    Myalgia (muscle aches/pain)
	    Myositis (muscle aches/pain and weakness)

Serosal	Pleuritis (pleuritic chest pain, shortness of breath) Pericarditis (chest pain, rarely associated with hemodynamic compromise) Peritoneal inflammation (often presents with diffuse abdominal pain)
Cardiovascular	Raynaud's phenomenon Myocarditis/endocarditis (chest pain, shortness of breath, peripheral edema) Vasculitis—small vessel (variable presentation depending on organs involved)
Pulmonary	Interstitial disease/"shrinking lung syndrome" (cough, shortness of breath) Pneumonitis/pulmonary hemorrhage (shortness of breath, cough, hemoptysis) Pulmonary hypertension (shortness of breath, syncope)
Hematologic	Lymphadenopathy (swollen glands) Thrombocytopenia (easily bruised, purpuric skin rash) Hemolytic anemia (fatigue, weakness, pallor)
Renal/Urologic	Lupus nephritis (peripheral edema, dark urine) Lupoid cystitis (urgency, frequency, and dysuria with sterile urine)

Neuropsychiatric	Neurologic
	    Headache (particularly refractory migraine-like headaches)
	    Seizures
	    Cerebral vascular accidents
	    Peripheral neuropathy
	    Cranial neuropathy
	    Transverse myelitis
	Psychiatric
	    Cognitive dysfunction
	    Depression
	    Psychosis

Physical Examination

Because so many organ systems may be involved, it is important to conduct a thorough physical examination (Table 2).

Constitutional signs may include fever, tachycardia, bradycardia, tachypnea, and conjunctival pallor. Skin rashes include the typical maculopapular erythematous malar or "butterfly" rash and discoid and other rashes, including purpura. Oral/nasal ulcerations, lymphadenopathy, heart murmur, pleural and/or pericardial rub and other signs of heart failure and pleural effusion, diffuse abdominal tenderness, hepatosplenomegaly, stigmata of deep vein thrombosis and/or arterial thrombosis including pulmonary embolism, and peripheral edema can be detected during physical examination.

The musculoskeletal system is commonly involved and may cause stiffness, swelling, pain in joints and periarticular structures, and weakness of muscles from acute and chronic inflammation. Examination may reveal symmetric swelling, tenderness, warmth, erythema, and decreased range of motion of joints.

Although the arthritis in SLE is usually non-erosive, damage of periarticular structures can lead to tendon rupture and/or reducible joint deformities/subluxation (Jacoud's arthropathy) and may compromise hand function. The joints usually lack the exuberant synovitis seen in rheumatoid arthritis, and quite often, joint tenderness is out of proportion to physical and radiologic findings. Muscle tenderness and weakness and fibromyalgia tender points can also be seen.

Focal neurologic signs and change in mental status may indicate central nervous system involvement by SLE.

Functional Limitations

Functional limitations vary widely depending on the severity of the disease and which organ systems are involved. Some patients may have no limitations. If musculoskeletal or joint involvement is present, pain, weakness, and loss of range of motion can limit hand, arm, and leg function. Typically, patients have difficulty dressing, bathing, doing household chores, working, and participating in recreational activities. Mobility, including walking and running, might also be affected. Cardiac and/or pulmonary involvement may affect endurance. Central nervous system sequelae can be particularly devastating, and limitations depend on the part of the brain affected.

Diagnostic Studies

The wide variation in the manifestation of SLE often makes both the diagnosis and management of the condition a challenge. Diagnosis of SLE requires a careful, elaborate history; a meticulous physical examination; and diagnostic studies that depend on disease manifestations. The classification criteria (see Table 1) can also be a useful guide in making the diagnosis.

Some of the common but non-specific laboratory findings include anemia; positive Coomb's test; elevated erythrocyte sedimentation rate (ESR), C-reactive protein, transaminases, creatine phosphokinase (CPK), aldolase, amylase, lipase, blood urea nitrogen (BUN), and creatinine levels. Proteinuria, dysmorphic red blood cells (RBCs), RBC and white blood cell (WBC) casts in urinalysis, indicate kidney involvement. When suspicion for SLE is high on clinical grounds, some of the following more specific tests are usually ordered to establish the diagnosis of SLE[3,4]:

- ANA and antibodies to ENA ([extractable nuclear antigens], which include Ro, La, Sm, and U1RNP) (Table 3)
- Anticardiolipin antibodies, lupus anticoagulant, and false-positive non-specific tests for syphilis (e.g., VDRL)—may confirm the presence of SLE associated antiphospholipid antibody syndrome.

TABLE 3. Commonly Used Serologic Tests for SLE

Antibody	Sensitivity for SLE*	Specificity for SLE[†]	Clinical Correlation
ANA	95	+	Screening test; specificity 60%; also present in other autoimmune/rheumatic/inflammatory disorders, infections, and approximately 8% of normal population; patterns of ANA are usually non-specific except for certain antibodies (e.g., peripheral nuclear pattern [anti-dsDNA] seen in SLE, centromere pattern [anticentromere], seen in 75% of patients with CREST [calcinosis, Raynaud's phenomenon, esophageal dysmotility, sclerodactyly, and telangiectasia] syndrome, nucleolar pattern [antinucleolar, usually seen in scleroderma])
Anti-dsDNA	60–90	++	Glomerulonephritis; titres may correlate with disease activity
AntiHistones	50–70	+	Drug-induced lupus
Anti-Ro (SS-A)	20–60	+	Subacute cutaneous lupus; neonatal SLE and congenital heart block; anti-Ro in 60% and anti-La in 50% of patients with Sjögren's disease; "ANA (-) SLE"
Anti-La (SS-B)	15–40	+	
Anti-Sm	10–30	++	Nephritis, CNS involvement; titres may correlate with disease activity[‡]
Anti-RNP	10–30	+	Mixed connective tissue disease[‡]
Anti-U1RNP	10	+	Mixed connective tissue disease[‡]
Anti-P	10–15	++	CNS lupus, lupus psychosis
Anti-Cardiolipin	10–30	–	Thrombosis, fetal loss, thrombocytopenia

* The sensitivity of the test depends on the frequency at which the antibodies are detected in patients with SLE.
[†] ++ = highly specific; + = antibody present in other autoimmune disorders; – = antibody present in other inflammatory diseases.
[‡] An overlap syndrome of SLE, polymyositis, and scleroderma occurs in higher frequency in patients with anti-RNP and anti-Sm antibodies. The presence of anti-U1RNP antibodies is a requirement for the diagnosis of mixed connective tissue disease .

- Elevated serum concentrations of immune complexes and evidence of complement consumption (e.g., decreased serum concentrations of complement split products such as C4b, C5a, and sC5b-9) can be a good indicator of SLE disease actitivity.

Radiographs of involved joints may reveal periarticular osteopenia without bony erosion and may also show signs of advanced osteonecrosis. Radiographs of the chest can show pleural effusion, increased interstitial markings, prominent pulmonary vessels, consolidations, and cardiomegaly. High resolution computerized tomography (CT) scan of the chest may be needed when pulmonary hemorrhage or active interstitial lung disease is suspected. CT scan and ultrasound studies may help diagnose lupoid hepatitis and pancreatitis. MRI can detect early osteonecrosis.

Biopsy of involved tissues (commonly the skin and kidneys), lumbar puncture, and cultures are often needed to rule out other possible diagnoses.

Differential Diagnosis

Other autoimmune disorders and overlap syndrome (e.g., mixed connective rissue disease (MCTD), polymyositis/dermatomyositis, scleroderma, Raynaud's disease, spondyloarthropathies, rheumatoid arthritis)

Dermatitis

Hematologic disorders (e.g., idiopathic thrombocytopenic purpura)

Neurologic disorders (e.g., epilepsy, multiple sclerosis)

Psychiatric disorders

Treatment

Initial

Treatment depends on the particular manifestations for a given patient (see Table 2), but there are some general principles of management, including patient education and psychosocial interventions, avoidance of sun exposure (which is well known to cause exacerbation of SLE), assiduous treatment of hypertension, treatment of clotting diatheses, and prompt evaluation of unexplained fever (since these patients are immunocompromised either due to disease activity or the medication used to treat SLE). Immunizations with influenza and pneumococcal vaccines and antibiotic prophylaxis for any invasive procedures such as dental work (if the patient is taking immunosuppressive medications. Finally, a reliable means of family planning is needed since pregnancy can cause flare up of disease. These patients need close monitoring by a high risk obstetrician, especially because these patients are often taking medications for which safety in pregnancy has not been established. Patients with musculoskeletal symptoms or serositis frequently respond to NSAIDS. Analgesics may also be used for pain control.

Antimalarials, especially hydroxychloroquine, are the most commonly used second line agent for such symptoms and are also used for SLE skin lesions. Ideally, corticosteroids should be reserved for major organ system involvement and life threatening situations; they are, however, widely used for many manifestations of SLE. For skin disease, topical steroid preparations may suffice. For patients who require high doses of steroids for long periods, immunosuppressive drugs such as cyclophosphamide, azathioprine, methotrexate, cyclosporin, and mycophenolate mofetil may be used as steroid-sparing agents. Depending on disease manifestations, hormonal therapies (danazol, prolactin secretion inhibition by bromcriptine, DHEA [dehydroepiandrosterone], plasma exchange and intravenous immunoglobulin (IVIG) [for thrombocytopenia and pulmonary hemorrhage], and dapsone [cutaneous disease] may also be useful.

Rehabilitation

Depending on the manifestations of the disease, patients may benefit from skilled physical and occupational therapy.

Although the arthropathy of SLE is usually mild and non-aggressive and can be adequately controlled by general medical treatment, therapists can assist with fabricating splints and performing gentle range of motion and strengthening exercises. In an acutely inflamed joint, aggressive movement is avoided and strengthening is typically done statically. Modalities such as paraffin baths can also help decrease pain and improve range of motion. Even with treatment, non-erosive SLE arthropathy can still lead to reducible subluxation/deformities with ulnar deviation and swan-neck deformities of the hands (Jacoud's type arthropathy) that resembles rheumatoid arthritis.

Patients with severe involvement of their hands may benefit from adaptive equipment such as elastic (no tie) shoelaces and reacher and wide handled tools (e.g., scissors, knives). For indivudals who use the computer, voice activated software or a foot computer mouse may be beneficial.

Patients with severe pulmonary and cardiac manifestations and extreme fatigue may also benefit from physical or occupational therapy to learn pacing strategies, breathing exercises, and relaxation techniques. Gentle conditioning exercises may be appropriate in some individuals to improve cardiovascular endurance.[5,13–18]

If mobility is affected, physical therapy can be ordered to specifically address walking and transfers. Appropriate assistive devices such as canes and walkers can be provided by the physical therapist, who will also instruct the patient on how to use the device. Patients who have siginificant lower extremity weakness may benefit from bracing. In some cases, wheelchairs or scooters may be necessary.

Procedures

Depending on disease manifestation, patients may benefit from corticosteroid injections of joints, bursae, tendons sheaths, and tender points. Patients may also require thoracentesis, pericardiocentesis, pleuradesis and pleural stripping, pericardial window, bronchoscopy, lumbar puncture, and biopsy of involved tissue for both diagnostic and therapeutic purposes. Patients with end stage lupus nephropathy are managed with dialysis or kidney transplantation.[5–12]

Surgery

SLE is a multisystem organ disease and rarely may require surgery to manage the disease manifestations or complications (e.g., ischemic bowels).

Potential Disease Complications

Depending on disease manifestations, complications may range from reducible joint deformities/subluxations (Jacoud's arthropathy) to life threatening renal, pulmonary, cardiac, vasculitic, thrombotic, GI, and CNS complications—some of which could be irreversible.

Potential Treatment Complications

Side effects of commonly used medications in SLE are listed in Table 4.[5–12]

TABLE 4. Side Effects of Commonly Used Medications in SLE

Medication	Side Effects	Medication	Side Effects
Traditional NSAIDs	Dyspepsia Peptic ulcer GI bleeding Platelet dysfunction Renal insufficiency Hepatotoxicity Rash Aseptic meningitis	Cyclophosphamide	Dyspepsia/diarrhea Myelosupression Myeloproliferative disorders/ other malignancies Hemorrhagic cystitis Infertility Alopecia
COX-2 selective NSAIDs	Dyspepsia Renal insufficiency Hepatotoxicity Rash	Azathioprine	Myelosuppression Hepatotoxicity Pancreatitis Lymphoproliferative disorders (long-term risk)
Gluocorticoids	Increased appetite/weight gain Cushingoid habitus Acne Fluid retention Hypertension Diabetes Glaucoma/cataracts Atherosclerosis Avascular necrosis Osteoporosis Impaired wound healing Increased susceptibility to infection	Methotrexate Mycophenolate mofetil	Hepatic fibrosis/cirrhosis Pneumonitis Myelosuppression Mucositis Dyspepsia Alopecia Dyspepsia Diarrhea/vomiting Myelosuppression Leukopenia Infection/sepsis Hypertension Tremor
Antimalarials	Dyspepsia Macular damage Abnormal skin pigmentation Neuromyopathy Rash	Cyclosporin A	Renal insufficiency Hypertension Anemia Hirsutism Tremor Gum hyperplasia

References

1. Tan EM, Cohen AS, Fries JF, et al: The 1982 revised criteria for the classifaction of systematic lupus erythematosus (SLE). Arthritis Rheum 1982;25:1271–1277.
2. Boumpas DT, Austin HA, Fessler BJ, et al: Systemic lupus erthematosus: Renal, neuorpsychiatric, cardiovascular, pulmonoary, and hematologic disease. Ann Intern Med 1995;122:940–950.
3. Maddison PJ: Autoantibody profile. In Maddison PJ, Isenberg DJ, Woo P, Glass DN (eds): Oxford Textbook of Rheumatology, 2nd ed. Oxford, Oxford University Press, 1998, pp 665–676.
4. Elkon KB: Autoantibodies in SLE. In Klippel JH, Dieppe PA (eds): Rheumatology, 2nd ed. Philadelphia, Mosby, 1998, pp 7.5.1.
5. Di Cesare PE, Zuckerman JD: Articular manifestations of systemic lupus erythematosus. In Lahita RG (ed): Systemic Lupus Erythematosus, 3rd ed. New York, Academic Press, 1999, p 793.
6. Spalton DJ, Verdon Roe GM, Hughes GRV: Hyrdoxychlorquine, dosage parameters and retinopathy. Lupus 1993;2:355–358.
7. Wilson K, Abeles M: A 2 year open-ended trial of methotrexate in systemic lupus erythematosus. J Rheumatol 1994;21:1674–1677.
8. Waltz-LeBlanc BA, Dagenais P, Urowitz MB, Gladman DD: Methotrexate in systemic lupus erythematosus. J Rheumatol 1994;21:836–838.
9. Klippel JH: Is aggressive therapy effective for lupus? Rheum Dis Clin North Am 1993;19:249–261.
10. Wang CL, Wang F, Bosco JJ: Ovarian failure in oral cyclophosphamide treatment for systemic lupus erythematosus. Lupus 1995;4:11–14.
11. Khamashta MA, Ruiz-Irastorza G, Hughes GR: Therapy of systemic lupus erythematosus: New agents and new evidence. Expert Opin Investig Drugs 2000;9(7):1581–1593.
12. Chan TM, Li FK, Tang CS, et al: Efficacy of mycophenolate mofetil in patients with diffuse proliferative lupus nephritis. Hong Kong-Guangzhou Nephrology Study Group. N Engl J Med 2000;343(16):1156–1162.
13. Forte S, Carlone S, Vaccaro F, et al: Pulmonary gas exchange and exercise capacity in patients with systemic lupus erythematosus. J Rheumatol 1999;26(12):2591–2594.
14. Kipen Y, Briganti EM, Strauss BJ, et al: Three year follow-up of body composition changes in pre-menopausal women with systemic lupus erythematosus. Rheumatology (Oxford) 1999;38(1):59–65.
15. Daltroy LH, Robb-Nicholson C, Iversen MD, et al: Effectiveness of minimally supervised home aerobic training in patients with systemic rheumatic disease. Br J Rheumatol 1995;34(11):1064–1069.
16. Robb-Nicholson LC, Daltroy L, Eaton H, et al: Effects of aerobic conditioning in lupus fatigue: a pilot study. Br J Rheumatol 1989;28(6):500–505.
17. Jonsson H, Nived O, Sturfelt G, et al: Lung function in patients with systemic lupus erythematosus and persistent chest symptoms. Br J Rheumatol 1989;28(6):492–499.
18. Labowitz RJ, Challman J, Palmeri S: Aerobic exercise in the management of rheumatic diseases. Del Med J 1988;60(11):659–662.

144 Transverse Myelitis

Deborah Reiss Schneider, MD

Synonyms

Transverse myelitis

Idiopathic transverse myelitis

Myelitis

Myelopathy

ICD-9 Code

323.9
Unspecified cause of encephalitis

Definition

Myelitis refers to inflammation of the spinal cord. Transverse myelitis indicates inflammation across one or several levels. Idiopathic transverse myelitis implies no specific viral or bacterial agent or any known inflammatory cause can be found.[2]

The incidence of transverse myelitis in the United States is approximately 4.6 cases per million per year.[4,5] The onset of transverse myelitis is variable. Up to 45% of cases may worsen maximally within the first 24 hours, whereas other cases take as long as a few weeks to fully present.[1,3] Presentations may be categorized into three groups: (1) smoothly progressive onset with ascending symptoms, (2) subacute gradually progressive onset, and (3) hyperacute catastrophic onset. The hyperacute onset often results in a more profound illness and a poorer outcome.[6] Recovery is commonly complete and may take anywhere from 1 to 3 months. If no recovery has occurred by 2 to 3 months, then complete recovery is less likely.[4-6]

Infectious causes may present more acutely and may be more likely to present with spinal shock than other causes, such as multiple sclerosis. In one study, the infectious group tended to have more back pain, ascending dysfunction over more segments, and spinal cord swelling on MRI. Seventy-three percent of the infectious associated group had a preceding upper respiratory tract illness.[4]

Symptoms

Patients with transverse myelitis may present with back or neck pain, pain or girdle sensations around the trunk, fever, flu-like sensations, weakness in the arms or legs (often more pronounced on one side initially), sensory abnormalities (temperature, pain, light touch, position, vibration), and difficulty with bowel or bladder function.

Inflammation of the spinal cord may cause partial or complete paralysis. Presentation can be as a posterior column syndrome, anterior spinothalamic tract syndrome, hemicord syndrome, non-specific pattern, or complete spinal cord injury. Bowel and bladder dysfunction commonly occurs. The level of the inflammation determines which limbs or which part of the trunk may be affected. In one study, transverse myelitis affected the cervical region most commonly, followed by the upper thoracic region.[7] Individuals may commonly complain of sensations of tight bands and dysesthesias around the trunk at the levels of the lesion.[3] Involvement of cognitive function or cranial nerves is generally not seen with idiopathic transverse myelitis and suggests another diagnosis.

The history should also include a complete review about symptoms associated with infection, autoimmune diseases, space occupying lesions, multiple sclerosis, immunizations, and vitamin deficiencies. Each infection, autoimmune disease, or compressive myelopathy has unique characteristics, and these should be explored. The season may determine which virus is more likely.[2] An individual's exposure to certain environments, pets, and travel; past medical history; and family history can all provide clues as to the cause. A full review of systems will help clarify possible systemic causes. Questions regarding upper respiratory tract illnesses, recent vaccines, animal bites, tick bites, joint aches, vision changes, muscle pain, rashes, cough, chest pains, problems with breathing, nausea, constipation, and difficulty with voiding should all be asked. Individuals with transverse myelitis from any cause may complain of back, leg, or arm pains, so this information is explored in detail to rule out reversible conditions. A complete social history may reveal an exposure to an infection or reveal chronically traumatic exercise routines to the back or nerves.

Physical Examination

Most infections or autoimmune illnesses affecting the spinal cord also affect other systems. Therefore, the physical examination must be complete and systematic in its exploration for possible etiologies. Since spinal cord inflammation may be devastating to an individual's functioning, no treatable cause should be missed.

Vital signs may indicate a problem with oxygenation or blood flow to the spinal cord. Temperature elevations may indicate an infection. Complete evaluation of the lungs, heart, gastrointestinal system, genitourinary system, and joints may provide clues to an autoimmune disease, vitamin deficiency, or infection. Clearly, an in-depth neurologic examination is essential. Cognitive dysfunction or abnormalities of the cranial nerves may exclude the diagnosis of idiopathic transverse myelitis. Full evaluation of motor weakness or coordination; reflexes; and sensory loss of pinprick, light touch, vibration, position sense, or temperature will help determine the level of involvement and the focus of diagnostic testing.[3]

Functional Limitations

As with any spinal cord injury, functional limitations depend on the level of the injury. If an individual is not severely debilitated from other illnesses, possible function is determined by which muscles continue to be innervated. Individuals with C4 as their maximum functioning level remain dependent for most self-care. Some environmental control can be created by sip-and-puff devices, head or cheek or tongue controls, or voice activation. A functioning C5 level allows for some self-feeding. Independent use of a power wheelchair and driving is possible. C6 innervation allows for some self-care in dress, independent transferring, use of a manual wheelchair, and self-catheterization with assistive devices. T1 innervation allows an individual to function with partial standby physical assistance, independent use of a manual wheelchair, and in most cases self-catheterization. Upper thoracic musculature allows for easier use of manual wheelchairs, and individuals are independent in self-care of their bladder and bowels. Some ambulation with knee-ankle-foot-orthoses (KAFOs) may be attempted for exercise, but independent bipedal ambulation is not realistic unless the patient has some upper lumbar innervation.[8] Each level of additional lumbar and sacral innervation increases the ease of ambulation with an appropriate orthosis. Incomplete injuries will present with a mixture of possible functions. Since significant recovery may occur in transverse myelitis, the patient may want to wait a few months before investing in expensive durable medical equipment or alterations of the home.

Diagnostic Studies

MRI is generally performed when transverse myelitis is suspected to rule out a tumor or other lesion that may be causing a compressive myelopathy.[3]

Although not absolutely definitive, MRI has features that help differentiate transverse myelitis from other disorders, such as multiple sclerosis. Transverse myelitis is more likely to have high signals of intensity on T2 weighted images extending longitudinally over more segments.[7,9] The number of segments involved may be anywhere from one or two to as many as 11,[7–9] or may involve the entire cord (as described in lupus),[10] or sometimes the medulla.[7,12] However, in transverse myelitis the lesion appears more likely to affect the central region of the cord and involve more than two thirds of the cord diameter. In multiple sclerosis, the lesion appears more peripheral and generally involves less than one half of the diameter of the cord.[9] Also, the lesion in transverse myelitis is more likely to resemble a spinal cord tumor and may be mistakenly biopsied.[7,9] Contrast is commonly given to help highlight lesions that may be due to compression.[9]

MRI of the brain is often performed, in conjunction with the aforementioned procedure, to determine whether the patient's condition is a prelude to multiple sclerosis. Various statistics have been given in an attempt to assess the likelihood of multiple sclerosis as the cause of "idiopathic" transverse myelitis. If a study shows no brain lesions, the likelihood of multiple sclerosis is as low as 5% to 15%.[1,3] When brain abnormalities are seen, the chance of multiple sclerosis being the cause increases to 50% to 60%.[1,3] Myelogram may be done if MRI is not available.[3]

Other testing may include blood work, such as basic chemistries and blood counts; ANA; erythrocyte sedimentation rate; immunoglobulins; rapid plasmin reagin or VDRL; lyme titers; *Mycoplasma pneumoniae;* mycobacterium cultures; titers for various viruses, including HIV, West Nile virus, poliomyelitis, hepatitis, Epstein-Barr virus, cytomegalovirus, and enteric cytopathic human orphan virus; vitamin B_{12} level, or an SS-A antibody for Sjögren's disease. A spinal tap may be performed to check for pressures in the central nervous system, cell count, protein, glucose, immunoglobulins, and protein electrophoresis. In one study, oligoclonal bands were found in 3/5 specimens of patients found to have multiple sclerosis and 0/4 specimens of patients with parainfectious associated causes.[4] Vascular flow studies or clotting parameters may be needed if hematoma, thrombosis, or vasculitis is thought to be the cause.

Electrodiagnostic studies, including somatosensory and motor evoked potentials, may be useful for both diagnostic purposes and to monitor treatment progress.

Cardiac stress testing may be appropriate for some patients because of the enormous stress placed on the heart when mobility is impaired. Urinary evaluation may include cystograms, voiding cystourethrograms, cystoscopy, or urodynamic studies. Bowel evaluation may require x-rays or scans to rule out obstruction.

Differential Diagnosis[1–5,9–22]

Multiple sclerosis

Systemic lupus erythematosus

Sarcoidosis

Behçet's mixed connective tissue syndrome

Space-occupying lesions

    Herniated nucleus pulposus
    Spinal stenosis
    Spinal abscess
    Hematoma

Postvaccination

Infection
  Viral: Epstein-Barr virus, herpes simplex, herpes zoster, cytomegalovirus, HIV, enteroviruses
    (poliomyelitis, coxsackievirus, enteric cytopathic human orphan virus), mumps, adenovirus,
    rubeola, measles, angiotrophic large cell lymphoma, leukemia virus, influenza, rabies, West
    Nile virus
  Bacteria: lyme borreliosis, syphilis, tuberculosis, *M. pneumoniae*, cat-scratch disease (*Bartonella
    henselae*), histoplasmosis
Vascular
  Vasculitis secondary to heroine abuse
  Thrombosis of spinal arteries
  Arteriovenous malformations
  B_{12} vitamin deficiency

Treatment

Initial

Initial hospitalization is common to monitor vital signs and manage respiratory status, bowel and
bladder complications, etc.[3,8,24,25] Various medications have been tried for idiopathic transverse
myelitis without much success in changing the course. Intravenous methylprednisolone has been
advocated to prevent further damage to the spinal cord as a result of swelling.[3,11,12] Cyclophosphamide
in combination with methylprednisolone has had some success on lesions related to lupus.[13]
Treatment regimens have been followed-up using sensory and motor evoked potentials.[23]

Treatment of compressive myelopathies or bacterial infections may immediately reverse the
disease course.[3] Immunosuppressive agents, antiviral agents, antibacterial agents, and surgical
decompression may be useful, depending on whether a specific etiology is identified.[11]

Rehabilitation

Rehabilitation is a crucial component of any spinal cord injury (see Chapters 138–140). Physical
and occupational therapists can assist patients with mobility issues and work on strengthening,
range of motion, reconditioning, and activities of daily living. If pain is present, modalities may be
helpful. Therapists can also help educate the patient about proper skin care, particularly for
insensate areas. If bracing is necessary, referral to a qualified orthotist can greatly improve
mobility. Bowel, bladder, and sexual function should be addressed by qualified health care
providers who specialize in these aspects of spinal cord injuries.

It is important to keep in mind that transverse myelitis may or may not be a transient condition.
Recovery may occur, so it is particularly important to minimize the effects of temporary
denervation. All muscles and joints should be kept as active as possible. Putting joints through a
full range of motion daily will help prevent contractures. Checking the skin thoroughly on a daily
basis can prevent major infections and skin breakdown. Insensate areas of high pressure should
be padded. If respiration is compromised, exercises for muscles of inspiration may be started,
glossopharyngeal breathing may be taught, or electrical stimulation of the diaphragm may be
considered.[24] Passive and active exercises and, occasionally, electrical stimulation are methods to
keep muscle as flexible and strong as possible. Spasticity may become problematic, as with all
upper motor neuron lesions. Proper stretching and medical management can minimize this
complication and diminish joint contractures. Bowel and bladder programs should be started
immediately. Non-functioning bowels or bladder may lead to bowel obstruction or kidney damage
if not addressed. Initially, a Foley catheter may be used for voiding management, but intermittent
catheterization is commonly used when possible. In some cases, a patient with a C6 lesion and
appropriate aids may, self-catheterize. Significant independence is gained by self-catheterization.
Bowels are managed by mechanical or medical stimulation for evacuation. A program of daily
bowel training is often started in the hospital but may be extended to every 2 to 3 days once an

individual returns home. Being dependent for this function is difficult for many people to accept. Care, both physically and psychologically, must be taken when teaching the regimen.

Individuals who require assistive devices receive training in the use of a wheelchair, walker, crutches, or cane. Independently maneuvering steps and curbs with an assistive device can provide a new level of freedom. If transferring requires assistance, training of family members or assistants becomes crucial. Properly trained care providers will be more inclined to assist and less likely to injure themselves or the patient.

Independence in self-care is also important to individuals. For patients with transverse myelitis at the cervical level, various temporary or permanent orthoses can be provided to help with self-care. Proper bathroom equipment can create independence. Adjusting the height of the toilet seat or grab bar placement in the bathroom may make the difference between dependence and independence.

The selection of appropriate aids is essential to maximize function. Many of these are expensive. Timing of the purchases also becomes a factor, particularly in a possibly transient condition. Despite a prognosis for recovery, it is important to keep an individual as functionally independent as possible throughout the entire recovery period.

Procedures

Procedures in transverse myelitis are also determined by which systems have been affected by the spinal cord injury. Procedures may include implantation of diaphragmatic electrodes if respiration has been affected. Some patients may receive training in functional electrical stimulation to help maintain fitness or increase ambulatory function.

Surgery

Surgery is not done specifically for idiopathic transverse myelitis. If a compressive abnormality is found, such as an abscess, herniated nucleus pulposus, spinal stenosis, or tumor, surgery will be performed as soon as possible to relieve pressure from the spinal cord. Complications stemming from spinal cord injury may require surgery, including skin breakdown, inadvertent injury to skin, from lack of sensation in muscles and joints, kidney stones or infections, and tendon transfers, to increase an individual's functioning.

Potential Disease Complications

The etiology of the spinal cord trauma does not alter the potential disease complications, which can result from permanent cord injury. Common complications include deep venous thrombosis, and pulmonary embolism, and pressure ulceration of skin if pressure relief is not done regularly. Respiratory complications, other than pulmonary emboli, may include weakness of respiratory musculature of varying degrees. Severe weakness may require mechanical ventilatory assistance. Patients are at increased risk for pneumonia or sleep apnea from the illness or sedating medications. Spasticity and joint contracture over time may result. Heterotopic ossification may surround a joint, further promoting contracture. Gastrointestinal complications may begin with an acute ileus, followed by chronic constipation. Ulceration, inflammation, and hemorrhage may occur due to the injury in combination with the use of methylprednisolone to prevent acute swelling of the spinal cord. Urinary tract infections are also common since retained urine and instrumentation both increase the likelihood of infection. Pain is a common complaint after spinal cord injury and in some studies has affected more than 90% of individuals. This is often attributed to "central pain" or is believed to have a psychogenic component. Treatments initiated for this pain often include tricyclic antidepressants, anticonvulsants, local anesthetics, and nonsteroidal anti-inflammatory drugs. Overuse syndromes can also result in pain; muscles and joints are commonly overused in trying to maintain or learn new functions. Shoulder pain specifically is a dominant issue, and the specific problem (tendinitis, arthritis, rotator cuff tear, impingement, contracture) must be identified and properly rehabilitated. Often, proper transfer techniques or specific adaptive equipment may be helpful. Pressure from resting too long on superficial nerves can also cause pain. Relief of pressure is the key. If difficulty with reproduction is an issue, techniques for sexual fulfillment as well as fertility issues, need to be addressed.

Potential Treatment Complications

Treatment complications may result from side effects of medications required to treat the disease. Skin complications may result from any ill-fitting device or poorly applied bandage. The skin of the patient with spinal cord injury may not have the same resistance to pressure as "normal" skin, and this is exacerbated when the skin is fully insensate. Autonomic dysreflexia may occur. If mechanical ventilation is required, failure of equipment can result in hypoxia, strictures, or tracheal inflammation. Respiratory infection may occur with or without mechanical ventilation in higher levels of tetraplegia. High dose steroids used to treat initial inflammation may cause gastritis, ulceration, or hemorrhage in the gastrointestinal tract. Deep venous thrombosis prophylaxis may exacerbate bleeding complications. Catheterization may cause urinary tract infections or false passages in the urethra, making further catheterization more difficult and possibly resulting in strictures. Bowel programs may cause anal irritations and if not well controlled, skin maceration around the sensitive sacral region.

References

1. Fauci AS, et al: Harrison's Principles of Internal Medicine, 14th ed. New York, McGraw-Hill, 1998, pp 2483–2485.
2. Gorbach SL, et al: Infectious Diseases, 2nd ed. Philadelphia. W.B. Saunders,. 1998, pp 1378–1379.
3. Transverse Myelitis web site. Transverse Myelitis. available at http://www.myelitis.org/tm.htm (accessed 10/23/00).
4. Jeffery DR, Mandler RN, Davis LE: Transverse myelitis: retrospective analysis of 33 cases, with differentiation of cases associated with multiple sclerosis and parainfectious events. Arch Neurol 1993;50:532.
5. Berman M, Feldman S, Alter M, et. al: Acute transverse myelitis: incidence and etiological considerations. Neurology 1981;31:966.
6. Ropper AH, Poskanzer DC: The prognosis of acute and subacute transverse myelopathy based on early signs and symptoms. Ann Neurol 1978;4:451–459.
7. Bakshi R, Kinkel PR, Mechtler LL, et al: Magnetic resonance imaging findings in 22 cases of myelitis: Comparison between patients with and without multiple sclerosis. Eur J Neurol 1998;5(1):35–48.
8. Grabois M, et al: Physical Medicine and Rehabilitation. Malden, MA, Blackwell Science, 2000, pp 1306–1318.
9. Murthy JM, Reddy JJ, Meena AK, Kaul S: Acute transverse myelitis: MR characteristics. Neurol India 1999;47(4):290–293.
10. Manabe Y, et al: Sjögren's syndrome with acute transverse myelopathy as the initial manifestation. J Neurol Sci 2000;176(2):158–161.
11. Andersen O, et al: Myelitis. Curr Opinion Neurol 2000;13(3):311–316.
12. Kovacs B, Lafferty TL, Brent LH, et al: Transverse myelopathy in systemic lupus erythematosus: An analysis of 14 cases and review of the literature. Ann Rheum Dis 2000;59(2):120–124.
13. Neumann-Andersen G, Lindgren S: Involvement of the entire spinal cord and medulla oblongata in acute catastrophic-onset transverse myelitis in SLE. Clin Rheumatol 2000;19(2):156–160.
14. Wakatsuki T et al: Sjögren's syndrome with primary biliary cirrhosis, complicated by transverse myelitis and malignant lymphoma. Intern Med 2000; 39(3):260–265.
15. Weatherby SJ, Davies MB, Hawkins CP, Dawes P: Transverse myelopathy, a rare complication of mixed connective tissue disease: Comparison with SLE related transverse myelopathy [letter]. Neurol Neurosurg Psychiatry 2000;68(4):532–533.
16. Nomura Y, Takatsu R, Fujisawa K, et al: A case of transverse myelitis caused by primary antiphospholipid antibody syndrome. Rinsho Shinkeigaku 1999;39(9):976–978.
17. Muranjan MN, et al: Acute transverse myelitis due to spinal epidural hematoma—first manifestation of severe hemophilia. Indian Pediatr 1999;36(11):1151–1153.
18. Renard JL, Guillamo JS, Ramirez JM, et al: Acute transverse cervical myelitis following hepatitis B vaccination. Evolution of anti-HBs antibodies.Presse Med 1999;10;28(24):1290–1292.
19. Bohr L, Paerregaard A, Valerius NH: Acute transverse myelitis caused by enterovirus. Ugeskr Laeger 1999;161(19):2817–2818.
20. Giobbia M, Carniato A, Scotton PG, et al: Cytomegalovirus-associated transverse myelitis in a non-immunocompromised patient. Infection 1999;27(3):228–230.
21. Wong M, Connolly AM, Noetzel MJ. Poliomyelitis-like syndrome associated with Epstein-Barr virus infection. Pediatr Neurol 1999;20(3):235–237.
22. Smith R, Eviatar L: Neurologic manifestations of Mycoplasma pneumoniae infections: Diverse spectrum of diseases. A report of six cases and review of the literature. Clin Pediatr 2000;39(4):195–201.
23. Kalita J, Guptar PM, Misra UK: Clinical and evoked potential changes in acute transverse myelitis following methyl prednisolone. Spinal Cord 1999;37(9):658–662.
24. Braddom RL: Physical Medicine and Rehabilitation. Philadelphia, W.B. Saunders, 1996, pp 674–685.
25. Cheng W, et al: Residual bladder dysfunction 2 to 10 years after acute transverse myelitis. Paediatr Child Health 1999;35(5):476–478.
26. Braddom RL, Randall L: Physical Medicine and Rehabilitation. Philadelphia, W.B. Saunders, 1996, pp 1149–1179.

145 Traumatic Brain Injury

David T. Burke, MD

Synonyms

Head injury

Acquired brain injury

Concussion

ICD-9 Codes

854.0
Intracranial injury of other and unspecified nature without mention of open intracranial wound

854.1
Intracranial injury of other and unspecified nature with open intracranial wound

907.0
Late effect of intracranial injury without mention of skull fracture

Definition

Traumatic brain injury is an insult to the brain, stemming from an external physical force and resulting in either temporary or permanent impairment, functional disability, or psychosocial maladjustment. There are approximately 1.5 million to 2 million brain injuries each year in the United States. Brain injuries usually occur as a consequence of motor vehicle accidents, falls, violence, and sports. Brain injuries are twice as frequent in males as in females. There is a peak incidence among those 15 to 24 years old and again among those 75 years old and older.[1]

The pathophysiology of brain injury is usually divided into *primary injury*, which is the injury to the brain that results at the time of the insult, and *secondary injury*, which can be thought of as the biochemical or physiologic related damage that develops over a period of hours, days, weeks, and perhaps months after the primary injury. Secondary insults include intracranial hemorrhage, swelling, hypoxia, brain shift, herniation, as well as numerous neurochemical and cellular events.[2,3] Some of the latter have yet to be well described or their significance well elucidated.

Symptoms

Symptoms may vary according to the severity of the injury and the stage of recovery. The history should include a detailed summary of the injury; co-morbid conditions; the initial Glasgow coma scale score (Table 1); the length of the coma, if any; and the length of post-traumatic amnesia. A review of important relationships both in the home and in the community is helpful in

TABLE 1. Glasgow Coma Scale

Patient Response	Score
Eyes opening	
Eyes open spontaneously	4
Eyes open when spoken to	3
Eyes open to painful stimuli	2
Eyes do not open	1
Motor	
Follows commands	6
Makes localized movements to painful stimuli	5
Makes withdrawl movements to painful stimuli	4
Demonstrates flexor posturing to painful stimuli	3.
Demonstrates extensor posturing to painful stimuli	2
No motor response to pain	1
Verbal	
Oriented to place and date	5
Converses but is disoriented	4
Utters inappropriate words, though not conversing	3
Makes incomprehensible nonverbal sounds	2
Not vocalizing	1

determining the prognosis for the patient's recovery. If regression in function has occurred since the injury, the clinician should review for potential metabolic insults, including infection, side effects of medications, or hydration/nutrition.

Patients with severe injury and extremely altered levels of arousal often have no symptoms. After the acute phase of recovery, the clinician might expect symptoms to include seizures, contractures, spasticity, altered vision, vertigo or dizziness, and altered sense of smell. These may be the result of cranial nerve injuries or of central processing dysfunction. Symptoms of dysautonomia may still be seen at outpatient followup and may be characterized by increased body temperatures, tachycardia, tachypnea, increased posturing, and profuse sweating.[4]

Common late symptoms may include memory deficits, especially those of short-term memory to long-term memory transfer, higher level executive dysfunction, headaches, difficulty with sleep/wake cycles, labile mood, depression, apathy, difficulty with attention, social disinhibition, sexual dysfunction, anxiety, impulsivity, fatigue, and difficulties with fine and gross motor control.[1]

Physical Examination

A thorough neurologic examination, including a neuropsychologic evaluation, is important to assess the consequences of a brain injury. The neurologic examination should include an assessment of mental status, a review of cranial nerve function, vision, hearing, deep tendon reflexes, and abnormal reflexes. The examination should also include muscle strength, tone, and coordination and an assessment of gait or mobility in a wheelchair. It is important to make a thorough assessment of the patient's neuropsychologic profile with the assistance of a neuropsychologist. This should be done to determine both physical abilities and the cognitive and emotional issues, which would reduce the patient's function.

Functional Limitations

Motor

Patients may have difficulty with mobility and self-care as a result of isolated motor weakness and/or coordination. Safe mobility may also be impeded by poor cognition, including deficits with planning or poor impulse control.

Behavior

Individuals often experience subtle or dramatic personality changes that alter relationships with others. These may include problems in the initiation of responses, verbal or physical aggression, altered emotional control, social disinhibition, depression, decreased sense of self-worth, and altered sexual function.

Social

Patients often are unable to return to work at their previous level of function. As a consequence, they may suffer significant economic strain and may have difficulty with their relationships, including their marriage. Family members may be helpful in pointing out issues of social isolation, depression, and anger.

Diagnostic Studies

Imaging Studies

As a rule the use of computed tomography (CT) and/or magnetic resonance imagery (MRI) is helpful for the initial assessment of intracranial bleeding as well as the shifting of fluids and tissues, but these studies are rather poor in their ability to estimate the actual volume and location of injured tissue.[5] More sophisticated testing has been introduced, including SPECT and PET, but for the most part are of little use in assessing the functional limitations caused by the injury. At the time of outpatient follow-up, it may be necessary to remind the patient and his or her caregivers of the extreme limitations of the films and to focus on that patient's functional abilities as the more important measure of the extent of the patient's injuries. In general, followup radiologic examinations are often beneficial if the patient has excessively slow progress or has demonstrated a decline in function. Otherwise, these are of limited utility.

Functional Assessment Tools

One of the best diagnostic tools is the Glasgow Coma Scale, which is used for the initial evaluation of the severity of the patient's injury (see Table 1). A review of this initial score will help in the determination of the extent of the injury and thus with prognostication. Later, as a review of function in the outpatient setting, progress can be measured by the Glasgow Outcome Scale (GOS). Post-traumatic amnesia is important for prognostication as well and can be assessed using the Galveston Orientation Assessment Test (GOAT). To characterize the current level of functional recovery, the Rancho Los Amigos scale is helpful in characterizing the patient's awareness and interaction with the environment.

Neuropsychologic Testing

This battery of tests, performed by a neuropsychologist, is the best means of determining the full spectrum of cognitive, affective, and emotional function of the individual. This may be done early in the course of recovery but should be repeated at times when a change in function needs to be documented. This testing may provide the clinician with critical information needed to progress the patient toward more independence or responsibility at home or at work. This also may be a critical assessment tool for the documentation of the injury for payers of a disability policy.

Differential Diagnosis

Anoxic brain injury	Delirium	Affective disorder
Metabolic encephalopathy	Multi-infarct dementia	Depression
Dementia	Thought disorder	Whiplash associated disorder

Treatment

Initial

The initial focus of treating a patient with a brain injury is to reduce the magnitude of the secondary head injury. If the initial injury is of sufficient severity, a CT or MRI is needed to determine the need for surgical intervention. The scans are reviewed for signs of excessive bleeding or shifting of the brain. If absent, medical intervention should address the possible secondary injury that may result. While it is still unclear as to how long a window of opportunity exists to affect the extent of secondary injury, it is generally accepted that this opportunity likely exists only during the time of the initial acute hospitalization.[2] For this reason, there is likely no opportunity to affect this process in the outpatient setting.

Initially, the metabolic issues such as blood pressure, electrolytes, hydration/nutrition, infectious processes, and medications need to be addressed. Any imbalance in these might inhibit the potential of the surviving brain tissue. Hydration and nutrition should be well maintained. An individual with a brain injury may be unable or unwilling to take nutrients by mouth, and this may necessitate either intravenous or direct gastrointestinal feedings. This may be a significant issue well into the postacute phase of recovery.

A survey for possible infectious processes should include at a minimum the pulmonary and genitourinary systems. It is important to recognize that even infections that a clinician might otherwise label as subclinical can disrupt the function of a damaged brain. For this reason all such infections should be treated as symptomatic.

Medications can have exaggerated effects among those with a brain injury and thus need to be reviewed carefully to eliminate any that may interfere with cognitive function. While the list is long, the most common offenders include antiseizure medications, antihypertensive medications, antispasticity medications, neuroleptics, and gastrointestinal medications. Some of these might be unnecessary, whereas others might have less disruptive alternatives.

In addition to neuropsychologic testing of the cognitive performance of the patient, psychologic services are important in the assessment and treatment of affective disorders, which may include depression and post-traumatic stress disorder. It is important to consider psychology services as being useful for the family and support system because the stress on these individuals may be tremendous. Psychologists and behavior specialists may be helpful for the intervention into behavior issues.

After the metabolic status has been optimized, the clinician should focus on the remaining physical and cognitive deficits to determine whether medications might be useful to enhance the function of the individual.

Arousal

Arousal will fluctuate throughout the day for a person with brain injury. Fatigue and endurance will be longstanding issues. Frequent rests and naps may be needed, even at more than 1 year after injury. Medical intervention may be initiated for hypoarousal and excessive fatigue. This includes amantadine, bromocriptine, carbidopa/levodopa, methylphenidate, provigil, amphetamine, nortriptyline, and protriptyline.[3]

Attention

Neuropharmacologic agents for attention are similar to those used for arousal. These include neurostimulants such as methylphenidate; pemoline; modafinil; and dopaminergic agents, including amantadine, bromocriptine, and carbidopa/levodopa. Antidepressants may be useful, including a long list of mixed as well as selective serotonin reuptake inhibitors (SSRIs). These will be especially useful if there is an element of depression interfering with cognition.

Agitation

Since agitation is a common and often troubling issue among those recovering from a brain injury, a careful selection of agents is important to prevent injury, to allow focus on rehabilitation, and to reduce the stress on caregivers. In general the agents that are preferred help control behavior while producing the least reduction in cognition. Because benzodiazepines are thought to have the potential of interfering with the recovery of the injured brain, these are certainly not recommended in the early stages of recovery. Other medications are therefore used as first line agents. As an anxiolytic, burpirone seems preferable. A clinician might use antiseizure medications (e.g., divalproex sodium, carbamazepine), newer antipsychotic medications (e.g., risperidone), as well as antidepressants for anxious or agitated patients. Since poor attention to the environment might result in behavioral agitation, stimulants such as amantadine and methylphenidate should also be considered as useful agents.

Memory

Since memory requires both arousal and attention, the medications previously discussed might produce improvements in the ability to learn. In addition there have been limited reports of positive results through the use of donepezil and other similar medications. Memory can be more certainly enhanced, however, through the use of compensatory strategies and services. Speech pathologists can be useful for the introduction of and training in some of these strategies. There are portable computers that can be preprogrammed with important information, and these memory aides can be frequently updated for individuals whose brain injury precludes the programming of the electronic memory aides.

Seizures

There is a reasonable body of literature to suggest that the use of antiseizure medications is not warranted if no seizure occurs within the first week after the brain injury. If the patient experiences a seizure after 1 week, then the use of anticonvulsant agents is probably warranted for an extended period. Recommended agents depend on seizure type and usually include carbamazepine, valproic acid, and gabapentin[9,10]

Spasticity

Spasticity is a common problem among patients with brain injury. Patients may also have problems with hyperactive muscle stretch reflexes and clonus. The modified Ashworth scale (page 787) can be used to measure the degree of spasticity. As a first step of intervention, the clinician should look for noxious stimuli, including anything that may produce pain. Infectious issues, positioning, and seating should be addressed as potential offenders. Stretching should be initiated and may necessitate the use of casting and splinting. If medications are needed, these may include tizantidine, clonidine, dantrolene, diazepam, and baclofen. All of these agents are thought to have potential side effects and should be used judiciously.

Rehabilitation

The rehabilitation of patients with brain injury begins during the acute stage of treatment when the issues of secondary brain injury are the greatest. After the acute phase, it is important that the clinician review the potential pharmacologic management and combine this with an interdisciplinary group of therapies, depending on what specific deficits the patient has.

Physical Therapy

Physical therapy is important for the restoration of range of motion of the lower extremities and, if needed, through the use of serial casting. This may be aided by the use of neurolysis or blocks at the neuromuscular junction. Later, issues of wheelchair preparation and propulsion may be important for those with sufficient impairment of mobility. Ambulation training with the appropriate assistive device should be frequently reviewed as the patient progresses with ambulation. Safety must always be considered because the patient with brain injury may be endangered by impulsivity or poor planning and judgment.

Occupational Therapy

Occupational therapy should address the preservation of joints when a lack of strength or an excess in tone or spasticity threatens a joint. The issues of self-care, including daily activities such as dressing, bathing, and grooming, must be addressed and emphasize the need for a planning strategy for the patient. Cooking and driving evaluations may be needed to advise the patient prior to his or her return to the home.

Speech Pathology

Early in the care of the patient, the ability to swallow safely may need to be addressed. Additionally, the speech pathologist should ideally work with the neuropsychologist to identify focal cognitive needs of the patient and to address these over a length of time. These often involve memory strategies and pragmatics.

Vocational Rehabilitation

Many patients will have difficulty returning to their previous level of employment. Vocational rehabilitation counselors can evaluate the patient to determine a patient's skills and the need for training.

Procedures

For spasticity, local injections may be preferable to oral medications and can include nerve root blocks, nerve blocks, motor unit blocks (all with phenol), and neuromuscular junction blocks (with botulism toxin). When spasticity is severe and not responsive to these interventions, a baclofen pump may be considered for continuous infusion of baclofen into the CSF. (Refer to Chapter 136.)

Surgery

Patients with new onset hydrocephalus may necessitate the placement of a shunt placed to reduce the pressure load at the brain. If medications and other measures fail to control spasticity, then surgery may be an option.

Potential Disease Complications

Seizures can result from a brain injury. The risk is highest early after the injury but persists for years. Soon after the injury, patients are at risk for aspiration pneumonia and, if their swallowing is impaired, for malnutrition and dehydration. As with all trauma patients, there is a risk for deep venous thrombosis. This must be treated with prophylactic heparin, or if hemorrhage is a risk, with pneumatic compression devices.

Potential Treatment Complications

Medications that are used to treat attention and arousal may lead to excess arousal and agitation. This may manifest with somatic complaints or delirium. Medications for agitation may slow the patient's recovery over time and may reduce the patient's function while the medications are taken. Refer to Table 2.

TABLE 2.   Medications Used to Treat Patients with Traumatic Injury

Symptoms	Medication	Initial Dose	End Dose
Arousal	Amantadine	50 mg bid	100 mg bid
	Bromocriptine*	1.25 mg bid	50 mg bid
	Carbidopa/levodopa*	10/100 tid	25/100 tid
	Methylphenidate	2.5 mg AM and 2 PM	20 mg AM and 2 PM
	Provigil	100 mg qd	100 mg bid
	Dextroamphetamine (Dexedrine)	5 mg qd	30 mg AM and PM
	Nortriptyline	10 mg tid	25 mg tid
	Protriptyline	5 mg tid	20 mg tid
Attention	Methylphenidate	2.5 mg AM and 2 PM	20 mg AM and 2 PM
	Pemoline	37.5 mg AM	100 mg bid
	Modafinil	100 mg AM	200 mg AM and PM
	Amantadine	100 mg AM	150 mg AM and 2 PM
	Bromocriptine*	1.25 mg AM	50 mg bid
	Carbidopa/levodopa*	10/100 tid	25/100 tid
	Sertraline (Zoloft)	50 mg qd	200 mg qd
	Citalopram (Celexa)	20 mg qd	60 mg qd
Agitation	Buspirone	7.5 mg bid	30 mg bid
	Carbamazepine	200 mg bid	600 mg bid
	Risperidone	1 mg bid	16 mg/day
	Morphine	10 mg q 4 hrs	10 mg q 4 hrs

* Limited by hypotension.

References

1. Rehabilitation of persons with traumatic brain injury. NIH Consensus Statement. 1998;16(1):1–41.
2. Burke DT, Kamath A: Management of post-traumatic seizure disorders. In Woo BH, Nesathurai S (eds): The Rehabilitation of People with Traumatic Brain Injury. Malden, MA, Blackwell Science, 2000.
3. Novack TA, Dillon MC, Jackson WT: Neurochemical mechanisms in brain injury and treatment: A review. J Clin Exp Neuropsychol 1996;18(5):685–706.
4. Baguley IJ, Nicholls JL, Felmingham KL, et al: Dysautonomia after traumatic brain injury: a forgotten syndrome? J Neurol Neurosurg Psychiatry 1999;67(1):39–43.
5. Chesnut RM, Carney N, Maynard H, et al: Rehabilitation for traumatic brain injury. Evidence report No. 2. Rockville, MD, Agency for Healthcare Policy and Research, 1999.
6. Kaplan M: Neuropharmacology after traumatic brain injury. In Woo BH, Nesathurai S (eds): The Rehabilitation of People with Traumatic Brain Injury. Malden, MA Blackwell Science, 2000.
7. Sandel ME, Mysiw WJ: The agitated brain injured patient. Part 1: Definitions, differential diagnosis, and assessment. Arch Phys Med Rehabil 1996;77(6):617–623.
8. Mysiw WJ, Sandel ME: The agitated brain injured patient. Part 2: Pathophysiology and treatment. Arch Phys Med Rehabil 1997;78(2):213–220.
9. Brain Injury Special Interest Group of the American Academy of Physical Medicine and Rehabilitation: Practice parameter: Antiepileptic drug treatment of posttraumatic seizures. Arch Phys Med Rehabil 1998;79(5):594–597.
10. Massagli TL: Neurobehavioral effects of phenytoin, carbamazepine, and valproic acid: Implications for use in traumatic brain injury [see comments]. Arch Phys Med Rehabil 1991;72(3):219–226.

Index

Page numbers in **boldface type** indicate complete chapters.

Ankle
    anatomy of, 398
    arthritis of, **394–396**
    bursitis of, **397–399**
    chronic instability of, **409–413**
    ganglia of, **420–422**
    lateral, ligaments of, 400
    pronated, as iliotibial band syndrome
        risk factor, 329
    rheumatoid arthritis of, 395, 729
    sprains of, **400–404**
        as ankle instability cause, 409, 410,
            412
        definition of, 400
        recurrent lateral, 412
        severity grading of, 400, 401
    total replacement (arthroplasty) of,
        396
Ankle brachial index (ABI), 543
Ankle impingement syndrome, 412
Ankylosing spondylitis, **475–478**
Ankylosis
    collateral ligament injury-related,
        315
    psoriatic arthritis-related, 697
Anterior cruciate ligament
    anatomy of, 301, 346, 367
    laxity of, 346
    sprains of, **301–307**
    tears of, 346
Anterior interosseous syndrome,
    119–120, 121, 122, 123, 124, 125
Antiadrenergics, as smooth sphincter
    dyssynergia treatment, 629
Antibiotic prophylaxis, in systemic
    lupus erythematosus patients, 797
Anticardiolipin antibodies, as systemic
    lupus erythematosus indicator, 795,
    796
Anticholinergics
    as bladder detrussor instability
        treatment, 780
    as dystonia treatment, 597
    as hyperreflexic bladder treatment,
        629, 633
    as movement disorder treatment, 597
    as Parkinson's disease treatment, 654
    as pulmonary disease treatment, 709,
        716
    side effects of, 780
Anticoagulants
    as cerebral hemorrhage risk factor,
        780
    as deep venous thrombosis
        treatment, 533–534
    as olecranon bursitis risk factor, 126
Anticonvulsants
    use in brain injury patients, 810
    as pain treatment
        in brachial plexopathy, 668, 669
        in chronic pain syndrome, 515
        in occipital neuralgia, 41
        in phantom sensation pain,
            472–473
        in repetitive strain injuries, 724

Anticonvulsants (*cont.*)
    as pain treatment (*cont.*)
        in stroke patients, 780
        in thoracic outlet syndrome, 221,
            223
        in thoracic radiculopathy, 226, 227,
            668
    side effects of, 227, 669, 782, 809
Antidepressants. *See also* Tricyclic
    antidepressants
    as brain injury treatment, 809
    as phantom sensation pain
        treatment, 472–473
    use by stroke patients, 789, 790
Antiestrogens, as osteoporosis
    prophylaxis, 649
Antihypertension drugs, side effects of,
    in brain injury patients, 809
Antiinflammatory drugs. *See also*
    Nonsteroidal anti-inflammatory
    drugs
    gastrointestinal side effects of, 452
Antimalarial drugs
    as psoriatic arthritis treatment, 698
    as rheumatoid arthritis treatment,
        733
    side effects of, 698, 733, 798
    as systemic lupus erythematosus
        treatment, 797, 798
Antinuclear antibodies
    HIV infection-associated, 461
    systemic lupus erythematosus-
        associated, 793, 795, 796
Antioxidants, as amyotrophic lateral
    sclerosis treatment, 589
Anti-Parkinson drugs, 597, 652
    side effects of, 598
Antiphospholipid antibody syndrome,
    795
Antiplatelet agents
    as cerebral hemorrhage risk factor,
        780
    as stroke prophylaxis, 780
Antishock garments, as compartment
    syndrome cause, 316
Antiviral therapy
    for AIDS/HIV infection, 462, 463
    for Parkinson's disease, 654
Anxiety
    chronic pain syndrome-related, 512
    motor neuron disease-related, 590
    psychostimulants-related, 782
    stroke-related, 785, 787, 789–790
Aphasia, 747, 748, 749–750, 751
    stroke-related, 778, 779, 785
        effect on motor vehicle driving
            ability, 788
Apley grind/compression test, 347, 348
Apprehension test, 77, 78, 85
Apraxia, of speech, 747, 748–749, 750,
    751
Aprosodia, motor, stroke-related, 785
Ardeparin, 534
Arnold-Chiari malformations, 620–621,
    622, 625

Arteriography, for thoracic outlet
    syndrome evaluation, 221
Arteriovenous grafts, for dialysis
    vascular access, 517, 521, 522, 523
Arthralgia, mallet toe-related, 434
Arthritis. *See also* Arthropathy;
        Osteoarthritis; Rheumatoid
        arthritis
    of ankle, **394–396**
    of distal interphalangeal joint, 167
    of elbow, **107–114**
    enteropathic, **552–558**
    inflammatory, as osteoarthritis risk
        factor, 638
    pisiohamate, 203
    posterior cruciate ligament
        instability-related, 371
    psoriatic, **694–698**
    systemic lupus erythematosus-
        related, 795, 797
    triscaphe, 204, 205
Arthritis mutilans, 694, 695
Arthrocentesis
    in anterior cruciate ligament injury,
        303, 304, 306
    in meniscal tears, 350
    in total knee replacement
        (arthroplasty) patients, 386
Arthrodesis
    as claw toe deformity treatment, 416
    as hammer toe deformity treatment,
        429–430
    of hand
        as osteoarthritis treatment, 173
        as rheumatoid arthritis treatment,
            178
    of knee, as osteoarthritis treatment,
        338
    as mallet toe deformity treatment,
        433–434
    as posterior tibial dysfunction
        treatment, 451
    of wrist
        as osteoarthritis treatment, 206–207
        as rheumatoid arthritis treatment,
            178, 212, 213
Arthrography
    in adhesive capsulitis, 63
    cervical, 10
    in glenohumeral instability, 79
    in lumbar facet arthropathy, 241
Arthropathy
    of facets
        cervical, **9–11**
        lumbar, **240–242**
    Jacoud's, 795, 798
Arthroplasty
    of ankle, 396
    complications of, 396
    of elbow, as arthritis treatment,
        112–113
    as hammer toe deformity treatment,
        429
    of hand, as osteoarthritis treatment,
        173

Arthroplasty (*cont.*)
of hip, 272–273, **290–296**
heterotopic ossification associated
with, 572, 573
implant loosening in, 292, 293
with radiation therapy, 574
side effects of, 478
of knee, 338, **383–390**
prosthesis loosening in, 384, 385,
389–390
treatment complications of,
388–390
of wrist
as osteoarthritis treatment,
206–207
as rheumatoid arthritis treatment,
212, 213
Arthroscopy
of adhesive capsulitis, 63
of biceps tendinitis, 69
as deep venous thrombosis risk
factor, 338
of elbow, in arthritis, 112
of knee, in meniscal injury, 351
of posterior cruciate ligament injury,
370
of shoulder, in osteoarthritis, 106
Ashworth Scale, for spasticity
measurement, 787
Aspiration. *See also* Arthrocentesis
of Baker's cyst, 309, 310
of bursa, as olecranon bursitis
treatment, 129–120
of ganglion cysts, 166, 421–422
of knee
for meniscal tear diagnosis, 348
in total knee replacement
(arthroplasty) patients, 386
in motor neuron disease patients, 587
silent, 548
tracheal, 548
Aspirin
as deep venous thrombosis
prophylaxis, 533
as stroke therapy, 780, 782
Asterixis, 518, 594
"Asymmetrical adult flat foot"
deformity, 449
Ataxia, 597, 598, 602
Atenolol, as phantom pain treatment,
467
Atherosclerosis, 542
as stroke cause, in young adults, 784
Athetosis, 594, 595
Athletes
ankle bracing in, 411
chronic ankle instability in, 410, 411,
412
female, menstrual abnormalities in,
379, 380, 381, 382
glenohumeral instability in, 79, 82
hamstring strains in, 323–327
knee bursitis in, 341
meniscal tears in, 346
patellar tendinitis in, 353–357

Athletes (*cont.*)
quadriceps contusions in, 287–289
quadriceps tendinitis in, 372, 373
shin splints in, **375–378**
Atlantoaxial subluxation, 730
Attention deficits
brain injury-related, 809, 811
stroke-related, 780
Autonomic dysreflexia
thoracic spinal cord injury-related,
763, 764, 770
transverse myelitis-related, 805
Azathioprine, as peripheral neuropathy
treatment, 662

Babinski's sign, 214, 232, 587, 743
Back, cerebral palsy-related deformities
of, 499–500
Baclofen
as movement disorder treatment, 597
as pain treatment, in multiple
sclerosis, 604
side effects of, 777
as spasticity treatment, 744–745
in multiple sclerosis, 604
in spinal cord injury, 757–758, 760,
761, 774
as stroke treatment, 780
Baclofen pump, 745, 746, 811
"Bamboo spine" radiographic
appearance, of ankylosing
spondylitis, 476, 477
Barium swallow, 549, 683
Bath Ankylosing Spondylitis
Functional Index, 476
Bed rest
as contracture cause, 525
by post-polio syndrome patients, 686
Benign prostatic hyperplasia, 628
Benzodiazepines
as detrusor-sphincter dyssynergia
treatment, 629
as movement disorder treatment, 597
as spasticity treatment, 744–745
Benzopyrones, as lymphedema
treatment, 577
Benztropine, as Parkinson's disease
treatment, 654
Beta blockers, as phantom pain
treatment, 467
Bethanechol, as areflexic bladder
treatment, 629
Biceps tendon
rupture of, **72–75**
tendinitis of, **67–71**
Bicipital groove, palpation of, 68
Bicyclists, iliotibial band syndrome in,
329, 330, 332
Bier block, as reflex sympathetic
dystrophy treatment, 720–721
Bilevel positive airway pressure
(BiPAP)
use in amyotrophic lateral sclerosis
patients, 592
use in post-polio syndrome patients, 684

Bisphosphonates
as osteoporosis prophylaxis, 649
as Paget's disease treatment, 583
as premature osteoporosis treatment,
382
side effects of, 382, 585
Bladder, innervation of, 626–627
Bladder cancer, 630, 636
Bladder dysfunction. *See also* Urinary
incontinence
areflexic bladder, 627, 629, 632
cerebral palsy-related, 499–500
cervical spondylitic myelopathy-
related, 5, 7
multiple sclerosis-related, 606
neurogenic bladder, **626–627**
spinal cord injury-related, 763, 766,
769
stroke-related, 780
transverse myelitis-related, 803
Bladder pressure, high, adverse effect
on renal function, 632
Blood transfusion, in total knee
replacement (arthroplasty)
patients, 385
Blurred vision, ankylosing spondylitis-
related, 475
Bone density
measurement of
in amenorrhea, 380
in osteoporosis, 646–647
menstrual abnormality-related
decrease in, 379
Bone disease, metabolic, **579–585**
Bone metabolism, chronic renal failure-
related abnormalities of, 523
Bone mineral density
exercise-related increase in, 648
osteoporosis-related decrease in, 645,
647
Bone scan
of chronic ankle instability, 410–411
of heterotopic ossification, 570, 571,
572
of reflex sympathetic dystrophy, 719
of stress fractures, 380
of tarsal tunnel syndrome, 455
of thoracic compression fractures, 215
Borg's rating of perceived exertion,
711–712
Botulinum toxin injections
as detrusor-sphincter dyssynergia
treatment, 629
as epicondylitis treatment, 117
as focal dystonia treatment, 597
side effects of, 503, 598–599, 746
as spasticity treatment, 744, 745
in brain injury, 811
in cerebral palsy, 503
in cervical spinal cord injury,
759–760
in neural tube defects, 624
in stroke, 781, 791
as trapezius muscle strain treatment,
53

Mineral metabolism, chronic renal failure-related abnormalities of, 523

Mineral supplementation, as pressure ulcer treatment, 702

Mini Mental State Examination, 787

Minnesota Multiphasic Personality Inventory, 513

Mitral valve, chronic renal failure-related calcification of, 523

Mitral valve prolapse, as stroke cause, in young adults, 784

Modafinil
as brain injury treatment, 809
as fatigue treatment, in post-polio syndrome, 684, 685
side effects of, 685

Mononeuritis multiplex, rheumatoid arthritis-related, 727

Mononeuropathy, burn-related, 480, 481

Monoplegia, cerebral palsy-related, 499

Morning stiffness, rheumatoid arthritis-related, 208, 694, 726

Morphine
as chronic pain syndrome treatment, 515
as lumbar radiculopathy-related pain treatment, 246–247

Morphine metabolites, 670

Morton's foot, 435

Morton's neuroma, 436, **439–443**

Motor impairment, traumatic brain injury-related, 807

Motor neuron disease, **586–593**
definition of, 586
diagnosis of, 587–589
dysphagia associated with, 548, 587, 591
lower, 586, 587, 589
treatment and rehabilitation of, 589–593
upper, 586, 587, 588, 589, 743

Motor neurons, in post-polio syndrome, 679–680

Motor vehicle accidents, rear-end, as temporomandibular joint dysfunction cause, 45

Mouth guards, contraindication in temporomandibular joint dysfunction, 48

Movement disorders, **594–599**

MS Contin, 246–247

Mulder's sign/click, 440

Multiple sclerosis, **600–607**

Multisystem atrophy (Shy-Drager syndrome), 594

Muscle atrophy
progressive, 586
ulnar neuropathy-related, 201

Muscle relaxants
as cervical myelopathy treatment, 15
as cervical sprain/strain treatment, 28, 29
as cervical stenosis treatment, 32

Muscle relaxants (cont.)
as cervicogenic vertigo treatment, 36, 37
as piriformis syndrome treatment, 285
as radial neuropathy treatment, 135
as thoracic compression fracture treatment, 215–216
as thoracic strain/sprain treatment, 230

Muscular dystrophy, 613
fascioscapulohumeral, 616, 714

Musicians, instrumental, thoracic outlet syndrome in, 220

Musician's cramp, 598

Myalgia, post-polio, 684

Myelitis, transverse, **800–805**

Myelography, computed tomographic
of cervical spondylosis, 14–15
of lumbar degenerative disease, 233–234

Myelomalacia, 6

Myelomeningocele, 622

Myelopathy
cervical, **12–18**, 20
spondylitic, **3–8**
rheumatoid arthritis-related, 727

Myelotomy, Bischof's, 606

Myoclonus, 594, 595

Myofascial pain and dysfunction syndrome, **608–612**
thoracic strains/sprains-related, 230

Myokymia, facial, multiple sclerosis-related, 602

Myopathies, **613–619**
oxygen saturation decrease associated with, 709–710

Myositis
systemic lupus erythematosus-related, 796
trapezius, 50

Myositis ossificans traumatica, 289

Napping
by brain injury patients, 809
by stroke patients, 790

Narcotics, as pain treatment
in AIDS, 462
in cervical myelopathy, 15
in phantom sensation pain, 472–473
side effects of, 23

Neck. *See also* Cervical spine
range of motion of, 20–21
sprains/strains of, **25–29**
occipital neuralgia associated with, 41

Necrosis
avascular
of hip, 268, 270, 292
HIV infection-related, 461
of lunate bone. *See* Kienbock's disease
oral steroids-related, 227

Nephropathies, chronic reflux, as chronic renal failure cause, 517

Nerve blocks
as phantom limb pain treatment, 469
as radial neuropathy treatment, 137

Nerve compression test, for carpal tunnel syndrome diagnosis, 187

Nerve conduction studies
of hamstring strains, 326
of lumbosacral plexopathy, 674
of Morton's neuroma, 441
of myopathies, 617
of peripheral neuropathies, 661
of pronator teres syndrome, 122
of ulnar neuropathy, 141, 202

Nerve palsy, in stroke patients, 785–786

Nerve tension testing, in lumbar facet arthropathy, 240–241

Neuralgia, occipital, **38–43**

Neural tube defects, **620–625**

Neuritis, brachial, 664, 666

Neuroleptics, side effects of, 595, 809

Neurologic disorders, rheumatoid arthritis-related, 727

Neurologic examination
in cancer, 495
in cervical radiculopathy, 21
in cervical spinal cord injury, 754, 755
in cervical sprains/strains, 26
in chronic fatigue syndrome, 506
in chronic pain syndrome, 512–513
in chronic renal failure, 518
in dementia, 538
in dysphagia, 548
in knee osteoarthritis, 335
in lumbar spinal stenosis, 258
in lumbosacral plexopathy, 674
in metatarsalgia, 436
in movement disorders, 595
in multiple sclerosis, 601
in peroneal neuropathy, 364
in post-concussion syndrome, 689
in posterior cruciate ligament injury, 369
in scapular winging, 98
in stroke, 778
in temporomandibular joint dysfunction, 46
in thoracic compression fractures, 214–215
in traumatic brain injury, 807
in trigger finger, 191–192

Neuroma
Morton's, 436, **439–443**
"stump," 441, 442

Neurontin
as pain treatment, in AIDS patients, 462
as spasticity treatment, in young stroke patients, 790

Neuropathies
AIDS antiviral therapy-related, 463
femoral, **274–278**
lateral femoral cutaneous, **279–282**

Tics, 594, 595, 597
Tinel's sign, 108, 187, 220, 454
Tinnitus, temporomandibular
    dysfunction-related, 44
Tizanidine
    as chronic pain syndrome treatment,
        515
    as spasticity treatment, 744–745
        in brain injury, 810
        in multiple sclerosis, 604
        in spinal cord injury, 758, 761, 774
        in stroke, 780, 790
Toenail deformities
    claw toe-related, 416
    hammer toe-related, 430
    mallet toe-related, 434
Toes, bunion-related stress fractures of,
    407
"Too-many-toes" sign, 450
Topiramate, as peripheral neuropathy
    treatment, 662
Torticollis, 596
Total ankle replacement (arthroplasty),
    396
Tourette's syndrome, 595
Tracheostomy
    in amyotrophic lateral sclerosis
        patients, 592
    complications of, 593
    in pulmonary disease patients, 713,
        714
Traction
    cervical
        as cervical facet arthropathy
            treatment, 10
        as cervical sprain/strain treatment,
            28
        on femoral nerve, 276
        as myelopathy treatment, 15, 16, 17
Traction injuries, as brachial plexus
    lesion cause, 664–665
Tramadol, 216, 462
Trancutaneous electrical stimulation
    (TENS), as pain treatment
    in AIDS, 462
    in cervical facet arthropathy, 10
    in cervical myelopathy, 16
    in cervical radiculopathy, 22
    in cervical stenosis, 32
    in femoral neuropathy, 277
    in lumbosacral plexopathy, 676
    in occipital neuralgia, 41
    in osteoarthritis, 642
    in peripheral neuropathy, 662
    in phantom pain sensations, 467
    in piriformis syndrome, 285
    in radial neuropathy, 135
    in stroke, 791
    in thoracic radiculopathy, 226
Transverse myelitis, **800–805**
Trapezius muscles
    anatomy of, 51, 97
    strains of, **50–54**
Trauma
    as compartment syndrome cause, 316

Trauma (*cont.*)
    as Kienbock's disease, 181
    as lower-limb amputation cause, 470
    as temporomandibular dysfunction
        cause, 44, 45
    as upper-limb amputation cause, 465,
        467
Traumatic brain injury, **806–812**
    heterotopic ossification-related, 569,
        570, 572–573
    mild, sequelae of, 687–693
    primary and secondary, 806
Trazodone, as pain treatment, in AIDS
    patients, 462
Tremor, 594–595, 596
    chronic renal failure-related, 518
    non-Parkinsonian, 594
    Parkinson's disease-related, 594, 595,
        652, 653, 655, 656
    treatment and rehabilitation of, 597,
        598
Trendelenburg position, as acute
    compartment syndrome risk factor,
    316
Trendelenburg's sign, 291
Trendelenburg test. for osteoarthritis
    evaluation, 639
Triceps muscle, evaluation of, in radial
    neuropathy, 133
Tricyclic antidepressants
    as bladder dysfunction treatment
        of hyperreflxic bladder, 629
        in stroke patients, 790
    cardiovascular disease as
        contraindication to, 223
    as pain treatment
        in AIDS, 462
        in brachial plexopathy, 668, 669
        in cervical myelopathy, 15
        in chronic pain syndromes, 515
        in fibromyalgia, 560, 562
        in multiple sclerosis, 604
        in peripheral neuropathy, 662, 663
        in pronator teres syndrome, 123
        in thoracic outlet syndrome, 221,
            223
        in thoracic radiculopathy, 226, 227
    side effects of, 227, 663, 669, 685, 769,
        777
    use by stroke patients, 789
Trigger finger, **191–194**
Trigger point injections
    as cervical sprain/strain treatment, 28
    as cervicogenic vertigo treatment, 36,
        37
    as lumbar sprain/strain treatment, 251
    as myofascial pain and dysfunction
        syndrome treatment, 611, 612
    as radial neuropathy treatment, 137
    as temporomandibular joint
        dysfunction treatment, 48
    as thoracic strain/sprain treatment,
        230
    as trapezius muscle strain treatment,
        53

Trigger points
    cervicogenic vertigo-related, 35
    chronic fatigue syndrome-related, 508
    fibromyalgia-related, 561
    iliotibial band syndrome-related, 329
    myofascial pain and dysfunction
        syndrome-related, 608–609
    occipital neuralgia-related, 39
    radial neuropathy-related, 134
Trihexyphenidyl, as Parkinson's disease
    treatment, 597
Triplegia, cerebral palsy-related, 499
Trochanters, greater, bursitis of,
    297–300
Tryptophan, as eosinophilia-myalgia
    syndrome cause, 597

Ulcers
    esophageal, bisphosphonates-related,
        382
    of foot
        bunion-related, 407
        claw toe deformity-related, 415, 416
        corns (clavus)-related, 418
        diabetes and peripheral vascular
            disease-related, 542–546
        hammer toe deformity-related, 427,
            428, 430
        mallet toe deformity-related, 432,
            434
        metatarsalgia-related, 438
        as toe loss cause, 427
    gastrointestinal, nonsteroidal anti-
        inflammatory drugs-related, 643
    pressure, **699–704**
        amputation-related, 470–471
        cerebral palsy-related, 501
        contracture-related, 526, 528
        heterotopic ossification-related, 574
        lumbosacral spinal cord injury-
            related, 773, 775, 776
        prevention of, 701
        spinal cord injury-related, 755, 756,
            757, 759, 760, 763, 765–766,
            769
Ulnar collateral ligaments, sprains of,
    195–197
Ulnar nerve
    entrapment of. *See* Neuropathies,
        ulnar
    neuropathy of, **139–142**
Ultrasound
    contraindications to, 299, 326, 342
    diagnostic
        in deep venous thrombosis, 532
        Doppler, in cervical spondylosis, 14,
            15
        in flexor tendon injuries, 158
        in heterotopic ossification, 571
        in Morton's neuroma, 441
        in neurogenic bladder, 630
        in patellar tendinitis, 355
        in plantar fasciitis, 445
        in posterior tibial dysfunction, 450
        in rotator cuff tears, 91